THE NETTER COLLECTION
of Medical Illustrations

2nd Edition

Reproductive System
Endocrine System
Respiratory System
Urinary System
Integumentary System
Musculoskeletal System
Digestive System
Nervous System
Circulatory System

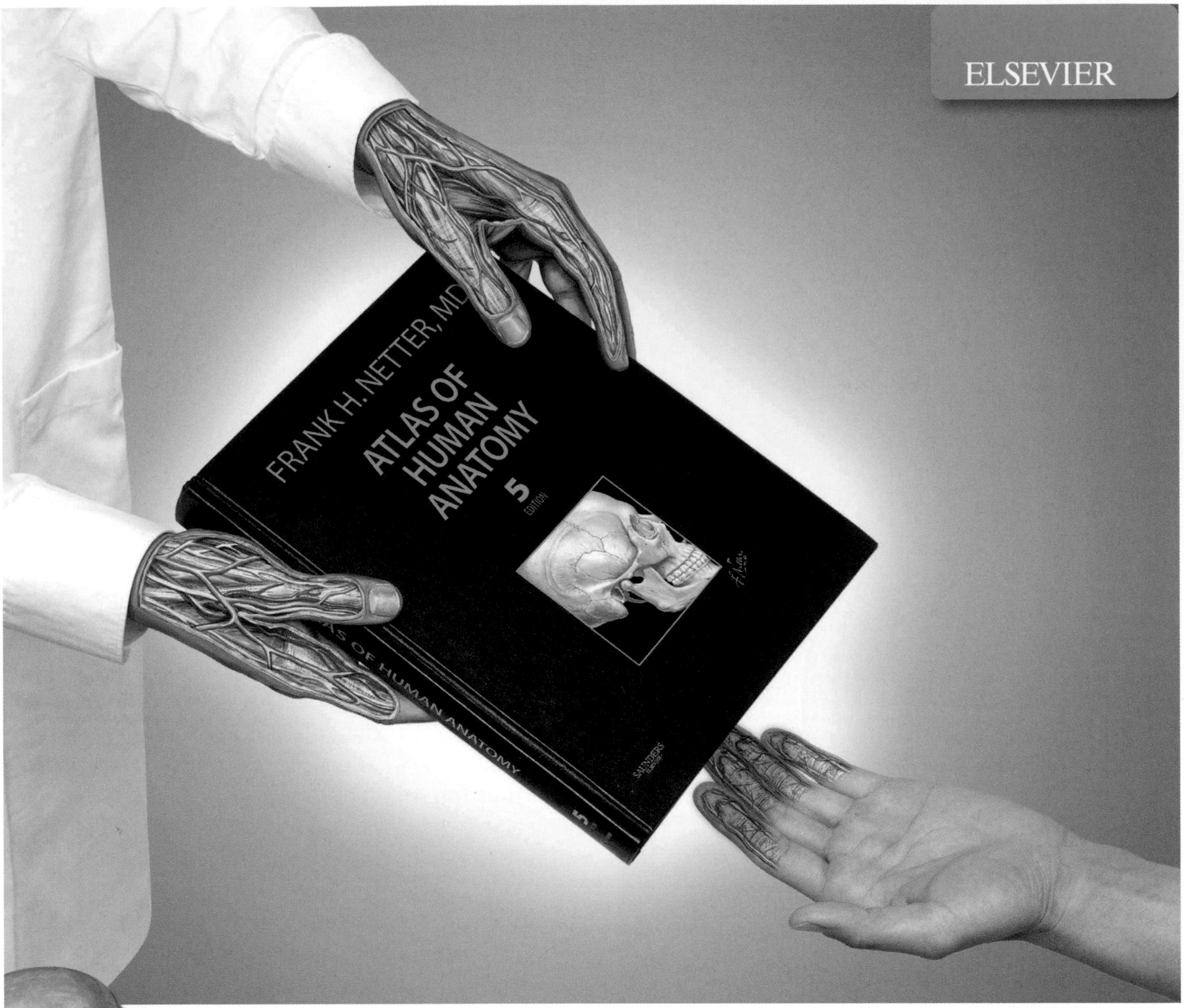

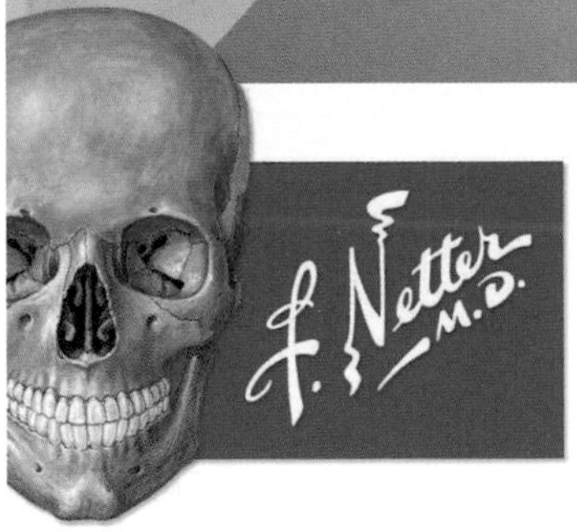

VOLUME 3

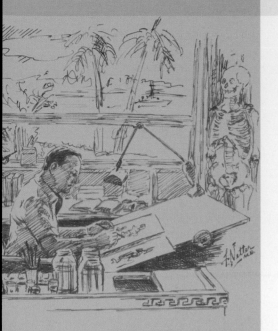

The Netter Collection
OF MEDICAL ILLUSTRATIONS:
Respiratory System

Second Edition

David A. Kaminsky, MD
Associate Professor
Pulmonary and Critical Care Medicine
University of Vermont
Burlington, Vermont

Illustrations by
Frank H. Netter, MD, and Carlos A.G. Machado, MD

CONTRIBUTING ILLUSTRATORS
John A. Craig, MD
James A. Perkins, MS, MFA
Kristen Wienandt Marzejon, MS, MFA
Tiffany S. DaVanzo, MA, CMI
Anita Impagliazzo, MA, CMI

ELSEVIER
SAUNDERS

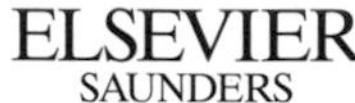

1600 John F. Kennedy Blvd.
Ste 1800
Philadelphia, PA 19103-2899

THE NETTER COLLECTION OF MEDICAL ILLUSTRATIONS: ISBN: 978-1-4377-0574-4
RESPIRATORY SYSTEM, Volume 3, Second Edition

Notices

Knowledge and best practice in this field are constantly changing. As new research and experience broaden our understanding, changes in research methods, professional practices, or medical treatment may become necessary.

Practitioners and researchers must always rely on their own experience and knowledge in evaluating and using any information, methods, compounds, or experiments described herein. In using such information or methods they should be mindful of their own safety and the safety of others, including parties for whom they have a professional responsibility.

With respect to any drug or pharmaceutical products identified, readers are advised to check the most current information provided (i) on procedures featured or (ii) by the manufacturer of each product to be administered, to verify the recommended dose or formula, the method and duration of administration, and contraindications. It is the responsibility of practitioners, relying on their own experience and knowledge of their patients, to make diagnoses, to determine dosages and the best treatment for each individual patient, and to take all appropriate safety precautions.

To the fullest extent of the law, neither the Publisher nor the authors, contributors, or editors, assume any liability for any injury and/or damage to persons or property as a matter of products liability, negligence or otherwise, or from any use or operation of any methods, products, instructions, or ideas contained in the material herein.

ISBN: **978-1-4377-0595-9**

Acquisitions Editor: Elyse O'Grady
Developmental Editor: Marybeth Thiel
Editorial Assistant: Chris Hazle-Cary
Publishing Services Manager: Patricia Tannian
Senior Project Manager: John Casey
Designer: Lou Forgione

Printed in China

Last digit is the print number: 9 8 7 6 5 4 3 2 1

ABOUT THE SERIES

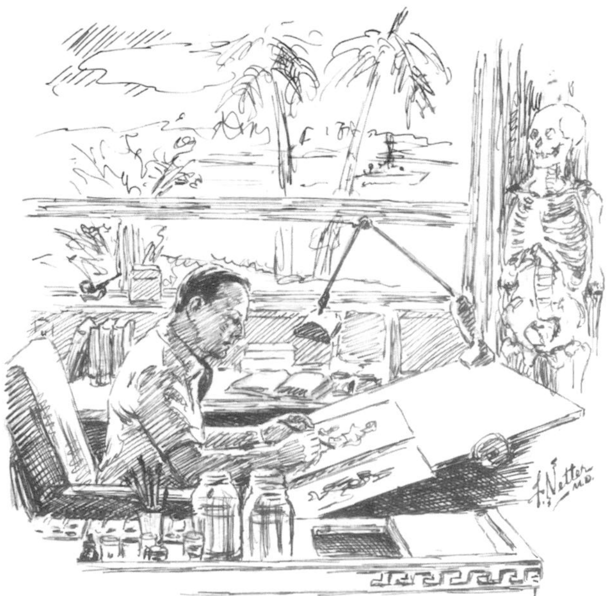

Dr. Frank Netter at work

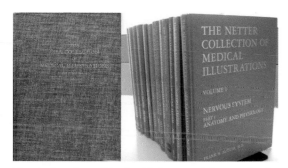

The single-volume "blue book" that paved the way for the multivolume *Netter Collection of Medical Illustrations* series, affectionately known as the "green books."

Dr. Frank H. Netter exemplified the distinct vocations of doctor, artist, and teacher. Even more important, he unified them. Netter's illustrations always began with meticulous research into the forms of the body, a philosophy that steered his broad and deep medical understanding. He often said, "Clarification is the goal. No matter how beautifully it is painted, a medical illustration has little value if it does not make clear a medical point." His greatest challenge—and greatest success—was chartering a middle course between artistic clarity and instructional complexity. That success is captured in this series, beginning in 1948, when the first comprehensive collection of Netter's work, a single volume, was published by CIBA Pharmaceuticals. It met with such success that over the following 40 years the collection was expanded into an eight-volume series—each devoted to a single body system.

In this second edition of the legendary series, we are delighted to offer Netter's timeless work, now arranged and informed by modern text and radiologic imaging contributed by field-leading doctors and teachers from world-renowned medical institutions and supplemented with new illustrations created by artists working in the Netter tradition. Inside the classic green covers, students and practitioners will find hundreds of original works of art—the human body in pictures—paired with the latest in expert medical knowledge and innovation, and anchored in the sublime style of Frank Netter.

Dr. Carlos Machado was chosen by Novartis to be Dr. Netter's successor. He continues to be the primary artist contributing to the Netter family of products. Dr. Machado says, "For 16 years, in my updating of the illustrations in the *Netter Atlas of Human Anatomy*, as well as many other Netter publications, I have faced the challenging mission of continuing Dr. Netter's legacy, of following and understanding his concepts, and of reproducing his style by using his favorite techniques."

Although the science and teaching of medicine endures changes in terminology, practice, and discovery, some things remain the same. A patient is a patient. A teacher is a teacher. And the pictures of Dr. Netter—he called them pictures, never paintings—remain the same blend of beautiful and instructional resources that have guided physicians' hands and nurtured their imaginations for over half a century.

The original series could not exist without the dedication of all those who edited, authored, or in other ways contributed, nor, of course, without the excellence of Dr. Netter, who is fondly remembered by all who knew him. For this exciting second edition, we also owe our gratitude to the authors, editors, advisors, and artists whose relentless efforts were instrumental in adapting these timeless works into reliable references for today's clinicians in training and in practice. From all of us at Elsevier, we thank you.

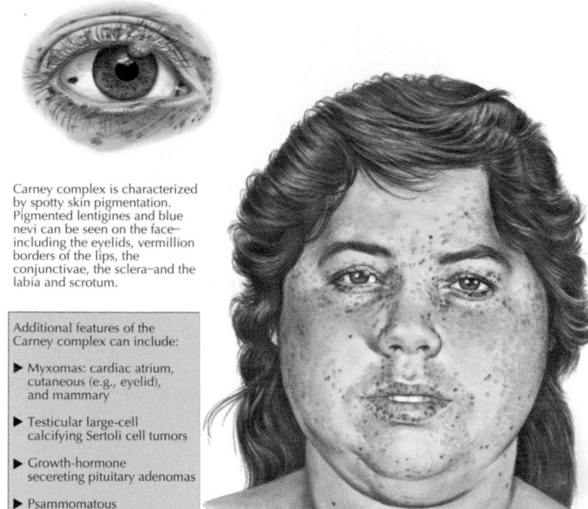

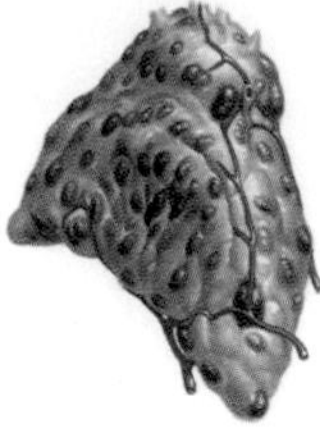

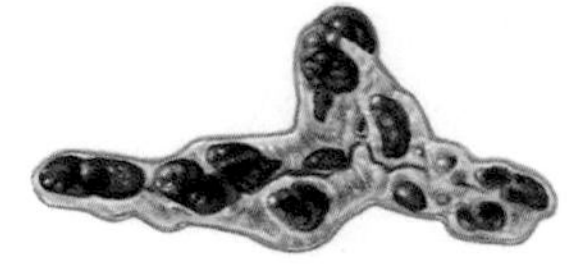

A brand new illustrated plate painted by Carlos Machado, MD, for *The Endocrine System*, Volume 2, ed. 2

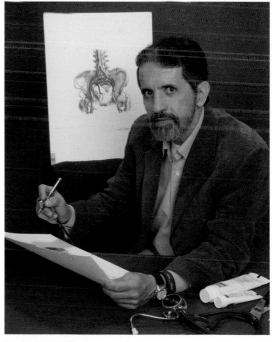

Dr. Carlos Machado at work

ABOUT THE EDITOR

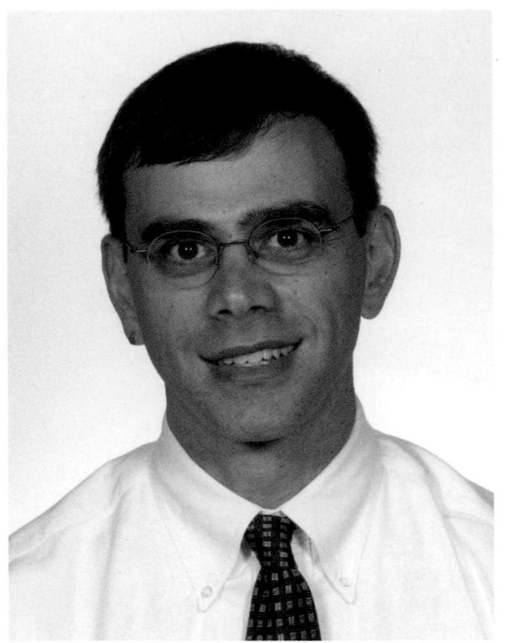

David A. Kaminsky, MD, is Associate Professor of Pulmonary and Critical Care Medicine at the University of Vermont College of Medicine. He received his undergraduate degree from Yale University, and medical degree from University of Massachusetts Medical School. He completed his residency training in Internal Medicine at Columbia Presbyterian Medical Center in New York City, and fellowship training in Pulmonary and Critical Care Medicine at the University of Colorado Health Sciences Center in Denver. He joined the faculty of the University of Vermont College of Medicine in 1995 and continues to work as a clinician, researcher, and educator. Dr. Kaminsky is the Clinical Director of the Pulmonary Function Lab, Program Director for the Fellowship Training Program in Pulmonary and Critical Care, and Associate Chair of the Institutional Review Board at University of Vermont. His areas of research interest include pulmonary physiology, lung mechanics, asthma, and COPD. His work has been funded by the National Institutes of Health, the American Lung Association, the Whittaker Foundation, and other agencies. Dr. Kaminsky has published nearly 40 original papers and a dozen book chapters and reviews. He lives in the Burlington, Vermont, area with his wife and two children, two cats, and dog. He enjoys many outdoor activities, including running, hiking, sailing, rowing, and ice hockey.

PREFACE

It has been an honor to be the editor of the second edition—first major revision in 30 years—of Netter's Respiratory System. The changes that have occurred over the past 3 decades in pulmonary medicine have been profound. The challenge of editing this edition has therefore been to include these updates while at the same time preserving the unique nature and artistic beauty of Netter's classic depiction of human health and disease. In addition to ensuring the accuracy and relevance of the timeless topics of anatomy and physiology, we have significantly revised the sections on airways, parenchymal and pleural diseases, lung cancer, infectious diseases, thromboembolic disease, inhalational diseases, acute respiratory distress syndrome, pharmacotherapy, radiology, mechanical ventilation, and trauma and surgery. New sections have been created on pulmonary immunology, pulmonary hypertension, lung manifestations of systemic disease, sleep medicine, exhaled breath analysis, endobronchial ultrasound, video-assisted thoracoscopic ultrasound, lung volume reduction surgery, and lung transplantation. I am indebted to the many outstanding contributors to this edition, who are each international experts in their field. Without their input, it would have been impossible to ensure that the most up-to-date, accurate information would be provided to bring Netter's Respiratory Disease into the 21st century. I would like to thank especially those contributors who have been my teachers and mentors over the years: Drs. David Badesch, Jason Bates, Gerry Davis, Barry Make, Ted Marcy, Polly Parsons, Charlie Irvin, Richard Irwin, Mike Iseman, and Talmadge King. Special thanks also go to Dr. Jeffrey Klein, who made extra efforts to provide radiographic images for many different sections of the book. Finally, I want to dedicate this work to my grandfather, Dr. Edward Budnitz, who shared with me his love of medicine and inspired me to pursue a career as a physician.

David Kaminsky
Burlington, Vermont
November 2010

ABOUT THE ARTIST FROM THE FIRST EDITION

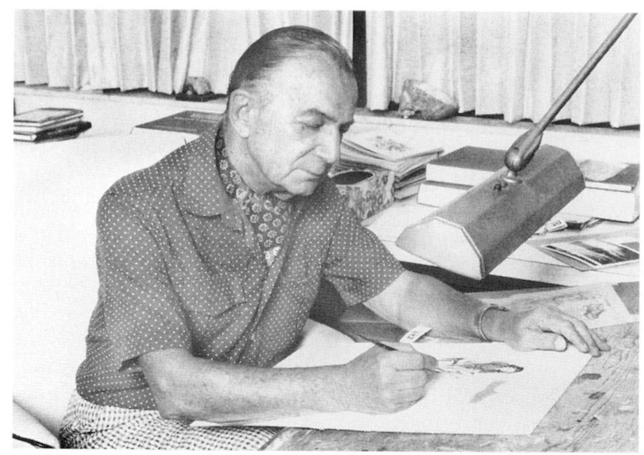

The medical paintings of Dr. Frank Netter have received such wide acclaim from physicians the world over for so long that the image of the man himself has begun to take on mythical proportions. And, indeed, it is easy to understand how such a transformation could take place. Yet, Dr. Netter is a real human being who breathes, eats and carries on a daily routine just like the rest of us and who, for that matter, stands a little in awe of the image which is so often ascribed to him.

In order to help affirm his reality as a man, we asked Dr. Netter to make the accompanying self-portrait of himself at work in his studio. The sketch portrays a number of elements which may be familiar to those who have seen photographs of Dr. Netter's studio in previous volumes of The Ciba Collection of Medical Illustrations or in other publications—the man himself, the drawing board, the paints, the brushes, the skeleton and other accoutrements. The difference is in the background. No longer is it the skyline of New York, which could be seen from his former studio window. Now it is the open sunny landscape of southern Florida, with waving palm trees and a boat traversing the waters of the intracoastal waterway.

Nevertheless, the Netters' move south from their long established New York home does not signify an intention to wind down a highly productive work schedule. Florida has meant a change in location and climate, but the intensity of Frank Netter's commitment to what has become his life's work continues undiminished. He is usually in his studio by 7:00 AM, where he concentrates on the project before him until about two o'clock. The afternoons are mostly devoted to golf, to swimming in the sea or pool, to fishing, to time with his family or friends, or to other diversions. At times he takes a "postman's holiday" to paint a landscape or a portrait just for the fun of it.

But not all of Dr. Netter's work is done at the drawing board. Much of it consists of intensive study and wide reading, observation of physicians at work in the clinic, hospital or laboratory, and long hours of discussion with a collaborator. Even during his hours of relaxation the concept of the illustrations is germinating in his mind. After these preliminaries he makes pencil sketches, composing the details and layout of the various elements of the illustrations, positioning x-rays and photomicrographs, and determining the exact dimensions and placing of the legends in order to achieve the maximum teaching effect. Only after the sketches are checked, double checked, and revised for accuracy and detail does he proceed with the finished painting. Most of his paintings are in water color, but at times he has used other media including casein paint, chalks, acrylics or oils. He maintains, however, that the medium is not very important. Good pictures can be made in any medium. He prefers water color only because through long use he feels more at home with it and because he can express himself more directly and work more rapidly with it.

Dr. Netter's great facility and skill at representative painting, gift though it may be, did not come to fruition without dedicated study and training—not only in drawing and painting but in graphic design, composition and layout as well. From the time he was a little boy he wanted to be an artist. He studied intensively at the National Academy of Design, the Art Students League of New York and other outstanding schools as well as with private teachers. He won many honors and, indeed, became a successful commercial artist in the heyday of that profession. But then, partly because of his own interest and partly because of urging by his family to do "something more serious" he decided to give up art and initiate a new career in medicine. Once in medical school, however, he found that because of his graphic training he could learn his subjects best by making drawings. So his early medical illustrations were made for his own education. But it was not long before his drawings caught the eyes of his professors, who then kept him busy in what little spare time he had making illustrations for their books and articles. Netter graduated from New York University School of Medicine and completed his internship and surgical residency at Bellevue Hospital in the depths of the great depression. It soon became evident that his art commissions from publishers and pharmaceutical manufacturers were a better source of income than his depression-stifled medical practice, and he made the decision to be a full-time medical artist.

Dr. Netter's association with the CIBA Pharmaceutical Company began in 1938 with his creation of a folder cut out in the shape of a heart. Paintings of the anterior and posterior (basal) surface of the heart were printed on the front and back and sections of the internal anatomy were depicted on the inside. An advertising message was overprinted both inside and out. The immediate response of physicians to this piece was to request that it be produced without the advertising message. This was done to great success, and thus was born a series of anatomy and pathology illustration projects, the demand for which was so great that it eventually led, in 1948, to the publication of the first book of The Ciba Collection of Medical Illustrations. The year 1978, then, is not only the year of introduction of Volume 7, Respiratory System, but is also the thirtieth anniversary of the first book of The Ciba Collection of Medical Illustrations. Coincidentally, it is also the thirtieth anniversary of the first issue of the Ciba Clinical Symposia series.

Dr. Netter is still preparing well over 100 paintings a year for The Ciba Collection of Medical Illustrations and Clinical Symposia. Even now he is well into the task of illustrating a new atlas on the musculoskeletal system. Much has been said and written in the past about the Netter "genius." Perhaps the most impressive aspect of all is not his "genius," but the use this remarkable artist-physician-teacher makes of his gifts. His collective works are monumental, and they continue to grow.

Philip B. Flagler

INTRODUCTION TO THE FIRST EDITION

Whenever a new atlas of mine appears, I feel as a woman must feel when she has just had a baby. The tediousness and travail of the long pregnancy and the pain of delivery are over, and it remains to be seen how my offspring will fare in the world.

In this case, there were a number of problems during the gestation. One of these was that interest in the respiratory system and its diseases has not only greatly increased in recent years but that its focus has been radically altered. The reasons for these changes are manifold. They include the great differences which have come about in the incidence of various lung diseases; the advent and better utilization of antibiotics; advances in radiologic technique and interpretation; the development of additional diagnostic techniques such as radioactive isotope scanning; expansion in the study of pulmonary physiology and application of pulmonary function tests; progress in understanding of pulmonary pathology; increased facility in thoracic surgery and the development of methods for predetermining operability, such as mediastinoscopy; the design or improvement of technical and diagnostic mechanisms such as oxygen and aerosol apparatus, mechanical ventilators, more efficient spirometers and surgical staplers; and alterations in the personal habits, environment and average age of the population.

All these factors, as well as others, are, however, interactive. For example, the great decrease in incidence of pulmonary tuberculosis is related to the advent of antibiotics: but it is also a consequence of improvement in living standards and habits, as well as of improved early diagnosis. These factors may also be responsible for the lesser incidence and morbidity of pneumococcal pneumonia. Whereas in former years these two diseases were major concerns of the chest physician, they are nowadays of much less significance. But this, on the other hand, has allowed more time and effort to be diverted to other lung disorders. The greatly increased incidence of lung cancer appears to have resulted in considerable measure from changes in personal habits (such as smoking), environmental pollution and occupational activity, and possibly also change in population age. But earlier discovery of tumors through greater public awareness and improved diagnosis, plus greater surgical facility, have led to increased interest in operability, and this in turn has stimulated study of pathologic classification in relation to malignancy. The increase in chronic bronchitis and emphysema, while largely real and attributable to the same etiologic factors as cancer, may to some extent be only apparent—due to better diagnostic methods and utilization of pulmonary function studies. But recognition of some of the etiologic factors and better understanding of the underlying pathologic processes, coupled with availability and utilization of such measures as aerosol medication, improved equipment for oxygen administration and mechanical ventilation, and postural drainage have greatly modified for the better the management of these distressing disorders. The current relatively high incidence of occupational diseases may likewise to some extent be only apparent, because of greater awareness and better diagnosis. Pulmonary embolus and infarction have also received increased attention in recent years as the common sources of emboli have been identified, and as the manifestations of pulmonary vascular obstruction have been more clearly defined.

In light of the foregoing examples of the changing emphasis in the field of pulmonary medicine, to which many more could be added, I have tried in this atlas to give to each topic its proper emphasis in relation to the subject as a whole, in accord with current concepts. In doing this, much consideration had to be given to space availability. A good public speaker must deliver the essentials of his message within the time allotted to him for if he rambles on and on, his audience is lost and his message ineffective. So, too, the artist must portray his subject matter as effectively as possible within the allotted pages. What to leave out becomes, at times, as important as what to include. Without such considerations, this volume might have grown to twice or three times its size and become unbalanced, or become so crowded with minutiae as to be dull and boring. In either event, the utility of the book would have been greatly impaired.

As in the preparation of all my previous atlases, my major efforts in this work were again necessarily directed towards gathering, absorbing and digesting the information about each subject so that I might properly portray it. Thus study, learning and analysis of the subject matter became as time consuming, or more so, than the actual painting of the pictures. One cannot intelligently portray a subject unless one understands it. My goal was to picture or diagram the essence of each subject, avoiding the incidental or inconsequential. In some instances I have, however, included topics which, at present, do not seem to have great practical application but which, in the future, may give important clues to pathogenesis, diagnosis or treatment. All this was greatly facilitated, indeed made possible, through the devoted cooperation of the many distinguished consultants who are listed individually on other pages of this volume. I herewith express my appreciation to each and every one of them for the time, effort and guidance which they gave me, and for the knowledge which they imparted to me. I also thank the many others who, although not officially consultants, nevertheless helped me with advice or information or by supplying reference material to me. They are also credited elsewhere in this book. I especially thank Dr. Matthew B. Divertie for his careful and thorough review of both the pictorial and text material and for his many constructive suggestions.

The production of this book involved a tremendous amount of organizational work, such as assembling and compiling the material as it grew in volume, correlating illustrations and text, grammatical checking, reference checking, type specification, page layout, proofreading, and a multitude of mechanical and practical details incidental to publication. I tremendously admire the efficiency with which these matters were handled by Mr. Philip Flagler and his staff at CIBA, including Ms. Gina Dingle, Ms. Barbara Bekiesz, Ms. Kristine Bean and Mr. Pierre Lair. Finally, I once more give praise to the CIBA Pharmaceutical Company and its executives for their vision in sponsoring this project and for the free hand they have given me in executing it. I have tried to do justice to it.

FRANK H. NETTER, MD

ADVISORY BOARD

CONTRIBUTORS

Steven H. Abman, MD
Professor
Department of Pediatrics, Section of Pulmonology
University of Colorado School of Medicine and The Children's Hospital
Aurora, Colorado
Plates 1-33 to 1-43

David B. Badesch, MD
Professor of Medicine
Division of Pulmonary Sciences and Critical Care Medicine and Cardiology
Clinical Director, Pulmonary Hypertension Center
University of Colorado Denver
Aurora, Colorado
Plates 4-114 to 4-126

Peter J. Barnes DM, DSc, FRCP, FMedSci, FRS
Head of Respiratory Medicine
National Heart and Lung Institute
Imperial College
London, England, UK
Plates 2-22 to 2-24, 5-1 to 5-10

Jason H.T. Bates, PhD, DSc
Professor of Medicine, Physiology, Biophysics
University of Vermont College of Medicine
Burlington, Vermont
Plates 2-14 to 2-21

Kevin K. Brown, MD
Professor of Medicine
Vice Chairman, Department of Medicine
Director, Interstitial Lung Disease Program
National Jewish Medical and Research Center
Denver, Colorado
Plates 4-157 to 4-162

Vito Brusasco, MD
Professor of Respiratory Medicine
University of Genoa
Genoa, Italy
Plates 2-8 to 2-13

Nancy A. Collop, MD
Professor of Sleep Medicine and Neurology
Director, Emory Sleep Program
Emory University
Atlanta, Georgia
Plates 4-165 and 4-166

Bryan Corrin, MD, FRCPath
Professor Emeritus of Pathology
London University
Honorary Senior Clinical Research Fellow
National Heart and Lung Institute
Imperial College
Honorary Consultant Pathologist
Royal Brompton Hospital
London, England, UK
Plates 1-1 to 1-16

Gerald S. Davis, MD
Professor of Medicine
Pulmonary Disease and Critical Care Medicine
University of Vermont College of Medicine
Fletcher Allen Health Care
Burlington, Vermont
Plates 4-103 to 4-113

Malcolm M. DeCamp, MD
Fowler-McCormick Professor of Surgery
Northwestern University Feinberg School of Medicine
Chief, Division of Thoracic Surgery
Northwestern Memorial Hospital
Chicago, Illinois
Plates 3-26, 5-25 to 5-33

Raed A. Dweik, MD
Director, Pulmonary Vascular Program
Department of Pulmonary and Critical Care Medicine
Cleveland Clinic
Cleveland, Ohio
Plate 3-20

David Feller-Kopman, MD
Director, Interventional Pulmonology
Associate Professor of Medicine
The Johns Hopkins Hospital
Baltimore, Maryland
Plates 3-21 to 3-25, 5-15 to 5-17, 5-20 to 5-23

Alex H. Gifford, MD
Fellow, Pulmonary and Critical Care Medicine
Dartmouth-Hitchcock Medical Center
Lebanon, New Hampshire
Plates 2-25 to 2-31

Curtis Green, MD
Professor of Radiology and Cardiology
University of Vermont College of Medicine
Staff Radiologist
Fletcher Allen Health Care
Burlington, Vermont
Plates 3-4 to 3-19

Anne Greenough MD (Cantab), MB BS, DCH, FRCP, FRCPCH
Division of Asthma Allergy and Lung Biology, MRC, and Asthma
UK Centre in Allergic Mechanisms of Asthma
King's College London
Neonatal Centre
King's College Hospital
Denmark Hill
London, England, UK
Plates 4-1 to 4-9, 4-144, 4-145

Charles G. Irvin, PhD
Vice Chairman for Research
Department of Medicine
Director, Vermont Lung Center
Professor, Departments of Medicine and Molecular Physiology & Biophysics
University of Vermont College of Medicine
Burlington, Vermont
Plates 2-1 to 2-7

Richard S. Irwin, MD
Professor of Medicine
University of Massachusetts Medical School
Chair, Critical Care
UMass Memorial Medical Center
Worcester, Massachusetts
Plate 4-10

Michael Iseman, MD
Professor of Medicine
National Jewish Medical and Research Center
Denver, Colorado
Plates 4-93 to 4-102

James R. Jett, MD
Professor of Medicine
National Jewish Medical and Research Center
Denver, Colorado
Plates 4-48 to 4-63

Marc A. Judson, MD
Professor of Medicine
Division of Pulmonary and Critical Care Medicine
Medical University of South Carolina
Charleston, South Carolina
Plates 4-155 and 4-156

David A. Kaminsky, MD
Associate Professor
Pulmonary and Critical Care Medicine
University of Vermont College of Medicine
Burlington, Vermont
Plates 3-1 to 3-3, 5-18

Greg King, MB, ChB, PhD, FRACP
Head of Imaging Group
The Woolcock Institute of Medical Research
Department of Respiratory Medicine
Royal North Shore Hospital
St. Leonards, Australia
Plates 4-163 and 4-164

Talmadge E. King, Jr., MD
Julius R. Krevans Distinguished Professorship in Internal Medicine
Chair, Department of Medicine
University of California, San Francisco
San Francisco, California
Plates 4-147 to 4-154

Jeffrey Klein, MD
Director, Thoracic Radiology
Fletcher Allen Health Care
Professor
University of Vermont College of Medicine
Burlington, Vermont
Plates 3-4 to 3-19

Kevin O. Leslie, MD
Professor of Pathology
Mayo Clinic Arizona
Scottsdale, Arizona
Plates 1-17 to 1-31

Donald A. Mahler, MD
Professor of Medicine
Pulmonary and Critical Care Medicine
Dartmouth Medical School
Dartmouth-Hitchcock Medical Center
Lebanon, New Hampshire
Plates 2-25 to 2-31

Barry Make, MD
Professor of Medicine
National Jewish Medical and Research Center
Denver, Colorado
Plates 5-11 to 5-14

Theodore W. Marcy, MD, MPH
Professor of Medicine
Pulmonary Disease and Critical Care Medicine Unit
University of Vermont College of Medicine
Burlington, Vermont
Plates 4-127, 4-128, 5-24

James G. Martin, MD, DSc
Director, Meakins Christie Laboratories
Professor of Medicine
McGill University
Montreal, Quebec, Canada
Plate 1-32

Deborah H. McCollister, RN
University of Colorado Health Sciences Center
Denver, Colorado
Plates 4-114 to 4-126

Meredith C. McCormack, MD, MHS
Assistant Professor of Medicine
Division of Pulmonary and Critical Care Medicine
Johns Hopkins University
Baltimore, Maryland
Plates 4-28 to 4-42

Ernest Moore, MD
Professor and Vice Chairman
Department of Surgery
University of Colorado Denver
Bruce M. Rockwell Distinguished Chair in Trauma
Chief of Surgery
Denver Health
Denver, Colorado
Plates 4-135 to 4-143

Michael S. Niederman, MD
Chairman, Department of Medicine
Winthrop-University Hospital
Mineola, New York;
Professor of Medicine
Vice-Chairman, Department of Medicine
SUNY at Stony Brook
Stony Brook, New York
Plates 4-64 to 4-83

Paul M. O'Byrne, MB, FRCPI, FRCPC
E.J. Moran Campbell Professor and Chair
Department of Medicine
McMaster University
Hamilton, Ontario, Canada
Plates 4-14 to 4-27

Polly E. Parsons, MD
E. L. Amidon Professor of Medicine
Chair, Department of Medicine
Director, Pulmonary and Critical Care Medicine
University of Vermont College of Medicine
Medicine Health Care Service Leader
Fletcher Allen Health Care
Burlington, Vermont
Plate 4-146

Elena Pollina, MD
Department of Histopathology
King's College Hospital
London, England, UK
Plates 4-1 to 4-9

Catheryne J. Queen
Mycobacterial and Respiratory Diseases Division
National Jewish Health Medical and Research Center
Denver, Colorado
Plates 4-93 to 4-102

Margaret Rosenfeld, MD, MPH
Medical Director, Pulmonary Function Laboratory
Seattle Children's
Associate Professor of Pediatrics
University of Washington School of Medicine
Seattle, Washington
Plates 4-43 to 4-47

Steven Sahn, MD
Professor of Medicine
Division of Pulmonary, Critical Care, Allergy, and Sleep Medicine
Medical University of South Carolina
Charleston, South Carolina
Plates 4-129 to 4-134

Sanjay Sethi, MD
Professor, Department of Medicine
Chief, Division of Pulmonary, Critical Care, and Sleep Medicine
University at Buffalo, SUNY
Section Chief, Division of Pulmonary, Critical Care and Sleep Medicine
Western New York VA HealthCare System
Buffalo, New York
Plates 4-84 to 4-92

Damon A. Silverman, MD
Assistant Professor of Otolaryngology
University of Vermont College of Medicine
Director, The Vermont Voice Center
Fletcher Allen Health Care
Burlington, Vermont
Plates 4-11 to 4-13, 5-19

Robert A. Wise, MD
Professor of Medicine and Environmental Health Sciences
Division of Pulmonary and Critical Care Medicine
Johns Hopkins University
Johns Hopkins Asthma & Allergy Center
Baltimore, Maryland
Plates 4-28 to 4-42

CONTENTS

Contents

SECTION 1

ANATOMY AND EMBRYOLOGY

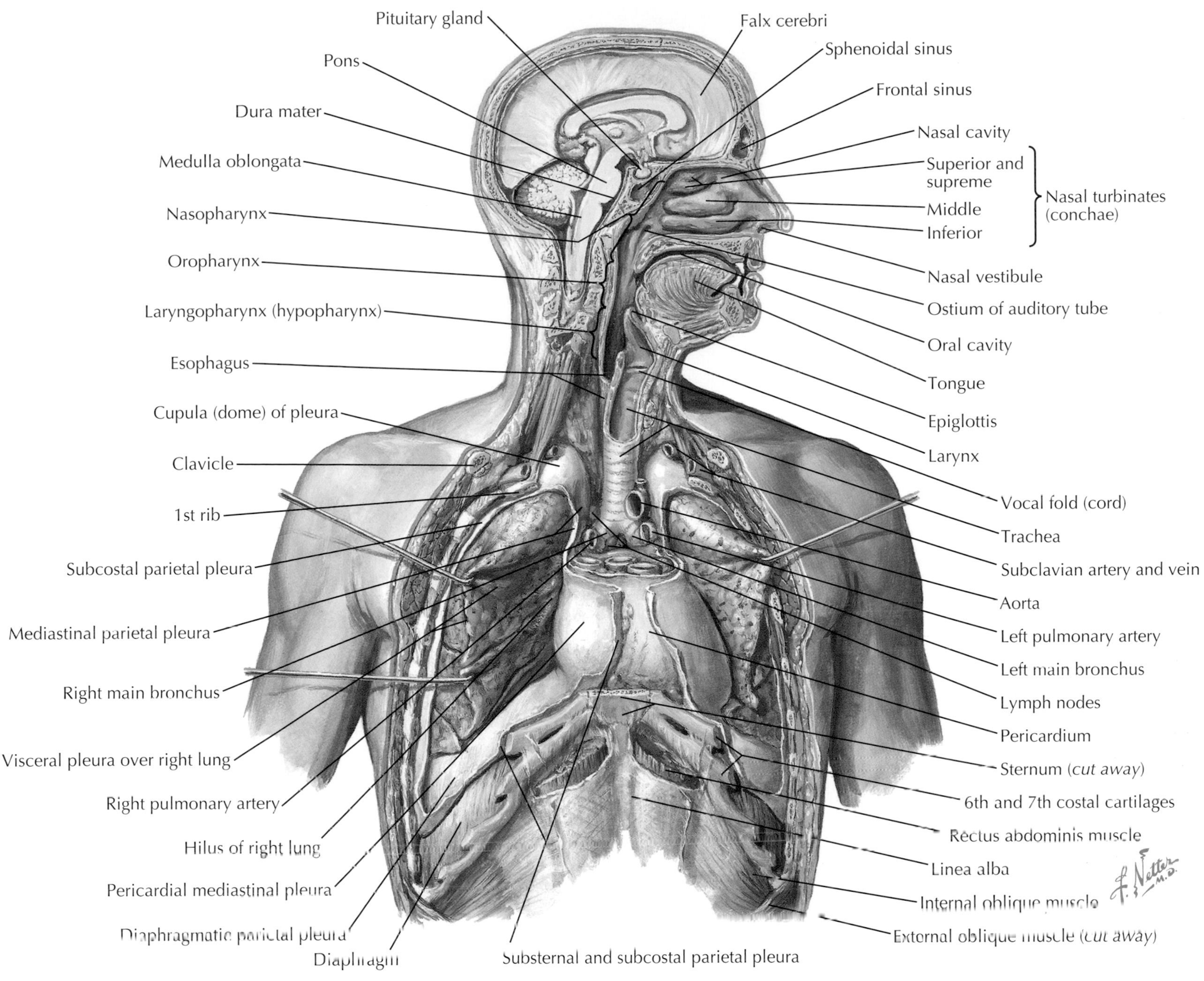

Respiratory System

The respiratory system is made up of the structures involved in the exchange of oxygen and carbon dioxide between the blood and the atmosphere, so-called *external respiration*. The exchange of gases between the blood in the capillaries of the systemic circulation and the tissues in which these capillaries are located is referred to as *internal respiration*.

The respiratory system consists of the external nose, internal nose, and paranasal sinuses; the pharynx, which is the common passage for air and food; the larynx, where the voice is produced; and the trachea, bronchi, and lungs. Accessory structures necessary for the operation of the respiratory system are the pleurae, diaphragm, thoracic wall, and muscles that raise and lower the ribs in inspiration and expiration. The muscles of the anterolateral abdominal wall are also accessory to *forceful* expiration (their contraction forces the diaphragm upward by pressing the contents of the abdominal cavity against it from below) and are used in "abdominal" respiration. Certain muscles of the neck can elevate the ribs, thus enlarging the anteroposterior diameter of the thorax, and under some circumstances, the muscles attaching the arms to the thoracic wall can also help change the capacity of the thorax.

In Plates 1-1 through 1-16, the anatomy of the respiratory system and significant accessory structures is shown. It is important not only to visualize these structures in isolation but also to become familiar with their blood supply, nerve supply, and relationships with both adjacent structures and the surface of the body. One should keep in mind that these relationships are subject to the same degree of individual variation that affects all anatomic structures. The illustrations depict the most common situations encountered. No attempt is made to describe all of the many variations that occur.

An important and clinically valuable concept that is worth emphasizing at this point is the convention of subdividing each lung into lobes and segments on the basis of branching of the bronchial tree. From the standpoint of its embryologic development, as well as of its function as a fully established organ of respiration, the lung is indeed the ultimate branching of the main bronchus that leads into it. Knowledge of the subdivision of the lung on this basis is essential to anatomists, physiologists, pathologists, radiologists, surgeons, and chest physicians because without this three-dimensional key, there is no exact means of precisely localizing lesions within the respiratory system.

Bony Thorax

The skeletal framework of the thorax—the bony thorax—consists of 12 pairs of ribs and their cartilages, 12 thoracic vertebrae and intervertebral discs, and the sternum. The illustration also includes one clavicle and scapula because these bones serve as important attachments for some of the muscles involved in respiration.

The sternum is made up of three parts—the manubrium, body, and xiphoid process. The manubrium and body are not in quite the same plane and thus form the *sternal angle* at their junction, a significant landmark at which the costal cartilage of the second rib articulates with the sternum. The superior border of the manubrium is slightly concave, forming what is called the *suprasternal notch*.

The costal cartilages of the first through seventh ribs ordinarily articulate with the sternum and are called *true ribs*. The costal cartilages of the eighth through tenth ribs (*false ribs*) are usually attached to the cartilage of the rib above, and the ventral ends of the cartilages of the eleventh and twelfth ribs (*floating ribs*) have no direct skeletal attachment.

All of the ribs articulate dorsally with the vertebral column in such a way that their ventral end (together with the sternum) can be raised slightly, as occurs in inspiration. The articulations of the costal cartilages with the sternum, except those of the first rib, are true or synovial joints that allow more freedom of movement than there would be without this type of articulation.

The deep surface of the scapula (the subscapular fossa) fits against the posterolateral aspect of the thorax over the second to seventh ribs, where, to a great extent, it is held by the muscles that are attached to it. The acromion process of the scapula articulates with the lateral end of the clavicle; this acts as a strut to hold the lateral angle of the scapula away from the thorax. On the dorsal surface of the scapula, a spine protrudes and continues laterally into the acromion process. At its vertebral end, the spine flattens into a smooth triangular surface with the base of the triangle at the vertebral border. The spine separates the supraspinous fossa from the infraspinous fossa. Three borders of the scapula are described—superior, lateral, and medial or vertebral. On the superior border is a notch or incisura, and lateral to this, the coracoid process protrudes anteriorly.

The lateral angle of the scapula presents a slight concavity, the glenoid fossa, for articulation with the head of the humerus. At the superior end of the glenoid fossa is the supraglenoid tuberosity, and at its inferior margin is the infraglenoid tuberosity.

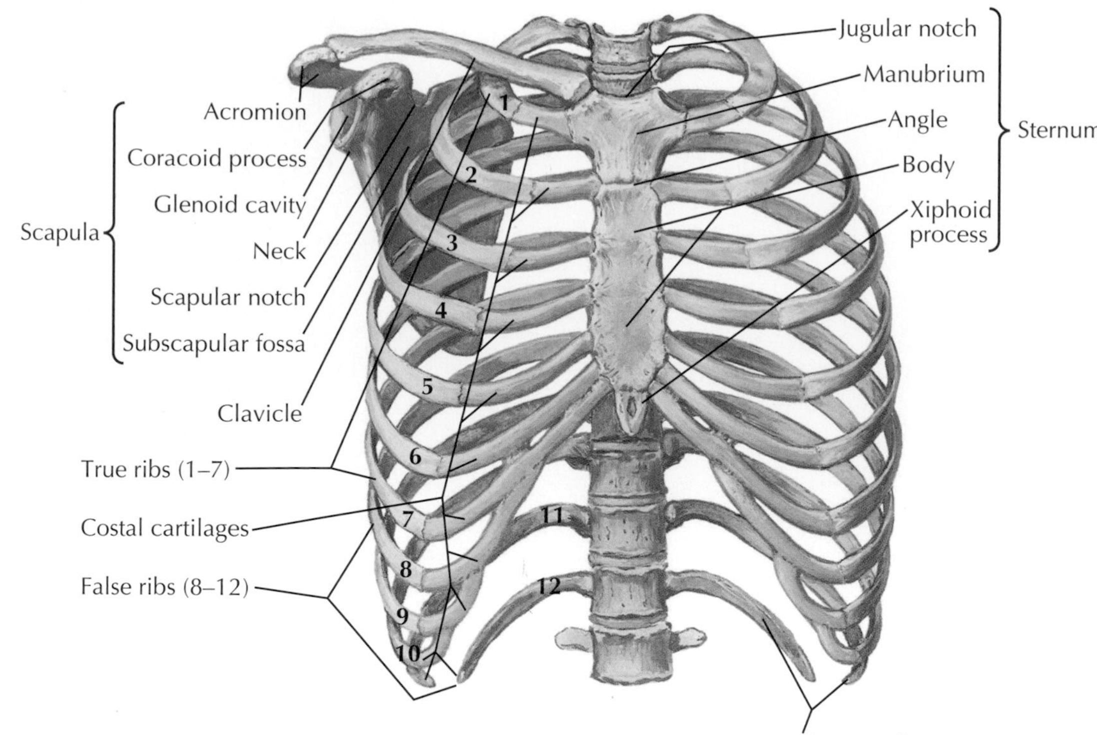

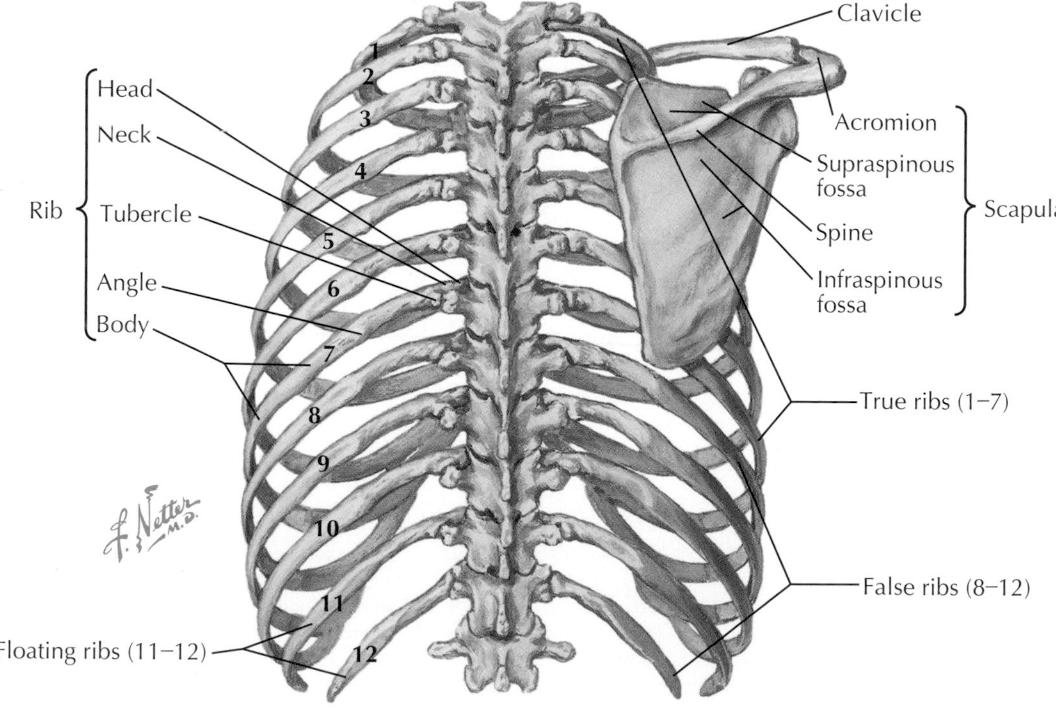

The clavicle articulates at its medial end with the superolateral aspect of the manubrium of the sternum and at its lateral end with the medial edge of the acromion process of the scapula. Its medial two-thirds are curved slightly anteriorly, and its lateral third is curved posteriorly. Muscular attachments to the medial and lateral parts of the clavicle leave its middle portion less protected and thus readily subject to fracture.

The vertebral levels of the bony landmarks on the ventral aspect of the thorax are variable and differ somewhat with the phase of respiration. In general, the upper border of the manubrium is at the level of the second to third thoracic vertebrae, the sternal angle opposite the fourth to fifth thoracic vertebrae, and the xiphisternal junction at the level of the ninth thoracic vertebra.

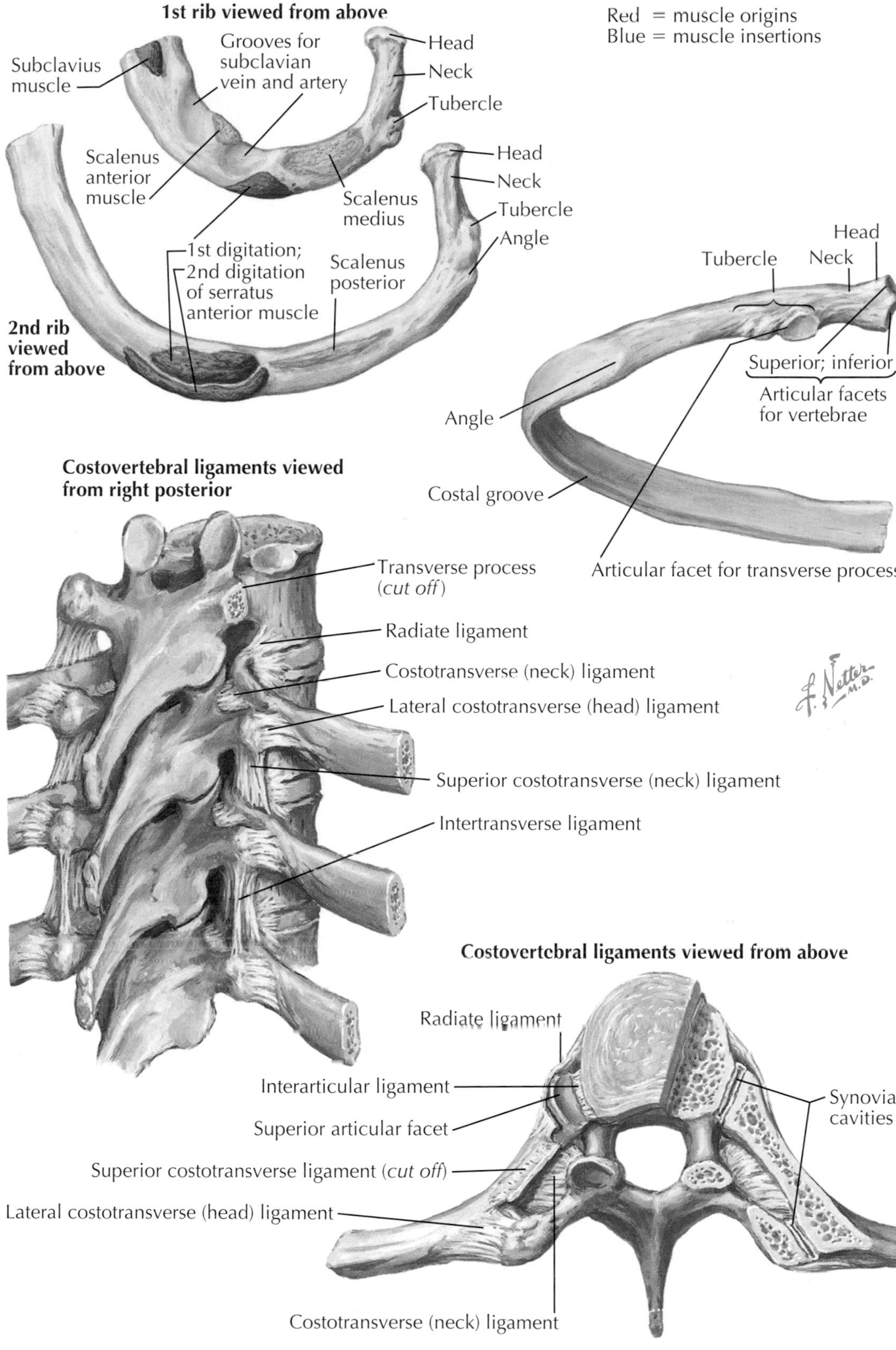

Rib Characteristics and Costovertebral Articulations

A typical rib has a head, a neck, and a body. The head articulates with one or two vertebral bodies (see below). A tubercle at the lateral end of the relatively short neck articulates with the transverse process of the lower of the two vertebrae with which the head of the rib articulates. As the body is followed anteriorly, the "angle" of the rib is formed. At the inferior border of the body is the costal or subcostal groove, partially housing the intercostal artery, vein, and nerve. Each rib is continued anteriorly by a costal cartilage by which it is attached either directly or indirectly to the sternum, except for the eleventh and twelfth ribs, which have no sternal attachment.

The first and second ribs differ from the typical rib and therefore need special description. The first rib—the shortest and most curved of all the ribs—is quite flat, and its almost horizontal surfaces face roughly superiorly and inferiorly. On its superior surface are grooves for the subclavian artery and subclavian vein, separated by a tubercle for the attachment of the scalenus anterior muscle.

The second rib is a good deal longer than the first, but its curvature is very similar to the curvature of the first rib. The angle of the second rib, which is close to the tubercle, is not at all marked. Its external surface faces to some extent superiorly but a bit more outward than that of the first rib.

The typical articulation of a rib with the vertebral column involves both the head and tubercle of the rib. The head has two articular facets—the superior facet making contact with the vertebral body above and the inferior one with the vertebral body below. Between these, the head of the rib is bound to the intervertebral disc by the intraarticular ligament. The articular facet on the tubercle of the rib contacts the transverse process of the lower of the two vertebrae. These are true or synovial joints, with articular cartilages, joint capsules, and synovial cavities. The articulations of the first, tenth, eleventh, and twelfth ribs are each with only one vertebra, the vertebra of the same number.

The ligaments related to the typical articulation of a rib with the vertebral column are as follows: for articulation of the head of the rib, the intraarticular ligament and the capsular ligament, with a thickening of its anterior part forming the radiate ligament; and for the costotransverse joint, the thin capsular ligament, the lateral costotransverse ligament between the lateral part of the tubercle of the rib and the tip of the transverse process, and the superior costotransverse ligament attached to the transverse process of the rib above.

The first and the last two (or three) ribs each has a single articular facet that makes contact with an impression on the side of the thoracic vertebra of the same number. No intraarticular ligament is present, so there is just a single synovial cavity, in contrast to the two synovial cavities present for the, typical rib. The lowest ribs do not have synovial joints between their tubercles and the transverse processes of the related vertebrae.

ANTERIOR THORACIC WALL

The anterior thoracic wall is covered by skin and the superficial fascia, which contains the mammary glands. Its framework is formed by the anterior part of the bony thorax, described and illustrated in Plate 1-2.

The muscles here belong to three groups: muscles of the upper extremity, muscles of the anterolateral abdominal wall, and intrinsic muscles of the thorax (see Plates 1-4, 1-5, and 1-6).

MUSCLES OF THE UPPER EXTREMITY

These muscles include the pectoralis major, pectoralis minor, serratus anterior, and subclavius.

The *pectoralis major* is a thick, fan-shaped muscle that has three areas of origin: clavicular, sternocostal, and abdominal. The clavicular origin is the anterior surface of roughly the medial half of the clavicle. The sternocostal origin is the anterior surface of the manubrium and body of the sternum and the costal cartilages of the first six ribs. The small and variable abdominal origin is the aponeurosis of the external abdominal oblique muscle. The pectoralis major inserts onto the crest of the greater tubercle of the humerus.

The *pectoralis minor* is a thin triangular muscle that lies deep to the pectoralis major. It arises from the superior margins and external surfaces of the third, fourth, and fifth ribs close to their costal cartilages and from the fascia covering the intervening intercostal muscles. The pectoralis minor inserts onto the coracoid process of the scapula. The pectoralis major and minor muscles are supplied by the medial and lateral anterior thoracic (pectoral) nerves, which are branches of the medial and lateral cords of the brachial plexus.

The *serratus anterior* is a large muscular sheet that curves around the thorax. It arises by muscular digitations from the external surfaces and superior borders of the first eight or nine ribs and from the fascia covering the intervening intercostal muscles. It inserts onto the ventral surface of the vertebral border of the scapula. Its nerve supply is the long thoracic nerve, a branch of the brachial plexus (fifth, sixth, and seventh cervical nerves), which courses inferiorly on the external surface of the muscle.

The *subclavius* is a small triangular muscle tucked between the clavicle and the first rib. It has a tendinous origin from the junction of the first rib and its costal cartilage, and it inserts into a groove toward the lateral end of the lower surface of the clavicle. It receives its nerve supply from the subclavian branch of the brachial plexus.

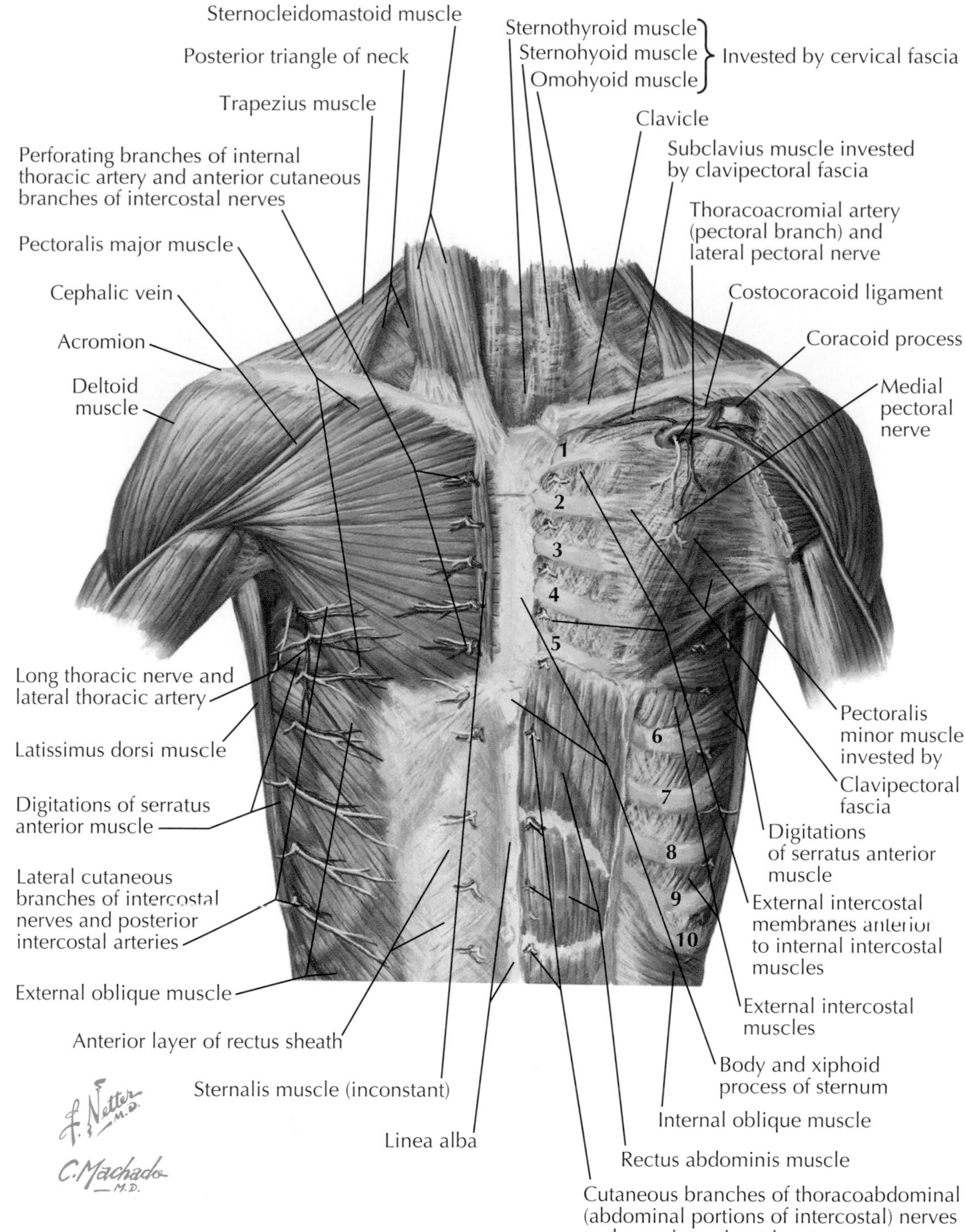

MUSCLES OF THE ANTEROLATERAL ABDOMINAL WALL

These muscles, which are partially on the anterior thoracic wall, are the external abdominal oblique and the rectus abdominis.

The *external abdominal oblique muscle* originates by fleshy digitations from the external surfaces and inferior borders of the fifth to twelfth ribs. The fasciculi from the last two ribs insert into the iliac crest, and the remaining fasciculi end in an aponeurosis that inserts in the linea alba.

The superior end of the *rectus abdominis muscle* is attached primarily to the external surfaces of the costal cartilages of the fifth, sixth, and seventh ribs. The rectus abdominis muscle is enclosed in a sheath formed by the aponeuroses of the external oblique, the internal oblique, and the transverse abdominis muscles. Its inferior end is attached to the crest of the pubis.

The muscles of the anterolateral abdominal wall are supplied by the thoracoabdominal branches of the lower six thoracic nerves.

INTRINSIC MUSCLES OF THE THORAX

These muscles, which help to form the anterior thoracic wall, are the external and internal intercostal muscles and the transversus thoracis muscle.

The *external intercostal muscles* each arise from the lower border of the rib above and insert onto the upper border of the rib below. Their fibers are directed downward and medially. They extend from the tubercles of

Anterior Thoracic Wall

(Continued)

the ribs to the beginnings of the costal cartilages, from which they continue medially as the anterior intercostal membranes. The *internal intercostal muscles* each arise from the inner lip and floor of the costal groove of the rib above and from the related costal cartilage. They insert onto the upper border of the rib below. These muscles extend from the sternum to the angles of the ribs, from which they continue to the vertebral column as the posterior intercostal membranes. The fibers of the internal intercostal muscles are directed downward and laterally. The *innermost intercostal muscles* are deep to the internal intercostals, of which they were once regarded a constituent. They attach to the internal aspects of adjoining ribs and their fibers run in the same direction as those of the internal intercostals. The intercostal muscles are supplied by the related intercostal nerves.

A muscle occasionally present, the *sternalis*, lies on the origin of the pectoralis major muscle parallel to the sternum. Its variable attachments are to the costal cartilages, sternum, rectus sheath, and sternocleidomastoid and pectoralis major muscles.

On the inner surface of the anterior thoracic wall lies a thin sheet of muscular and tendinous fibers called the *transversus thoracis muscle*. This muscle arises from the posterior surfaces of the xiphoid process, the lower third of the body of the sternum, and the sternal ends of the related costal cartilages. It is inserted by muscular slips onto the inner surfaces of the second or third to the sixth costal cartilages.

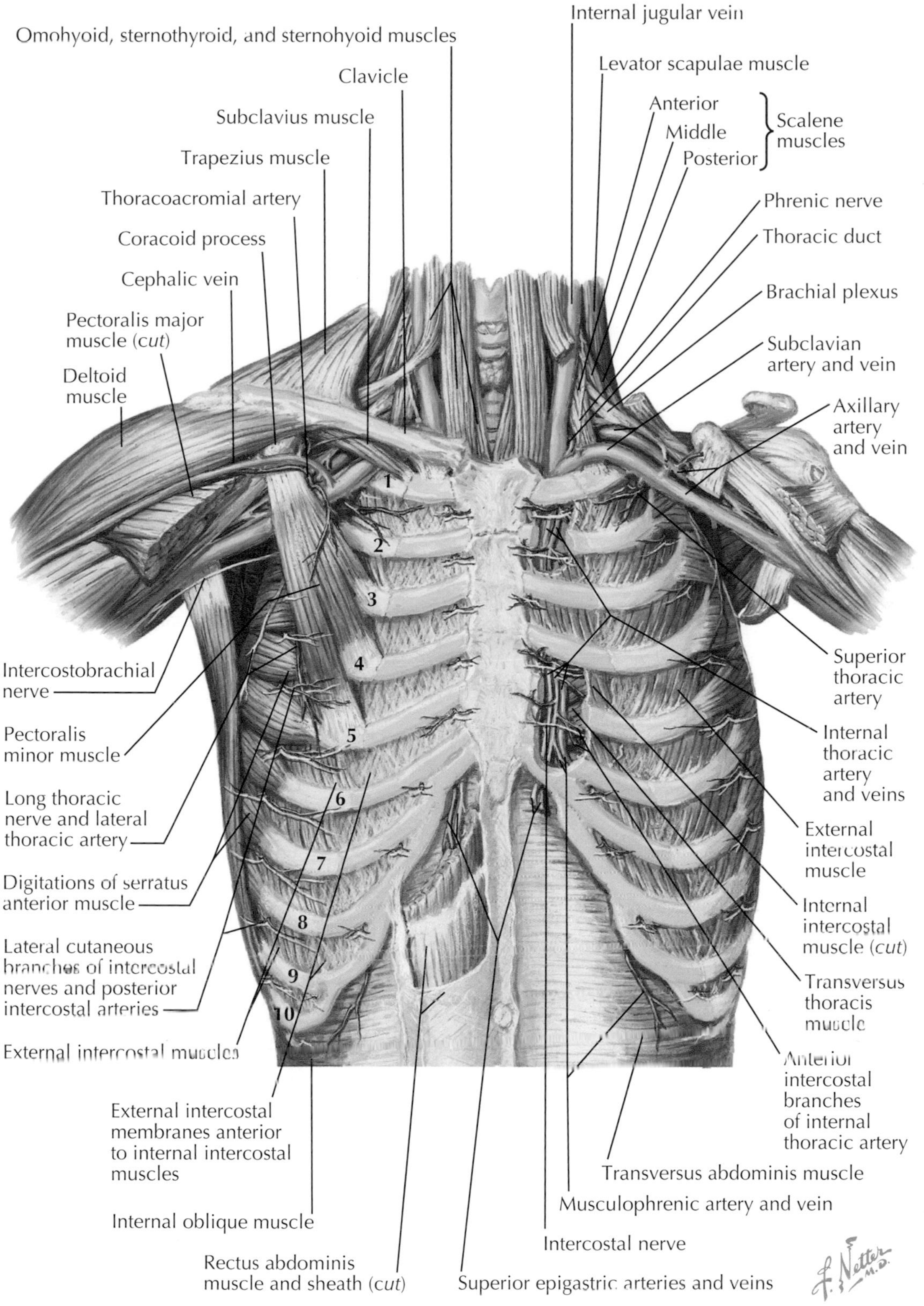

NERVES OF THE ANTERIOR THORACIC WALL

The nerve supply of the skin of the anterior thoracic wall has two sources: the anterior and middle supraclavicular nerves (branches of the cervical plexus made up mostly of fibers from the fourth cervical nerve) cross over the clavicle to supply the skin of the infraclavicular area; the anterior and lateral cutaneous branches of the related intercostal nerves pierce the muscles to supply the skin of the remainder of the anterior thoracic wall.

ARTERIES OF THE ANTERIOR THORACIC WALL

Arteries supplying the anterior thoracic wall come from several sources. There is typically an artery in the upper part of the intercostal space and one in the lower part of the space. Posteriorly, nine pairs of intercostal arteries come from the back of the aorta and run forward in the lower nine intercostal spaces. Also posteriorly, the first intercostal space receives the highest intercostal branch of the costocervical trunk from the subclavian artery. This same artery anastomoses with the highest aortic intercostal artery, contributing to the supply of the second intercostal space. Near the angle of the rib, each aortic intercostal artery gives off a collateral intercostal branch that descends to run forward along the upper border of the rib below the intercostal space. These arteries anastomose with the intercostal branches of the internal thoracic (internal mammary) artery, of which there are two in each of the upper five or six spaces.

VEINS OF THE ANTERIOR THORACIC WALL

Similar to venous drainage elsewhere, that of the anterior thoracic wall exhibits considerable variation. The most frequent pattern involves the veins accompanying the internal thoracic (internal mammary) arteries and

ANTERIOR THORACIC WALL
(Continued)

the azygos, hemiazygos, and accessory hemiazygos veins. The veins accompanying the internal thoracic arteries receive tributaries corresponding to the arterial branches and empty into the brachiocephalic (innominate) veins of the same side. The first posterior intercostal vein usually empties into either the brachiocephalic (innominate) or the vertebral vein. The right highest intercostal vein usually drains blood from the second and third intercostal spaces and passes inferiorly to empty into the azygos vein. The left highest intercostal vein also receives the second and third posterior intercostal veins and empties into the lower border of the left brachiocephalic vein.

The fourth to the eleventh posterior intercostal veins on the right side empty into the azygos vein, which is ordinarily formed by the junction of the right ascending lumbar vein and the right subcostal vein. The latter courses superiorly on the right side of the thoracic vertebrae to the level of the fourth posterior intercostal vein, where it passes in front of the root of the lung to empty into the superior vena cava just before this vessel enters the pericardial sac. On the left side, the ascending lumbar vein and the subcostal vein form the hemiazygos vein, which usually receives the lower four posterior intercostal veins as it runs superiorly to the left of the vertebral column. Here it crosses at about the level of the ninth thoracic vertebra to empty into the azygos vein. The accessory hemiazygos vein receives the fourth to the eighth posterior intercostal veins as it courses inferiorly to the left of the vertebral column before crossing at about the level of the eighth thoracic vertebra, also emptying into the azygos vein.

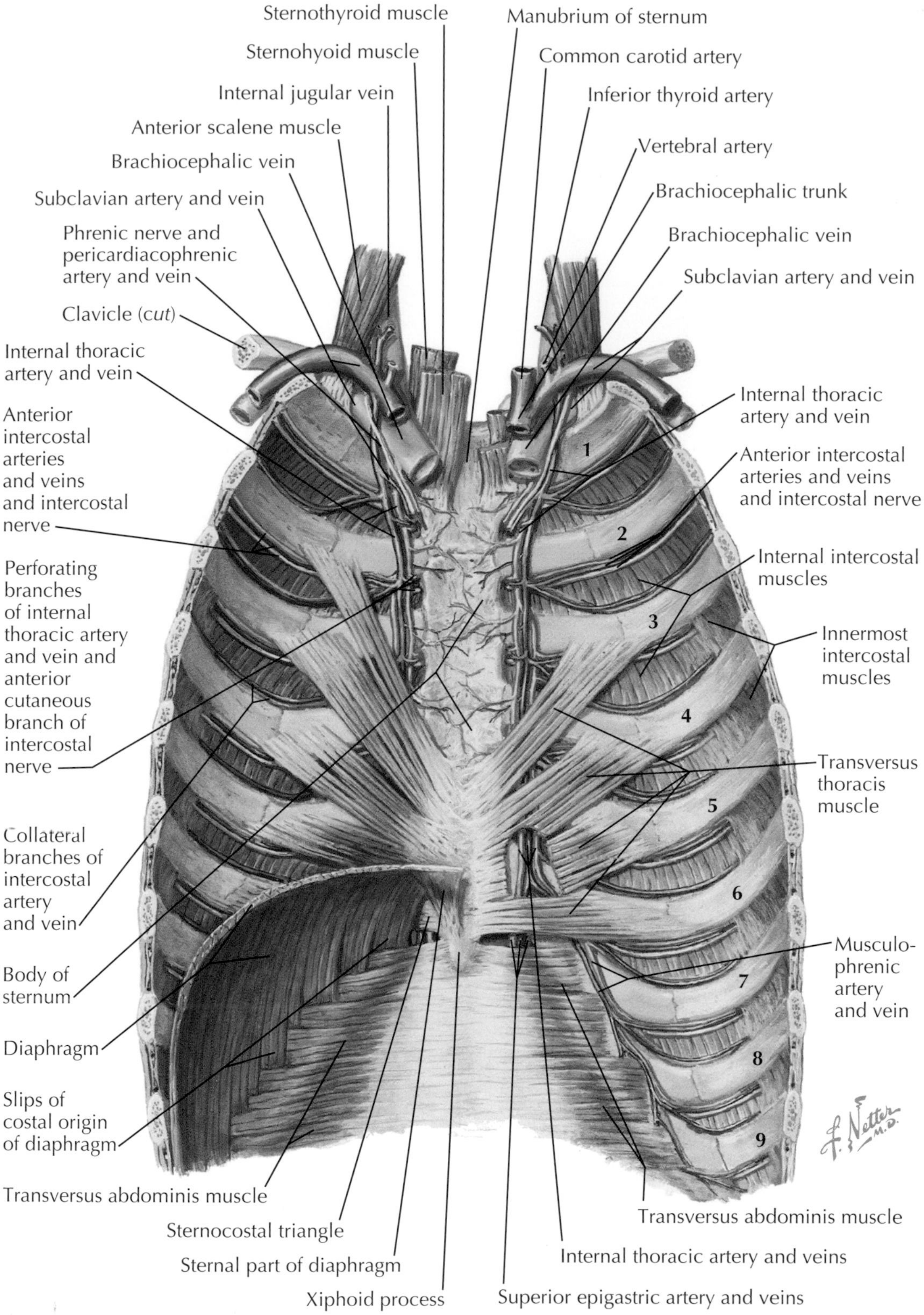

LYMPHATIC DRAINAGE OF THE ANTERIOR THORACIC WALL

The lymphatic drainage of the anterior thoracic wall involves three general groups of lymph nodes: sternal (internal thoracic), phrenic (diaphragmatic), and intercostal. The sternal nodes lie along the superior parts of the internal thoracic arteries. There are several groups of phrenic nodes on the superior surface of the diaphragm, and there is an intercostal node or two at the vertebral end of each intercostal space. The efferents of the sternal nodes usually empty into the bronchomediastinal trunk. The efferents of the phrenic nodes ordinarily go to the sternal nodes. The upper intercostal nodes send their efferents to the thoracic duct, and the lower ones on each side drain into a vessel that courses inferiorly into the cisterna chyli.

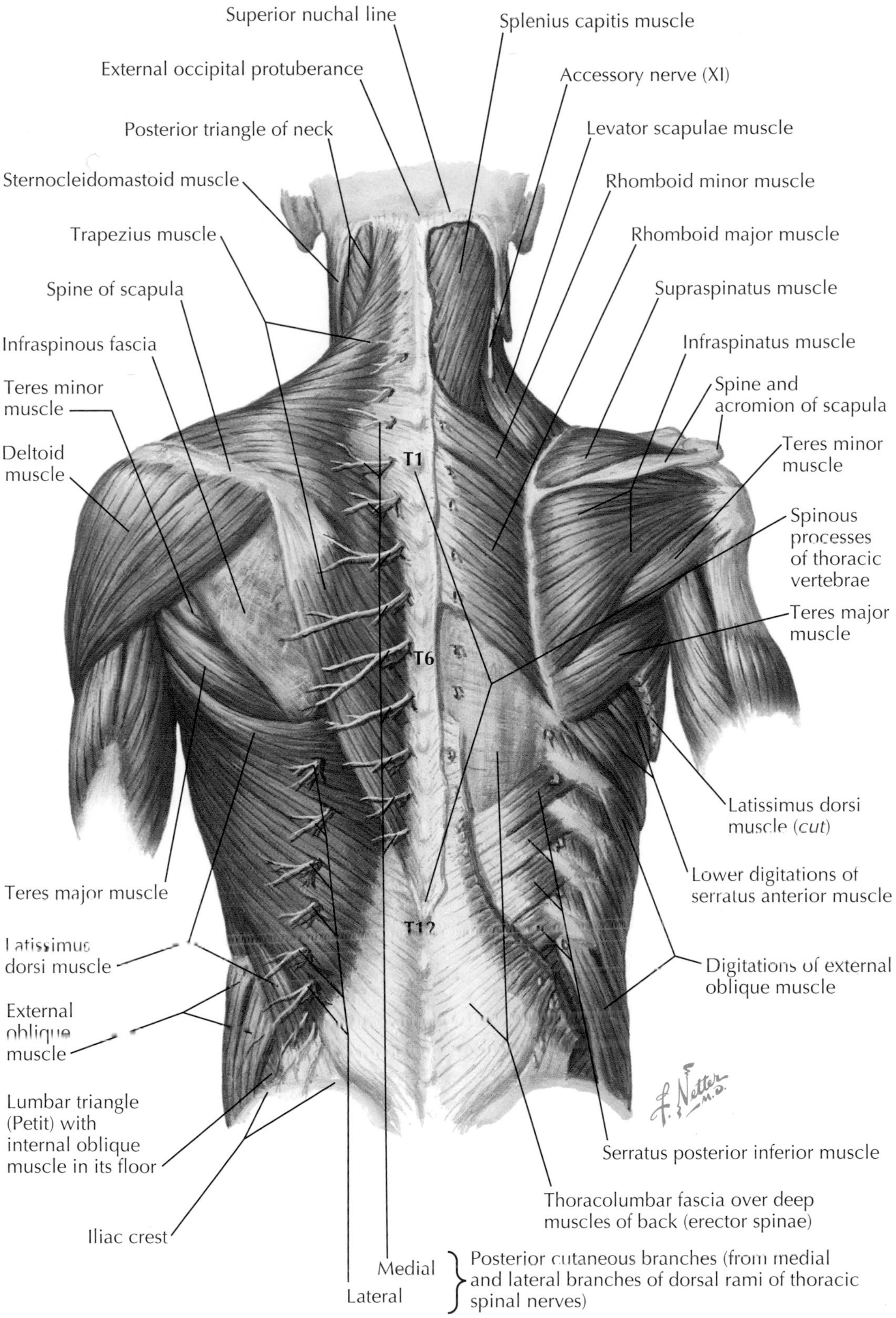

Dorsal Aspect of the Thorax

The dorsal aspect of the thorax is also covered by skin and superficial fascia, with the cutaneous nerves to the skin of the back ramifying in the latter. These cutaneous nerves are branches of the posterior primary divisions (dorsal rami) of the thoracic nerves—for the upper six thoracic levels the medial branch and for the lower six the lateral branch.

The more superficial muscles on the posterior aspect of the thorax belong to the group connecting the upper extremity to the vertebral column. They are the trapezius, latissimus dorsi, rhomboideus major, rhomboideus minor, and levator scapulae.

The *trapezius muscle* arises from about the medial third of the superior nuchal line, the external occipital protuberance and the posterior margin of the ligamentum nuchae, and the spinous processes of the seventh cervical and all of the thoracic vertebrae and the related supraspinous ligaments. The lower fibers converge into an aponeurosis that slides over the triangular area at the medial end of the spine of the scapula and is attached at the apex of this triangle. The middle group of fibers is inserted on the medial margin of the acromion and the upper margin of the posterior border of the spine of the scapula. The upper group of fibers ends on the posterior border of the lateral third of the clavicle. The trapezius is supplied by the spinal part of the eleventh cranial nerve and branches from the anterior divisions (ventral rami) of the third and fourth cervical nerves. When contracting, the muscle tends to pull the scapula medially while at the same time rotating it, thus carrying the shoulder superiorly. If the shoulder is fixed, the upper fibers tilt the head so that the face goes upward toward the opposite side.

The *latissimus dorsi muscle* has a broad origin—by a small muscular slip from the outer lip of the iliac crest just lateral to the sacrospinalis muscle and by an extensive aponeurosis attached to the spinous processes of the lower six thoracic vertebrae, the lumbar and sacral vertebrae, and the related supraspinous ligaments. This muscle is inserted into the depth of the intertubercular groove of the humerus. Its nerve supply comes from the sixth, seventh, and eighth cervical nerves by way of the thoracodorsal branch of the brachial plexus. This muscle helps with extension, adduction, and medial rotation at the shoulder joint and helps to depress the raised arm against resistance.

The *rhomboideus major and minor muscles* are often difficult to separate. The rhomboideus major arises from the tips of the spinous processes and supraspinous ligaments of the second to fifth thoracic vertebrae. Its insertion is into the vertebral border of the scapula via a tendinous arch running from the lower angle of the smooth triangle at the root of the spine to the inferior angle. The rhomboideus minor muscle arises from the spinous processes of the first thoracic and last cervical vertebrae and the lower part of the ligamentum nuchae and is inserted into the vertebral border of the scapula at the base of the triangle, forming the root of the scapular spine. The rhomboideus muscles are supplied by fibers from the fifth and sixth cervical nerves by way of the dorsoscapular branch of the brachial plexus. The rhomboideus major and minor muscles tend to

Dorsal Aspect of the Thorax *(Continued)*

draw the scapula toward the vertebral column and slightly superiorly, with the lower fibers of the major muscles helping to rotate the scapula so that the shoulder is depressed.

The *levator scapulae muscle* originates in four tendinous slips attached to the transverse processes of the first four cervical vertebrae. Its insertion is the vertebral border of the scapula from its superior angle to the smooth triangle at the medial end of the spine scapula. Its nerve supply is primarily by cervical plexus branches from the ventral rami of the third and fourth cervical nerves. The levator scapulae, as the name indicates, elevates the scapula, drawing it medially and rotating it so that the tip of the shoulder is depressed.

Just deep to the group of muscles connecting the upper extremity to the vertebral column lie the serratus posterior superior and serratus posterior inferior muscles.

The *serratus posterior superior muscle* has an origin via a thin aponeurosis attached to the lower part of the ligamentum nuchae and to the spinous processes and related supraspinous ligaments of the seventh cervical and upper two or three thoracic vertebrae. It is inserted by fleshy digitations into the upper borders of the second to fifth ribs lateral to their angles. This muscle helps to increase the size of the thoracic cavity by elevating the ribs. The *serratus posterior inferior muscle* arises by means of a thin aponeurosis from the spinous processes and related supraspinous ligaments of the last two thoracic vertebrae and the first two or three lumbar vertebrae. This muscle inserts by fleshy digitations into the lower borders of the last four ribs, just beyond their angles. It tends to pull the last four ribs downward and outward. The serratus posterior muscles receive branches of the ventral rami of the thoracic nerves at the levels at which they are located.

Just deep to the serratus posterior superior muscle lie the thoracic portions of the splenius cervicis and capitis muscles.

The *splenius cervicis muscle* has a tendinous origin from the spinous processes of the third to sixth thoracic vertebrae and wraps around the deeper muscles to insert by tendinous fasciculi onto the transverse processes of the upper two or three cervical vertebrae. The *splenius capitis muscle* arises from the inferior half of the ligamentum nuchae and the spinous processes of the seventh cervical and the first three or four thoracic vertebrae. It is inserted onto the occipital bone just inferior to the lateral third of the superior nuchal line. The splenius muscles tend to pull the head and neck backward and laterally and to turn the face toward the same side. They are supplied by branches of the posterior primary divisions of the middle and lower cervical nerves.

The groove lateral to the spinous processes of the thoracic vertebrae is filled by the *sacrospinalis muscle*, which is covered by the thoracic part of the lumbodorsal fascia. Deep to the sacrospinalis muscle lie the short vertebrocostal and intervertebral muscles; they are not described here.

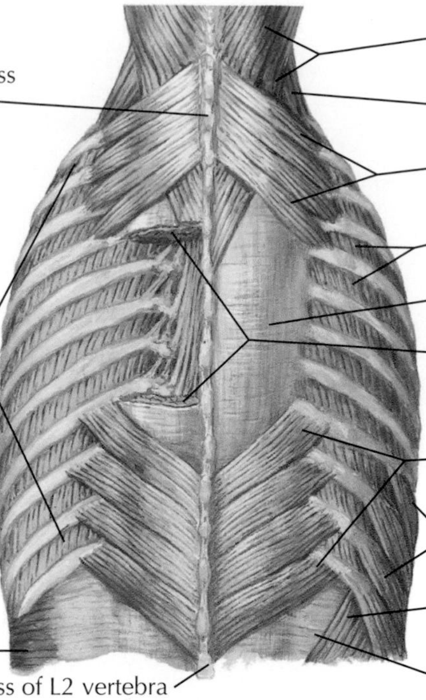

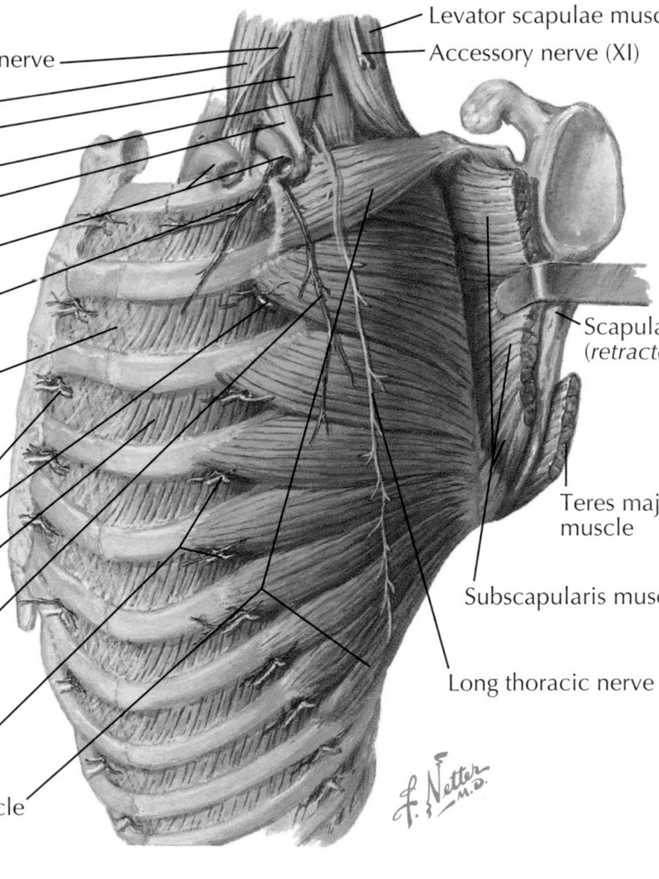

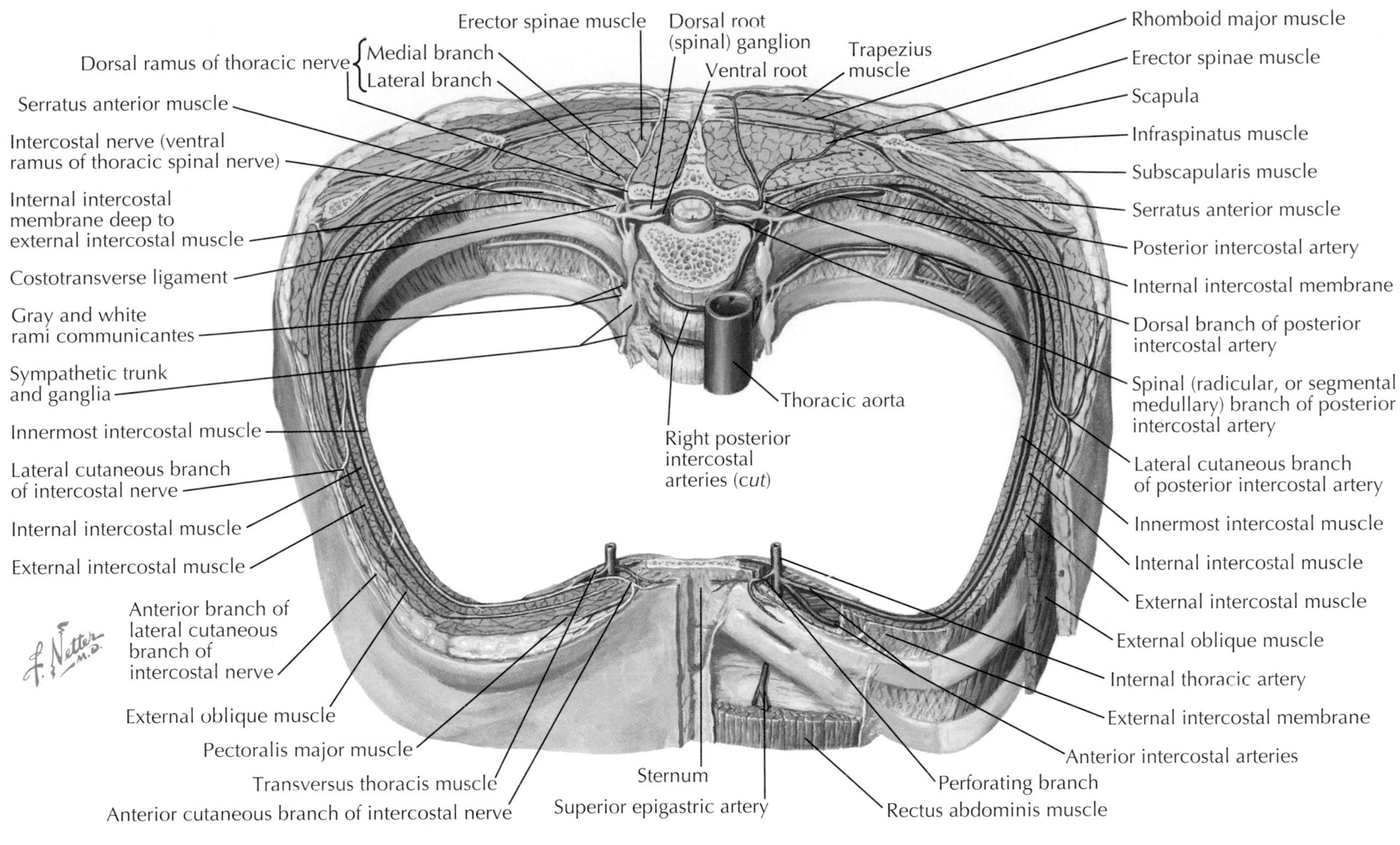

Intercostal Nerves and Arteries

The typical thoracic spinal nerve is formed by the junction of a dorsal root and a ventral root near the intervertebral foramen below the vertebra having the same number as the nerve. The *dorsal root* is made up of a series of rootlets that emerge from one segment of the spinal cord between its dorsal and lateral white columns; it contains the nerve cell bodies of the afferent neurons that enter the spinal cord through it. This collection of nerve cell bodies causes a swelling of the root, named the *dorsal root ganglion.* A series of rootlets composed of axons of ventral-born gray cells leaves the same segment of the cord between the lateral and ventral white columns to form the *ventral root* of the spinal nerve.

The dorsal and ventral roots join near the intervertebral foramen to make up the very short *common trunk* of the spinal nerve, which divides almost immediately into the dorsal ramus (posterior primary division) and the ventral ramus (anterior primary division). The white and gray rami communicantes, which connect the ganglia of the sympathetic trunk and the thoracic nerves of the same level, join the ventral ramus near its origin.

The *dorsal ramus* of the thoracic nerve, passing posteriorly, pierces the erector spinae muscle (which it supplies), the trapezius muscle, and the other superficial muscles of the back (depending on the level) to reach the superficial fascia. There it divides into a smaller medial branch and a longer lateral cutaneous branch, which supply the skin.

The *ventral ramus* of the thoracic nerve is the intercostal nerve of that particular level (for the twelfth thoracic nerve, the subcostal nerve). From the seventh to the eleventh thoracic levels, the ventral rami of the thoracic nerves continue from the intercostal spaces into the anterior abdominal wall. The intercostal nerve runs forward in the thoracic wall between the innermost intercostal muscle and the internal intercostal muscle. It lies inferior to the intercostal vein and intercostal artery and gives off a collateral branch to the lower part of the space, as do the vein and artery. The intercostal nerve has a lateral cutaneous branch at the lateral aspect of the thorax that pierces the overlying intercostal muscles to reach the subcutaneous tissue. There it divides into an anterior (mammary) and a posterior branch. At the anterior end of the intercostal space, the intercostal nerve ends by becoming the anterior cutaneous nerve, which divides into a lateral branch and a shorter and smaller medial branch.

The aorta, lying on the anterior aspect of the vertebral bodies, gives off pairs of posterior (aortic) intercostal arteries. The right posterior intercostal arteries lie on the anterior aspect and the right side of the vertebral bodies as they travel to reach the intercostal spaces of the right side. The right and left posterior intercostal arteries course forward in the upper part of the intercostal spaces between the intercostal vein above and the intercostal nerve below to anastomose with the anterior intercostal branches of the internal thoracic and musculophrenic arteries. Collateral branches run in the inferior parts of the intercostal space.

To reach the pleural cavity from the outside at the anterolateral aspect of the thorax, a needle would pass through the following layers: skin, superficial fascia, intercostal muscles and related deep fascial layers, subpleural fascia, and parietal layer of the pleura. If the needle is carefully inserted near the lower part of the intercostal space (i.e., above the rib margin), one is reasonably sure of avoiding the intercostal nerve and vessels.

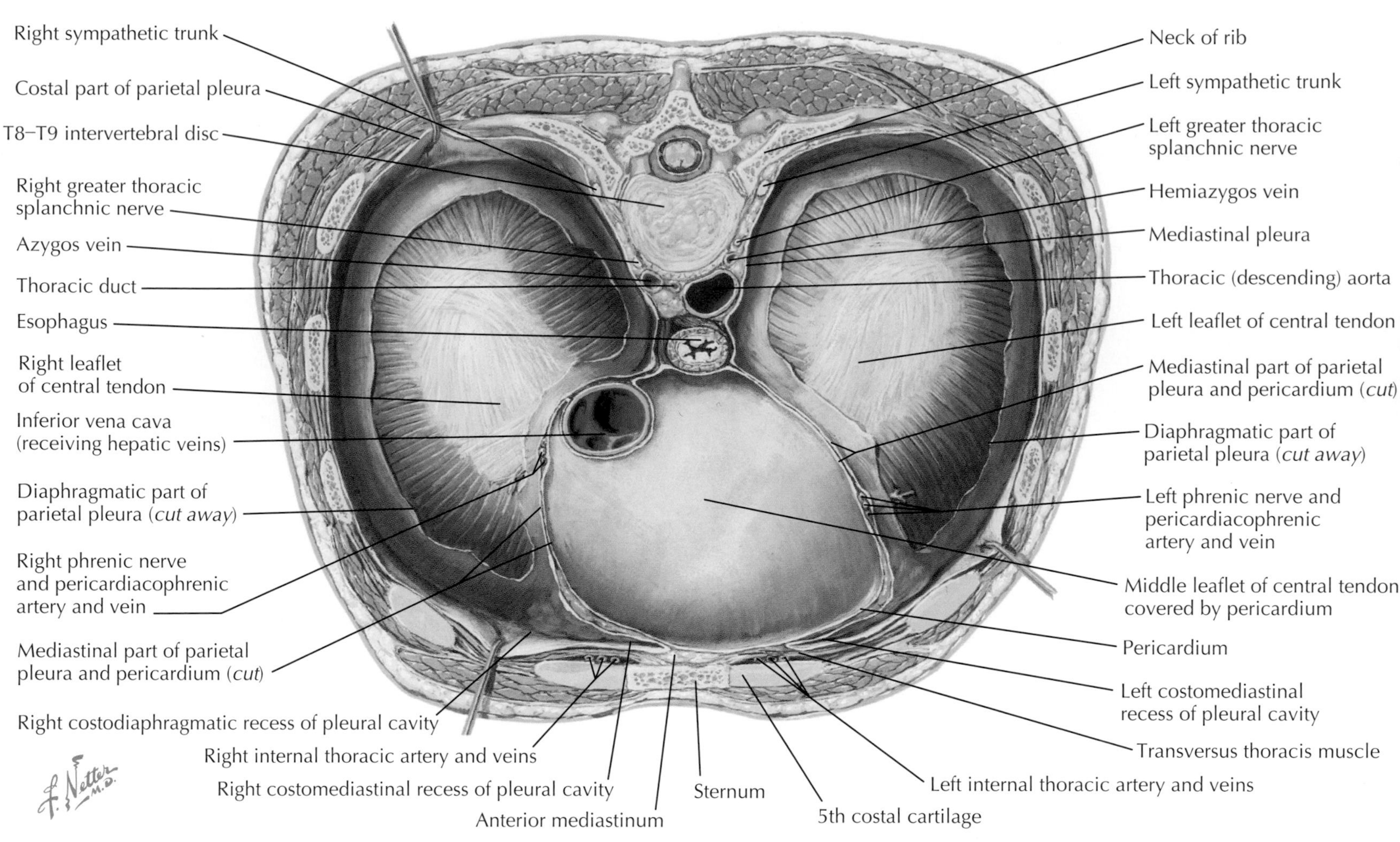

DIAPHRAGM (VIEWED FROM ABOVE)

The diaphragm is a curved musculotendinous septum separating the thoracic from the abdominal cavity, forming the floor of the thoracic cavity with its convex upper surface facing the thorax. The dome of the diaphragm on the right side is as high as the fifth costal cartilage (varying with the phase of respiration) and on the left is only slightly lower, so that some of the abdominal viscera are covered by the thoracic cage.

The origin of the diaphragm is from the outlet of the thorax and has three parts: sternal, costal, and lumbar.

The *sternal origin* is by two fleshy slips from the back of the xiphoid process. The *costal origin* is by fleshy slips that interdigitate with the slips of origin of the transversus abdominis muscle and arise from the inner surfaces of the costal cartilages and adjacent parts of the last six ribs on each side. The *lumbar portion* of the origin is by a right and a left crus and right and left medial and lateral lumbocostal arches (sometimes termed arcuate ligaments). The tendinous crura blend with the anterior longitudinal ligament of the vertebral column and are attached to the anterior surfaces of the lumbar vertebral bodies and related intervertebral discs—to the first three on the right and the first two on the left. The medial lumbocostal arch, a thickening of the fascia covering the psoas major muscle, extends from the side of the body of the first or second lumbar vertebra to the front of the transverse process of the first (sometimes also the second) lumbar vertebra. The lateral lumbocostal arch, passing across the quadratus lumborum muscle, extends from the transverse process of the first lumbar vertebra to the tip and lower border of the twelfth rib.

From the extensive origin just described, the fibers converge to insert in a three-leafed central tendon. Contraction of the muscular portion of the diaphragm pulls the central tendon downward, thus increasing the volume of the thoracic cavity and bringing about inspiration.

The diaphragmatic nerve supply is by way of the right and left phrenic nerves, which are branches of the right and left cervical plexuses and receive their fibers primarily from the fourth cervical nerves, with some contribution from the third and fifth cervical nerves.

Several structures pass between the thoracic and abdominal cavities, mainly through apertures in the diaphragm.

The *aortic aperture* is at the level of the twelfth thoracic vertebra situated between the diaphragm and the vertebra. It transmits the aorta, azygos vein, and thoracic duct.

The *esophageal aperture* is located at the level of the tenth thoracic vertebra in the fleshy part of the diaphragm. It transmits the esophagus, the right and left vagus nerves, and small esophageal arteries and veins.

The *inferior vena caval aperture* is situated at the level of the disc between the eighth and ninth thoracic vertebrae at the junction of the right and middle leaflets of the central tendon. It is traversed by the inferior vena cava and some branches of the right phrenic nerve.

The right crus is pierced by the right greater and lesser splanchnic nerves, and the left crus is pierced by the left greater and lesser splanchnic nerves and the hemiazygos vein. The sympathetic trunks usually do not pierce the diaphragm but pass behind the medial lumbocostal arches.

The base of the fibrous pericardial sac is partially blended with the middle leaflet of the central tendon of the diaphragm. The diaphragmatic portions of the parietal pleura are closely blended with the upper surfaces of the right and left portions of the diaphragm. Where the diaphragmatic pleura reflects at a sharp angle to become the costal pleura, the costodiaphragmatic recess or costophrenic sulcus is formed. Where the costal pleura reflects to become pericardial pleura, the costomediastinal recess is formed.

TOPOGRAPHY OF THE LUNGS (ANTERIOR VIEW)

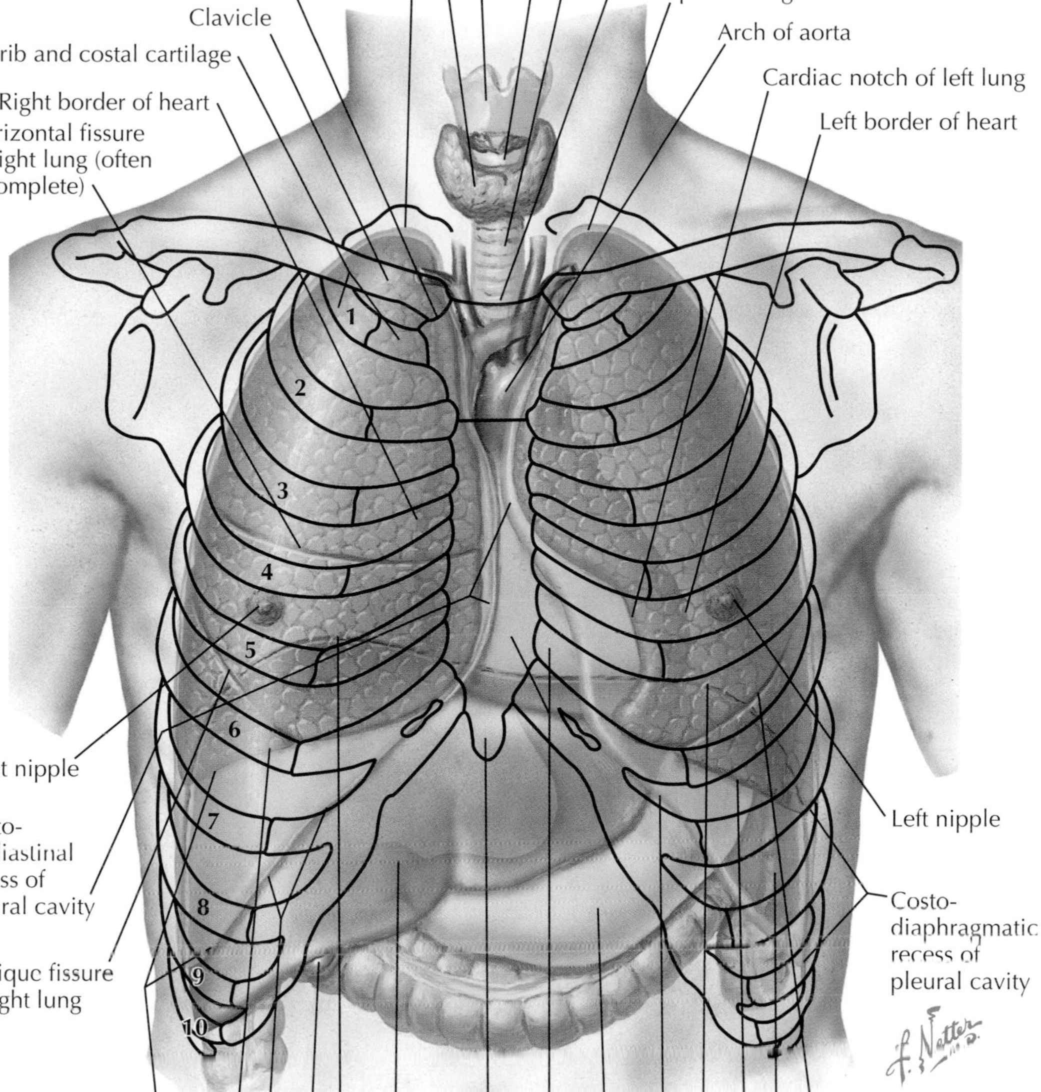

Because the apex of each lung reaches as far superiorly as the vertebral end of the first rib, the lung usually extends about 1 inch above the medial third of the clavicle when viewed from the front. Thus, the lung projects into the base of the neck.

The anterior border of the right lung descends behind the sternoclavicular joint and almost reaches the midline at the level of the sternal angle. It continues inferiorly posterior to the sternum to the level of the sixth chondrosternal junction. There the inferior border curves laterally and slightly inferiorly, crossing the sixth rib in the midclavicular line and the eighth rib in the midaxillary line. It then runs posteriorly and medially at the level of the spinous process of the tenth thoracic vertebra. These levels are, of course, variable and apply to the lung in expiration. In inspiration, the levels for the inferior border are roughly two ribs lower.

The anterior border of the left lung is similar in position to that of the right lung. However, at the level of the fourth costal cartilage, it deviates laterally because of the heart, causing a cardiac notch in this border of the lung. The inferior border of the left lung is similar in position to that of the right lung except that it extends farther inferiorly because the right lung is pushed up by the liver below the diaphragm on the right side.

The oblique fissure of the right lung, separating the lower lobe from the upper and middle lobes, ends at the lower border of the lung near the midclavicular line. The horizontal fissure separating the middle from the upper lobe begins at the oblique fissure and runs horizontally forward to the lung's anterior border, which it reaches at about the level of the fourth costal cartilage.

The oblique fissure of the left lung is similar in its location to the corresponding fissure of the right side. The left lung ordinarily has only two lobes, and there is usually no horizontal fissure in this lung. Extra fissures may occur in either lung, usually between bronchopulmonary segments and, in the left lung, between the superior and inferior divisions of the upper lobe, giving rise to a three-lobed left lung.

The lungs seldom extend as far inferiorly as the parietal pleura, so some of the diaphragmatic parietal pleura is usually in contact with costal parietal pleura. This area—which, of course, varies in size with the phase of respiration—is called the *costodiaphragmatic recess* of the pleura or the *costophrenic sulcus*. A similar but much less extensive area is present where the anterior border of the lung does not extend to its limits medially—especially in expiration—and the costal and mediastinal parietal pleurae are in contact. This area is called the *costomediastinal recess*.

The diaphragm separates the liver from the right lung and, depending on the size of the liver, from the left lung. The left lung is also separated by the diaphragm from the stomach and the spleen.

The nipple in males usually overlies the fourth intercostal space in approximately the midclavicular line. In females, its position varies, depending on the size and functional state of the breast.

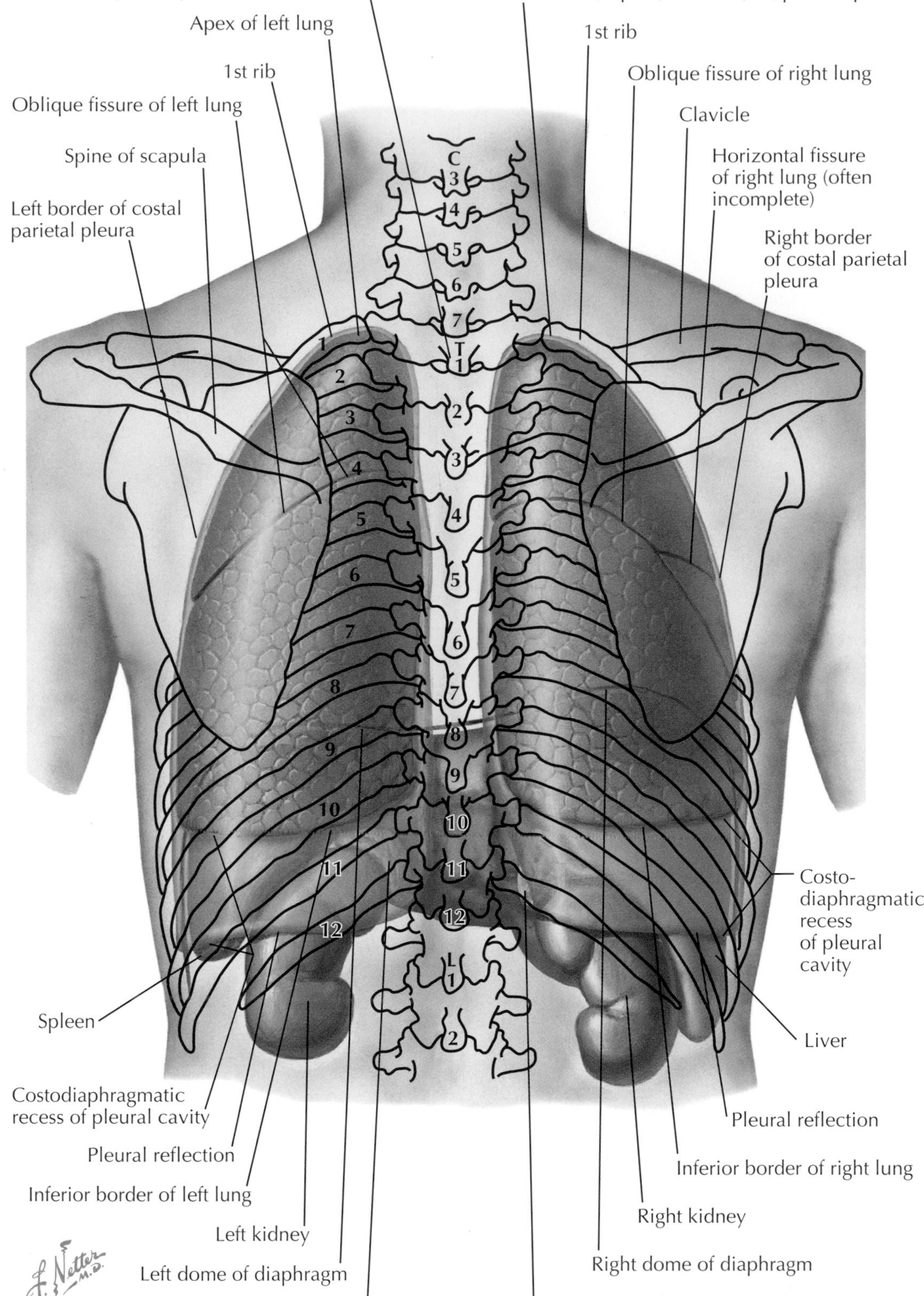

Topography of the Lungs (Posterior View)

The apex of the lung extends as far superiorly as the vertebral end of the first rib and therefore as high as the first thoracic vertebra. From there, the lung extends inferiorly as far as the diaphragm, with the base of the lung resting on the diaphragm and fitted to its superior surface. Because of the diaphragm's domed shape, the level of the highest point on the base of the right lung is about at the eighth to ninth thoracic vertebrae. The highest point on the base of the left lung is a fraction of an inch lower. From these high points, the bases of the two lungs follow the curves of the diaphragm to reach the levels described earlier for the inferior borders of the lungs.

The highest point on the oblique fissure of the two lungs is on their posterior aspects, at about the level of the third to fourth thoracic vertebrae, a little over 1 inch from the midline.

If the arm is raised over the head, the vertebral border of the scapula approximates the position of the oblique fissure of the lung. If the shoulder is brought forward as far as possible, the scapula is carried laterally, so that the area in which auscultation can be satisfactorily carried out on the posterior aspect of the chest is significantly widened.

The parietal pleura is separated from the visceral pleura by a potential space (the pleural cavity), which under normal circumstances contains only a minimal amount of serous fluid. Caudal to the inferior margin of the lung, the costal parietal pleura is in contact with the diaphragmatic parietal pleura, forming the costodiaphragmatic recess (costophrenic sulcus). This allows for the caudal movement of the inferior margin of the lung on inspiration.

Under abnormal circumstances, the pleural cavity may contain air, increased amounts of serous fluid, blood, or pus. The accumulation of a significant amount of any of these in the pleural cavity compresses the lung and causes respiratory difficulties.

The diaphragm separates the base of the left lung from the fundus of the stomach and the spleen. Because of this relationship, if the stomach is distended by food or gas, it may push the diaphragm upward and embarrass respiratory activity.

The diaphragm similarly separates the base of the right lung from the liver, which, if enlarged, elevates the diaphragm and pushes against the lung, possibly limiting its expansion. A hepatic abscess may rupture through the diaphragm to involve the related pleural cavity and lung.

In this illustration, the lungs are shown in relation to the bony thorax, scapula, and diaphragm, but overlying the structures shown are the deep and superficial muscles of the back in addition to the superficial fascia and skin.

MEDIAL SURFACE OF THE LUNGS

The medial (mediastinal) surfaces of the right and left lungs present concave mirror images of the right and left sides of the mediastinum so that in addition to the structures forming the root of the lung, the medial lung surface presents distinct impressions made by the structures constituting the mediastinum (see Plates 1-18 and 1-19).

MEDIAL SURFACE OF THE RIGHT LUNG

The oblique and horizontal fissures (if complete) divide the right lung into upper, middle, and lower lobes. The pleura reflects directly from the parietal to the visceral surface around the root of the lung except where it forms the pulmonary ligament, which extends from the inferior aspect of the root vertically down to the medial border of the base of the lung.

The main structures forming the root of the right lung are the superior and inferior pulmonary veins, which are situated anterior and inferior to the pulmonary artery, and the bronchus, which is posterior in position. A number of lymph nodes are also present.

Much of the ventral and inferior portions of the mediastinal surface show the impression caused by the heart. Superior to this is the groove caused by the superior vena cava, with the groove for the right brachiocephalic (innominate) vein above that. Near the apex of the lung is the groove for the right subclavian artery. Arching over the root of the lung is the groove caused by the azygos vein. Superior to this are the areas for the trachea (anteriorly) and the esophagus (posteriorly). The area for the esophagus continues inferiorly posterior to the root of the lung.

Because the inferior margin of the outer, costal surface of the lung extends downward farther than the lower margin of the medial surface, the diaphragmatic surface of the lung can also be seen when the medial aspect of the lung is observed.

MEDIAL SURFACE OF THE LEFT LUNG

The oblique fissure (if complete) divides the left lung into upper and lower lobes. The relationship of the pleura to the root of the left lung is similar to that on the right.

Structures forming the root of the left lung are the pulmonary artery superiorly, the bronchus posteriorly, and the superior and inferior pulmonary veins anteriorly and inferiorly. Some lymph nodes are also present.

A large impression caused by the heart is present anterior and inferior to the root of the lung. It is responsible for a rather marked "cardiac notch" in the anterior border of the upper lobe of the left lung. Inferior to this notch is a projection of the upper lobe, the lingula.

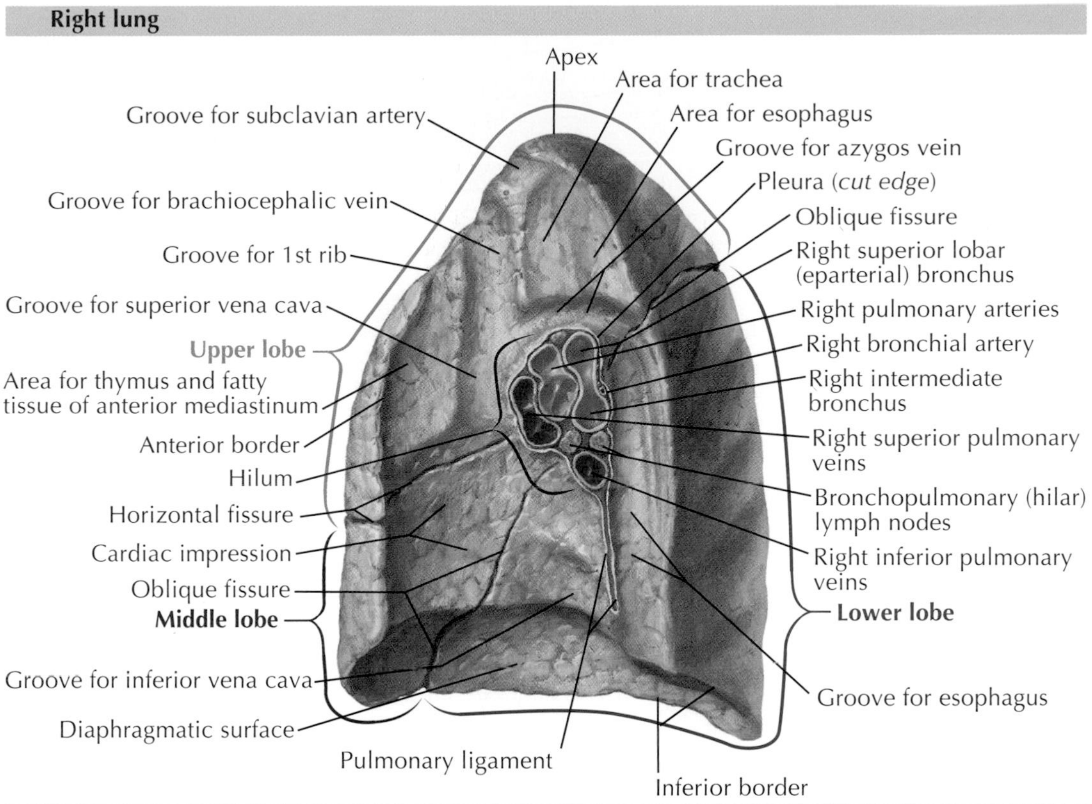

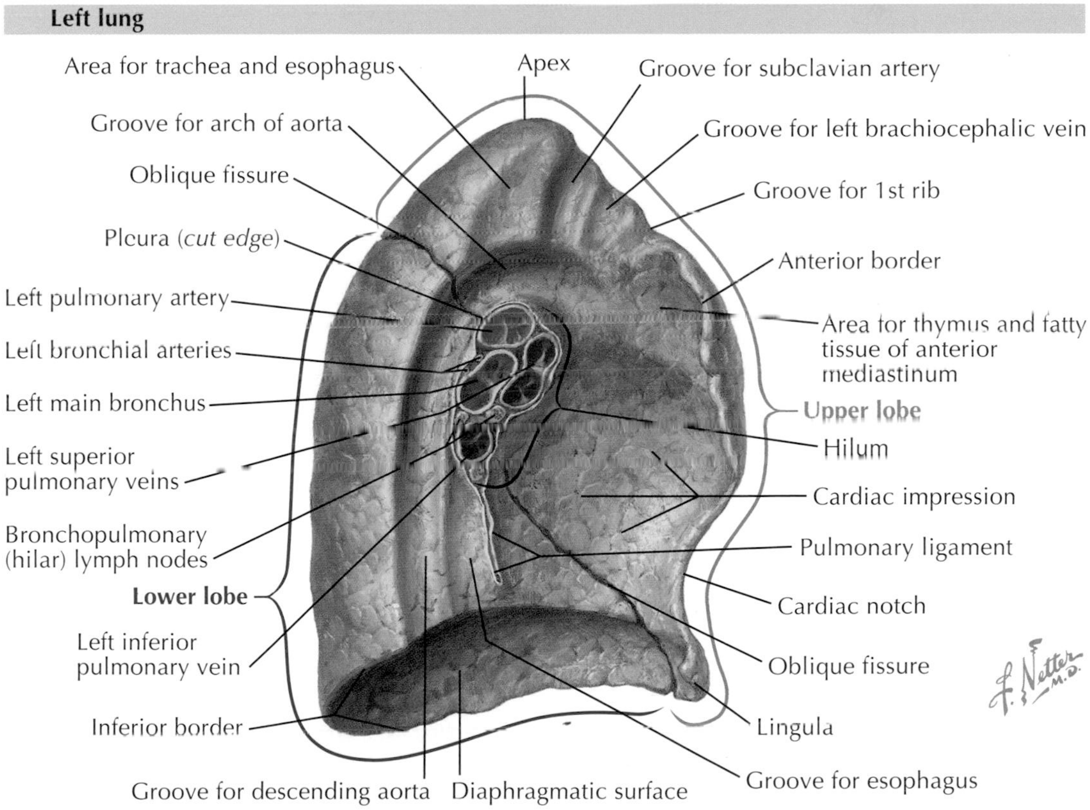

Right lung

Apex
Area for trachea
Groove for subclavian artery
Area for esophagus
Groove for azygos vein
Pleura (*cut edge*)
Groove for brachiocephalic vein
Oblique fissure
Groove for 1st rib
Right superior lobar (eparterial) bronchus
Groove for superior vena cava
Right pulmonary arteries
Upper lobe
Right bronchial artery
Area for thymus and fatty tissue of anterior mediastinum
Right intermediate bronchus
Anterior border
Right superior pulmonary veins
Hilum
Horizontal fissure
Bronchopulmonary (hilar) lymph nodes
Cardiac impression
Right inferior pulmonary veins
Oblique fissure
Middle lobe
Lower lobe
Groove for inferior vena cava
Groove for esophagus
Diaphragmatic surface
Pulmonary ligament
Inferior border

Left lung

Area for trachea and esophagus
Apex
Groove for subclavian artery
Groove for arch of aorta
Groove for left brachiocephalic vein
Oblique fissure
Groove for 1st rib
Pleura (*cut edge*)
Anterior border
Left pulmonary artery
Area for thymus and fatty tissue of anterior mediastinum
Left bronchial arteries
Left main bronchus
Upper lobe
Hilum
Left superior pulmonary veins
Cardiac impression
Bronchopulmonary (hilar) lymph nodes
Pulmonary ligament
Lower lobe
Cardiac notch
Left inferior pulmonary vein
Oblique fissure
Inferior border
Lingula
Groove for descending aorta
Diaphragmatic surface
Groove for esophagus

F. Netter M.D.

Arching over the root of the left lung and continuing inferiorly—posterior to the root—to the base of the lung is a groove for the aortic arch and the descending aorta.

Superior to the groove for the aortic arch are, from behind forward, areas for the esophagus and trachea, the groove for the left subclavian artery, the groove for the left brachiocephalic (innominate) vein, and a groove caused by the first rib.

The portion of the medial surface of the left lung posterior to the areas for the descending aorta and esophagus is in contact with the thoracic vertebral bodies and the vertebral ends of the ribs except where separated from them by structures lying in the position described above.

As on the right side, the diaphragmatic surface of the left lung can be seen as the medial aspect of the lung is observed.

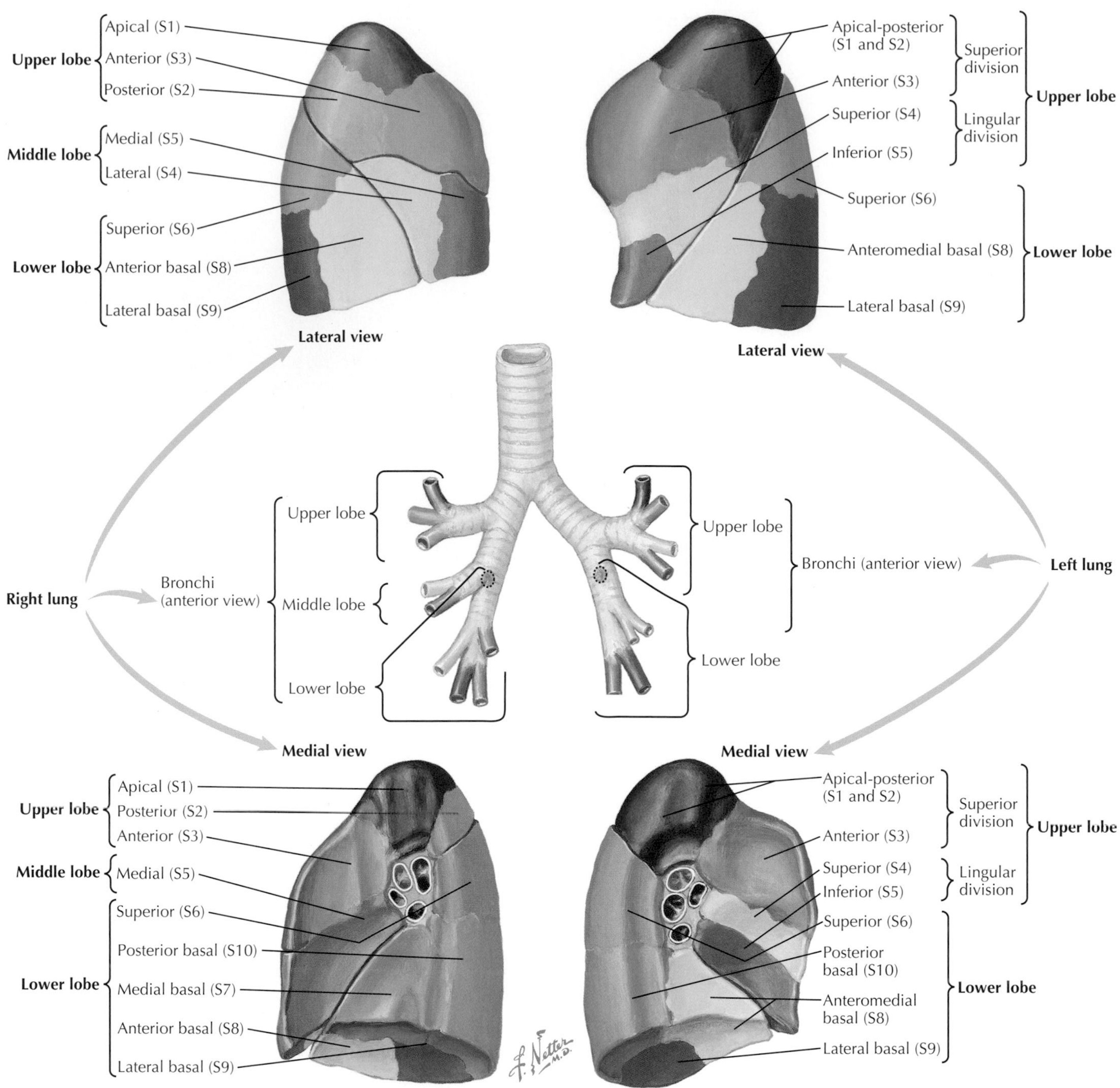

BRONCHOPULMONARY SEGMENTS

A bronchopulmonary segment is that portion of the lung supplied by the primary branch of a lobar bronchus. Each segment is surrounded by connective tissue that is continuous with visceral pleura and forms a separate, functionally independent respiratory unit. The artery supplying a segment follows the segmental bronchus but the segmental veins are at the periphery of the segment and thus can be helpful in delineating it.

RIGHT LUNG

The right main bronchus gives rise to three lobar bronchi: upper, middle, and lower. Any two of these may occasionally have a common stem.

Right Upper Lobe

The *apical segment* (S1) of the right upper lobe forms the apex of the right lung. It extends into the root of the neck as high as the vertebral end of the first rib. Toward the lateral aspect of the lung, the apical segment dips downward slightly between the posterior and anterior segments. This boundary line is roughly at the level of the first rib anteriorly and almost down to the second rib posteriorly.

The *posterior segment* (S2) extends from the apical segment down to the lateral portion of the horizontal fissure and the upper part of the oblique fissure.

The *anterior segment* (S3) extends from the apical segment above down to the horizontal fissure at about the level of the fourth rib.

Right Middle Lobe

The middle lobe bronchus branches into two segmental bronchi, the complete branchings of which become the *lateral segment* (S4) and *medial segment* (S5) of the lobe. These segments are separated by a vertical plane extending from the hilum out to the costal surface of the lung and reaching its inferior border just anterior to the lower end of the oblique fissure. The segments are related to the anterior parts of the fourth and fifth ribs and their costal cartilages.

Right Lower Lobe

The lower lobe bronchus gives off a posteriorly directed superior segmental bronchus just below the level of the orifice of the middle lobe bronchus. The *superior*

Pulmonary Segments in Relationship to Ribs

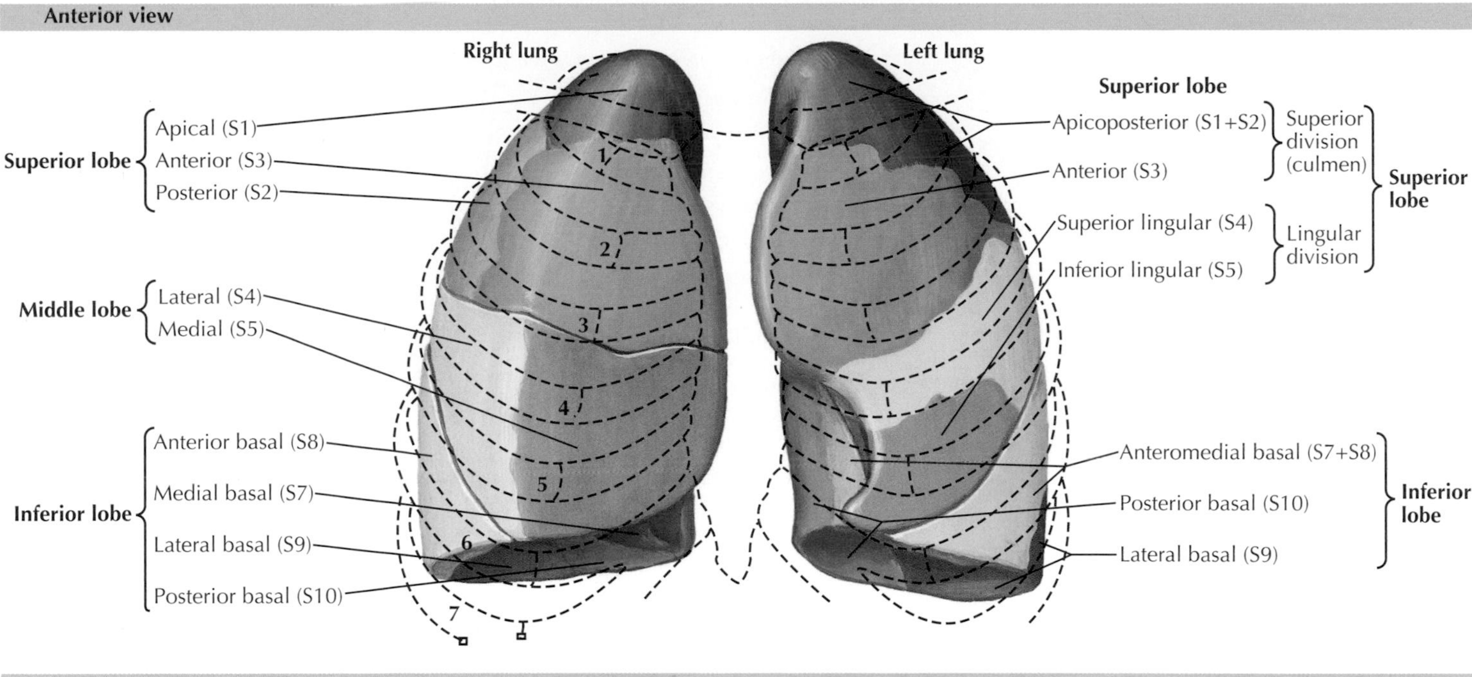

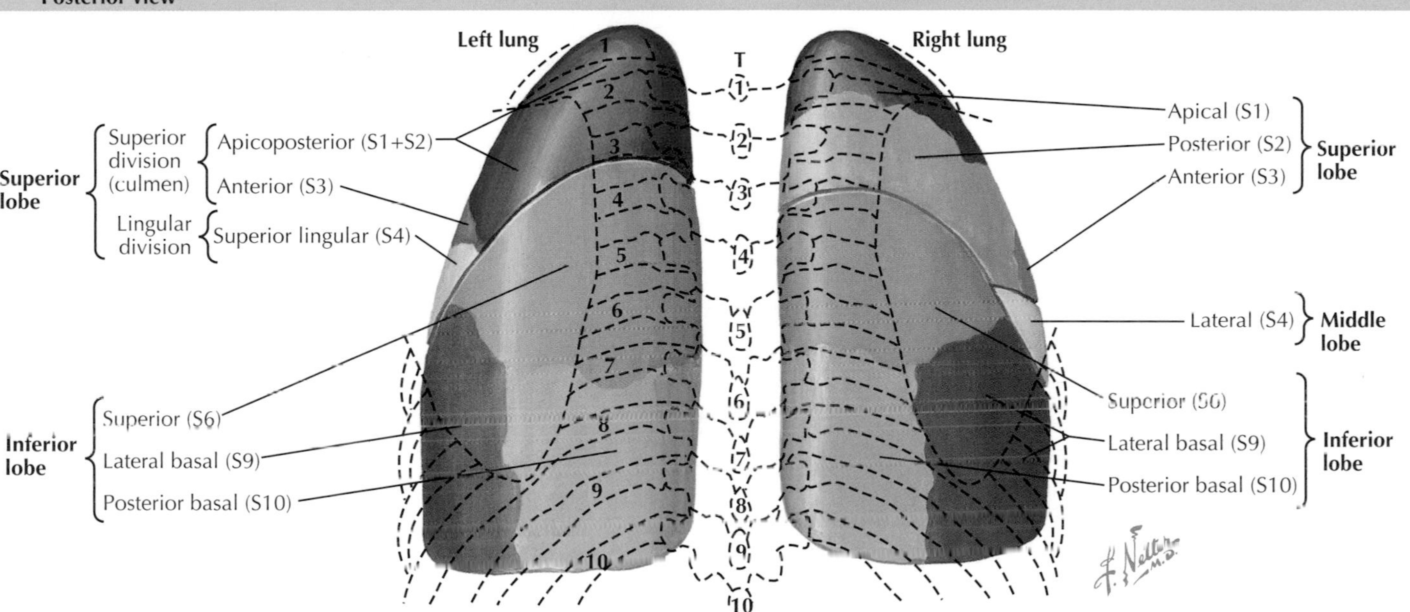

Bronchopulmonary Segments *(Continued)*

segment (S6) of the lower lobe occupies the entire superior part of the lower lobe and extends from the upper part of the oblique fissure at about the level of the vertebral end of the third rib to the level of the vertebral end of the fifth or sixth rib.

Inferior to the level at which the superior segmental bronchus arises, the lower lobe divides into four basal segmental bronchi: *medial* (S7), *anterior* (S8), *lateral* (S9), and *posterior* (S10). The basal segments of the lower lobe form the base of the lung and rest on the diaphragm. The medial basal segment is sometimes partially separated from other basal segments by an extra fissure; in this event, it has sometimes been called the *cardiac lobe* of the lung.

LEFT LUNG

The left main bronchus is longer than the right and not in such direct a line with the trachea. Foreign bodies, therefore, are somewhat more likely to enter the right than the left bronchus.

Left Upper Lobe

The upper lobe bronchus subdivides into a superior division bronchus and an inferior or lingular division bronchus. The superior division can be thought of as corresponding to the right upper lobe, with the lingular division corresponding to the right middle lobe; there is usually no fissure separating the two, and their segmental subdivisions are not the same.

Unlike the situation on the right, the superior division of the left upper lobe has only two segments: the *apicoposterior segment* (S1 and S2), which corresponds to a combination of the right apical and posterior segments, and the *anterior segment* (S3). The inferior or lingular division also has two segments, the *superior* (S4) and *inferior* (S5) segments.

Left Lower Lobe

The segments here are similar to those of the right lower lobe except that the portion corresponding to the right anterior basal and medial basal segments is supplied on the left by two bronchi that have a common stem and thus forms a single *anteromedial basal* (S8) segment. Other left lower lobe segments are *superior* (S6), *lateral basal* (S9), and *posterior basal* (S10).

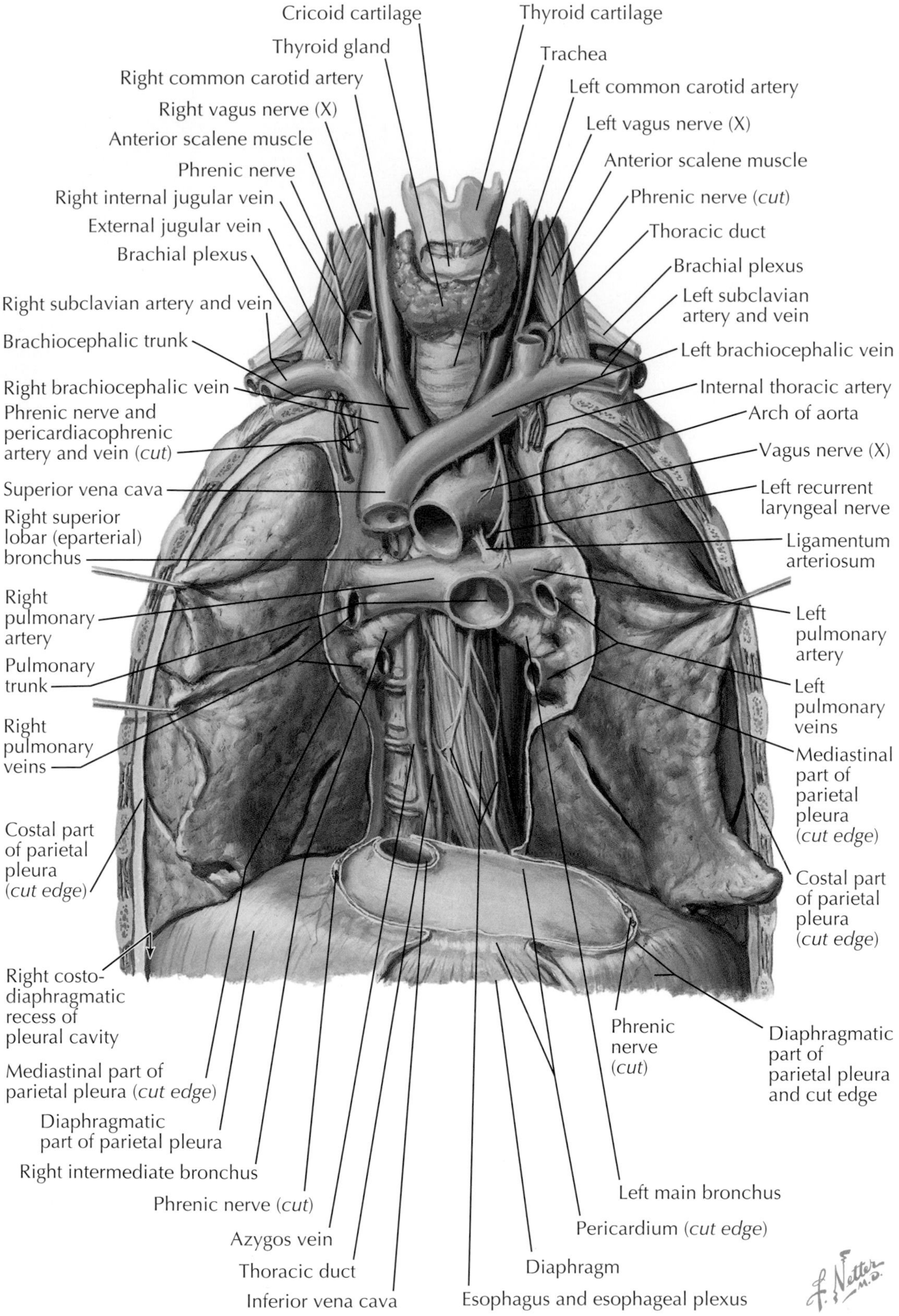

Relationships of the Trachea and Main Bronchi

The trachea begins at the lower border of the larynx (just below the cricoid cartilage) at about the level of the sixth cervical vertebra and ends at about the level of the upper border of the fifth thoracic vertebra, where it divides into the two main bronchi. The thyroid gland lies on the anterior and both lateral aspects of the highest part of the trachea.

As the aorta arches over the root of the left lung, it first lies anterior to the trachea and then on its left side. The major arteries arising from the aortic arch are in close relationship with the trachea. The brachiocephalic (innominate) artery at first is anterior to the trachea and then is on its right side before dividing into the right common carotid and right subclavian arteries. The left common carotid artery is first anterior to and then on the left lateral aspect of the trachea.

The left brachiocephalic (innominate) vein crosses from left to right, anterior to the trachea and partly separated from it by the major branches of the aortic arch. The right brachiocephalic vein is separated from the trachea by the right brachiocephalic artery.

The beginning of the right main bronchus lies anterior to the esophagus. As it courses inferiorly and laterally to divide into the lobar bronchi, it is posterior to the right pulmonary artery. The bronchus crosses in front of the azygos vein and is separated from the thoracic duct by the esophagus. The relationship to other structures at the root of the lung is shown in Plate 1-13.

The beginning of the left main bronchus also lies anterior to the esophagus, from which it runs laterally and inferiorly to reach the hilum of the left lung. Because its course is less vertical than that of the right main bronchus (less in a direct line with the trachea), foreign bodies are a little more likely to enter the right bronchus than the left.

The left recurrent laryngeal nerve arises from the left vagus nerve as it crosses the arch of the aorta and swings posteriorly to loop around the aortic arch just lateral to the ligamentum arteriosum. This nerve then runs cranially in the groove between the trachea and the esophagus to reach the larynx.

The esophagus starts as a continuation of the pharynx at the lower border of the larynx and continues through the thorax. It then passes through the esophageal aperture of the diaphragm to enter the abdominal cavity and terminate at the stomach.

The ligamentum arteriosum, the remnant of the ductus arteriosus, runs from the beginning of the left pulmonary artery to the undersurface of the arch of the aorta. In fetal life, the ligamentum arteriosum shunts blood from the pulmonary artery to the aorta, so that fetal blood does not pass through the pulmonary circulation.

The vagus nerves split into several bundles below the root of the lung and form the esophageal plexus on the surface of the esophagus. Other contributions to the plexus come from the sympathetic trunks and splanchnic nerves. At the lower end of the plexus, two trunks are formed, which pass through the esophageal aperture of the diaphragm. The anterior trunk is mostly derived from the left vagus and the posterior trunk mostly from the right vagus.

Also worthy of note are the pulmonary veins, shown cut at the roots of the right and left lungs; the parietal pleura, cut to expose the lungs, each of which is covered by visceral pleura; the cut edge of the pericardium; and the inferior vena cava passing through the diaphragm.

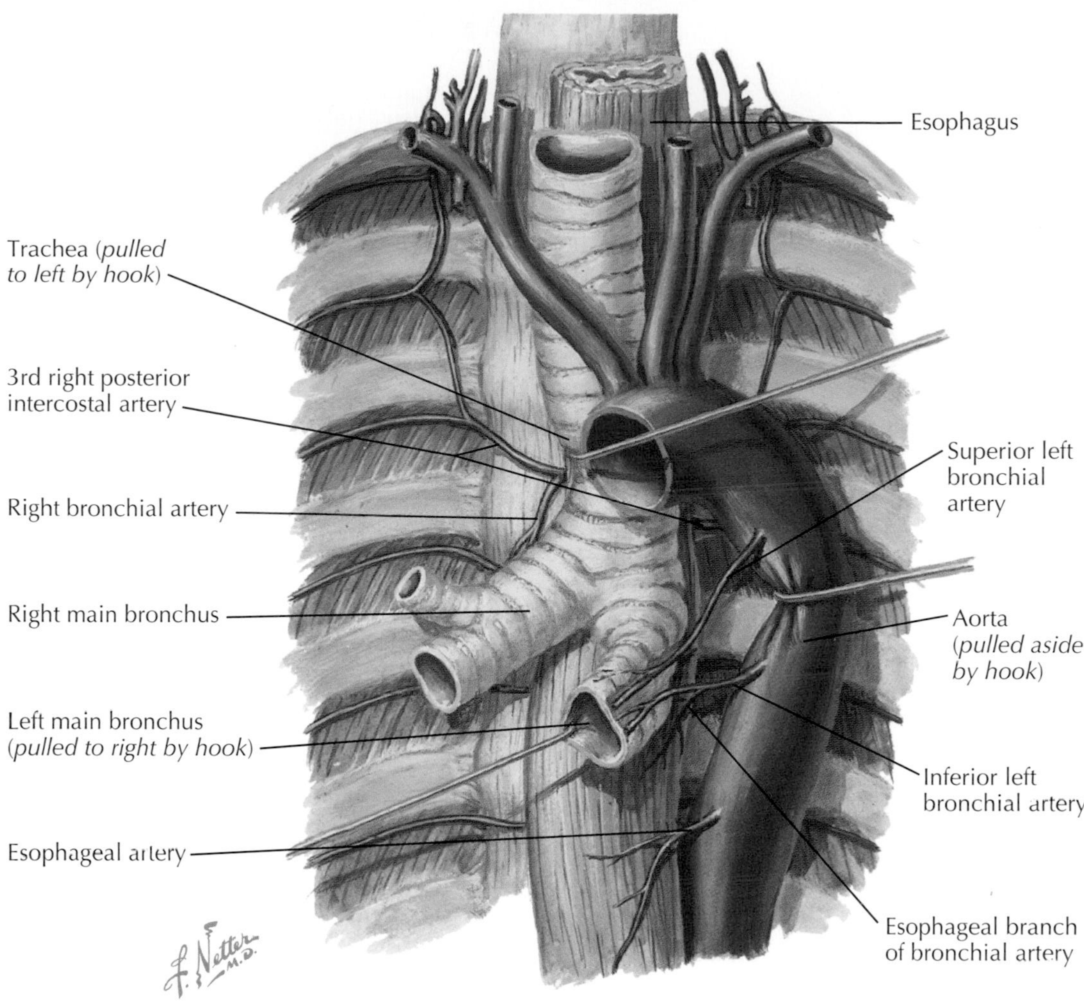

BRONCHIAL ARTERIES

The lungs receive blood from two sets of arteries. The *pulmonary arteries* follow the bronchi and ramify into capillary networks that surround the alveoli, allowing exchange of oxygen and carbon dioxide. The *bronchial arteries* derive from the aorta. They supply oxygenated blood to the tissues of the lung that are not in close proximity to inspired air, such as the muscular walls of the larger pulmonary vessels and airways (to the level of the respiratory bronchioles) and the visceral pleurae.

The origin of the right bronchial artery is quite variable. It arises frequently from the third right posterior intercostal artery (the first right aortic intercostal artery) and descends to reach the posterior aspects of the right main bronchus. It may arise from a common stem with the left inferior bronchial artery, which originates from the descending aorta slightly inferior to the point where the left main bronchus crosses it. Or it may arise from the inferior aspect of the arch of the aorta and course behind the trachea to reach the posterior wall of the right main bronchus.

On the left side, two arteries are typically present, one superior and one inferior. The superior artery tends to arise from the inferior aspect of the aortic arch as it becomes the descending aorta. The inferior artery most often arises near the beginning of the descending aorta toward its posterior aspect. The left bronchial arteries come to lie on the posterior surface of the left main bronchus and follow the branching of the bronchial tree into the left lung.

Some of the more common variations of the bronchial arteries are shown in the lower part of the illustration. The right bronchial artery and the inferior left bronchial artery may come from a common stem arising from the descending aorta. There may be only a single bronchial artery on the left. Supernumerary bronchial arteries may be present, going to either bronchus or both bronchi.

The majority of those who have studied the blood supply of the lungs seem to agree that precapillary anastomoses are present between the bronchial and pulmonary arteries, which can enlarge when either of these two systems becomes obstructed (an event that more commonly affects the pulmonary arteries). Whether these anastomoses are able to maintain full oxygenation of an involved area of lung has not been completely established but would seem likely given the surprisingly low rate of infarction in otherwise normal individuals who experience pulmonary embolism.

Branches of the bronchial arteries spread out on the surface of the lung beneath the pleura where they form a capillary network that contributes to the pleural blood supply.

Variations in bronchial arteries

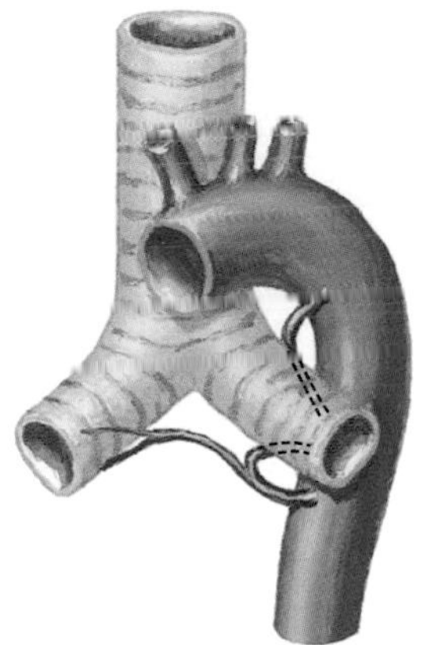

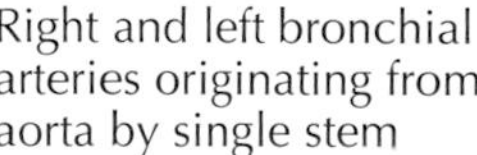
Right and left bronchial arteries originating from aorta by single stem

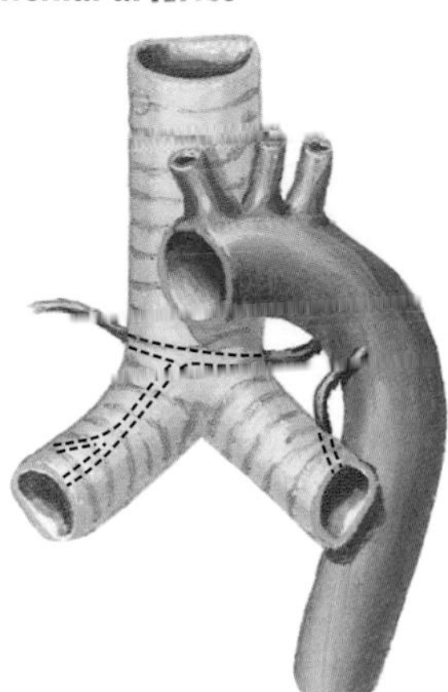
Only single bronchial artery to each bronchus (normally, two to left bronchus)

Bronchial veins

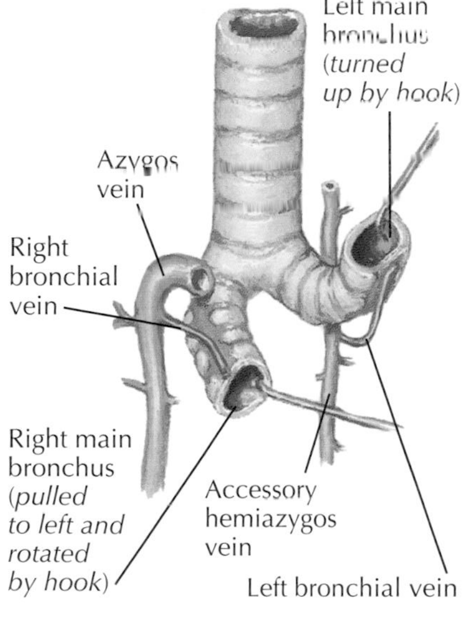

MEDIASTINUM

The mediastinum is that portion of the thorax that lies between the right and left pleural sacs and is bounded ventrally by the sternum and dorsally by the bodies of the thoracic vertebrae. The superior boundary of the mediastinum is defined by the thoracic inlet, and its inferior boundary is formed by the diaphragm. By convention, the mediastinum is divided into *superior* and *inferior* parts by a plane extending horizontally from the base of the fourth vertebral body to the angle of the sternum. The superior mediastinum contains the aortic arch; the brachiocephalic (innominate) artery; the beginnings of the left common carotid and left subclavian arteries; the right pulmonary artery trunk; the right and left brachiocephalic (innominate) veins as they come together to form the superior vena cava; the trachea with right and left vagus, cardiac, phrenic, and left recurrent laryngeal nerves; the esophagus and the thoracic duct; most of the thymus; the superficial part of the cardiac plexus; and a few lymph nodes.

The anterior mediastinum lies below the superior mediastinum in the area bordered by the pericardium posteriorly and the body of the sternum anteriorly. The anterior mediastinum contains a small amount of fascia, the sternopericardial ligaments, a few lymph nodes, and variable amounts of the thymus.

The middle mediastinum contains the heart and pericardium, the beginning of the ascending aorta, the lower half of the superior vena cava with the azygos vein opening into it, the bifurcation of the trachea into right and left bronchi, the pulmonary artery dividing into right and left branches, the terminal parts of the right and left pulmonary veins, and the right and left phrenic nerves.

The posterior mediastinum is bordered anteriorly by the tracheal bifurcation and posteriorly by the vertebral column. The posterior mediastinum contains the thoracic portion of the descending aorta, esophagus, azygos and hemiazygos veins, right and left vagus nerves, splanchnic nerves, thoracic duct, and many lymph nodes.

The relationships among compartments and their included structures are of great clinical importance because a space-occupying lesion in any one of these may affect neighboring structures. These relationships can be appreciated through careful scrutiny of Plates 1-18 and 1-19.

The esophagus passes through the posterior mediastinum immediately ventral to the thoracic vertebral bodies and is separated from these by the right intercostal arteries, thoracic duct, and hemiazygos vein. It partially overlaps the azygos vein to its right side. The right and left vagus nerves form a plexus around the esophagus, with the left vagus trunk on its anterior surface and the right vagus trunk on its posterior surface. The trachea passes through the superior mediastinum anterior to the esophagus. This relationship continues as the trachea passes into the middle mediastinum to bifurcate.

In the superior and anterior mediastinum, the remnants of the thymus gland are present in adults. The right and left brachiocephalic veins and the superior vena cava are the most anterior of the major structures in the mediastinum followed in sequence (from anterior to posterior) by the aortic arch, the brachiocephalic artery, and the beginnings of the left common carotid and left subclavian arteries.

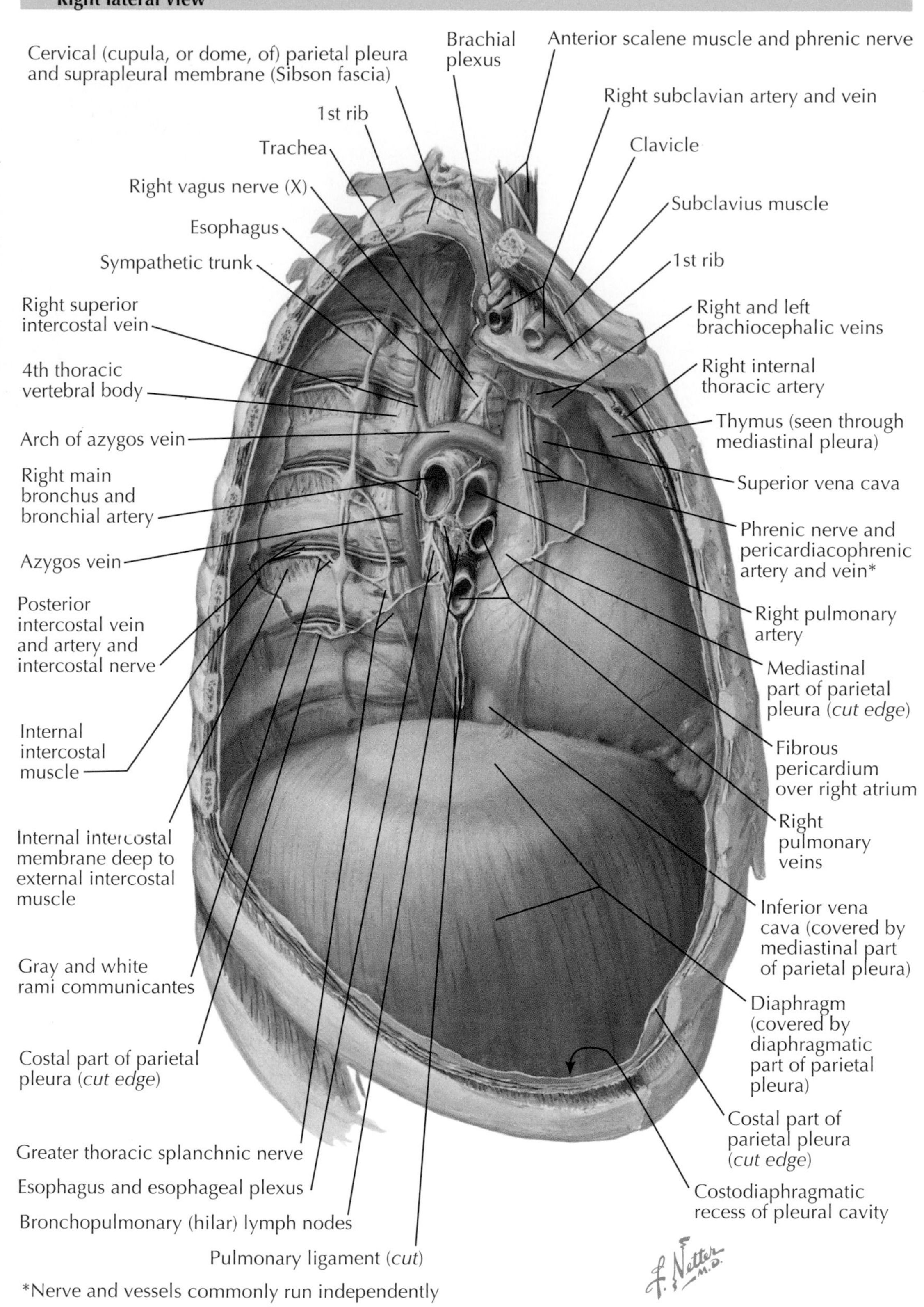

RIGHT THORACIC CAVITY

The hilum of the right lung contains the right main bronchus with the right pulmonary artery trunk anterior and the right pulmonary veins anteriorly and inferiorly. The azygos vein arches over the root of the right lung at the hilum to empty into the superior vena cava. As the azygos vein begins to arch, it receives the right superior intercostal vein, which accepts blood from the upper three or four intercostal spaces.

The visceral pleurae reflect onto the parietal mediastinal surface immediately below the hilum of the right lung to form the pulmonary ligament.

The thoracic portion of the right ganglionated sympathetic trunk courses vertically near the necks of the ribs and is connected with each intercostal nerve by a

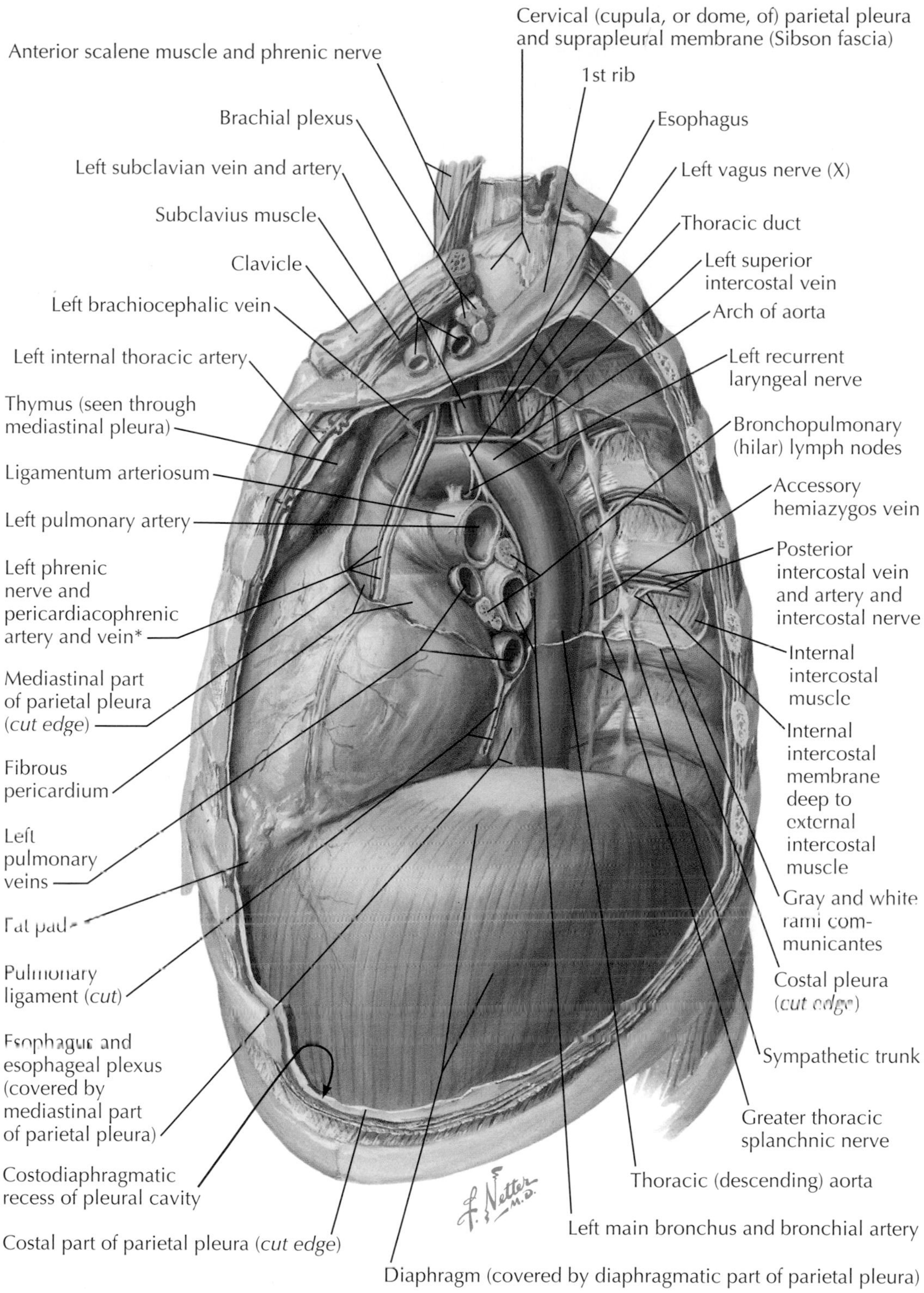

*Nerve and vessels commonly run independently

MEDIASTINUM *(Continued)*

gray and a white ramus communicans. The splanchnic nerves branch from the fifth (or sixth) to the twelfth ganglia and course medially and inferiorly to pierce the crus of the diaphragm and enter the abdominal cavity.

The right phrenic nerve and the pericardiacophrenic artery and vein pass vertically between the mediastinal parietal pleura and the pericardial sac to supply the diaphragm.

The medial "wall" of the right thoracic cavity is formed by the thoracic vertebral bodies posteriorly and anteriorly by the mediastinum, dominated by the pericardial sac containing the heart. The posterior, lateral, and anterior walls of the right thoracic cavity comprise the thoracic cage, which is limited inferiorly by the diaphragm.

LEFT THORACIC CAVITY

The structures forming the hilum of the left lung are the left main bronchus, left pulmonary artery, and left pulmonary veins. The pulmonary artery is located superior to the left main bronchus with the left pulmonary veins posterior and inferior.

The aorta arches over and descends posterior to the left hilum. As it descends, it lies at first to the left of the thoracic vertebral bodies (starting with the lower border of the fourth vertebra); it then approaches the anterior aspect of the vertebral bodies, where it lies as it pierces the diaphragm. The aorta gives off nine pairs of intercostal arteries. They supply the lower nine intercostal spaces.

The ligamentum arteriosum (the remnant of the embryonic ductus arteriosus) runs between the left pulmonary artery and the aortic arch.

The thoracic portion of the left ganglionated sympathetic trunk is similar to the portion on the right side and does not need special description here.

The left phrenic nerve and the left pericardiacophrenic artery and vein cross the aortic arch and descend between the mediastinal parietal pleura and the pericardial sac to pass through the muscular part of the diaphragm.

The left vagus nerve passes in front of the arch at the aorta, giving off its recurrent branch, which passes under the arch to course upward to the larynx. The vagus nerve continues caudally on the posterior aspect of the root of the lung to enter the esophageal plexus, from which the left vagal trunk emerges to follow the esophagus into the abdomen.

The left superior intercostal vein typically drains blood from the upper three or four intercostal spaces. It crosses the aortic arch and the beginnings of the left subclavian and left common carotid arteries and empties into the left brachiocephalic vein, often anastomosing with the accessory hemiazygos vein.

The medial wall of the left thoracic cavity is formed by the thoracic vertebral bodies posteriorly and the mediastinum containing the pericardial sac and the heart. As with the right thoracic cavity, the posterior, lateral, and anterior walls of the left thoracic cavity are formed by the thoracic cage and limited inferiorly by the diaphragm.

Innervation of the Lungs and Tracheobronchial Tree

The tracheobronchial tree and lungs are innervated by the autonomic nervous system. Three types of pathways are involved: *autonomic afferent, parasympathetic efferent, and sympathetic efferent*. Each type of fiber is discussed here; the neurochemical control of respiration is covered later in the section on physiology (see Plates 2-25 and 2-26).

Autonomic Afferent Fibers

Afferent fibers from stretch receptors in the alveoli and from irritant receptors in the airways travel via the pulmonary plexus (located around the tracheal bifurcation and hila of the lungs) to the vagus nerve. Similarly, fibers from irritant receptors in the trachea and from cough receptors in the larynx reach the central nervous system via the vagus nerve. Chemoreceptors in the carotid and aortic bodies and pressor receptors in the carotid sinus and aortic arch also give rise to afferent autonomic fibers. Whereas the fibers from the carotid sinus and carotid body travel via the glossopharyngeal nerve, those from the aortic body and aortic arch travel via the vagus nerve. Other receptors in the nose and nasal sinuses give rise to afferent fibers that form parts of the trigeminal and glossopharyngeal nerves. In addition, the respiratory centers are controlled to some extent by impulses from the hypothalamus and higher centers as well as from the reticular activating system.

Parasympathetic Efferent Fibers

All parasympathetic preganglionic efferent fibers to the tracheobronchial tree are contained in the vagus nerve, originating chiefly from cells in the dorsal vagal nuclei that are closely related to the medullary respiratory centers. The fibers relay with short postganglionic fibers in the vicinity of (or within the walls of) the tracheobronchial tree. This parasympathetic efferent pathway carries motor impulses to the smooth muscle and glands of the tracheobronchial tree. The impulses are cholinergically mediated and produce bronchial smooth muscle contraction, glandular secretion, and vasodilatation.

Sympathetic Efferent Fibers

The preganglionic efferent fibers emerge from the spinal medulla (cord) at levels T1 or T2 to T5 or T6 and pass to the sympathetic trunks via white rami communicantes. Fibers carrying impulses to the larynx and upper trachea ascend in the sympathetic trunk and synapse in the cervical sympathetic ganglia with postganglionic fibers to those structures. The remainder synapse in the upper thoracic ganglia of the sympathetic trunks, from where the postganglionic fibers pass to the lower trachea, bronchi, and bronchioles, largely via the pulmonary plexus. The postganglionic nerve endings are adrenergic. Sympathetic stimulation relaxes bronchial and bronchiolar smooth muscle, inhibits glandular secretion, and causes vasoconstriction. Pharmacologic studies indicate that there are two types of adrenergic receptors, α and β. The α receptors are located primarily in smooth muscle and exocrine glands. The β receptors have been differentiated pharmacologically into β_1, located in the heart, and β_2, located in smooth muscle throughout the body, including bronchial and vascular smooth muscle. Generally, α stimulation is excitatory. β Stimulation may be inhibitory (relaxation of bronchial smooth muscle) or excitatory (increase in both heart rate and force of contraction). β Stimulation also tends to mobilize energy by glycogenolysis and lipolysis.

Certain tissues contain both α and β receptors. The result of stimulation depends on the nature of the stimulating catecholamine and the relative proportion of the two types of receptors. In the lungs, β_2 stimulation (there are no β_1 receptors there) cause bronchodilatation and possibly decreased secretion of mucus; α-adrenergic stimulation by pharmacologic agents causes bronchoconstriction.

Innervation of Tracheobronchial Tree: Schema

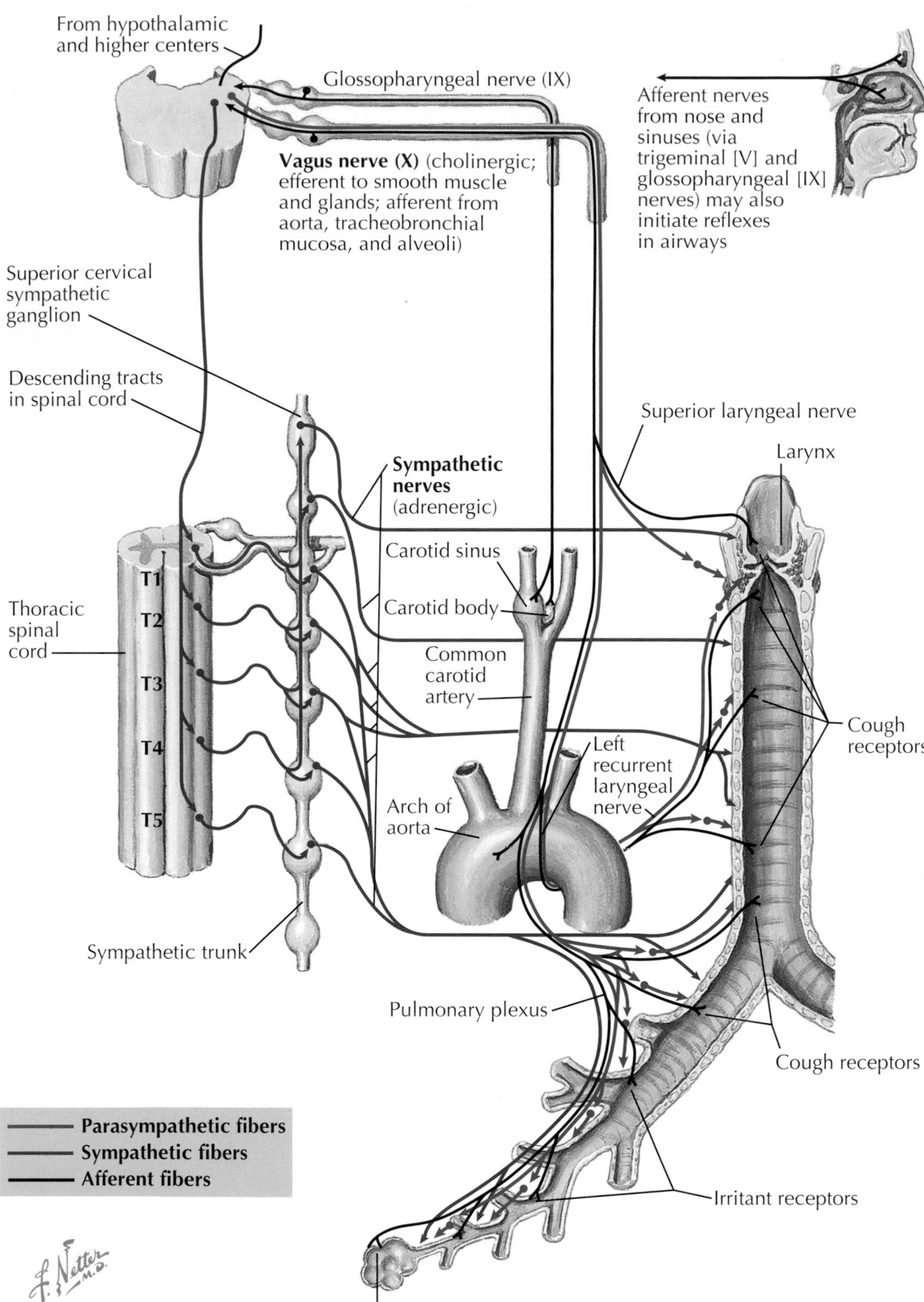

STRUCTURE OF THE TRACHEA AND MAJOR BRONCHI

The trachea or windpipe passes from the larynx to the level of the upper border of the fifth thoracic vertebra, where it divides into the two main bronchi that enter the right and left lungs. About 20 C-shaped plates of cartilage support the anterior and lateral walls of the trachea and main bronchi. The posterior wall, or *membranous* trachea, is free of cartilage but does have interlacing bundles of muscle fibers that insert into the posterior ends of the cartilage plates. The external diameter of the trachea is approximately 2.0 cm in men and 1.5 cm in women. The tracheal length is approximately 10 to 11 cm.

Mucous glands are particularly numerous in the posterior aspect of the tracheal mucosa. Throughout the trachea and large airways, some of these glands lie between the cartilage plates, and others are external to the muscle layers with ducts that penetrate this layer to open on the mucosal surface. Posteriorly, elastic fibers are grouped in longitudinal bundles immediately beneath the basement membrane of the tracheal epithelium, and these appear to the naked eye as broad, flat bands that give a rigid effect to the inner lining of the trachea; they are not so obvious anteriorly. More distally, the bands of elastic fibers are thinner and surround the entire circumference of the airways.

Just above the point at which the main bronchus enters the lung, the cartilage plates come together to completely encircle the airway. Posteriorly, the ends of the plates meet, and the membranous region disappears. The plates are no longer C-shaped but are smaller, more irregular, and arranged around the entire bronchial wall. At the hilum of the lung, the main bronchus divides into lobar bronchi, at which point the plates of cartilage are larger and saddle shaped to support this region of branching.

At the level where cartilage completely surrounds the circumference of the airway, the muscle coat undergoes a striking rearrangement. It no longer inserts into the cartilage (as in the trachea) but forms a separate layer of interlacing bundles internal to it. From this point and more distally, the airways can now be completely occluded by contraction of the muscle; however, the trachea is never subjected to such complete sphincteric action. The right main bronchus is shorter and less sharply angled away from the trachea than the left. For this reason, foreign bodies may lodge in the right main bronchus more often than the left when aspiration takes place while sitting or standing.

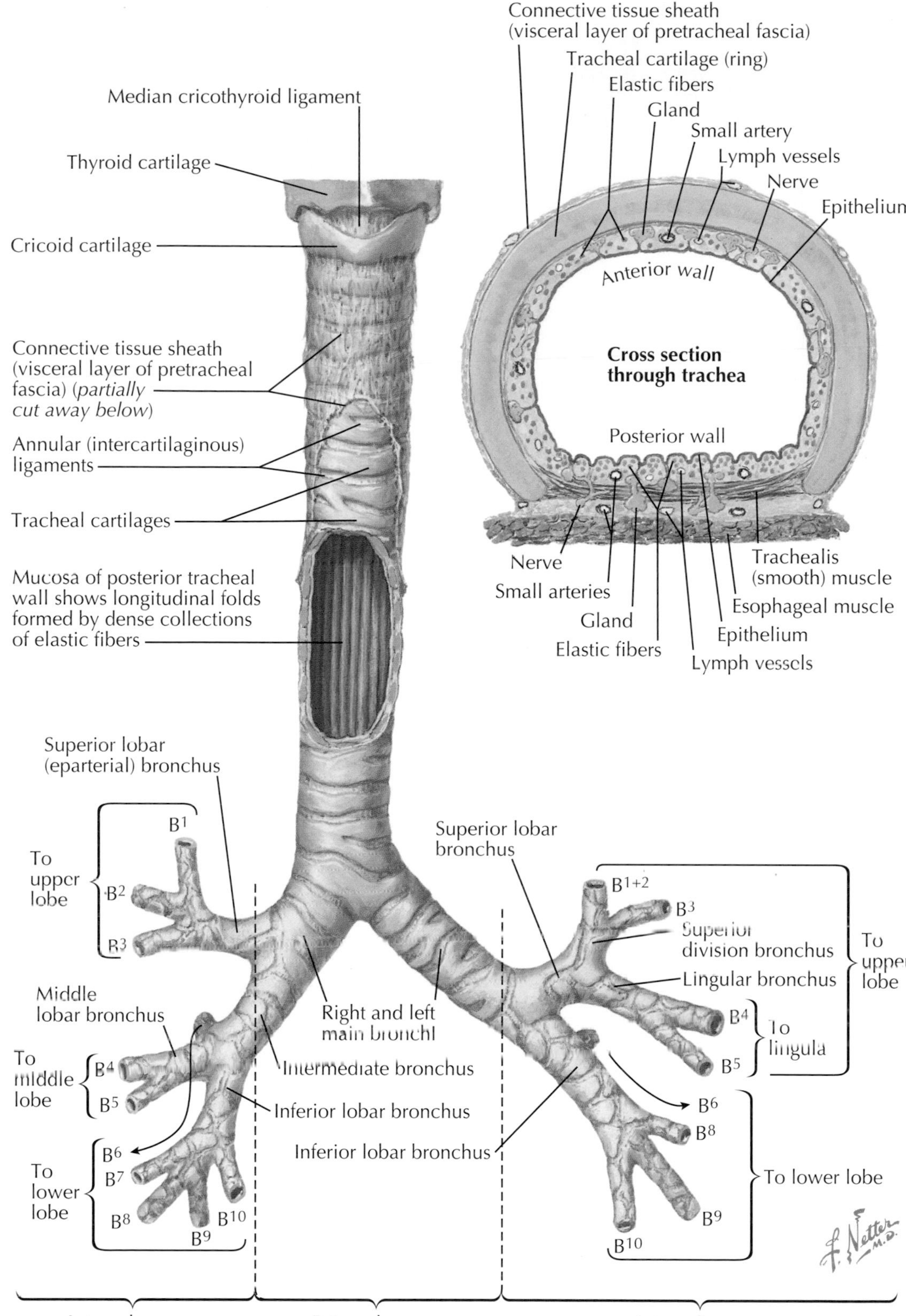

LOBES AND SEGMENTS

The right lung has three lobes and the left has two, although the lingula of the left lung is analogous to the right middle lobe.

The bronchopulmonary segments are the topographic units of the lung and are a means of identifying regions of the lung either radiologically or surgically; there are eight bronchopulmonary segments in the left lung but 10 in the right lung (see Plate 1-14). A segment is not a functional end unit in the lung because it is not isolated by connective tissue. Neighboring segments share common venous and lymphatic drainage and, by collateral ventilation, air passes across segmental boundaries. The pleura isolates one lobe from another, but because the main or oblique fissure is complete in only about 50% of subjects, even a lobe is not always an end unit.

For counting orders or generations of airways, it is sometimes appropriate to count the trachea as the first generation, the main bronchi as the second generation, and so on. To compare features within a segment, it is better to count the segmental bronchi as the first generation of airways.

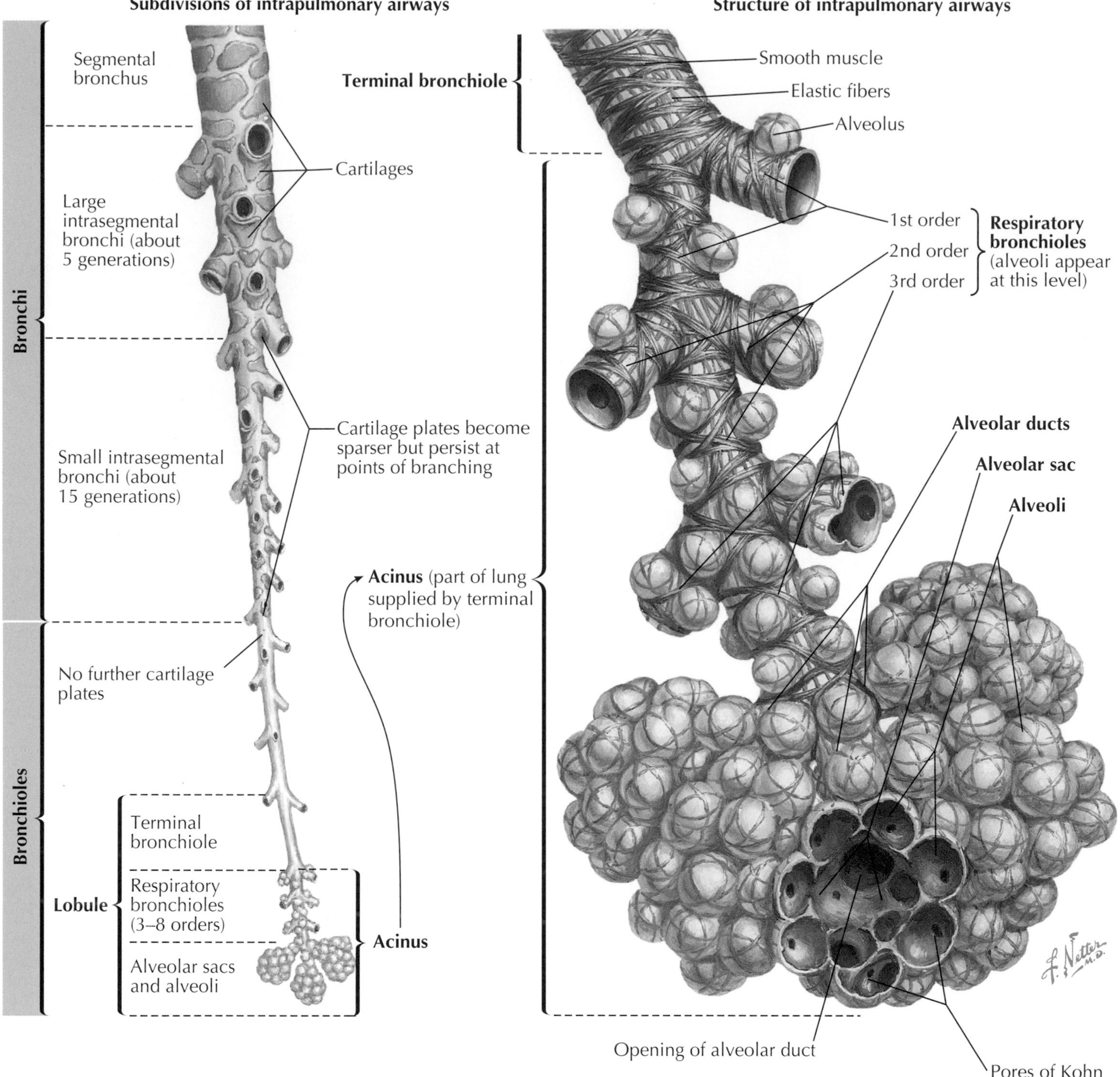

Intrapulmonary Airways

According to the distribution of cartilage, airways are divided into bronchi and bronchioles. *Bronchi* have cartilage plates as discussed earlier. *Bronchioles* are distal to the bronchi beyond the last plate of cartilage and proximal to the alveolar region. Cartilage plates become sparser toward the periphery of the lung, and in the last generations of bronchi, plates are found only at the points of branching. The large bronchi have enough inherent rigidity to sustain patency even during massive lung collapse; the small bronchi collapse along with the bronchioles and alveoli. Small and large bronchi have submucosal mucous glands within their walls.

When any airway is pursued to its distal limit, the *terminal bronchiole* is reached. Three to five terminal bronchioles make up a *lobule*. The *acinus*, or respiratory unit, of the lung is defined as the lung tissue supplied by a terminal bronchiole. Acini vary in size and shape. In adults, the acinus may be up to 1 cm in diameter. Within the acinus, three to eight generations of *respiratory bronchioles* may be found. Respiratory bronchioles have the structure of bronchioles in part of their walls but have alveoli opening directly to their lumina as well. Beyond these lie the alveolar ducts and alveolar sacs before the alveoli proper are reached.

None of these units is isolated from its neighbor by complete connective tissue septa. Collateral air passage occurs between acinus and acinus and between lobule and lobule through the pores of Kohn in the alveolar wall and through respiratory bronchioles between adjacent alveoli.

Connective tissue forms a sheath around airways and blood vessels. It also forms septa that are relatively numerous in some parts of the edges of the lingula and middle lobe and parts of the costodiaphragmatic and costovertebral edges. These septa impede collateral ventilation but do not prevent collateral air drift because they never completely isolate one unit from its neighbor in humans.

Section of large bronchus

Higher magnification of epithelium

Ciliated columnar epithelium with many goblet cells

Basal cells

Basement membrane

Smooth muscle

Mucous glands

Stroma with many elastic fibers

Artery

Nerve fiber

Perichondrium

Cartilage

Fibroelastic layer

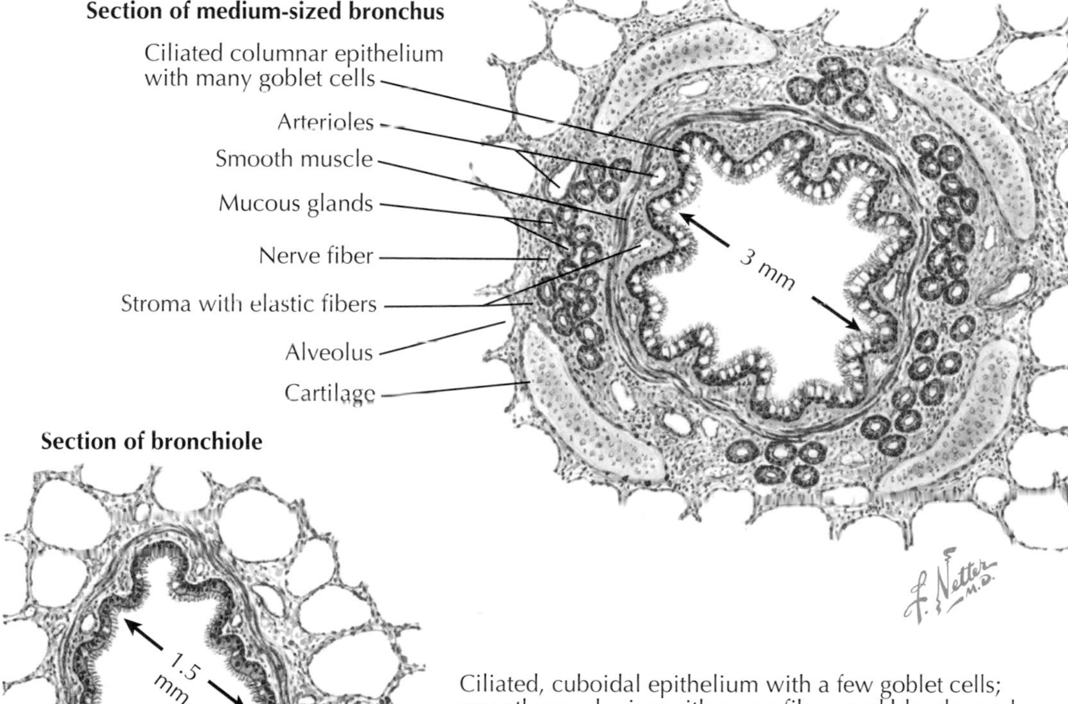

Ciliated, cuboidal epithelium with a few goblet cells; smooth muscle ring with nerve fibers and blood vessels; stroma contains many elastic fibers. Cartilage plates and glands absent.

Structure of Bronchi and Bronchioles—Light Microscopy

The airways are the hollow tubes that conduct air to the respiratory regions of the lung. They are lined throughout their length by pseudostratified, ciliated, columnar epithelium (also referred to as *respiratory epithelium*) supported by a basement membrane (see Plate 1-24 for details of cell types and their arrangement). The remainder of the wall includes a muscle coat and accessory structures such as submucosal glands, together with connective tissue. In the bronchi, cartilage provides additional support.

In adults, the diameter of the main bronchus is similar to that of the trachea (~2 cm), and the diameter of a terminal bronchiole is about 1 mm. These measurements vary with age and the size of the individual and with the functional state of the airway. For reference purposes, it is helpful to designate airways by their order or generation along an axial pathway. The epithelium is thicker in the larger airways and gradually thins toward the periphery of the lung.

Immediately beneath the basement membrane, elastic fibers are collected into fine bands that form longitudinal ridges. In cross-section, the fiber bundles are at the apices of the bronchial folds. The rest of the wall is made up of loose connective tissue containing blood vessels, nerves, capillaries, and lymphatics.

BLOOD SUPPLY

The bronchial arteries supply the capillary bed in the airway wall, forming one plexus internal and another external to the muscle layer (see also Plate 1-26).

VENOUS DRAINAGE

The capillary bed of the bronchi and bronchioles drains into the pulmonary veins. At each point of airway bifurcation, two venous tributaries join. Only at the hilum is there some drainage to the azygos system through veins referred to as the *true bronchial veins*.

LYMPHATICS

Lymphatic channels lie internal to and between the plates of cartilage and internal and external to the muscle layer. Lymphatics are numerous in airway walls. They are not found in alveolar walls but start in the region of the respiratory and terminal bronchioles.

NERVE SUPPLY

Large nerves—both myelinated and nonmyelinated—are seen in the wall of the airway. Motor nerves supply the glands and the muscles of the airway. Intraepithelial nerve endings that are almost certainly sensory fibers have also been described, but whether there are also motor nerve endings at the epithelial level is uncertain.

As the lumen tapers toward the periphery and the airway wall becomes thinner, the small airways are more intimately related to the surrounding alveoli. Functional interaction between the two is probably very important at this level, and inflammation spreads easily through the walls of the small airways.

ULTRASTRUCTURE OF THE TRACHEAL, BRONCHIAL, AND BRONCHIOLAR EPITHELIUM

The lining of the respiratory airways is predominantly a pseudostratified, ciliated, columnar epithelium in which all cells are attached to the basement membrane but not all reach the lumen. In the smaller peripheral airways, the epithelium may be only a single layer thick and cuboidal rather than columnar because basal cells are absent at this level.

Ciliated cells are present in even the smallest airways and respiratory bronchioles, where they are adjacent to alveolar lining cells. The "ciliary escalator" starts at the most distal point of the airway epithelium. In smaller airways, the cilia are not as tall as in the more central airways. Eight epithelial cell types can be identified in humans, although ultrastructural features and cell kinetics have been studied mainly in animals. The following classification is based on studies in the rat: the (1) basal and (2) pulmonary neuroendocrine cells are attached to the basement membrane but do not reach the lumen; (3) the intermediate cell is probably the precursor that differentiates into (4) the ciliated cell, (5) the brush cell, or one of the secretory cells—(6) the mucous (goblet) cell, (7) the serous cell, or (8) the Clara cell.

The *basal cell* divides and daughter cells pass to the superficial layer.

The pulmonary neuroendocrine cell (PNEC), previously referred to as the *Kulchitsky cell*, contains numerous neurosecretory granules and is a rare, but likely important, functional cell of the airway epithelium. The PNEC neurosecretory granules contain serotonin and other bioactive peptides such as gastrin-releasing peptide (GRP). PNECs are more numerous before birth and may play a role in the innate immune system.

The *intermediate cell* is columnar. It has electron-lucent cytoplasm and no special features. It is probably the cell that differentiates into the others.

The *ciliated cell* carries the cilia of the respiratory epithelium. The cilium has nine double pairs of axonemes and a special axoneme in the center. The arrangement is modified at the base and at the apex, where a coronet of small claws has been identified. The feet of the axonemes are arranged so that a cilium "plugs" into the cytoplasm. The axonemes are attached to each other by "arms" of dynein, a contractile protein, and these provide the mechanism for ciliary motion.

The *brush cell* resembles a similar cell type found in the gut and in the nasal sinuses. Its function in the respiratory tract remains unknown, but hypotheses regarding its function include immune surveillance, cell regeneration, chemoreceptor, sensor of alveolar fluid or air tension, and regulator of capillary resistance and perfusion.

The *mucous (goblet) cell* is a secretory cell containing numerous large and confluent secretory granules. Electron microscopic studies have shown that confluence represents fusion of the two trilaminar membranes of adjacent granules to produce a pentilaminar layer.

The *serous cell* resembles the serous cell of the submucosal gland and contains small, discrete, electron-dense secretory granules. Its cytoplasm is also more electron dense than that of the Clara cell.

The *Clara cell* also contains small, discrete, electron-dense granules, but compared with the serous cell, the cytoplasm is electron lucent, and there is relatively more smooth than rough endoplasmic reticulum.

The serous cell is mainly found centrally; the Clara cell is found only distally. These are the more common secretory cells of the airways, but irritation, drug reaction, or infection may lead to an increase in the number of secretory cells. The serous and Clara cells then develop into mucous cells. Differentiated cells are seen in mitosis, but this is probably not the main way that cell numbers increase.

The basement membrane is well defined and becomes thinner in small airways. In certain diseases—notably asthma—the reticular basement membrane (lamina reticularis) increases in thickness, although its structure remains normal.

Nerve fibers are seen within the epithelium. They are nonmyelinated and without a Schwann cell sheath. Their vesicle content suggests that the fibers are sensory or motor and either cholinergic or adrenergic in type.

Electron micrograph of bronchial epithelium

Goblet cell
Ciliated columnar cell
Basal cell
Basement membrane

Light micrograph of respiratory epithelium

Microtubule B
Microtubule A
Microtubule doublet (9 total)
Cell membrane
Axial filament complex

Shaft of cilium

Mucus
Nerve
Ciliated cells
Goblet (mucous) cell
Basement membrane
Basal cell
Brush cell
Basal cell
Nerve
Goblet cell (discharging)
Serous cell
Pulmonary neuroendocrine cell (PNEC) (Kulchitsky cell)

Trachea and large bronchi. Ciliated and goblet cells predominant, with some serous cells and occasional brush cells and Clara cells. Numerous basal cells and occasional Kulchitsky cells are present.

F. Netter M.D.
JOHN A.CRAIG—AD

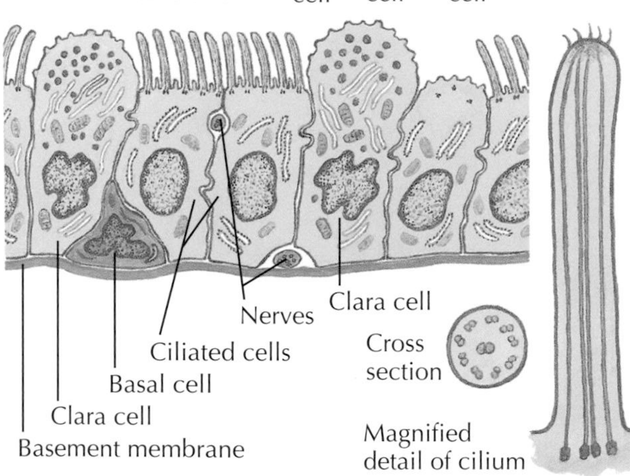

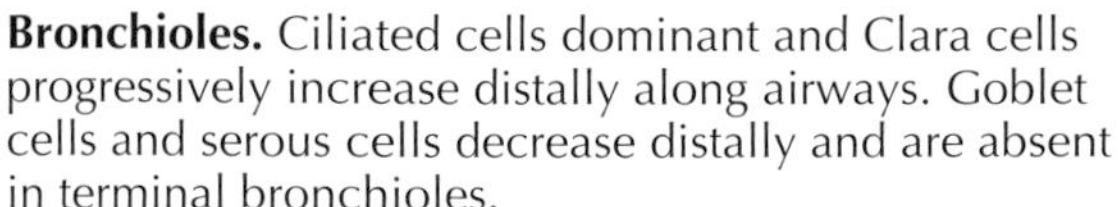

Bronchioles. Ciliated cells dominant and Clara cells progressively increase distally along airways. Goblet cells and serous cells decrease distally and are absent in terminal bronchioles.

Electron micrograph of cilia

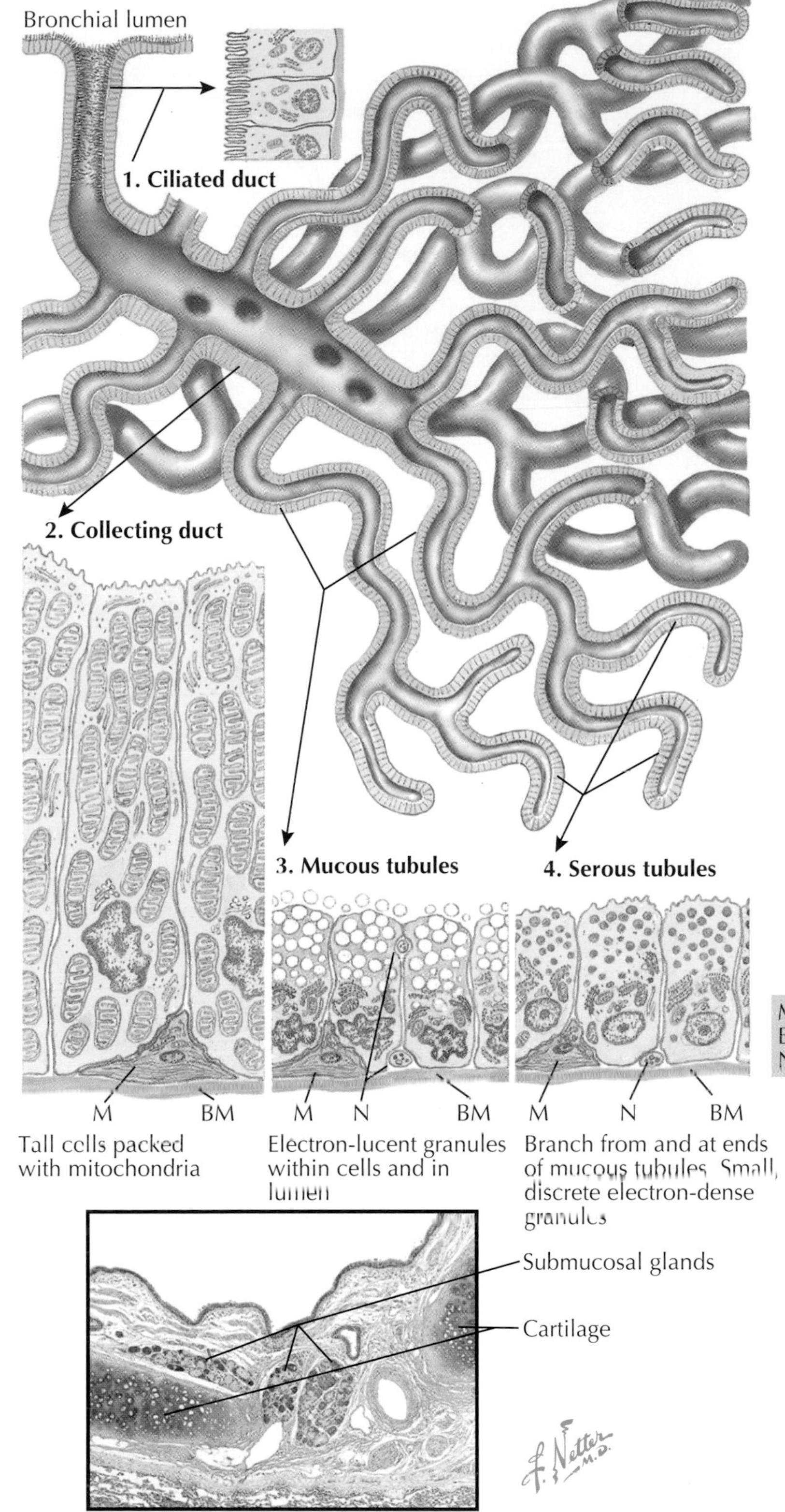

Light micrograph of submucosal glands

M = myoepithelial cell
BM = basement membrane
N = nerve

Bronchial Submucosal Glands

The submucosal glands of the human airways are of the branched tubuloacinar type: *tubulo* refers to the main part of the secretory tubule and *acinar* to the blind end of such a tubule.

Three-dimensional reconstruction of the gland reveals its various zones:

1. The origin is referred to as the *ciliated duct* and is lined by bronchial epithelium with its mixed population of cells. With the naked eye, the origin of the gland is seen as a hole of pinpoint size in the surface epithelium of the bronchus.
2. The second part of the duct expands to form the *collecting duct* and is lined by a columnar epithelium in which the cells are eosinophilic after staining with hematoxylin and eosin. Ultrastructural examination shows these cells to be packed with mitochondria, resembling the cells of the striated duct of the salivary gland (except that they lack the folds of membrane responsible for the appearance of striation). The collecting duct may be up to 0.25 mm in diameter and 1 mm long. It passes obliquely from the airway lumen, so the usual macroscopic section does not include the full length of the duct. It is usually seen as a rather large "acinus" composed of cells without secretory granules.
3. About 13 tubules rise from each collecting duct. These may branch several times and are closely intertwined with each other. The secretory cells lining these tubules are of two types: mucous and serous. Mucous cells line the central or proximal part of a tubule; serous cells line the distal part. Outpouchings or short-sided tubules may arise from the sides of the mucous tubules, and these are lined by serous cells. The peripheral portion of a tubule usually branches several times, and each of the final blind endings is lined with serous cells.

The gland tissue is internal to a basement membrane. In addition to the cell types described above, the following are found: (1) myoepithelial cells; (2) "clear" cells; and (3) nerve fibers, including motor fibers. Outside the basement membrane, there are rich vascular and lymphatic networks and the nerve plexus.

In histologic cross-sections, the submucosal gland is seen as a compact structure. In a main bronchus of an adult, the gland is about 0.2 mm in diameter or less than one-third the thickness of the airway wall (measured from the luminal surface to the cartilage layer). This ratio is similar in both children and adults and is consistent throughout airways at various levels of branching. The ratio of gland size to wall thickness (sometimes referred to as the *Reid index*) is a useful way of assessing abnormalities in gland size because gland hypertrophy is a hallmark of a number of inflammatory diseases of the large airways.

In humans, the secretory tubules of the mucous and serous cells contain mainly an acid glycoprotein, either sialic acid or its sulfate ester.

The concentration of bronchial submucosal openings in the trachea is on the order of one gland opening per mm^2. The glands become sparser towards the periphery of the lung, their decrease in number and concentration being parallel to the diminution in the amount of cartilage in the airway.

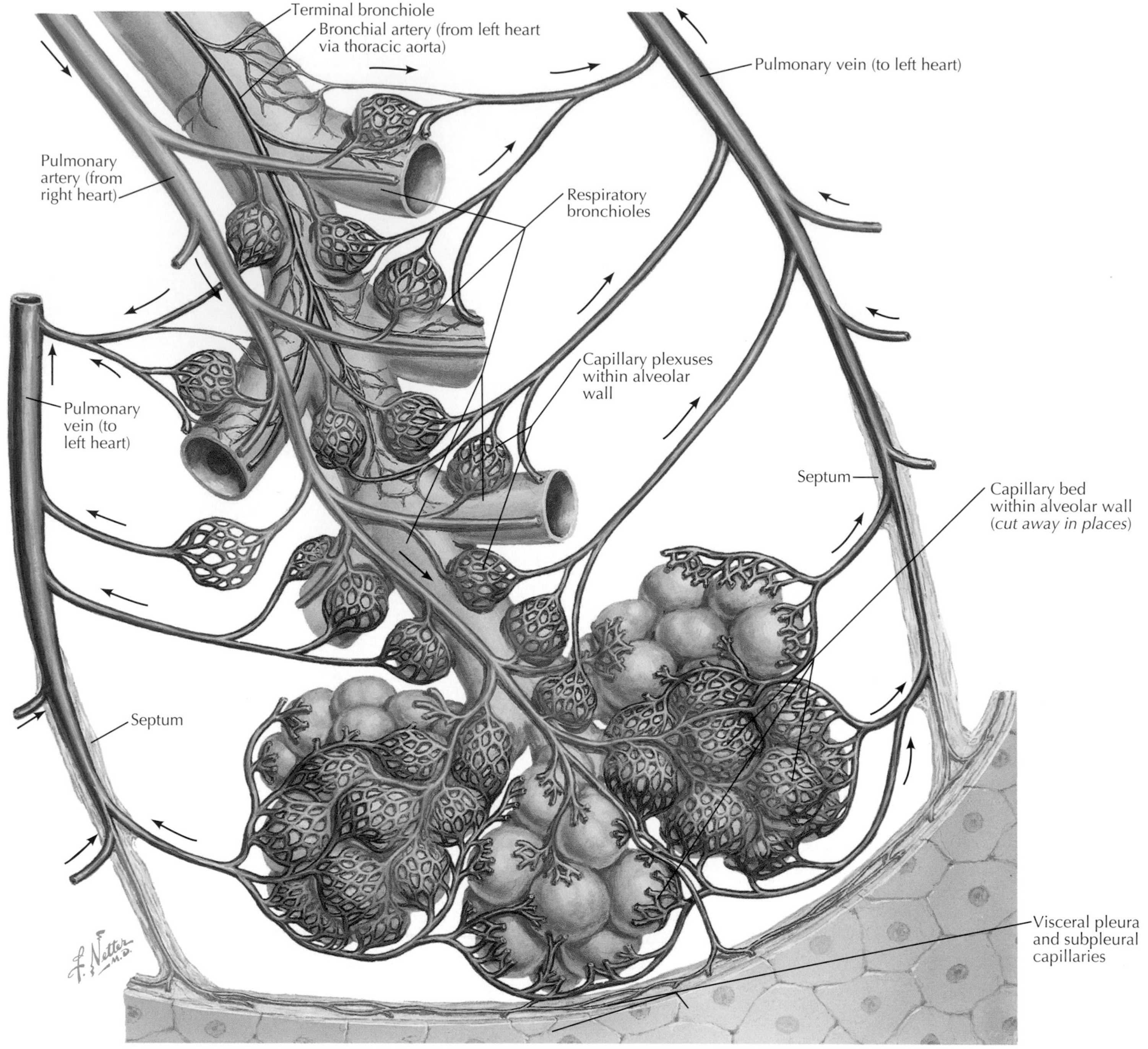

Pulmonary arteries and their branches distribute segmentally with the bronchi. Pulmonary veins and their tributaries drain intersegmentally.

Intrapulmonary Blood Circulation

The human lung is supplied by two arterial systems referred to as *pulmonary* and *bronchial*, each originating from a different side of the heart. Blood from the lungs is drained by two venous systems, *pulmonary* and *true bronchial*. The pulmonary veins drain oxygenated blood from the regions supplied by the pulmonary artery and deoxygenated blood from the airways within the lung that are supplied by the bronchial artery. The true bronchial veins serve only the perihilar region, supplied mainly by the bronchial artery, and this blood drains to the azygous system and right atrium.

Arteries

The *bronchial arteries* arise from the aorta and supply the capillary plexus of the airway walls from the hilum to the respiratory bronchiole.

The *pulmonary artery* branches run with airways and their accompanying bronchial arteries in a single connective tissue sheath referred to as the *bronchoarterial* or *bronchovascular* bundle. The pulmonary artery transforms into a capillary bed only when it reaches the alveoli of the respiratory bronchiole. It supplies all capillaries in the alveolar walls that constitute the respiratory surface of the lung.

Veins

All intrapulmonary blood drains to the pulmonary veins. The veins lie at the periphery of any unit—acinus, lobule, or segment. Veins receive tributaries from the alveolar capillary network, the pleura, and the airways.

Precapillary Anastomosis

Pulmonary and bronchial arteries, and hence the right and left sides of the heart, communicate through the capillary bed in the region of the respiratory bronchiole and through the intrapulmonary venous bed. Pulmonary-to-bronchial artery anastomoses are present in the walls of the larger airways but normally are closed. They open if blood flow is interrupted in either system and in certain disease states such as pulmonary arteriovenous malformation.

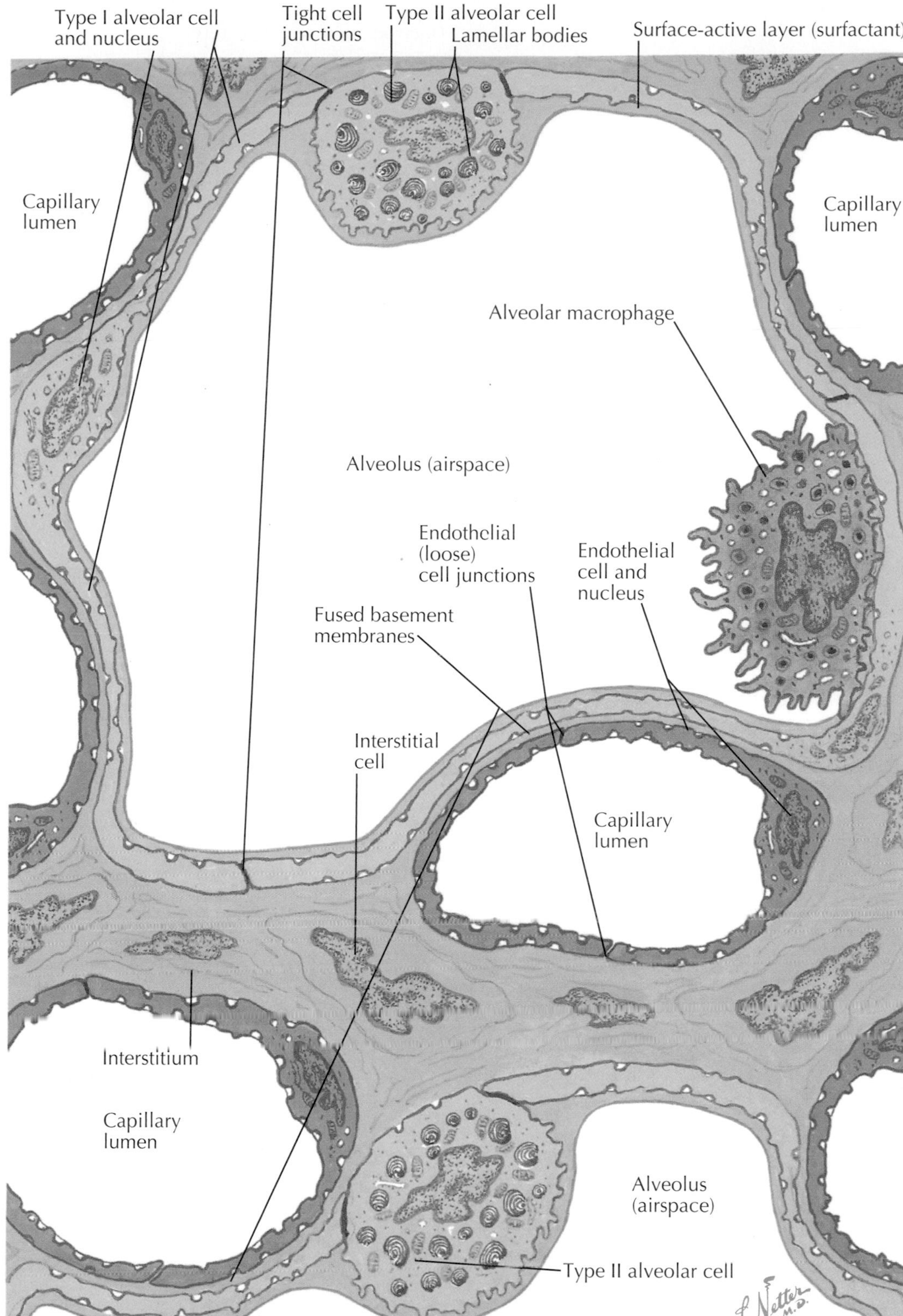

FINE STRUCTURE OF ALVEOLAR CAPILLARY UNIT

The cellular composition of the alveolar capillary unit was not recognized until the era of electron microscopy. Before that time, it was thought that a single membrane separated blood and air at the level of the terminal airspace. We now know that, even at its narrowest, the boundary between blood and air is composed of at least two cell types (the type I alveolar epithelial cell and the endothelial cell) and extracellular material, namely, the surfactant lining of the alveolar surface, the basement membranes, and the so-called "endothelial fuzz." The last is composed of mucopolysaccharides and proteoglycans (or glycocalyx) that may be involved in signal transduction, including mechanotransduction or shear stress at the endothelial surface. Plate 1-27 shows part of a terminal airspace and cross sections of surrounding capillaries. In humans, the diameter of the alveoli varies from 100 to 300 µm. The capillary segments are much smaller in diameter (10-14 µm) and may be separated from each other by even smaller distances. Each alveolus (there are 300 million alveoli in the adult human lungs) may be associated with as many as 1000 capillary segments.

The thinness of the cellular boundary between the blood and the air presents enormous surface area to air on one side and to blood on the other (~70 m^2 for both lungs). Given the paucity of organelles, the cells at this location likely play mainly passive roles in physiologic and metabolic events involved in the management of airborne or bloodborne substrates.

Ninety-five percent of the alveolus is lined by epithelial type I cells. The remaining cells are larger polygonal type II cells. These two cell types form a complete epithelial layer sealed by tight junctions. The cellular layer lining the alveoli is remarkably impermeable to salt-containing solutions, but little is known about specific metabolic activities of type I alveolar cells. Growing evidence suggests a more important role in the maintenance of alveolar homeostasis than previously thought, evidenced by the expression a large number of proteins such as aquaporin (AQP-5), T1α, functional ion channels, caveolins, adenosine receptors, and multidrug-resistant genes. Type II cells and endothelial cells have long been known to play active roles in the metabolic function of the lung by producing surfactant and processing circulating vasoactive substances, respectively. In addition, recent research suggests more complex roles for both of these cell types.

ALVEOLAR CELLS AND SURFACE-ACTIVE LAYER

As illustrated in Plate 1-28, in addition to being larger, the type II alveolar cell is distinguished from the type I alveolar cell by having short, blunt projections on the free alveolar surface and lamellar inclusion bodies. The intracellular origins of the lamellar bodies (LBs) and the exact mechanism for lipid transport into them

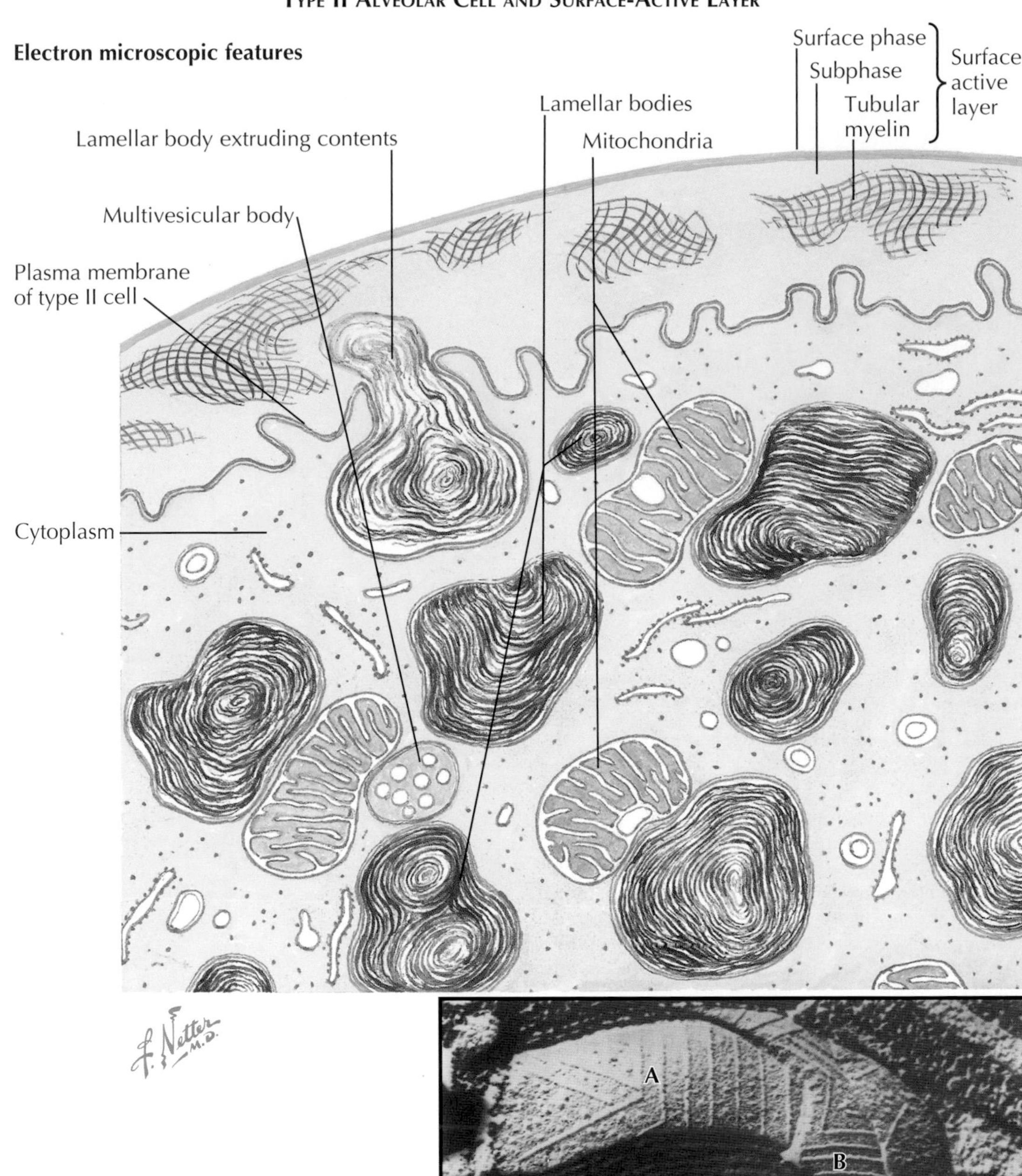

Freeze-fracture preparation of a lamellar body with closely apposed, fractured lamellae. Series of parallel ribs, each ca. 80 Å in width evident on lamellae A and B, the series angled to each other. Particles or knobs, ca. 100 Å in diameter, are prominent on lamella C but also apparent between ribs.

Fine Structure of Alveolar Capillary Unit *(Continued)*

are not known with certainty, although lipid translocation across the LB membrane is facilitated by the ABCA subfamily of adenosine triphosphate–binding cassette transporters. The LB contains the phospholipid component of surfactant and two small hydrophobic surfactant polypeptide proteins (SP-B and SP-C) that are coreleased from the type II cell by a process similar to exocytosis. Two additional components of surfactant (large hydrophilic proteins SP-A and SP-D) are synthesized and released independent of LBs.

After release into the airspace, surfactant forms a lipid monolayer on the alveolar surface, greatly reducing surface tension. Although surfactant production, release, and recycling are critical type II cell functions, these cells are now known to have many additional functions, including repopulation of type I cells, clearance, repair, migration to areas of lung injury, and host defense (including the expression of Toll-like receptors). Type II cells also secrete and respond to an array of cytokines and chemokines and have been shown to regulate monocyte transmigration across the epithelium.

Alveolar macrophages are migratory cells and, after fixation for microscopy, they are usually seen free in the alveolar space or closely applied to the surface of type I cells. Alveolar macrophages are characterized by irregular cytoplasmic projections and large numbers of lysosomes. Alveolar macrophages are important in the defense mechanisms of the lungs.

The cellular components of the blood-air barrier frequently consist only of the extremely flattened extensions of endothelial cells and type I alveolar cells. In other regions, the wall contains such cell types as smooth muscle cells, pericytes, fibroblasts, and occasional mononuclear cells (including plasma cells). Smooth muscle cells are found around the mouth of each alveolus in humans. Pericytes ensheathed in basement membrane occur around pulmonary alveolar capillaries but less frequently than on systemic capillaries. The pericytes are characterized by having finely branched cytoplasmic processes that approach the endothelial cells and a web of cytoplasmic filaments that run along the membrane close to the endothelium. Pericytes can be distinguished from fibroblasts in that the latter are free of a basement membrane sheath.

ENDOTHELIAL CELL STRUCTURE

Details of the fine structure of pulmonary capillary endothelial cells are shown in Plate 1-29. The endothelium is of the continuous type (not fenestrated), and the cells are frequently linked by tight junctions. Alveolar epithelial cells and alveolar capillary endothelial cells are uniquely interactive and highly codependent during lung development. The ultrastructural features of the

Fine Structure of Alveolar Capillary Unit *(Continued)*

capillary endothelial cell are in keeping with their primary roles as fluid barriers and gas transfer facilitators. The thickest portion of the cell is in the vicinity of the nucleus, where the majority of cytoplasmic organelles, such as mitochondria, Golgi apparatus, rough endoplasmic reticulum, multivesicular bodies, microtubules, microfilaments, and Weibel-Palade bodies, reside. However, the more peripheral slender extensions of these cells are practically devoid of organelles, and may be as thin as 0.1 μm in some regions.

A growing body of evidence indicates that the endothelium plays a large number of important physiologic roles at the alveolar level, many of which appear to be mediated by the *caveolae intracellulare*. The caveolae are a subset of membrane (lipid) rafts, present as flask-shaped invaginations of the plasma membrane. When the pulmonary capillary endothelial cell membrane is freeze fractured, the caveolae appear as pits on the inner fracture face and as domes on the outer fracture face. Intramembranous particles, about 80 to 100 Å in diameter, are randomly scattered on both faces, except in association with caveolae, where they occur in rings or plaques. These rings correspond to the skeletal rim seen in thin sections. The intramembranous particles also occur on the curved faces of the caveola membrane.

The caveolae contain caveolin proteins, which serve as organizing centers for signal transduction. Caveolin proteins have cytoplasmic N and C termini, palmitoylation sites, and a scaffolding domain that facilitates interaction with signaling molecules. Caveolae are implicated in a wide variety of cell transport events, including transcytosis and cholesterol trafficking. Many of the caveolae intracellulares directly face the vascular lumen, but they are also found on the abluminal surface as vesicles, vastly increasing the surface of the endothelium. The luminal stoma of the caveola is spanned by a delicate diaphragm composed of a single lamella (by contrast with the unit membrane construction of the endothelial plasma membrane and caveola membrane) that helps create a specialized microenvironment within the caveola.

In addition to the caveolae, the endothelial surface has numerous fingerlike projections, which are best demonstrated in scanning electron micrographs. The size (250-350 nm in diameter; 300 to ≥3000 nm long) and density of the projections are such that they may prevent the formed elements of blood from approaching the endothelial surface and have the effect of directing an eddy flow of plasma along the cells. Their function is not entirely known, but they vastly increase the cell surface area for interaction with soluble elements in the blood.

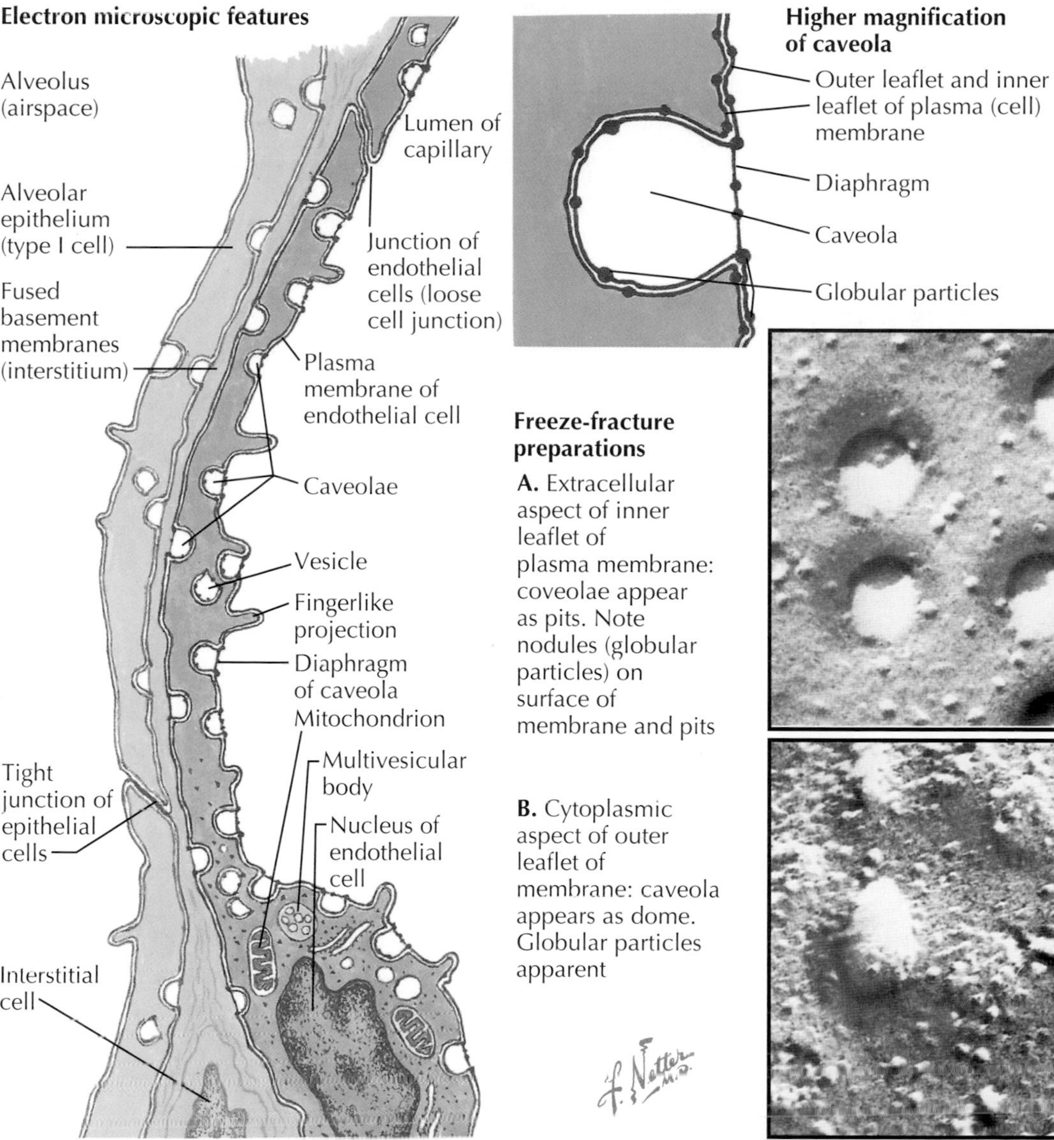

Scanning electron micrograph

Luminal surface of pulmonary artery. The endothelial projections range from 250 to 350 nm in diameter and 300 to 3000 nm in length. They may be simple knobs or longer arms, some of which branch or bud. They are densest over main body of cells but extend laterally to overlap adjacent cells

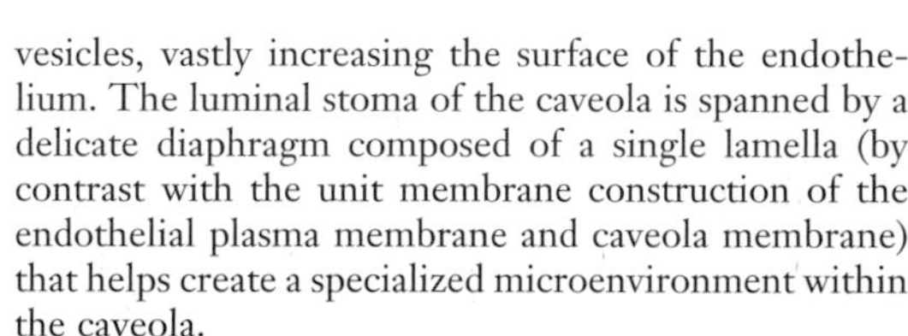

Lymphatic Drainage of the Lungs and Pleura

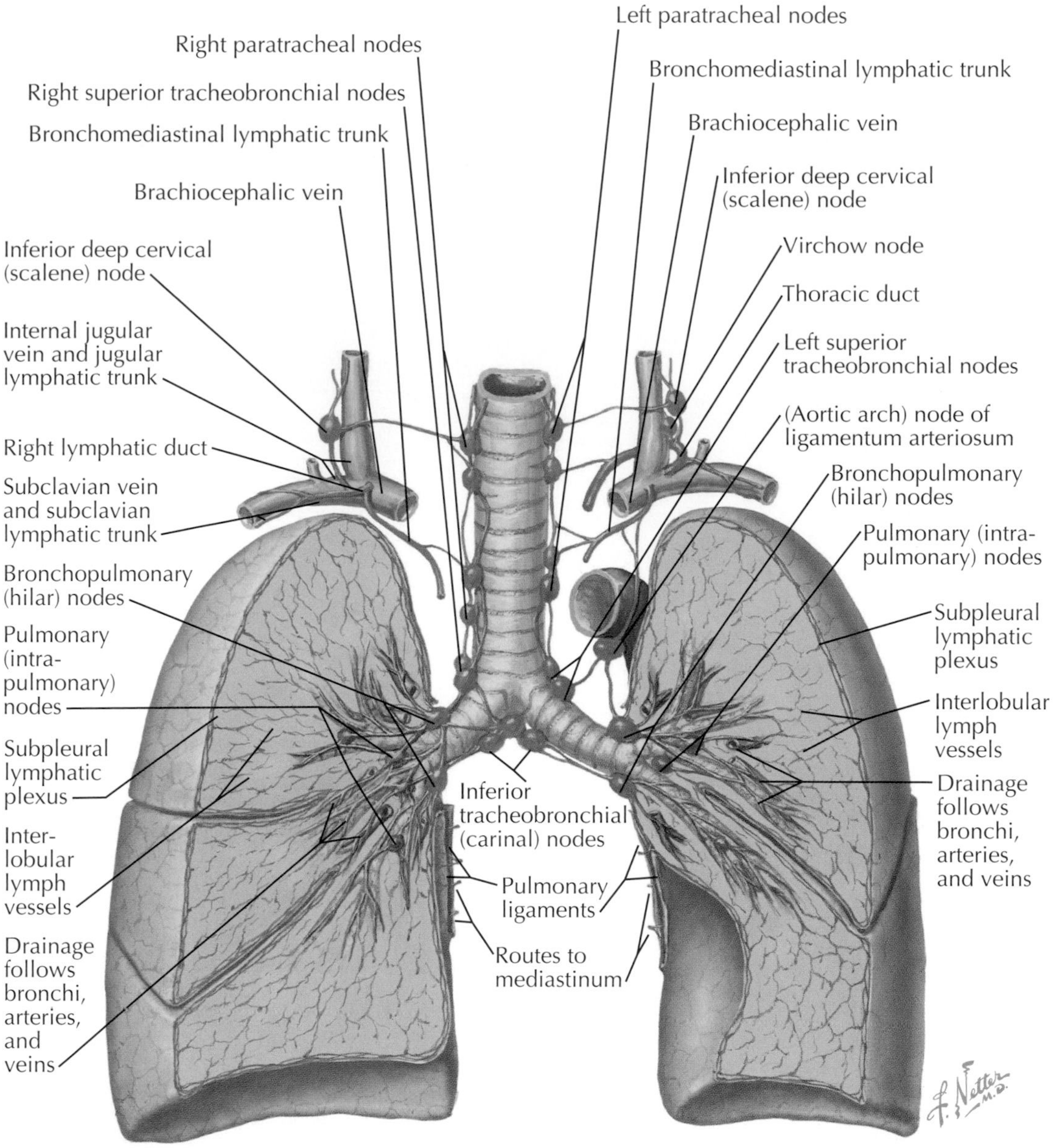

The lymphatic drainage of the lung plays critical roles in the removal of excess interstitial fluid and particulate matter (free or within macrophages) deposited in the airspaces and in lymphocyte trafficking and immune surveillance. Discrepancies exist between the terminology of the *Nomina Anatomica* adopted by anatomists for lung lymphatic routes and the terms commonly and conveniently used by clinicians, surgeons, and radiologists. For this reason, in the illustrations, the terms in common usage are included in parentheses after the official *Nomina Anatomica* designations.

As the lymphatic channels approach the hilum, lymph nodes are present in the following distributions:

1. The pulmonary (intrapulmonary nodes) within the lung, located chiefly at bifurcations of the large bronchi
2. The bronchopulmonary (hilar) nodes situated in the pulmonary hilum at the site of entry of the main bronchi and vessels
3. The tracheobronchial nodes, which anatomists subdivide into two groups: a *superior* group situated in the obtuse angles between the trachea and bronchi and an *inferior* (carinal) group situated below or at the carina (i.e., at the junction of the two main bronchi)
4. The tracheal (paratracheal) group situated alongside and to some extent in front of the trachea throughout its course; these are sometimes subdivided into *lower* tracheal (paratracheal) nodes and an *upper* group in accordance with their relative positions
5. The inferior deep cervical (scalene) nodes situated in relation to the lower part of the internal jugular vein, usually under cover of the scalenus anterior muscle
6. The aortic arch nodes situated under the arch of the aorta

Beginning centrally, the major lymph channels on the *right* side are (1) the bronchomediastinal lymph trunk, which collects lymph from the mediastinum, and (2) the jugular lymph trunk. The latter commonly unites with (3) the subclavian trunk to form a right lymphatic duct, which in turn joins the origin of the right brachiocephalic vein. In some cases, however, these three major lymphatic channels join the brachiocephalic vein independently. On the *left* side, the thoracic duct curves behind the internal jugular vein to enter the right brachiocephalic vein at the junction of the subclavian vein and internal jugular veins. There may or may not be a separate right bronchomediastinal lymph trunk; if present, it may join the thoracic duct or enter the brachiocephalic vein independently.

Within the lung, lymphatic plexuses course as two separate arcades, one along the bronchovascular sheath (beginning at the level of the respiratory bronchiole) and the other along the pulmonary veins coursing through the interlobular planes, connective tissue septa, and the pleura. In the bronchi, fine lymph channels in the submucosa communicate with much larger lymphatic vessels in the adventitia. Beyond this point, the lymph is collected by the interlobular lymphatics. The bronchial pathways communicate with the lymph vessels along the accompanying pulmonary arteries. The pulmonary veins that lie at the edge of the respiratory units—whether acinus, lobule, or segment—are surrounded by connective tissue and have lymphatic plexuses in their walls. They are separated from the bronchi and arteries, but at least centrally, communicating channels connect the various lymphatic systems that form a fine network beneath the pleural surface over the surface of the lungs and the interlobar fissures.

Drainage routes

Right lung: All lobes drain to pulmonary and bronchopulmonary (hilar) nodes, then to inferior tracheobronchial (carinal) nodes, right superior tracheobronchial nodes, and right paratracheal nodes on the way to the brachiocephalic vein via the bronchomediastinal lymphatic trunk and/or the inferior deep cervical (scalene) node

Left lung: Superior lobe drains to pulmonary and bronchopulmonary (hilar) nodes, inferior tracheobronchial (carinal) nodes, left superior tracheobronchial nodes, left paratracheal nodes and/or (aortic arch) node of ligamentum arteriosum, then to brachiocephalic vein via left bronchomediastinal trunk and thoracic duct. Left inferior lobe also drains to pulmonary and bronchopulmonary (hilar) nodes and to inferior tracheobronchial (carinal) nodes but then mostly to right superior tracheobronchial nodes, where it follows same route as lymph from right lung

DISTRIBUTION OF LYMPHATICS IN LUNGS AND PLEURA

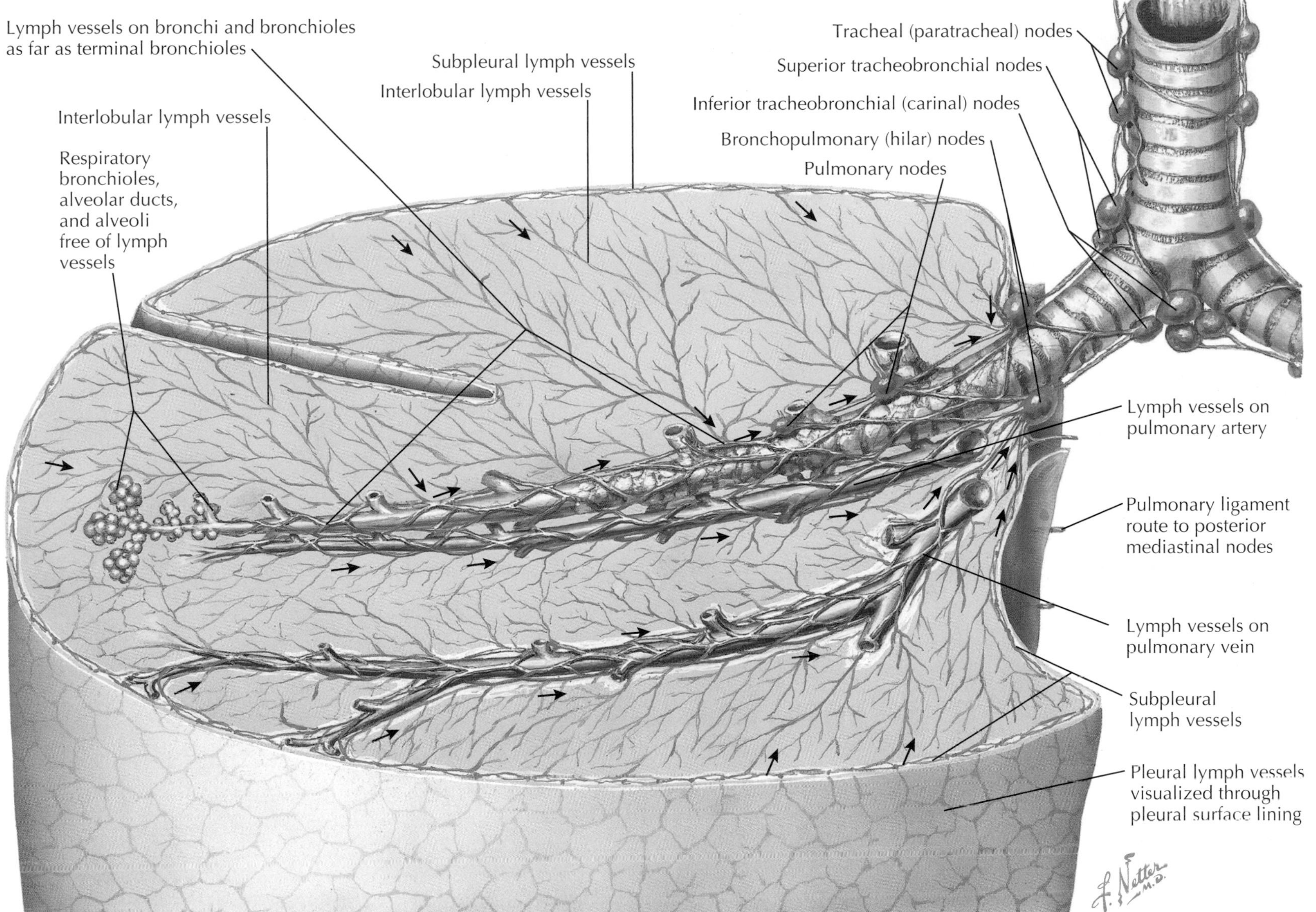

LYMPHATIC DRAINAGE OF THE LUNGS AND PLEURA

(Continued)

The network was formerly thought to drain it its entirety to the hilar nodes, but it has now been shown to communicate not only with the arterial and venous channels but with the interlobular plexuses as well. Only the portion of the pleural drainage close to the hilum supplies the nodes there. The interlobular vessels pass to the bronchial, arterial, and venous pulmonary plexuses and to the pulmonary and bronchopulmonary nodes.

Almost all the lymph from the lungs eventually reaches the bronchopulmonary (hilar) lymph nodes, with or without passing through pulmonary lymph nodes on its way. Some lymph may bypass the hilum and go directly to the tracheobronchial lymph nodes. From the *right* lung, drainage from the bronchopulmonary (hilar) group is to the superior and inferior (carinal) tracheobronchial and the right tracheal (paratracheal) nodes. From there, lymph goes either by the way of the bronchomediastinal trunk to the right brachiocephalic vein, via the inferior deep cervical (scalene) lymph nodes to the same vein, or through both of these channels. On the *left* side, the course is somewhat different. There, either most or all of the drainage from the *upper* lobe, after passing through the bronchopulmonary (hilar) lymph nodes, moves either by way of the tracheobronchial and tracheal (paratracheal) lymph nodes, bronchomediastinal trunk, scalene nodes, and thoracic duct to the brachiocephalic vein or by way of the aortic arch nodes to the same termination. From the *left lower* lobe and usually from the lingula, lymph flows to the right after passing through the bronchopulmonary (hilar) nodes and goes mostly to the lower tracheobronchial (carinal) lymph nodes. It then follows the same course as the lymph from the right lung by way of the right tracheal (paratracheal) nodes—an important point in disease, especially tumors of the left lower lobe.

A number of factors may cause deviation from these major pathways of lymph drainage. The pulmonary lymphatic vessels contain many valves that normally direct the flow toward the hilum. Obstruction in parts of the system, however, may cause a "backing up" effect with incompetence of the valves, reversal of flow, and opening of collateral channels. It is noteworthy that in pulmonary edema, the pulmonary lymph vessels have been found to be greatly distended (see Plate 4-127).

Some lymph may leave the lungs through vessels that emerge in the pulmonary ligaments and pass to the posterior mediastinal lymph nodes. Nagaishi's textbook states that some of the pulmonary drainage may even reach intraabdominal lymph nodes, although a specific transit route is not described. Finally, there are probably cross-connections between the right and left tracheal (paratracheal) nodes, a situation that may further alter the drainage pathways.

Clinically, the nodal positions are described by the regional lymph node classification for lung cancer staging as detailed in Plate 4-49. This classification is anatomically based and validated, allowing for consistent lymph node mapping used in staging lung cancer.

Pulmonary Immunology: Lymphocytes, Mast Cells, Eosinophils, and Neutrophils

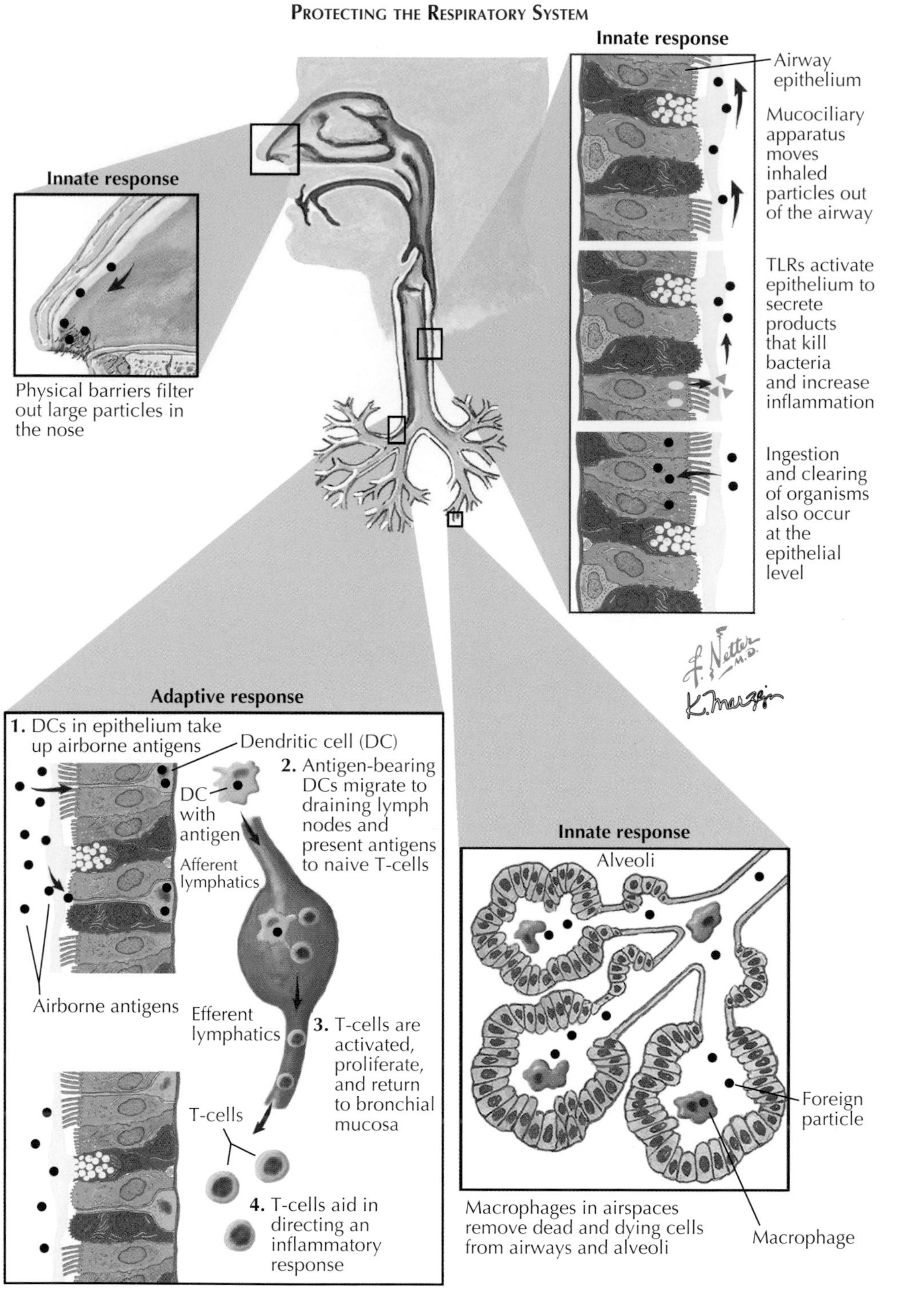

The respiratory system is in intimate contact with the environment through the inhalation of large volumes of air every day (~10,000 L). Protecting the respiratory system from pathogens and toxins while avoiding unnecessary inflammation when harmless proteins are inhaled is a challenge. Physical barriers such as the filtration of air by the nose and upper airways and the mucociliary apparatus, which moves inhaled particles, organisms, and cells toward the pharynx, where they can be swallowed, provide the first line of defense. Ingestion of organisms and particulate material by macrophages resident within the lung is another important line of defense. Ingestion of silica particles or asbestos fibers by macrophages may fail to clear these particles and may lead to persistence of inflammation and ultimately lung tissue damage.

The airway epithelial cells have the capacity to ingest bacteria and have a variety of receptors, such as Toll-like receptors, on their surface that may lead to activation of the epithelium on exposure to bacterial or viral products (e.g., DNA, RNA, lipopolysaccharide). Activated epithelium secretes chemoattractant molecules that will attract neutrophils, eosinophils, and lymphocytes, depending on the particular need. Cytokines secreted by the epithelium may also promote inflammation. Defensins are proteins that are secreted by epithelial cells that may bind to microbial cell membranes and create pores that assist in killing organisms. Epithelial cells also produce surfactant proteins that may assist in the elimination of pathogenic organisms.

Adaptive immune responses to pathogenic organisms and foreign proteins involve lymphocyte populations. Intraepithelial lymphocytes are usually CD8 + T cells, which are well placed to exert cytotoxic effects on infected epithelial cells. Indeed, the epithelial cells are the primary target for a variety of respiratory viruses such as rhinovirus and adenovirus. After infection, cells may present antigen on their surface that leads to activation of CD8+ T cells and cell killing through release of perforin and granzyme or by Fas-Fas ligand interactions. However, the common cold rhinovirus infects epithelial cells without inducing killing of these cells and triggers inflammation. Other viruses that target the airway epithelium such as respiratory syncytial virus (RSV) may cause severe inflammation of the small airways in infants. Both rhinovirus and RSV are associated with asthma attacks.

PROTECTING THE RESPIRATORY SYSTEM
Innate response
Physical barriers filter out large particles in the nose
Innate response
Airway epithelium
Mucociliary apparatus moves inhaled particles out of the airway
TLRs activate epithelium to secrete products that kill bacteria and increase inflammation
Ingestion and clearing of organisms also occur at the epithelial level
Adaptive response
1. DCs in epithelium take up airborne antigens
Dendritic cell (DC)
2. Antigen-bearing DCs migrate to draining lymph nodes and present antigens to naive T-cells
DC with antigen
Afferent lymphatics
Airborne antigens
Efferent lymphatics
3. T-cells are activated, proliferate, and return to bronchial mucosa
T-cells
4. T-cells aid in directing an inflammatory response
Innate response
Alveoli
Foreign particle
Macrophages in airspaces remove dead and dying cells from airways and alveoli
Macrophage

Under the epithelium, there is a network of dendritic cells. These large cells have projections that protrude between epithelial cells into the airway lumen and may sample foreign antigenic substances. After ingestion of foreign protein, these cells migrate to regional lymph nodes, where they present an antigenic fragment of the protein to CD4+ T cells with a T-cell receptor with a high affinity for the antigenic peptide. The subsequent T-cell reaction may lead to the clonal expansion of the cells and their differentiation into one of several subsets of CD4+ cells. These cells recirculate and may home to the site of origin of the dendritic cell, where they may now produce cytokines that play a key role in directing the type of inflammation. Whereas Th1 type cells are associated with delayed-type hypersensitivity reactions, Th2 cells may lead to typical eosinophil-rich allergic inflammation, immunoglobulin E synthesis (IgE), mucous cell differentiation, and airway hyperresponsiveness. These are all characteristic features of allergic asthma. Coating of mast cells in the airways, which are recruited after exposure to aeroallergens, with IgE renders these cells susceptible to activation by allergens. Release of histamine, growth factors, and cytokines occurs, and the synthesis de novo of leukotrienes and prostaglandins contributes to bronchoconstriction and inflammation. Bronchoconstriction is often biphasic; an early response occurs within minutes and resolves within 1 or 2 hours, and a secondary wave of airway narrowing called the *late response* occurs after several hours. This latter reaction is also T-cell dependent.

Several other T-cell subsets are of importance in controlling inflammation and host defense. Regulatory T cells may prevent, limit, or participate in terminating inflammation. Other newly described T-cell subsets such as Th17 cells are associated with inflammation that has a strong neutrophilic component, and these cells may be implicated in more severe forms of asthma. T cells bearing an alternative TCR, the $\gamma\delta$ TCR, are important in host defense against certain infectious agents, including *Mycobacterium tuberculosis* and *Pneumocystis jiroveci*. Natural killer (NK) cells and invariant NKT (*i*NKT) cells participate in immunologic responses. NK cells are required for protection against several viral infections, *Bordetella pertussis*, and *Mycobacterium tuberculosis*.

Development of the Lower Respiratory System

The development of the respiratory system in humans is an interesting demonstration of ontogeny recapitulating phylogeny. The embryology of the system goes through the fish, amphibian, reptilian, and mammalian evolutionary stages of humans' ancestry. In the change from an aqueous to an aerobic environment, many basic structures were modified but retained as parts of the respiratory system, and others became nonrespiratory structures. At the same time, entirely new respiratory structures evolved. The olfactory organ of aqueous forms was incorporated into the respiratory system of terrestrial forms, and the simple sphincter mechanism of the swim bladder of fish became the larynx of air breathers, which also took on the function of phonation. In contrast, the part of the respiratory system involved in the gas exchange vital to life has essentially not changed throughout vertebrate evolution. Exchange of oxygen and carbon dioxide between the external environment and the circulating bloodstream occurs through a wet epithelium in both gills and lungs.

The respiratory system in humans differs from the other major body systems in that it is not operational until birth. Therefore, development of the antenatal respiratory system is genetically determined independently of the functional demands of the growing embryo and fetus. The system's physiologic development is mainly one of preparation for instant action at birth, a feat unmatched by any other system. When the fetus passes from the uterine aquatic environment, the partially collapsed, fluid-filled lungs immediately function efficiently to sustain life. The chief cause of perinatal death of human infants is failure of the respiratory system to work properly. In the majority of perinatal deaths, all other body systems are functioning normally.

PRIMITIVE RESPIRATORY TUBE

During the fourth gestational week, the first indication of the future respiratory tree is a groove that runs lengthwise in the floor of the pharynx just caudal to the pharyngeal pouches. From the outside, this laryngotracheal groove appears as a ridge. The ridge grows caudally to become a tube, the lung bud, and the cranial or upper part of the tube becomes the larynx. The caudal part becomes the future trachea, which soon develops two knoblike enlargements at its distal end, the bronchial buds (Plate 1-33).

TRACHEA

As the trachea lengthens, anterior to and parallel with the esophagus, the bronchial buds are carried progressively more caudal in the body until they reach their definitive position in the thorax. During this growth period, mesenchymal cells from the splanchnic mesoderm surround the tracheal tube of entoderm and give rise to the connective tissue, smooth muscle, and cartilage of the tracheal wall. By and during the eighth gestational week, the rudiments of the 16 to 20 C-shaped tracheal cartilages appear (see Plate 1-36). These mesenchymal rudiments transform into cartilage in a

Developing Respiratory Tract and Pharynx

Respiratory tract at 4 to 5 weeks

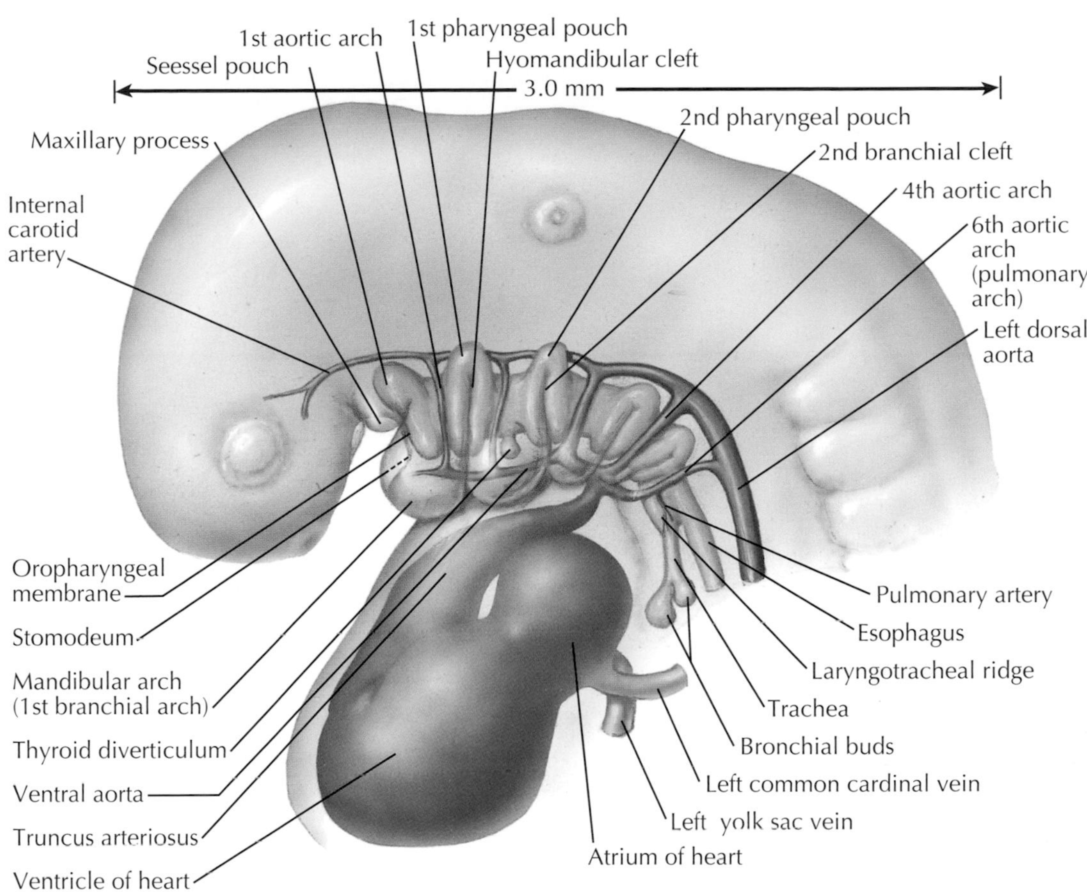

Pharynx at 4 to 5 weeks (ventral view)

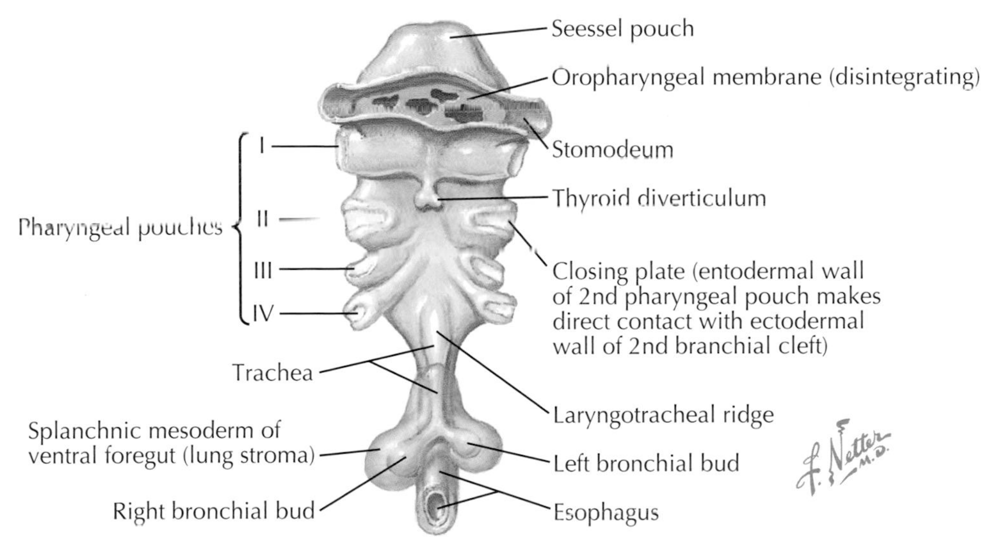

Development of the Lower Respiratory System

(Continued)

cranial to caudal direction up to the tenth week. Only the epithelial lining and glands of the trachea are derived from entoderm. The lining starts to become ciliated at 10 weeks, with the cilia beating toward the larynx. By 12 weeks, the mucosal glands begin to appear in a cranial to caudal direction. All major microscopic features are recognizable by the end of the fifth month. However, the infantile trachea differs grossly from the adult form because it is short and narrow compared with a relatively very large larynx. This size difference continues for several months after birth.

BRONCHI

The bronchial buds of the trachea become the two main bronchi. As soon as the right bronchus appears, it is a little larger than the left one and tends to be more vertically oriented (see Plates 1-33 and 1-36). These differences become more pronounced up to and after the time the bronchi mature, accounting for the fact that foreign bodies enter the right main bronchus much more often than the left.

During the fifth week, each main bronchus gives rise to two bronchial buds. These buds develop secondary branches to the future lobes: the upper, middle, and lower lobes on the right side and the upper and lower lobes on the left (Plate 1-34). By the seventh week, tertiary branches appear (see Plate 1-35), 10 in the right lung and nine in the left. These tertiary branches will supply the clinically important bronchopulmonary segments, which become separated from each other by tenuous connective tissue septa (see Plate 1-36). The tenuous connective tissue surrounding each segment delineates a separate respiratory unit of the lung, but some collateral ventilation does occur between segments. A branch of the pulmonary artery accompanies each segmental bronchus to serve as the independent blood supply to a bronchopulmonary segment. Again, some collateral circulation occurs across segments. The pulmonary veins do not accompany the segmental bronchi and arteries but run chiefly through the substance of the lung between the segments, as do the lymphatic vessels.

Respiratory System at 5 to 6 Weeks

Sagittal section

4.0 mm
Stomodeum
Oronasal membrane
Olfactory (nasal) pit
Primitive palate
Tongue (*cut surface*)
Mandibular arch (1st branchial arch)
Truncus arteriosus
Atrium of heart
Ventricle of heart
Pericardial cavity
Gallbladder
Foregut
Rathke pouch
Opening of 1st pharyngeal pouch (auditory tube)
Foramen cecum of tongue (site of origin of thyroid gland)
Openings of 2nd, 3rd, and 4th pharyngeal pouches
Epiglottis
Laryngotracheal opening
Trachea
Esophagus
Left pleuropericardial fold (future mediastinal tissue between pleural and pericardial cavities)
Left lung bulging into pleural canal, which connects pericardial and peritoneal cavities
Pleuroperitoneal fold (future posterior portion of left side of diaphragm)
Transverse septum (mesenchymal tissue; future anterior portion of diaphragm)
Peritoneal cavity
Liver developing in mesenchymal tissue, which forms transverse septum

Bronchi and lungs

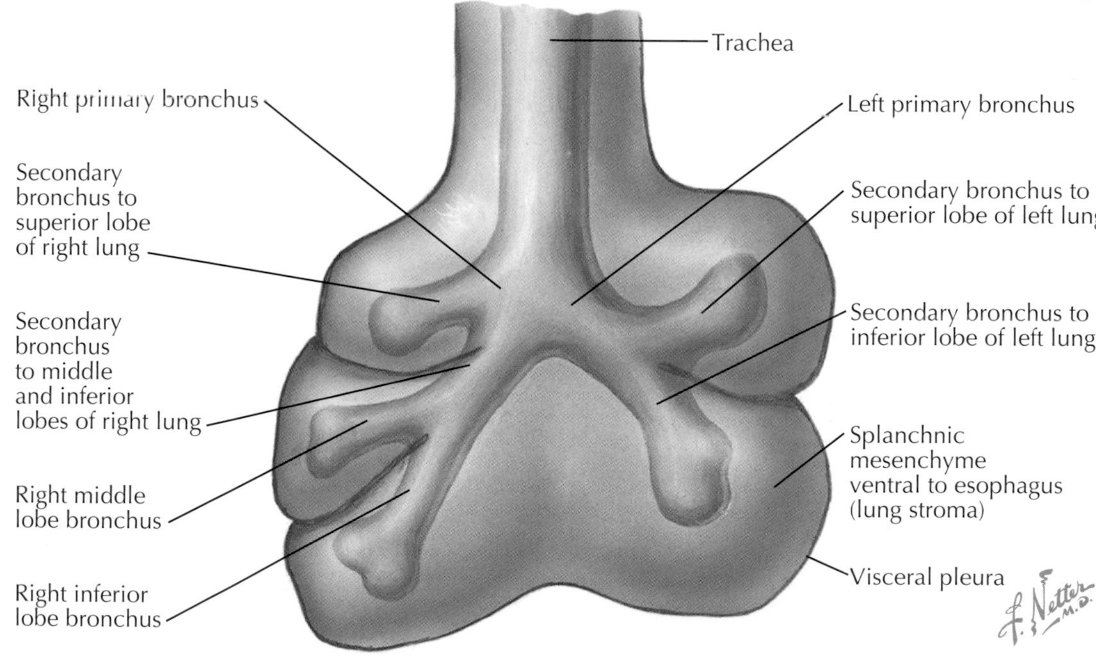

Branching of the segmental bronchi continues until, by the sixth month, about 17 orders of branching have been formed. Additional branching continues postnatally and until puberty, when about 24 orders of branches have been established. After the full complement of branches has appeared, no new ones will form to replace any lost through trauma or disease. The mature lung makes up for any branches lost by enlarging the remaining functional segments, which then do more work (compensatory hyperinflation).

CARTILAGE, SMOOTH MUSCLE, AND CONNECTIVE TISSUE

Cartilage is present in the main bronchi by the tenth week and in the segmental bronchi by the twelfth week.

DEVELOPMENT OF THE LOWER RESPIRATORY SYSTEM

(Continued)

Cilia appear in the lining of the main bronchi at 12 weeks and in the segmental bronchi at 13 weeks. At birth, the ciliated epithelium extends to the terminal bronchioles.

Mucous glands appear in the bronchi at 13 weeks and actively produce mucus by 14 weeks. At 28 weeks, seven-eighths of the potential adult number of mucous glands is present in the respiratory tubes.

By the third gestational month, smooth muscle cells differentiate to form the posterior wall of the trachea and extrapulmonary main bronchi, which permanently lack cartilage. Smooth muscle cells form bundles arranged obliquely and circularly around the bronchioles, including the terminal bronchioles, whose entire walls have no cartilage. The smooth muscle that extends to the alveolar ducts acts as a sphincter. In an allergic reaction, such as bronchial asthma, smooth muscle spasm greatly increases airway resistance. High surface tension in the terminal airways containing a large accumulation of mucus then further reduces the smaller than normal bronchiolar diameter during expiration. Because inspiration is affected by contraction of powerful muscles and is associated with widening and lengthening of the bronchial tree muscles, individuals with asthma can usually inspire adequately. But these individuals have great difficulty exhaling because expiration normally results from passive recoil of the stretched thoracic wall and lungs. To overcome the increased airway resistance of an asthmatic attack, muscles of the anterior abdominal wall must be contracted and stabilized, thus allowing the diaphragm to push with greater force and drive air out of the lungs with maximum effort.

Autonomic innervation of the lungs is not extensive; all effects of both sympathetic and parasympathetic innervation are mild. Parasympathetic stimulation can cause moderate contraction of smooth muscle of the respiratory tubes and perhaps some dilatation of the blood vessels. In contrast, sympathetic stimulation may mildly dilate the tubes and mildly constrict the vessels. Therefore, sympathomimetic drugs may be helpful in inhibiting the spasmodic contraction of the respiratory tube smooth muscle during an asthmatic attack.

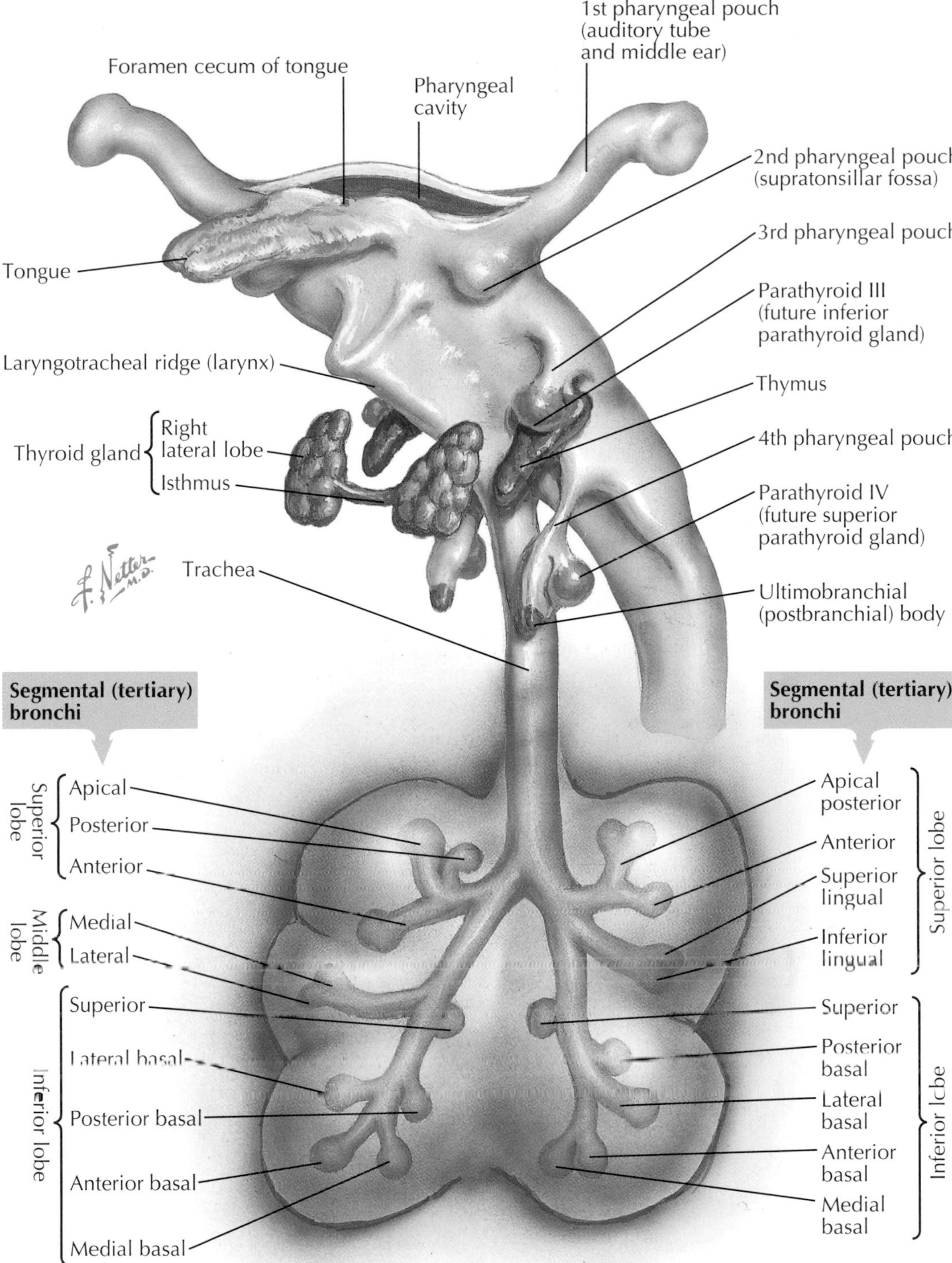

Note that although the left anterior basal and the left medial basal bronchi are shown as separate structures here at this early stage of development, they are considered together as the left anteromedial basal bronchus (LB8) at full development.

PLEURAL CAVITIES

The pericardial, pleural, and peritoneal cavities develop as subdivisions of two primitive coelomic cavities that extend along the length of the embryo. Normally, each is only a potential space with serous lining that produces a slimy secretion. This reduces friction as the ordinarily apposed surfaces rub against each other. After trauma or other forms of pathology, the cavities may become actual spaces containing proteinaceous exudate, air, or blood.

During the second week of life, the two coelomic cavities in the region of the developing heart fuse into a single pericardial coelom. While the pericardial cavity is becoming established, it is in open communication caudally on each side with the still paired primitive coeloms in the embryo's future abdominal region. Partitioning of the pericardial coelom from these primitive

Development of the Lower Respiratory System
(Continued)

coeloms starts by the establishment of a shelf of mesenchyme, the transverse septum, into which the liver becomes incorporated as it is developing (see Plate 1-34). This transverse septum grows in from the anterior body wall toward the dorsal or posterior body wall but never reaches it and finally becomes part of the diaphragm. Therefore, the two channels of communication between the pericardial coelom and the two primitive coelomic cavities persist to become the pleural canals.

Pleural Canals

In the fish stage of vertebrate evolution, the transverse septum completely separates the pericardial and peritoneal cavities. Whereas in lungfish the air bladder projects directly into a common pleuroperitoneal space, in amphibians and reptiles the lungs are found in a similar space caudal to the pericardial cavity. In humans, the amphibian and reptilian evolutionary stage of lung development occurs when the growing lungs project into the pleural canals. Each pleural cavity then becomes isolated by the growth of the pleuropericardial and pleuroperitoneal folds. These in turn become associated with the transverse septum (see below).

Pleuropericardial and Pleuroperitoneal Folds

The vertically oriented pleuropericardial folds arise on each side from the body walls where the common cardinal veins swing around to enter the sinus venosus, which subsequently becomes the right atrium. These body-wall folds bulge into the pleural canals between the lungs and the heart (see Plates 1-34 and 1-38). When the free borders of the pleuropericardial folds fuse with midline mesenchymal tissue at the base of the heart, they completely separate what is now the pericardial cavity from the pleuroperitoneal coelom (see Plate 1-38). At this time, the latter space contains the lungs as well as the abdominal and pelvic viscera.

The pleuroperitoneal folds are actually two horizontally oriented ridges of the dorsolateral body wall where the common cardinal veins are located (see Plate 1-34). Each fold grows anteriorly and medially to fuse with the transverse septum and mesenchymal tissue surrounding the aorta, esophagus, and inferior vena cava.

Larynx, Tracheobronchial Tree, and Lungs at 7 to 10 Weeks

Tertiary branches of bronchi to bronchopulmonary segments

Right lung		Left lung		
Upper lobe	Apical (Ap), posterior (P), anterior (A)	Upper lobe	Superior division	Apical-posterior (Ap-p), Anterior (A)
Middle lobe	Medial (M), lateral (L)		Lingular division	Superior (S), inferior (I)
Lower lobe	Superior (S), anterior basal (A-b), posterior basal (P-b), medial basal (M-b), lateral basal (L-b)	Lower lobe		Superior (S), anterior basal (A-b), medial basal (M-b), posterior basal (P-b), lateral basal (L-b)

The two pleural canals are then walled off from the newly formed peritoneal cavity, and the formation of the pleural cavities and diaphragm is completed (see Plates 1-37 and 1-39).

DIAPHRAGM

A diaphragm is lacking in fish, amphibians, reptiles, and birds. In mammals, it is the principal respiratory muscle. Although there are numerous accessory respiratory muscles, they cannot support life to a normal degree without a functioning diaphragm. Reptiles have a dual muscular respiratory mechanism: the action of the trunk muscles creates negative pressure, and the floor of the mouth pushes air into the lungs under positive pressure. The reptilian action of the muscles of the floor of the mouth is also the chief respiratory muscular mechanism in amphibians (“frog breathing”).

Sagittal Section at 6 to 7 Weeks

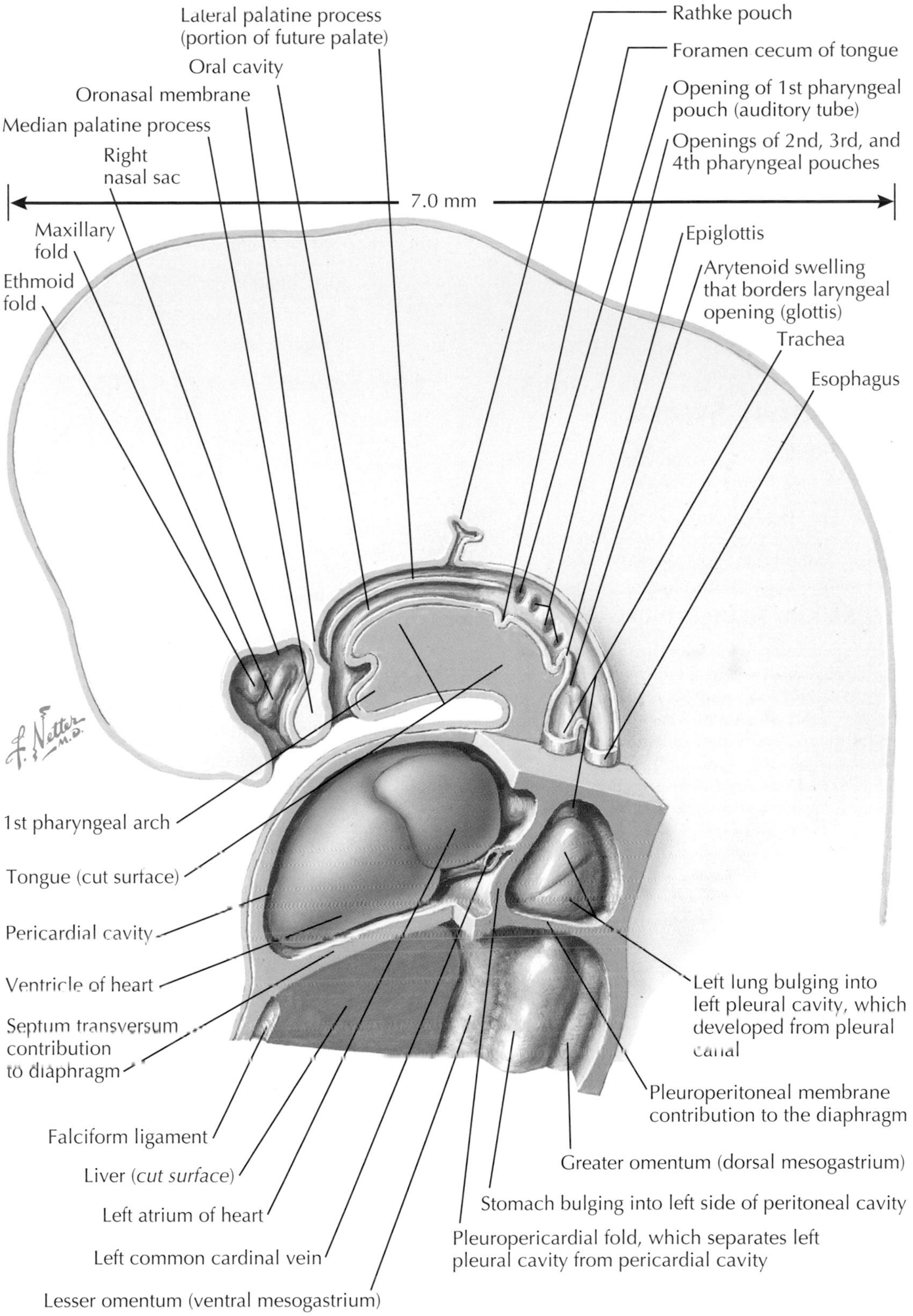

Development of the Lower Respiratory System
(Continued)

In birds, which like mammals evolved from reptiles, respiration is accomplished chiefly by the intercostal trunk muscles that move the ribs, to which the lungs are attached.

In the evolutionary transition from gill breathing to lung breathing, original muscles from the mandibular arch gave rise to the musculature of the floor of the mouth, especially the mylohyoid muscle. In amphibians and reptiles, air brought in through the nares is forced into the lungs by the musculatory action of the floor of the mouth. In mammals, a new respiratory muscle—the diaphragm—evolved from structures lacking muscle in certain reptiles, specifically, the transverse septum and two unfused coelomic folds that are the pleuroperitoneal folds in mammalian development.

Diaphragmatic musculature in mammals develops from a common mass of mesoderm at the posterior region of the branchial arches from which the tongue and infrahyoid muscles are also derived (see Plate 1-39). The transverse septum, the largest single contribution to the diaphragm, develops in the neck or cervical region of the embryo (see Plates 1-34 and 1-39). The diaphragmatic striated musculature migrates to the transverse septum along with branches of the third, fourth, and fifth cervical spinal nerves, which become its exclusive motor nerve through the phrenic nerve. By differential growth, especially an increase in size of the thoracic region, there is a so-called migration and descent of the diaphragm to a much more caudal position. At the end of the eighth gestational week, the diaphragm is attached to the dorsal body wall at the level of the first lumbar segment. The phrenic nerves, which are located in the body wall where the pleuropericardial folds develop, lengthen as the diaphragm descends. They are, therefore, relocated to a position between the pericardium and the pleurae as the pleural cavities increase in size (see Plate 1-38).

After the transverse septum, the two pleuroperitoneal folds and the numerous other minor folds unite to complete the diaphragm at or during the seventh gestational week, the diaphragmatic musculature becomes peripherally positioned (see Plate 1-39), and its domelike central area remains tendinous. As soon as the diaphragm is completely developed, it begins to contract at irregular intervals. Near term, these contractions, which are essentially hiccups, become more vigorous and more frequent. They exercise the muscles for the time when air breathing begins at birth.

During inhalation, the diaphragm flattens as it contracts. This action reduces the intrathoracic pressure by enlarging the thoracic cavity and with it the intrapulmonary space. The vocal folds are separated, and thus air rushes into the lungs at atmospheric pressure. Normal inspiration is caused chiefly by the contraction of the diaphragm. Other powerful striated muscles that assist the diaphragm are in the neck and chest region and are attached to the skull, clavicle, ribs, vertebral column, and upper limbs. Therefore, whereas inspiration is effected by the contraction of powerful muscles, expiration is largely a passive action caused by recoil of the stretched tissues of the thoracic wall and lungs.

The diaphragm is subject to developmental defects that permit herniation of abdominal viscera into the

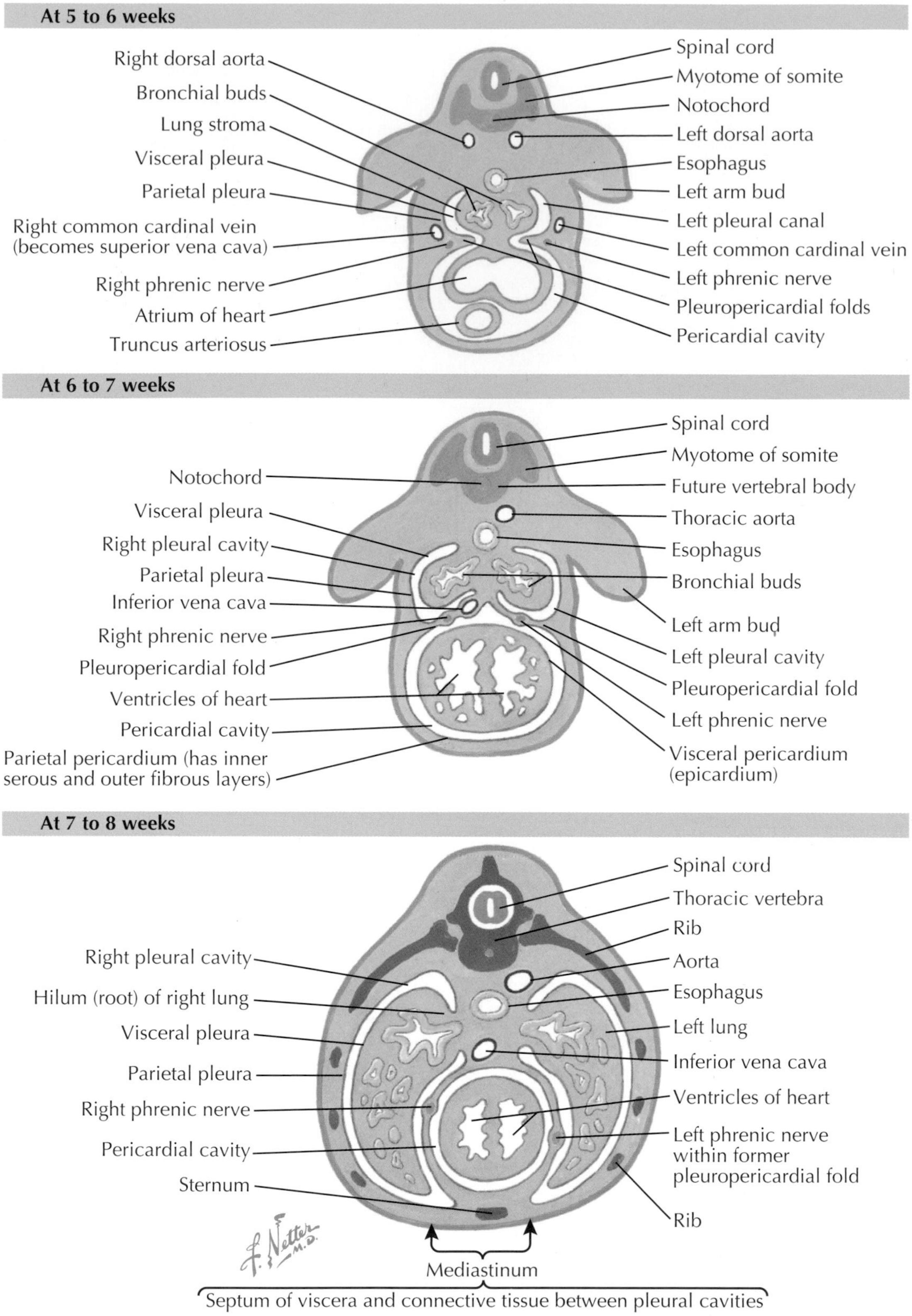

Development of the Lower Respiratory System

(Continued)

thorax. The most common diaphragmatic congenital hernia is related to defective development of the left pleuroperitoneal fold (see Plate 1-39).

PLEURA AND MEDIASTINUM

The lungs develop much later than the heart, as was the case throughout their evolutionary history. The small lungs, posterior to a relatively very large heart, grow in an anterior direction on each side of it (Plate 1-38). The pleural cavities open in advance of the growing lungs so they are already prepared to receive them. By the eighth gestational week, the lungs are larger than the heart and nearly surround it. The pleural cavities now occupy the two sides of the thoracic cavity. All other thoracic viscera, including the heart, great vessels, esophagus, and associated connective tissue, are now between the two pleural cavities, from the vertebral column to the sternum. This broad medial septum of viscera and connective tissue is known as the mediastinum.

As the lungs protrude into the pleural canals (see Plate 1-34), they are invested by the lining mesothelium of these spaces, which becomes the visceral pleura (Plate 1-38). Before the pleuropericardial folds wall off the pleural canals from the pericardial coelom, the mesothelium lining the walls of these thoracic subdivisions is continuous (see Plates 1-34 and 1-38). As soon as the pleural canals become the pleural cavities, the lining of the walls of the canals becomes the parietal pleura. The region where the visceral pleura reflects off the lungs and becomes continuous with the parietal pleura shifts medially and becomes smaller to envelop the structures that constitute the root of the lung.

Throughout human development, the right lung is larger than the left, as is the case with the right and left pleural cavities. This size differential is related to the shift of the heart to the left side of the thorax. In adult mammals and reptiles, the right lung is also larger than the left lung. In adult humans, the space occupied by the heart produces the cardiac notch of the left lung.

TERMINAL RESPIRATORY TUBES

The amphibian stage of development of portions of the respiratory tubes occurs at 4 to 5 weeks when the bronchial buds are present (see Plate 1-33). Amphibian lungs are essentially two air sacs, each with a large single lumen. In reptilians, segmental bronchi are present at 7 to 8 weeks (see Plate 1-36). The reptilian lung has branching respiratory tubes ending in terminal sacs that are similar to mammalian primitive alveoli. They add greatly to the surface area where gas exchange occurs; in contrast, the amphibian lung has only rudimentary alveoli.

Alveolar development does not begin in human fetuses until airway development is complete at 16 weeks. Between the fourth and sixth months of gestation, the last airway is transformed to a terminal or respiratory bronchiole. Generally, each respiratory bronchiole divides into three to six alveolar ducts (see Plate 1-40). Each alveolar duct first ends in a bulging terminal sac lined by cuboidal or columnar epithelium that ultimately evolves into definitive alveoli. Capillaries multiply so that the region of terminal airspaces becomes highly vascularized.

Development of the Lower Respiratory System
(Continued)

During the sixth gestational month, the epithelium of the terminal sacs thins where it is in contact with a capillary (see Plate 1-40). The epithelial cells become so thin when the alveoli fill with air that, before the advent of electron microscopy, there seemed to be breaks in the lining where only capillary endothelium separated the blood from the alveolar air (see Plate 1-41). The capillaries, covered by the thin epithelial cells, line the alveolar spaces (see Plate 1-41). These very thin cells, constituting the major part of the alveolar surface, are known as type I pneumocytes. Other cells, scattered along the lining of the alveoli, are cuboidal, have microvilli on their luminal surfaces, and contain osmiophilic inclusions of surfactant or its precursors. These cells are known as type II pneumocytes, and they also appear during the sixth gestational month.

The original mesenchyme that gives rise to the pulmonary capillaries and lymphatics is also the source of the fibrocytes that produce an abundance of elastic fibers in the lungs (see Plate 1-40). After the lungs become inflated with air, the elastic fibers are constantly stretched and, by attempting to contract, contribute to the normal recoil or collapsing tendency of the lungs. On the other hand, the natural tendency of the chest wall is to expand. The resulting negative pressure in the pleural cavities helps to keep the lungs expanded. The visceral pleurae continually absorb fluid so that only a small amount of it remains in the potential intrapleural space at all times. Because the elastic fibers of the lungs are stretched even more during inspiration, they are the chief structures responsible for returning the enlarged alveoli and bronchioles to their more contracted resting dimensions during normal passive expiration.

Alveolar-Capillary (Respiratory) Membrane

By the 28th week, the lung has lost its glandular appearance. The respiratory airways end in a cluster of large thin-walled sacs separated from one another by a matrix of loose connective tissue. At this stage, respiration can be supported because gas exchange can occur at the terminal sacs, and surfactant is present to maintain alveolar stability. The primitive alveoli do not become definitive as true alveoli until after birth, at which time they are only shallow bulges of the walls of the terminal sacs and respiratory bronchioles. Even so, the thickness of the blood-air barrier, which is also known as the *respiratory* or *alveolar-capillary membrane*, is about 0.4 μm. This is within the range found in adults—that is, 2.5 μm to smaller than 0.1 μm (1 μm is 0.001 mm). The lungs of a newborn infant contain 24 million primitive alveoli (see Plate 1-41).

During the first 3 years of life, the increase in lung size is caused by alveolar multiplication rather than by greater alveolar size. From the third to the eighth year, the alveoli increase in size as well as in number until there are 300 million in the two lungs. After the eighth year, alveoli become larger only until the chest wall stops growing. At age 8 years, the diameter of the mature alveolus is 100 to 300 μm. Physical diffusion of oxygen from the alveolus into the red blood cell and of carbon dioxide in the opposite direction occurs through the respiratory membrane, which consists of an alveolar type I pneumocyte and a capillary endothelial cell and

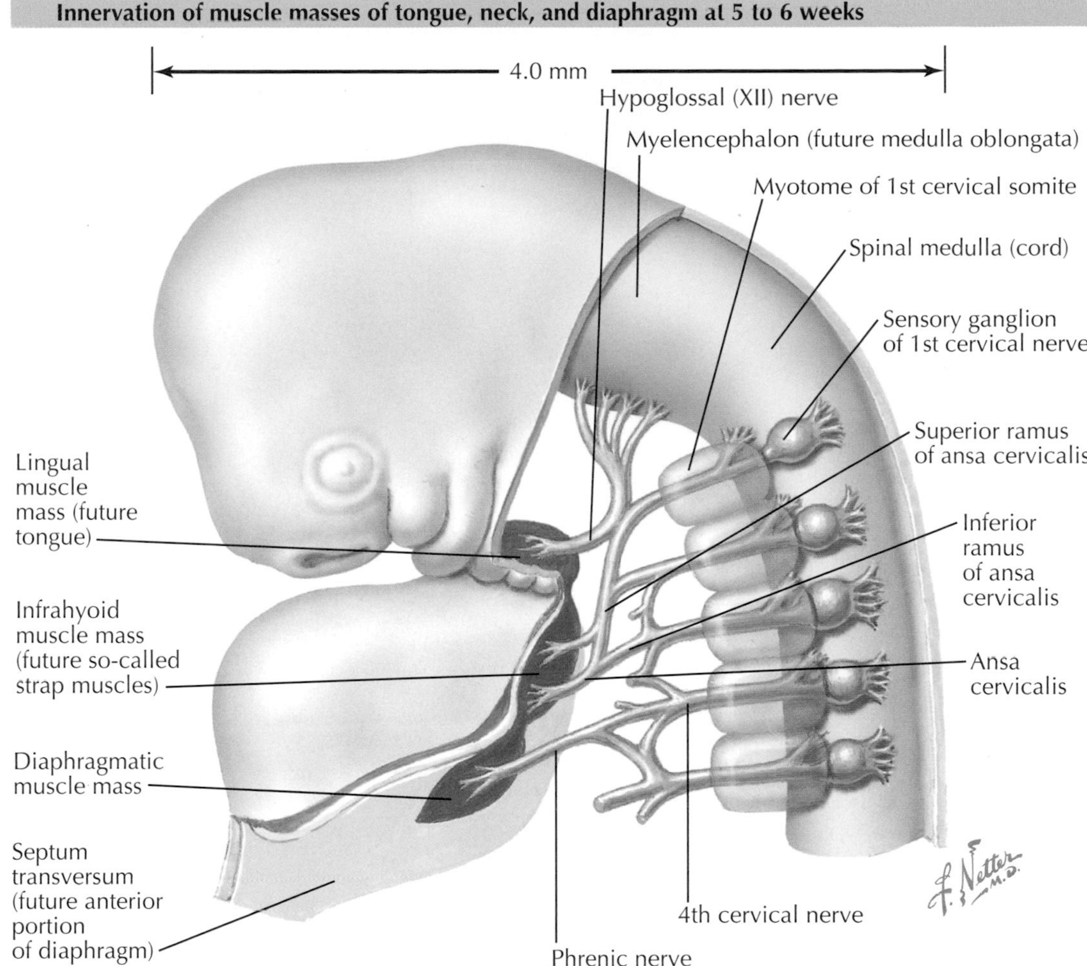

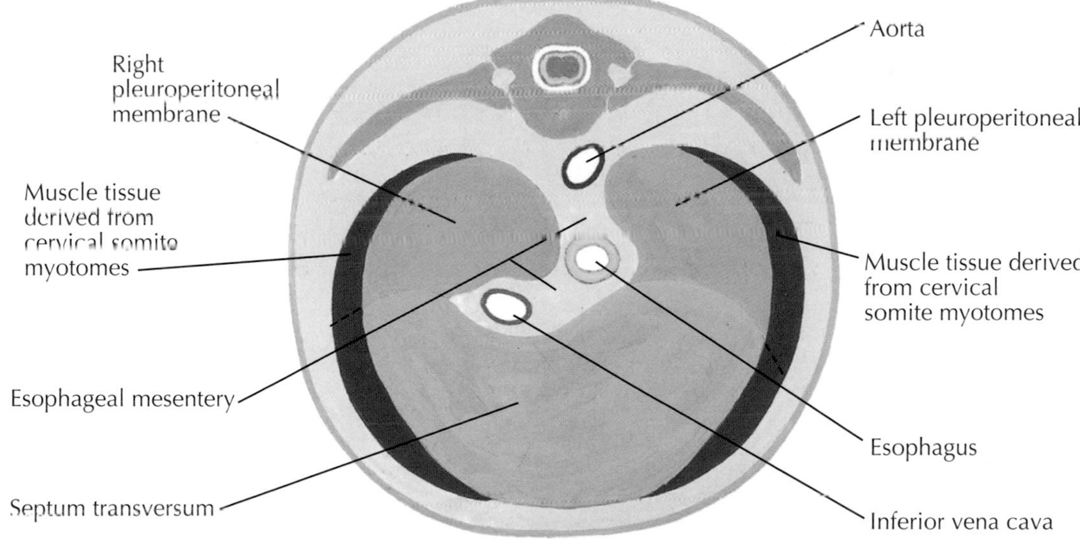

Development of the Lower Respiratory System
(Continued)

their respective basement membranes. Consequently, oxygen and carbon dioxide do not have to pass across a great distance between the erythrocyte and the alveolus, and gas diffusion can be accomplished very rapidly. The total surface area of the respiratory membrane of both lungs is about 70 m^2, which is vast when compared with the 1.7 m^2 of total body surface of an adult. The average diameter of a pulmonary capillary is only about 7 μm (see Plate 1-41). The extensive alveolar and associated capillary endothelial surface is also responsible for a large water vapor loss during respiration; adult lungs eliminate about 800 mL of water a day in expired air.

SURFACTANT

No matter how complete the development of the respiratory system at birth, one factor that determines whether it will support life is the presence of a substance known as pulmonary surfactant. Therefore, because of its functional implications, the most important morphologic event is the appearance at about the twenty-third week of lamellar inclusion bodies in the type II pneumocytes of the lining of the terminal sacs. These bodies are precursors of surfactant, a lipoprotein mixture rich in phospholipids, especially dipalmitoyl lecithin. Surfactant has a "detergent" property of lowering surface tension in the fluid layer that lines the primitive alveoli after air enters the lungs, and it acts as an antiatelectasis factor to maintain patency of terminal airspaces (see Plate 1-41).

Surface tension of fluid is measured in dynes per centimeter. A drop of water on a sheet of glass tends to round up into a compact mass because of its surface tension of about 72 dynes/cm at the air-water interface. If household detergent is added to the drop of water, its surface tension is reduces to about 20 dynes/cm, and it spreads into a very thin film on the glass (see Plate 1-42). In a similar manner, surfactant reduces surface tension of the fluid layer lining the alveolus to about 5 dynes/cm. Its ability to form a monomolecular layer at the interface between air and the alveolar lining fluid (see Plate 1-41) allows some air to be retained within the alveolus at all times.

Although surfactant is present in the lungs as early as the twenty-third gestational week, the lungs at this stage are unable to retain air after inflation, and they collapse completely before 28 to 32 weeks. The quantity of surfactant within the lungs increases markedly toward term; this is one of the most important reasons why older fetuses have a better chance of survival as air breathers. Surfactant must be produced continually because it has a half-life of 14 to 24 hours. A deficiency of surfactant is associated with the infant respiratory distress syndrome (RDS), also known as hyaline membrane disease (see Plates 4-144 and 4-145). This is caused by the relative instability of the immature lung because of failure to produce surfactant in amounts sufficient for neonatal respiration. Death from the disease occurs within a few hours to a few days after birth. The alveoli of the dead infants are filled with a proteinaceous fluid that resembles a glassy or hyaline membrane.

The high incidence of RDS in premature infants is caused by their low initial concentrations of surfactant.

Terminal Air Tube

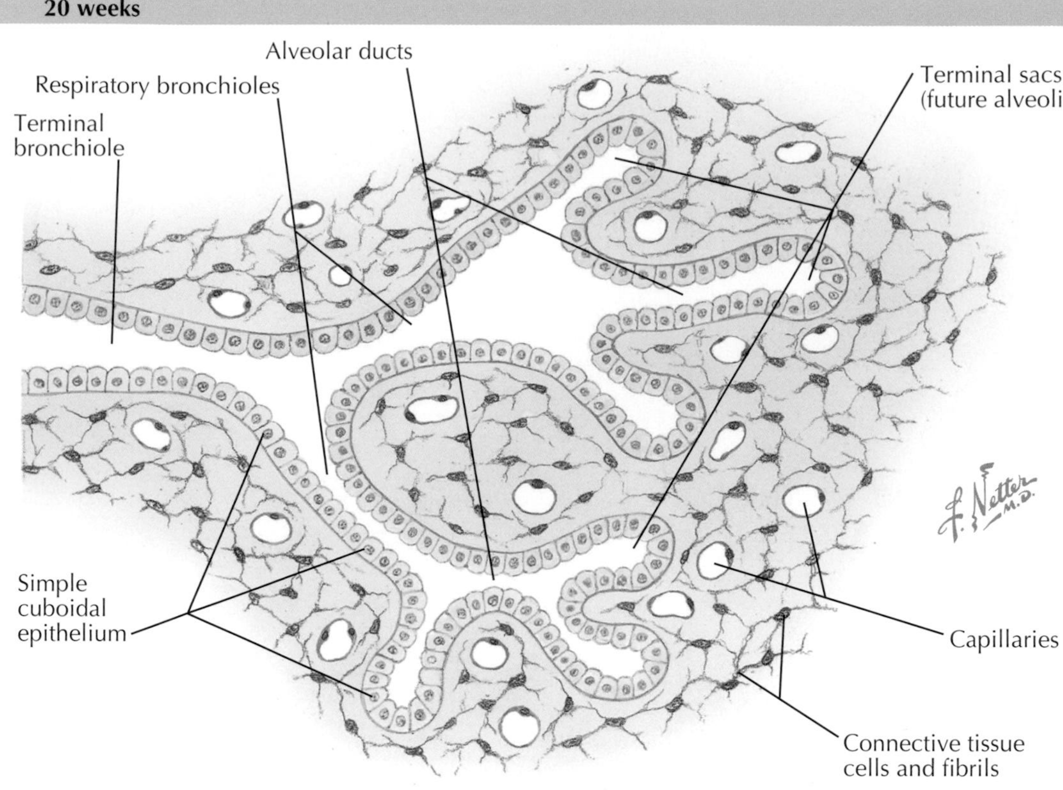

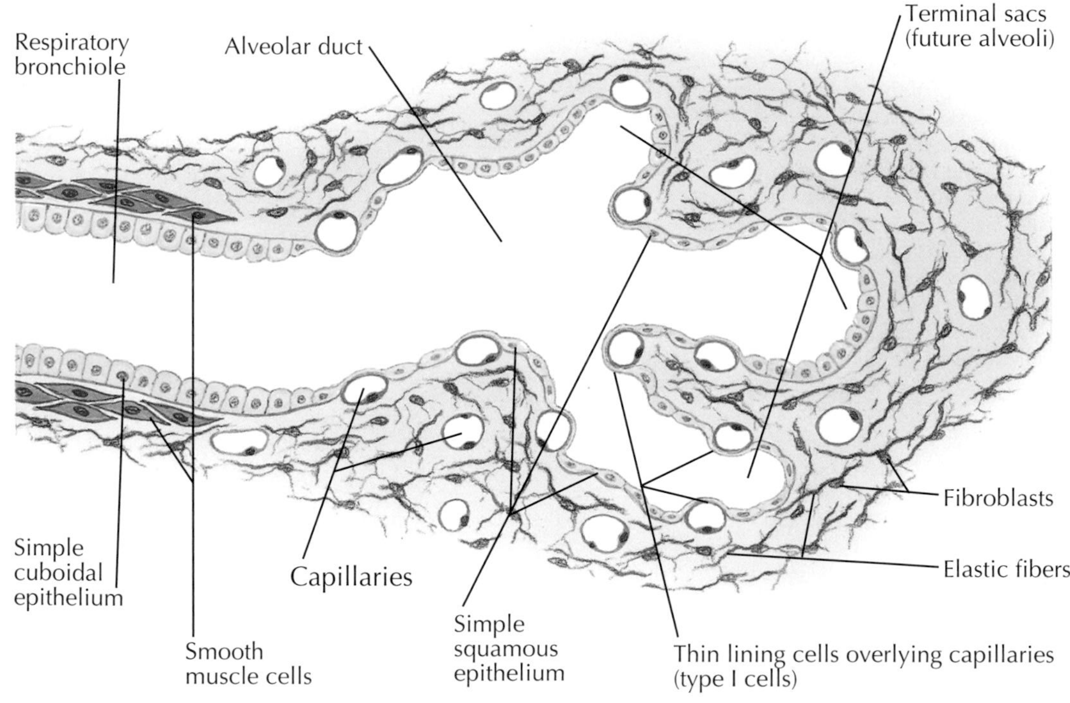

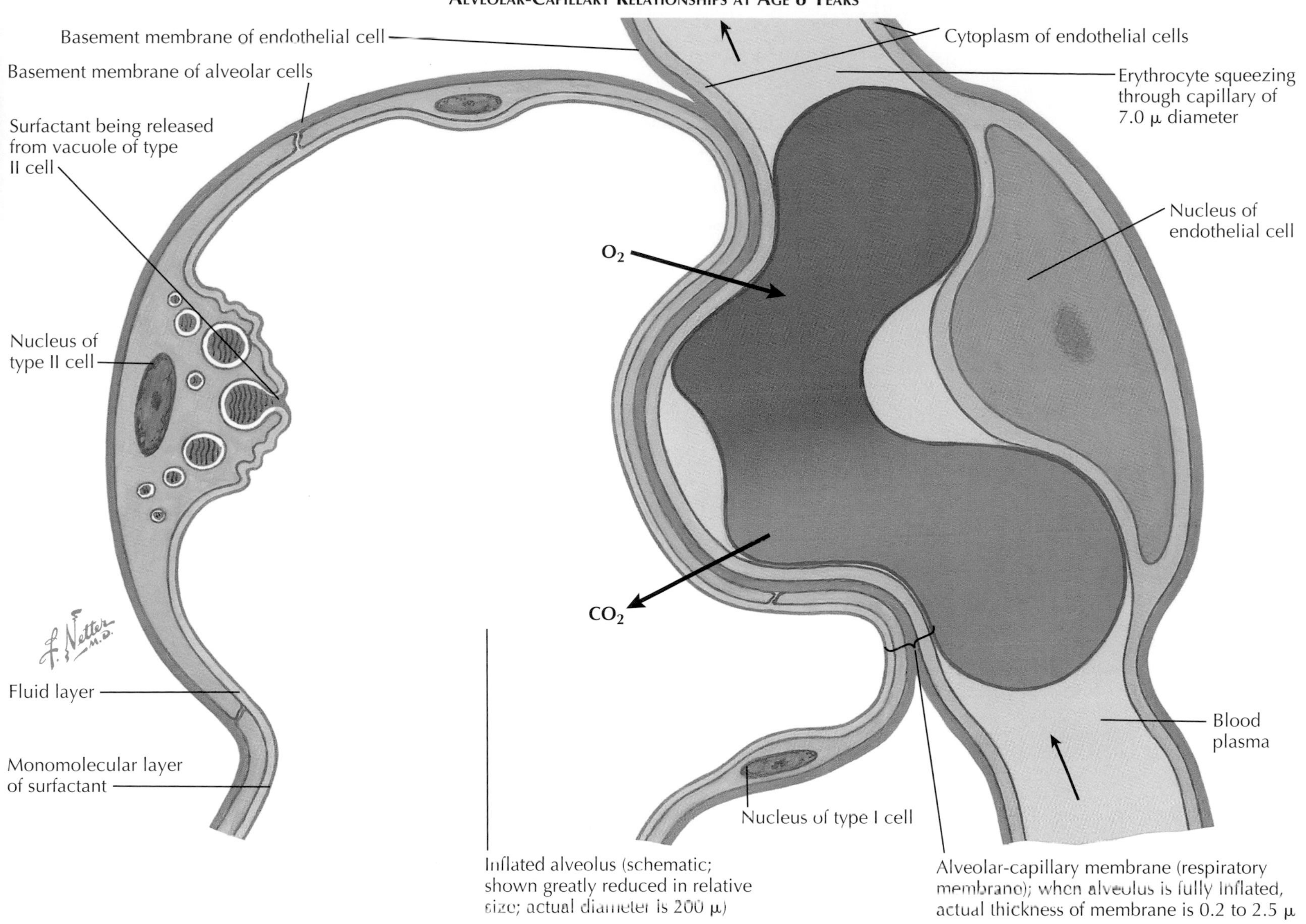

Development of the Lower Respiratory System

(Continued)

Prematurity, cesarean section, and perinatal asphyxia are recognized predisposing factors. Surface tension of lung extracts of newborn infants with birth weights of 1200 g or more is only about 5 dynes/cm. In extracts from infants with birth weights less than 1200 g who have hyaline membrane disease, it may be four times that value.

Before birth, the respiratory tubes are filled with fluid, some of it amniotic fluid brought in by "practice" inspiratory movements. However, most of the fluid is produced by the lining of the respiratory tubes (as much as 120 mL/h near term). This pulmonary fluid passes through the oral and nasal cavities to mix with the amniotic fluid. Amniotic fluid contains phospholipids, and amniocentesis before the thirty-fifth week usually shows that the ratio of lecithin to sphingomyelin is less than or equal to 1 because the latter remains constant as gestation advances. Such a ratio indicates that the fetus is immature in regard to surfactant production. A ratio of more than 2:1 indicates that the fetal lungs are sufficiently mature to prevent the development of RDS.

The role of thyroxine and adrenal corticosteroids in stimulating lung maturation and surfactant production has not yet been settled and is still under investigation. Surfactant is present in the lungs of all vertebrate air breathers. The amount of surfactant correlates well with alveolar surface area and with the amount of certain saturated phospholipids in the lung tissue in a stepwise fashion up the phylogenetic scale from amphibians through reptiles to mammals.

FIRST BREATH

Before the first breath, the lungs are filled with fluid. Therefore, the lungs of a stillborn infant who has not taken a breath of air differ from those of an infant who has. The lungs of a stillborn infant are firm; do not crepitate when handled; and because they contain no air, sink in water. Some of the fluid normally within the lungs at birth is extruded from the mouth; most of it is removed through the lymphatic vessels in the region of the primitive alveoli. The pleural lymphatic vessels are relatively larger and more numerous in fetuses and newborn infants than in adults, and lymph flow is high during the first few hours after birth. The flow is less 2 days later but is still higher than in adults.

A certain amount of fluid must of necessity always remain in the alveoli, but in the partially atelectatic (collapsed) primitive alveoli, the surface tension of the viscid fluid tends to hold the walls of the alveoli together. Therefore, the first breath of some 30 to 40 mL in volume requires a tremendous physical effort, and a negative intrathoracic pressure—as much as 40 to 100 cm of water—is needed for expansion. This is about 14 times the pressure required to produce breaths of a similar volume subsequently (see Plate 1-42).

Contraction of the diaphragm is mainly responsible for the first breath that is often associated with the first good cry, but the accessory muscles of respiration offer little assistance at this time. Expansion of the chest wall is slight in the days just after birth. In fact, the thoracic skeleton contains so much flexible cartilage that the chest wall tends to collapse with each inspiration, especially in premature infants.

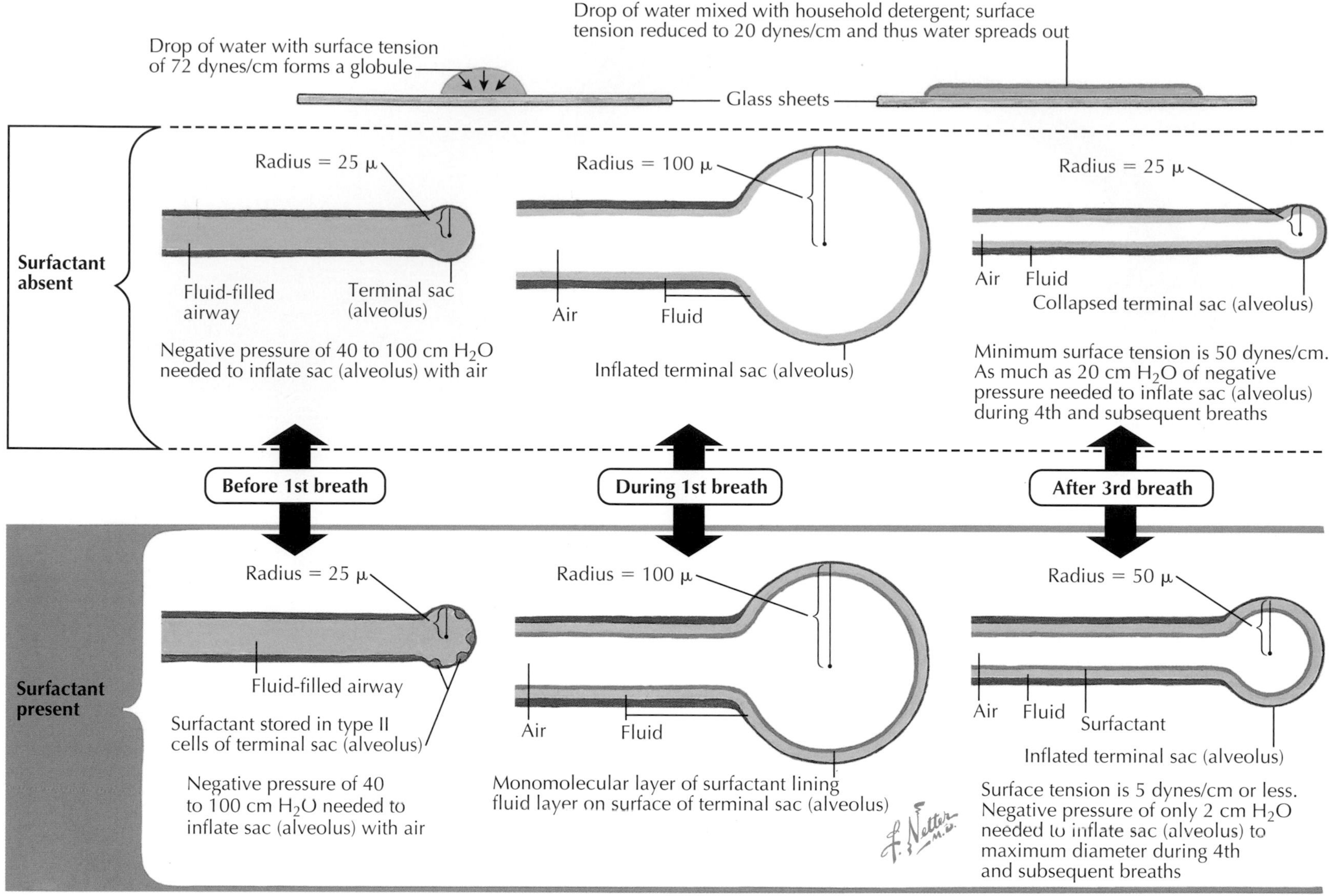

SURFACTANT EFFECTS
Drop of water with surface tension of 72 dynes/cm forms a globule
Drop of water mixed with household detergent; surface tension reduced to 20 dynes/cm and thus water spreads out
Glass sheets
Surfactant absent
Radius = 25 μ
Fluid-filled airway
Terminal sac (alveolus)
Negative pressure of 40 to 100 cm H2O needed to inflate sac (alveolus) with air
Radius = 100 μ
Air
Fluid
Inflated terminal sac (alveolus)
Radius = 25 μ
Air
Fluid
Collapsed terminal sac (alveolus)
Minimum surface tension is 50 dynes/cm. As much as 20 cm H2O of negative pressure needed to inflate sac (alveolus) during 4th and subsequent breaths
Before 1st breath
During 1st breath
After 3rd breath
Surfactant present
Radius = 25 μ
Fluid-filled airway
Surfactant stored in type II cells of terminal sac (alveolus)
Negative pressure of 40 to 100 cm H2O needed to inflate sac (alveolus) with air
Radius = 100 μ
Air
Fluid
Monomolecular layer of surfactant lining fluid layer on surface of terminal sac (alveolus)
Radius = 50 μ
Air
Fluid
Surfactant
Inflated terminal sac (alveolus)
Surface tension is 5 dynes/cm or less. Negative pressure of only 2 cm H2O needed to inflate sac (alveolus) to maximum diameter during 4th and subsequent breaths
F. Netter M.D.

DEVELOPMENT OF THE LOWER RESPIRATORY SYSTEM

(Continued)

When air expands the primitive alveolus during the first breath, surfactant (or its precursors stored in type II pneumocytes) is rapidly discharged into the alveolar space (Plate 1-42). This monomolecular layer prevents the development of an air-water interface that otherwise would have seven to 14 times as much surface tension as does the air-surfactant interface.

According to the Laplace equation, the pressure required to prevent collapse of a bubble caused by surface tension is inversely proportional to the bubble's radius. Because the radii of primitive alveoli are very small, the collapsing forces are correspondingly high. Therefore, as the lungs deflate, the alveolar radii are further reduced, and the collapsing forces are proportionately increased. Alveoli lacking surfactant thus cannot retain air after expiration, and they collapse (Plate 1-42); infants in whom hyaline membrane disease develops have so little air in their nonexpanded alveoli that at autopsy, the lungs immediately sink when placed in water. Surfactant has the fortunate property of increasing its activity as its surface area is reduced. Therefore, on expiration, the surfactant effectively lowers the alveolar surface tension so that air can be retained.

Without sufficient surfactant, all breaths after the first would require great physical effort. A negative pressure as great as 20 cm of water is required to reinflate a collapsed primitive alveolus with a radius of 25 μm and a minimal surface tension of 50 dynes/cm. By contrast, with surfactant present, the alveolus of a deflated lung would have a radius of 50 μm, and its minimal surface tension would be only 5 dynes/cm or less. Thus, a negative pressure of only 2 cm of water is all that would be needed to maximally reinflate it under these conditions (Plate 1-42). The physical effort a premature infant lacking surfactant requires to breathe is so great that exhaustion of the infant will soon result unless mechanical support is provided.

Although the second breath is much easier for a normal full-term infant, breathing is usually not completely normal until about 40 minutes after birth. The entire lung does not become fully inflated as soon as respiration begins, and for the first week to 10 days after birth, small parts of the lungs may still remain underinflated.

The onset of breathing at birth is accompanied by important and immediate circulatory system readjustments that allow adequate blood flow through the lungs. During fetal life, only about 12% of the cardiac output goes to the lungs because most of the flow from the right ventricle is shunted away from the pulmonary artery to the aorta through the large ductus arteriosus. The fluid-filled atelectatic lungs create a high resistance in the pulmonary circulation by compressing the blood vessels. Expansion of the lungs induces vasodilation of the pulmonary vessels and results in a sudden increase in blood flow—up to 200% or more. This increased pulmonary blood flow, coupled with the cutting off of the large placental circulation when the umbilical cord is tied, actually means that a smaller quantity of blood is propelled a shorter distance within the infant. Therefore, the most crucial event at birth is the expansion of the lungs with the first breath of air, rather than the alterations occurring in the vascular system. After respiration has been established, the normal vascular system is well prepared to meet the functional demands imposed on it after birth.

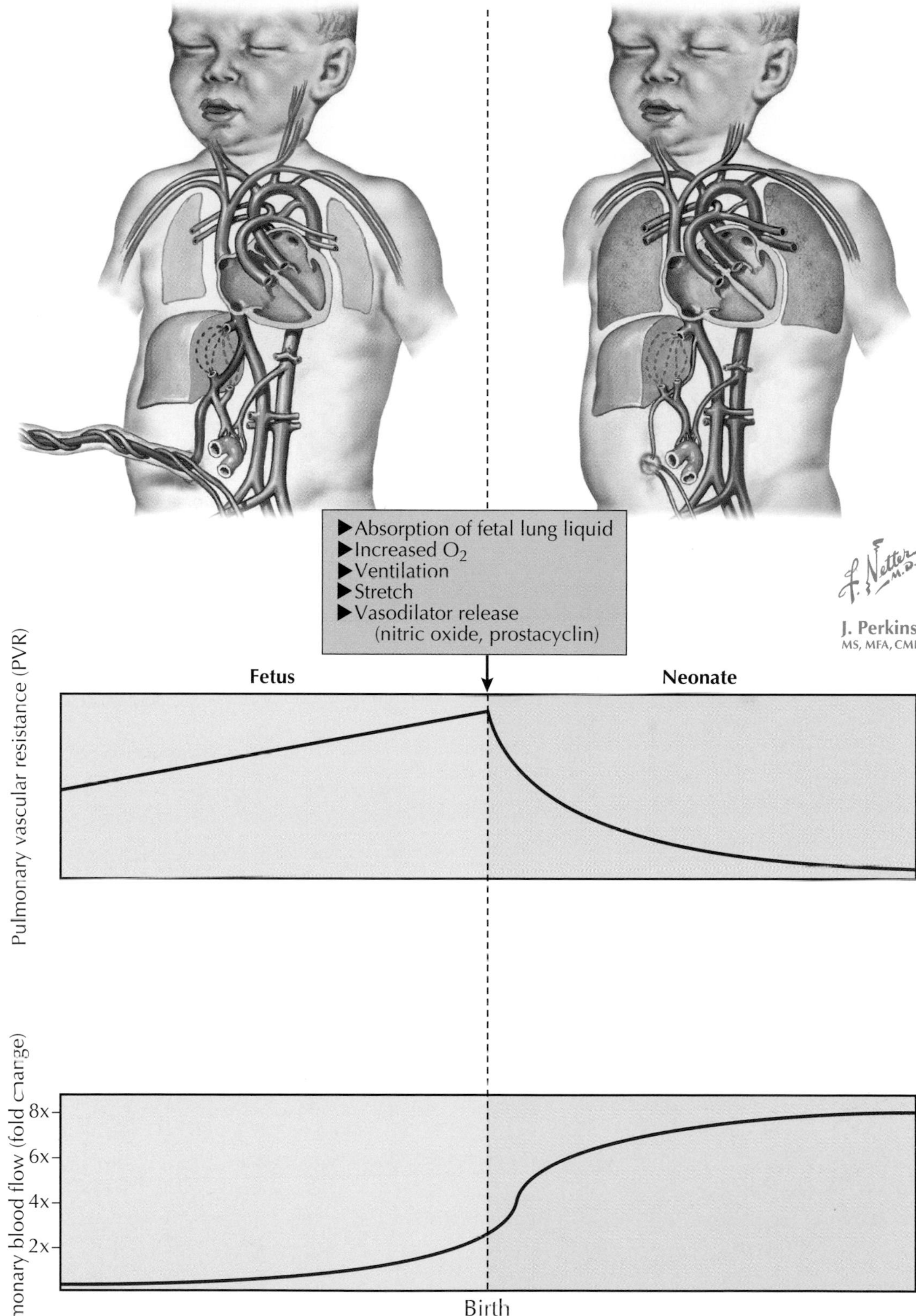

PHYSIOLOGY OF THE PERINATAL PULMONARY CIRCULATION

Pulmonary vascular resistance (PVR) is high throughout fetal life, especially compared with the low resistance of the systemic circulation. As a result, the fetal lung receives less than 3% to 8% of combined ventricular output, with most of the right ventricular output crossing the ductus arteriosus to the aorta. In addition to structural maturation and growth of the developing lung circulation, the vessel wall also undergoes functional maturation, leading to enhanced vasoreactivity during fetal life. Mechanisms that contribute to high basal PVR in fetuses include low oxygen tension, relatively low basal production of vasodilator products (e.g., prostacyclin [PgI_2] and nitrous oxide [NO]), increased production of vasoconstrictors (including endothelin-1), and altered smooth muscle cell reactivity (e.g., enhanced myogenic tone). During development, the fetal pulmonary circulation is characterized by a progressive increase in responsiveness to vasoactive stimuli, including changes in oxygen tension.

Postnatal survival depends on the successful transition of the fetal pulmonary circulation from its high resistance state in utero to a low-resistance, high-flow vascular bed within minutes after delivery. This decrease in PVR allows for the eightfold increase in pulmonary blood flow that is necessary for the lungs to serve their postnatal function for gas exchange (see Plate 1-43). Mechanisms that contribute to the normal decrease in PVR at birth include vasodilation caused by birth-related stimuli, such as increased oxygen tension, ventilation, and shear stress, and altered production of several vasoactive products, especially the enhanced release of NO and prostacyclin. In addition, high pulmonary blood flow abruptly causes a structural reorganization of the vascular wall that includes flattening of the endothelium and thinning of smooth muscle cells and matrix. Thus, the ability to accommodate this marked increase in blood flow requires rapid functional and structural adaptations to ensure the normal postnatal decrease in PVR.

Some infants fail to achieve or sustain the normal decrease in PVR at birth, leading to severe respiratory distress and hypoxemia, which is referred to as *persistent pulmonary hypertension of the newborn* (PPHN). PPHN is a major clinical problem, contributing significantly to high morbidity and mortality in both full-term and premature neonates.

SECTION 2

PHYSIOLOGY

Pulmonary Mechanics and Gas Exchange

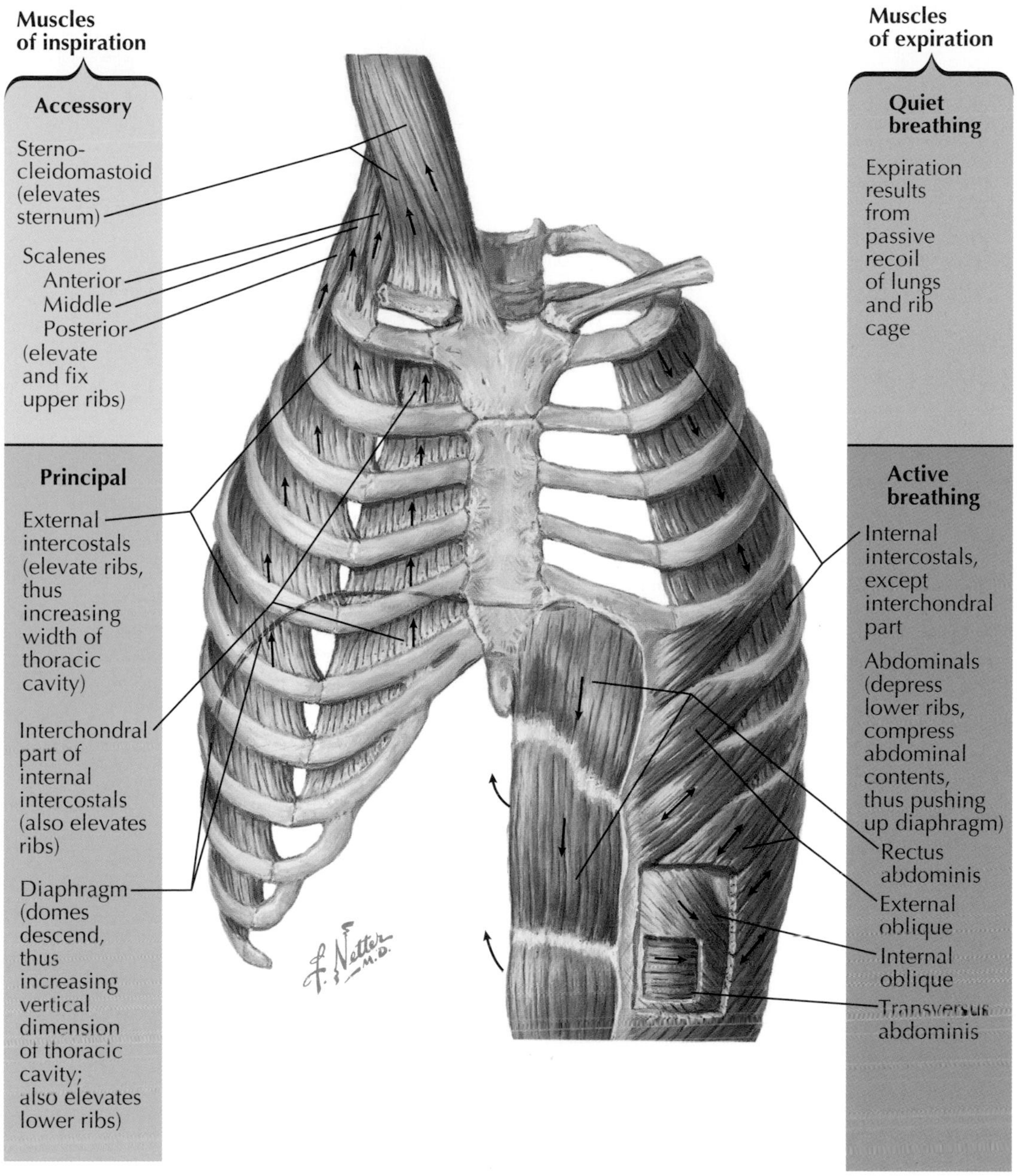

The major function of the lung is to deliver oxygen to and remove carbon dioxide from the blood as it passes through the pulmonary capillary bed. This function is achieved through a series of complex and highly integrated series of processes. The first step in this essential gas exchange process is the contraction of the inspiratory muscles, producing the force (pressure decrease or pressure difference) to overcome the resistance of the lung and chest wall and resulting in the passage of air down a negative pressure gradient from the airway opening (mouth or nose) along the tracheobronchial tree into the alveoli of the lung. The exchange of respiratory gases with the blood and pulmonary capillaries is aided by an ultrathin alveolar-capillary membrane where oxygen diffuses across the membrane into the blood. Carbon dioxide passes in the opposite direction. The adequacy of gas exchange can be determined from the tensions of oxygen and carbon dioxide in the blood leaving the lungs that supply the organs of the body.

Assessment of the mechanical properties of the lung and chest wall and evaluation of the efficiency of gas exchange in the lungs are clinically important. When abnormalities are revealed early, impairment may still be reversible or at least treatable. Pulmonary function testing is also helpful in elucidating the basis for breathlessness, a common symptom of pulmonary disease, as well as important in characterizing the pathophysiology and providing a measure of the severity of pulmonary diseases. Pulmonary function testing is also an excellent measure of general health and the risk of mortality from all causes. The range of pulmonary function tests, their accepted symbols, techniques of performance, and interpretation are summarized in Plates 3-1 and 3-2.

RESPIRATORY MUSCLES

The chest expands and the lungs are filled with air by the contraction of the inspiratory muscles that create a negative pressure within the chest cavity and a negative pressure gradient down the airways (see Plate 2-1). The diaphragm is the principal muscle of inspiration and provides the pressure gradient for the movement of much of the air that enters the lungs during quiet breathing. Contraction of the diaphragm causes the left and right domes to descend downward and the chest to expand upward and outward. At the same time, because of the vertically oriented attachments of the diaphragm to the costal margins, diaphragmatic contraction also serves to elevate the lower ribs.

Contraction of the intercostal muscles, the external intercostal muscles, and the parasternal intercartilaginous muscles raises the ribs during inspiration. As the ribs are elevated, the anteroposterior and transverse dimensions of the chest enlarge because of the anatomic movement of the ribs around the axis of their necks. This is commonly referred to as the *bucket handle effect*. Upward displacement of the upper ribs is accompanied by an increase in the anteroposterior dimension similar to the motion of a "water pump handle," and elevation of the lower ribs is associated with an increase in the transverse dimension of the chest.

In addition to the diaphragm and intercostal muscles, other accessory inspiratory muscles contribute to the movement of the chest in other situations. The scalene muscles make their major contribution during high levels of ventilation when the upper parts of the chest are maximally enlarged. These muscles arise from the transverse processes of the lower five cervical vertebrae and insert into the upper aspect of the first and second ribs. Contraction of these muscles elevates and fixes the uppermost part of the rib cage.

Another accessory muscle, the sternomastoid (sternocleidomastoid), normally also becomes active only at high levels of ventilation. Contraction of the sternomastoid muscle is frequently apparent during severe asthma and with other disorders that obstruct the movement of air into the lungs. The sternomastoid muscle elevates the sternum and slightly enlarges the anteroposterior and longitudinal dimensions of the chest.

In contrast to inspiration, expiration during quiet breathing occurs as a more passive process as a result of recoil of the lung. However, at higher levels of ventilation or when movement of air out of the lungs is impeded, expiration becomes active. Muscles involved in active expiration include the internal intercostal muscles, which depress the ribs; the external and internal oblique abdominal muscles; and the transversus and rectus abdominis muscles, which compress the abdominal contents, depress the lower ribs, and pull down the anterior part of the lower chest. These expiratory muscles also play important and complex roles in regulating breathing and lung volume during talking, singing, coughing, defecation, and parturition.

The strength of the respiratory muscles can be determined from maximal static respiratory pressures (i.e., maximal pressure generated during a forced inspiratory or expiratory maneuver against a manometer or pressure gauge). Pressure developed during an isometric contraction of the respiratory muscles is a function of the length of those muscles and is therefore related to the lung volume at which the maneuver is performed. Maximal inspiratory static pressure is measured when the inspiratory muscles are optimally lengthened after a complete expiration to residual volume (RV). Similarly, maximal static expiratory pressure is determined

PULMONARY MECHANICS AND GAS EXCHANGE *(Continued)*

SPIROMETRY: LUNG VOLUME AND MEASUREMENT

Volume displacement

Flow measurement

Spirometry performed before and after inhalation of short-acting bronchodilator

Automated spirometry measures forced expiratory volume in 1 second (FEV_1) and forced vital capacity (FVC) and calculates FEV_1/FVC ratio

Printout of FVC, FEV_1, and FEV_1/FVC ratio

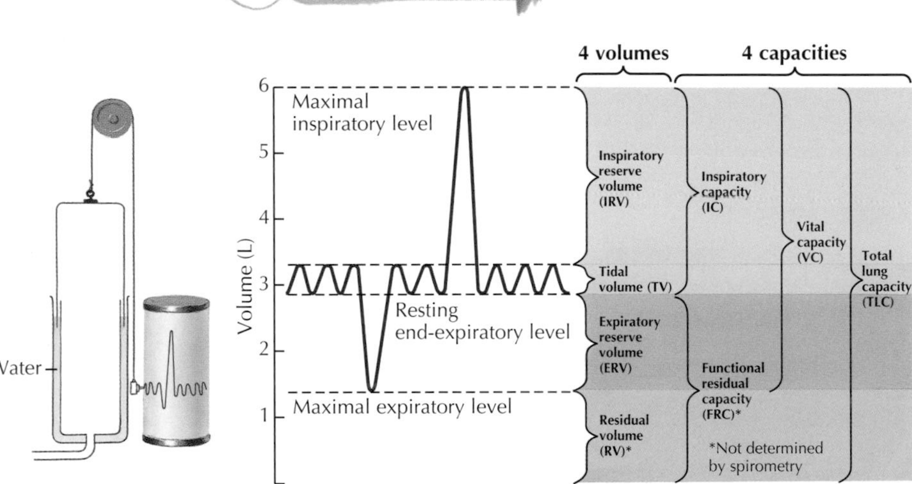

after a full inspiration to total lung capacity (TLC) when the expiratory muscles are in their most mechanically advantageous position.

Measurement of maximal static respiratory pressures can be clinically useful in the evaluation of patients with neuromuscular disorders. Respiratory muscle weakness, when severe, can reduce the ventilatory capacity and result in breathlessness, even when lung function is otherwise normal.

LUNG VOLUMES AND SUBDIVISIONS

Lung Volumes and Capacities

The forced expiratory volume in 1 second (FEV_1) (see Plate 3-1) is largely determined by size of the forced vital capacity (FVC), which in turn is determined by the factors that determine TLC and RV; hence, the size of the lung is important. There is significant correlation between the size of the FVC and respiratory disease progression as well as death from all causes.

Determination of the size of the lung is made by measuring lung volumes and lung capacities. A lung capacity is defined as two or more lung volumes. There are four lung capacities: TLC, inspiratory capacity (IC), functional residual capacity (FRC), and vital capacity (VC). There are four separate lung volumes: RV, expiratory reserve volume (ERV), tidal volume (TV), and inspiratory reserve volume (IRV).

TLC is the maximal amount of air in the lung after a full inspiration. TLC is made up of four lung volumes: RV + ERV + TV + IRV or two capacities FRC + IC and other combinations.

IC is the maximal volume of air inhaled from the end of a normal breath (FRC) to TLC. IC = TV + IRV.

FRC is the volume of air in the lung at the end of a normal breath. FRC = ERV + RV.

VC is the volume of air exhaled after a complete expiration from TLC. This effort ends when the RV is reached. VC = IRV + TV + ERV or IC + ERV. When the effort is done with a maximal force, it is termed the FVC.

IRV is the volume of air inhaled from the end of a normal tidal breath to TLC.

TV (or V_T) is the volume of air that is inhaled and exhaled during normal breathing.

ERV is maximal volume of air exhaled from the end of a normal breath and is terminated when the RV is reached.

RV is the volume of air that remains in the lung at the end of a maximal expiration. A spirometer is a device that measures the volume of air inhaled into and exhaled out of the lung (see Plate 2-2).

Spirometers come in two general types; based on the measurement principle used, they can measure either volume or flow. In the volume-type spirometer, air is captured as a displacement of some physical container (e.g., the vertical displacement of a bell in a water seal or displacement of a dry bellows). With the flow-type spirometer, volume is determined by the electrical integration of a flow signal (Plate 2-2). Other types of instruments measure flow or volume in a variety of ways such as using temperature probes, turbines, or vanes. To measure lung volumes and specifically the VC, the patient sits and breathes into the spirometer. A technician then instructs the patient to inhale and exhale maximally with either a slow effort or a maximally generated effort. The volume of air inhaled and exhaled is at ambient temperature, pressure, saturated (ATPS) but by convention is expressed to body temperature, pressure, saturated (BTPS). A spirometer can only measure three volumes (IRV, ERV, and TV) and two capacities (IC and VC), but in practice, usually only the VC is measured. A low VC is often observed in patients with either restrictive or obstructive diseases, so other volumes and capacities must be measured, but to measure the TLC, FRC, and RV, the FRC needs to be determined.

FRC is generally measured by two very different techniques: inert gas dilution or applying Boyle's law during gas compression.

MEASURING LUNG VOLUMES (see Plate 2-3)

The *inert gas dilution* method involves the measurement of FRC be determining the dilution of an inert gas. The inert gas helium is used most often, but other inert gases can be used as well. Helium is both inert and insoluble. A breathing circuit is filled with a gas mixture that contains oxygen and a known percentage of helium. The patient is switched to this gas mixture at end expiration (FRC). As the helium or other inert gas in the circuit mixes with the air in the lung, the concentration of helium falls to a new or diluted level. Because helium does not cross the alveolar-capillary membrane, the total amount of helium in the system does not change during the test period. Consequently, the initial concentration of helium ($He_{initial}$) multiplied by the volume of gas in the spirometer at the start of the test ($V_{spirometer}$) equals the final concentration of helium (He_{final}) multiplied by the volume of gas in the spirometer at the end of the test plus the volume of air in the lung (i.e., FRC). The equation can be written as follows:

$$He_{initial} \times V_{spirometer} = He_{final}\,(V_{spirometer} + FRC)$$

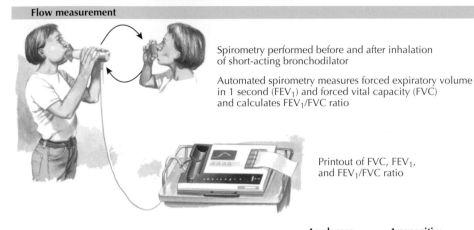

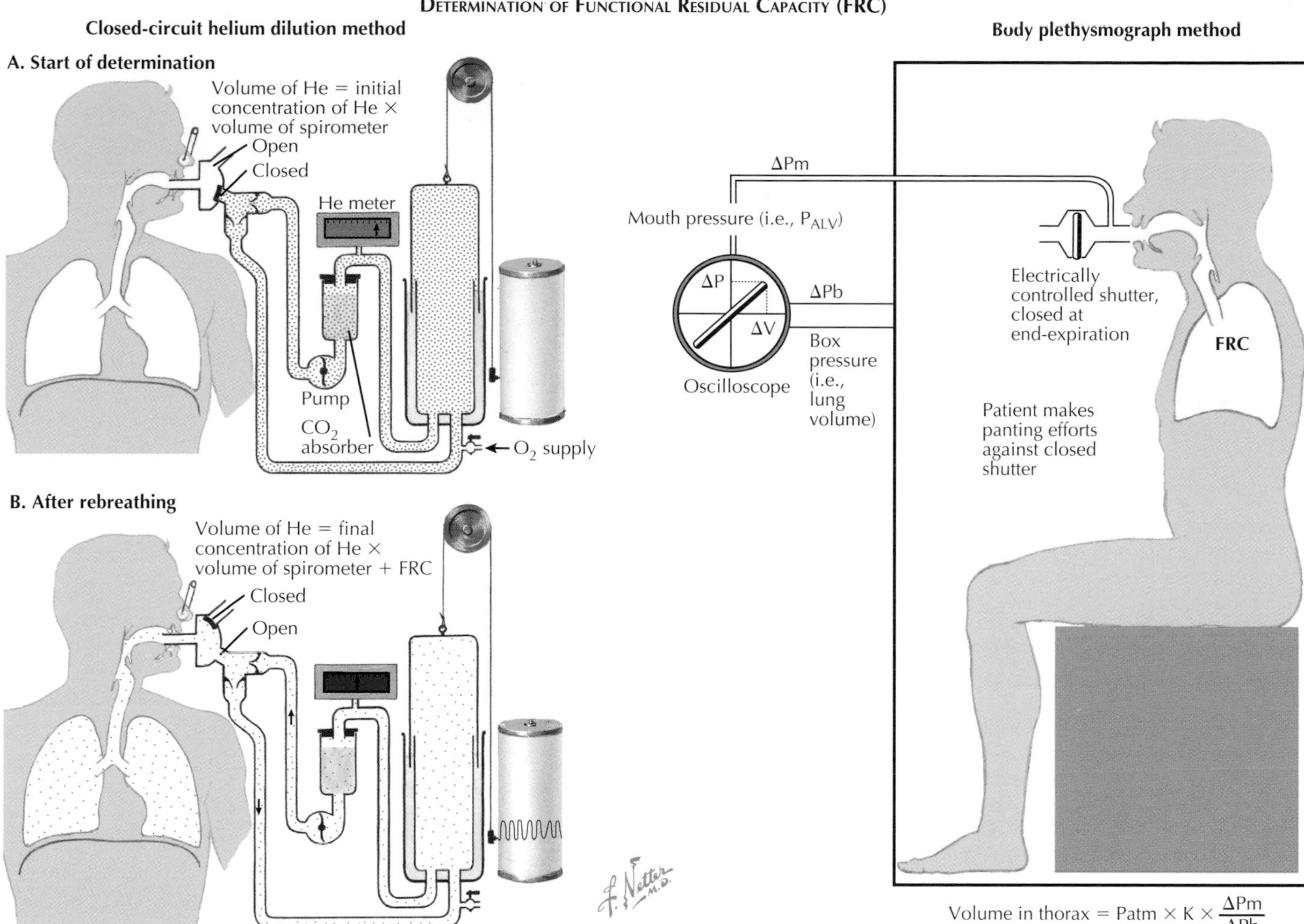

Pulmonary Mechanics and Gas Exchange *(Continued)*

Solving for FRC, the equation becomes

$$FRC = \frac{V_{spirometer} \times (He_{initial} - He_{final})}{He_{final}}$$

The *open-circuit nitrogen washout* technique is another inert gas dilution method in which nitrogen is completely displaced from the lungs during a period of 100% oxygen breathing. All expired air is collected, and the volume and nitrogen concentration of the sample are measured. Because the total volume of nitrogen in the expired air equals the volume of nitrogen in the lung before the start of the test, the volume of expired air multiplied by the nitrogen concentration of the expired air equals the volume of air in the lung (FRC) multiplied by the initial concentration of nitrogen in the lung.

Both of these inert gas dilution techniques measure the gas (FRC) that communicates with the room air. What is not measured is the gas trapped in the lung behind closed or obstructed airways. For example, in a patient with emphysema, this trapped gas can be quite large (>1 L) and represents the gas trapped in the emphysematous bullae.

The *body plethysmograph technique*, or Boyle's law technique, uses a closed chamber within which the patient is seated (see Plate 2-3).

At the end of a normal breath (FRC), a shutter closes, and the patient gently pants against the closed shutter. During the subsequent inspiratory and expiratory efforts against the closed shutter, the pressure in the airways and alveoli falls or rises below atmospheric levels, and the gas in the lung undergoes decompression and compression. Because the plethysmograph is sealed, the resulting increase and decrease in lung volume is reflected by an increase or decrease in the pressure within the plethysmograph.

Thoracic gas volume is then determined by applying Boyle's law, which states that for a gas at a constant temperature, the product of pressure and volume in two different states (compressed or decompressed) is constant. $PV = P^1 V^1$. Boyle's law can also be expressed as follows:

$$P \times V = (P + \Delta P) \times (V + \Delta V)$$

where P = initial pressure, V = initial volume, ΔP is a change in pressure, and ΔV is a corresponding change in volume. This expression can be simplified, solving for V:

$$V = (P + \Delta P) \times \frac{\Delta V}{\Delta P}$$

With respect to the respiratory system, V represents the initial volume of gas in the thorax (i.e., FRC), P represents the pressure in the alveoli at the end of a normal expiration (i.e., atmospheric pressure), ΔP represents the change in alveolar pressure during breathing efforts against a closed shutter, and ΔV represents the change in thoracic gas volume resulting from gas expansion or compression during obstructed breathing. Changes in alveolar pressure are determined from changes in mouth pressure (ΔP = ΔPm), and changes in the volume of thoracic gas are reflected by changes in the pressure within the plethysmograph (ΔV = ΔPp). Because changes in alveolar pressure during the gentle breathing maneuver against a closed shutter are extremely small as compared with atmospheric pressure, FRC can be calculated from the following simplified equation:

$$FRC = \text{atmospheric pressure} \times \frac{\Delta Pb}{\Delta Pm}$$

FRC measured by the body plethysmograph measures all the gas within the lung whether it communicates with the atmosphere or not. So in the situation of excessive trapped gas, the FRC determined by the body plethysmograph is greater than the FRC determined by inert gas dilution.

Mechanics of Ventilatory Apparatus (see Plate 2-4)

The respiratory system or ventilatory apparatus consists of the lungs and surrounding chest wall. The chest wall

PULMONARY MECHANICS AND GAS EXCHANGE *(Continued)*

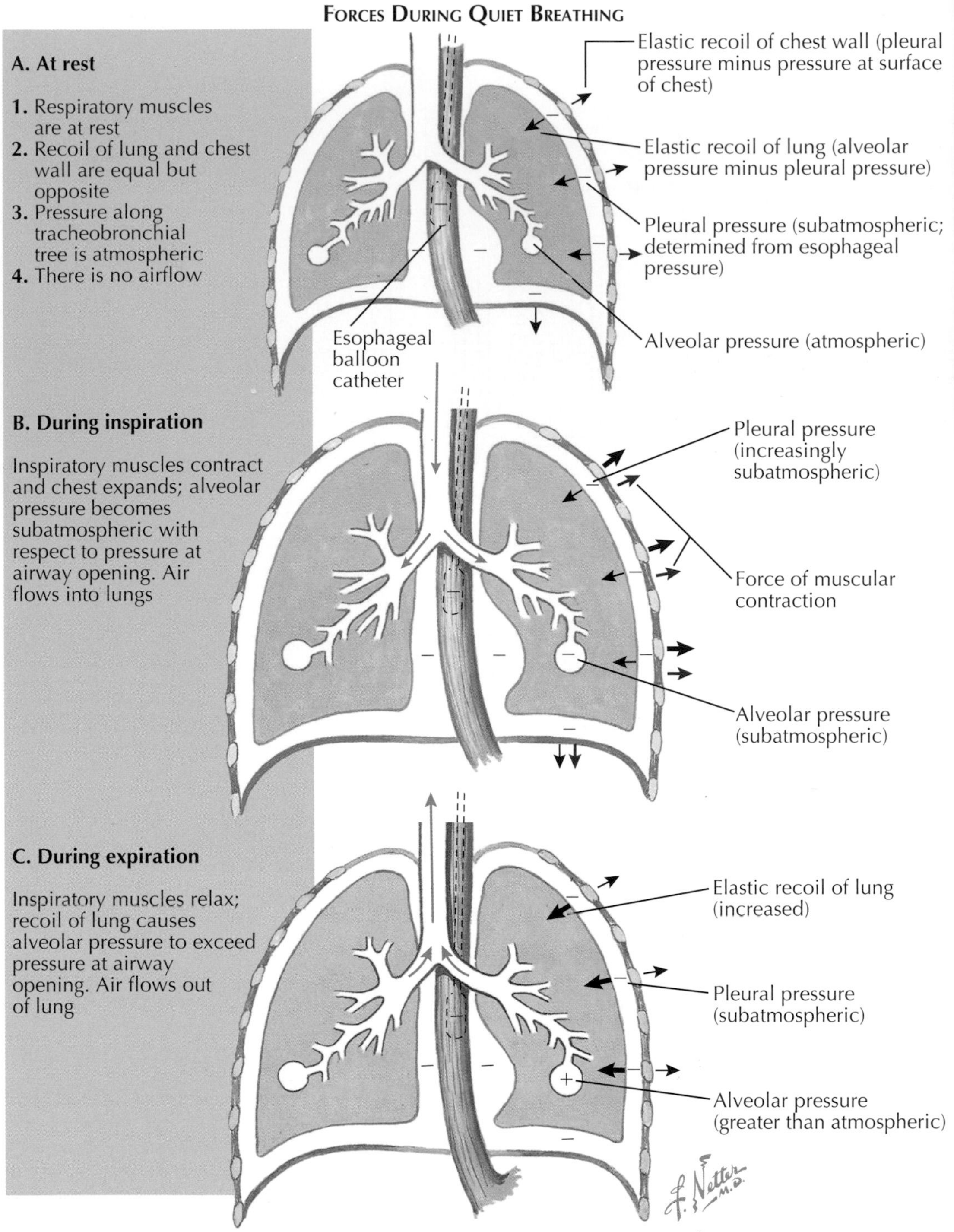

includes not only the rib cage but also the diaphragm and abdominal wall. The lungs fill the chest such that the visceral pleurae are in contact with the parietal pleurae of the chest cage where the pleural space is filled with a small amount of liquid and is therefore really only a potential space. As a result of their close physical contact, the lungs and chest wall act in unison. From a mechanical point of view, the respiratory system or ventilatory apparatus may be regarded as a pump that can be characterized by its elastic (E), flow-resistive (R), and inertial (I) properties (see Plates 2-4 and 2-5). Dynamically, the total pressure developed by the contracting muscles must overcome three resistances:

$$\Delta P = P_E + P_R + P_I$$

where P_E is pressure attributable to elastic resistance (E), P_R is pressure attributable to flow-resistance (R), and P_I is pressure attributable to inertia (I).

In terms of flow and volume:

$$\Delta P = EV + R\dot{V} + I\ddot{V}, \text{ where } V = \text{volume},$$

$$\dot{V} = \text{flow, and } \ddot{V} = \text{acceleration.}$$

At the end of a normal expiration, the respiratory muscles are at rest. The elastic recoil of the lung, which is inward and favors deflation, is balanced by the elastic recoil of the chest, which is directed outward and favors inflation, and these opposing forces generate a subatmospheric pressure of approximately 5 cm H_2O in the pleural space between the visceral and parietal pleurae. At the point of no flow, the pressure along the entire airway from the mouth to the alveoli is at atmospheric level. The difference between alveolar and pleural pressure or the pressure difference across the lung structures is the transpulmonary pressure (P_{TP}).

As the inspiratory muscles contract during inspiration and the chest expands, the pleural pressure becomes increasingly negative or subatmospheric. Because of the resistance (Raw) offered by the tracheobronchial tree to the flow of air into the lung, the alveolar pressure also becomes subatmospheric. At a given rate of airflow, the difference between alveolar pressure and the pressure at the airway opening, which remains at atmospheric level, is used to measure of the flow resistance of the airways:

$$\text{Raw} = \frac{\text{Patm} - \text{Palv}}{\dot{V}}$$

or

$$\text{Airway resistance} = \frac{\text{Alveolar pressure} - \text{Airway opening pressure}}{\text{Rate of airflow}}$$

Movement of air into the lungs continues until the alveolar pressure again reaches or equilibrates with atmospheric level or the alveolar pressure minus the airway opening pressure equals zero, which is when the pressure difference between the alveoli and the airway opening no longer exists.

Elastic Properties of the Lung
(see Plate 2-5)

The compliance or distensibility of the lungs is determined from the relationship between changes in lung volume and changes in transpulmonary pressure.

FORCES DURING QUIET BREATHING

A. At rest

1. Respiratory muscles are at rest
2. Recoil of lung and chest wall are equal but opposite
3. Pressure along tracheobronchial tree is atmospheric
4. There is no airflow

B. During inspiration

Inspiratory muscles contract and chest expands; alveolar pressure becomes subatmospheric with respect to pressure at airway opening. Air flows into lungs

C. During expiration

Inspiratory muscles relax; recoil of lung causes alveolar pressure to exceed pressure at airway opening. Air flows out of lung

At the end of inspiration, when flow is zero, the volume of air in the lungs is greater, and the pleural pressure is more subatmospheric than at FRC when the breath begins. At this point, the difference between alveolar and pleural pressure—the transpulmonary pressure—is increased. This change in transpulmonary pressure required to effect a given change in the volume of air in the lungs is a measure of the elastic resistance of the lungs:

$$E = \frac{\Delta P_{TP}}{\Delta Vol}$$

or:

$$\text{Lung elastic resistance (or elastance)} = \frac{\text{Change in transpulmonary pressure}}{\text{Change in lung volume}}$$

The inverse of which is lung compliance:

$$C = \frac{\Delta Vol}{\Delta P_{TP}}$$

The forces required to overcome elastic resistance are stored within the elastic elements; expiration then occurs when these forces are released. When the respiratory muscles stop contracting and start relaxing, the recoil of the lung causes the alveolar pressure to exceed the pressure at the mouth, the pressure gradient is reversed, and air flows out of the lung.

The elastic properties of the lungs (see Plate 2-5) are determined statically when airflow is stopped. Under these no-flow conditions, alveolar pressure equals the pressure at the mouth; pleural pressure is determined indirectly from the pressure in the lower third of the esophagus by means of a balloon catheter. In practice,

PULMONARY MECHANICS AND GAS EXCHANGE *(Continued)*

the subject inhales to TLC and then slowly exhales, airflow is then periodically interrupted, and static measurements are made of lung volume and transpulmonary pressure. From the measurements of volume and transpulmonary pressure, lung compliance ($C_L = \Delta V/\Delta P_{TP}$) or its inverse elastance ($E_L + \Delta P_{TP}/\Delta Vol$) is determined.

Pressure-volume characteristics of the lung are nonlinear. Thus, compliance of the lung is decreased at high volumes and greatest as RV is approached. Forces favoring further collapse of the lung can be demonstrated throughout the range of VC, even at low lung volumes. If the inflationary forces of the chest wall on the lung are eliminated by removing the lung from the thorax or by opening the chest (pneumothorax), the lung will collapse to a virtually airless state upon reaching an equilibrium position.

Lung tissue elasticity arises in part from the fibers of elastin and collagen that are present in the alveolar walls and that surround both the bronchioles and pulmonary capillaries. The elastin fibers can approximately double their resting length; in contrast, the collagen fibers are poorly extensible and act primarily to limit expansion at high lung volumes. Lung expansion occurs through an unfolding and geometric rearrangement of the fibers analogous to the way a nylon stocking is easily stretched even though the individual fibers are elongated very little.

The distensibility of the lungs increases (compliance increases) with advancing age as a result of alterations in the elastin and collagen fibers in the lung. Pulmonary emphysema, which destroys alveolar walls and enlarges alveolar spaces, similarly increases lung compliance. In contrast, compliance of the lung is reduced by disorders such as pulmonary fibrosis, which affect the interstitial tissues of the lung, and by diffuse alveolar consolidation and edema, which also interfere with expansion of the lung.

SURFACE TENSION (see Plate 2-6)

The elastic behavior of the lung also depends on the surface tension of the film lining the alveoli. The attractive forces between molecules of the liquid film are stronger than those between the film and the gas in the alveoli. Consequently, the area of the surface film shrinks. The behavior of the surface film has been examined in experimental animals by comparing pressure-volume relationships of air-filled lungs with those of saline-filled lungs. Because saline eliminates the liquid-air interface without affecting tissue elasticity, lungs distended with liquid require a substantially lower transpulmonary pressure to maintain a given lung volume than do lungs inflated with air. Thus, surface forces make a major contribution to the retractive forces of the lung.

Surface forces can be characterized by Laplace's law (see Plate 2-6). Laplace's law states that the pressure inside a spherical structure such as an alveolus is directly proportional to the tension in the wall and inversely proportional to the radius of curvature. When the liquid-air interface and surface tension forces are abolished by instillation of saline into the alveolar spaces, the pressure required to maintain a given lung volume is markedly reduced.

MEASUREMENT OF ELASTIC PROPERTIES OF THE LUNG

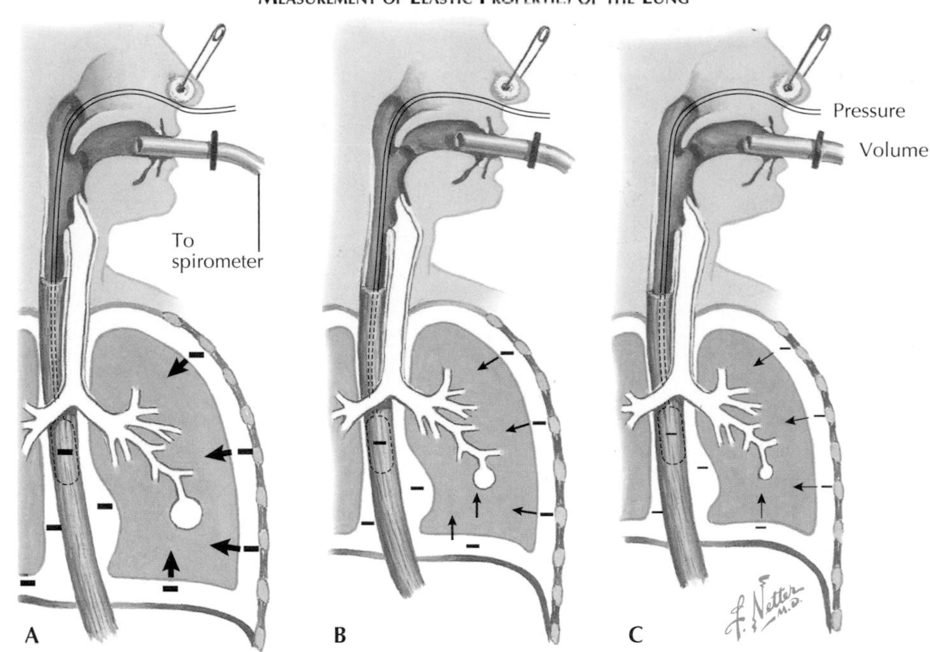

During a slow expiration from TLC, flow is periodically interrupted, and measurements are made of lung volume and transpulmonary pressure. Transpulmonary pressure is the difference between alveolar and pleural pressures. Pleural pressure is determined from pressure in the esophagus. Because there is no airflow, alveolar pressure is the same as the pressure at the airway opening.

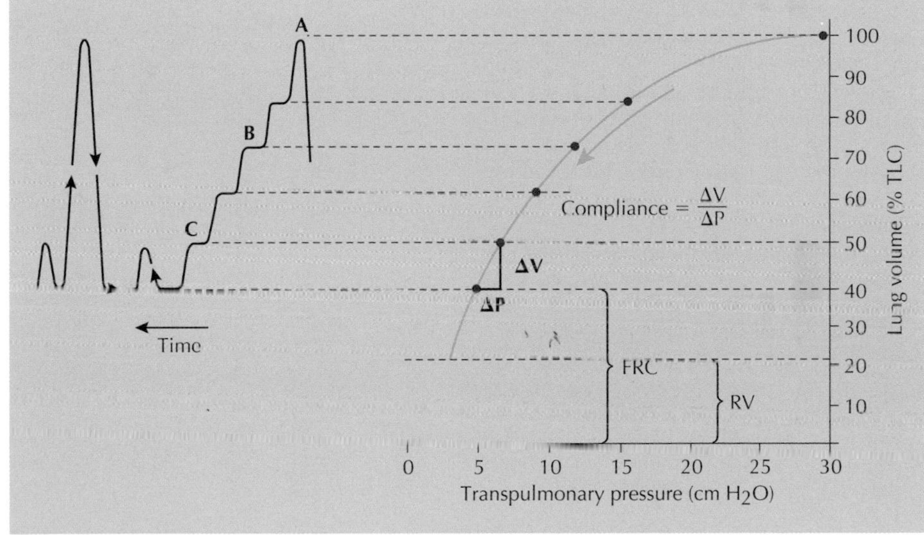

The surface tension of the film lining the alveolar walls depends on lung volume; surface tension is high when the lungs are inflated and low at small lung volumes. These variations in surface tension with changes in lung volume require that the surface film contain a unique type of surface-active material. If the surface tension remained constant instead of changing with lung volume, a greater pressure would be required to keep an alveolus open as its radius of curvature diminished with decreasing lung volume. The surface-active material lining the alveoli, or *surfactant*, is a product of the type II granular pneumocyte and has dipalmitoyl lecithin as an important constituent. Surfactant serves a number of important functions. Without surfactant, small alveoli would empty into communicating larger ones, and atelectasis would occur. Indeed, this is the situation in premature infants who lack surfactant. Surfactant's low surface tension, particularly at low lung volumes, increases the compliance of the lung and facilitates expansion during the subsequent breath; hence, the stability of alveoli at low lung volumes is maintained.

Elastic Properties of the Chest Wall and Total Respiratory System (see Plate 2-7)

The elastic recoil of the chest wall is outward and favors inflation. If the chest is unopposed by the lungs, it enlarges to approximately 70% of the TLC, and this point represents the equilibrium or resting position of the chest wall. At this point, the pressure across the chest wall (the difference between pleural pressure and the pressure at the surface of the chest when the respiratory muscles are completely at rest) is zero. If the thorax expands beyond this equilibrium point, the chest wall, similar to the lung, will recoil inward, resisting expansion and favoring a return to the equilibrium position.

PULMONARY MECHANICS AND GAS EXCHANGE *(Continued)*

On the other hand, at all volumes less than 70% of TLC, the recoil of the chest is opposite to that of the lung such that it is directly outward and favors inflation.

The lung and chest wall are considered to be in series, so that the recoil pressure of the total respiratory system (P_{RS}) is the algebraic sum of the pressures exerted by the recoil of the lung (P_L) and the recoil of the chest wall (P_W).

$$P_{RS} = P_L + P_W$$

The P_L is determined from the difference between alveolar pressure (Palv) and pleural pressure (Ppl). The P_W when the respiratory muscles are at rest is determined from the difference between pleural pressure (Ppl) and the pressure at the external surface of the chest (Patm). Thus, the recoil of the entire respiratory system can be expressed as follows:

$$P_{RS} = (\text{Palv} - \text{Ppl}) + (\text{Ppl} - \text{Patm})$$

When the respiratory muscles are completely at rest and the pressure at the surface of the chest is at atmospheric levels:

$$P_{RS} = \text{Palv}$$

The elastic properties of the total respiratory system can be evaluated in a number of ways. Each method requires that a given lung volume be maintained during complete relaxation of all the respiratory muscles and is generally accomplished by application of external forces such as positive pressure to the airways or negative pressure around the chest or through voluntary relaxation of the respiratory muscles while the airway opening is occluded.

FRC therefore represents the unique equilibrium or resting position where the recoil pressure is zero. At this one point (FRC), the increased (deflation) recoil pressure of the lung is equal but opposite to the outward (inflation) recoil pressure of the chest wall. At any volume above FRC, the recoil pressure exceeds atmospheric levels, favoring a decrease in lung volume; at volumes below FRC, the recoil pressure is less than atmospheric pressure and the respiratory system tends to retract outward in an attempt to increase lung volume. FRC is therefore a measure of the elastic forces of the respiratory system.

Elastic recoil properties of the chest wall, which play an important role in determining the subdivisions of lung volume, may be rendered abnormal by disorders such as marked obesity, kyphoscoliosis, and ankylosing spondylitis.

Distribution of Airflow Resistance
(see Plate 2-8)

The motion of gas from the alveoli to the airway opening requires pressure dissipation. The ratio of transpulmonary pressure (difference between pleural and mouth pressures) to flow defines *pulmonary resistance*, which is the sum of the viscous resistance caused by the gas movement through the airways (*airway resistance*) and the viscoelastic resistance offered by lung tissue displacement (*tissue resistance*).

Pulmonary resistance is inversely related to breathing frequency, attributable to the frequency dependence of tissue resistance, and to lung volume, attributable to the volume dependence of airway resistance.

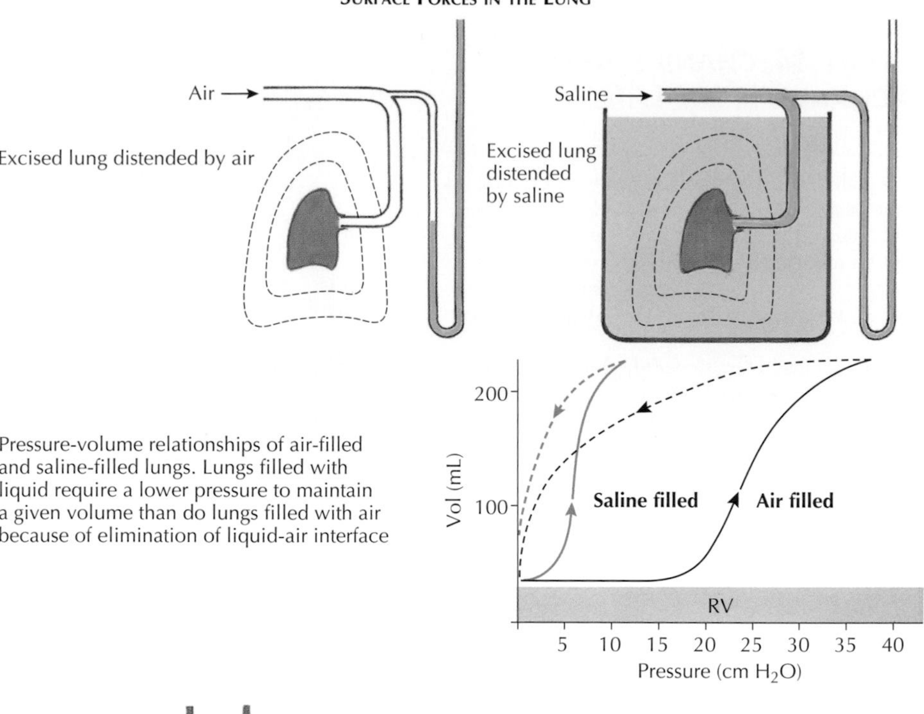

Pressure-volume relationships of air-filled and saline-filled lungs. Lungs filled with liquid require a lower pressure to maintain a given volume than do lungs filled with air because of elimination of liquid-air interface

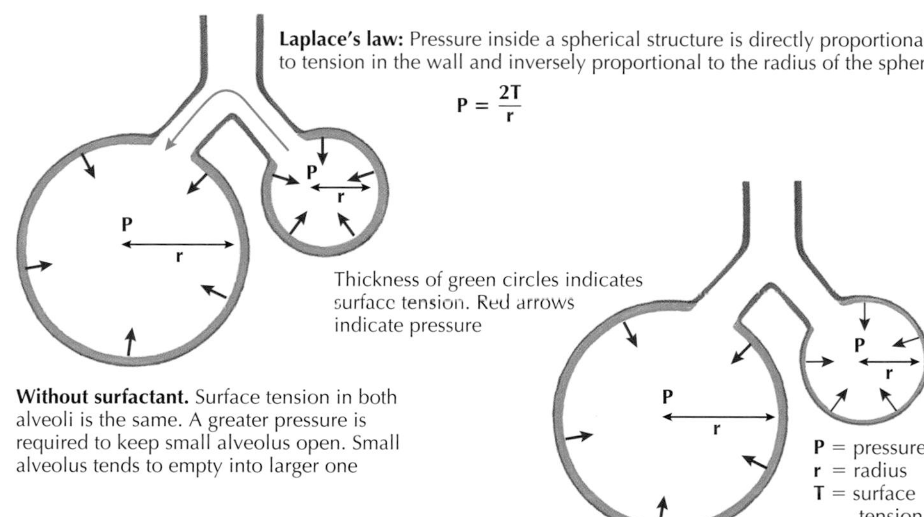

Laplace's law: Pressure inside a spherical structure is directly proportional to tension in the wall and inversely proportional to the radius of the sphere

$$P = \frac{2T}{r}$$

Without surfactant. Surface tension in both alveoli is the same. A greater pressure is required to keep small alveolus open. Small alveolus tends to empty into larger one

With surfactant. Surface tension reduced in small alveolus. Pressure distending both alveoli is approximately the same. Alveoli are stabilized, and the tendency for small alveolus to empty into larger one is reduced

During normal tidal breathing at rest, tissue resistance represents a major component of pulmonary resistance, and it may be further increased in diseases affecting the lung parenchyma, such as pulmonary fibrosis. Tissue resistance is defined as the ratio of the pressure difference between pleural surface and alveoli to airflow and thus cannot be directly measured in vivo.

The driving pressure producing airflow along the airways is the difference between alveolar (Palv) and airway opening (Pao) pressures. Airway resistance (Raw) is thus defined as the ratio of this driving pressure to airflow ($\dot{V}$) according to the equation:

$$\text{Raw} = \frac{\text{Palv} - \text{Pao}}{\dot{V}}$$

Airway resistance can be readily determined in vivo by whole-body plethysmography, which allows measurement of changes in Palv while mouth flow is simultaneously measured by a pneumotachograph. In normal subjects, a large proportion of airway resistance is offered by the upper respiratory tract. During tidal breathing at rest, the contributions of nose and larynx to airway resistance sum up to 40% to 60%, a variability likely attributable to anatomical differences. The larynx contributes to resistance more on expiration than inspiration because the vocal cords are abducted during the latter, and the nose contributes more on inspiration than expiration.

The resistance of intrathoracic airways is mainly attributable to bronchi proximal to the seventh airway generation. With more distal branching, the number of airways increases exponentially much more than their diameter decreases. Thus, the total cross-sectional area of the tracheobronchial tree is also exponentially increasing toward the periphery. As a consequence, the

Pulmonary Mechanics and Gas Exchange *(Continued)*

airways with a diameter smaller than 2 mm contribute to about 10% of the total airway resistance of a normal lung. In diseased conditions, the resistance of these peripheral airways may increase considerably, but it should be more than doubled to result in an increase of total airway resistance exceeding 10%.

The airways are nonrigid structures and are compressed or distended when a pressure difference exists between their lumina and the surrounding space (*transmural pressure*). The pressure surrounding the intrathoracic airways approximates pleural pressure because these airways are exposed to the force required to distend the lung (*transpulmonary pressure*). Thus, the transmural pressure of a given airway varies directly with transpulmonary pressure, and its diameter changes in proportion to the cube root of lung volume changes. Because the resistance of a given airway is inversely proportional to the fourth power of its radius, a hyperbolic inverse relationship exists between airway resistance and lung volume. In normal individuals, the product of airway resistance and lung volume (*specific airway resistance*) and its inverse (*specific airway conductance*) are relatively constant and are used to correct airway resistance for the volume at which it is measured. If the lung elastic recoil is reduced, as in pulmonary emphysema, both transmural pressure and airway caliber decrease, and airway resistance increases.

The effects of changes in transmural pressure on airway caliber also depend on the airway wall compliance; this in turn depends on the structural support of a given airway. The trachea has a cartilage layer in its anterior and lateral walls that prevents complete collapse even when transmural pressure is negative. Whereas the bronchi are less supported by incomplete cartilaginous rings and plates, bronchioles have no cartilage. Nevertheless, their excessive narrowing upon maximal airway smooth muscle activation is, in normal subjects, prevented by internal and external elastic loads, the former being represented by airway wall structures, the latter by the force of interdependence provided by the alveolar attachments to the outer airway walls. If alveolar attachments are destroyed, such as in emphysema, the force of interdependence is reduced, and the airway caliber is less for any given airway smooth muscle tone.

Airway caliber may also be reduced and airway resistance increased in patients with lung disease such as asthma and chronic bronchitis (chronic obstructive pulmonary disease) because of mucosal edema, hypertrophy or hyperplasia of mucous glands, changes in mucus properties, or hypertrophy or hyperplasia of bronchial smooth muscle.

Patterns of Airflow (see Plate 2-9)

The relationship between driving pressure and the resulting airflow along the tracheobronchial tree is extremely complicated because the airways are a system of irregularly branching tubes that are neither rigid nor perfectly circular.

The driving pressure required to overcome friction depends on the rate and pattern of airflow. There are two major patterns of airflow. *Laminar flow* is characterized by streamlines that are parallel to the sides of the tube and sliding over each other. The streamlines at the center of the tube move faster than those closest to the walls so that the flow profile is parabolic. The pressure-flow characteristics of laminar flow depend on length (l) and radius (r) of the tube and the viscosity of gas (μ) according to the Poiseuille equation:

$$\frac{P}{\dot{V}} = \frac{8\mu l}{\pi r^4}$$

where P is driving pressure and $\dot{V}$ is flow. The above equation shows that driving pressure is directly proportional to flow ($\Delta P \propto \mu\dot{V}$) and highly dependent on tube radius. If the radius of the tube is halved, the pressure required to maintain a given flow rate must be increased 16 times. Laminar flow dominates in the periphery of the lung, where $\dot{V}$ is low because the airway caliber is small but the total cross-section area is large. *Turbulent flow* occurs at high flow rates and is characterized by a complete disorganization of streamlines. The molecules of gas may then move laterally, collide with each other, and change their velocities. Under these circumstances, the pressure-flow relationships change. The airflow is no longer directly proportional to the driving pressure as with laminar flow; rather, the driving pressure to produce a given rate of airflow is proportional to the square of flow ($\Delta P \propto \rho\dot{V}^2$). Also, the driving pressure is dependent on gas density but is little affected by viscosity. Turbulent flow dominates in the more central airways, where $\dot{V}$ is high because airway caliber is large but the total cross-section area is small.

Whether the pattern of flow is laminar or turbulent is determined from the Reynolds number (Re), a dimensionless number that depends on the rate of airflow ($\dot{V}$), the density (ρ) and viscosity (μ) of gas, and the radius of the tube (r), according to the equation:

$$Re = \frac{2\dot{V}\rho}{\pi r \mu}$$

Elastic Properties of the Respiratory System: Lung and Chest Wall

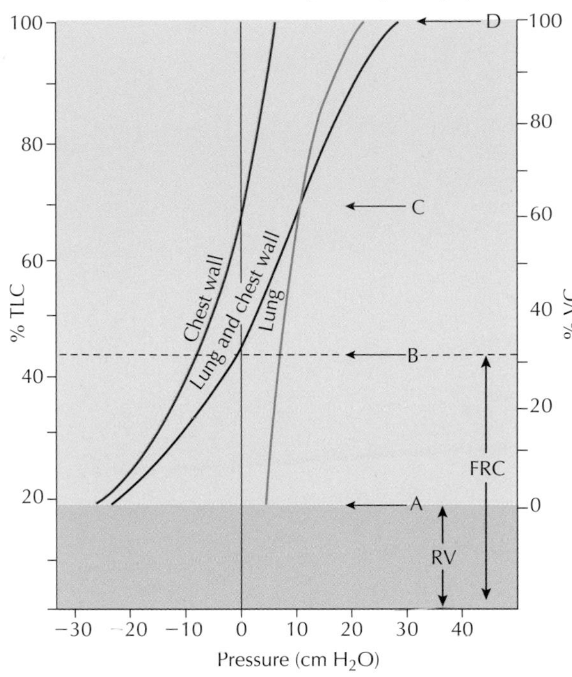

Elastic recoil pressure of respiratory system is algebraic sum of recoil pressures of lung and chest wall

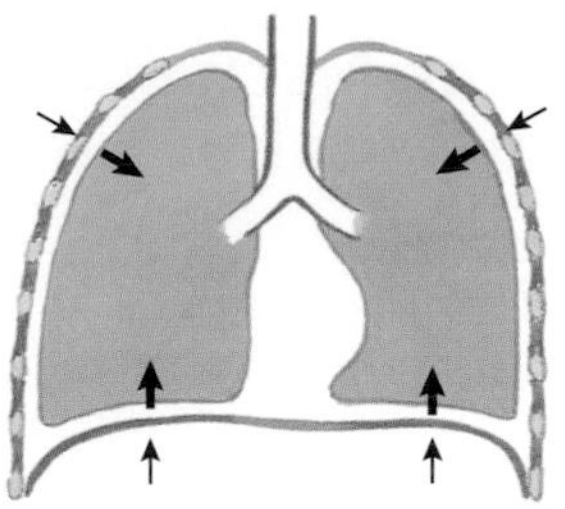

D. At total lung capacity Elastic recoil of both lung and chest wall directed inward, favoring decrease in lung volume

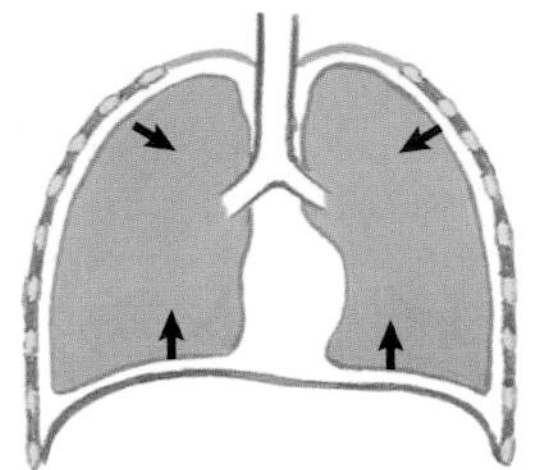

C. At approximately 70% of total lung capacity Equilibrium position of chest wall (its recoil equals zero)

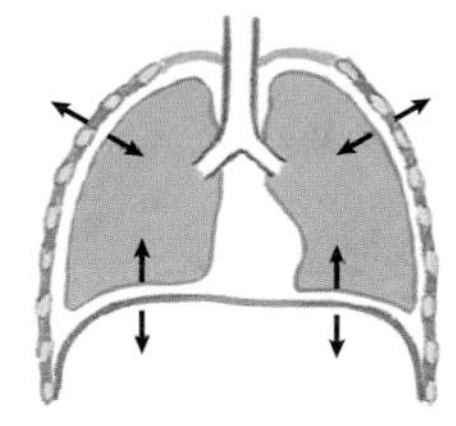

B. At functional residual capacity Elastic recoils of lung and chest wall are equal but opposite

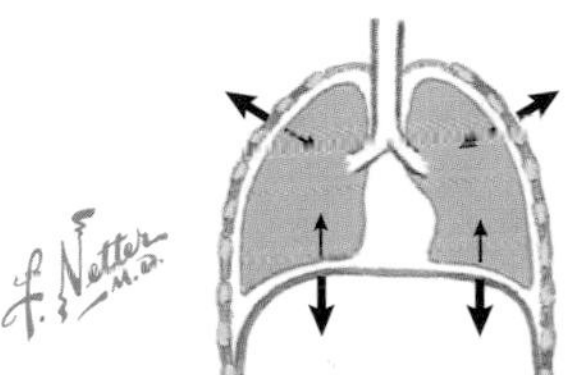

A. At residual volume Elastic recoil of chest wall directed outward is large. Recoil of lung directed inward is very small

Pulmonary Mechanics and Gas Exchange *(Continued)*

In straight, smooth, rigid tubes, turbulence results when the Reynolds number exceeds 2000. It is apparent that turbulence is most likely to occur when the rate of airflow and the gas density are high, the viscosity is low, and the tube radius is small. However, even at low flow during expiration, particularly at branches in the tracheobronchial tree where flow in two separate tubes comes together into a single one, the parabolic profile of laminar flow may become blunted, the streamlines may separate from the walls of the tube, and minor eddy formations may develop. This is referred to as a mixed or *transitional flow* pattern. With a mixed flow pattern, the driving pressure to produce a given flow depends on both the viscosity and the density of the gas.

In addition to pressure dissipation to generate flow, expiration requires some energy to accelerate the gas moving from the large cross-sectional area of the respiratory zone to the smaller cross-sectional area of conducting zone (bronchi, trachea). The ΔP caused by convective acceleration is described by the Bernoulli equation, $\Delta P = \frac{1}{2}\rho(\dot{V}/A)^2$, where A is cross-section area.

In a normal lung, the laminar flow pattern occurs only in the very small peripheral airways, where the flow through any given airway is extremely low. In the remainder of the tracheobronchial tree, flow is transitional, and in the trachea, turbulence regularly occurs.

Determinants of Maximal Expiratory Flow (see Plate 2-10)

An assessment of the flow-resistive properties of the airways is obtained from the flow-volume relationship during a forced expiratory maneuver. An individual inhales maximally to TLC and then exhales to RV as rapidly as possible. During this maneuver, the airflow rises quickly to a maximal value at a lung volume close to TLC. As lung volume decreases, its recoil pressure decreases, the intrathoracic airways narrow, the airway resistance increases, and the airflow decreases almost linearly.

A family of flow-volume curves can be obtained by repeating full expiratory maneuvers over the entire VC at different levels of effort. At lung volumes close to TLC, the airflow increases progressively with increasing effort. At intermediate and low lung volumes, expiratory flow reaches maximal levels with moderate efforts and thereafter increases no further despite increasing efforts. If pleural pressure is measured during such maneuvers, the relationship among lung volume, effort, and expiratory airflow can be explored by plotting a family of *isovolume pressure-flow curves*. At all lung volumes, pleural pressure becomes less subatmospheric and subsequently exceeds atmospheric pressure as the expiratory effort is progressively increased. Correspondingly, the airflow increases. At lung volumes greater than 75% of VC, the airflow increases continuously with increasing pleural pressure and is thus considered to be effort dependent. In contrast, at volumes below 75% of VC, flow levels off as pleural pressure exceeds atmospheric pressure but does not increase further with increases in effort and is thus considered to be effort independent. Because airflow remains constant despite an increase in driving pressure, it follows that the resistance to airflow must also be increasing proportionally with pleural pressure, probably because of compression and narrowing of intrathoracic airways.

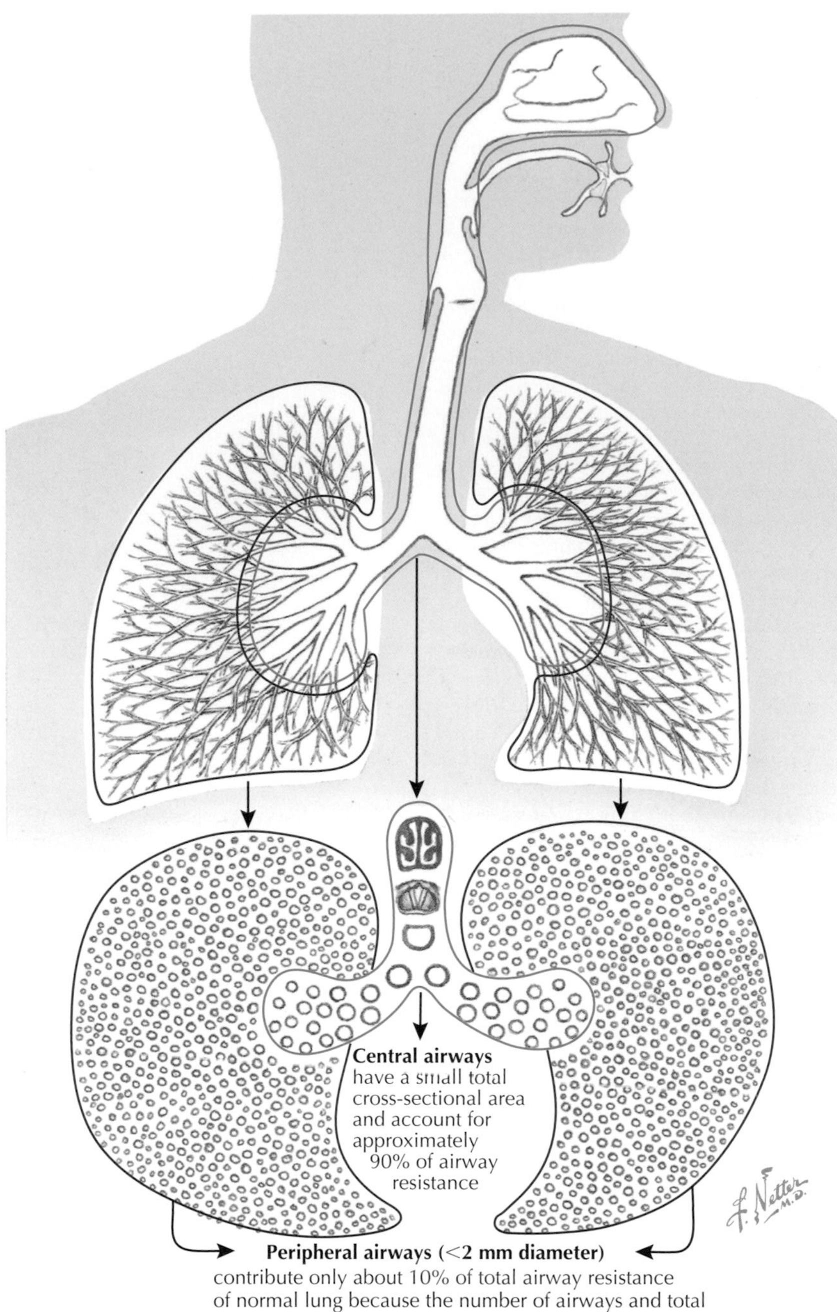

Distribution of Airway Resistance
Central airways have a small total cross-sectional area and account for approximately 90% of airway resistance
Peripheral airways (<2 mm diameter) contribute only about 10% of total airway resistance of normal lung because the number of airways and total cross-sectional area in any generation are very large

An explanation of this phenomenon is illustrated by a simple model of the lung. Alveoli are represented by an elastic sac and intrathoracic airways by a compressible tube, both enclosed within a pleural space. At a given end-inspiratory lung volume, when airflow is arrested, pleural pressure is subatmospheric and counterbalances the elastic recoil pressure of the lung. The alveolar pressure (i.e., the sum of the elastic recoil pressure of the lung and pleural pressure) is zero. Because airflow has ceased, pressures along the entire airway are also at atmospheric levels. During a forced expiration, pleural pressure increases above atmospheric pressure and increases alveolar pressure. Airway pressure decreases progressively from the alveolus toward the airway opening to overcome viscous resistance. At a point along the airway, referred to as the *equal pressure point*, the decrease in airway pressure from that in the alveolus equals the recoil pressure of the lung. At this point, the intraluminal pressure equals the pressure surrounding the airways (i.e., the pleural pressure). Downstream, the intraluminal pressure decreases below pleural pressure, thus resulting in a negative transmural pressure, and the airways are dynamically compressed.

The airways can be divided into two segments arranged in series, one upstream (i.e., from alveoli to the equal pressure point) and one downstream (i.e., from the equal pressure point to the airway opening). As soon as maximal expiratory flow is achieved, further increases in pleural pressure with increasing expiratory force simply produce more compression of the downstream segment but do not affect airflow through the upstream segment.

The driving pressure of the upstream segment (i.e., the pressure decrease from alveoli to equal pressure

PULMONARY MECHANICS AND GAS EXCHANGE *(Continued)*

point) equals the lung elastic recoil pressure. Consequently, the airflow during forced expiration ($\dot{V}_{max}$) represents the ratio of lung elastic recoil pressure (P_L) to the resistance of the upstream segment (Rus), according to the equation:

$$\dot{V}_{max} = \frac{P_L}{Rus}$$

However, because the caliber of a given airway at the flow-limiting site also depends on airway wall stiffness, the maximal flow ($\dot{V}_{max}$) during forced expiration will be:

$$\dot{V}_{max} = A(A/\rho \cdot \Delta P/\Delta A)^{1/2}$$

The quantity $(A/\rho \cdot \Delta P/\Delta A)^{1/2t}$ is the speed that a small wave propagates in a compressible tube and is related to tube area (A), gas density (ρ), and tube wall stiffness (ΔP/ ΔA). The *wave speed theory* of flow limitation thus demonstrates that maximal flow is increased for airways with greater area or greater wall stiffness and gases of lower density.

Forced Expiratory Maneuver
(see Plate 2-11)

The magnitude of airflow during a forceful expiration from TLC to RV provides an indirect measure of the flow-resistive properties of the lung. This is because a maximal effort is not required to achieve maximal flow at intermediate and low lung volumes. Thus, parameters measured over most of a forced expiratory maneuver are little affected by suboptimal efforts and are good, albeit indirect, indexes of airway resistance. This so-called FVC maneuver is usually recorded as volume exhaled against time (*spirogram*). For clinical purposes, the volume exhaled during the first second (i.e., FEV_1) is measured and expressed as a ratio to FVC.

The FEV_1/FVC ratio is generally taken as an index of airway function; a decrease in FEV_1 below the normal range with less or no change in FVC is consistent with an obstructive disorder, (e.g., bronchial asthma, chronic bronchitis, emphysema). A normal FEV_1/FVC ratio in the presence of similar decrements of both FEV_1 and FVC may be taken as suggestive of a restrictive disorder (pulmonary fibrosis, obesity, neuromuscular disease), but it may occasionally occur in airflow obstruction, when the only abnormality is an increase in RV caused by airway closure. Therefore, the diagnosis of restrictive abnormality requires the measurement of TLC. The reduction of FEV_1 is generally taken as an estimate of severity for either obstructive or restrictive abnormalities as determined by spirometry.

A forced expiratory VC maneuver can be also displayed as airflow against expired volume. This plot, called *maximal expiratory flow-volume curve*, is particularly useful for quality control of forced expiratory maneuver. In obstructive disorders, the descending limb of the expiratory flow-volume curve shows an upward concavity, a shape that can be numerically described by taking instantaneous flows at specific lung volumes, such as 75%, 50%, and 25% of FVC, but their clinical significance is debated, and they should not be used for diagnosis.

Comparing tidal with forced expiratory flow-volume curves allows one to estimate the occurrence of expiratory flow limitation during breathing. This mechanism is responsible for dynamic lung hyperinflation, which is an increase of FRC above the relaxation volume of the system. When maximal flow is attained during tidal breathing because of bronchoconstriction or exercise hyperpnea, the only way to maintain or increase minute ventilation is to breathe at increased lung volume, at which greater expiratory flows can be generated. Occurrence or relief of dynamic lung hyperinflation and expiratory flow limitation during tidal breathing can be simply inferred from changes in inspiratory capacity (difference between FRC and TLC).

Flow limitation during tidal expiration may be present either in obstructive disorders because maximal flows are reduced or in restrictive disorders because breathing occurs at low lung volume. In restrictive disorders, all lung volumes are reduced, and flow is low throughout expiration even if, with respect to absolute lung volume, it may be greater than normal.

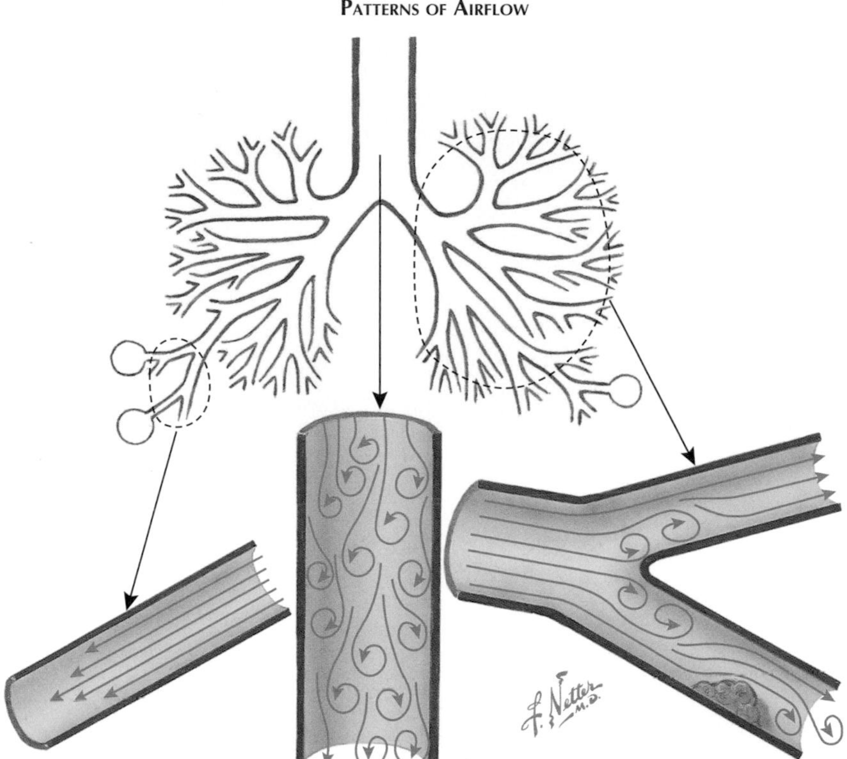

Laminar flow occurs mainly in small peripheral airways where rate of airflow through any airway is low. Driving pressure is proportional to gas viscosity

Turbulent flow occurs at high flow rates in trachea and larger airways. Driving pressure is proportional to square of flow and is dependent on gas density

Transitional flow occurs in larger airways, particularly at branches and at sites of narrowing. Driving pressure is proportional to both gas density and gas viscosity

Poiseuille's law. Resistance to laminar flow is inversely proportional to tube radius to the 4th power and directly proportional to length of tube. When radius is halved, resistance is increased 16-fold. If driving pressure is constant, flow will fall to one sixteenth. Doubling length only doubles resistance. If driving pressure is constant, flow will fall to one half

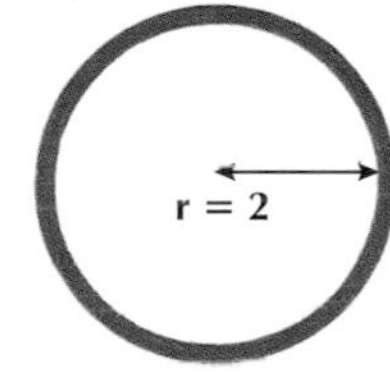

Resistance ~1

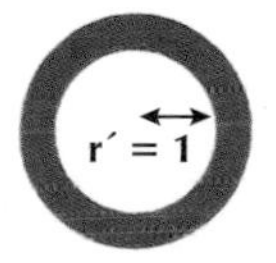

Resistance ~16

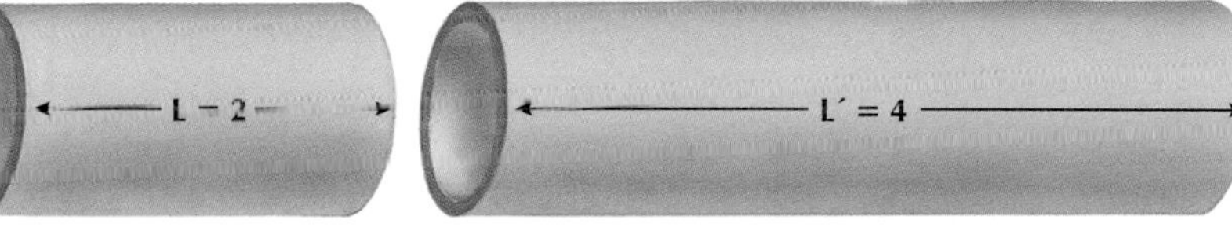

Resistance ~2

Resistance ~4

Dynamic Lung Compliance and Work of Breathing (see Plate 2-12)

Changes in lung volume and pleural pressure during a breathing cycle, displayed as a *pressure-volume loop*, describe elastic and flow-resistive properties of the lung as well as the work performed by the respiratory muscles on the lung.

At the end of both expiration and inspiration, airflow is zero; the difference in pleural pressure between these two points reflects the increasing elastic recoil as lung volume enlarges. The slope of the line connecting end-expiratory and end-inspiratory points on the pressure-volume loop provides a measure of *dynamic lung compliance*. In addition, during inspiration, the change in pleural pressure at any given lung volume reflects not only the pressure needed to overcome lung elastic recoil but also the pressure required to overcome airway and lung tissue resistances.

EXPIRATORY FLOW

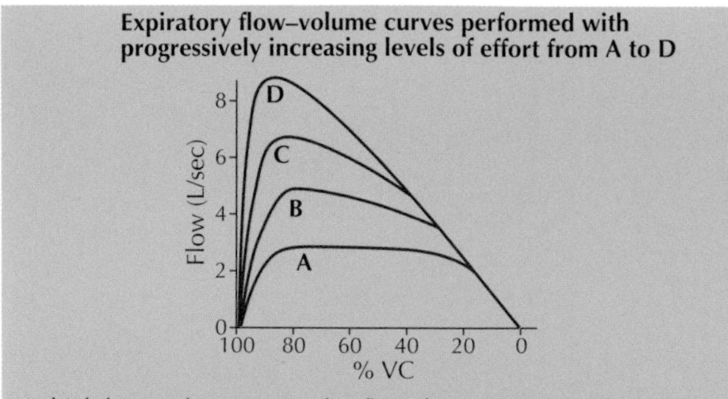

At high lung volumes, rate of airflow during expiration increases progressively with increasing effort. At intermediate and low lung volumes, airflow reaches maximal levels after only modest effort is exerted and thereafter increases no further despite increasing effort

Isovolume pressure–flow curves

At lung volumes greater than 75% of VC, airflow increases progressively with increasing pleural pressure. Airflow is effort dependent. At volumes below 75% of VC, airflow levels off as pleural pressure exceeds atmospheric pressure. Thereafter, airflow is effort independent because further increases in pleural pressure result in no further increase in rate of airflow

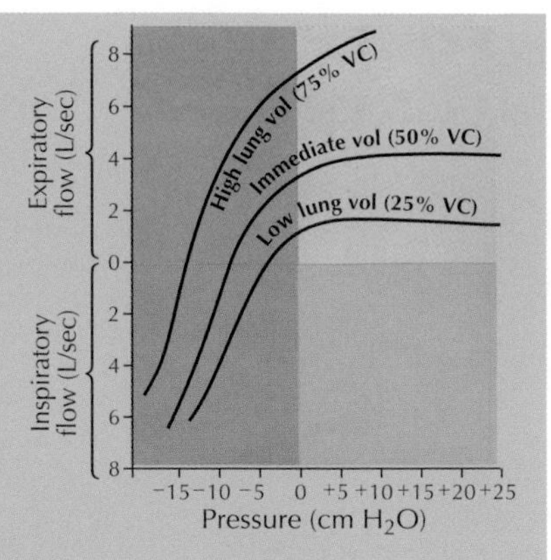

Determinants of maximal expiratory flow

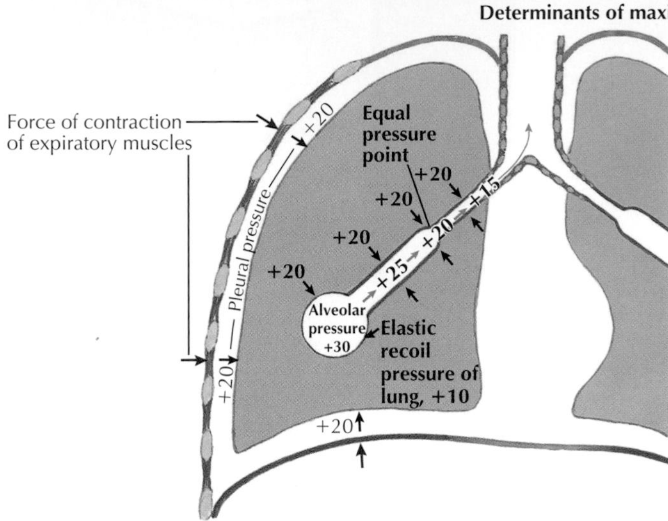

At onset of maximal airflow, contraction of expiratory muscles at a given lung volume raises pleural pressure above atmospheric level (+20 cm H_2O). Alveolar pressure (sum of pleural pressure and lung recoil pressure) is yet higher (+30 cm H_2O). Airway pressure falls progressively from alveolus to airway opening in overcoming resistance. At equal pressure point of airway, pressure within airway equals pressure surrounding it (pleural pressure). Beyond this point, as intraluminal pressure drops further below pleural pressure, airway will be compressed

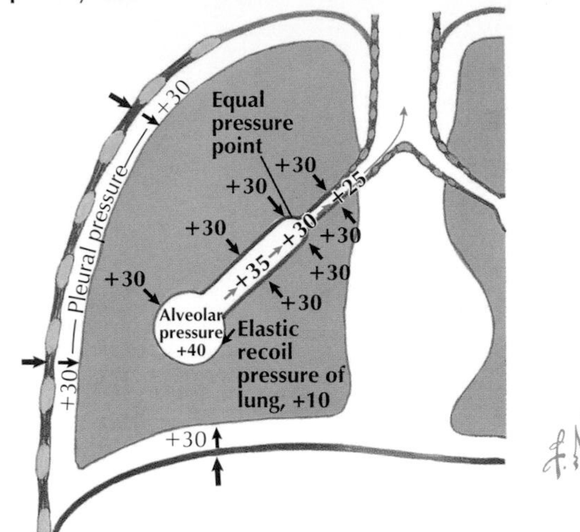

With further increases in expiratory effort, at same lung volume, pleural pressure is greater and alveolar pressure is correspondingly higher. Fall in airway pressure and location of equal pressure point are unchanged, but beyond equal pressure point, intrathoracic airways will be compressed to a greater degree by higher pleural pressure. Once maximal airflow is achieved, further increases in pleural pressure produce proportional increases in resistance of segment downstream from equal pressure point, so rate of airflow does not change

PULMONARY MECHANICS AND GAS EXCHANGE *(Continued)*

In normal individuals, dynamic lung compliance closely approximates static lung compliance and remains essentially unchanged when breathing frequency is increased up to 60 breaths/min. This is because lung units in parallel with each other normally fill and empty evenly and synchronously, even when airflow is high and lung volume changes rapidly. For the distribution of ventilation to parallel lung units to be independent of airflow, their time constants (i.e., the products of resistance and compliance) must be approximately equal. In the presence of uneven distribution of time constants, a given change in pleural pressure produces a smaller overall change in lung volume, and dynamic compliance decreases. However, because the time constants of lung units distal to airways with 2-mm diameter are on the order of 0.01 second, fourfold differences in time constants are necessary to cause dynamic compliance to decrease with increasing frequency. The frequency dependence of dynamic compliance is a time-consuming and technically difficult test, but it is sensitive to changes in peripheral airways when conventional measurements of lung mechanics (i.e., static compliance, overall airway resistance) are still within normal limits.

The mechanical *work of breathing* (W) performed by the respiratory muscles can be readily evaluated during spontaneous breathing from changes in pleural pressure (P) and lung volume (V) according to the equation:

$$W = \int PdV$$

During quiet breathing, lung elastic recoil is sufficient to overcome nonelastic forces during expiration, which is therefore passive. At high levels of ventilation or when airway resistance is increased, additional mechanical work may be required to overcome nonelastic forces during expiration; pleural pressure must exceed atmospheric pressure, and expiration is no longer passive.

The work of breathing at any given level of ventilation depends on the pattern of breathing. Whereas large TVs increase the elastic work of inspiration, high breathing frequencies increase the work against flow-resistive forces. During quiet breathing and exercise, individuals tend to adjust TV and breathing frequency at values that minimize the work of breathing. Patients with pulmonary fibrosis and increased elastic work of breathing tend to breathe shallowly and rapidly. Patients with airway obstruction tend to breathe at increased lung volume (dynamic lung hyperinflation) to minimize airway resistance, although this is associated with increased elastic work on inspiration.

From the point of view of energy requirements, the work of breathing can be considered as oxygen cost of breathing. In normal individuals, this is approximately 1 mL oxygen per liter of ventilation, which is less than 5% of total oxygen consumption but increases with increasing ventilation. Thus, the oxygen consumed by respiratory muscles can be inferred from the increase in total oxygen consumption when ventilation is increased, either voluntarily or in response to breathing carbon dioxide. Patients with pulmonary disorders demonstrate an increased oxygen cost of quiet

PULMONARY MECHANICS AND GAS EXCHANGE *(Continued)*

breathing as well as a disproportionate increase at elevated levels of ventilation.

Pleural Pressure Gradient and Closing Volume *(see Plate 2-13)*

In the upright position, pleural pressure is more negative with respect to atmospheric pressure at the apex of the lung than at the base. Pleural pressure increases by approximately 0.25 cm H_2O per centimeter of vertical distance from the top to the bottom of the lung because of the weight of the lung and the effects of gravity. Because of these differences in pleural pressure, the transpulmonary pressure is greater at the top than at the bottom of the lung, so at most lung volumes, the alveoli at the lung apices are more expanded than those at the lung bases.

At low lung volumes approaching RV, the pleural pressure at the bottom of the lung actually exceeds intraluminal airway pressure and leads to closure of peripheral airways at the lung bases. The first portion of a breath taken from RV thus enters alveoli at the lung apex. However, in the TV range and above, because of regional variations in lung compliance, ventilation per alveolus is greater at the bottom than at the top of the lung.

The distribution of ventilation and volume at which airways at the lung bases begin to close can be assessed by the *single-breath nitrogen washout and closing volume test* (see Plate 2-13). The concentration of nitrogen at the mouth is measured and plotted against expired lung volume after a single full inspiration of 100% oxygen from RV to TLC. The initial portion of the inspiration, which consists of dead-space gas rich in nitrogen, goes to the upper lung zones, and the remainder of the breath, containing only oxygen, is distributed preferentially to the lower lung zones. The result is that the concentration of oxygen in the alveoli of the lung bases is greater than in those of the lung apices.

During the subsequent expiration, the initial portion of the washout consists of dead space and contains no nitrogen (*phase I*). Then, as alveolar gas containing nitrogen begins to be washed out, the concentration of nitrogen in the expired air rises to reach a plateau. The portion of the curve where the concentration of nitrogen rises steeply is called *phase II*, and the plateau is referred to as *phase III*. Provided gas enters and leaves all regions of lung synchronously and equally, phase III will be flat. When the distribution of ventilation is nonuniform, gas coming from different alveoli will have different nitrogen concentrations, producing an increasing nitrogen concentration during phase III.

At low lung volumes, when the airways at the lung bases close, only the alveoli at the top of the lung continue to empty. Because the concentration of nitrogen in the alveoli of the upper lung zones is higher, the slope of the nitrogen-volume curve (*phase IV*) abruptly increases. The volume at which this increase in slope occurs is referred to as the *closing volume*.

With pathologic changes occurring in peripheral airways less than 2 to 3 mm in diameter, the closing volume and the slope of phase III increase. Although the single-breath nitrogen test is considered sensitive for early diagnosis of small airway disease, its specificity is low because loss of lung elastic recoil also increases the closing volume. This feature accounts for the progressive increase in closing volume seen with advancing age in normal individuals.

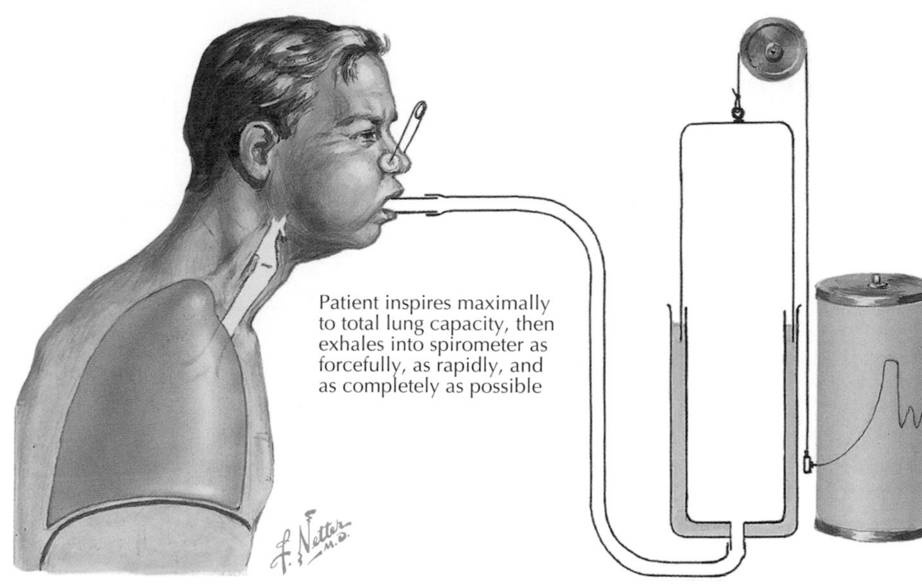

Forced Expiratory Vital Capacity Maneuver
Patient inspires maximally to total lung capacity, then exhales into spirometer as forcefully, as rapidly, and as completely as possible
F. Netter M.D.

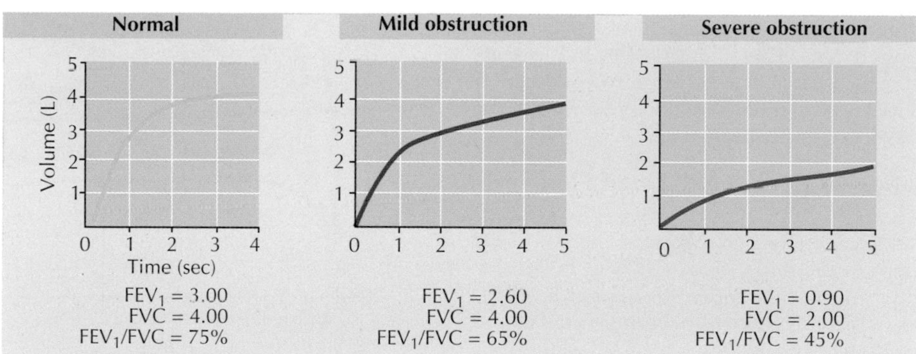

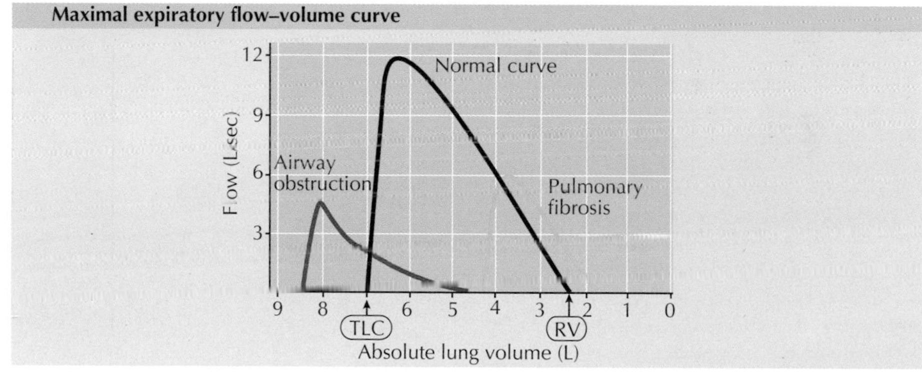

PULMONARY CIRCULATION

Mixed venous blood from the systemic circulation is collected in the right atrium and passes to the right ventricle (see Plate 2-14). Contraction of the right ventricle delivers the entire cardiac output along the pulmonary arteries to the capillary bed where gas exchange takes place. The pulmonary capillaries consist of a fine network of thin-walled vessels, but because the surface area of the capillary bed is approximately 70 m^2, it may be regarded as a sheet of flowing blood rather than as individual channels. At any one moment, the pulmonary capillary bed holds only about 100 mL of blood; most of the remainder of the blood in the pulmonary circulation is contained in the compliant pulmonary venules and veins which, along with the left atrium, serve as a reservoir for the left ventricle.

Intravascular Pressure

The systemic circulation distributes blood flow to various organs such as the muscles, kidneys, and gastrointestinal tract in response to their specific requirements. By contrast, the pulmonary circulation is concerned only with blood flow through the lungs. Pulmonary vascular pressures are very low compared with those in the systemic circulation; systolic pulmonary artery pressure is approximately 25 mm Hg, diastolic pressure is 8 mm Hg, and mean arterial pressure is about 14 mm Hg. Pressure in the left atrium is 5 mm Hg, only slightly less than the pressure in the large pulmonary veins. The pressure decrease across the entire pulmonary circulation—the difference

PULMONARY MECHANICS AND GAS EXCHANGE *(Continued)*

WORK OF BREATHING

A. Normal

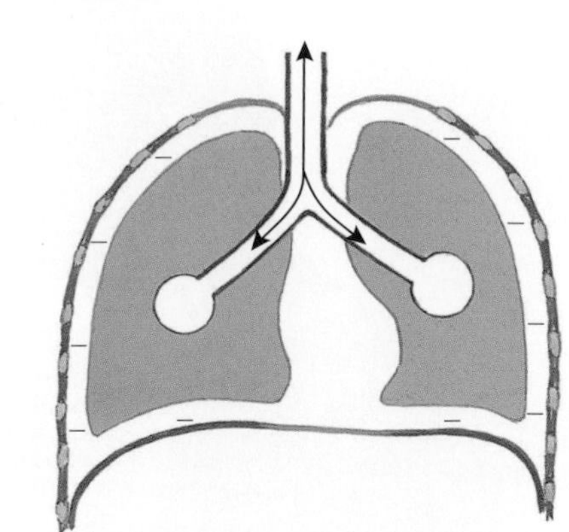

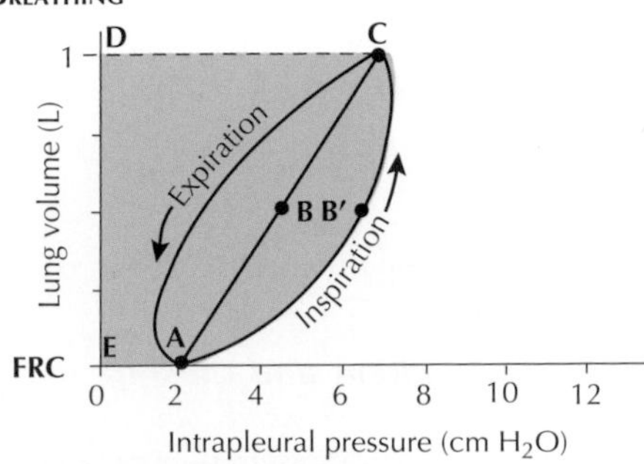

Work performed on lung during breathing can be determined from dynamic pressure–volume loop. Work to overcome elastic forces is represented by area of trapezoid EABCD. Additional work required to overcome flow resistance during inspiration is represented by area of right half of loop AB′CBA

B. Obstructive disease

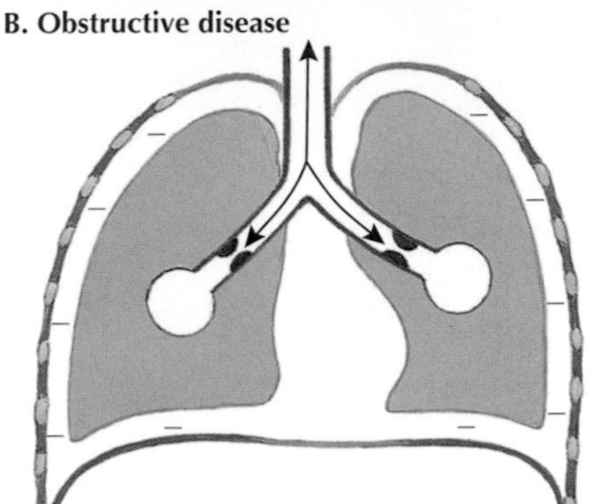

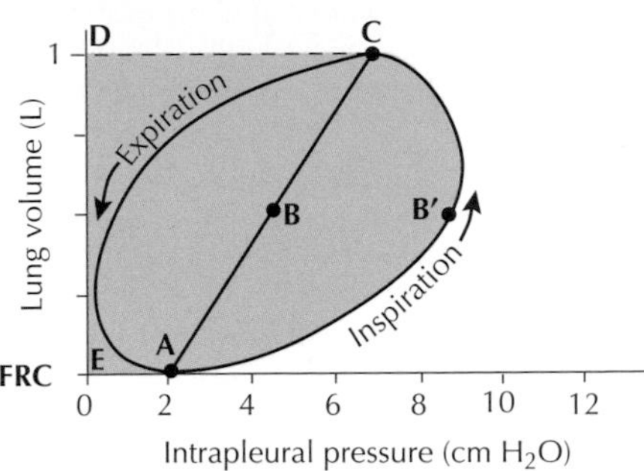

In disorders characterized by airway obstruction, work to overcome flow resistance is increased; elastic work of breathing remains unchanged

C. Restrictive disease

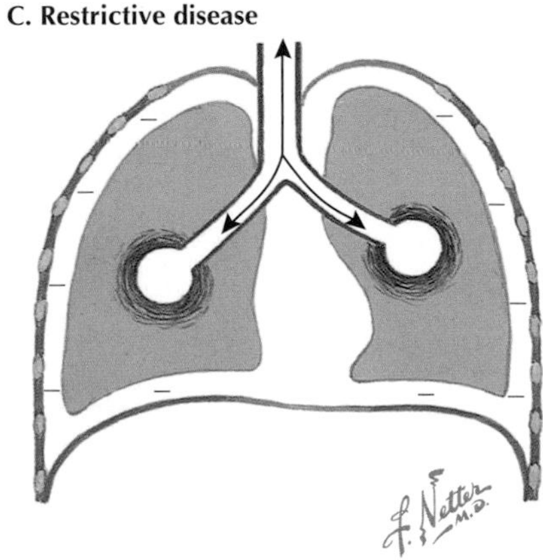

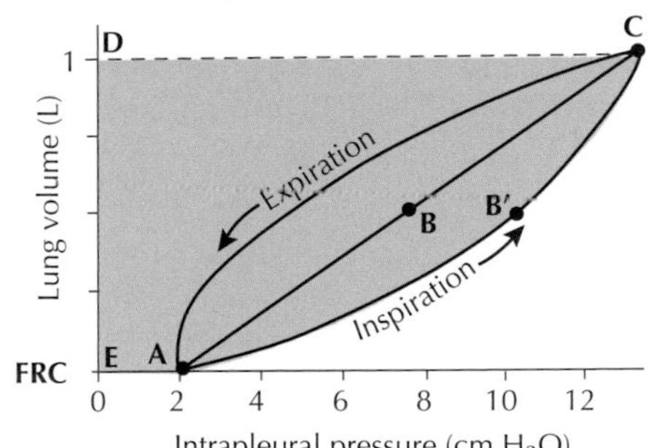

Restrictive lung diseases result in increase of elastic work of breathing; work to overcome flow resistance is normal

between mean pulmonary artery pressure and mean left atrial pressure—constitutes the driving pressure that produces blood flow through the lungs.

Blood Flow

Pulmonary capillary blood flow ($\dot{Q}c$) can be determined in a number of ways. The Fick method makes use of the principle that the rate of oxygen taken up by the blood ($\dot{V}_{O_2}$) as it passes through the lungs is given by the product of $\dot{Q}c$. The difference in oxygen content between arterial and mixed venous blood (Ca_{O_2} and Cv_{O_2}, respectively) $\dot{Q}c$ can thus be calculated as:

$$\dot{Q}c = \frac{\dot{V}_{O_2}}{Ca_{O_2} - Cv_{O_2}}$$

$\dot{Q}c$ can also be measured by the thermodilution and indicator dilution techniques, in which a tracer substance is injected into the venous system, and its concentration in the arterial blood is recorded as a function of time. The Fick and dilution methods measure blood flow averaged over many heartbeats.

Distribution of Pulmonary Blood Flow

(see Plate 2-14)

Gravity has a major effect on the distribution of blood flow throughout the lungs, causing flow to be greater at the bottom than at the top in the upright position. Blood flow is also influenced by the resistance of the vascular pathway it must traverse in moving from artery to vein, and this resistance tends to increase with path length. This causes the pattern of blood flow distribution to decrease with distance from the hilum of the lung. Blood flow becomes more evenly distributed in the supine position and during exercise.

Normally, pulmonary artery pressure is just sufficient to deliver blood to the lung apices at rest. Consequently, a decrease in hydrostatic pressure produced by hemorrhage or shock may lower intravascular pressure at the lung apex below alveolar pressure, causing the highly compliant alveolar blood vessels to become compressed even to the point of complete occlusion. Under these circumstances, this area at the lung apex is called zone 1. Farther down the lung, there is a region called zone 2 within which pulmonary artery pressure is greater than alveolar pressure because of the hydrostatic gradient, but where alveolar pressure is still greater than venous pressure. Still farther down the lung, gravity increases hydrostatic vascular pressures to the point that venous pressure exceeds alveolar pressure. Within this region, known as zone 3, blood flow is determined principally by the difference between pulmonary arterial and venous pressures. Descending through zone 3, the transmural pressure across the capillary wall increases, which causes distension of already open vessels and recruitment of new ones, leading to an increase in flow. Finally, at the very bottom of the lung, these effects are offset by a decrease in the outward elastic recoil forces exerted by the parenchyma on the extraalveolar vessel walls, and overall pulmonary vascular resistance increases again.

Pulmonary Vascular Resistance

Pulmonary vascular resistance (see Plate 2-15) is calculated from the decrease in blood pressure across the pulmonary circulation (i.e., the difference between mean pulmonary artery pressure and mean left atrial pressure) and $\dot{Q}c$ according to the vascular equivalent of Ohm's law for electric circuits. That is:

$$\text{Pulmonary vascular resistance} = \frac{\text{Pressure drop}}{\dot{Q}_c}$$

Blood flow through the pulmonary circulation is essentially the same as that through the systemic circulation, yet the pressure drop across the pulmonary circulation is only one-tenth that across the systemic circulation. It follows that pulmonary vascular resistance is one-tenth of the systemic resistance. The major sites of pulmonary vascular resistance are the arterioles and capillaries.

The pulmonary circulation is able to accommodate several fold increases in $\dot{Q}_c$, such as occur during exercise, with only small changes in pulmonary artery pressure. This means that as $\dot{Q}c$ increases, pulmonary vascular resistance must decrease. There are two principal mechanisms by which this occurs; blood vessels already conducting blood increase their caliber, and vessels that were previously closed are recruited to increase the number of vessels transporting blood in parallel.

Pulmonary blood vessels are extremely thin walled and compliant, so their caliber is greatly influenced by transmural pressure (i.e., the difference in pressure inside and outside the vessel wall). The smallest pulmonary capillaries are surrounded by alveoli and thus are subjected externally to alveolar pressure. Increases in alveolar pressure produced, for example, by positive-pressure mechanical ventilation can compress these vessels to the point of closure. Even increases in lung volume during spontaneous breathing tend to increase the resistance of these alveolar vessels because the

Pulmonary Mechanics and Gas Exchange *(Continued)*

longitudinal stretching that occurs causes the vessel walls to approach each other. By contrast, larger blood vessels are tethered outwardly by the lung parenchyma, which acts like a spring to hold the vessels open. The parenchymal attachments effectively apply pleural pressure to the outside of the vessel wall. Consequently, as lung volume increases, the outward pull on these extraalveolar vessels also increases, causing the vessels to dilate and their resistance to decrease. Overall pulmonary vascular resistance is probably lowest at FRC.

Factors Affecting the Pulmonary Vascular Bed

A variety of neural stimuli as well as chemical and humoral substances can affect the pulmonary vascular bed (see Plate 2-15). Pulmonary blood vessels are innervated by both sympathetic and parasympathetic nerves, but under normal circumstances in humans, the autonomic nervous system has virtually no role in determining pulmonary vascular resistance. Hypoxemia, on the other hand, is a potent stimulus that constricts both precapillary and postcapillary vessels. This effect is independent of neural and humoral mechanisms because it can be demonstrated even in the isolated lung. The effects of hypercapnia on the pulmonary vasculature are variable and appear to depend on changes in hydrogen ion concentration. Acidosis, whether respiratory or metabolic, increases pulmonary vascular tone, and acidosis and hypoxemia together are considered to act synergistically in constricting pulmonary vessels and increasing pulmonary vascular resistance. Chemical and humoral agents that produce pulmonary vasoconstriction include epinephrine, norepinephrine, histamine, angiotensin, and endothelin-1. Bradykinin, acetylcholine, nitric oxide, and prostacyclin cause vasodilatation.

Pulmonary vascular resistance may be increased by various cardiopulmonary disorders. Pulmonary fibrosis, characterized by a diffuse increase in fibrous tissue in the lung, obliterates and compresses pulmonary capillaries. Pulmonary emboli directly obstruct pulmonary arteries and arterioles and may produce secondary vasoconstriction through the release of vasoactive substances. Idiopathic pulmonary arterial hypertension leads to remodeling of pulmonary blood vessels, thickening their walls and decreasing luminal caliber. These disorders cause the heart to have to exert increased forces of contraction to maintain blood flow through the lungs, which can lead eventually to hypertrophy, strain, and ultimately failure of the right ventricle.

DIFFUSION

Oxygen and carbon dioxide pass between the alveoli and the pulmonary capillary blood by *diffusion*, the passive tendency of molecules to move down a partial pressure gradient (see Plate 2-16). This tendency is a manifestation of the second law of thermodynamics, which states, in essence, that nature always wants to spread energy and matter around in the most even way possible.

Partial Pressure

When a gas is composed of a mixture of different molecules, each molecular species contributes to the total gas pressure in proportion to its relative number of molecules. Thus, for example, in a gas at a pressure of 760 mm Hg (1 atm) in which 80% of the molecules are nitrogen and 20% are oxygen, the partial pressure of nitrogen is $0.8 \times 760 = 608$ mm Hg, and the partial pressure of oxygen is the remainder at $760 - 608 = 152$ mm Hg. When molecules of a gas are dissolved in a liquid, they obviously do not exert a physical pressure by impacting against the walls of the container as when they are in the gas phase. Nevertheless, a dissolved gas still has a partial pressure, which is defined as its partial pressure in the gas phase when the liquid and gas phases have come into dynamic equilibrium.

Transport to the Blood-Gas Barrier

After air enters the mouth and nose during inspiration, it moves through the conducting airways of the lung by convection. That is, bulk gas flow is driven along the airways under the influence of a pressure gradient. The airways continue to divide as they progress into the lung, which increases their combined cross-section at a geometric rate. Eventually, at about the level of the alveolar duct, the effective airway cross is so large that bulk flow becomes negligible. Thereafter, inspired gas molecules mix with resident alveolar gas and make their way to the blood-gas barrier largely by diffusion. The diffusion rate in the gas phase is inversely proportional to molecular weight because light molecules move more quickly, so they experience more frequent collisions than do heavy molecules. Gaseous diffusion of oxygen (molecular weight, 32) is thus faster than that of carbon dioxide (molecular weight, 44).

The distance over which gases have to diffuse to reach the blood-gas barrier is small in normal alveoli, and complete mixing of newly inspired air with resident gas occurs within a fraction of a second. This

Pleural Pressure Gradient and Closing Volume

Pleural pressure gradient. Pleural pressure in upright position is more subatmospheric at top of lung and increases down lung consequent to weight of lung and force of gravity

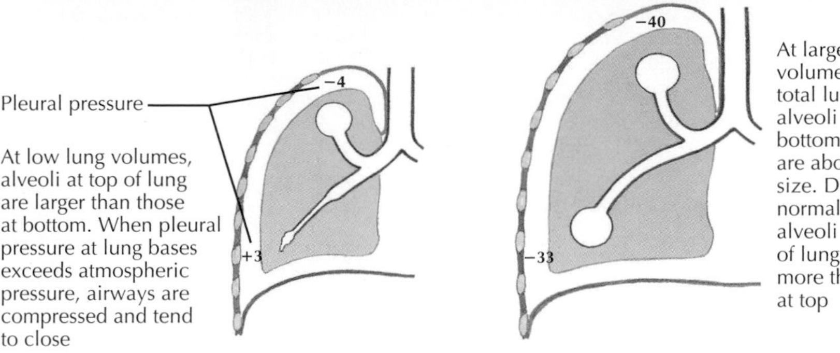
Pleural pressure
−4
+3
At low lung volumes, alveoli at top of lung are larger than those at bottom. When pleural pressure at lung bases exceeds atmospheric pressure, airways are compressed and tend to close
−40
−33
At large lung volumes near total lung capacity, alveoli at top and bottom of lung are about same size. During normal breathing, alveoli at bottom of lung expand more than those at top

Closing volume. A single full breath of 100% O_2 is inhaled from residual volume to total lung capacity. Initial portion of breath (dead-space air, rich in N_2) enters alveoli in upper lung zones. Remainder of breath (O_2 only) preferentially goes to lower lung zones, so concentration N_2 is lower in alveoli of lung bases. During subsequent expiration, concentration of N_2 at mouth is plotted against expired lung volume

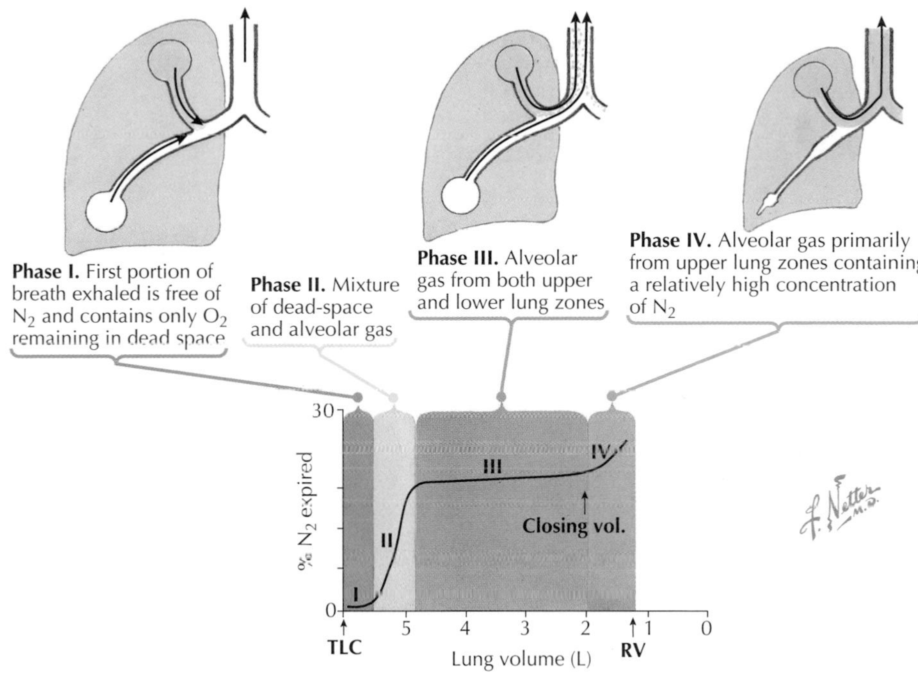
Phase I. First portion of breath exhaled is free of N2 and contains only O2 remaining in dead space
Phase II. Mixture of dead-space and alveolar gas
Phase III. Alveolar gas from both upper and lower lung zones
Phase IV. Alveolar gas primarily from upper lung zones containing a relatively high concentration of N2
30
0
% N2 expired
I
II
III
IV
Closing vol.
TLC
5
4
3
2
1
0
RV
Lung volume (L)
F. Netter M.D.

Pulmonary Mechanics and Gas Exchange *(Continued)*

is effectively instantaneous over the time scale of breathing. By contrast, when the alveolar spaces are enlarged as occurs in emphysema, the diffusive transport time may be prolonged to the point of becoming a limiting factor in gas transfer.

Membrane Diffusion

Gas transfer across the alveolar-capillary membrane involves diffusion between gas and liquid phases, as well as diffusion within the liquid phase. The rates at which these processes occur depends on the solubility of the gas in the liquid. As a result, carbon dioxide diffuses across the blood-gas barrier approximately 20 times more rapidly than oxygen because, despite its greater molecular weight, carbon dioxide is considerably more soluble in water than is oxygen.

Barriers to Diffusion

There are a sequence of barriers that oxygen and carbon dioxide must cross to move between alveolus and blood. These are collectively known as the blood-gas barrier and include the fluid layer that lines the alveoli, the alveolar epithelium and its underlying basement membrane, a region of interstitial fluid, the capillary endothelium, a layer of plasma in the capillary blood, and the red blood cell membrane. Oxygen traverses these individual barriers in the order just cited, and carbon dioxide crosses them in reverse.

Alveolar-Capillary Partial Pressure Gradients

The rate at which gas molecules move by diffusion, either in the gas phase or when dissolved in a liquid, is proportional to the local partial pressure gradient of the gas. The difference in the partial pressures of oxygen (Po_2) between alveolar air and pulmonary capillary blood is greatest at the beginning of the capillary where venous blood enters with a Po_2 of about 40 mm Hg. Oxygen moves down its concentration gradient from alveolus to capillary blood, causing the Po_2 of the blood to increase as it moves past the blood-gas barrier. The alveolar Po_2 does not fall at the same rate because the combined oxygen storage capacity of the alveoli is much greater than that of the blood adjacent to the blood-gas barrier. The transit time of blood through the pulmonary capillaries is brief (only 0.75 sec). However, in normal lungs, the diffusion of oxygen across the blood-gas barrier is so rapid that the Po_2 of the blood reaches that of the alveolar air before the blood has passed even halfway along the alveolar capillaries. For this reason, oxygen transport in healthy lungs is not diffusion limited.

Physical activity increases pulmonary blood flow and decreases the transit time of blood through the pulmonary capillaries. Normally, the diffusion reserve of the lung is so great that the alveolar air and capillary blood reach virtual equilibrium with respect to Po_2 even in the reduced time available for gas transfer during heavy exercise. Certain diseases, however, may compromise the diffusive capacity of the blood-gas barrier, either by thickening it such as occurs in pulmonary edema and fibrosis or by decreasing its total area as occurs in emphysema. Exchange of oxygen may then become diffusion limited during exercise and even at rest in extreme cases.

Distribution of Pulmonary Blood Flow

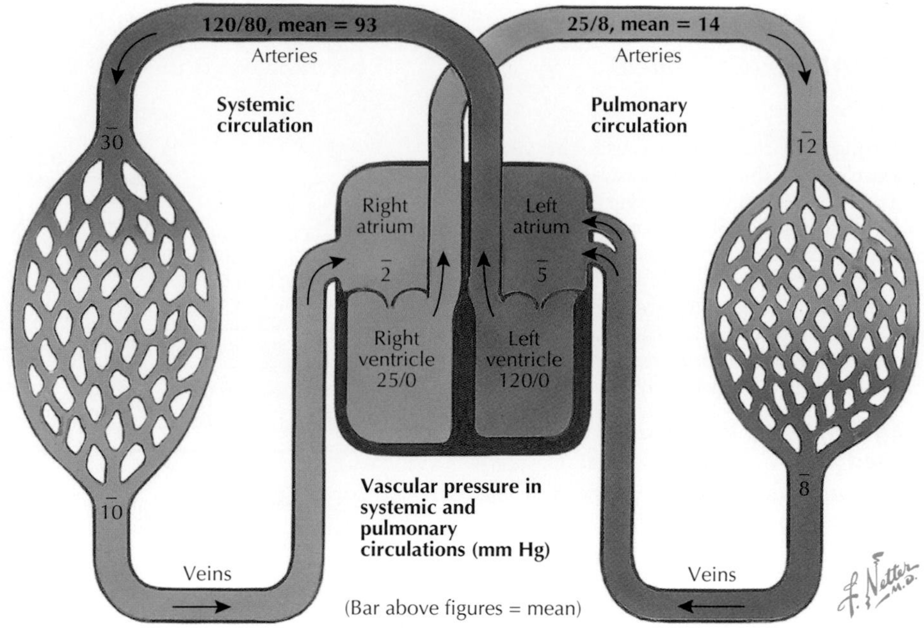

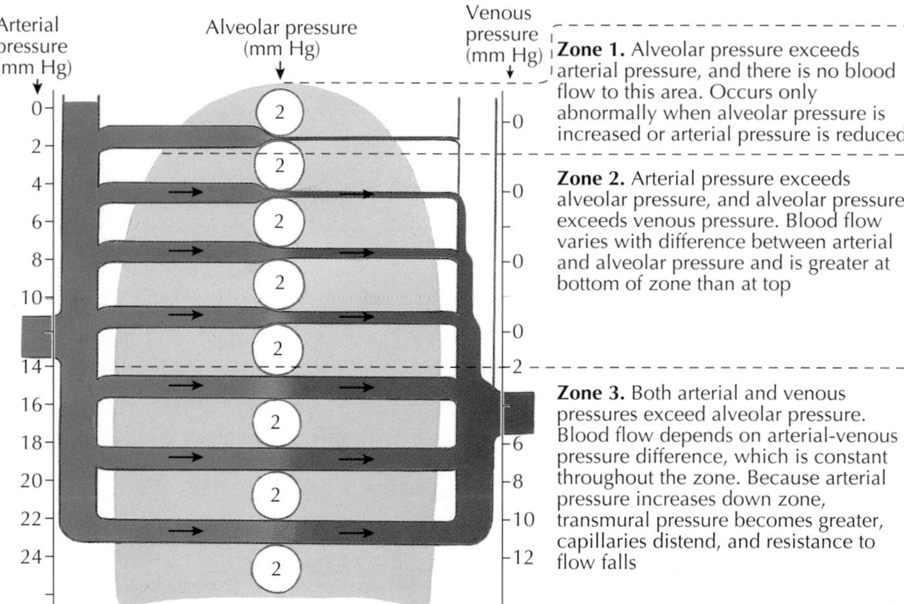

Arterial pressure (mm Hg)
Alveolar pressure (mm Hg)
Venous pressure (mm Hg)
0
2
4
6
8
10
14
16
18
20
22
24
2
0
2
6
8
10
12
Zone 1. Alveolar pressure exceeds arterial pressure, and there is no blood flow to this area. Occurs only abnormally when alveolar pressure is increased or arterial pressure is reduced
Zone 2. Arterial pressure exceeds alveolar pressure, and alveolar pressure exceeds venous pressure. Blood flow varies with difference between arterial and alveolar pressure and is greater at bottom of zone than at top
Zone 3. Both arterial and venous pressures exceed alveolar pressure. Blood flow depends on arterial-venous pressure difference, which is constant throughout the zone. Because arterial pressure increases down zone, transmural pressure becomes greater, capillaries distend, and resistance to flow falls

The diffusion rate of carbon dioxide across the blood-gas barrier greatly exceeds that of oxygen, so the time required for equilibrium between alveolar air and capillary blood is correspondingly less. Thus, even when diffusion is considerably impaired, the alveolar-arterial partial pressure gradient for carbon dioxide remains small.

Diffusing Capacity and Its Components

The diffusing capacity of the lung is a measure of the ease with which a gas is able to move from the alveoli to the capillary blood and is defined as the flow of gas normalized to its mean partial pressure gradient across the blood-gas barrier. As explained above, the diffusion of oxygen and carbon dioxide across the blood-gas barrier is so efficient that under almost all conditions, the partial pressure gradients of both gases are obliterated by the time the pulmonary blood leaves the alveolar capillaries. This means that the diffusing capacity for these gases only becomes a rate-limited step in gas transport in cases of extreme pathology, such as severe emphysema or pulmonary edema. Consequently, monitoring the rate of uptake of oxygen into the lungs or the rate of production of carbon dioxide provides essentially no information about pathologic processes that may be starting to affect the physical properties of the blood-gas barrier, such as early emphysema. Thus, neither oxygen nor carbon dioxide is limited by its rates of diffusion across the blood-gas barrier and so cannot be used to measure the diffusing capacity of the lungs. There is, however, another gas that can be used for this purpose, namely carbon monoxide.

Hemoglobin has such an enormous affinity for carbon monoxide that its stores are never saturated, which means that when carbon monoxide is inhaled

PULMONARY MECHANICS AND GAS EXCHANGE *(Continued)*

into the lungs, its partial pressure (P_{CO}) in the pulmonary capillary blood never increases to the point of obliterating the alveolar-capillary partial pressure gradient. In fact, P_{CO} in the blood remains so low that it can essentially be ignored. This property is what makes carbon monoxide so dangerous, but here it can be used to advantage. Specifically, the diffusing capacity of the lung for carbon monoxide ($D_{L_{CO}}$) is reflected only in the rate of uptake of carbon monoxide into the lungs ($\dot{V}_{CO}$) and its mean alveolar partial pressure ($P_{\bar{A}_{CO}}$) according to the equation:

$$D_{L_{CO}} = \frac{\dot{V}_{CO}}{P_{\bar{A}_{CO}}}$$

$D_{L_{CO}}$ can be measured by having a subject take a single full inspiration of a very low concentration of carbon monoxide followed by a 10-second breath-hold and then a full expiration. The partial pressure of carbon monoxide measured during expiration gives $P_{\bar{A}_{CO}}$, and the difference between inspired and expired concentrations multiplied by the total expired volume gives $\dot{V}_{CO}$ relative to the duration of the maneuver. This method is relatively simple, but breath-holding may be difficult for patients with lung disease who are dyspneic. An alternative approach is to have the subject breathe quietly and continuously from a very dilute mixture until the rate of uptake of carbon monoxide into the lungs is constant, as determined from continuous measurement of P_{CO} at the mouth. The accuracy of the measurement of $D_{L_{CO}}$ depends on how accurately the alveolar carbon monoxide concentration is determined and is improved if measurements are made during exercise.

$D_{L_{CO}}$ has units of conductance (the inverse of resistance), so it provides a measure of the ease with which carbon monoxide can diffuse from the alveolus into the blood. The resistance to this diffusion (inverse of $D_{L_{CO}}$) has two components, a membrane component and an intravascular component. The *membrane component* of diffusion resistance increases when the alveolar walls are damaged (emphysema) or when pulmonary blood flow is obstructed (pulmonary embolism, vascular disease) because these conditions reduce the effective area across which diffusion can occur. Diffusion resistance is also increased by increases in the thickness of the blood-gas barrier. This thickening may occur within the tissue portion of the barrier caused by conditions such as interstitial pulmonary edema, fibrosis, intraalveolar edema, and consolidation. Effective tissue thickening may also occur within the blood portion if the diffusion distance across the plasma increases because of either dilatation of the pulmonary capillaries or scarcity of red blood cells (hemodilution). The *intravascular component* of the resistance to diffusion results from the finite reaction time required for oxygen to bind to hemoglobin and depends on the density of red blood cells in the pulmonary capillaries and their hemoglobin concentration (see Plate 2-20).

GAS EXCHANGE

Properties of Gases

Gases in the lung, including oxygen, carbon dioxide, and nitrogen, obey the perfect gas law:

PULMONARY VASCULAR RESISTANCE

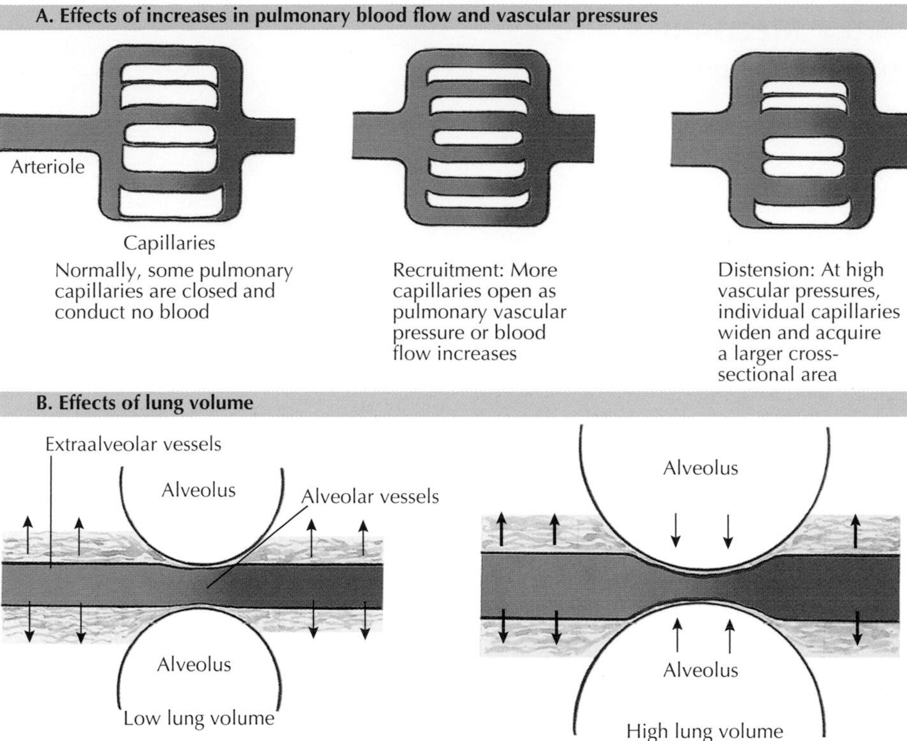

As lung volume increases, increasing traction on extraalveolar capillaries produces distension, and their resistance falls. Alveolar vessels, in contrast, are compressed by enlarging alveoli, and their resistance increases

C. Effects of chemical and humoral substances

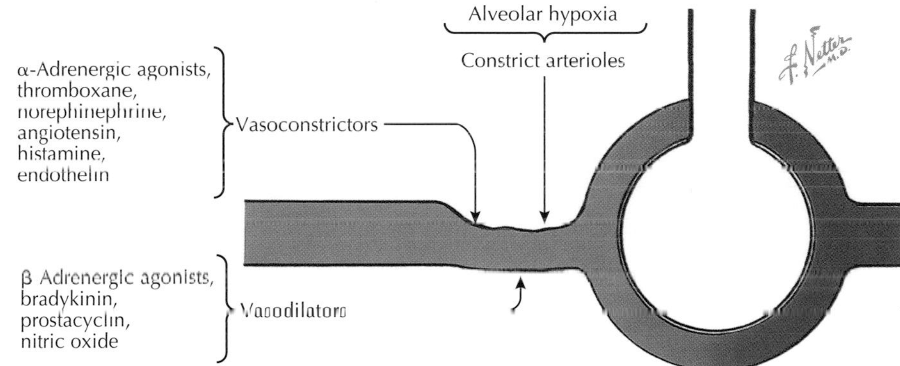

$$PV = nrT$$

where P is pressure, V is volume, n is the number of gas molecules, r is the gas constant, and T is the absolute temperature. The perfect gas law is the general expression from which, for a fixed value of n, three other famous laws of gases follow. For example, if T is kept constant, then V varies inversely with P, a relationship known as Boyle's law. Similarly, if P is held fixed, then V is proportional to T, which is Charles' law. Finally, Gay-Lussac's law is obtained by holding V constant and seeing that P varies directly with T.

At sea level, the total pressure of atmospheric air is 760 mm Hg. The major constituents of air are nitrogen with a partial pressure of about 593 mm Hg and oxygen with a partial pressure of about 160 mm Hg. The remaining approximately 1% of air is comprised of carbon dioxide (<1 mm Hg), water vapor, and inert gases such as argon and neon.

Inspired atmospheric air is warmed and humidified as it passes through the nasopharynx and tracheobronchial tree. These structures are very efficient exchangers of heat and water vapor so that by the time inspired air reaches the alveoli, it has been heated to body temperature and become fully saturated. At body temperature, regardless of barometric pressure, the saturated partial pressure of water vapor is 47 mm Hg. Thus, if the air entering the trachea is completely dry, by the time it reaches the alveoli, it will have a partial pressure of 760 − 47 = 713 mm Hg, the remainder being the 47 mm Hg of water vapor.

Ventilation, Oxygen Uptake, and Carbon Dioxide Output

When inspired gas reaches the alveoli, it is separated from the pulmonary capillary blood only by the extremely thin blood-gas barrier across which diffusive transfer of oxygen and carbon dioxide occurs (see Plate

PULMONARY MECHANICS AND GAS EXCHANGE *(Continued)*

2-16). Oxygen is continuously removed from the alveolar gas, and carbon dioxide is continuously added. Ventilation serves to maintain alveolar gas composition by replenishing oxygen from and eliminating carbon dioxide to the atmosphere. The composition of alveolar gas thus depends on the balance between alveolar ventilation ($\dot{V}_E$) and pulmonary capillary blood flow ($\dot{Q}_c$) and varies slightly over the breathing cycle. Normally, mean alveolar P_{CO_2} and P_{O_2} are approximately 100 mm Hg and 40 mm Hg, respectively.

Pulmonary capillary blood normally removes oxygen from the lungs at a greater rate than it delivers carbon dioxide to the lungs. The ratio of carbon dioxide output to oxygen uptake is called the *respiratory exchange ratio* and is normally about 0.8. A related quantity is the ratio of the rate at which carbon dioxide is produced to the rate at which oxygen is used by the body's cells, known as the *respiratory quotient*. Whereas the respiratory quotient is determined by cellular metabolism and is affected by the nature of the diet, the respiratory exchange ratio is affected by the pattern of breathing. The two ratios may be different transiently, but under steady-state conditions, they must be identical to maintain the oxygen and carbon dioxide stores of the body constant.

The quantity of carbon dioxide in inspired air is normally negligible, so the amount of carbon dioxide eliminated per minute ($\dot{V}_{CO_2}$) can be calculated considering only the expired minute ventilation ($\dot{V}_E$) and the fraction of carbon dioxide in the expired air (F_{ECO_2}) according to the equation:

$$\dot{V}_{CO_2} = \dot{V}_E \times F_{ECO_2}$$

In contrast, significant quantities of oxygen are present in both inspired and expired air, so oxygen uptake is determined from the difference in the amounts of oxygen in inspired and expired air by means of the equation:

$$\dot{V}_{O_2} = (\dot{V}_I \times F_{IO_2}) - (\dot{V}_E \times F_{EO_2})$$

where $\dot{V}_{O_2}$ is the oxygen uptake per minute, F_{IO_2} is the fraction of oxygen in inspired air, and F_{EO_2} is the concentration of oxygen in mixed expired air.

Dead Space

The minute ventilation ($\dot{V}_E$) (i.e., the total volume of air inspired into the lungs each minute) is the product of the tidal volume (V_T) and the breathing frequency (f) in breaths per minute,

$$\dot{V}_E = V_T \times f$$

The entire $\dot{V}_E$, however, does not participate in gas exchange. A portion of each V_T remains in the mouth, nose, pharynx, larynx, trachea, bronchi, and bronchioles, so it does not make it all the way down to the alveoli. This volume is called the *anatomic dead space* and is numerically approximately equal in milliliters to an individual's ideal body weight in pounds (i.e., about 150 mL in a typical adult). In addition, some inspired air reaches alveoli that are not in contact with pulmonary capillary blood. This volume of air does not participate in gas exchange and is called the *alveolar dead space*. The sum of the anatomic and alveolar dead spaces is termed the *physiologic dead space*, with volume V_D. In a normal lung, the alveolar dead space is very small, so the anatomic and physiologic dead spaces are virtually identical and equal about one-third of V_T at rest. The remaining two-thirds of V_T, the alveolar component (V_A), ventilates alveoli perfused by pulmonary capillary blood and so participates directly in gas exchange and contributes to maintaining alveolar gas composition. V_T thus consists of two components according to:

$$V_T = V_D + V_A$$

Alveolar minute ventilation is then the volume of fresh gas reaching the alveoli each minute, given by:

$$\dot{V}_A = (V_T - V_D) \times f$$

The partial pressure of carbon dioxide in the dead-space gas is the same as that in inspired air and is virtually zero. Consequently, when the gas from an entire expiration is collected in a single container, the dead-space gas dilutes the alveolar gas. This causes the mole fraction (ratio of partial pressure to total gas pressure) of carbon dioxide in mixed expired air ($F_{\bar{E}CO_2}$) to be lower than the fraction in alveolar gas (F_{ACO_2}). $F_{\bar{E}CO_2}$ can be determined by analyzing the mixed expired gas, and F_{ACO_2} can be determined from the gas exiting the lungs at the end of an expiration. The total amount of carbon dioxide (measured as volume of pure gas at standard temperature and pressure) leaving the lungs in a single expiration can thus be calculated in two ways—as the product of V_T and $F_{\bar{E}CO_2}$ or as the product of (V_T − V_D) and F_{ACO_2}. The Bohr method for estimating dead space equates these two products to give:

$$V_D = V_T\left(\frac{F_{ACO_2} - F_{\bar{E}CO_2}}{F_{ACO_2}}\right)$$

PATHWAYS AND TRANSFERS OF O_2 AND CO_2

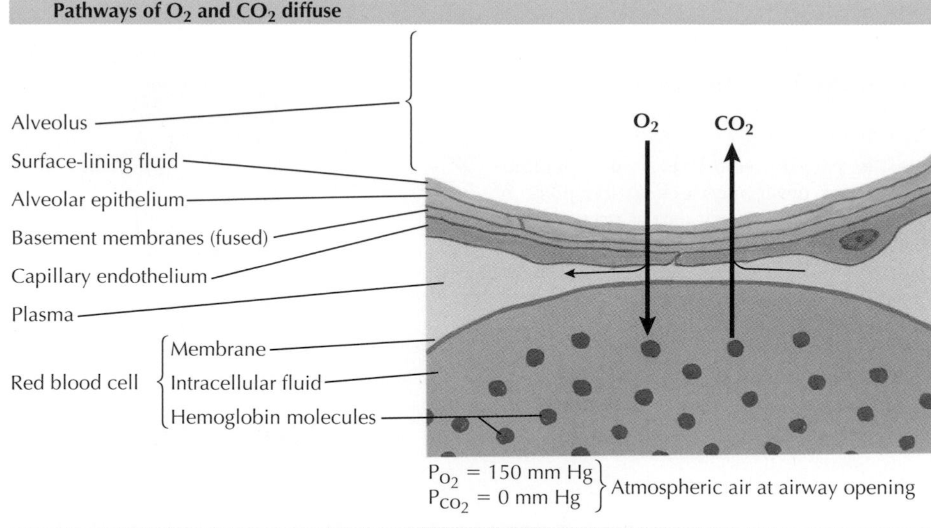

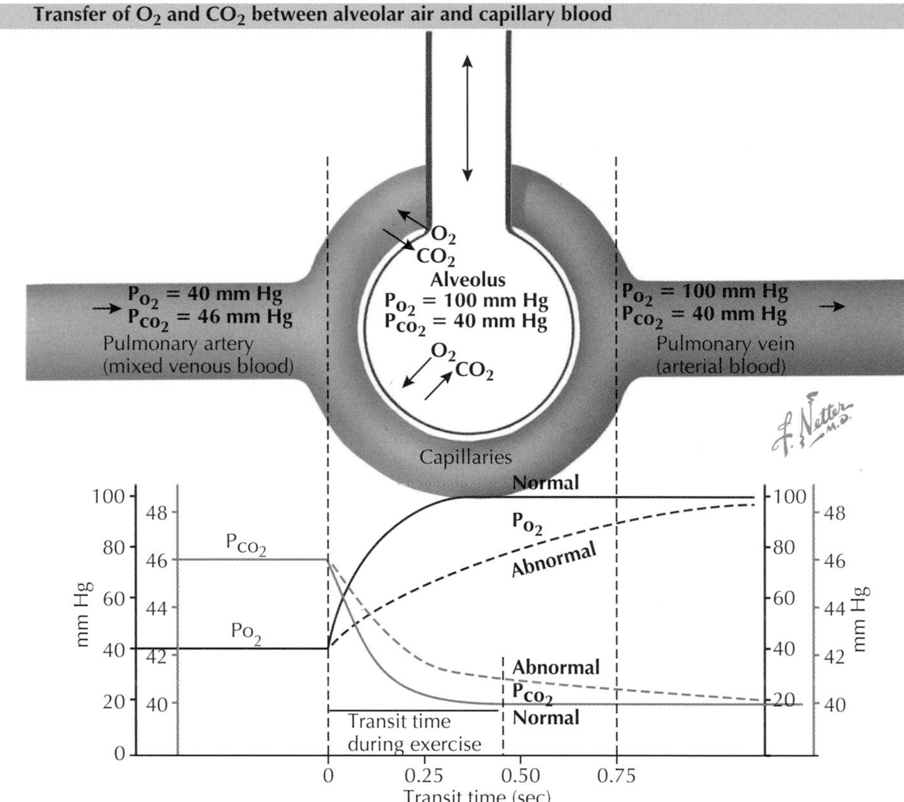

PULMONARY MECHANICS AND GAS EXCHANGE *(Continued)*

Because dead-space gas contains no carbon dioxide, the volume of carbon dioxide eliminated from the lungs each minute ($\dot{V}_{CO_2}$) can be expressed in terms of $\dot{V}_A$ and F_{ACO_2} thus:

$$\dot{V}_{CO_2} = \dot{V}_A \times F_{ACO_2}$$

Finally, F_{ACO_2} is proportional to the partial pressure of carbon dioxide in alveolar gas, which is essentially the same as that in arterial blood (P_{aCO_2}). This means that P_{aCO_2} is determined by the balance between metabolic activity and alveolar ventilation.

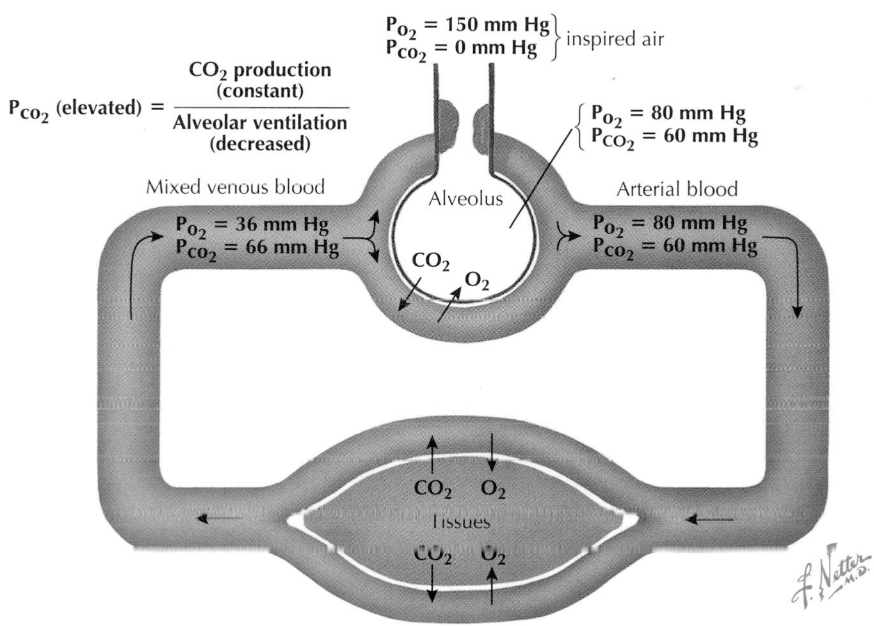

ALVEOLAR HYPOVENTILATION

When $\dot{V}_A$ decreases below that required by the metabolic activity of the body, the result is a condition known as alveolar hypoventilation (see Plate 2-17). When this happens, the rates of transfer of oxygen to the blood and carbon dioxide from the blood are not sufficient to maintain normal partial pressures within the alveolar gas, so P_{AO_2} decreases and P_{ACO_2} increases. The most immediate consequence of alveolar hypoventilation is an increase in the carbon dioxide content of the blood. The oxygen-carrying capacity of the blood is less sensitive to decreased alveolar ventilation, but oxygen content also decreases if hypoventilation is severe enough.

Alveolar hypoventilation can be produced for brief periods of time by a conscious decision to suppress breathing. In pathologic situations, it can be caused by a variety of factors. Trauma to the lungs or chest, for example, may render the respiratory pump ineffectual. Hypoventilation may also result when the central nervous system is depressed by the administration of narcotics, sedatives, or anesthetics or by disorders of the brain such as stroke, meningitis, and increased intracranial pressure. Even when central respiratory activity is normal, the respiratory muscles may not be capable of generating the pressures necessary for proper ventilation because of disorders such as amyotrophic lateral sclerosis, myasthenia gravis, and polymyositis.

Alveolar Gas Composition

The adequacy of gas exchange in the lung is reflected in the arterial partial pressures of oxygen and carbon dioxide, (P_{aO_2} and P_{aCO_2}, respectively). In a healthy lung, ventilation and pulmonary blood flow are distributed reasonably uniformly throughout the lungs, and the resistance to gaseous diffusion across the blood-gas barrier is small. As a result, there is little difference in partial pressure between arterial blood and alveolar gas for both oxygen and carbon dioxide. However, a number of lung diseases can affect the efficiency of gas exchange to the point where arterial-alveolar partial pressure differences for these gases may become substantial. Thus, a thorough evaluation of pulmonary gas exchange necessitates the determination of both alveolar and arterial partial pressures.

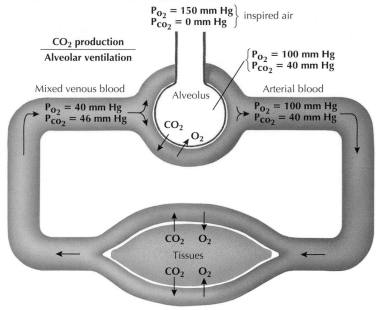

In normal individuals, particularly at rest, the gas leaving the mouth at the end of an expiration is gas that was previously in the alveolar regions of the lung. The partial pressures of oxygen and carbon dioxide in this end-tidal gas thus give a measure of P_{AO_2} and P_{ACO_2}. When lung disease affects the matching of ventilation and blood flow, however, the alveolar gas composition may vary markedly from one region to another. Furthermore, well-ventilated alveoli fill and empty easily, so they tend to contribute to the early portions of expiration, but poorly ventilated alveoli empty later in expiration. As a result, significant changes in expired P_{O_2} and P_{CO_2} may continue throughout expiration in the diseased lung; therefore a single sample of end-tidal gas may not reflect mean alveolar gas composition. Under these conditions, mean P_{AO_2} and P_{ACO_2} can be determined indirectly by assuming that arterial P_{aCO_2} approximates mean P_{ACO_2} (this is only justified for carbon dioxide on the basis of its great solubility compared to oxygen). P_{AO_2} can then be calculated according to the alveolar air equation:

$$P_{AO_2} = F_{IO_2}(P_B - P_{AH_2O}) - P_{ACO_2}\left[F_{IO_2} + \frac{1 - F_{IO_2}}{R}\right]$$

where F_{IO_2} is the inspired oxygen fraction, P_B is the atmospheric pressure, and P_{AH_2O} is the saturated partial pressure of water in alveolar gas. In other words, P_{AO_2} is determined from the difference between the inspired partial pressures of oxygen and the alveolar partial pressure of carbon dioxide, corrected for a non-unity value of the respiratory exchange ratio (R).

VENTILATION-PERFUSION RELATIONSHIPS (see Plate 2-18)

Efficient gas exchange requires that both alveolar ventilation and pulmonary capillary blood flow (perfusion) be distributed uniformly and in appropriate proportions to each of the numerous gas-exchanging units in the lung. Overall, the ratio of ventilation to perfusion ($\dot{V}_A/\dot{Q}_c$) is about 0.8, giving rise to a P_{AO_2} of approximately 100 mm Hg and a P_{ACO_2} of 40 mm Hg.

Pulmonary Mechanics and Gas Exchange *(Continued)*

When an individual is at FRC in the upright position, the top of the lung is more distended than the bottom of the lung because the top has to support the weight of the bottom. As a result, a greater portion of inspired air goes to the more distensible bottom regions. $\dot{V}_A$ thus decreases from the bottom to the top of the lung. $\dot{Q}_c$ also decreases from the bottom to the top of the lung, again largely as a result of gravity, but the vertical gradient in $\dot{Q}_c$ is greater than the gradient in $\dot{V}_A$. Consequently, the local $\dot{V}_A/\dot{Q}_c$ ratio increases from the base to the apex. At the top of the lung $\dot{V}_A/\dot{Q}_c$ is about 3.0 and decreases to approximately 0.6 at the bottom.

The normal differences in regional $\dot{V}_A/\dot{Q}_c$ throughout the lung cause only minor derangements in gas exchange. Pathologic abnormalities in airway resistance, lung compliance, and blood vessel caliber, however, can produce functionally compromising variations in $\dot{V}_A/\dot{Q}_c$. In the most extreme cases, local $\dot{V}_A/\dot{Q}_c$ may range from zero (shunt) to infinity (alveolar dead space). This can markedly reduce the efficiency of gas exchange and cause hypoxemia, as is conveniently demonstrated with a two-compartment model of the lung (see Plate 2-18).

For example, heterogeneities in the distribution of $\dot{V}_A$ may result from bronchial narrowing. In terms of the two-compartment model, this results in one compartment's receiving only a fraction of the ventilation of the other compartment. If $\dot{Q}_c$ remains evenly distributed, the $\dot{V}_A/\dot{Q}_c$ of the poorly ventilated but well-perfused compartment is low as compared with that of the normal compartment. Accordingly, P_{AO_2} and P_{aO_2} will be lower than normal in the poorly ventilated compartment, and P_{ACO_2} and P_{aCO_2} will be higher than normal. In the extreme case in which ventilation to the abnormal compartment falls to zero, P_{ACO_2} and P_{aCO_2} will approximate the P_{CO_2} of mixed venous blood.

The mean alveolar gas composition is the volume-weighted average of the compositions in each compartment. For example, if the P_{AO_2} of the poorly ventilated compartment is 60 mm Hg and this compartment receives only one-quarter of the ventilation of the normal lung unit, which itself has a P_{AO_2} of 100 mm Hg, the mean alveolar P_{O_2} will be $\frac{(3\times 100)+60}{4}$, or 90 mm Hg. Similarly, if the P_{ACO_2} of the normal compartment is 40 mm Hg and that of the poorly ventilated compartment is 44 mm Hg, the mean alveolar P_{ACO_2} will be $\frac{(3\times 40)+44}{4}$, or 41 mm Hg. Mean P_{aCO_2} can then be calculated under the assumption that it is proportional to mean P_{ACO_2}. This is not exactly true, but between the typical values of P_{CO_2} in the arterial blood (40 mm Hg) and the mixed venous blood (46 mm Hg), the relationship between partial pressure and content of carbon dioxide is essentially linear. Thus, even when a large fraction (1/4) of the lung is poorly ventilated, the resulting P_{ACO_2} and P_{aCO_2} (41 mm Hg) are still quite close to normal (40 mm Hg).

The same does not apply to oxygen, however, because the oxyhemoglobin dissociation curve has a very nonlinear shape. To determine how $\dot{V}_A/\dot{Q}_c$ mismatch affects the average oxygen content of arterial blood, it is first necessary to ascertain the oxygen content (or saturation) of the end-capillary blood leaving each of the two compartments. For example, if the end-capillary blood leaving the poorly ventilated compartment has a P_{aO_2} of 60 mm Hg (i.e., the same as the P_{AO_2} of that compartment), its saturation is approximately 90%. End-capillary blood from the normal unit with a typical P_{aO_2} of 100 mm Hg is 98% saturated with oxygen. The mixed arterial blood thus will have an oxygen saturation of $\frac{90+98}{2}$, or 94%. According to the oxyhemoglobin dissociation curve, however, an oxygen saturation of 94% corresponds to a P_{aO_2} of approximately 70 mm Hg, which is considerably lower than the value provided by the volume-weight mean of the compartmental P_{AO_2} values. The P_{aO_2} of the mixed arterial blood (70 mm Hg) is therefore much lower than normal (100 mm Hg), in contrast to the situation with carbon dioxide. Consequently, disorders of the lungs characterized by gas exchanging units with low $\dot{V}_A/\dot{Q}_c$ produce large alveolar-arterial P_{O_2} differences, but alveolar-arterial P_{CO_2} differences remain relatively small.

Lung units with very high $\dot{V}_A/\dot{Q}_c$ typically result from disorders that constrict, obstruct, or obliterate pulmonary blood vessels, leading to abnormally low blood flow to those units. Such units contribute little to overall gas exchange, so they have relatively high values of P_{ACO_2} and P_{aCO_2}. In the extreme case when blood flow is zero, P_{ACO_2} and P_{aCO_2} approximate the partial pressure of oxygen in the atmosphere. Ventilation to poorly perfused or nonperfused alveoli is thus wasted insofar as it contributes little or nothing to the arterialization of mixed venous blood. This wasted

Ventilation-Perfusion Relationships

A. Conditions with low ventilation-perfusion ratio

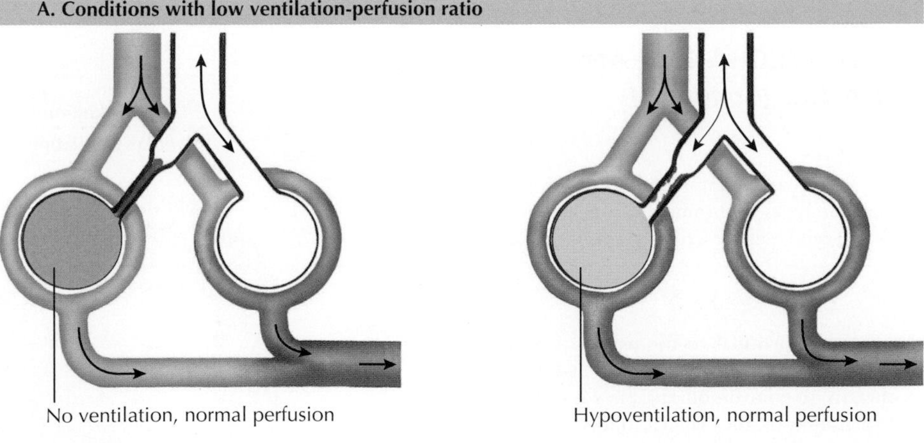

B. Conditions with high ventilation-perfusion ratio

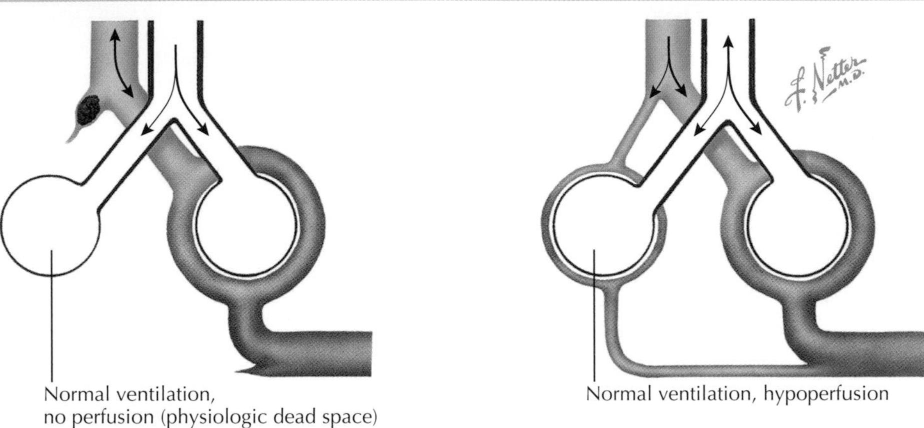

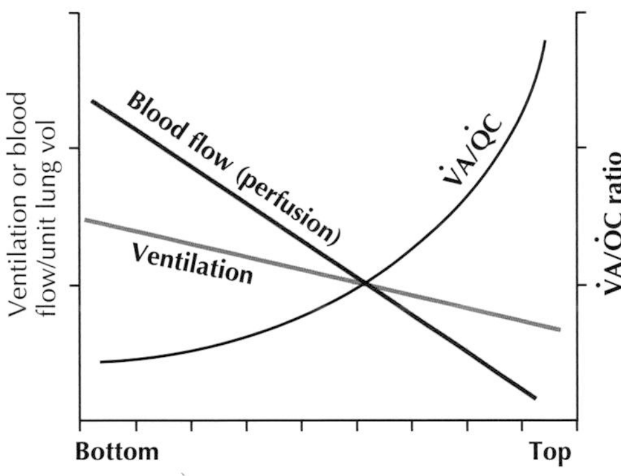

Both ventilation and blood flow are gravity dependent and decrease from bottom to top of lung. Gradient of blood flow is steeper than that of ventilation, so ventilation-perfusion ratio increases up lung

PULMONARY MECHANICS AND GAS EXCHANGE *(Continued)*

portion of $\dot{V}_A$ thus contributes to the physiologic dead space. The presence of high $\dot{V}_A/\dot{Q}_c$ does not directly produce arterial hypoxemia because the remaining well-perfused regions of the lung are able to oxygenate the blood that they receive. High $\dot{V}_A/\dot{Q}_c$, however, results in large alveolar-arterial Pco_2 differences.

Shunts (see Plate 2-19)

Blood flowing through bronchial veins, which empty directly into pulmonary veins, and through thebesian veins of the ventricular myocardium, which drain into the left ventricle, constitute right-to-left shunts, normally carrying up to 5% of the cardiac output. Right-to-left shunting of blood is increased in the presence of abnormal anatomic pathways such as intracardiac septal defects and pulmonary arteriovenous fistulas. Blood flow through regions of the lung with $\dot{V}_A/\dot{Q}_c$ of zero also adds to the right-to-left shunt. This condition occurs when gas exchanging units are perfused by pulmonary capillary blood but receive absolutely no ventilation because of bronchial obstruction or atelectasis or because the alveoli are filled with fluid or inflammatory secretions.

Right-to-left shunting results in the admixture of mixed venous blood ($P_{\bar{v}O_2}$, 40 mm Hg; $P_{\bar{v}CO_2}$, 46 mm Hg) with fully arterialized end-capillary blood ($P_{\bar{v}O_2}$, 100 mm Hg; $P_{\bar{v}CO_2}$, 40 mm Hg). The major consequence is a decrease in the overall arterial P_{aO_2}. Changes in P_{aCO_2} tend to be insignificant because the difference between mixed venous and arterialized end-capillary Pco_2 is small. Furthermore, any increase in arterial Pco_2 stimulates respiratory chemoreceptors to increase the level of ventilation, which restores the P_{aCO_2} toward normal values.

A right-to-left shunt corresponds to a lung region with a $\dot{V}_A/\dot{Q}_c$ of zero and can be quantified from the alveolar-arterial Po_2 difference during 100% oxygen breathing. Breathing pure oxygen for long enough will eventually remove all the nitrogen from even the most poorly ventilated regions of the lung, replacing it with oxygen. The alveoli will thus contain only oxygen (PA_{O_2}, ~673 mm Hg) and carbon dioxide (PA_{CO_2}, ~40 mm Hg). With such a high PA_{O_2}, pulmonary capillary blood perfusing lung units receiving any ventilation at all will become oxygenated and achieve a P_{aO_2} virtually the same as PA_{O_2}. Mixed venous blood partaking in a true right-to-left shunt, however, picks up no oxygen whatsoever, so it remains at the mixed venous Po_2. The Po_2 of the mixed arterial blood is thus reduced by the contribution from the shunted blood, producing an alveolar-arterial Po_2 difference.

The fraction of the cardiac output constituting the right-to-left shunt can be calculated from the shunt equation:

$$\dot{Q}s/\dot{Q}t = \frac{Cc_{O_2} - Ca_{O_2}}{Cc_{O_2} - C\bar{v}_{O_2}}$$

where $\dot{Q}s$ is shunt flow; $\dot{Q}t$ is total cardiac output; and Cc_{O_2}, Ca_{O_2} and $C\bar{v}_{O_2}$ are the oxygen contents of end-capillary blood, arterial blood, and mixed venous blood, respectively. Cc_{O_2} can be calculated from the end-capillary Po_2, which itself is considered equal to PA_{O_2}. Mixed venous Po_2 can be measured directly or determined by assuming an arterial–venous oxygen content difference of 5 mL/100 mL.

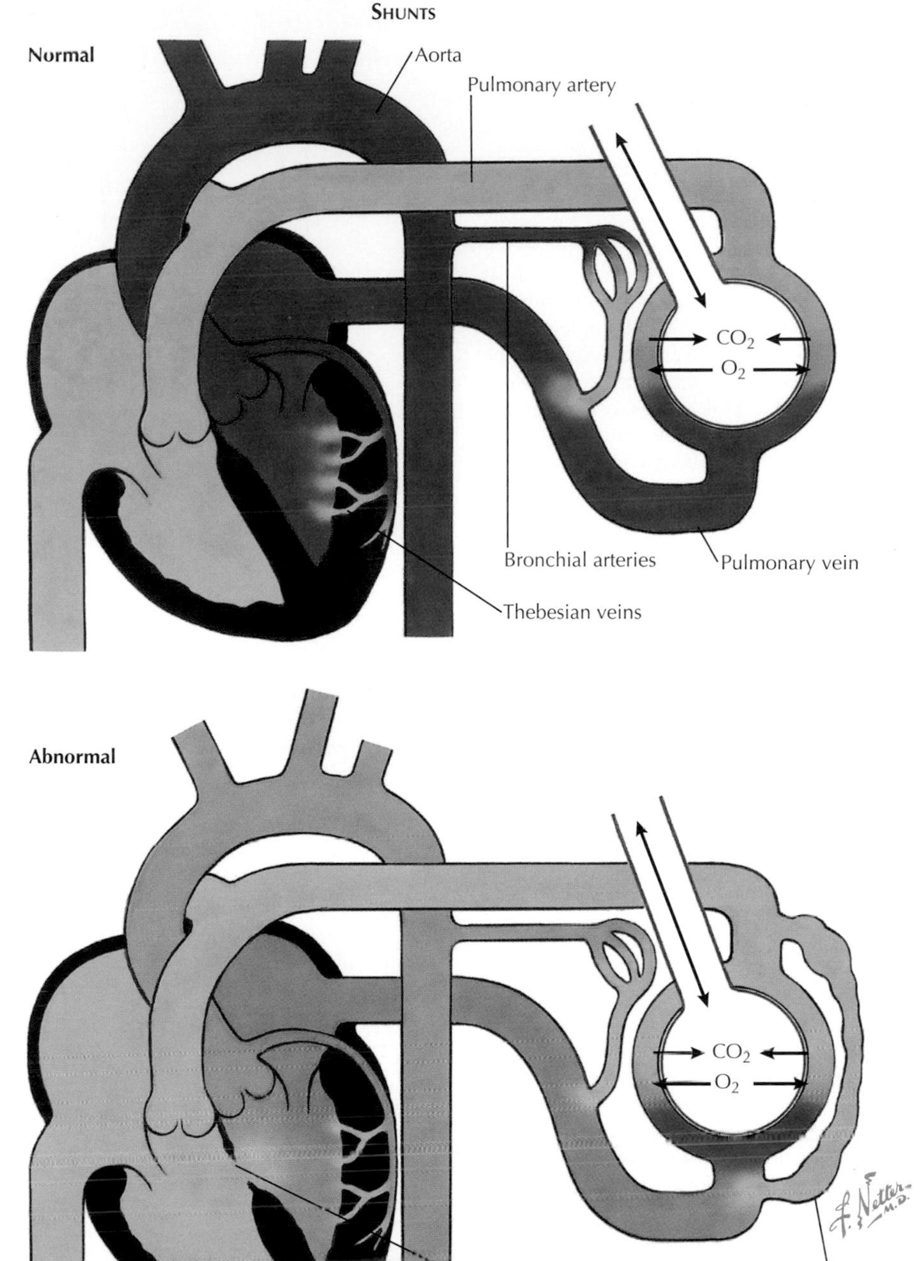

OXYGEN TRANSPORT

After oxygen has diffused from the alveoli of the lungs into the plasma of the pulmonary capillary blood and then entered the red blood cells, it must be stored for transport around the body. Oxygen is stored in two ways: in physical solution in plasma and in chemical combination with hemoglobin in the red blood cells (see Plate 2-20).

Physical Solution

The amount of oxygen dissolved in plasma is determined by its solubility and is directly proportional to the partial pressure of oxygen in the plasma. Whereas arterial blood with a Po_2 of 100 mm Hg contains 0.30 mL of oxygen (volume of gas at 0°C and 1 atm) dissolved in each 100 mL of plasma, mixed venous blood with a Po_2 of 40 mm Hg contains only 0.12 mL of dissolved oxygen per 100 mL of plasma. In other words, 0.18 mL of dissolved oxygen is delivered to the body tissues from every milliliter of blood that makes its way around the systemic circulation. This volume is nowhere near enough to meet the metabolic needs of the peripheral tissues.

Chemical Combination with Hemoglobin

More than 60 times more oxygen is carried in the blood in chemical combination with hemoglobin. The amount of oxygen that combines with hemoglobin increases with the partial pressure of oxygen but in a very nonlinear manner. The relationship between Po_2 and the

PULMONARY MECHANICS AND GAS EXCHANGE *(Continued)*

content of oxygen bound to hemoglobin is sigmoidal in shape, being almost flat at high Po_2 values typical of arterial blood and very steep at intermediate Po_2 values typical of venous blood. Hemoglobin in the blood has a maximum storage capacity for oxygen, which is achieved when all four oxygen-binding sites on every molecule of hemoglobin are occupied. A single gram of hemoglobin can hold up to 1.34 mL of oxygen. The normal hemoglobin concentration of an adult male is about 15 g Hb/100 mL of blood, so the maximum amount of oxygen that can combine with hemoglobin is 15 × 1.34, or 20.1 mL O_2/100 mL of blood. The actual amount of oxygen in chemical combination with hemoglobin relative to the maximal amount possible is expressed as the percentage saturation (S_{O_2}%), given by

$$S_{O_2}\% = \frac{\text{Oxygen combined with hemoglobin}}{\text{Maximum oxygen capacity}} \times 100$$

Whereas the S_{O_2}% of arterial blood with a Po_2 of 100 mm Hg is approximately 98%, that of venous blood with a Po_2 of 40 mm Hg is about 75%.

Oxyhemoglobin Dissociation Curve

The relationship between S_{O_2}% and Po_2 is called the *oxyhemoglobin dissociation curve*, and its highly nonlinear shape has a number of crucial physiologic advantages. The upper, flat portion of the curve ensures that S_{O_2}% remains close to 100% even when Po_2 becomes reduced below its normal value of 100 mm Hg by the demands of severe exercise, travel to high altitude, or even as a result of cardiopulmonary disorders. Conversely, when the oxygenated arterial blood travels to the periphery of the body and meets metabolically active tissues with a Po_2 typically of about 40 mm Hg, hemoglobin must desaturate by about 25% to bring the Po_2 of the blood and tissues into equilibrium. The sigmoidal shape of the dissociation curve thus ensures that blood always leaves the lungs fully loaded with oxygen and yet is able to deposit large quantities of oxygen to the tissues that need it.

The position of the oxyhemoglobin dissociation curve can be shifted to the right or left by factors that alter the oxygen requirements of the body. For example, during exercise, the peripheral tissues have an increased need for oxygen and produce increased amounts of carbon dioxide. The resulting increases in temperature, intracellular hydrogen ion concentration, and Pco_2 shift the dissociation curve to the right. This lowers the value of S_{O_2}% at the Po_2 of the peripheral tissues, resulting in greater release of oxygen to the tissues.

The affinity of hemoglobin for oxygen decreases when temperature is reduced and when the intracellular hydrogen ion concentration and Pco_2 are lowered. The result is a shift of the oxyhemoglobin dissociation curve to the left. This is the condition existing in the pulmonary capillaries when the hydrogen ion concentration decreases as carbon dioxide passes into the alveoli. The resulting increase in affinity for oxygen enhances its uptake by hemoglobin in the pulmonary capillaries. The position of the dissociation curve can be determined by measuring the arterial Po_2 corresponding to 50% saturation of hemoglobin. This normally occurs at about 26 mm Hg and is known as the P50 value.

The affinity of hemoglobin for oxygen is also influenced by the presence in the red blood cell of 2,3-diphosphoglycerate (DPG). This organic phosphate, an intermediate product of anaerobic glycolysis, decreases the affinity of hemoglobin for oxygen and promotes the increased release of oxygen that takes place in the peripheral tissues. The amount of DPG in red blood cells is increased when tissue oxygen delivery is compromised by anemia or hypoxemia and thus serves an important adaptive function for maintaining tissue oxygenation.

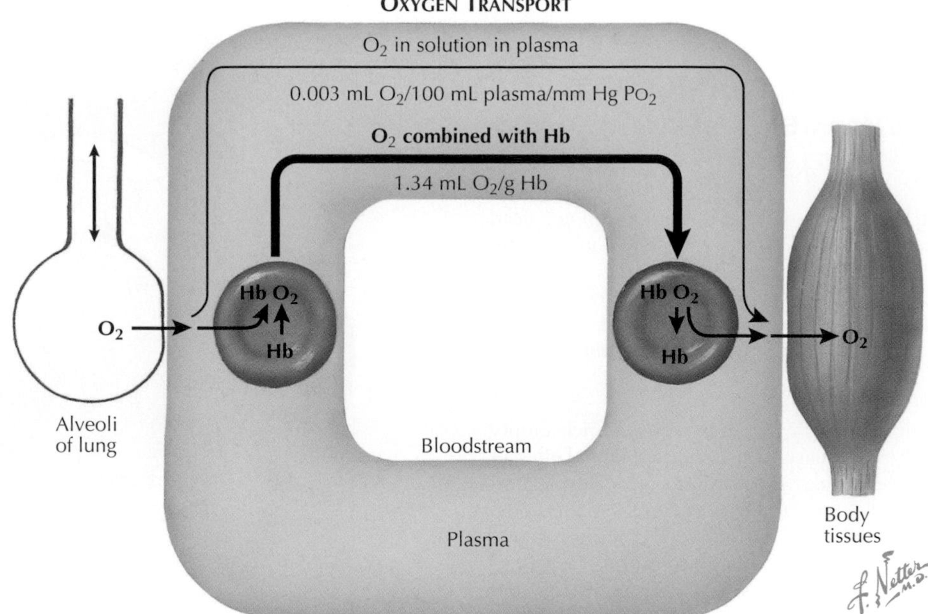

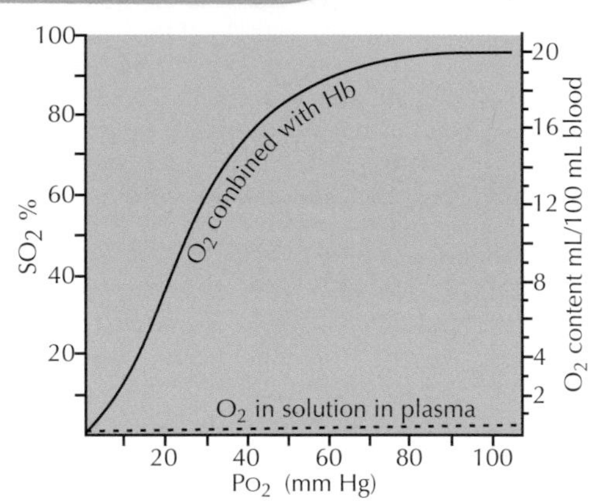

Oxyhemoglobin dissociation curve (at pH 7.4, Pco_2 40 mm Hg, 37°C)

Upper flat portion of curve allows Hb saturation to remain relatively constant during considerable changes in Po_2. At low Po_2 levels, where curve is steep, small changes in Po_2 result in marked changes in saturation. Increased Pco_2, lowered pH, and increased temperature shift curve to right and facilitate release of O_2 to tissues. Opposite changes in Pco_2, pH, and temperature shift curve to left

Effects of Pco_2, pH, and temperature on O_2 dissociation curve

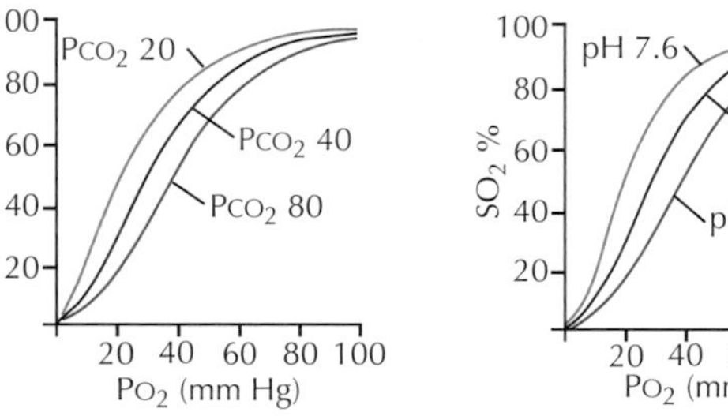

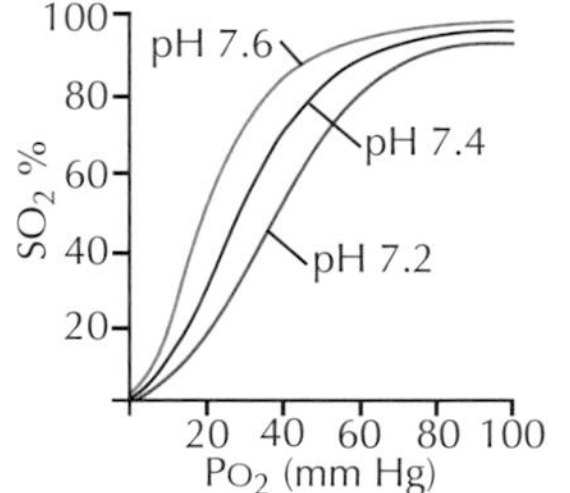

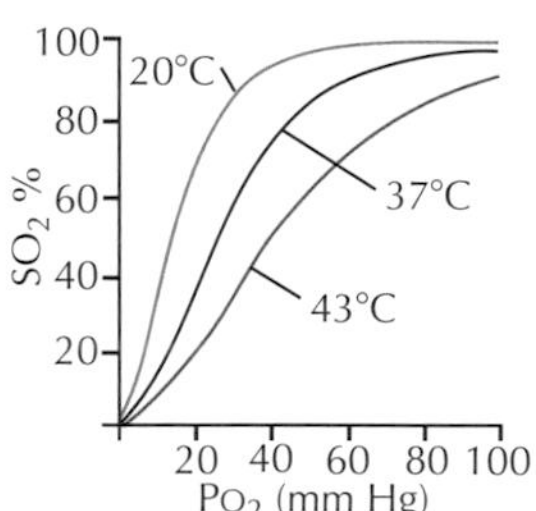

CARBON DIOXIDE TRANSPORT

Carbon dioxide is carried in the blood in a number of ways. About 10% is carried in solution, both in the plasma and the red blood cells, the precise amount depending linearly on the Pco_2. This is a much larger fraction than for oxygen because of the much greater solubility of carbon dioxide. Carbon dioxide is also carried in the red blood cells bound to hemoglobin as carbamino-hemoglobin.

The majority of the carbon dioxide in the blood is transported in the form of bicarbonate, which is produced from dissolved carbon dioxide according to the equation:

$$CO_2 + H_2O \Leftrightarrow H_2CO_3$$

In the plasma, this reaction favors the lefthand side, so that at equilibrium the concentration of carbon dioxide remains about 1000 times greater than that of carbonic acid. The red blood cells, however, contain an enzyme called carbonic anhydrase that catalyzes the hydration reaction so that carbonic acid is formed at a much higher rate. Carbonic acid partially dissociates into hydrogen ions (H^+) and bicarbonate ions (HCO_3^-) according to:

PULMONARY MECHANICS AND GAS EXCHANGE *(Continued)*

$$H_2CO_3 \Leftrightarrow H^+ + HCO_3^-$$

Some of the large amount of bicarbonate formed within the red blood cells then diffuses out of the cells into the plasma.

ACID-BASE REGULATION

A key consequence of the transport of carbon dioxide in the blood is the formation of large numbers of hydrogen ions, so the elimination of carbon dioxide by respiration is vitally important for controlling the pH of the blood. In fact, this mechanism is used to eliminate much of the metabolically produced acid from the body. The respiratory system is thus of great importance in acid-base regulation (see Plate 2-21).

The hydrogen ion concentration ($[H^+]$) in the blood is determined by the relationship between dissolved carbon dioxide, which is dependent on the P_{CO_2}, and the bicarbonate ion concentration ($[HCO_3^-]$). This relationship is embodied in the Henderson-Hasselbalch equation:

$$pH = pK + \log \frac{[HCO_3^-]}{0.03\ P_{CO_2}}$$

where pK is the dissociation constant (6.1) for the overall reaction between carbon dioxide and H_2O and the factor 0.03 is the solubility coefficient for carbon dioxide in the plasma. Variations in the ratio of $[HCO_3^-]$ and P_{CO_2}, produced by either metabolic or respiratory disturbances, result in changes in pH from the normal value of 7.4, leading to *acidemia* (i.e., low pH and high hydrogen ion concentration) or to *alkalemia* (i.e., high pH and low hydrogen ion concentration). The arterial P_{CO_2} is a measure of the *respiratory* component, and $[HCO_3^-]$ defines the *metabolic* or nonrespiratory contribution to the acid-base status. It is possible to measure hydrogen ion concentration directly, the normal value in blood being 35 to 45 nm/L.

Respiratory Disturbances

Respiratory acidosis is seen with alveolar hypoventilation and is characterized by an elevated P_{CO_2} and a low pH. Alveolar hypoventilation may occur when central nervous system function is depressed by sedatives, narcotics, or anesthetic agents. It can also occur as a consequence of disorders of the brain or when diseases affect the respiratory neuromuscular apparatus. Patients with severe lung disease, in whom the physiologic dead space is markedly increased, may also develop alveolar hypoventilation even though the overall level of ventilation remains normal.

Persistent carbon dioxide retention and acidosis promote the renal retention of bicarbonate. This compensatory action, which reaches maximal levels in 5 to 7 days, increases the bicarbonate ion concentration in the blood and tends to restore the pH toward normal, even though the P_{CO_2} remains unchanged.

Respiratory alkalosis results from alveolar hyperventilation, causing an excessive output of carbon dioxide that leads to hypocapnia and an elevated pH. Hyperventilation is seen in excessively anxious or apprehensive individuals and occurs secondary to fever and after the ingestion of drugs such as aspirin, which act as respiratory stimulants. Certain disorders of the central nervous system that interfere with respiratory control mechanisms also produce hyperventilation. In early stages of cardiopulmonary disorders, stimulation of pulmonary mechanoreceptors as well as hypoxemia can stimulate ventilation and induce respiratory alkalosis.

Renal adjustments to chronic respiratory alkalosis involve the excretion of bicarbonate ions by the kidney. Within several days, the bicarbonate ion concentration decreases and, despite the persistence of hypocapnia, the pH is restored to virtually normal values.

Metabolic Disturbances

Metabolic acidosis is caused by an accumulation of nonvolatile acids in the blood or by a loss of bicarbonate. Whereas levels of nonvolatile acids are increased in diabetes, uremia, and shock, loss of bicarbonate occurs in chronic renal insufficiency and with diarrhea. Transient increases in blood acid levels are also produced by accumulation of lactic acid caused by exercising above the anaerobic threshold. The resultant increase in hydrogen ion concentration is a strong respiratory stimulant. As the level of ventilation increases, the arterial P_{CO_2} decreases, and the change in pH is minimized.

Excessive loss of nonvolatile acids or increases in bicarbonate levels produce *metabolic alkalosis*. Circumstances under which this occurs include prolonged vomiting or gastric suction, ingestion of alkali, and administration of thiazide diuretics; these elevate the bicarbonate ion concentration and increase the pH. Because respiratory drive is diminished as the bicarbonate concentration increases and hydrogen ion accumulation decreases, ventilation is reduced, and the P_{CO_2} increases. These respiratory compensatory mechanisms, although relatively weak, lessen the change in pH. Accelerated renal excretion of bicarbonate also serves to restore the acid-base balance toward normal.

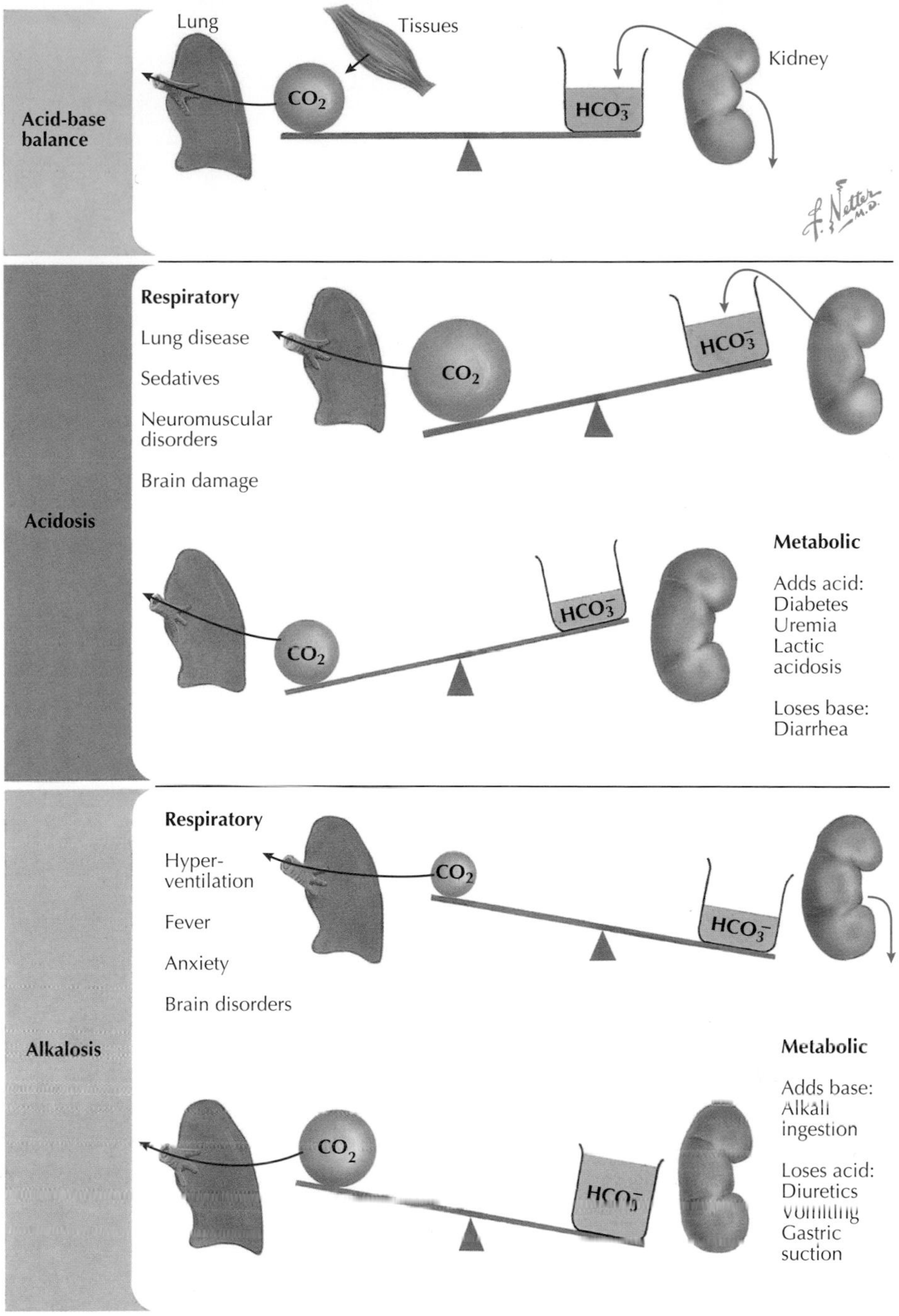

Pulmonary Defenses Against Oxidant and Other Noxious Injuries

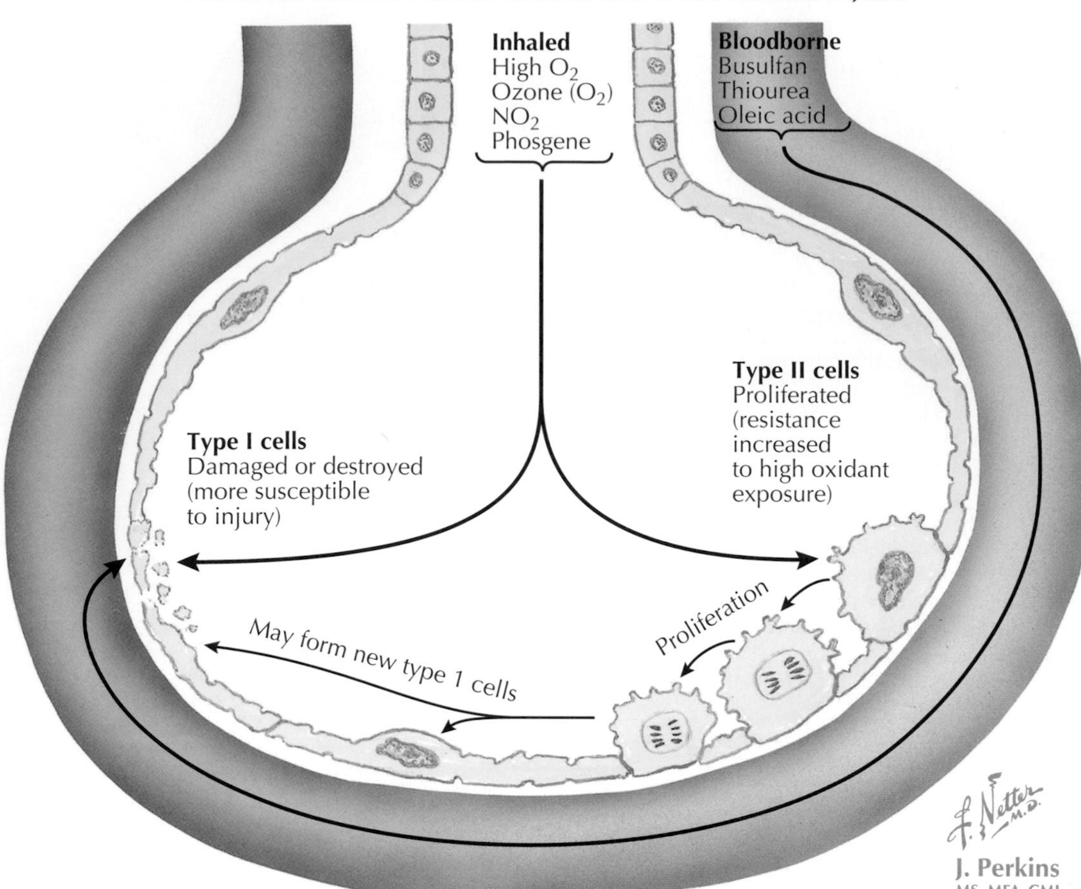

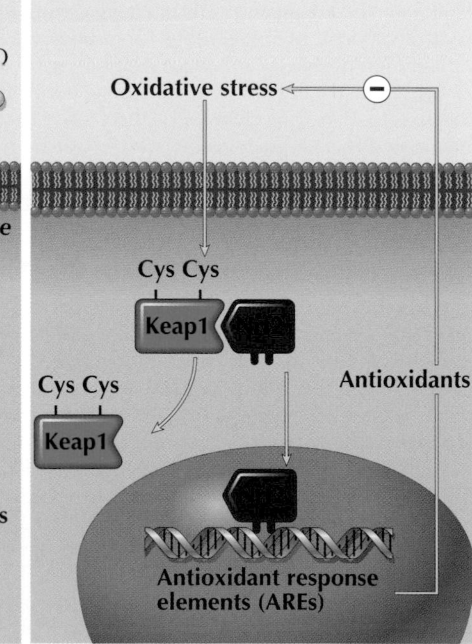

Response to Oxidant Injury

The lung is primarily designed for gas exchange between circulating blood and inhaled air. The delicate alveolar-capillary boundary where gas exchange takes place can be injured by inhaled or bloodborne noxious agents. The inhaled substances are either volatile chemicals such as phosgene, oxidants (especially oxygen at partial pressures above atmospheric), cigarette smoke, or ozone. Chemicals and a growing list of drugs reaching the lungs via the bloodstream can also cause injury. Among the tissue components of the lung, the type I or membranous pneumocyte, the predominant cell type lining the alveoli, is most susceptible to injury (see Plate 2-22). The type II cell, or granular pneumocyte, proliferates in response to injury in an apparent effort to repair the damage and replace the nonviable type I cell. A lung populated with a larger number of type II cells is more "tolerant" of continued exposure to the harmful effects of, for example, persistently high oxygen tensions.

An example of the response to injury of the lung by noxious agents is what happens after the inhalation of oxidants. Exposure to these compounds leads to the peroxidation of unsaturated lipids in membranes, which can eventually produce cell and tissue damage. The organism defends itself against the harmful effects of oxidant injury by mobilization of antioxidants such as α-tocopherol or by the conversion of lipid peroxides to hydroxy compounds, a reaction that is promoted by reduced glutathione. Reactive oxygen species, such as superoxide anions ($\cdot O_2^-$) and hydrogen peroxide (H_2O_2), are also generated endogenously from NADPH (nicotine adenine dinucleotide phosphate) oxidases (NOX1-6), from mitochondria, and from the endoplasmic reticulum via xanthine oxidase. Superoxide anions also combine avidly with nitric oxide to form peroxinitrite, which may impair the function of several proteins.

These endogenous oxidants may cause DNA damage by oxidation, lipid peroxidation, and the generation of several lipid mediators, and they may induce cell death through apoptosis. Oxidants also activate proinflammatory transcription factors, such as nuclear factor–κB (NF-κB) and activator protein-1 (AP-1), which switch on multiple inflammatory genes, leading to inflammation. Increased oxidative stress occurs when there is an imbalance between oxidants and antioxidants.

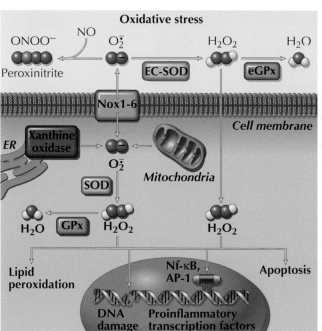

Antioxidants are important in defending against oxidative stress. Glutathione plays an important role as an endogenous antioxidant and is maintained in the reduced state by glutathione peroxidase (GPx) and glutathione reductase. Superoxide dismutase (SOD) is also important in removing superoxide anions, and three forms of this enzyme exist; copper-zinc SOD (SOD1) is found in the cytoplasm, manganese–SOD (SOD2) is found in mitochondria, and extracellular SOD (SOD3) is present in extracellular spaces. H_2O_2 is reduced by catalase to water. Several endogenous antioxidant genes are regulated by the transcription factor Nrf2 (nuclear erythroid 2–related factor 2), which is activated by oxidative stress, and this represents a feedback loop to limit the effects of reactive oxygen species. Several antioxidants, such as ascorbic acid (vitamin C) and α-tocopherol (vitamin E), are obtained from the diet. An antioxidant used in clinical practice is *N*-acetyl-cysteine, which results in increased synthesis of glutathione.

Inactivation of Circulating Vasoactive Substances

In 1924, Starling and Verney first noted in an isolated, perfused kidney preparation that vasoconstriction could be prevented if the lung was included in the perfusion system. They concluded that a vasoactive substance was removed during passage of the perfusate through the lung. The substance affecting the renal vasculature was later found to be serotonin, which was either removed or inactivated during its journey through the pulmonary circulation. It is now well established, in part because of the pioneering work of Vane, that the lung is intimately concerned with the inactivation and activation of circulating vasoactive substances, including catecholamines and prostaglandins (see Plate 2-23).

These intrapulmonary uptake mechanisms contribute to the control of peripheral vascular resistance and the "reconditioning" of blood before reentry into the arterial system. The structure of the lung and its location within the circulatory system are eminently suited to fulfilling this role. There, the entire blood volume has to pass through a single vascular bed and, although the intrapulmonary blood volume at any given moment is small (±60 mL), it is exposed to a large vascular surface area (±70 m^2), allowing intimate contact between substances within the blood and the endothelial cells.

The fate of serotonin in the lung is one example of the interaction between circulating vasoactive substances and the endothelium of the pulmonary vasculature. Serotonin (5-hydroxytryptamine) is a potent amine that affects the microcirculation in various areas of the body. It is generated in several cells, including platelets and certain neurones. Only a small fraction normally circulates free in the blood, most of the serotonin being bound by platelets. The pharmacologic action of this amine varies from tissue to tissue. In the lung, it causes constriction of pulmonary vessels. In animals, it also causes bronchoconstriction, but human airways show no response to this mediator.

Serotonin produced in the gastrointestinal tract reaches the liver via the portal circulation. In the liver, it is converted by means of a reaction that involves monoamine oxidase to 5-hydroxyin-doleacetic acid, a freely diffusible and water-soluble substance that does not have any known pharmacologic actions. Serotonin in blood reaching the lung is effectively removed by uptake into pulmonary endothelial cells. This process is dependent on a carrier mechanism that is saturable. After its uptake by tissue components of the lung, serotonin is oxidized to 5-hydroxyindoleacetic acid.

Serotonin Metabolism

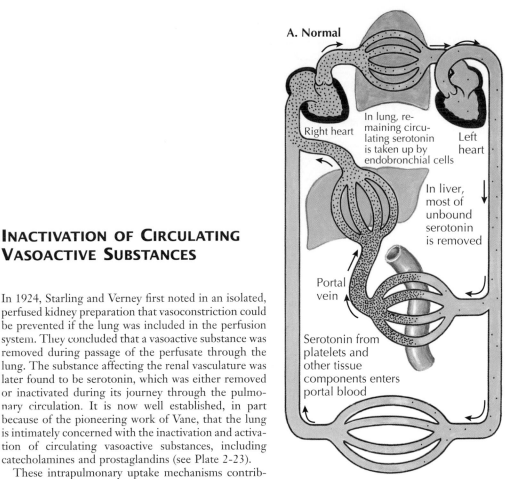

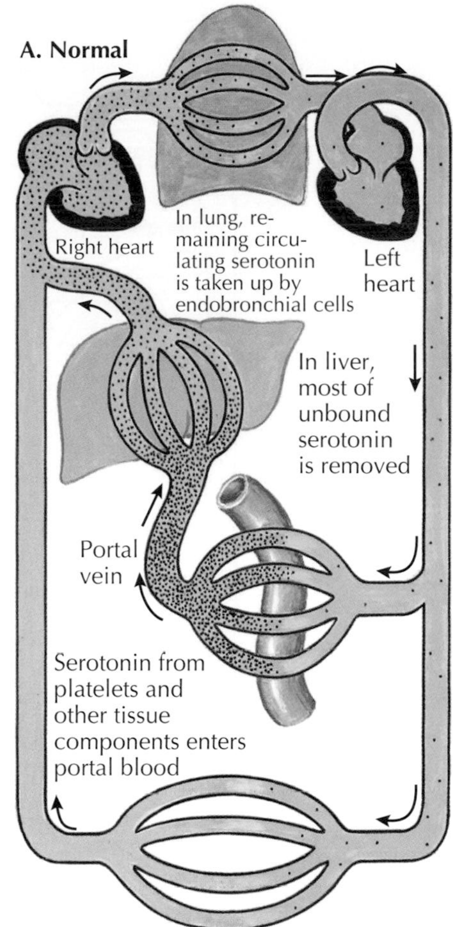
A. Normal
Right heart
In lung, remaining circulating serotonin is taken up by endobronchial cells
Left heart
In liver, most of unbound serotonin is removed
Portal vein
Serotonin from platelets and other tissue components enters portal blood

Remainder of circulation; relatively free of unbound serotonin

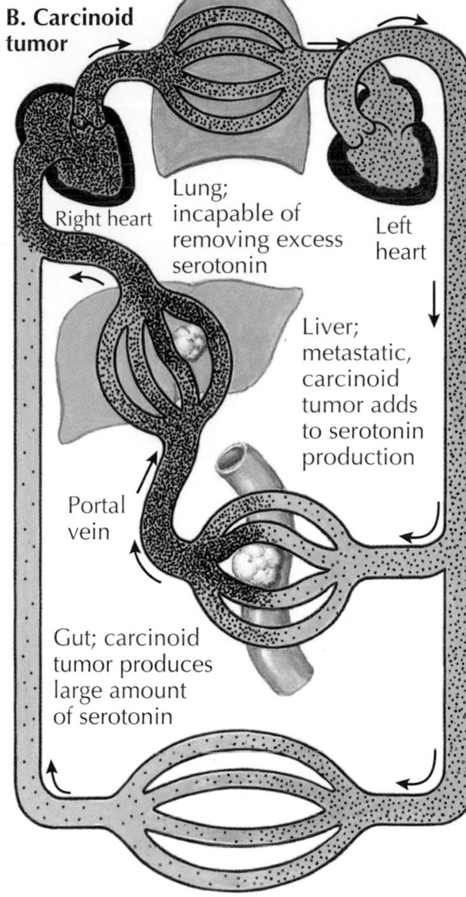
B. Carcinoid tumor
Right heart
Lung; incapable of removing excess serotonin
Left heart
Liver; metastatic, carcinoid tumor adds to serotonin production
Portal vein
Gut; carcinoid tumor produces large amount of serotonin

Remainder of circulation; pharmacologically active amount of serotonin present

Serotonin, if in excess, affects endothelium of right side of heart and pulmonary artery, causing pulmonary stenosis and tricuspid insufficiency

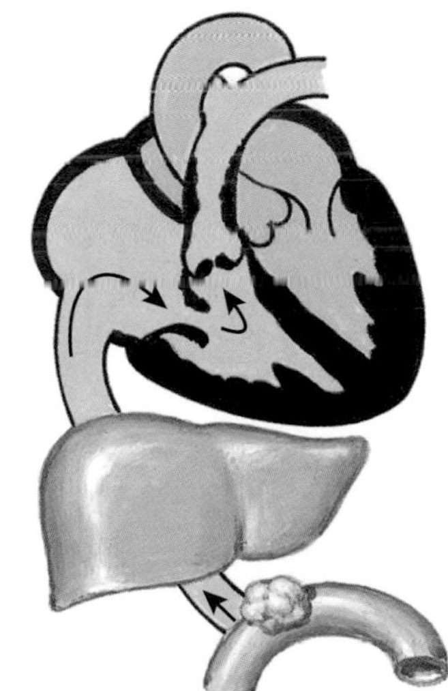

In presence of atrial septal defect, similar lesions appear in left heart

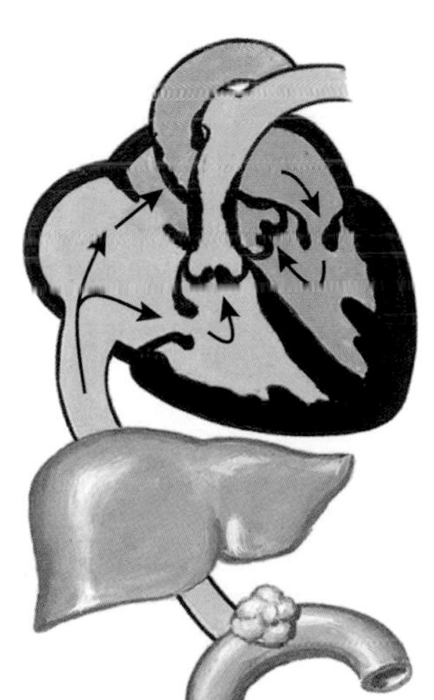
F. Netter M.D.

Excessive production of serotonin, or the appearance of serotonin-releasing tumor tissue (carcinoid) beyond the liver, leads to "overflow" of the amine into the hepatic veins and inferior vena cava. The amount of serotonin reaching the lung under these circumstances may exceed the capacity of the intrapulmonary removal system. Prolonged exposure of the endothelium of the pulmonary vasculature to excess serotonin leads to structural changes in the right side of the heart and large pulmonary vessels. The mechanism underlying these structural changes remains unknown. That the changes are caused by serotonin and not by its metabolites is suggested by the intriguing observation that in the presence of an atrial septal defect with a right-to-left shunt, when larger quantities of serotonin can "overflow" into the systemic circulation, structural changes also develop in the left side of the heart.

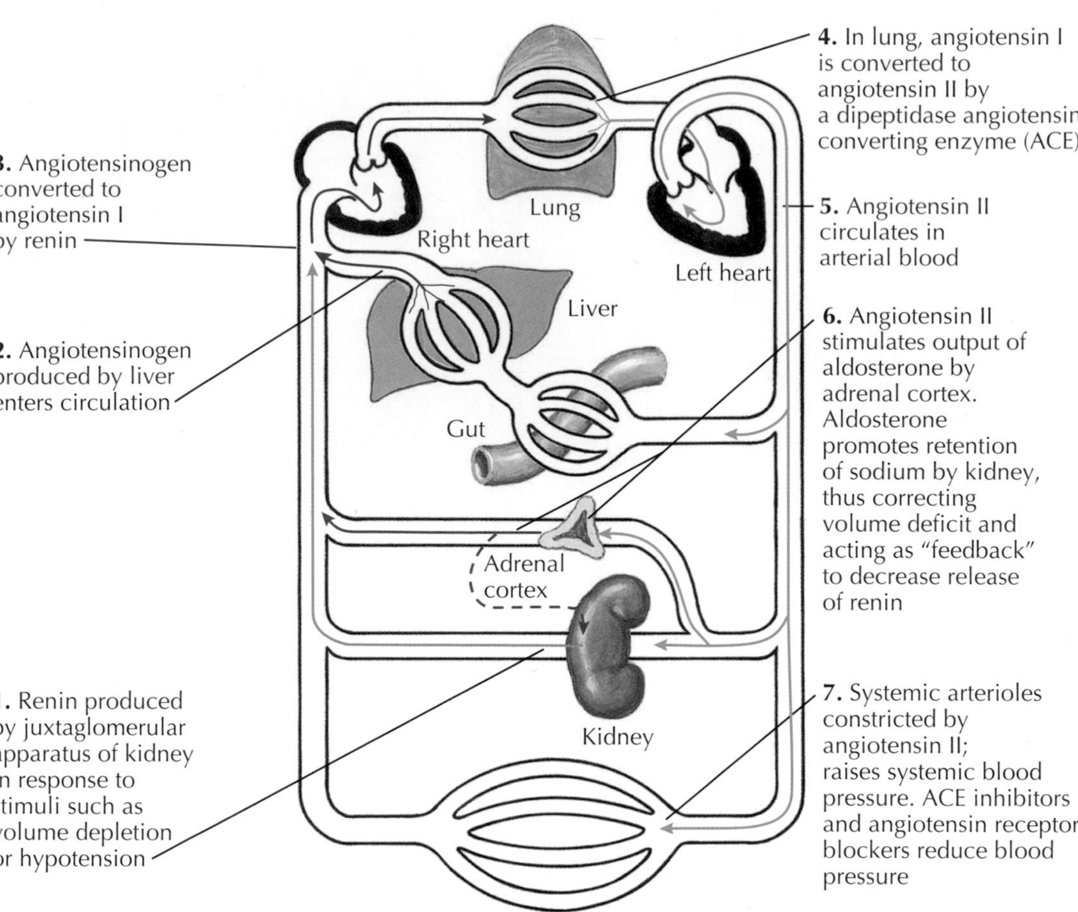

Renin-angiotensin system
4. In lung, angiotensin I is converted to angiotensin II by a dipeptidase angiotensin-converting enzyme (ACE)
3. Angiotensinogen converted to angiotensin I by renin
Lung
Right heart
5. Angiotensin II circulates in arterial blood
Left heart
Liver
2. Angiotensinogen produced by liver enters circulation
6. Angiotensin II stimulates output of aldosterone by adrenal cortex. Aldosterone promotes retention of sodium by kidney, thus correcting volume deficit and acting as "feedback" to decrease release of renin
Gut
Adrenal cortex
1. Renin produced by juxtaglomerular apparatus of kidney in response to stimuli such as volume depletion or hypotension
Kidney
7. Systemic arterioles constricted by angiotensin II; raises systemic blood pressure. ACE inhibitors and angiotensin receptor blockers reduce blood pressure

Activation of Circulating Precursors of Vasoactive Substances

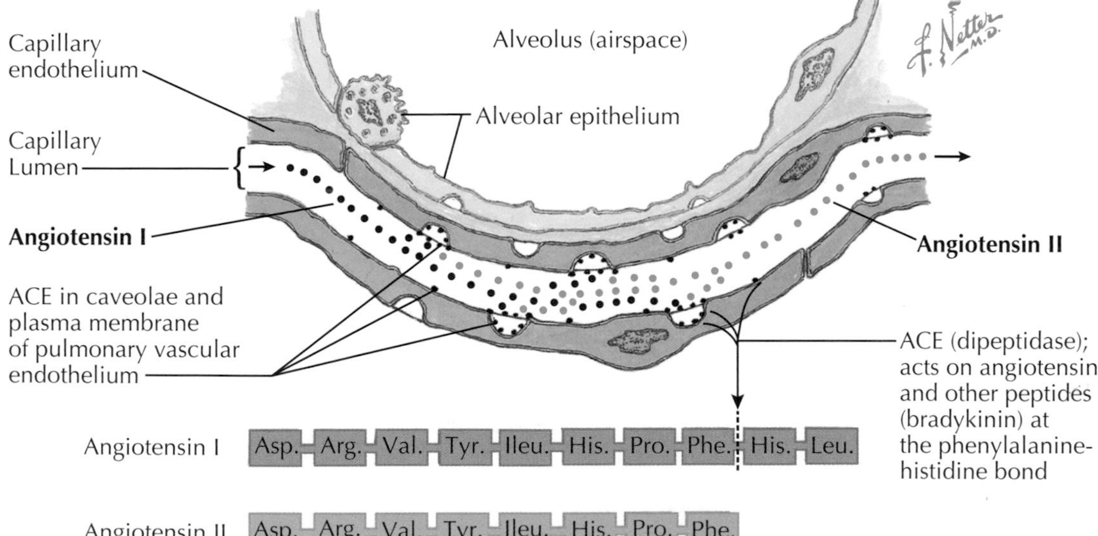

Intrapulmonary conversion of angiotensin
Capillary endothelium
Alveolus (airspace)
Alveolar epithelium
Capillary Lumen
Angiotensin I
Angiotensin II
ACE in caveolae and plasma membrane of pulmonary vascular endothelium
ACE (dipeptidase); acts on angiotensin and other peptides (bradykinin) at the phenylalanine-histidine bond
Angiotensin I Asp. Arg. Val. Tyr. Ileu. His. Pro. Phe. His. Leu.
Angiotensin II Asp. Arg. Val. Tyr. Ileu. His. Pro. Phe.

The fate of angiotensin in the lung is a paradigm for the conversion of an inactive precursor into a vasoactive substance. Angiotensin II is a potent vasoconstrictor derived from angiotensin I. This conversion is part of a more complex feedback loop originating in the kidneys where, in response to stimuli such as volume depletion or hypotension, renin is released into the bloodstream. Renin is a protease that acts on angiotensinogen (renin substrate), a globulin produced by the liver. The product of the interaction is the decapeptide angiotensin I. This polypeptide, in turn, is exposed to a dipeptidase angiotensin-converting enzyme (ACE) at the endothelial surface of the pulmonary vessels. ACE cleaves two amino acids from angiotensin I to form the octapeptide angiotensin II, which acts on angiotensin I receptors in systemic arterioles to increase peripheral vascular resistance. In addition, angiotensin II promotes the release of aldosterone from the adrenal cortex. Aldosterone is carried via the bloodstream to the kidneys, where it promotes the retention of sodium for correction of the original intravascular volume deficit. This action completes the feedback loop initiated by volume depletion or hypotension. Angiotensin II has a short half-life and is inactivated by several peptidases, collectively know as angiotensinases, which have been identified in many tissues. ACE inhibitors (such as captopril) and angiotensin I receptor antagonists (e.g., losartan) are used to treat hypertension.

ACE is located within or adjacent to the caveolae (small indentations on the endothelial surface layer of pulmonary capillaries) and has been isolated and purified. The enzyme also acts on another circulating vasoactive polypeptide, bradykinin, a nonapeptide that tends to lower systemic blood pressure. However, in contrast to the situation with angiotensin I, cleavage of amino acids from bradykinin abolishes its vasoactive properties. ACE has also been identified by fluorescein-labeled antibodies on vascular endothelial cells in many organs other than the lung (e.g., liver, spleen, kidneys, pancreas). Thus, the presence of ACE is not unique to the lung, although the structural arrangement in the lung does allow maximal conversion of angiotensin I to angiotensin II. The unique feature of the process in the lung is the efficiency of the enzymatic reaction caused by the strategic location of the enzyme within the pulmonary vasculature, where a small volume of blood is exposed to a large surface area before reentry into the high-pressure arterial system. Renin and angiotensin may also be generated locally within the pulmonary circulation.

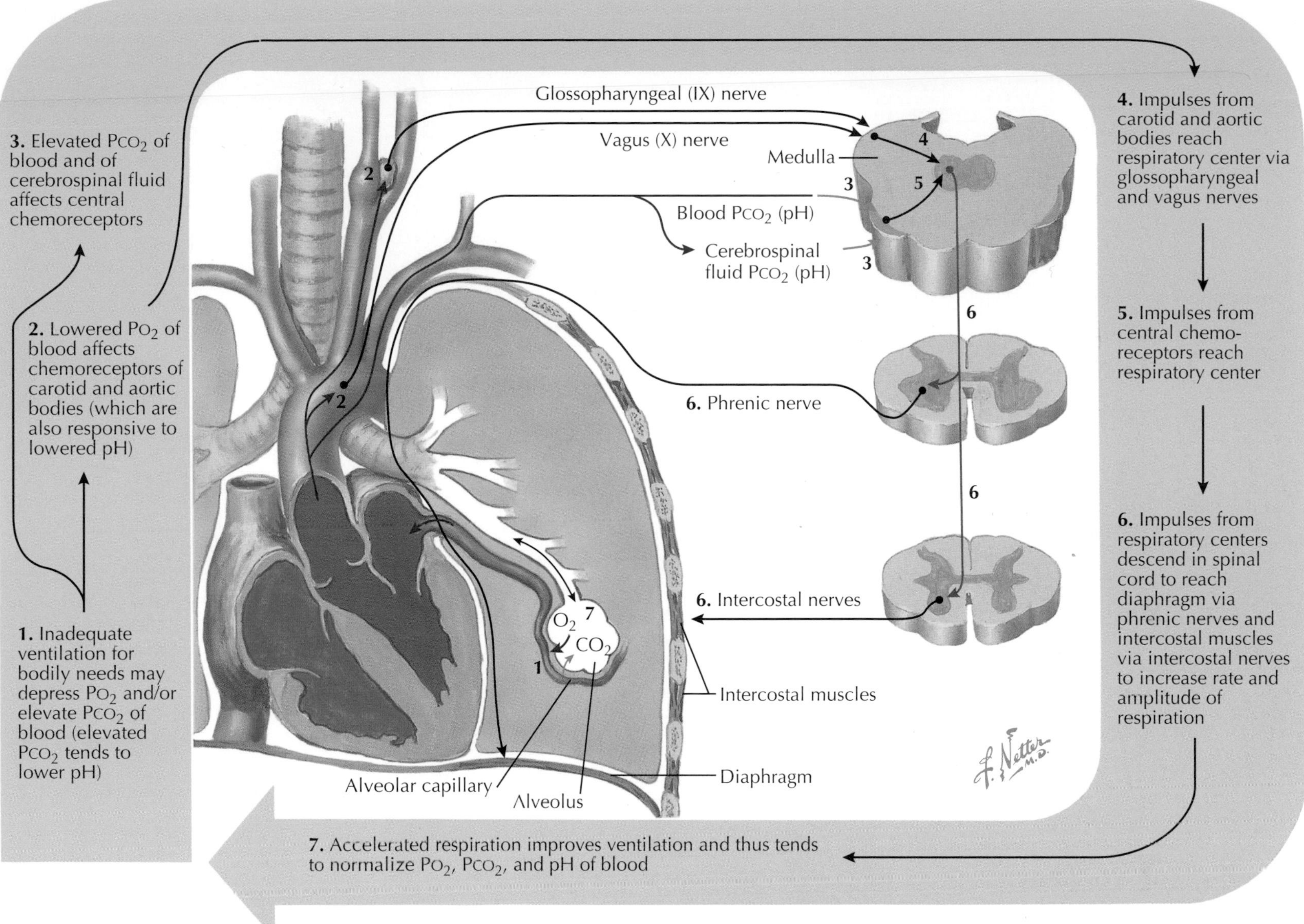

Chemical Control of Respiration (Feedback Mechanism)
Glossopharyngeal (IX) nerve
Vagus (X) nerve
Medulla
Blood PCO2 (pH)
Cerebrospinal fluid PCO2 (pH)
3. Elevated PCO2 of blood and of cerebrospinal fluid affects central chemoreceptors
2. Lowered PO2 of blood affects chemoreceptors of carotid and aortic bodies (which are also responsive to lowered pH)
1. Inadequate ventilation for bodily needs may depress PO2 and/or elevate PCO2 of blood (elevated PCO2 tends to lower pH)
4. Impulses from carotid and aortic bodies reach respiratory center via glossopharyngeal and vagus nerves
5. Impulses from central chemoreceptors reach respiratory center
6. Impulses from respiratory centers descend in spinal cord to reach diaphragm via phrenic nerves and intercostal muscles via intercostal nerves to increase rate and amplitude of respiration
6. Phrenic nerve
6. Intercostal nerves
Intercostal muscles
Diaphragm
Alveolar capillary
Alveolus
O2
CO2
7. Accelerated respiration improves ventilation and thus tends to normalize PO2, PCO2, and pH of blood

Control and Disorders of Respiration

Under normal circumstances, respiration is an unconscious activity. It consists of cyclic contraction and relaxation of the respiratory muscles controlled by groups of neurons in the medulla and pons. These respiratory centers integrate sensory input from chemical and neural receptors and provide neuronal drive to the respiratory muscles. This process drives the thoracic bellows to determine the appropriate level of ventilation to supply oxygen (O_2), eliminate carbon dioxide (CO_2), and contribute to acid-base balance. However, the respiratory system is also under the voluntary control of the motor and premotor cortices. Our understanding of the control of respiration is a result of investigations involving both humans as well as animals.

Chemical Receptors (see Plate 2-25)

Peripheral Chemoreceptors

The peripheral chemoreceptors include the carotid and aortic bodies that sense the partial pressure of arterial oxygen (PaO_2). These receptors also increase afferent discharge in response to hypercapnia or acidosis. Whereas the aortic chemoreceptors are active throughout infancy and childhood, the carotid chemoreceptors are more important in adults. The carotid bodies are located at the bifurcation of the common carotid arteries and are arranged like a cluster of glomeruli with neural type I and sustentacular type II cells. Neuronal impulses travel via the IX (glossopharyngeal) cranial nerve and increase when PaO_2 is below 75 mm Hg. These discharges reach the nucleus tractus solitarius (NTS), where excitatory neurotransmitters are released and stimulate ventilation. It is estimated that carotid bodies contribute approximately 15% of resting ventilation.

Central Chemoreceptors

The major purpose of the central nervous system (CNS) chemoreceptors is to adjust ventilation to maintain acid-base homeostasis. Of the various chemoreceptor sites located in the medulla and midbrain, the most important are found near the ventral surface of the medulla (VSM) and near the retrotrapezoid nucleus (RTN). These receptors respond vigorously and immediately to changes in pH within the CNS. Based in part on animal studies, it is believed that acetylcholine and the parasympathetic nervous system contribute to basal respiratory center rhythm and are important in the response to hypercapnia. Because CO_2 readily crosses the blood-brain barrier, changes in the partial pressure of arterial carbon dioxide ($PaCO_2$) are detected rapidly

NEURAL CONTROL OF BREATHING

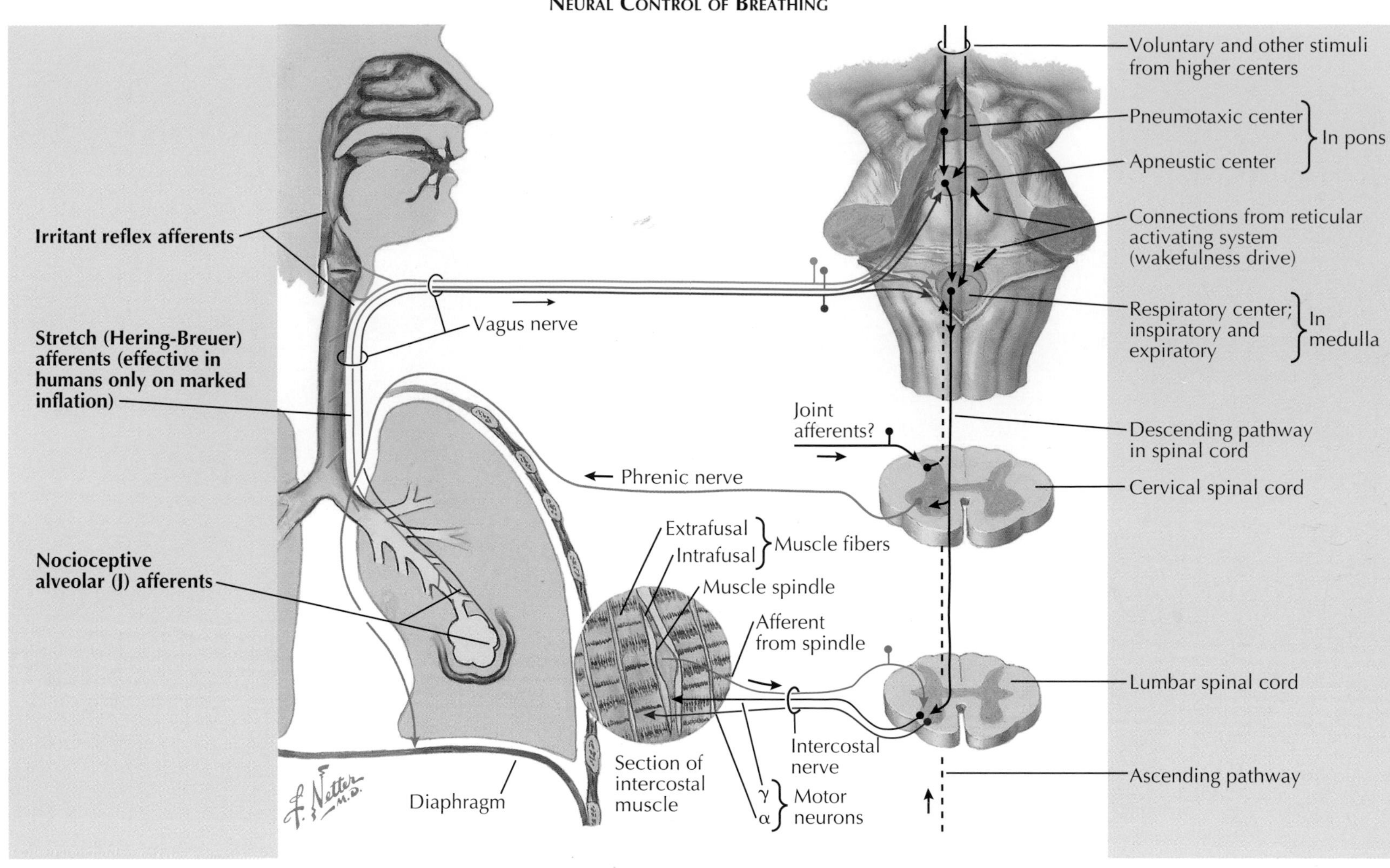

CONTROL AND DISORDERS OF RESPIRATION *(Continued)*

in the brain, leading to changes in ventilation and pH. In contrast, changes in the composition of electrolytes in the CNS occur over hours. The response rate of the central chemoreceptors is generally rapid with respiratory acid-base alterations and slow with metabolic abnormalities.

Neural Receptors *(see Plate 2-26)*

Various neural receptors are present in the upper airways, tracheobronchial tree, lung, chest wall, and pulmonary vasculature. The two major types of receptors are:

- Slowly adapting pulmonary stretch receptors and muscle spindles
- Rapidly adapting irritant receptors, including C-fibers

Both slowly and rapidly adapting receptors respond to changes in lung volume. In addition, irritant receptors are sensitive to chemicals and inhaled noxious agents (e.g., dust). The C-fiber nerve endings are located in the epithelium of the airways and respond to the local milieu.

When one or more of these receptors or fibers are stimulated, an afferent impulse is sent via the vagus nerve to the central respiratory centers. The response may increase respiratory rate or may produce cough or bronchoconstriction (or both) if an irritant is inhaled. It is believed that input from these neural receptors contributes to the hyperventilation (as evident by hypocapnia) that develops in patients with respiratory disorders (e.g., acute asthma, interstitial lung disease, pulmonary embolism, pneumonia) despite correction of hypoxemia by use of supplemental oxygen therapy.

Central Respiratory Centers *(see Plate 2-26)*

The central respiratory centers are located in the medulla and in the brainstem. These groups of neurons receive and process sensory information from central respiratory pacer cells, upper airway receptors, and chemical and neuronal receptors. Both stimulatory and inhibitory afferent impulses are integrated within these centers. Then the respiratory rhythm signals originating in the medulla are modified, and an efferent output is directed to the respiratory muscles. The overall neural outflow from the medulla drives the frequency of breathing as well as the pattern of breathing (i.e., inspiratory and expiratory flow and time). Typically, there is mild inhibitory input from the cerebral cortex to the central respiratory centers. However, the premotor and motor cortexes can exert voluntary respiratory system control via projections in the corticospinal tracts that synapse with the muscles of respiration. During sleep, the central motor command is reduced, which results in a slight increase (~3-4 mm Hg) in the partial pressure of arterial carbon dioxide ($PaCO_2$).

Medullary Centers

A series of inspiratory neurons in the ventrolateral nucleus tractus solitarius (NTS) referred to collectively as the dorsal respiratory group (DRG) has been shown to receive information from both slowly and rapidly adapting receptors in the lung by way of vagal afferents. The commissural nucleus of the NTS receives signals about rapid lung inflations and deflations via rapidly adapting afferents. The DRG serves as the initial relay and integration site for information from arterial baroreceptors, airway and lung stretch receptors, and cardiac receptors.

The ventral respiratory group (VRG) is composed of bilateral columns of respiratory neurons in the lateral medulla that extend from the C1 spinal cord level to just below the facial nucleus. Both the DRG and VRG cells project to the contralateral spinal motor neurons. The DRG cells drive phrenic motor neurons and the VRG. The major function of the VRG is to drive intercostal and abdominal respiratory motor neurons.

PONTINE CENTERS

Pacemaker neurons are located diffusely throughout the caudal pons. Neurons in the pontine respiratory group (PRG) respond through the vagus nerve to many sensory inputs, including (1) upper airway irritant

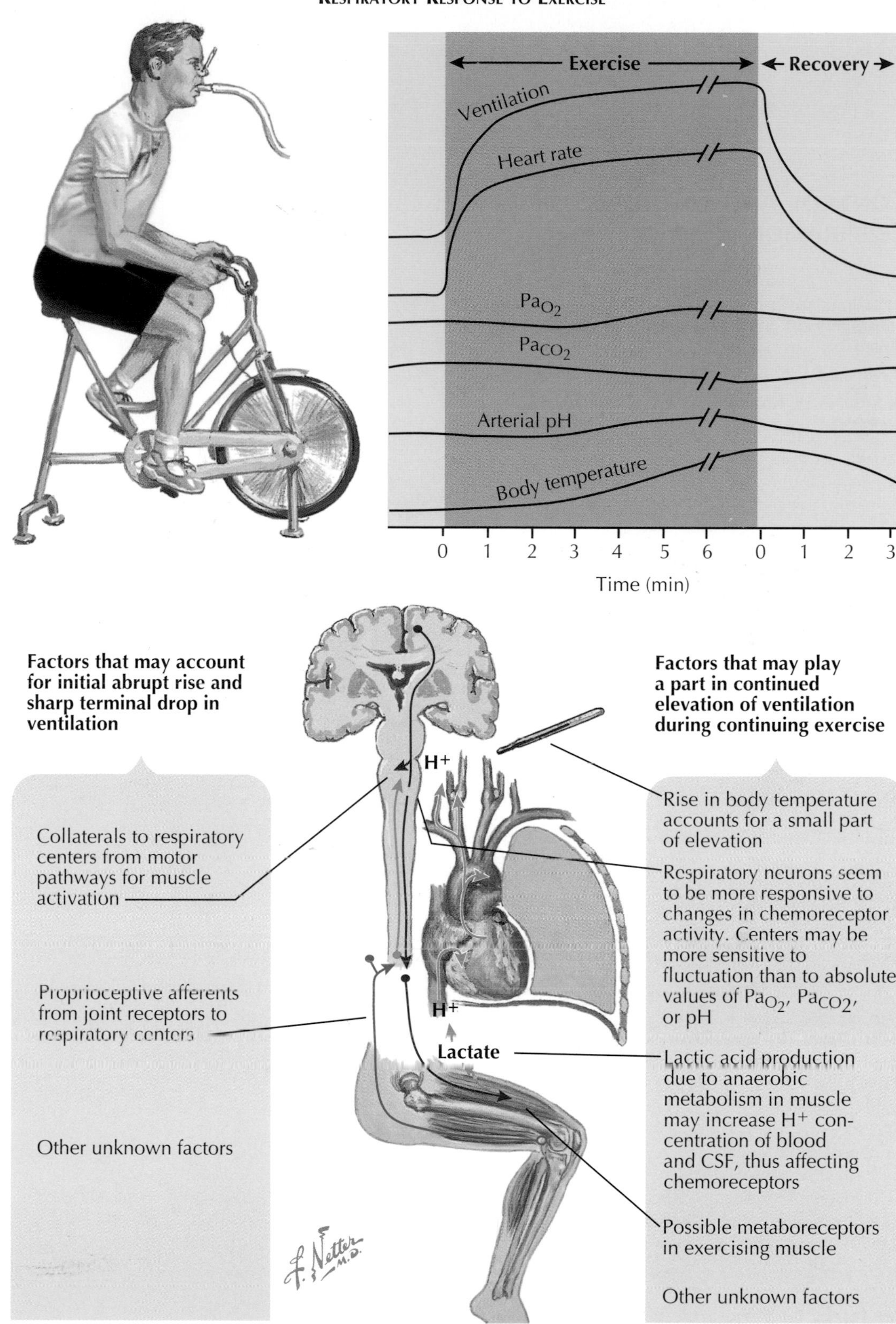
Respiratory Response to Exercise
Exercise
Recovery
Ventilation
Heart rate
Pa_{O_2}
Pa_{CO_2}
Arterial pH
Body temperature
0 1 2 3 4 5 6 0 1 2 3
Time (min)
Factors that may account for initial abrupt rise and sharp terminal drop in ventilation
Collaterals to respiratory centers from motor pathways for muscle activation
Proprioceptive afferents from joint receptors to respiratory centers
Other unknown factors
H+
H+
Lactate
Factors that may play a part in continued elevation of ventilation during continuing exercise
Rise in body temperature accounts for a small part of elevation
Respiratory neurons seem to be more responsive to changes in chemoreceptor activity. Centers may be more sensitive to fluctuation than to absolute values of Pa_{O_2}, Pa_{CO_2}, or pH
Lactic acid production due to anaerobic metabolism in muscle may increase H^+ concentration of blood and CSF, thus affecting chemoreceptors
Possible metaboreceptors in exercising muscle
Other unknown factors
F. Netter M.D.

Control and Disorders of Respiration *(Continued)*

receptors underlying the cough reflex; (2) aortic chemoreceptors, distal nociceptive fibers, and even articular proprioceptive elements that all stimulate ventilation; and (3) J-receptors in the lung parenchyma.

NEUROCHEMICAL CONTROL OF EXERCISE HYPERPNEA (see Plate 2-27)

Exercise performance requires the integrated coupling of the metabolic-cardiovascular-ventilatory systems to maintain stable levels of arterial pH, $PaCO_2$, and PaO_2 up to moderate intensities of exertion. The exact mechanism for exercise hyperpnea is unknown. Both feedforward and feedback mechanisms are thought to contribute to the hyperpneic response. At the initiation of constant work exercise, the responses of expired minute ventilation (V_E), oxygen consumption (VO_2), and carbon dioxide production (VCO_2) can be characterized by three phases:

- Phase I: An immediate increase at the start of exercise lasting 15 seconds
- Phase II: A slower increase to steady-state lasting 2 to 3 minutes
- Phase III: A steady-state level if below the onset of metabolic acidosis or a slow upward drift if metabolic acidosis ensues

The fast ventilatory response at exercise onset apparently stems from a combination of feedforward (central motor commands to working muscles) and feedback (from metaboreceptors and mechanoreceptors in exercising muscles) mechanisms. The feedforward ventilatory stimulation originates in the higher locomotor centers and stimulates phrenic, intercostal, and lumbar respiratory motor neurons. Animal studies demonstrate that electrical stimulation of motor neurons in the supramedullary CNS increases ventilation and cardiac output even when locomotor muscles are paralyzed. Current evidence suggests that both feedforward and feedback effects are synergistic for regulating exercise hyperpnea.

During steady-state conditions, alveolar ventilation increases during exercise in direct proportion to VCO_2. Because work rates generally exceed about 70% of peak VO_2, V_E increases out of proportion to VCO_2. This hyperventilation, which reduces $PaCO_2$, appears because of (1) feedback stimulation as lactic acid and heat accumulate in exercise muscles, (2) an increase in feedforward central command as more motor units are recruited to maintain muscle force as fatigue develops, and (3) stimulation from circulating catecholamines.

The PaO_2 is determined by two major factors during exercise: (1) the extent of alveolar ventilation at a certain level of metabolic demand and (2) the efficiency with which O_2 is transferred from alveolar gas to arterial blood, conceptualized as the alveolar-to-arterial PO_2 difference [(A-a) DO_2]. The oxygen content of arterial blood is directly related to the concentration of hemoglobin (grams of Hgb) and its fractional oxygen saturation (SaO_2). Oxygen dissociation from hemoglobin to respiring tissues is influenced by low pH (the Bohr effect), high PCO_2 (the Haldane effect), hyperthermia, and abundance of 2,3-diphosphoglycerate (DPG).

The ventilatory demands of high-intensity exercise require that airway flow rates may exceed 10 times resting levels and tidal volumes that approach five times values at rest. In healthy untrained individuals, the capacities for ventilation and alveolar-arterial oxygen transport are more than adequate at all exercise intensities. However, when highly trained individuals perform maximal exercise, mechanical limits of the lung (e.g., exercise flow limitation) and respiratory muscles may develop. In addition, many highly conditioned athletes experience significant arterial oxygen desaturation with exercise, especially with running, because of diffusion

CONTROL AND DISORDERS OF RESPIRATION *(Continued)*

limitation, an insufficient hyperventilatory response, and a rightward shift of the oxyhemoglobin dissociation curve.

RESPONSES AND ADAPTATION TO HYPOXIA (see Plate 2-28)

Responses to acute hypoxia as experienced with exposure to high altitude include increases in ventilation (primarily frequency of respiration), cardiac output, pulmonary artery pressure, and tissue extraction of oxygen. These responses are typically manifest by the symptom of breathlessness. The respiratory alkalosis caused by the hyperventilatory response decreases the sensitivity of both peripheral and central chemoreceptors. If the exposure to hypoxia continues (e.g., by residence at high altitude), ventilation increases further after the first few days.

The cardiovascular responses to acute hypoxia include increases in heart rate and in cardiac output; these changes subside with prolonged exposure to hypoxia. In high-altitude natives, pulmonary hypertension and systemic hypotension are common but reversible features. Recently, researchers have described a hypoxia-inducible family of transcription factors that is related to production of regulatory proteins that serve to redress cellular hypoxia, notably endothelin-1 (ET-1), vascular endothelial growth factor (VEGF), erythropoietin, and transferrin. VEGF and ET-1 appear to enhance pulmonary arterial tone, causing vasculopathy or remodeling.

An effect of chronic hypoxia is an increase in the concentration of red blood cells caused by the effects of erythropoietin on the bone marrow to stimulate red blood cell production. Usually, the increment is such that the oxygen content of arterial blood is maintained similar to that at sea level. Occasionally, an excessive increase in red blood cells may occur (secondary polycythemia). In addition, the red blood cells show a diminished hemoglobin affinity for oxygen because of an increase in organic phosphate (DPG) related to respiratory alkalosis and hemoglobin deoxygenation. Transferrin provides a repository for hemoglobin-building iron.

COMMON DISORDERS OF RESPIRATORY CONTROL (see Plate 2-29)

Equilibrium among blood gas tensions and pH can only be achieved when chemoreceptor feedback loops, neural processing structures, and ventilatory effector organs are closely integrated. The stability of this system can be affected by a number of abnormalities, including:

- Physical loss of mandated control elements
- Fluctuations in controller gain
- Unpredictable latency to restoration of the reference state

EFFECTS OF HIGH ALTITUDE ON RESPIRATORY MECHANISM

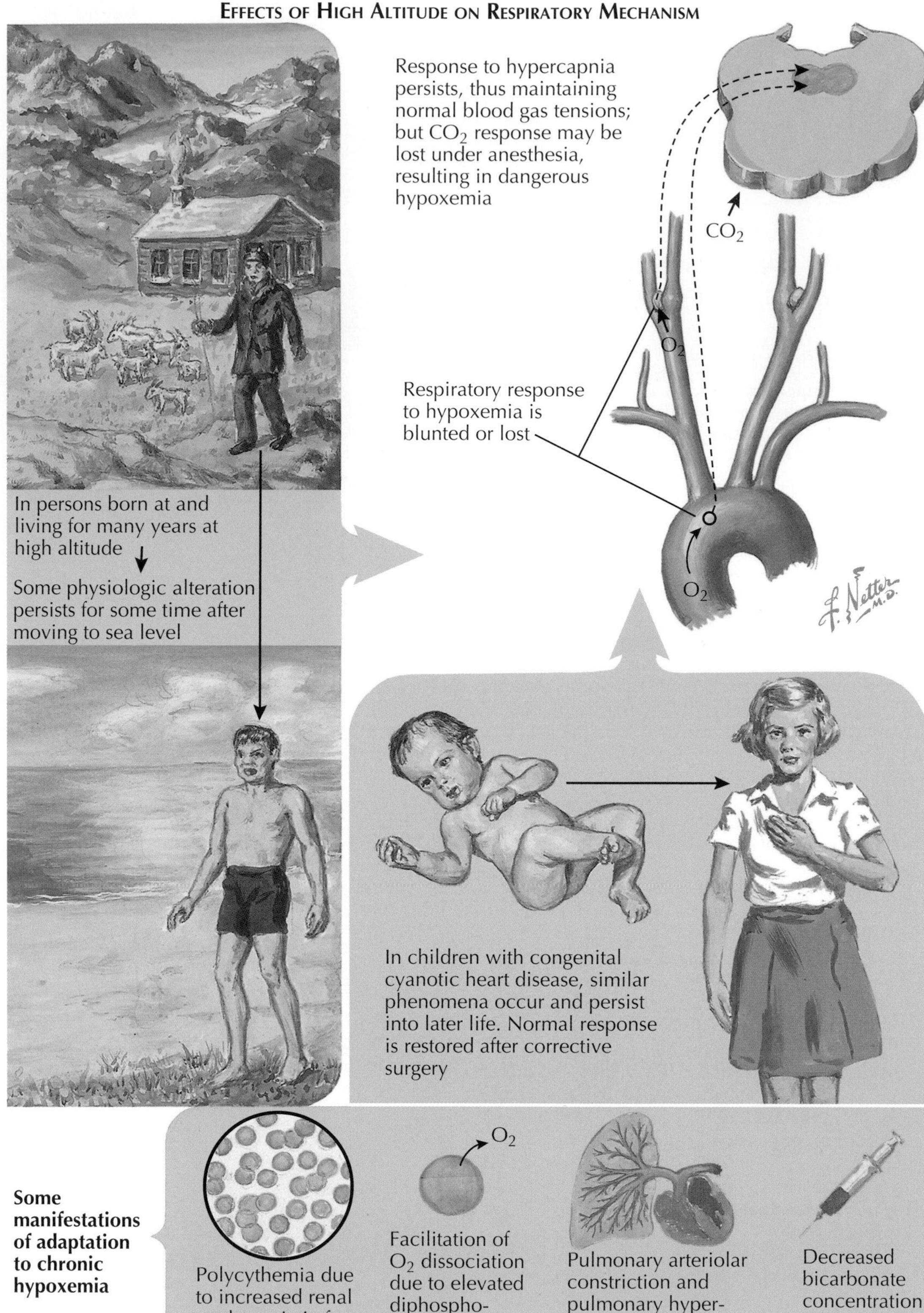

Response to hypercapnia persists, thus maintaining normal blood gas tensions; but CO_2 response may be lost under anesthesia, resulting in dangerous hypoxemia
CO_2
O_2
Respiratory response to hypoxemia is blunted or lost
O_2
In persons born at and living for many years at high altitude
Some physiologic alteration persists for some time after moving to sea level
In children with congenital cyanotic heart disease, similar phenomena occur and persist into later life. Normal response is restored after corrective surgery
Some manifestations of adaptation to chronic hypoxemia
Polycythemia due to increased renal erythropoietic factor
O_2
Facilitation of O_2 dissociation due to elevated diphosphoglycerate
Pulmonary arteriolar constriction and pulmonary hypertension with right heart hypertrophy
Decreased bicarbonate concentration in blood and in CSF
F. Netter M.D.

The manner in which $PaCO_2$ is regulated represents a classic negative-feedback control scenario in which variations of $PaCO_2$ precipitate ventilatory changes that serve to return this parameter to an equilibrium value. Hence, a brief hypopnea leading to a transient elevation in $PaCO_2$ would be detected by chemoreceptors, whose output would prompt an increase in ventilation to reinstate eucapnia. Because this compensatory action cannot happen instantaneously and must lag behind a given perturbation, the consequential brief hyperpnea then throws the system in the opposite direction. What ensues is an oscillatory rectifier, the magnitude and persistence of which relate to how much the signal from the original disturbance is amplified.

It is important to realize that the $PaCO_2$ regulatory schema is one determinant of ventilation, and other

HYPERVENTILATION AND HYPOVENTILATION

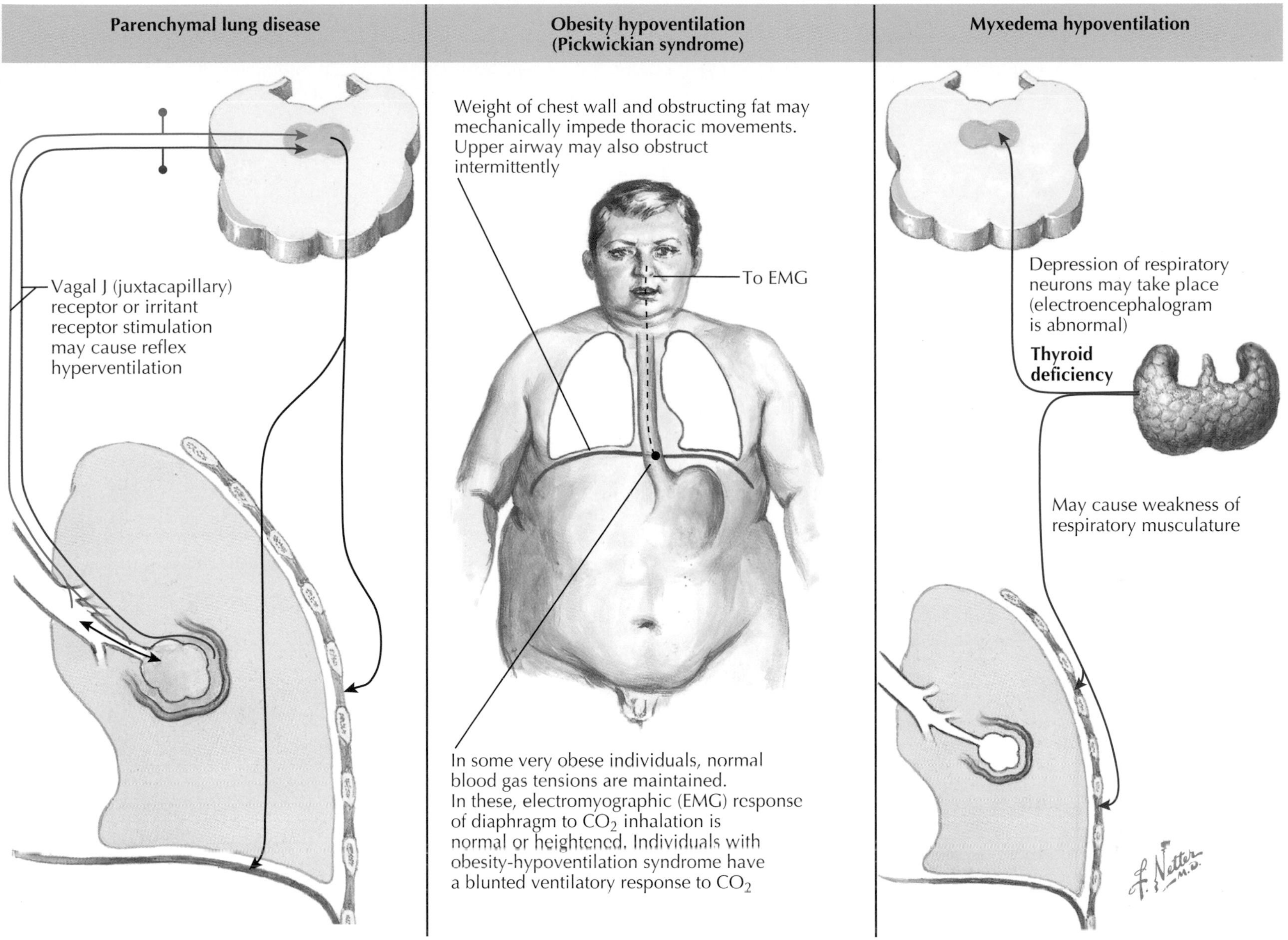

Parenchymal lung disease
Obesity hypoventilation (Pickwickian syndrome)
Myxedema hypoventilation
Vagal J (juxtacapillary) receptor or irritant receptor stimulation may cause reflex hyperventilation
Weight of chest wall and obstructing fat may mechanically impede thoracic movements. Upper airway may also obstruct intermittently
To EMG
In some very obese individuals, normal blood gas tensions are maintained. In these, electromyographic (EMG) response of diaphragm to CO_2 inhalation is normal or heightened. Individuals with obesity-hypoventilation syndrome have a blunted ventilatory response to CO_2
Depression of respiratory neurons may take place (electroencephalogram is abnormal)
Thyroid deficiency
May cause weakness of respiratory musculature

CONTROL AND DISORDERS OF RESPIRATION *(Continued)*

afferent circuits are important. As a result, there is tremendous variability in the patterns of breathing observed in healthy individuals. This variability is thought to reflect idiosyncratic sensory input to the central respiratory centers and longitudinal development of a homeostatic default system. Maladaptive or abnormal respiratory control can develop as evident by hyperventilation, hypoventilation, or unstable or irregular ventilation.

HYPERVENTILATION

Levels of progesterone increase throughout *pregnancy*, and this hormone is a known stimulant of respiratory drive. The increase in V_E is primarily caused by an increase in tidal volume. This causes chronic respiratory alkalosis for which renal bicarbonate excretion acts to preserve normal pH. Approximately 60% to 70% of women experience breathlessness during the course of pregnancy, which is thought to be related to elevated levels of progesterone.

The *hyperventilation syndrome* is characterized by a sensation of an inability to take a deep breath in, palpitations, paresthesias, and anxiety. These symptoms are typically episodic, occur at rest, and are unrelated to exercise. It is believed that the individual's anxiety alters voluntary control of the respiratory centers, thus causing hyperventilation.

HYPOVENTILATION

The *obesity-hypoventilation syndrome* (OHS) is related to an increased body mass index (usually >30 kg/m^2) and manifest by hypercapnia ($PaCO_2$ >45 mm Hg) during wakefulness in the absence of other possible causes for alveolar hypoventilation. Hypercapnia may be caused by impaired ventilatory mechanics as well as an abnormality in the control of respiration. The central adiposity decreases both chest wall compliance and the amount of work done by respiratory muscles for a given degree of respiratory drive. Patients with OHS breathe at low lung volumes with attendant closure of small airways. In addition, chemosensitivity to both hypoxia and to hypercapnia is blunted in those with OHS. Although sleep-disordered breathing is technically not part of the OHS, hypercapnia typically worsens during sleep in those with OHS. This may be a result of reduced central respiratory drive or upper airway obstructive events overnight.

Myxedema can cause hypoventilation in some patients with severe hypothyroidism. It is likely caused by both depression of ventilatory drive and possible respiratory muscle weakness.

Congenital central hypoventilation syndrome (CCHS) is associated with a nearly absent respiratory response to

Periodic Breathing (Cheyne-Stokes)

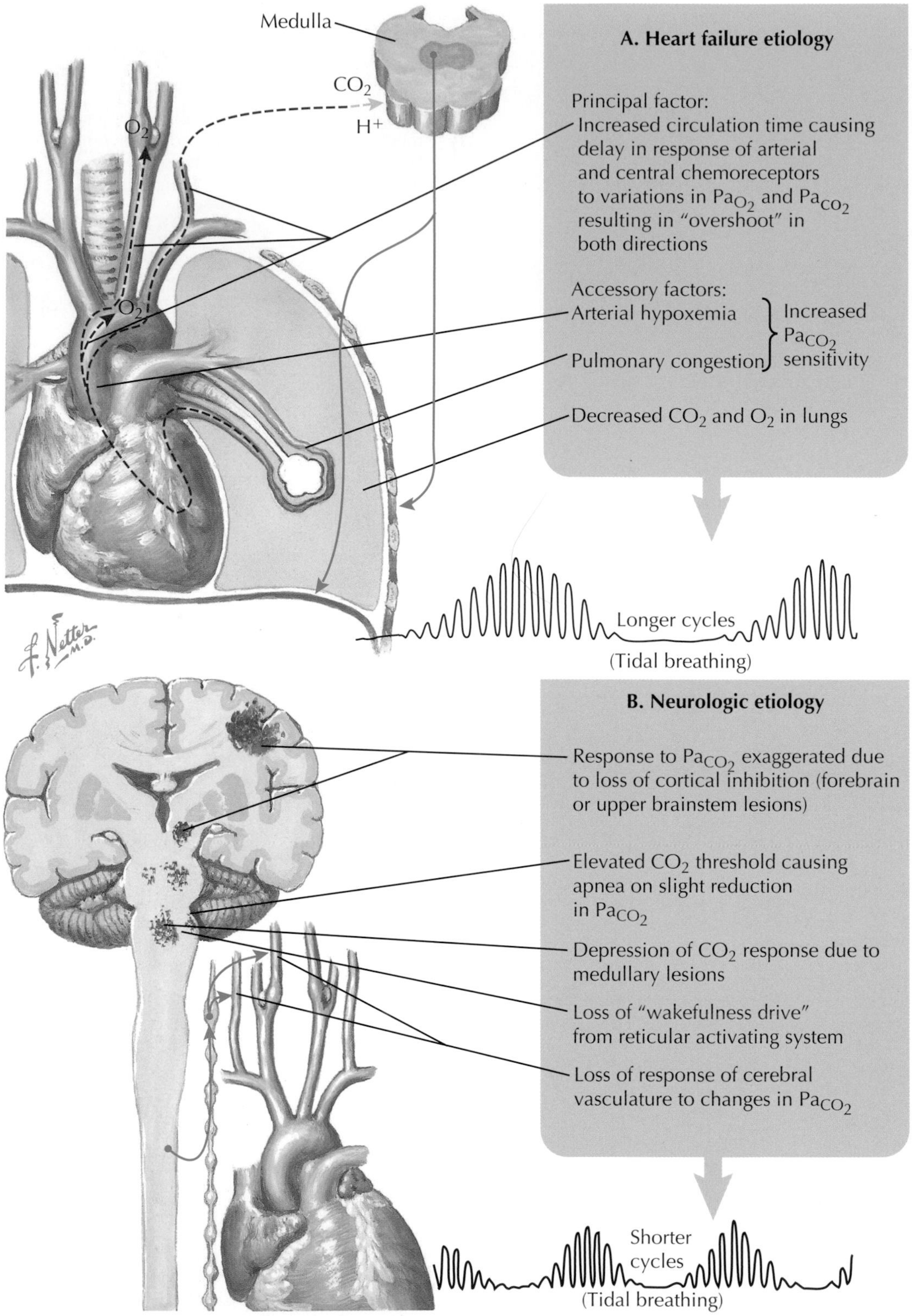

Medulla
CO_2
H^+
O_2
O_2

A. Heart failure etiology

Principal factor:
Increased circulation time causing delay in response of arterial and central chemoreceptors to variations in Pa_{O_2} and Pa_{CO_2} resulting in "overshoot" in both directions

Accessory factors:
Arterial hypoxemia
Pulmonary congestion
} Increased Pa_{CO_2} sensitivity

Decreased CO_2 and O_2 in lungs

Longer cycles
(Tidal breathing)

B. Neurologic etiology

Response to Pa_{CO_2} exaggerated due to loss of cortical inhibition (forebrain or upper brainstem lesions)

Elevated CO_2 threshold causing apnea on slight reduction in Pa_{CO_2}

Depression of CO_2 response due to medullary lesions

Loss of "wakefulness drive" from reticular activating system

Loss of response of cerebral vasculature to changes in Pa_{CO_2}

Shorter cycles
(Tidal breathing)

Control and Disorders of Respiration *(Continued)*

hypoxia and hypercapnia with mild elevations of $PaCO_2$ during wakefulness and marked elevations of $PaCO_2$ during sleep. However, patients with CCHS are able to increase V_E and maintain relatively normal $PaCO_2$ levels during exercise. CCHS may occur in association with Hirschsprung disease, a condition characterized by abnormalities of the cholinergic innervation of the gastrointestinal tract. This association, and the demonstration of subtle autonomic abnormalities in relatives of patients with CCHS, suggest that autonomic neuropathy, particularly of the parasympathetic system, is important in CCHS.

The *Ondine curse* is a rare condition in which patients experience alveolar hypoventilation caused by impaired autonomic control of ventilation, but their voluntary control remains intact. These individuals maintain relatively normal blood gases while awake, but "forget to breathe" when they fall asleep. This problem can develop after surgical incisions into the second cervical segment of the spinal cord (used to relieve intractable pain) and as a result of medullary infarction.

Carotid body resection, previously used as treatment for asthma, leads to depression of hypoxic ventilatory responsiveness. Bilateral endarterectomy as treatment for carotid artery disease may result in destruction of peripheral chemoreceptors with consequent reduction in hypoxic drive.

Hypoxic ventilatory response decreases by 40% in normal individuals after 10 days of *severe diet restriction*.

UNSTABLE OR IRREGULAR VENTILATION
(see Plate 2-30)

Cheyne-Stokes respiration (CSR) involves cyclic breathing in which apnea is followed by hyperpnea and then decreasing respiratory frequency followed by the next apneic period. This condition may occur in approximately 40% of patients with congestive heart failure and up to 50% of patients with an acute ischemic stroke. CSR is also associated with other neurologic diseases, sedation, normal sleep, acid-base disturbances, prematurity, and acclimatization to altitude. The mechanism for CSR appears to be a delay between changes in ventilation and detection of the resulting $PaCO_2$ by central chemoreceptors. This contributes to a cyclic pattern of respiration. In congestive heart failure, a prolonged lung to brain circulatory time introduces a lag between gas exchange at the alveolar-capillary membrane and registration of partial pressures at chemoreceptors. The increase in ventilatory drive may be caused, in part, by loss of effective damping factors ("underdampening"). In contrast to normal physiology, $PaCO_2$ tends to be highest and PaO_2 is lowest during hyperpnea.

Rett syndrome is a rare neurodevelopmental disorder that occurs almost exclusively in girls. Affected patients initially develop normally and then gradually lose speech and purposeful hand use. The syndrome is delineated by cognitive defects, stereotypical motor activity, microcephaly, seizures, and a disorganized breathing pattern during wakefulness characterized by periods of apnea alternating with periods of hyperventilation.

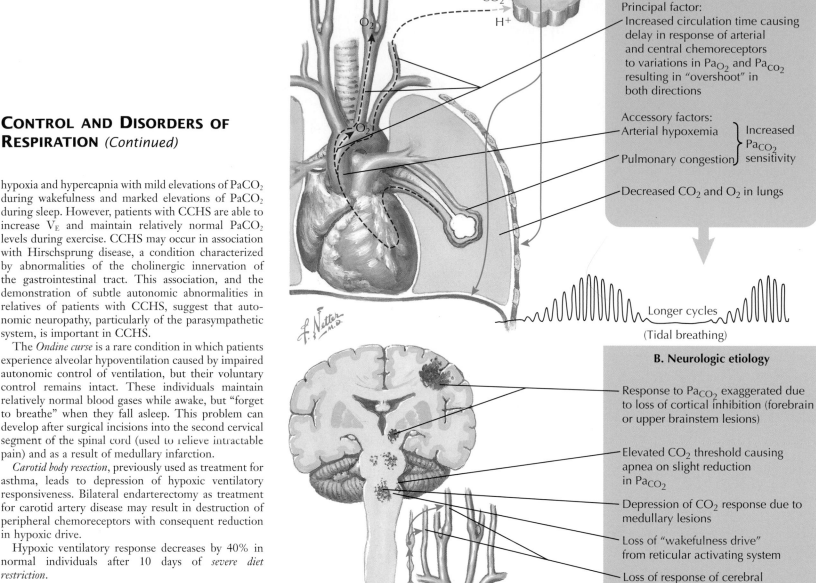

DRUGS THAT AFFECT VENTILATORY DRIVE

Central nervous depressants, such as opiates, barbiturates, and benzodiazepines, depress central respiratory drive. Those with preexisting hypoventilation are particularly susceptible to the deleterious effects of these medications.

Central nervous stimulants, such as caffeine, theophylline, medroxyprogesterone, and acetazolamide, enhance central respiratory drive.

SITES OF PATHOLOGIC DISTURBANCES IN CONTROL OF BREATHING

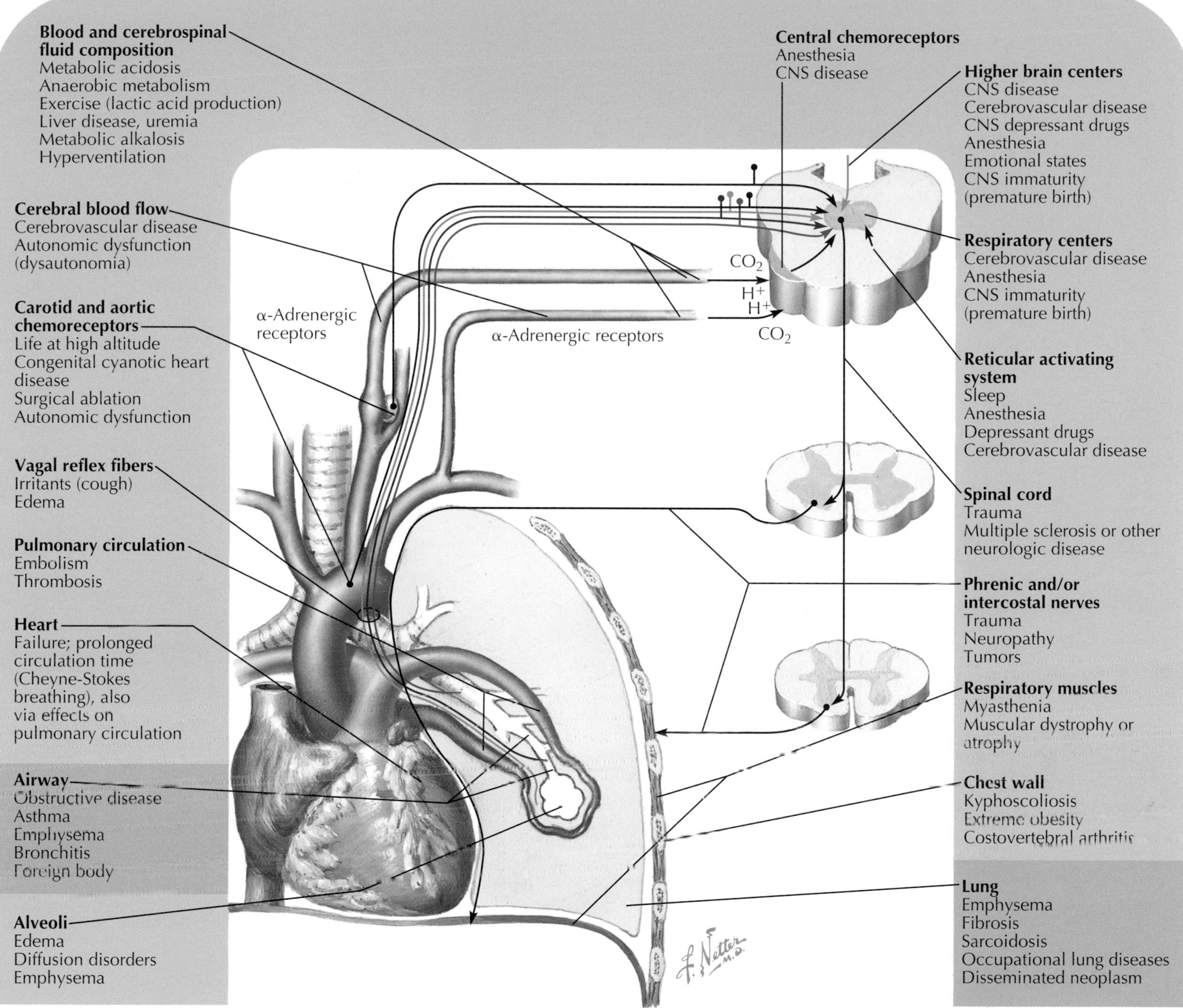

CONTROL AND DISORDERS OF RESPIRATION *(Continued)*

DISRUPTION OF NORMAL BREATHING CONTROL IN SELECTED DISEASES

(see Plate 2-31)

As evident in the above sections, the control of respiration is complex, and any number of diseases or exogenous variables can lead to impaired function. Diseases involving the airways, lung parenchyma, pulmonary circulation, and respiratory muscles can cause a decrease in PaO_2, usually caused by ventilation-perfusion inequalities.

In some patients with advanced *chronic obstructive pulmonary disease* (COPD), alveolar hypoventilation can develop, causing hypercapnia. This is more common in the chronic bronchitis phenotype of COPD. The rapid and shallow pattern of breathing in patients with COPD who develop CO_2 retention further contributes to an increase in dead-space ventilation.

Patients with a history of *near-fatal asthma* have been shown to have depressed ventilatory responses to both hypoxia and hypercapnia. Patients with asthma who have depressed chemosensitivity typically also exhibit low ratings of breathlessness in response to breathing through external respiratory loads. These features in some patients with asthma probably lead to a delay in seeking medical attention when an asthma attack ensues, thereby resulting in an increased risk of fatal asthma.

A variety of *neuromuscular diseases* can affect the ability of patients to ventilate adequately. For example, in those with mild to moderate respiratory muscle weakness, ventilatory drive is increased, leading to hyperventilation. With severe weakness of the respiratory muscles, hypercapnia can develop that may be greater than expected from respiratory mouth pressures. Alterations in the control of breathing may occur as manifest by reduced hypoxic or hypercapnic ventilatory drives. In patients with *poliomyelitis*, the primary ventilatory nuclei in the brainstem can be affected, leading to hypoventilation or apnea (or both), particularly during sleep.

DIAGNOSTIC PROCEDURES

Tests of Pulmonary Function

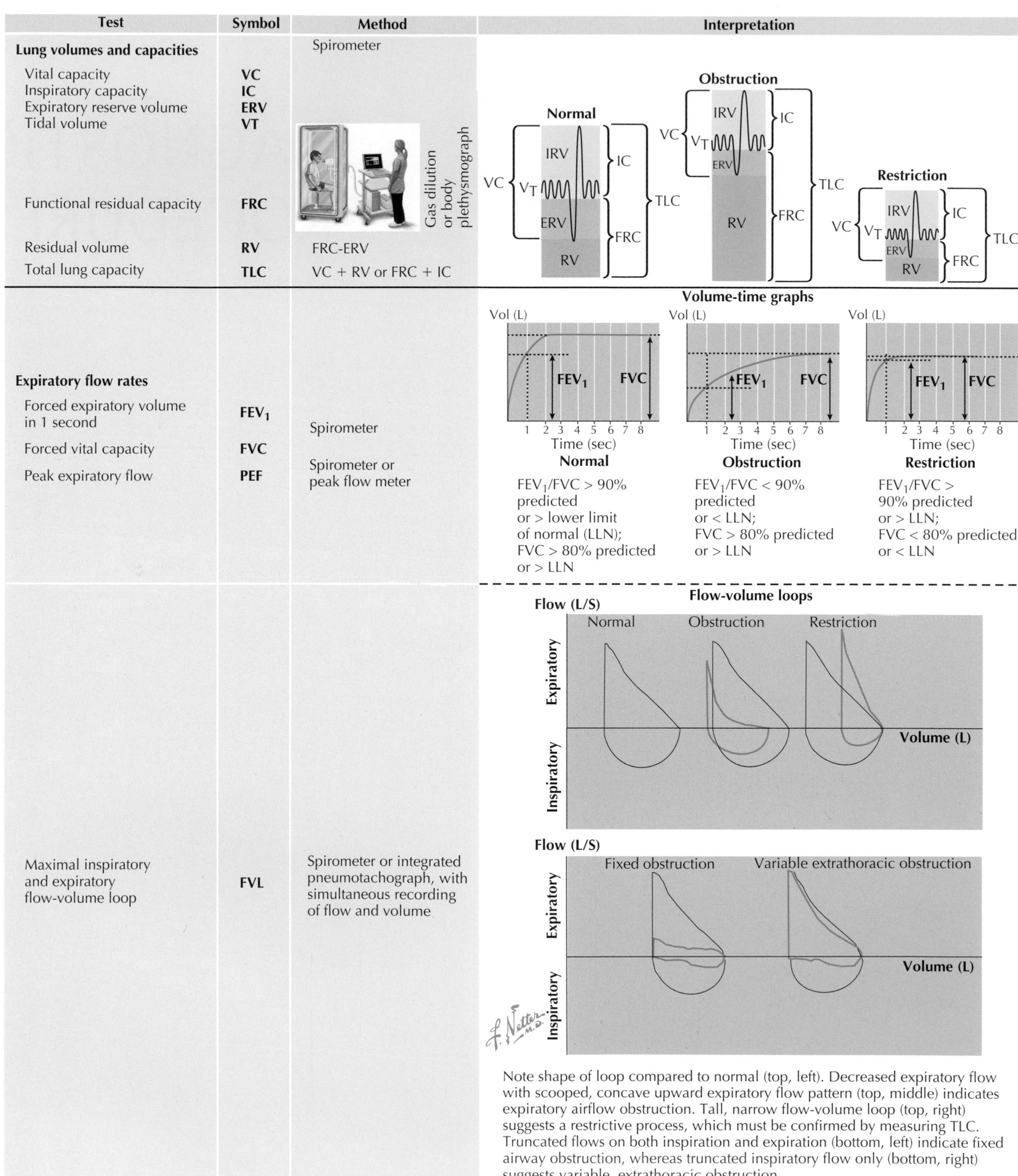

Test	Symbol	Method	Interpretation
Lung volumes and capacities		Spirometer	
Vital capacity	**VC**		
Inspiratory capacity	**IC**		
Expiratory reserve volume	**ERV**		
Tidal volume	**VT**		
Functional residual capacity	**FRC**	Gas dilution or body plethysmograph	
Residual volume	**RV**	FRC-ERV	
Total lung capacity	**TLC**	VC + RV or FRC + IC	
Expiratory flow rates			Volume-time graphs
Forced expiratory volume in 1 second	**FEV_1**		Normal: FEV_1/FVC > 90% predicted or > lower limit of normal (LLN); FVC > 80% predicted or > LLN
Forced vital capacity	**FVC**	Spirometer	Obstruction: FEV_1/FVC < 90% predicted or < LLN; FVC > 80% predicted or > LLN
Peak expiratory flow	**PEF**	Spirometer or peak flow meter	Restriction: FEV_1/FVC > 90% predicted or > LLN; FVC < 80% predicted or < LLN
Maximal inspiratory and expiratory flow-volume loop	**FVL**	Spirometer or integrated pneumotachograph, with simultaneous recording of flow and volume	Flow-volume loops

Note shape of loop compared to normal (top, left). Decreased expiratory flow with scooped, concave upward expiratory flow pattern (top, middle) indicates expiratory airflow obstruction. Tall, narrow flow-volume loop (top, right) suggests a restrictive process, which must be confirmed by measuring TLC. Truncated flows on both inspiration and expiration (bottom, left) indicate fixed airway obstruction, whereas truncated inspiratory flow only (bottom, right) suggests variable, extrathoracic obstruction.

Tests of Pulmonary Function *(Continued)*

Test	Symbol	Method	Interpretation
Lung elasticity Static recoil pressure Static compliance	P_{stat} C_{stat}	Pleural pressure (Ppl) is estimated as esophageal pressure measured with an esophageal balloon catheter, and alveolar pressure (Palv) is estimated as mouth pressure under conditions of no flow. Transpulmonary pressure (Ptp) is the difference of Palv – Ppl. Ptp is recorded at different lung volumes during expiration from TLC.	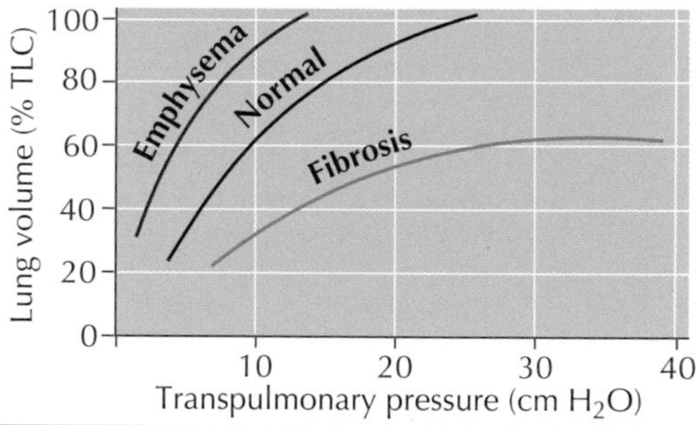 Static elastic recoil of lung is increased and static compliance reduced in diseases such as pulmonary fibrosis. Conversely, static lung compliance is increased and elastic recoil is reduced in emphysema
Airway resistance	**Raw**	Body plethysmograph to determine alveolar pressure and pneumotachograph to measure airflow	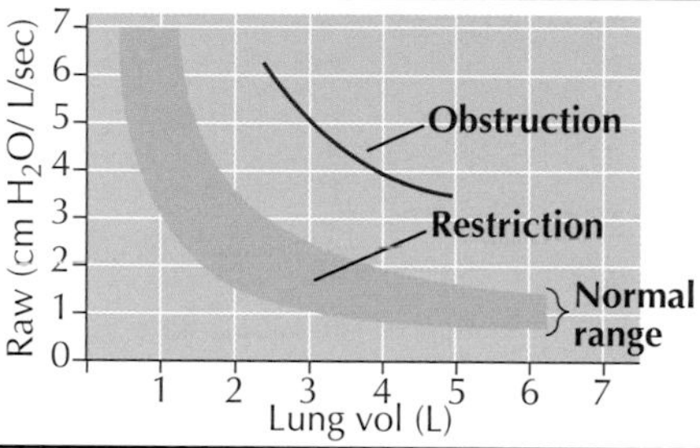 In obstructive lung disease airway resistance is increased. If obstruction involves only small airways (<2 mm diameter), only minimal changes in overall resistance may result. In restrictive disorders, resistance is often reduced because of increased traction on intrathoracic airway walls
Diffusing capacity	**DLCO**	Low concentration of CO inhaled; expired gas analyzed for CO	Diffusing capacity is reduced due to disruption of the alveolar-capillary membrane in such diseases as emphysema, diffuse interstitial lung disease, and pulmonary thromboembolic disease. It is also decreased in anemia. It may be increased in situations of increased intrathoracic hemoglobin, such as left-to-right shunt, erythrocytosis, alveolar hemorrhage, and occasionally asthma
Tests for small airway disease Closing volume Closing capacity	**CV** **CC**	Following a full inspiration of O_2, the expired lung volume from TLC to RV is plotted against the N_2 concentration	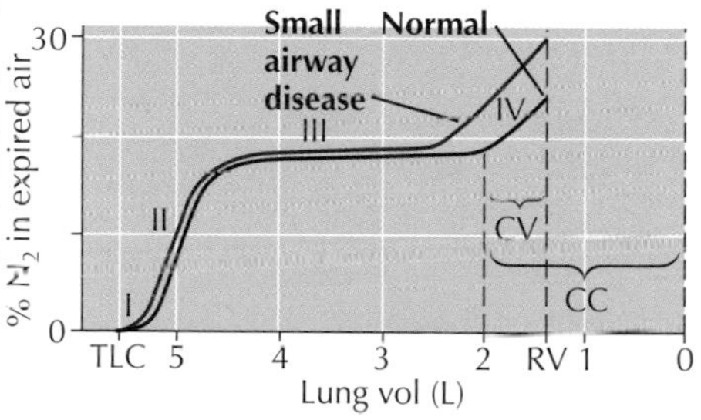 Airways in lower lung zones close at low lung volumes and only those alveoli at top of lungs continue to empty. Since concentration of N_2 in alveoli of upper zones is higher (most of inhaled O_2 goes to lower lung zones), slope of curve abruptly increases (phase IV) at point of airway closure (CV). Phase IV begins at larger lung volumes in individuals with even minor degrees of airway obstruction, increasing both CV and CC. See Plate 2-13 for further details.
Maximal expiratory flow-volume curve breathing 80% He and 20% O_2	$\Delta \dot{V}_{max, 50}$ $V \text{ iso } \dot{V}$	Spirometer or pneumotachograph to record flow and volume	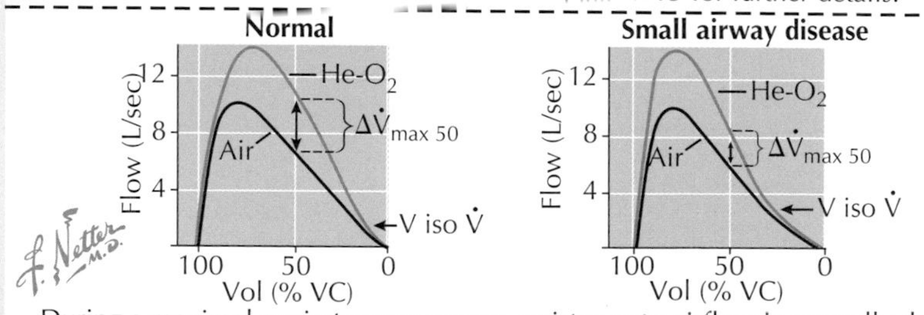 During a maximal expiratory maneuver, resistance to airflow is normally due to turbulence and convective acceleration. Breathing He, which is less dense than air, lowers resistance and increases flow at all but lowest volumes. In small airway disease, resistance to laminar flow makes up the larger portion of total resistance and airflow is relatively independent of gas density. Increase in expiratory flow at 50% of VC while breathing He-O_2 ($\Delta \dot{V}_{max, 50}$) will be less. Volume at which flows while breathing He-O_2 and while breathing air are identical ($V \text{ iso } \dot{V}$) will be higher in patients with small airway disease than in normal individuals
Frequency dependence of dynamic compliance	C_{dyn}	Esophageal balloon to measure pleural pressure and spirometer or pneumotachograph to record volume	Dynamic compliance is determined from changes in lung volume and difference in pleural pressure at end-inspiration and end-expiration. Normally C_{dyn} closely approximates C_{stat} and remains essentially unchanged as breathing frequency increases. Small airway disease may be characterized by patchy increases in airway resistance. During quiet breathing, ventilation may be evenly distributed throughout the lung but as breathing frequency increases, alveoli will fill and empty unevenly and asynchronously as air tends to go to those areas which offer least resistance. Change in pleural pressure for a given change in lung volume increases and dynamic compliance falls. In the setting of overall normal static compliance and normal overall airway resistance, such frequency dependent decreases in compliance reflect inhomogeneous small airways disease.

TESTS OF PULMONARY FUNCTION *(Continued)*

Test	Symbol	Method	Interpretation: Normal values	Interpretation: Abnormalities
Gas exchange				
Partial pressure of O_2 in arterial blood	Pa_{O_2}	Arterial blood is collected anaerobically in heparinized syringe	80 to 100 mm Hg breathing room air at sea level. Falls slightly with age.	Hypoxemia indicative of ventilation-perfusion abnormalities, shunts, diffusion defect, alveolar hypoventilation.
Partial pressure of CO_2 in arterial blood	Pa_{CO_2}		36 to 44 mm Hg	Pa_{CO_2} proportional to metabolic rate (CO_2 production) and inversely related to volume of alveolar ventilation
Arterial blood pH	pH		7.35 to 7.45 pH	Acidosis (pH <7.35) Respiratory (inadequate alveolar ventilation) Metabolic (gain of acid and/or loss of base) Alkalosis (pH >7.45) Respiratory (excessive alveolar ventilation) Metabolic (gain of base or loss of acid)
Alveolar-arterial O_2 difference, or A-a gradient	$A\text{-}aP_{O_2}$ A-aΔ		< 10 mm Hg breathing room air. Upper limit of normal approximated by (age/4) + 4	Primarily reflects mismatching of ventilation and perfusion and/or shunts. May also be affected by diffusion defects. Normal in hypoventilation.
Dead space-tidal volume ratio	Vd/VT	Determined from arterial and mixed expired P_{CO_2}	< 0.3- 0.4	Elevated ratio indicates wasted ventilation; *i.e.*, that volume of gas which does not take part in gas exchange
Shunt fraction	$\dot{Q}s/\dot{Q}T$	Determined from Pa_{O_2} after a period of breathing 100% O_2	< 5%	Elevation indicates increased amount of mixed venous blood entering systemic circulation without coming into contact with alveolar air, either because of shunting of blood past lungs to left side of heart or perfusion of regions of lung which are not ventilated
Muscle pressures				
Maximal inspiratory pressure	MIP	MIP measured as maximal pressure during inspiration from near RV. MEP measured as maximal pressure during expiration from near TLC.	MIP > −50 (F), −75 (M) cm H_20 MEP > 80 (F), 100 (M) cm H_20	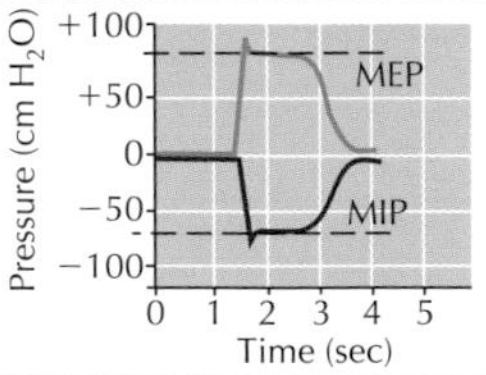 Reduced muscle pressures indicate neuromuscular weakness or suboptimal effort.
Maximal expiratory pressure	MEP			
Bronchial challenge				
Exercise	ΔFEV_1	Spirometry before and after 6–10 min of exercise to increase heart rate to >85% of predicted maximum, or to increase ventilation to 40–60% of predicted MVV.	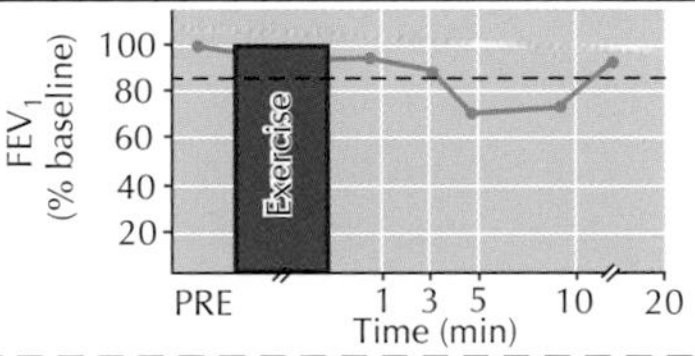	Positive response is decreased in FEV_1 from baseline by >15%
Methacholine	PC20	Spirometry before and after serially increasing doses of inhaled nebulized methacholine. PC20 = provocative concentration causing a fall in FEV_1 by 20%.	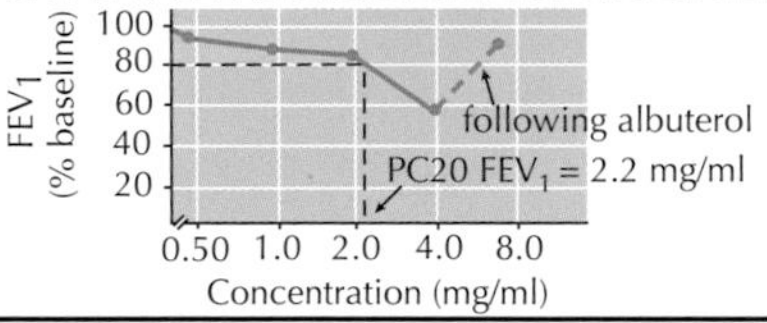	Positive response is decreased in FEV_1 by 20% at a dose of less than 8 mg/ml (PC20 < 8 mg/ml)
Cardiopulmonary exercise test		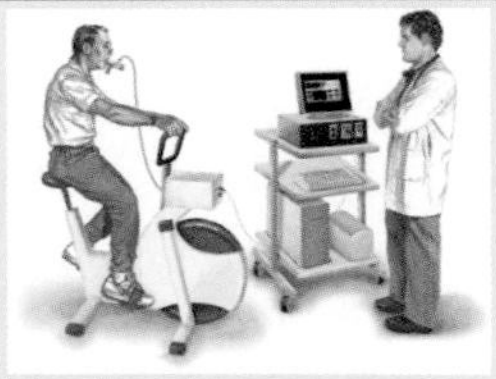	At maximal exercise:	
Maximal O_2 consumption	VO_2 max	Increasing work to exhaustion measured using a bicycle ergometer or treadmill, with breath-by-breath analysis and monitoring of RR, TV, HR, BP, ECG, pulse oximetry.	VO_2 max > 85% predicted (top left)	Cardiovascular limitation = ↑ HR reserve; ↓ O_2 pulse
CO_2 production	VCO_2			Ventilatory limitation = ↓ BR
Maximal predicted heart rate	HRmax		HRmax > 90% predicted (top right)	Gas exchange limitation = ↓ pO_2, ↑ A-aΔ
Heart rate reserve	HRR		HRR < 15 beats per minute	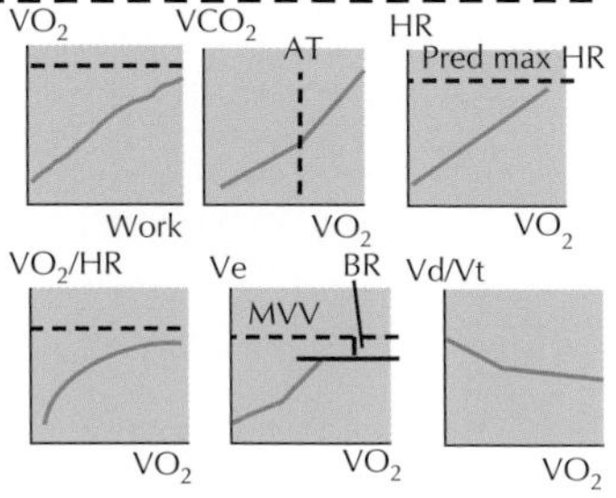
Oxygen pulse (VO_2/heart rate)	VO2/HR		O_2 pulse > 80% predicted (middle, left)	
Breathing reserve (BR)	MVV-Ve, or Ve/MVV		BR > 11 L, or Ve/MVV < 85% (middle, middle)	
Ventilatory equivalent for O_2 (minute ventilation/VO_2)	Ve/VO_2		Ve/VCO_2 at AT < 34 (bottom right)	
Ventilatory equivalent for CO_2 (minute ventilation/VCO_2)	Ve/VCO_2			
Dead space	Vd/VT		Vd/VT < 0.3–0.4, fall with exercise (middle, right)	
Arterial blood gases	pH, pCO_2, PO_2, A-a gradient (A-aΔ)		PaO_2 > 80 mmHg A-aΔ < 35 mmHg (bottom, left)	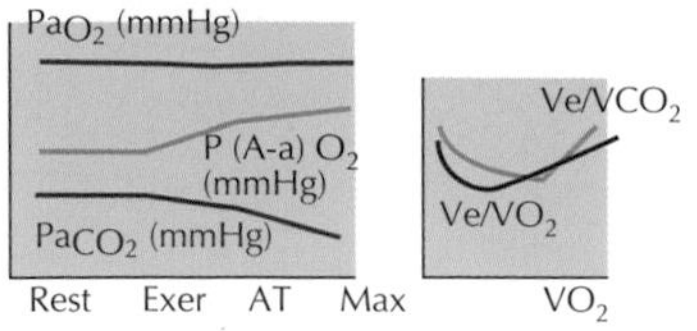
Anaerobic threshold	AT		AT > 40% max predicted VO_2 (top, middle)	

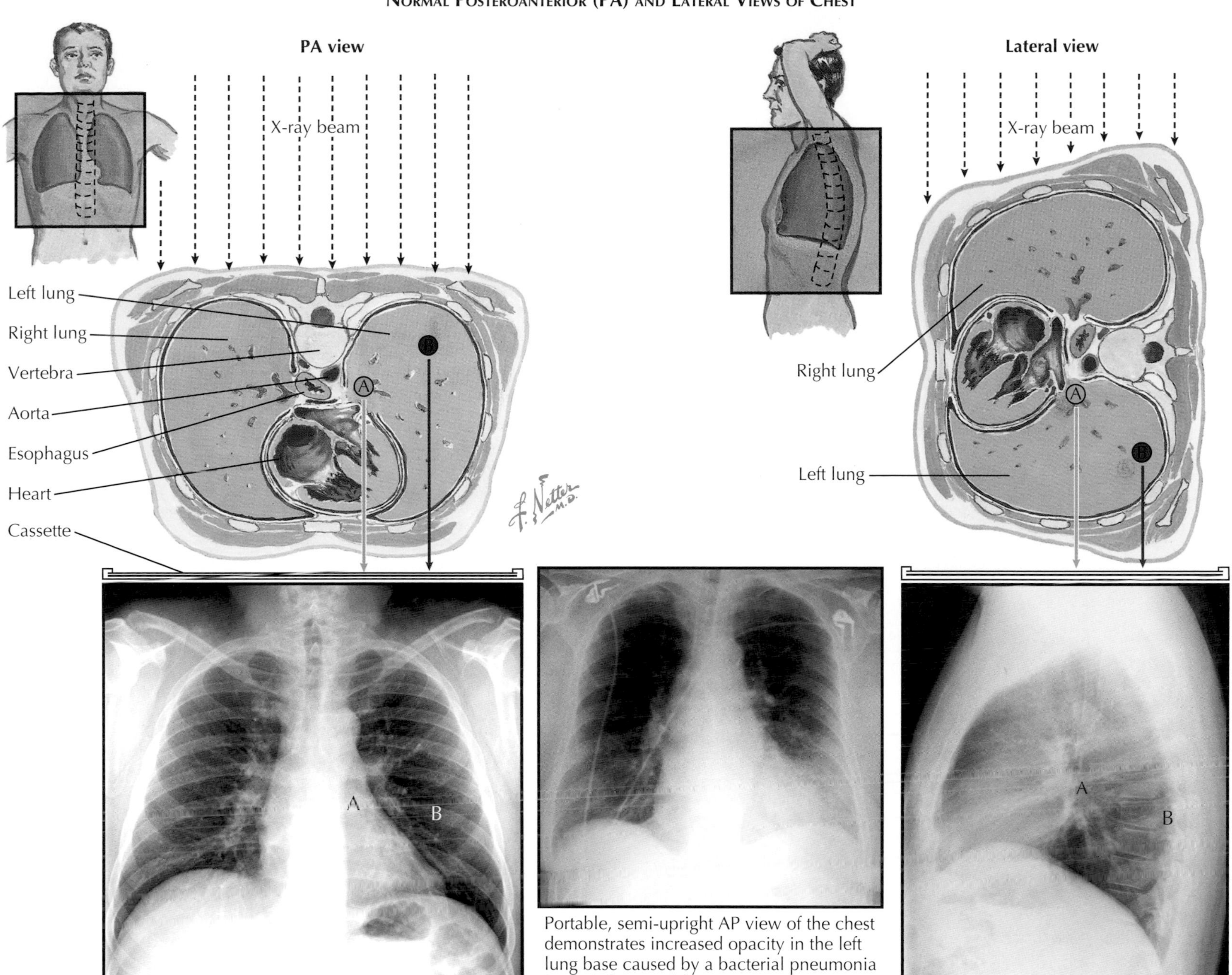

Portable, semi-upright AP view of the chest demonstrates increased opacity in the left lung base caused by a bacterial pneumonia in the left lower lobe

RADIOLOGIC EXAMINATION OF THE LUNGS

Chest radiography remains the primary imaging modality for initial evaluation of patients with suspected chest disease and in many cases not only identifies abnormalities but also allows a specific determination of the nature of the disease present.

ROUTINE EXAMINATION

(see Plates 3-4 to 3-6)

In most imaging centers, radiographs are no longer recorded on film but rather on digital imaging receptors. The imaging data can then either be transferred directly to a computer (digital radiography) or recorded on an imaging plate, similar in appearance to the traditional x-ray cassette. The data are placed into a "reader" and converted to an image (computed radiography). The images can then be printed on radiographic film but are more frequently stored in a digital database called a PACS (Picture Archiving and Communication System) and viewed on a computer monitor on which the contrast and brightness can be adjusted and the image magnified and annotated.

Frontal and lateral chest radiographs are the mainstay of chest radiography. Frontal radiographs are most frequently obtained with the patient facing the image receptor and the x-ray beam passing from posterior to anterior (PA projection). Almost all lateral chest radiographs are obtained with the patient's left side nearest the image receptor to minimize magnification of the heart. These are usually obtained with the image receptor 72 inches from the x-ray tube to decrease overall radiographic magnification. A relatively high beam energy of 125 to 140 kVp is usually used to increase film latitude (i.e., lengthen the gray scale). This makes the ribs less noticeable and lung pathology easier to see. In some instances, a frontal radiograph alone will suffice and has the advantage of decreasing radiation exposure because the lateral radiograph typically gives a higher radiation dose to the patient. Examples where one might choose to forego the lateral film include evaluating a patient for a positive purified protein derivative (PPD) result or after seeing a readily visible lesion. The lateral projection, however, may be very useful for lesion localization, evaluation of the spine, identification of pleural effusions, distinguishing a vessel seen on end from a nodule, and identification of calcium within the heart. Plate 3-4 demonstrates correct positioning for PA and lateral radiographs with corresponding images.

Lateral Decubitus View

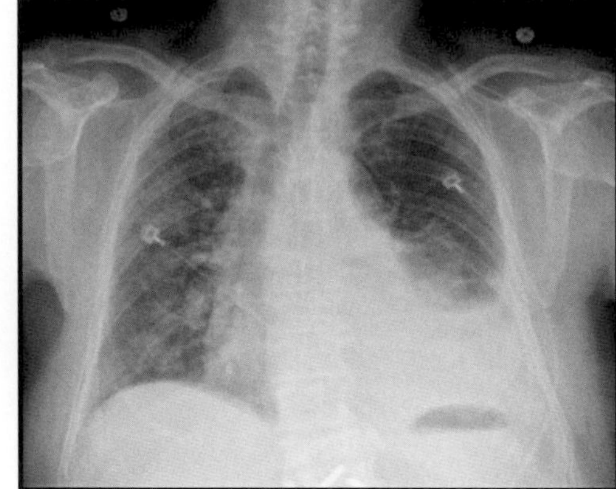

Pleural effusion. PA radiograph demonstrates blunting of the left costophrenic angle and separation of the stomach bubble from the lung base

X-ray film

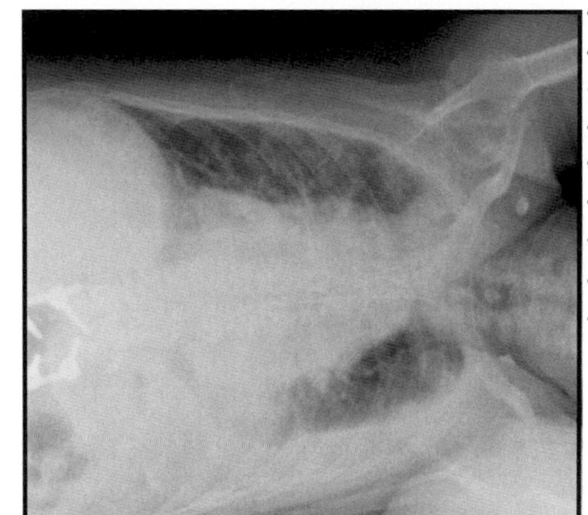

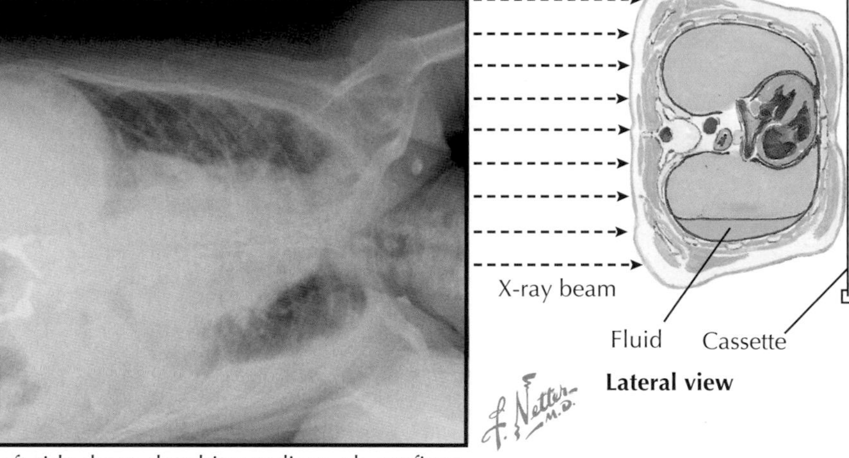

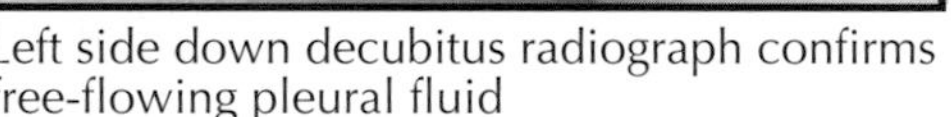

Left side down decubitus radiograph confirms free-flowing pleural fluid

Radiologic Examination of the Lungs *(Continued)*

Hospitalized patients, especially those in the intensive care unit, frequently cannot be readily brought to the radiology department for PA and lateral radiographs and are usually evaluated with a single portable anteroposterior (AP) radiograph where the cassette is placed behind the patient's back (see Plate 3-4). These studies are usually performed with the x-ray tube at a distance of 40 inches from the image receptor and at lower beam energy (80-90 kVp). The patient is rarely more than semi-upright and usually cannot take a deep breath, resulting in poorer image quality than studies performed in the radiology department. The AP projection and shorter source to image distance result in significant magnification of the cardiac silhouette and the lower beam energy makes the images have more contrast. Plate 3-4 demonstrates a standard supine AP chest radiograph.

Oblique views of the chest can serve to help localize lesions within the lung or determine whether a perceived lesion is inside the thorax or on the chest wall. In practice, however, they are rarely obtained except for evaluation of the rib cage.

Lateral decubitus chest radiographs are useful for evaluation of pleural fluid and can be used to identify the presence of even very small pleural effusions as well as to assess the amount of free-flowing fluid. In the lateral decubitus view, the patient lies on one side, and the x-ray beam passes horizontally through the patient (see Plate 3-5). As a general rule, both decubitus views should be obtained if possible because it may be difficult to determine how much free-flowing fluid there is on the down side when the effusion is large and to evaluate the underlying lung parenchyma on the up side when fluid shifts from lateral to medial. When an upright chest radiograph cannot be obtained, a lateral decubitus radiograph is the best way to look for a pneumothorax without resorting to computed tomography (CT). In this case, the side of interest is the up side of the chest. Plate 3-5 demonstrates proper positioning for a decubitus chest radiograph and a corresponding image.

The AP lordotic view of the chest was widely used in the past to evaluate the lung apices in patients in whom a suspicious opacity was seen on the standard PA view. By projecting the clavicles cephalad, the apices may be better visualized. In practice, however, the question of whether a perceived lesion is real is frequently not completely answered by the lordotic view, and in most places, it has been replaced by the more expensive but also more definitive CT scan. Furthermore, unless there is obvious calcium within a lesion, the lordotic view does not answer the question of what the lesion is.

Another imaging procedure that has largely been replaced is chest fluoroscopy, although it remains a quick way to confirm that a perceived lesion is actually a confluence of shadows, saving the patient from undergoing a CT scan. Chest fluoroscopy is also useful for evaluation of diaphragmatic motion and identifying a paralyzed diaphragm. If the diaphragm is paralyzed, it will move paradoxically when the patient forcefully sniffs.

Computed Tomography
(see Plate 3-6)

CT has revolutionized the diagnosis of thoracic disease not only by earlier detection of disease but also by much more accurate characterization of disease severity and extent. Modern units, termed *multidetector row (MDCT) scanners*, are capable of imaging the entire volume of the chest in less than 10 seconds, allowing 1-mm-thick high-resolution scans in a single breath-hold (see Plate 3-6). For this reason, virtually all CT scans performed on a MDCT scanner provide high-resolution detail of the parenchyma, although at a higher radiation dose

Radiologic Examination of the Lungs *(Continued)*

than the spaced scans of a high-resolution chest CT, which is still used to evaluate and monitor patients with diffuse parenchymal lung disease. This ability of the MDCT to provide thin sections of the entire lung provides detailed images for the evaluation of solitary pulmonary nodules. Because the reconstructed images from MDCTs in the sagittal and coronal planes are equal in resolution to the axial source images, these multiplanar reconstructions are especially useful for the evaluation of the aorta, the tracheobronchial tree, and the pulmonary vasculature (see Plate 3-6).

As a result of the rapid speed of scan acquisition during maximal intravascular contrast levels, CT has become the primary method for the evaluation of suspected pulmonary embolism. The ability to acquire the CT scan in correlation with the patient's electrocardiogram has allowed motion-free images of the heart and coronary arteries to be obtained noninvasively. An additional advantage of the rapid acquisition times possible with current MDCT scanners is the ability to image the chest dynamically during expiration, thereby providing an assessment of obstructive airways disease due to tracheobronchial or small airway pathology.

The radiation dose of a CT scan, however, is substantially greater than that of radiographs; therefore they should not be used unless the value of the information to be gained outweighs the potential harmful effects of ionizing radiation.

CONTRAST EXAMINATIONS

Contrast bronchography for the detection of tracheal and bronchial masses and in the evaluation for bronchiectasis has been completely supplanted by MDCT, but Plates 3-7 and 3-8 demonstrate the normal bronchial anatomy.

Pulmonary Angiography

Although still considered the gold standard in the radiologic evaluation of pulmonary vascular anatomy, catheter pulmonary angiography has all but been replaced by CT pulmonary angiography in the evaluation of acute pulmonary embolism. Conventional pulmonary angiography is performed by percutaneous catheterization of the pulmonary artery via a femoral or upper extremity venous access and still has a role, albeit somewhat limited, in the preoperative evaluation of chronic thromboembolic pulmonary hypertension and in the diagnosis and transcatheter embolization of pulmonary arteriovenous malformations. Rarely, pulmonary angiography is performed for the evaluation of congenital abnormalities such as agenesis, aplasia, or hypoplasia of the pulmonary arteries, as in the evaluation of the minority of patients who have massive hemoptysis thought to arise from a pulmonary arterial source, such as patients with suspected pulmonary artery aneurysms. Two- and three-dimensional reconstructions of the pulmonary vasculature obtained from MDCT scans provide equivalent information and have limited the use of pulmonary angiography for mostly therapeutic indications (see Plate 3-9).

Aortography

As with radiologic evaluation of the pulmonary arterial vasculature, conventional aortography performed via a retrograde catheterization of the aorta via the femoral or brachial artery has been largely supplanted by MDCT aortography, which provides diagnostic quality two- and three-dimensional reconstructions in the evaluation of traumatic aortic injury; aneurysm; dissection and its variants, including penetrating atherosclerotic ulcer and intramural hematoma; and aortitis. Plate 3-6 demonstrates reconstructed images of the aorta in a patient with an aortic dissection. In a patient with a mediastinal mass thought to be secondary to an aortic aneurysm, contrast CT aortography helps delineate the nature and extent of the aneurysm and

Technique of Helical Computed Tomography (CT)

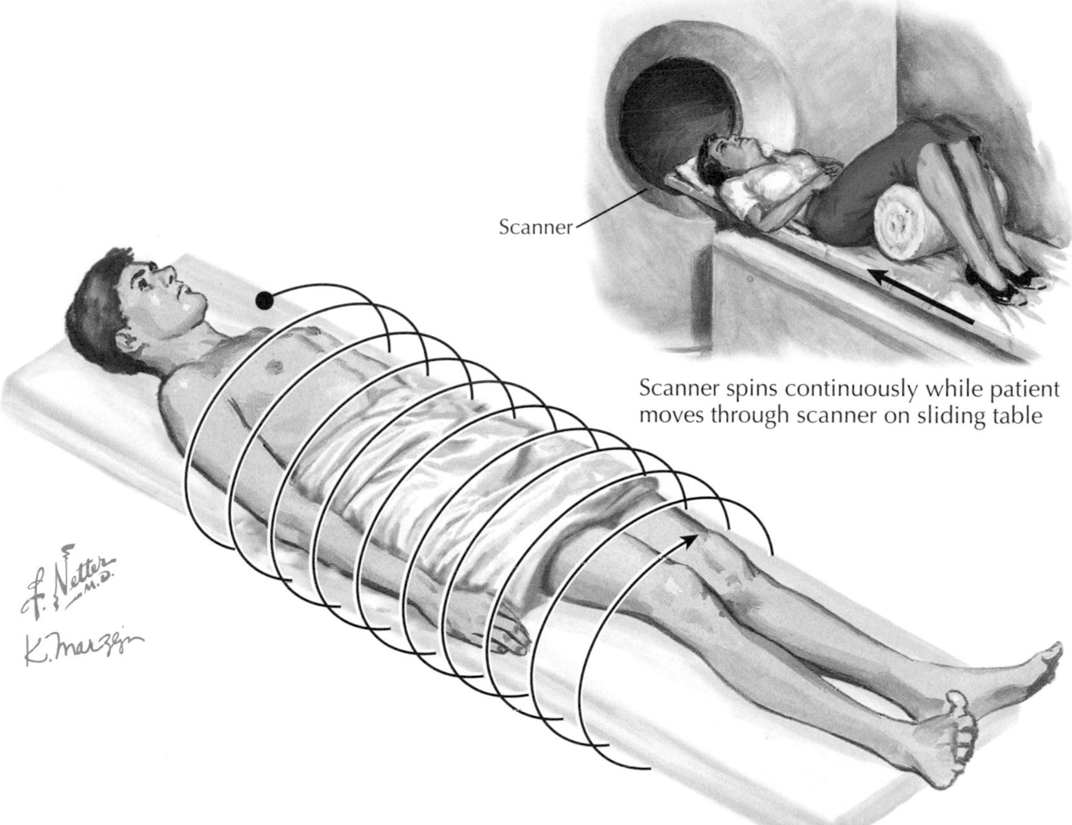

Scanner
Scanner spins continuously while patient moves through scanner on sliding table
F. Netter M.D.
K. Marzen

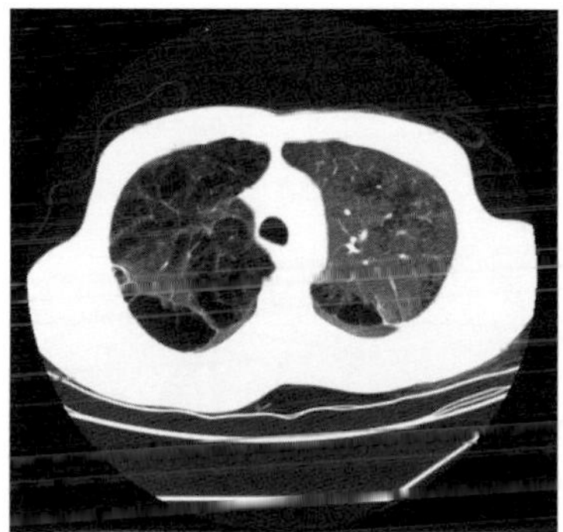
Axial CT scan of the upper thorax in a patient with severe centrilobular and paraseptal emphysema

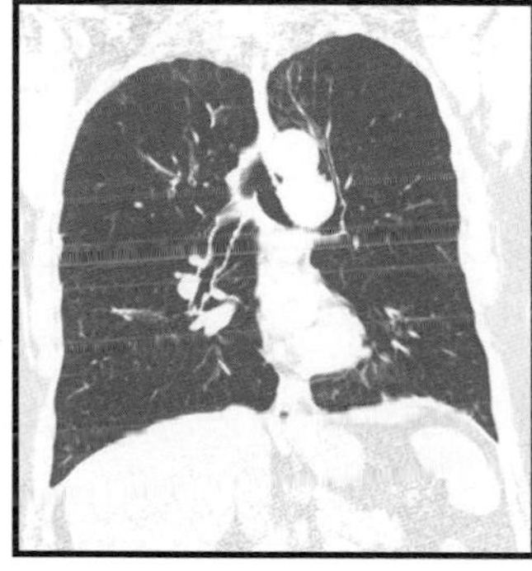
Coronal reconstruction of CT scan in a patient with severe emphysema causing extensive bilateral predominantly upper lobe lung destruction

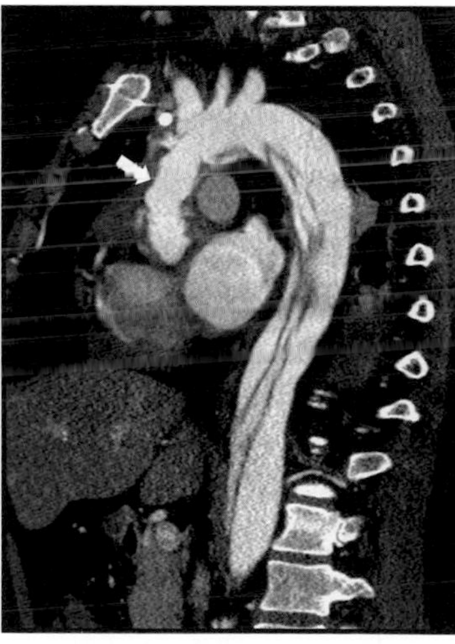
Parasagittal oblique reconstructed CT scan demonstrates multiple linear filling defects in the descending aorta representing intimal flaps from dissection. A graft is present in the ascending aortic graft (*arrow*).

Right Bronchial Tree as Revealed by Bronchograms

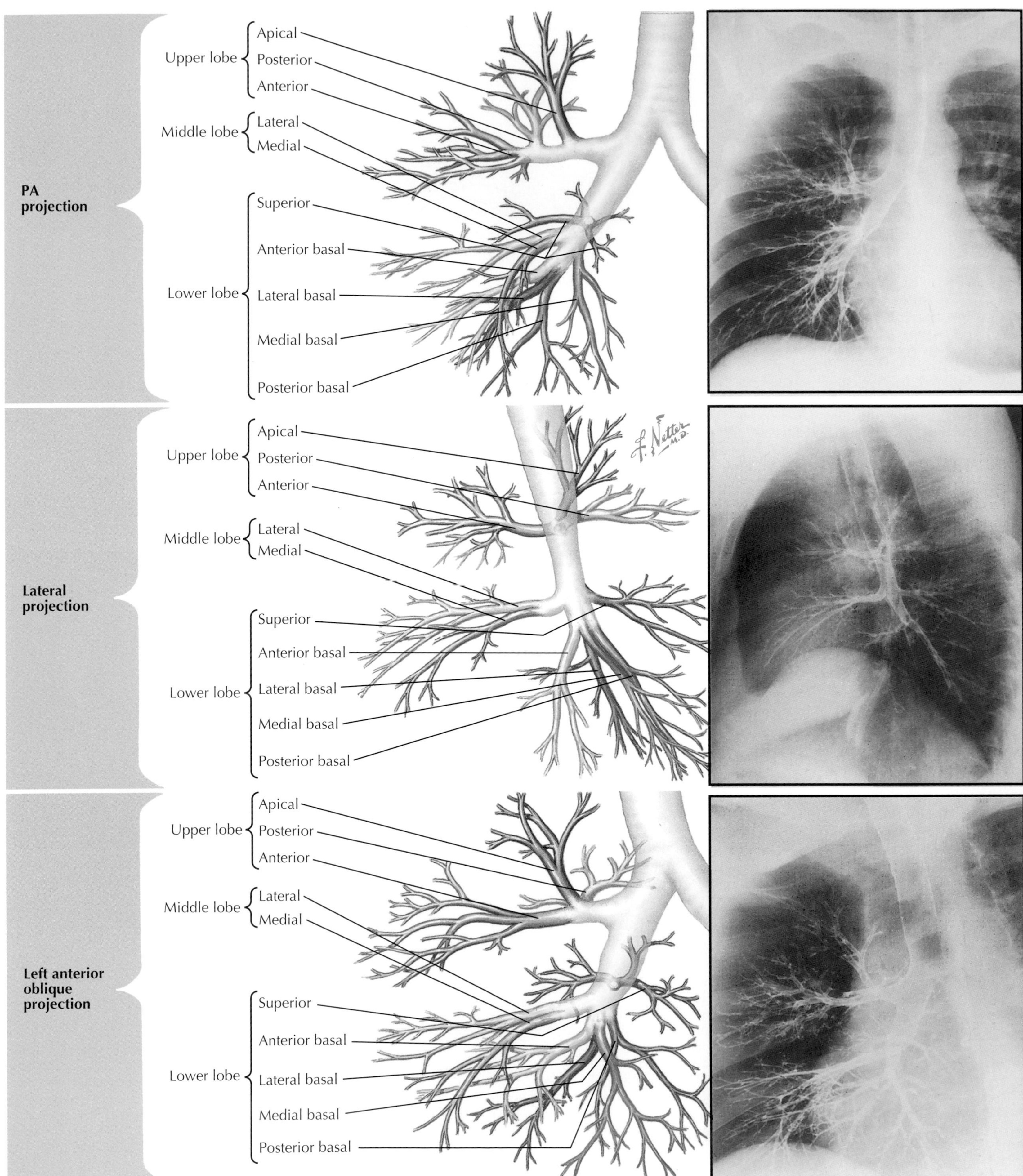

Left Bronchial Tree as Revealed by Bronchograms

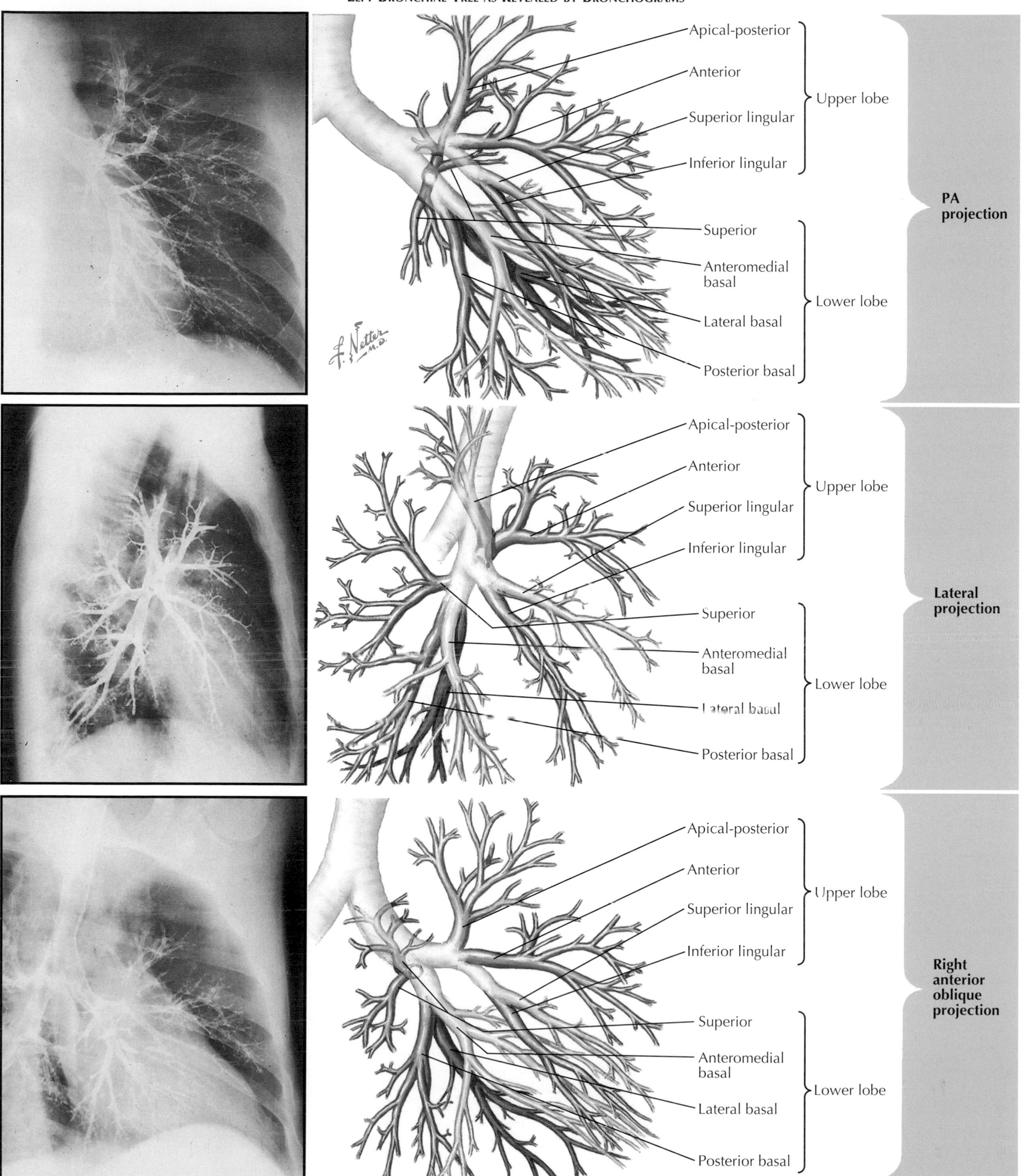

Pulmonary Angiography

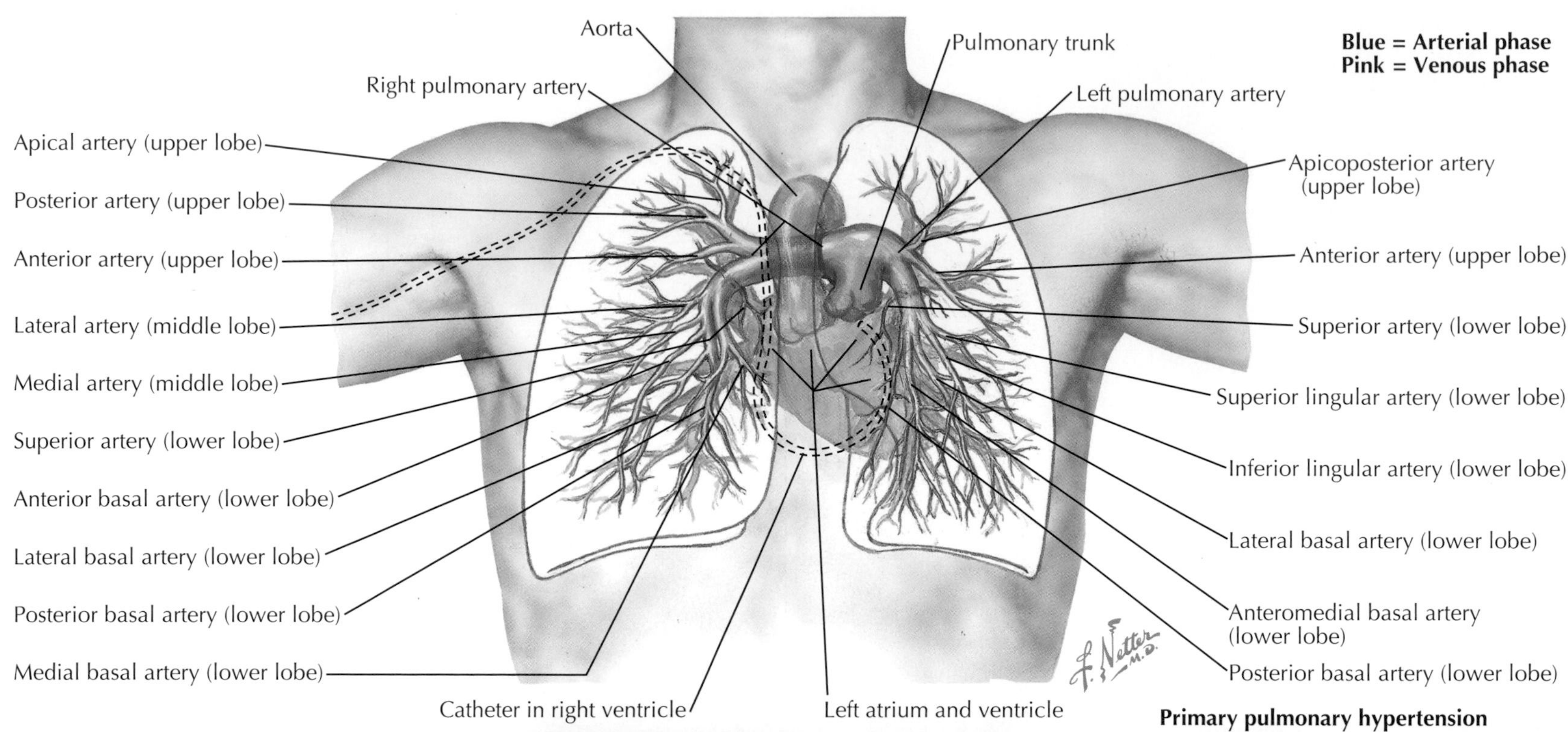

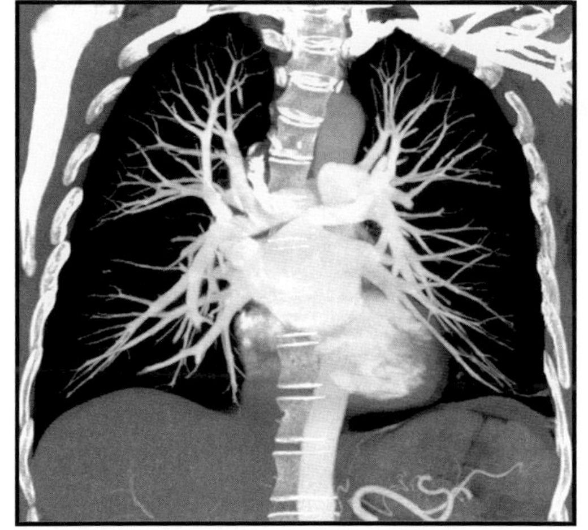
Normal pulmonary arterial anatomy demonstrated on a thick section maximum intensity projection coronal reconstruction of a CT performed to evaluate for pulmonary embolism

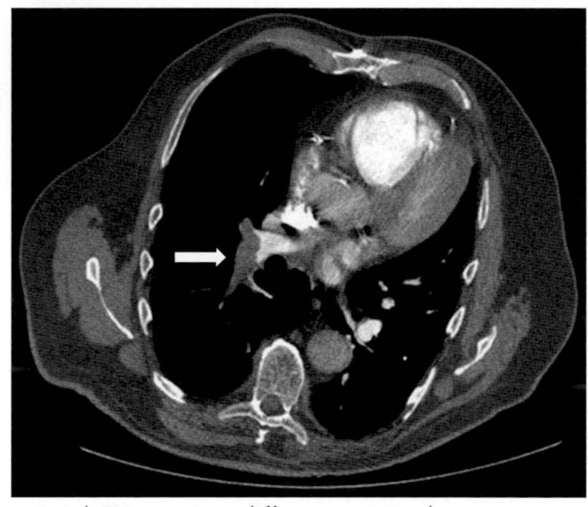
Axial CT scan in a different patient demonstrates a large embolus in the right lower lobe pulmonary artery (arrow)

Primary pulmonary hypertension

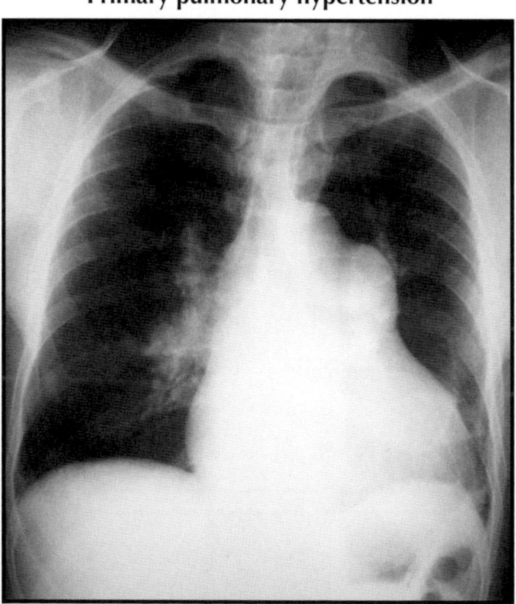
Marked enlargement of the central pulmonary arteries with diminution ("pruning") of the peripheral vessels

Radiologic Examination of the Lungs *(Continued)*

its relationship to the great vessels and adjacent mediastinal structures.

RADIONUCLIDE IMAGING

Ventilation-Perfusion Scintigraphy

Although CT pulmonary angiography has emerged as the primary imaging modality in the evaluation of suspected acute pulmonary embolism, ventilation-perfusion (V-Q) scanning remains a very sensitive method of evaluation for pulmonary embolism and is still used in selected situations for this indication. V-Q scanning after chest radiography remains of value in patients with contraindications to intravenous iodinated contrast administration and may be the more appropriate imaging study in younger individuals evaluated for possible pulmonary embolism because it subjects patients to a lower radiation dose than does CT. In patients with pulmonary hypertension who are being evaluated for possible chronic thromboembolic pulmonary hypertension, a normal lung perfusion scan can effectively exclude this diagnosis. Finally, V-Q scans are occasionally performed for the preoperative assessment of patients considered for lobar or lung resection because they can help assess the relative contribution of the affected lobe to overall pulmonary function, thereby accurately predicting the anticipated level of pulmonary disability after pulmonary resection.

Positron emission tomography (PET) (see Plate 3-10) using fluorine-18-labeled fluorodeoxyglucose (FDG) has high accuracy in the distinction of benign from malignant solitary pulmonary nodules. FDG-PET has a high sensitivity for malignant nodules larger than 10 mm in diameter, with most PET-negative lesions

Radiologic Examination of the Lungs *(Continued)*

requiring only follow-up imaging evaluation. Whole-body FDG-PET is now used routinely in the staging of lung cancer, with a higher accuracy for the detection of mediastinal and hilar lymph node involvement and high sensitivity for the detection of bone, liver, adrenal, and distant metastases.

Contrast Esophagography

In patients with suspected esophageal disease, barium or water-soluble esophagography is a rapid and accurate method of assessment, particularly for evaluation of mucosal diseases such as esophagitis or ulcer, esophageal diverticulae foreign body ingestion, esophageal masses, and perforation.

MAGNETIC RESONANCE IMAGING

Magnetic resonance imaging is a technique that does not require ionizing radiation but instead relies on the measurement of energy released by tissue protons that have been placed in an external magnetic field. Two essential characteristics of tissue, termed *T1* and *T2 relaxation times*, are used to evaluate tissues in health and disease. In general, whereas T1-weighted scans of the chest are useful for anatomic evaluation of the heart and mediastinum, providing excellent delineation of vascular from adjacent structures without the need for intravascular contrast, T2 weighted images are more useful for tissue characterization because they are sensitive to the greater water (i.e., proton) content of tumors. As with MDCTs, images in the direct axial, sagittal, and coronal planes are obtained.

SONOGRAPHY

The use of ultrasonography in the chest is limited by the inability of ultrasound to penetrate the lung. Sonographic examination of the chest has proven useful in the detection and characterization of pleural fluid collections. Sonographic guidance for thoracentesis and transthoracic biopsy of mediastinal, pleural, and chest wall lesions allows real-time visualization of tissue sampling without the use of ionizing radiation.

INTERPRETATION OF RADIOGRAPHIC PATTERNS

The scope of this section does not allow for a detailed discussion of all the pathologic processes that may be apparent on a chest radiograph. However, certain basic radiographic concepts are discussed.

Atelectasis

Atelectasis is loss of volume of a lung, lobe, or segment from any cause. Of the various mechanisms of atelectasis, the most important is obstruction of a major bronchus by tumor, foreign body, or bronchial plug. The other common causes of loss of lung volume are pneumonia, in which collapse occurs in the presence of patent bronchi, presumably secondary to abnormalities of surfactant, and passive, or compressive, atelectasis in which volume loss is directly caused by compression of the lung by extrinsic mass effect. Common causes of passive atelectasis include pleural fluid, pneumothorax, an elevated diaphragm, and a mass.

There are several radiographic signs of atelectasis. Felson divided these into direct and indirect signs. Direct signs are shift of a fissure; crowding of bronchovascular markings; and increased density of the involved portion of the lung, the most reliable being displacement of interlobar fissures (see Plates 3-11 and 3-12). A localized increase in density of the collapsed lobe is almost always present but is not specific for atelectasis. Indirect signs are (1) elevation of the ipsilateral diaphragm, (2) deviation of the trachea and other mediastinal structures toward the side of the atelectasis, (3) compensatory hyperaeration of the remainder of the ipsilateral lung and sometimes of the contralateral lung (which may occasionally cross the mediastinum), (4) displacement of a hilum toward the collapsed lobe or

Images from a PET-CT Scanner

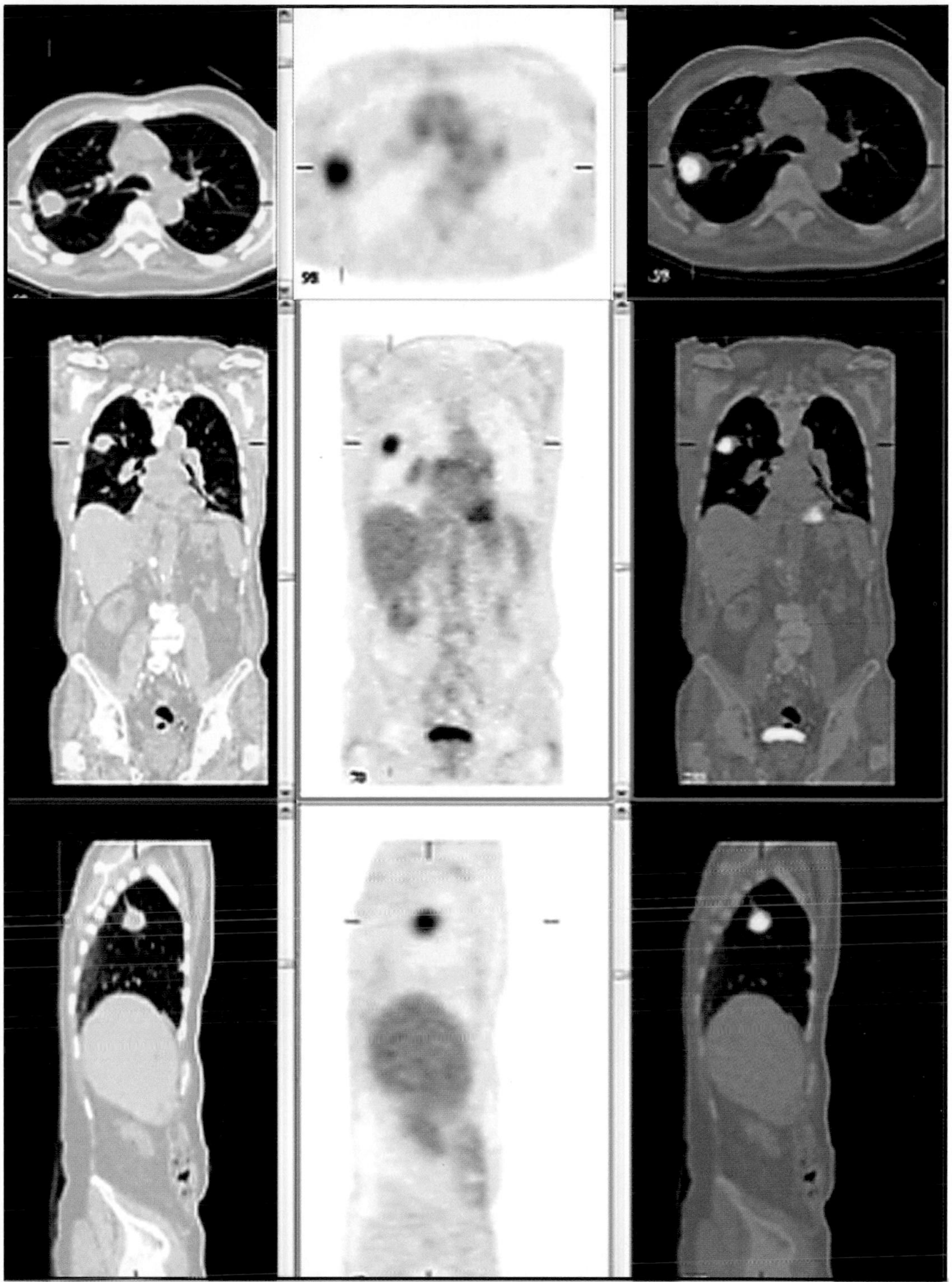

The images are obtained for both the CT (*left*) and PET (*middle*) components in axial (*top*), coronal (*middle*), and sagittal (*bottom*) planes. The PET and CT images are fused (*right*) for accurate localization of the foci of abnormal increased radiopharmaceutical uptake, which in the composite PET-CT image is seen in yellow. This patient had a biopsy-proven non–small cell carcinoma of the right upper lobe

Patterns of Lobar Collapse: Right Lung (after Lubert and Krause)

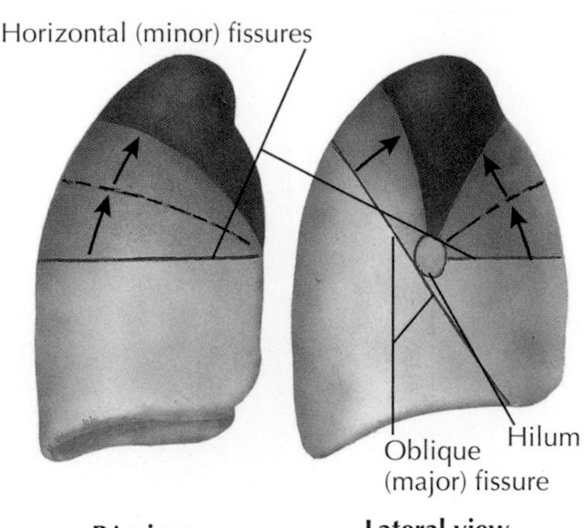

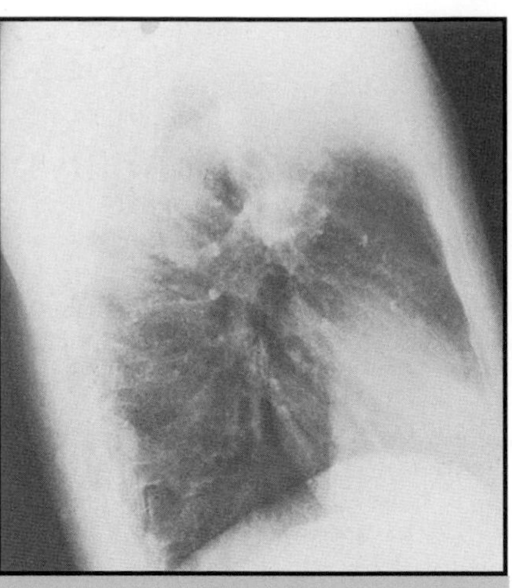

Right upper lobe collapse

PA and lateral radiographs demonstrating right upper lobe atelectasis and collapse secondary to an endobronchial carcinoma. Hilar adenopathy is also present as well as a metastasis in right 8th posterior rib

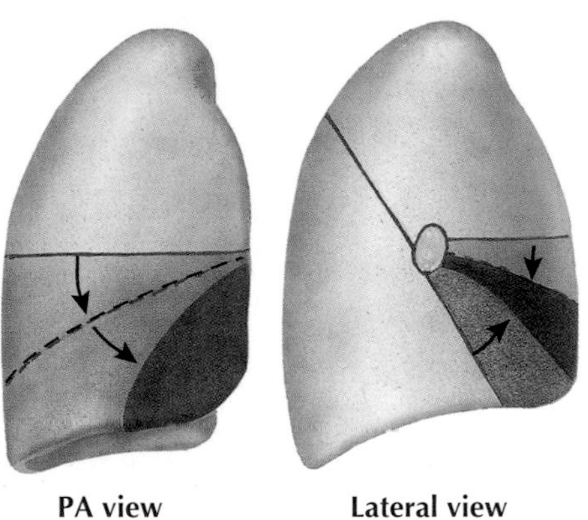

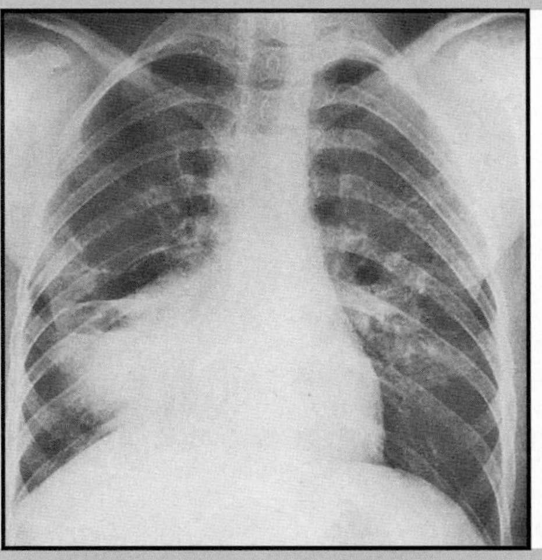

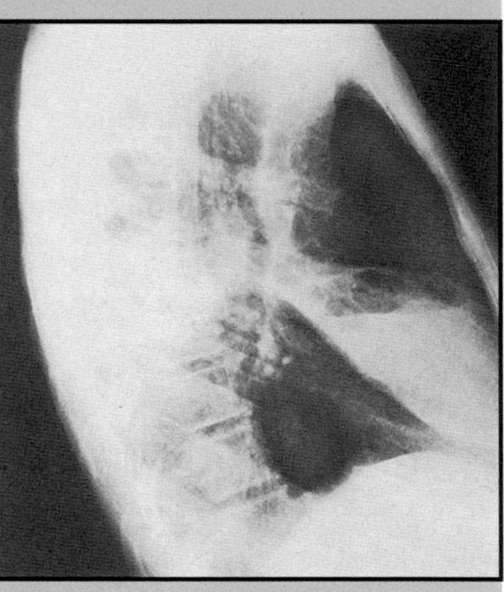

Right middle lobe collapse

PA and lateral radiographs demonstrating right middle lobe atelectasis and collapse secondary to allergic aspergillosis with bronchial obstruction by matted mycelia of aspergilli. There is an associated cavity in right middle lobe. Some consolidation in superior segment of left lower lobe is also present

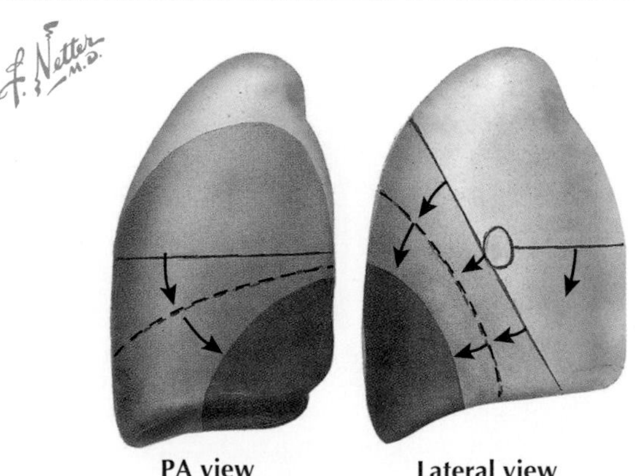

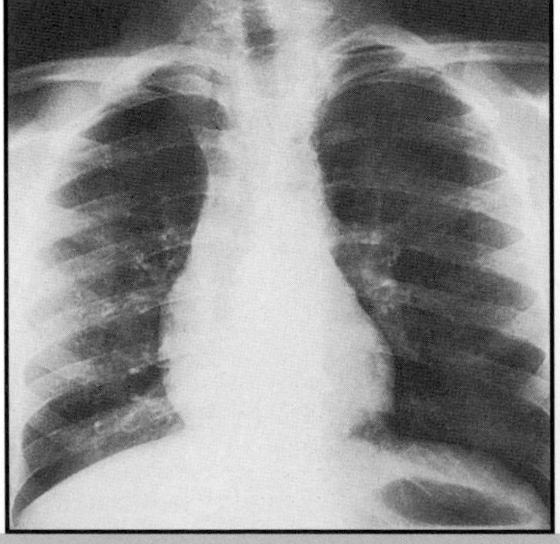

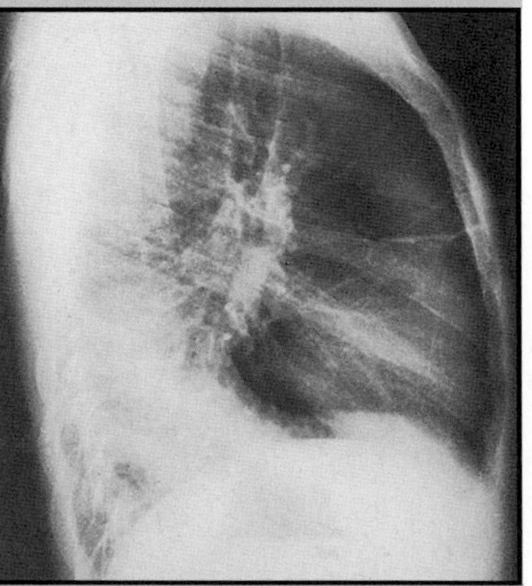

Right lower lobe collapse

PA and lateral radiographs demonstrating right lower lobe atelectasis and collapse secondary to bronchial plug in an asthmatic patient. On PA film, right lower lobe collapse lies primarily behind cardiac silhouette and is seen through heart shadow. On lateral radiograph, posterior displacement of major fissure and blurring of sharp margin of posterior part of right hemidiaphragm are seen. Both changes are indicative of consolidation and loss of volume of right lower lobe

Patterns of Lobar Collapse: Left Lung (after Lubert and Krause)

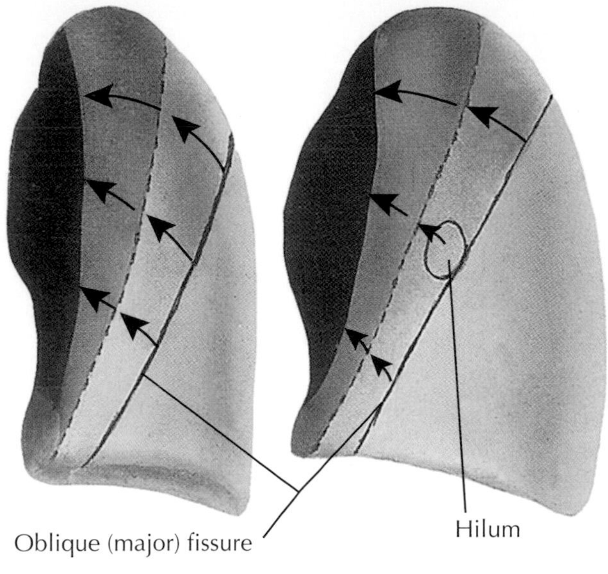

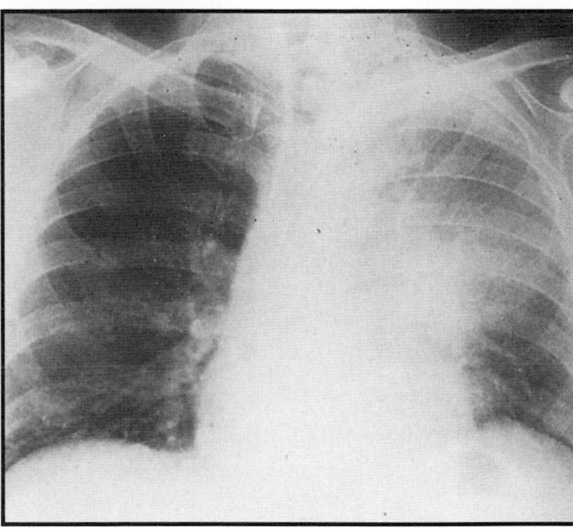

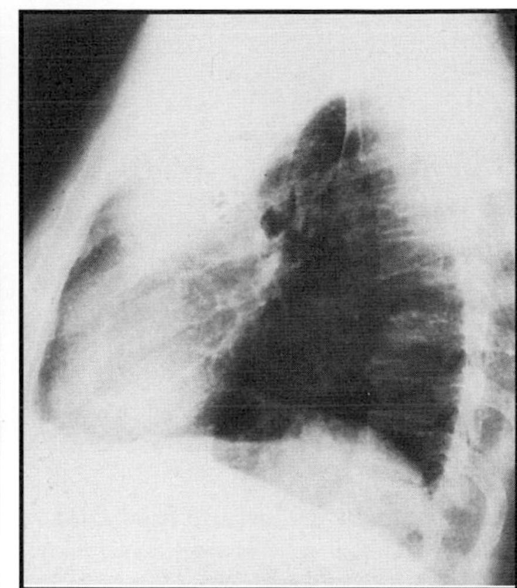

Left upper lobe collapse

PA and lateral radiographs demonstrating left upper lobe atelectasis and collapse secondary to bronchogenic carcinoma. Note loss of definition of aortic knob and left heart border (silhouette sign) caused by their relationship to atelectatic lung

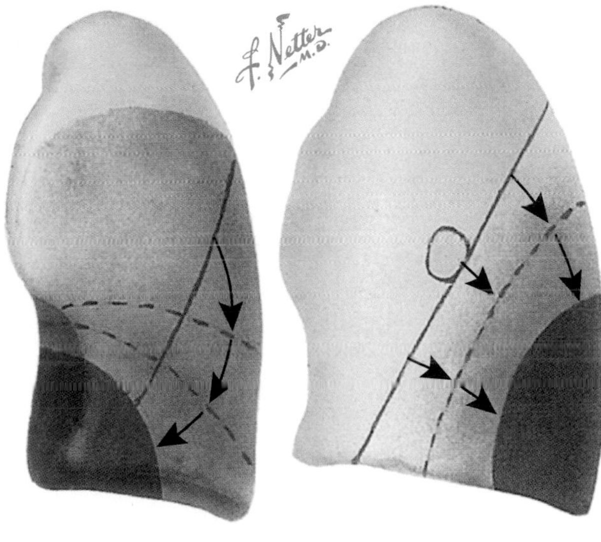

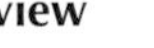

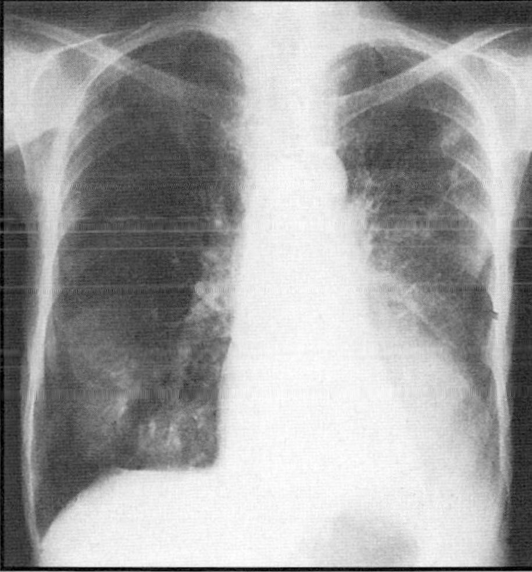

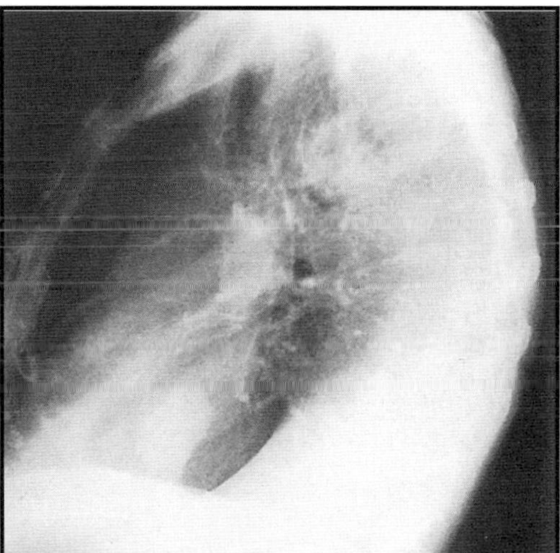

Right upper lobe collapse

PA and lateral radiographs demonstrating left lower lobe atelectasis and collapse secondary to endobronchial tumor. Other nodular lesions scattered through both lung fields represent additional metastases

Radiologic Examination of the Lungs *(Continued)*

segment, and (5) decrease in size of the thorax on the involved side. These indirect signs are ordinarily seen only with atelectasis of major lung segments. Except for perhaps hilar displacement, they are usually less reliable than the direct signs and can occasionally be simulated by normal and anatomic variations.

Certain fundamental observations can be made about lobar collapse: (1) the proximal portion of the lobe is tethered to the hilum, and consequently, the radiographic shadows of the collapsed lung will always point toward it; (2) lobar collapse is always toward the mediastinum on the PA study; and (3) on the lateral study, the upper lobe collapses anteriorly, the lower lobe collapses posteriorly, and the middle lobe symmetrically decreases in volume.

It is very important to recognize the patterns of lobar collapse because atelectasis is a major indicator of primary pulmonary pathology. Recognition of a collapsed lobe may be difficult, particularly if the collapse is almost complete. Of great help in identifying its presence is the silhouette sign, popularized by Felson. The silhouette sign may also be useful in identifying consolidation of the lung other than that caused by atelectasis. The sign is based on the premise that consolidation of lung will obliterate the interface between the lung and any structure adjacent to it. Frequently, obliteration of a heart border or fuzziness of the diaphragm is the first clue that leads

Radiologic Examination of the Lungs *(Continued)*

the observer to suspect the presence of an airspace abnormality.

Alveolar versus Interstitial Disease

Pulmonary pathology can be manifested by densities occurring in the pulmonary alveoli, in the interstitial spaces of the lungs, or in both. It is often useful to distinguish alveolar from interstitial disease, although in some instances, the distinction can be made only with great difficulty or not at all, and most diseases have components of both. In diseases that are predominantly either alveolar or interstitial in nature, certain radiographic signs may allow the investigator to distinguish one from the other. This task is considerably simpler on CT scans, although it may still be difficult.

Radiographic findings of alveolar disease are (1) coalescent densities, creating large shadows; (2) frequent presence of an air bronchogram (air in the more peripheral portions of the bronchial tree visualized because of fluid in surrounding alveoli; ordinarily, the bronchial air is not visible because there is no contrast between air in the bronchi and air in the surrounding alveoli); and (3) fluffy or irregular margins of localized areas of consolidation (see Plate 3-13). On chest radiographs, interstitial lung disease is typically characterized by (1) discrete, sharp opacities rather than fluffy and irregular opacities; (2) diffuse rather than localized disease; and (3) lack of coalescence.

Interstitial disease is also characterized by certain typical patterns—nodular, reticular, linear, and ground-glass opacities. Discrete, small interstitial nodules are seen in granulomatous diseases such as miliary tuberculosis and sarcoidosis; silicosis; and those with hematogenous metastases such as from thyroid, renal, breast, and colon carcinoma. The random distribution of nodules seen in infectious diseases such as tuberculosis and fungal infections, compared with the perilymphatic distribution of nodules characteristic for sarcoidosis and lymphangitic spread of carcinoma to the lungs, is most readily distinguished on thin-section CT analysis. Reticular interstitial disease typically represents one of three pathologic processes: interstitial fibrosis from any cause, the superimposition of innumerable thin-walled cysts as seen in diseases such as Langerhans cell histiocytosis and lymphangioleiomyomatosis, or thickened airway walls as seen classically in cystic fibrosis. Linear opacities are typically seen in acute interstitial lung disease, particularly hydrostatic interstitial pulmonary edema (see Plate 3-13); however, thickening of the interlobular septa (Kerley B lines) is a common finding in many interstitial lung diseases and may be seen in pneumonia secondary to viral and atypical organisms. Pulmonary lymphangitic carcinomatosis may also present with a linear pattern of disease, frequently associated with nodules (see Plate 3-13). *Ground-glass opacity* refers to a very fine reticular process that increases lung density as seen on either conventional radiographs or thin-section (i.e., 1-2 mm) CT scans, fails to obscure underlying vessels, and is not associated with an air bronchogram. Processes that produce ground-glass opacity include a broad spectrum of interstitial disease, although some airspace-filling diseases in which the alveoli are incompletely or nonuniformly filled with material can produce this pattern. Diseases typically associated with ground-glass opacity include atypical pneumonia such as from *Pneumocystis jiroveci* infection, pulmonary edema, hypersensitivity pneumonitis, and alveolar hemorrhage in a resolving phase. Coarse reticulation with discrete curvilinear opacities is most characteristic of usual interstitial pneumonia and the chronic phases of hypersensitivity pneumonitis and sarcoidosis (see Plate 3-13).

The distribution and thus likely cause of interstitial nodules is more accurately assessed by thin-section CT.

Alveolar Versus Interstitial Disease

Alveolar disease due to pneumonia

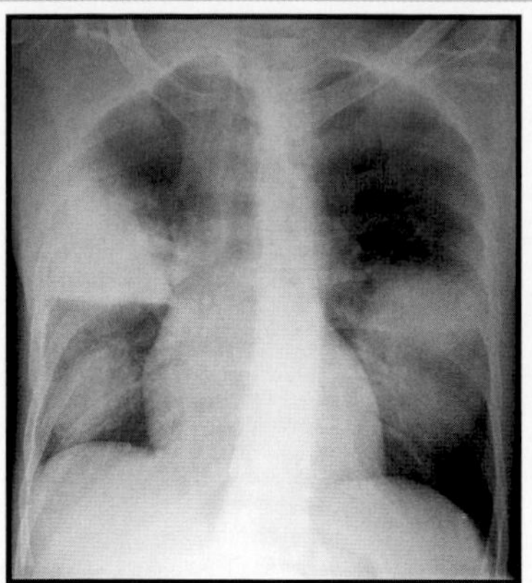

Chest radiograph demonstrating multifocal airspace opacities from bacterial pneumonia

Interstitial disease due to hydrostatic edema in a patient with left ventricular failure

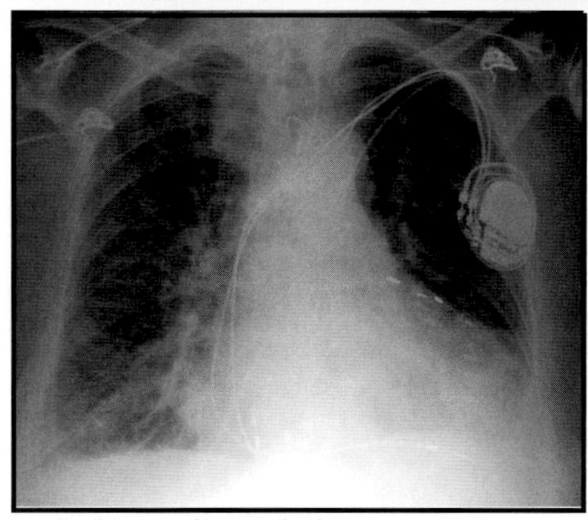

AP chest radiograph demonstrates cardiomegaly, indistinct pulmonary vessels, and thickened interlobular septa (Kerley B lines) in the right lung base

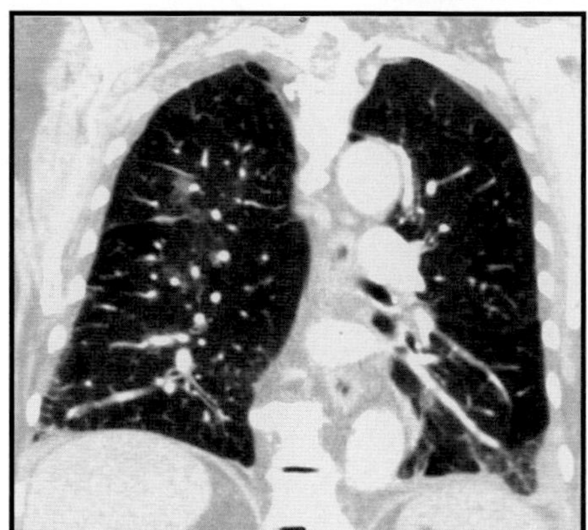

Coronal CT reconstruction demonstrates the Kerley lines and diffuse ground glass opacities in the right lung

Interstitial lung disease not due to hydrostatic edema

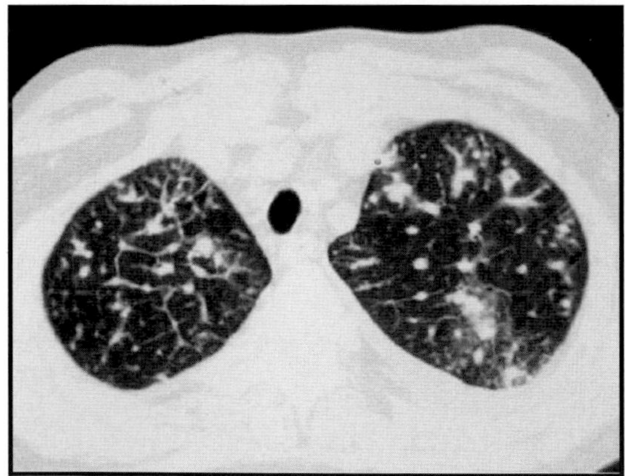

Axial CT scan of the upper lungs demonstrates multiple pulmonary nodules and nodular thickening of the interlobular septa from lymphangitic carcinomatosis

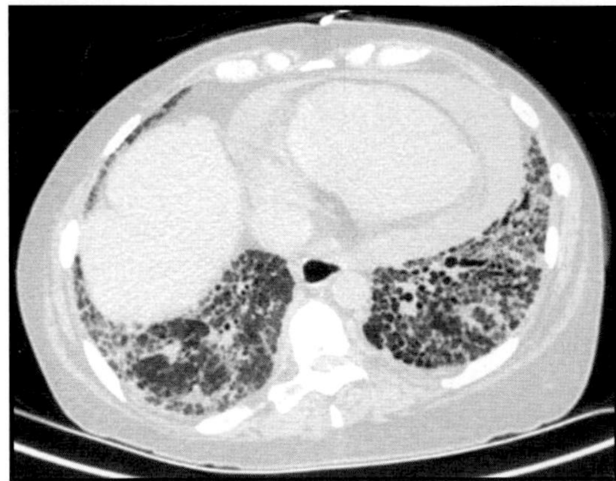

Usual interstitial pneumonia with end-stage pulmonary fibrosis. Axial CT lung bases demonstrates honeycomb cysts, reticulation, and traction bronchiectasis in a patient with progressive systemic sclerosis (scleroderma)

Radiologic Examination of the Lungs *(Continued)*

The common distributions of pulmonary nodules are centrilobular (common in subacute hypersensitivity pneumonitis, respiratory bronchiolitis, and some infections), perilymphatic (common in sarcoidosis and lymphangitic carcinomatosis), random or angiocentric (common in metastatic disease and infections), and "tree-in-bud" opacities caused by dilatation of the terminal bronchioles (almost always secondary to infection) (see Plate 3-14).

Causes of interstitial lung disease include:

1. Pneumoconiosis
   a. Silicosis
   b. Asbestosis
   c. Coal worker's pneumoconiosis
2. Infection
   a. Viral or atypical pneumonia (e.g., *Pneumocystis* spp. infection)
   b. Miliary tuberculosis or fungal infection
3. Malignancy (metastatic)
   a. Miliary metastases
   b. Lymphangitic carcinomatosis
4. Granulomatous diseases
   a. Sarcoidosis
5. Collagen vascular disease
   a. Scleroderma
   b. Rheumatoid lung disease
6. Interstitial pulmonary edema
7. Hypersensitivity pneumonitis
8. Chronic interstitial pneumonia
   a. Respiratory bronchiolitis interstitial lung disease or desquamative interstitial pneumonia
   b. Nonspecific interstitial pneumonia
   c. Usual interstitial pneumonia
9. Miscellaneous diseases
   a. Langerhans cell histiocytosis
   b. Amyloidosis

Localized Alveolar Disease

Pneumonia is the most common cause of localized alveolar infiltrates. Pneumonia may involve a single segment or several segments, a lobe, or occasionally almost all of both lungs (see Plate 3-15). Various other inflammatory lesions such as tuberculosis or fungal disease may present as a localized alveolar pattern. Tumors and inflammatory, noninfective alveolar diseases may also present in this way.

It may be helpful to recognize the pulmonary segment involved by localized disease. Knowledge of the bronchial anatomy of the lung allows one to localize the pulmonary segments. Plate 3-16 depicts the patterns seen on chest radiographs with consolidation of the individual segments. This is of some importance because, for example, reactivation tuberculosis almost exclusively involves the apical and posterior segments of the upper lobes and the superior segment of the lower lobe. Conversely, primary carcinoma of the lung occurs more frequently in the anterior segment of the upper lobe.

Diffuse Alveolar Disease

Although alveolar disease is characteristically an acute process and tends to be localized, it may be bilateral and diffuse. Diffuse alveolar disease often has a somewhat nodular pattern, but as a rule, the nodules are ill defined or fuzzy (see Plate 3-15). Some investigators believe these nodules represent the pulmonary acini. Acute, diffuse alveolar disease is most frequently the result of either hydrostatic pulmonary edema or lung injury causing capillary leakage edema. Chronic causes include pulmonary alveolar proteinosis, bronchoalveolar cell carcinoma, "alveolar" sarcoidosis, lymphoma, metastatic carcinoma (particularly from the breast), eosinophilic lung disease, desquamating interstitial pneumonitis, and various forms of vasculitis.

Distribution of Pulmonary Nodules

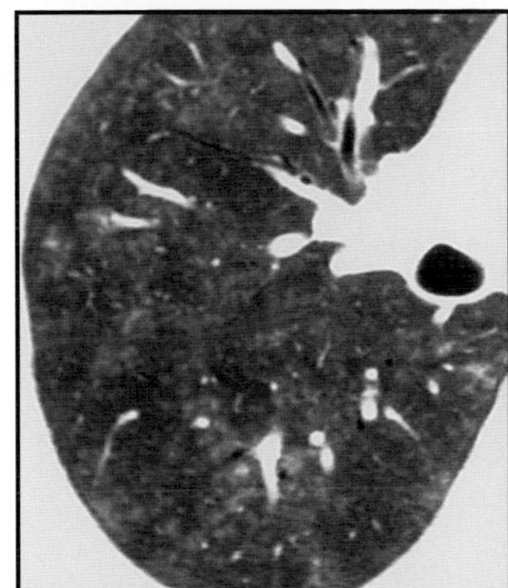

Ground-glass nodules in a regular pattern with prominence in the periphery consistent with a centrilobular distribution

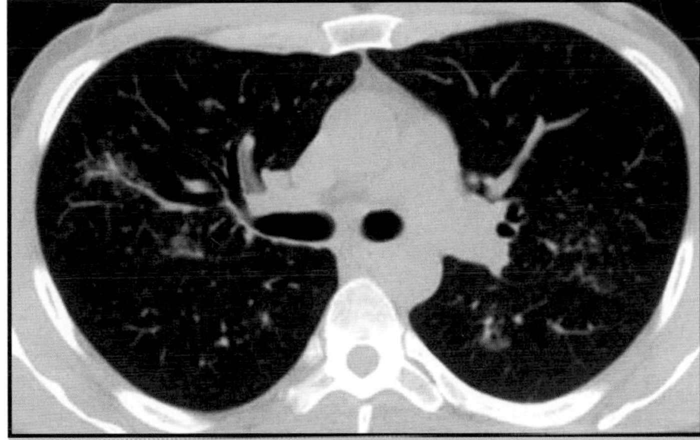

Perilymphatic nodules aligned along the bronchovascular bundles

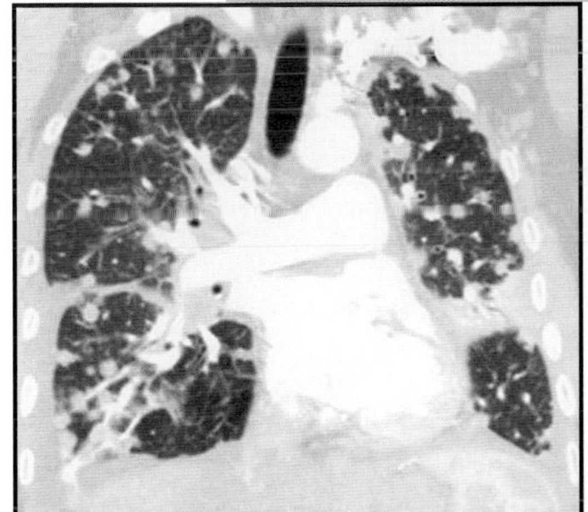

Random nodules dispersed throughout the lungs

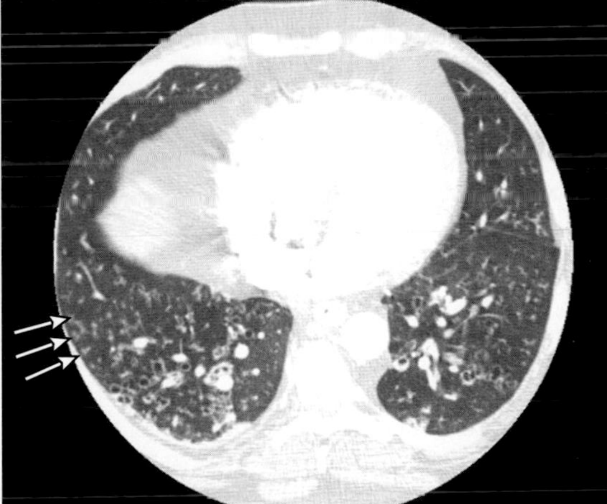

Tree-in-bud opacities (arrows) in the periphery of the lung in a patient who also has bronchiectasis

Radiologic Examination of the Lungs *(Continued)*

Solitary Pulmonary Nodule

Although localized densities with ill-defined margins (alveolar disease) are generally inflammatory, the well-circumscribed pulmonary nodule (coin lesion) is more likely to be a neoplasm, especially in patients older than age 35 years. A large number of benign diseases may also present as a well-circumscribed, solitary pulmonary nodule. A partial list includes granuloma (mycobacterial or fungal), hamartoma, bronchogenic cyst, arteriovenous, pulmonary sequestration, and necrobiotic nodules such as may occur in some patients with rheumatoid arthritis or Wegener granulomatosis.

Thin-section CT is usually very helpful in the identification and assessment of pulmonary nodules, although it cannot always distinguish benign from malignant disease. The most important CT features to evaluate include (1) the density of the nodule, such as whether it is solid, ground glass, or mixed attenuation; (2) assessment of the margins of the nodule; and (3) identification of calcium or fat within it. Benign and indeterminate patterns of nodule calcification are illustrated in Plate 3-17. Central calcification, concentric or lamellar calcification, multiple punctate calcifications, and multiple coarse (so-called "popcorn") calcifications are reliable signs of benignancy. Eccentric calcification is of no diagnostic value because it may also be seen in malignancy. Fat within a pulmonary nodule is virtually pathognomonic of a hamartoma. Irregular, speculated nodules are likely to be malignant. Plate 3-17 shows examples of hamartomas with "popcorn" calcification and fat and a spiculated bronchogenic carcinoma. Lesions that are completely composed of so-called ground-glass opacity may be either inflammatory or low-grade malignancy. Nodules that are of mixed solid and ground glass (see Plate 3-17) are usually malignant, and any nodule larger than 3 cm is likely malignant.

Cavitation of a pulmonary nodule is an indicator of activity and seldom helps to identify the underlying disease with certainty because either inflammatory nodules or tumors may cavitate.

If a nodule in the lung does not change over a long period of time, there is a strong likelihood that the lesion is benign. The physician can often obtain a previous radiograph and confirm that a lesion has not changed in more than 2 years, thus saving the patient an exploratory thoracotomy or CT scan. If no previous examination is available and the nodule is not obviously calcified, thin-section CT should be performed. If the nodule is clearly benign, no follow-up is necessary. If the nodule has features highly concerning for malignancy, a biopsy or resection should be performed. If the nodule is indeterminate and larger than 8 mm, a PET scan of the chest can be obtained to detect increased metabolic activity that is concerning for malignancy. Nodules larger than 8 mm that are negative on PET scans and nodules smaller than 8 mm are followed with thin-section CT for a least 2 years to confirm stability because not all lung cancers, notably bronchoalveolar cell carcinoma and carcinoid tumors, may be PET positive.

Interstitial lung disease is frequently chronic and diffuse.

Alveolar Disease

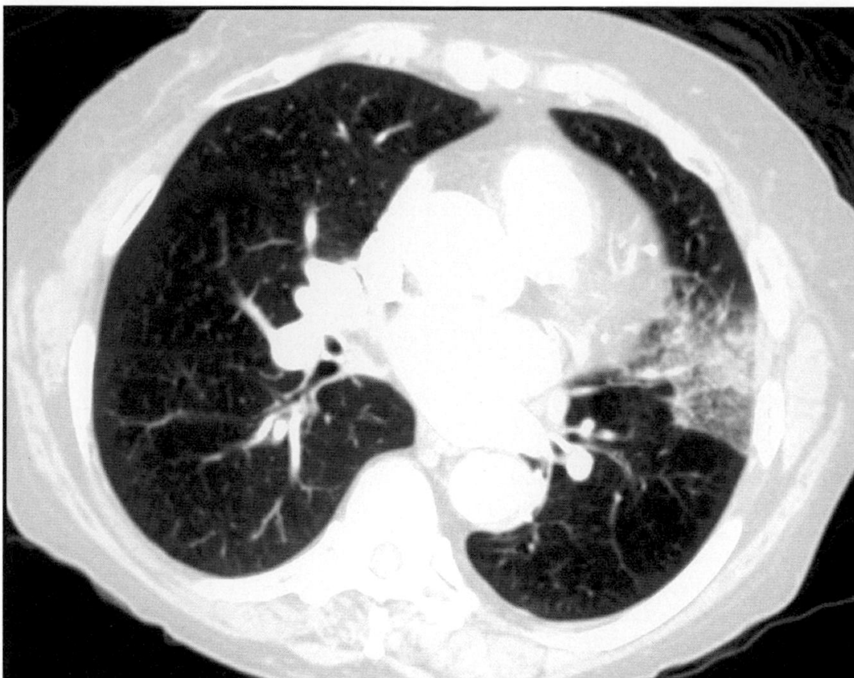

CT scan of the thorax demonstrates ill-defined airspace opacity in the lingula from pneumonia

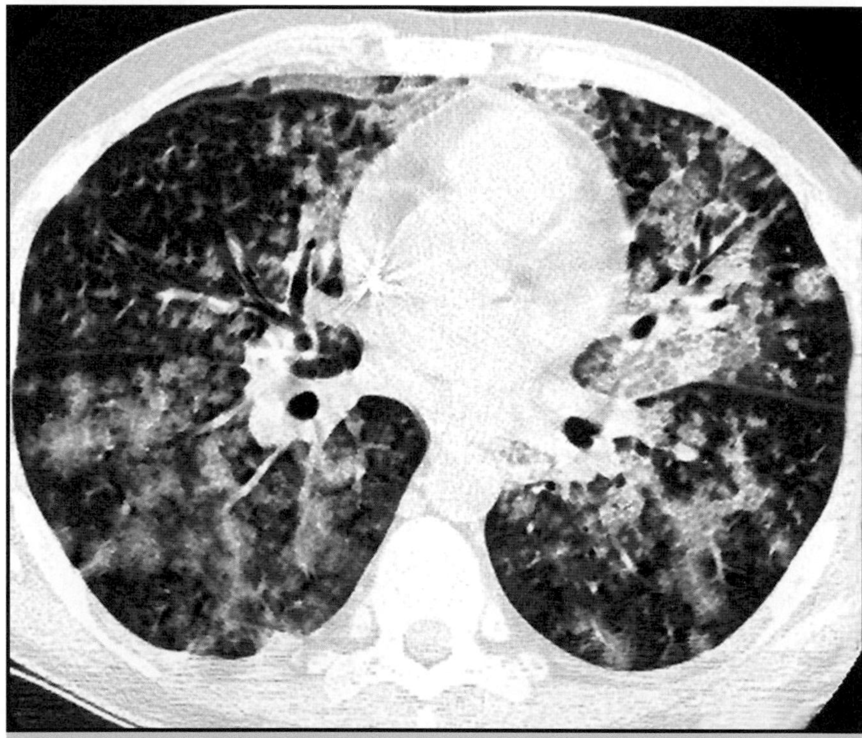

Multifocal nodular-appearing airspace opacities in a patient with viral pneumonia

Airways Disease

CT has replaced contrast bronchography in the evaluation of the tracheobronchial tree. Thin-section CT is a sensitive method of detecting bronchiectasis. Disease of the small airways is seen either directly as tree-in-bud opacities reflecting mucus-filled dilated bronchioles with peribronchiolar inflammation or indirectly by noting hyperlucency of involved lung with air trapping on expiratory scans. Problems of air distribution within

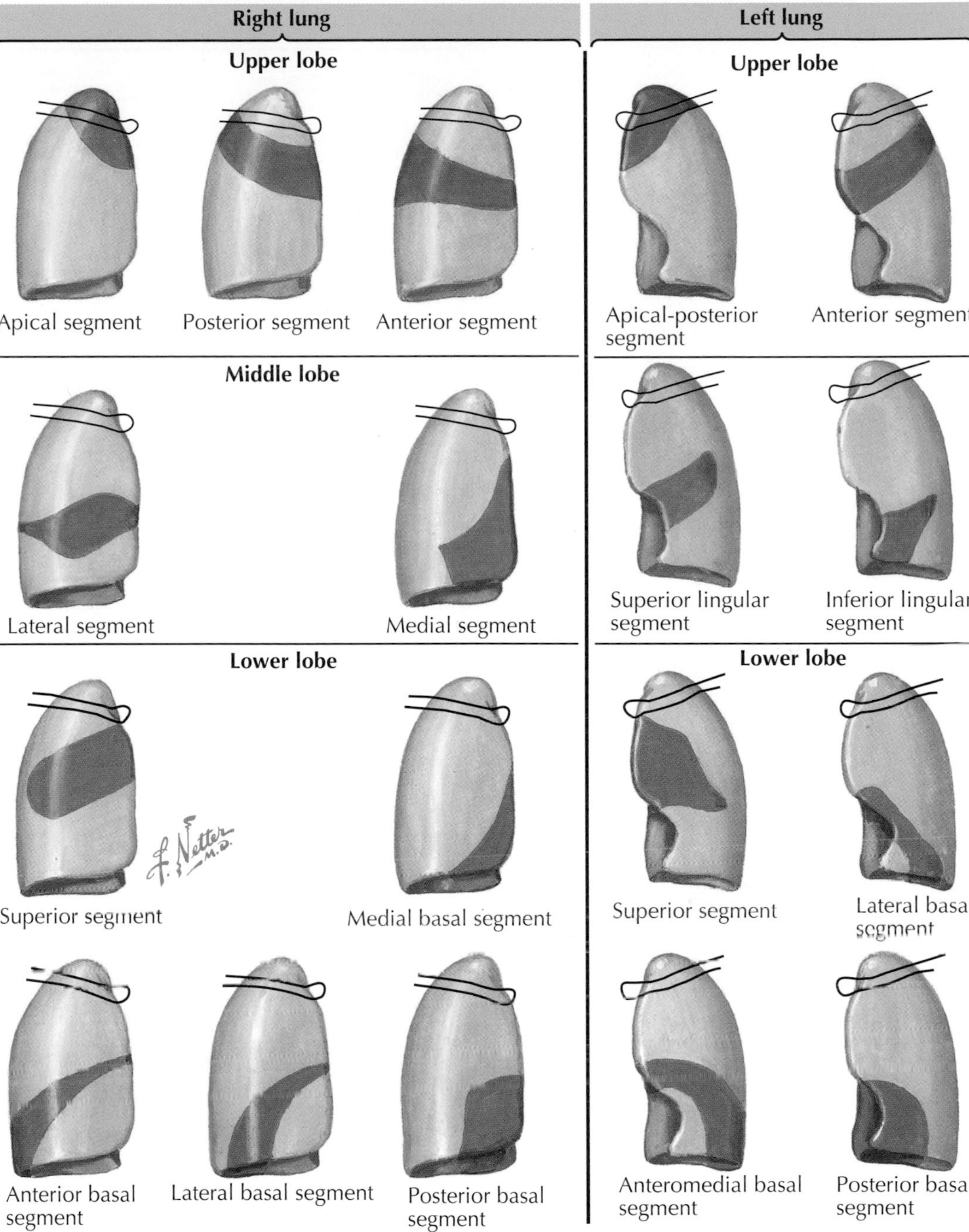

RADIOLOGIC EXAMINATION OF THE LUNGS *(Continued)*

the lungs are usually inapparent on radiographs, although they can frequently be suspected in patients with rather advanced disease. The most common of these is emphysema; in advanced cases, the lungs are hyperexpanded, resulting in flattening of the diaphragms; the pulmonary vasculature is attenuated; and there is an increase in the AP dimension of the thorax. Bullae are direct evidence of emphysema, although occasionally they are isolated abnormalities. In patients with asthma, the chest radiograph is generally normal unless the patient is in status asthmaticus, in which case the lung will be hyperinflated. Although most patients with chronic bronchitis have a normal chest radiograph, some patients are seen to have peribronchial cuffing and tram-tracks, reflecting thickened airway walls seen end-on or in length, respectively.

CT scans, especially with thin sections, can usually characterize the severity and distribution of emphysema quite well. Four anatomic forms of emphysema are well depicted on CT: centrilobular, panlobular, paraseptal, and paracicatricial types. Plate 4-31 demonstrates severe centrilobular and paraseptal emphysema caused by smoking. Plate 3-18 shows examples of panlobular and paracicatricial emphysema. CT scans performed during expiration are also useful for evaluating air trapping from small airways disease and central airways collapse from tracheobronchomalacia.

Evaluation of the Pulmonary Vasculature

The pulmonary arteries and veins are easily recognizable on chest radiographs, and the careful observer can frequently identify localized or generalized abnormalities of pulmonary blood flow. The pulmonary vascular bed has an extremely low resistance, allowing ready redistribution of its contents as resistance is increased locally.

Regional variations in pulmonary blood volume may result from airways or pulmonary vascular disease. Regional oligemia may result from obstruction of a bronchus by a foreign body, tumor, or mucous plug or from chronic obliteration of small airways as seen in patients with Swyer-James syndrome. Similar changes take place in pulmonary emphysema, although the redistribution that occurs in this disease is in greater part caused by actual destruction of the pulmonary vascular bed by the pathologic process. Processes that directly obstruct pulmonary arterial flow to the lung produce regional oligemia. These include congenital pulmonary arterial hypoplasia, hilar masses, and fibrosing mediastinitis. A central pulmonary embolism may produce a segment of oligemia distal to the obstructed pulmonary artery (termed the *Westermark sign*), but this is rarely appreciated radiographically.

Posture has a marked effect on flow distribution. In the erect position, the pulmonary vessels appear significantly larger in the bases than in the apices because of the effect of gravity. Alteration in posture obviously affects this distribution, and in the supine position, flow is relatively uniform from the apices to the bases in the frontal projection. Thus, it is of considerable importance when evaluating pulmonary vasculature to know the patient's position when the radiograph was obtained. On CT scans, a gradient is present from anterior to posterior with the vessels larger posteriorly when the patient is scanned in the supine position.

Disease processes that directly involve the pulmonary vasculature cause recognizable patterns of blood flow redistribution. In precapillary pulmonary hypertension, the peripheral vessels are small and the central vessels quite large, giving the characteristic "pruned tree" appearance (see Plate 3-9). In emphysema, local destruction of the capillary bed results in bizarre and unpredictable patterns of pulmonary blood flow. In patients with left-to-right shunts, severe anemia, or pregnancy, pulmonary blood flow may be significantly increased. This is recognizable as large vessels both centrally and peripherally. Patients with severe obstruction of pulmonary outflow, such as in tetralogy of Fallot, may develop connections between the systemic arteries and the pulmonary arteries, resulting in larger than normal peripheral vessels with small central arteries.

Pulmonary venous (postcapillary) hypertension is an abnormal elevation of the pulmonary venous pressure. This is most commonly measured indirectly as the pulmonary arteriole occlusion pressure (PAOP). Normal PAOP is below 14 mm Hg. Cardiac disease is the most familiar cause of pulmonary venous hypertension, although just as common is systemic volume overload

Radiologic Examination of the Lungs *(Continued)*

from renal failure or overhydration. In either case, elevation of left atrial pressure results in subradiographic edema in the dependent portions of the lungs. This increases vascular resistance in those regions, resulting in shunting of blood away from them and causing redistribution of the blood flow. In an erect patient, this causes engorgement of the upper lobe vessels. On a CT scan, the anterior vessels are enlarged. If venous pressure continues to increase, the patient will develop interstitial and then alveolar edema. Identical findings are present in patients with acute renal failure and acute systemic or pulmonary volume overload.

Pleural Disease

The parietal pleura is composed of a thin sheet of mesothelial cells that lines the inner surface of the ribs, and the visceral pleura that lines the lungs. Invaginations of visceral pleura form the interlobar fissures. Between the parietal and visceral pleurae is a space that may be involved in various disease processes. Pneumothorax is the accumulation of air in the pleural space, and it may result from spontaneous or traumatic causes. Pleural disease is typically manifested radiologically by the detection of pleural fluid, localized or diffuse pleural thickening, or a pleural nodule or mass.

Pleural fluid appears radiographically as homogeneous meniscoid opacity in the dependent part of the pleural cavity. Although small amounts of free fluid are difficult to detect, as little as 25 to 50 mL of fluid can be seen blunting the posterior costophrenic sulcus on upright lateral radiographs. A decubitus radiograph is the most sensitive method aside from sonography for detecting small amounts of pleural fluid, and it helps distinguish free-flowing from loculated collections. With larger (i.e., 200-300 mL) effusions, the lateral costophrenic sulcus is also blunted on the frontal radiograph. When a pleural effusion exceeds 500 mL, the hemidiaphragm becomes obscured. Loculated effusions as a result of intrapleural adhesions produce elliptical mass-like opacities along the costal pleura or when developing within an interlobar fissure appear as biconvex opacities termed *pseudotumors*.

Common causes of *unilateral* effusions are pneumonia; tuberculosis (which can produce right-sided or bilateral effusions); metastatic tumor; trauma; pulmonary infarction; lymphoma; and intraabdominal processes such as ascites (which can produce right-sided or bilateral effusions), subphrenic abscess, or pancreatitis. The most common cause of *bilateral* pleural effusion is congestive heart failure. Other frequent causes include the collagen vascular diseases, especially lupus erythematosus and rheumatoid arthritis; metastatic tumor; hypoproteinemia; and renal disease.

Solitary Pulmonary Nodule

Types and degrees of calcification that may be demonstrated in shadows by CT

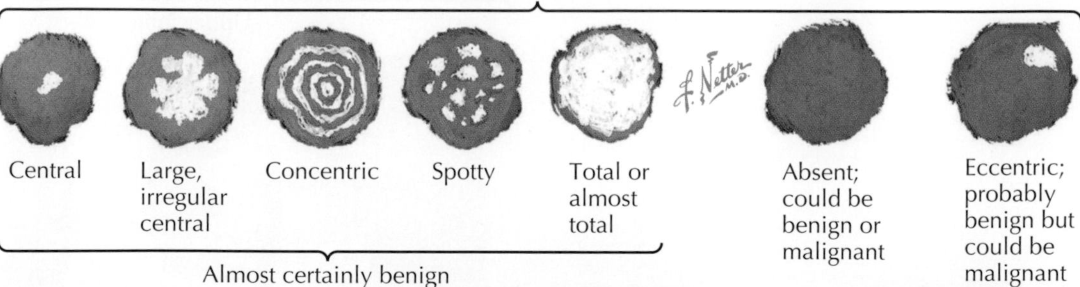

Pulmonary nodules in three different patients

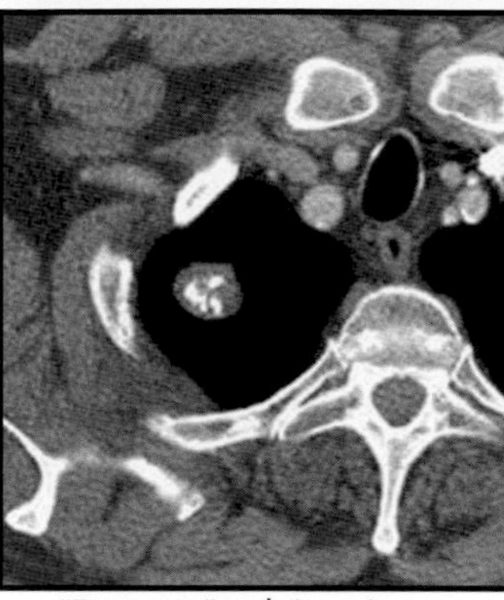

"Popcorn" calcium in a pulmonary hamartoma

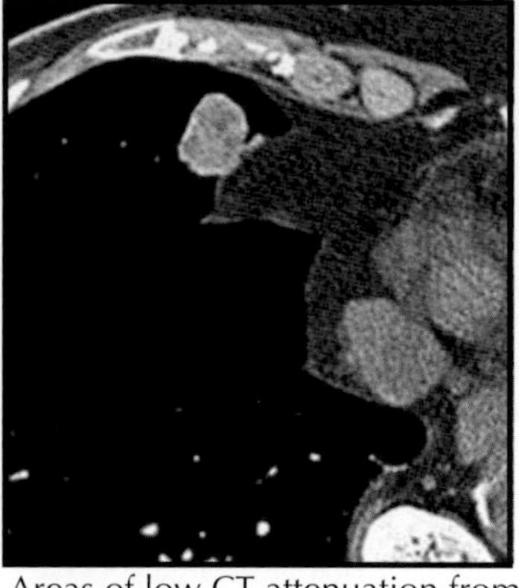

Areas of low CT attenuation from fat in a pulmonary hamartoma

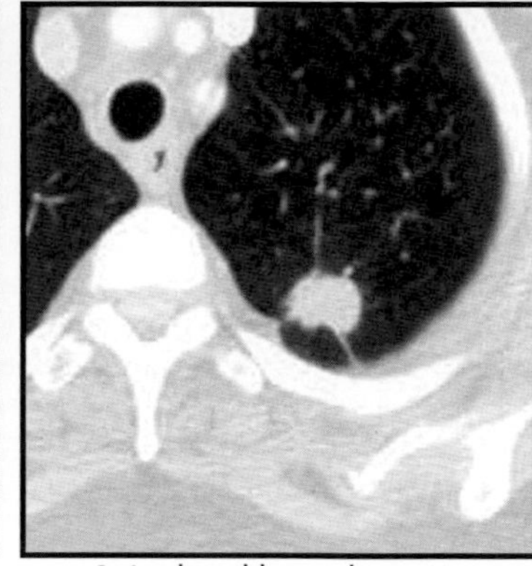

Spiculated bronchogenic carcinoma

Adenocarcinoma of the lung

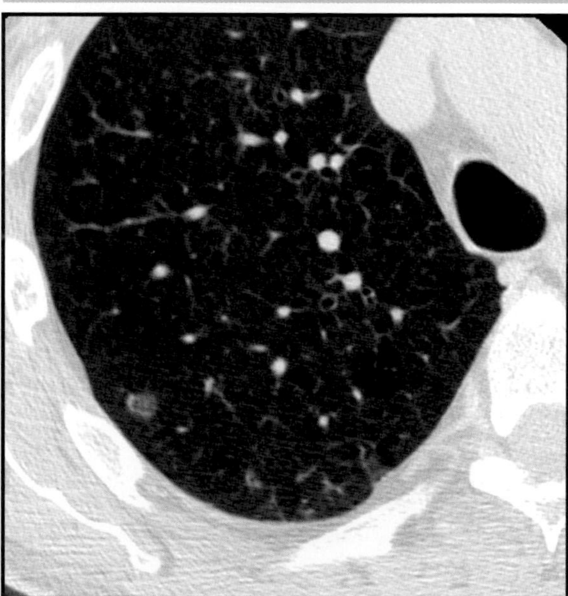

Original CT scan demonstrates a ground–glass attenuation nodule in the posterior right upper lobe

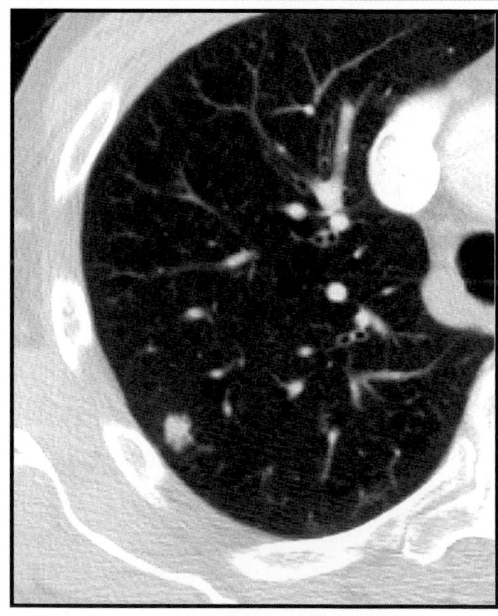

Repeat scan 1 year later demonstrates interval growth and development of more solid component in the nodule

Localized or diffuse pleural thickening may occur in a variety of conditions. *Localized* pleural thickening is commonly seen at the chest apices and actually reflects subpleural fibrosis in the apical lung. Common causes of focal pleural thickening include prior infection or infarction, pleural plaque formation, and extrapleural fat deposition. Blunting of the lateral costophrenic sulcus on a frontal radiograph in the absence of blunting of the posterior costophrenic sulcus usually indicates pleural fibrosis. Diffuse pleural thickening in one hemithorax is usually secondary to previous tuberculosis, empyema, or hemothorax. Bilateral diffuse pleural thickening tends to involve the costal pleural surfaces and is most often the result of asbestos-related pleural fibrosis, particularly if accompanied by pleural calcification. Nodular pleural thickening, particularly if involving the hemithorax circumferentially, is most typical of pleural malignancy caused by

Radiologic Examination of the Lungs *(Continued)*

metastatic disease or less commonly mesothelioma (see Plate 3-18).

A focal pleural nodule or mass is typically incompletely marginated by lung as it protrudes medially to create a smooth, sharp interface with tapered, obtuse borders at its edges (the "incomplete border sign"). The most common pleural mass is a loculated pleural effusion. Other causes of pleural masses include lipomas, metastatic and primary neoplasms, healing ribs fractures, pleural metastases, and (rarely) localized fibrous tumors of the pleura.

Abnormalities of the Diaphragm and Chest Wall

Anatomic variations of the diaphragmatic contour are common. Although each hemidiaphragm is generally a smooth, dome-shaped structure, localized bulges are common and are usually caused by a deficiency of muscle in that portion (partial eventration). Elevation of an entire hemidiaphragm may result from phrenic nerve paralysis or eventration of the entire hemidiaphragm, which are distinguished fluoroscopically by noting paradoxical superior movement of the diaphragm while the patient sniffs ("sniff test").

Foramina in the normal diaphragm may become enlarged and allow herniation of abdominal viscera into the chest. The paired foramina of Morgagni lie anteriorly and medially. Hernias occasionally occur through them and are more common on the right side than on the left. Most often, herniation develops through the centrally placed esophageal hiatus. The stomach is the usual viscus to herniate through this opening, but the colon and small bowel may also do so. Posterior and slightly lateral are the paired foramina of Bochdalek. Massive congenital hernias seen in newborns, although infrequent, generally bulge through a large foramen of Bochdalek, usually on the left side. In addition to diaphragmatic hernias, a tumor of the diaphragm sometimes presents as a mass on the chest radiograph.

Abnormalities of the chest wall may result from trauma, infection, or neoplasms. Rib fractures are common in adults after blunt trauma and are of limited clinical significance unless multiple contiguous segmental fractures result in paradoxical inward movement of the involved portion of the chest wall during inspiration (i.e., flail chest). Peripheral lung, pleural, or chest wall infections are identified by noting a mass on radiography or CT producing rib destruction. Most neoplasms arising primarily in the chest wall are metastatic tumors or myeloma, although primary bone and soft tissue tumors may occur. Extrapulmonary chest wall lesions typically produce rib erosion or destruction, and when protruding into the thorax, they produce a mass with smooth margins and tapered edges that form obtuse angles with the underlying lung, resulting in the "extrapleural sign" (see Plate 3-19).

Abnormalities of the Mediastinum

Mediastinal structures, with the exception of the trachea and air-filled portions of the esophagus, are indirectly visualized on chest radiographs as they interface with the adjacent lungs. Although mediastinal disease can be detected radiographically by noting abnormalities of mediastinal density, contour, or width, the superior contrast resolution of CT provides a more detailed analysis in the evaluation of mediastinal abnormalities.

The mediastinum is divided into superior and inferior compartments with the latter further divided into anterior, middle, and posterior subdivisions. The anterior compartment is bounded anteriorly by the sternum

Airway and Pleural Diseases

Cicatricial emphysema

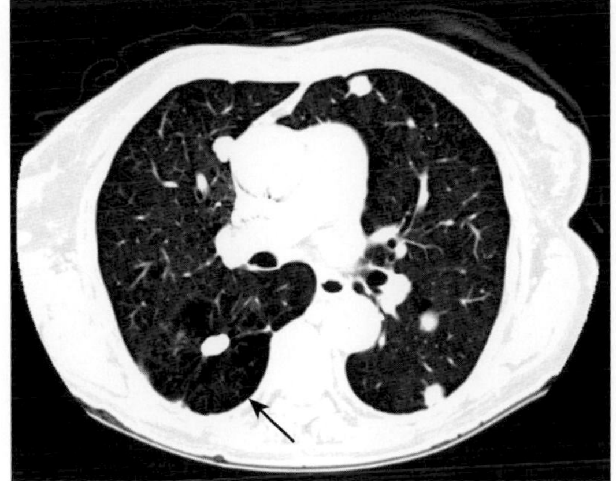

Cicatricial emphysema around a focus of granulomatous scarring in the right upper lobe

Panlobular emphysema

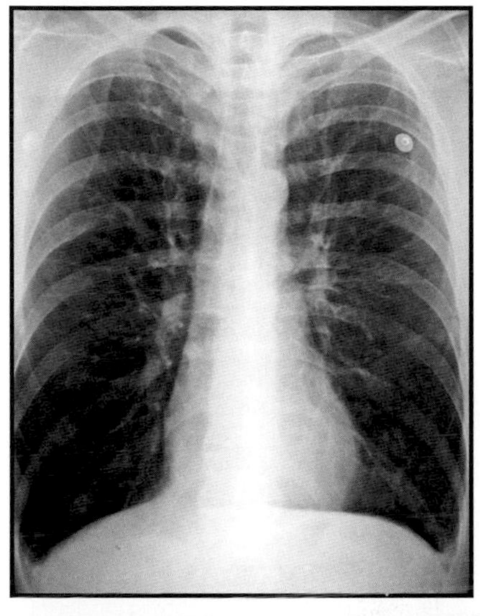

Panlobular emphysema from α_1-antitrypsin deficiency. There is marked bilateral lower lung hyperlucency

Mesothelioma

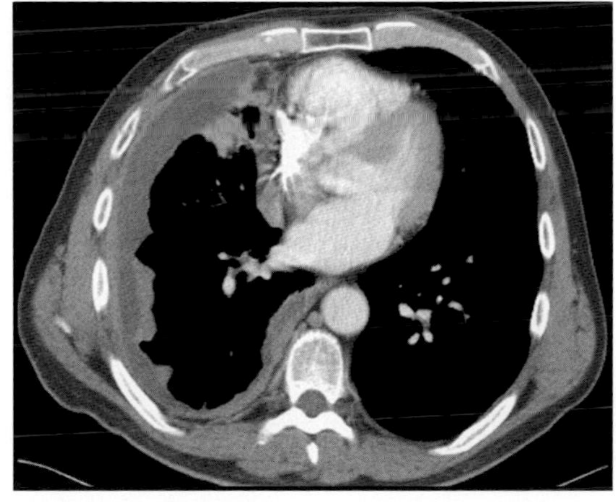

Axial CT demonstrates diffuse, nodular right-sided pleural thickening with contraction of the right hemithorax

Radiologic Examination of the Lungs *(Continued)*

and posteriorly by the heart, aorta, and great vessels. The middle compartment contains the heart, great vessels, and trachea and its branches; the hila are often included in this compartment. Structures situated posterior to the heart, including the vertebrae and paraspinal regions, esophagus, and descending aorta, lie in the posterior mediastinum.

Using this classification of mediastinal compartments, masses found in the *anterior mediastinum* are lymph node enlargement of any cause, thyroid goiters, and thymic and germ cell tumors. Thyroid masses almost invariably appear in the thoracic inlet and superior mediastinum and displace the trachea laterally. Lymph node enlargement is usually caused by lymphoma (see Plate 3-19), metastatic disease, or less often sarcoidosis or granulomatous infections, and can produce a smooth or lobulated mass and simultaneously involve the middle and posterior mediastinal compartments. Thymic and germ cell tumors lie below the aortic arch and typically present as a solitary, smoothly marginated mass.

In the *middle mediastinal compartment*, lymph node enlargement is a frequent cause of a mass and can present as a diffuse widening, often associated with enlargement of one or both hilar shadows. Anomalies or aneurysms of the aorta or great vessels and duplication cysts of the tracheobronchial tree may present as localized densities in this location (see Plate 3-19). Pericardial cysts or tumors also occur in the middle mediastinum.

The only common masses of the *posterior mediastinal compartment* are neurogenic tumors, particularly nerve sheath tumors and tumors of the sympathetic ganglia, including ganglioneuromas and neuroblastomas, but tumors or infections of the vertebral column may also occasionally present in a similar location. The esophagus itself may appear as a long tubular shadow, and tumors or diverticula of the esophagus may be seen as localized mediastinal masses. Aneurysms of the descending aorta and masses that extend through the esophageal hiatus, including hiatal hernias and pancreatic pseudocysts, are uncommon causes of posterior mediastinal masses.

The detection of mediastinal widening on frontal chest radiography is somewhat subjective but is most easily appreciated as a change in comparison with prior chest radiographs or the recognition of an outward convexity to the mediastinal contour. Mediastinal widening is commonly technical in nature because of patient rotation on the radiograph or as a result of diminished lung volumes. The most common cause of diffuse mediastinal widening is mediastinal lipomatosis, a condition that is easily recognized on CT as diffuse fatty infiltration of the mediastinum. Other more important causes of mediastinal widening include hemorrhage caused by aortic or great vessel injury, tumor infiltration as in lymphoma or small cell carcinoma of lung, and mediastinitis.

Occasionally, the only sign of the presence of mediastinal disease is a change in mediastinal density. Because conventional radiographs are unable to distinguish the differing tissue densities that comprise the mediastinum in health and disease, only the increased density of calcification and the lucency of air are readily detectable. Mediastinal calcification can be seen in treated lymphoma or as a result of prior granulomatous infection, most commonly histoplasmosis. Mediastinal lucency usually indicates pneumomediastinum and is seen as vertically oriented lucencies outlining the heart and mediastinal structures and typically extends superiorly into the thoracic inlet and neck.

Abnormalities of the Chest Wall and Mediastinum

Abnormalities of the chest wall

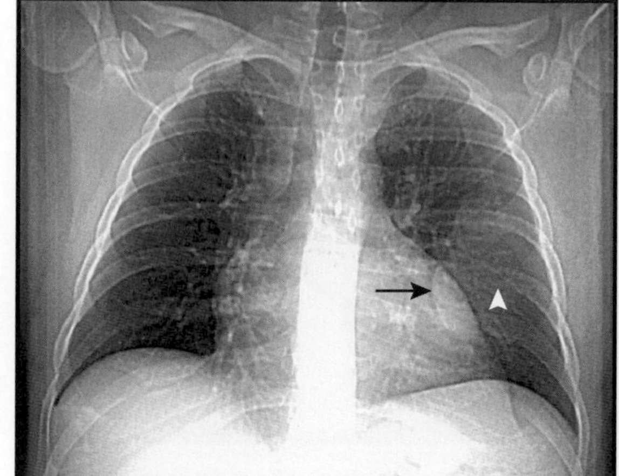

Primitive neuroectodermal (Askin) tumor of the left chest wall. Frontal scout view from a CT scan in a 36-year-old patient with left chest pain shows a lobulated left chest mass (arrow) with associated rib destruction (arrowhead)

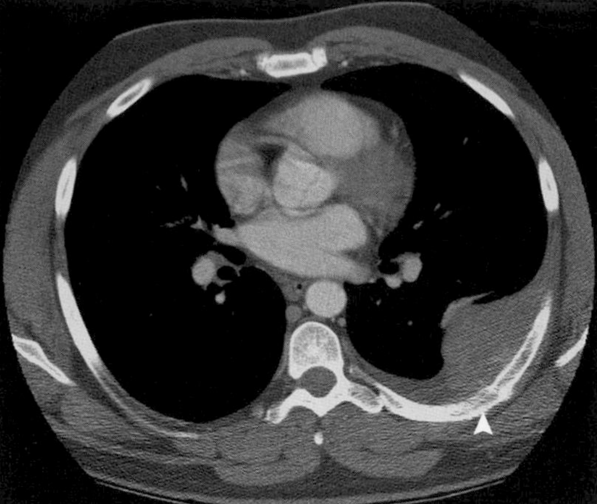

Contrast-enhanced CT in the same patient shows a soft tissue mass with partial destruction of an adjacent rib (arrowhead). En bloc surgical resection showed a small, round, blue cell tumor indicative of a primitive neuroectodermal tumor of the chest wall

Abnormalities of the mediastinum

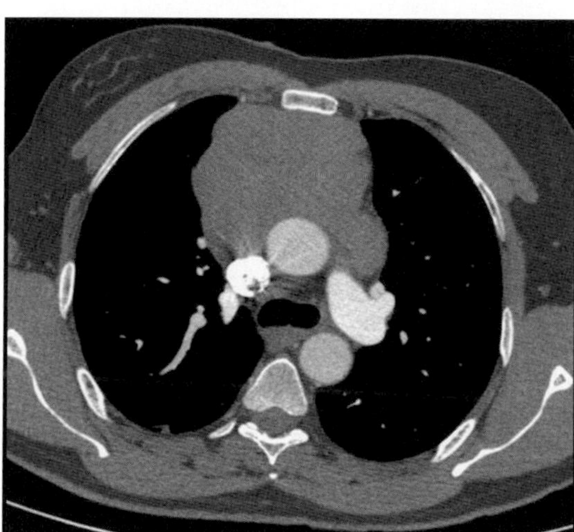

Anterior mediastinal mass secondary to non-Hodgkin lymphoma

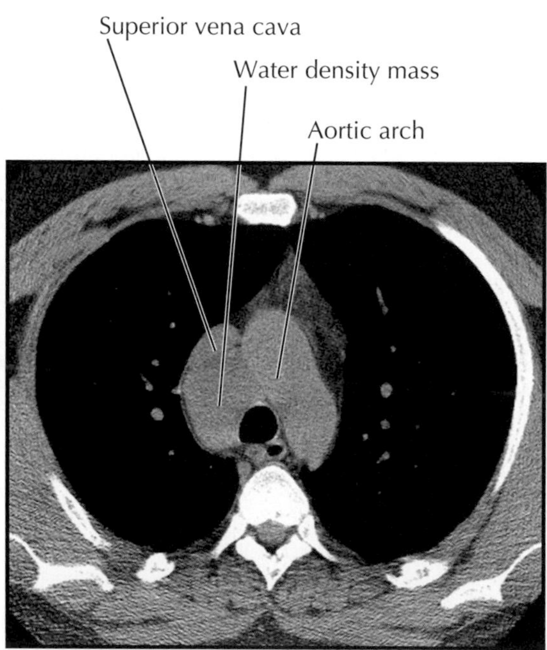

Bronchogenic cyst. A water density mass is situated between the aortic arch and superior vena cava

EXHALED BREATH ANALYSIS

Breath analysis offers a window on lung physiology and disease and is rapidly evolving as a new frontier in medical testing for disease states in the lung and beyond. Breath analysis is now used to diagnose and monitor asthma, to check for transplant organ rejection, and to detect lung cancer, among other applications.

With each breath we exhale, thousands of molecules are expelled in our breath, and each one of us has a "smellprint" that can tell a lot about our state of health. Hippocrates described *fetor oris* and *fetor hepaticus* in his treatise on breath aroma and disease. In 1784, Lavoisier and Laplace showed that respiration consumes oxygen and eliminates carbon dioxide. In the mid-1800s, Nebelthau showed that individuals with diabetes emit breath acetone. And in 1874, Anstie isolated ethanol from breath (which is the basis of breath alcohol testing today).

In addition to the known respiratory gases (oxygen and carbon dioxide) and water vapor, exhaled breath contains a multitude of other substances, including elemental gases such as nitric oxide (NO) and carbon monoxide (CO) and volatile organic compounds (VOCs). Exhaled breath also carries aerosolized droplets that can be collected as "exhaled breath condensate" (EBC), which contain nonvolatile compounds such as proteins dissolved in them as well.

A major breakthrough in the scientific study of breath started in the 1970s when Linus Pauling demonstrated the presence of 250 substances in exhaled breath. With modern mass spectrometry (MS) and gas chromatography mass spectrometry (GC-MS) instruments, we can now identify more than 1000 unique substances in exhaled breath. There are currently commercially available analyzers that can measure NO levels in exhaled breath to the parts per billion (ppb) range and CO to the parts per million (ppm) range. Sensitive mass spectrometers can measure volatile compounds on breath down to the parts per trillion (ppt) range.

Aerosolized droplets in exhaled breath can be captured by a variety of methods and analyzed for a wide range of biomarkers from metabolic end products to proteins to a variety of cytokines and chemokines, and the possibilities continue to expand.

Advances in the field of breath analysis require close multidisciplinary collaboration. One great example of how the collaboration between technical, medical, and commercial professionals has resulted in a clinically useful tool is the measurement of NO in exhaled breath for monitoring airway inflammation. The advent of chemiluminescence analyzers in the early 1990s allowed the detection of low (ppb) levels of NO in exhaled breath. This was quickly followed by the observation that patients with asthma had higher than normal levels of NO in their exhaled breath, which was later linked to eosinophilic airway inflammation. Standardization of the gas collection methods and measurement techniques allowed the industry to build the next generation of analyzers suitable for use in the clinical setting. In 2003, the Food and Drug Administration approved the first desktop NO analyzer for monitoring airway inflammation in individuals with asthma. The use of exhaled NO in monitoring asthma is useful for several reasons. It is noninvasive, it can be performed repeatedly, and it can be used in children and patients with severe airflow obstruction in whom other techniques are difficult or impossible to perform. Exhaled NO may also be more sensitive than currently available tests in detecting airway inflammation, which may allow more optimum therapy.

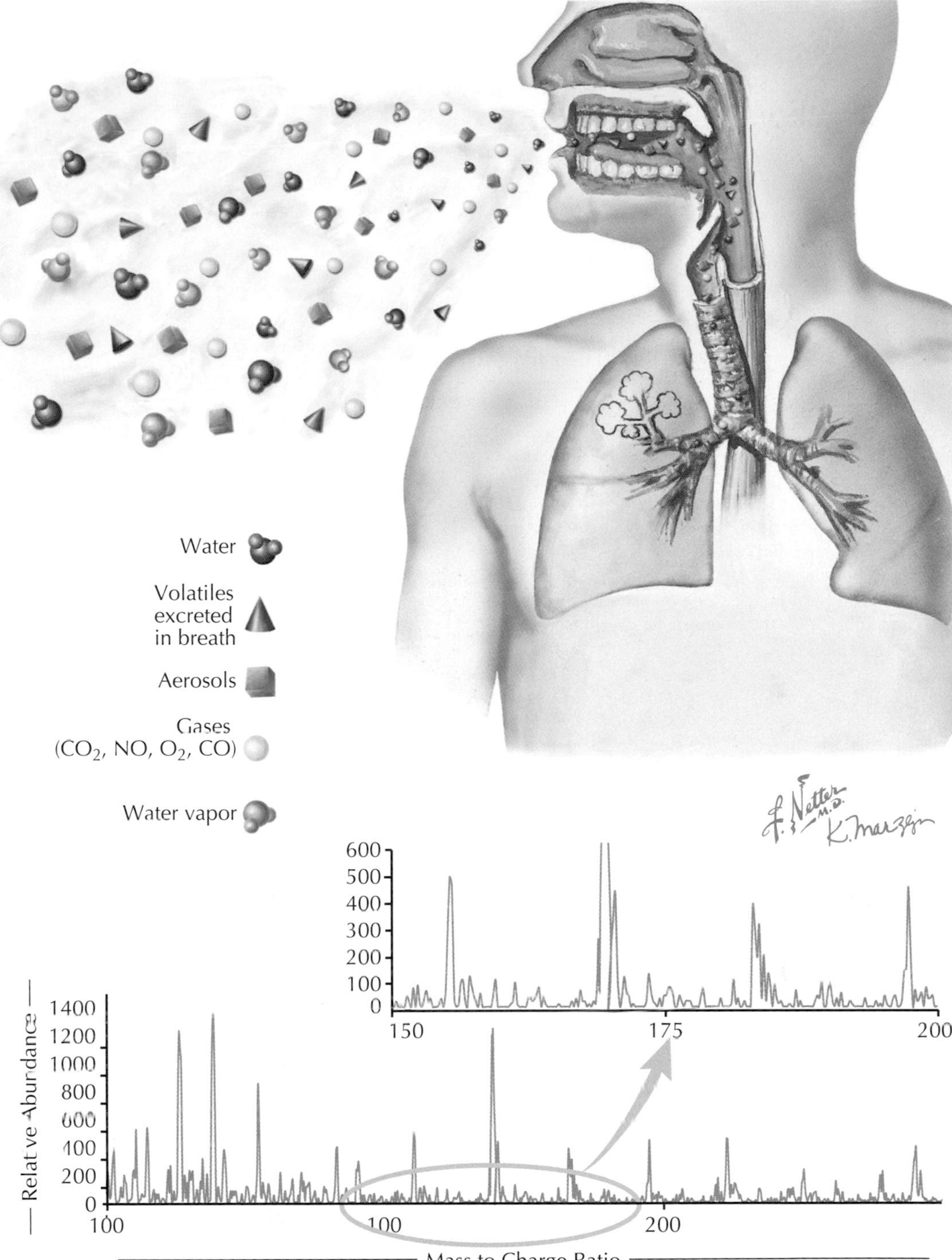

In addition to the known respiratory gases (oxygen and carbon dioxide) and water vapor, exhaled breath contains a multitude of other substances including elemental gases, volatile organic compounds (VOCs), and aerosolized droplets. Sensitive mass spectrometers can identify thousands of volatile compounds in exhaled breath. An example of a mass spectrometer tracing is shown depicting the distribution of volatile compounds in a sample of exhaled breath, with each spike representing the identification of a unique substance based on its mass to charge ratio. The upper tracing is a blow-up of a segment of the lower tracing.

FLEXIBLE BRONCHOSCOPY

Endoscopic examination of the tracheobronchial tree is an essential procedure in the diagnosis and treatment of patients with diseases of the lungs and airways. Although rigid bronchoscopy has been performed since 1897, the first flexible bronchoscope was introduced in 1968. Major advantages of the flexible bronchoscope are that it allows visualization and sampling of peripheral lesions that cannot be reached using a rigid instrument. Additionally, whereas flexible bronchoscopy can be performed with topical anesthesia and moderate sedation in the endoscopy suite or intensive care unit, rigid bronchoscopy requires general anesthesia and is typically performed in the operating room. Early flexible bronchoscopes used fiberoptic cables to send light in and out of the peripheral airways. With the miniaturization of electronic devices, the first video bronchoscope was introduced in 1987. Video technology offers an incredibly sharp image to be displayed on multiple monitors and allows the operator to capture both still images and video.

EQUIPMENT

The external diameter of the flexible bronchoscope varies from 2.7 mm to 6.3 mm in diameter. The diameter of the working channel ranges from 1.2 mm to 3.2 mm. A working channel 2.8 mm or larger is recommended for more therapeutic flexible bronchoscopy because it allows for better suction and the passage of larger instruments. It is important to note the relative anatomy at the tip of the bronchoscope. By convention, as viewed from the operator's perspective, the camera is at 9:00, and the instrument and suction channel are at 3:00. These landmarks play a role when navigating the airways, and the bronchoscope may need to be rotated to visualize the intended target.

As with all procedures, a careful history and physical examination are essential. The operator should have a plan as to what needs to be done and should communicate it to his or her support staff. Informed consent is required, and patients should be monitored as per local policy for moderate sedation. Because hypoxemia can be seen during bronchoscopy, all patients should receive supplemental oxygen. Adequate topical anesthesia is essential to reduce patient discomfort, and the total dose of lidocaine should be kept to less than 8 mg/kg in adults. Premedication with anticholinergic medications is not recommended.

The bronchoscope can be introduced transorally, transnasally, or through an endotracheal or tracheostomy tube. When passing the bronchoscope through the oropharynx, one should use a bite block to prevent damage to the bronchoscope.

The operator typically stands in front of the patient if he or she is seated or semi-recumbent or above the patient's head if he or she is supine. Knowledge of nasopharyngeal, oropharyngeal, and laryngeal anatomy is essential, as is a thorough understanding of the segmental bronchial anatomy. Familiarity with the controls of the bronchoscope is important to enable its tip to be properly directed without damage to the instrument or the mucosal lining. The bronchoscope should be kept straight because any curves will limit transmission of rotating the head of the bronchoscope to its tip.

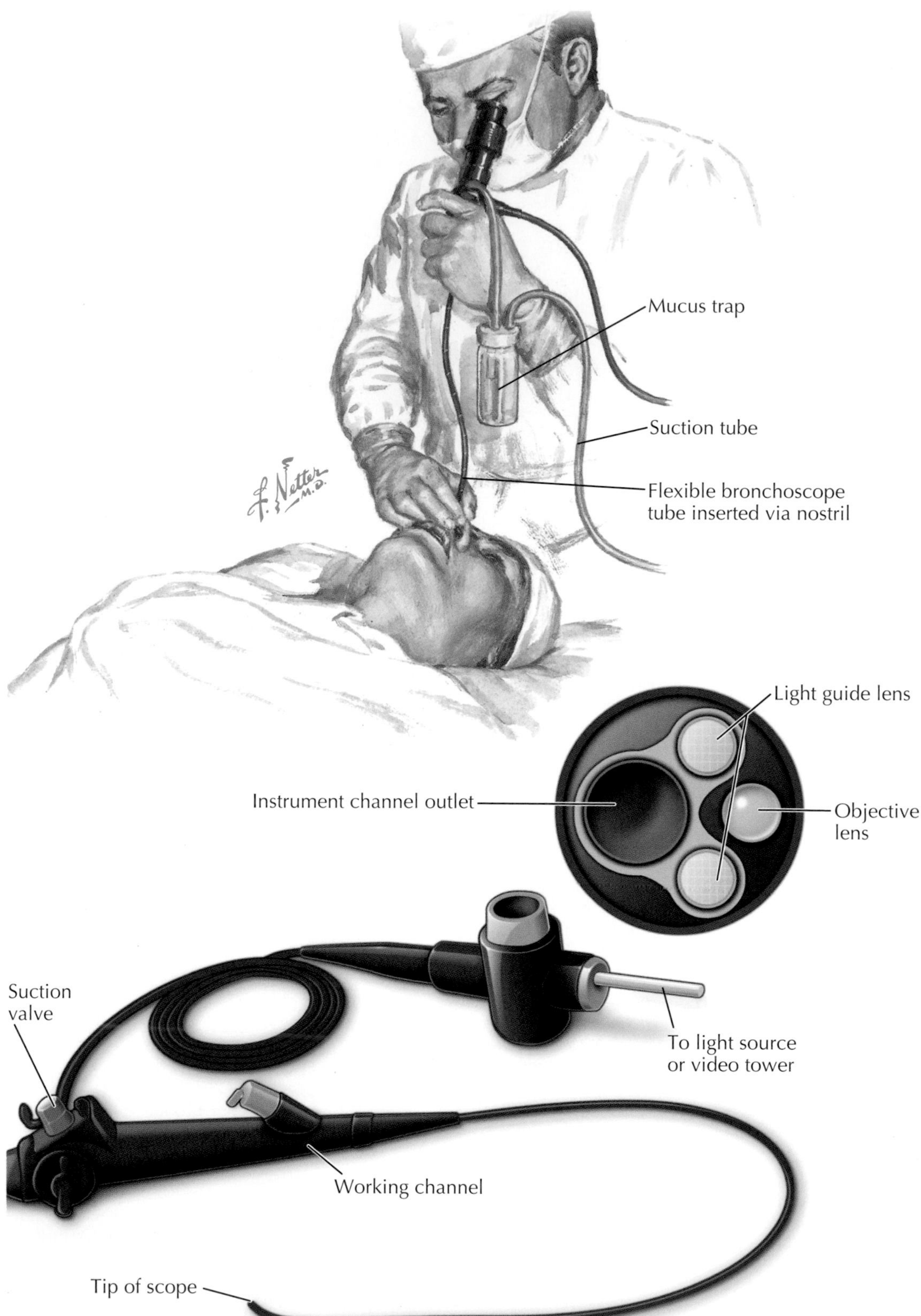

Many techniques are available during flexible bronchoscopy to sample both central and peripheral lesions. Endobronchial biopsies, brushings, washings, and needle aspiration can all be performed for visible lesions. Likewise, transbronchial needle aspiration, transbronchial biopsy, brushing, and bronchoalveolar lavage can be used to sample peripheral lesions. Advanced techniques such as endobronchial ultrasonography, virtual bronchoscopic navigation, and electromagnetic navigation may all increase the yield for sampling peripheral lesions.

Complications requiring immediate treatment include laryngospasm and bronchospasm and any bleeding that is more than mild in quantity. A pneumothorax, depending on its size, may call for placement of chest tubes. Severe hypoxemia and ventricular dysrhythmias usually require cessation of the procedure.

Typical bronchoscopic views

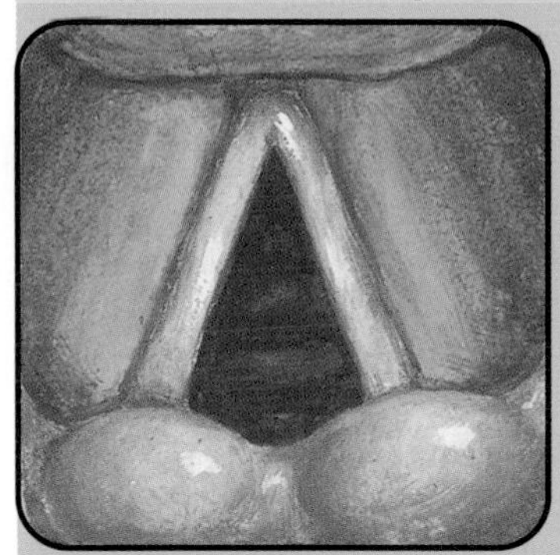
Vocal cords visualized during passage of bronchoscope. Anesthetic injected at this point to facilitate passage through glottis

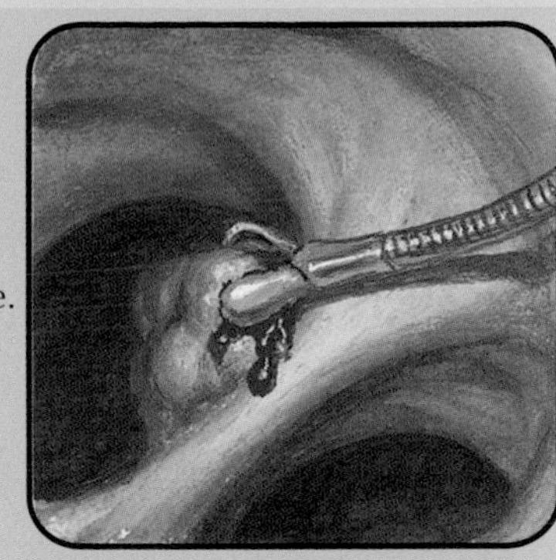
Tumor of superior segment of left lower lobe. Forceps about to take biopsy

Normal right upper lobe bronchus with openings of apical, posterior, and anterior segmental bronchi

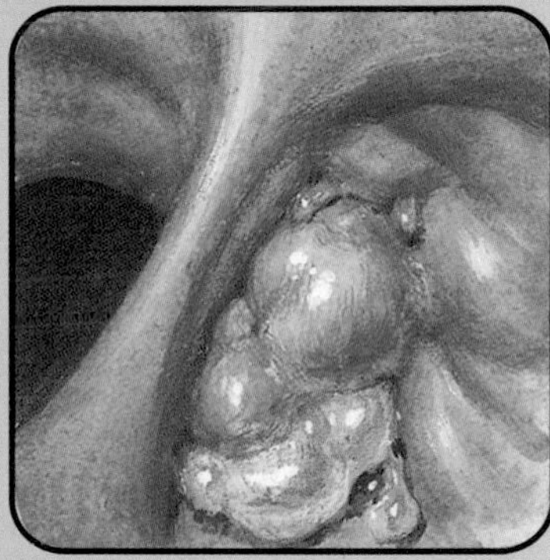
Bronchogenic carcinoma obstructing bronchus

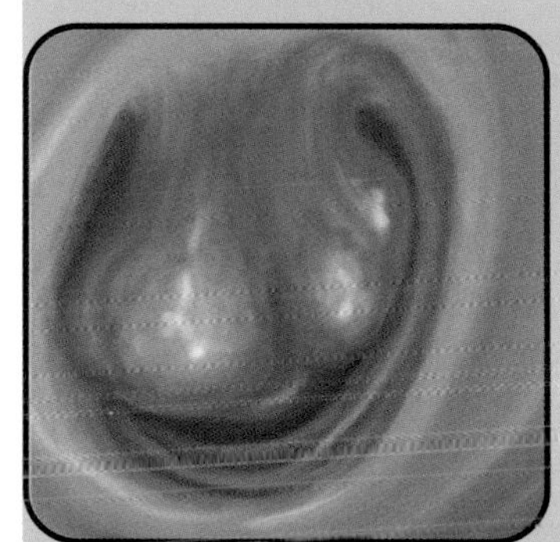
Carcinoid tumor

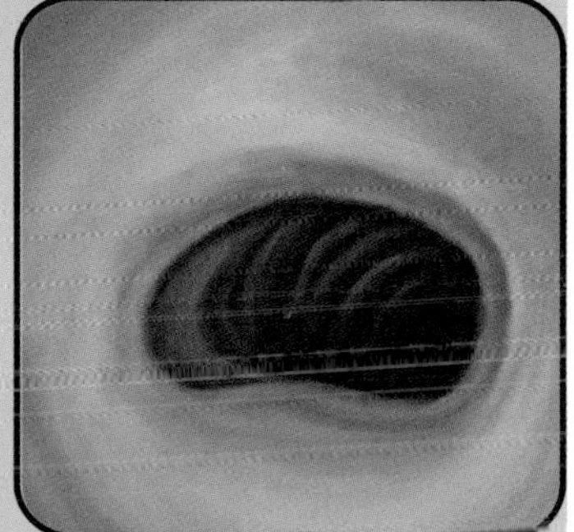
Tracheal stenosis

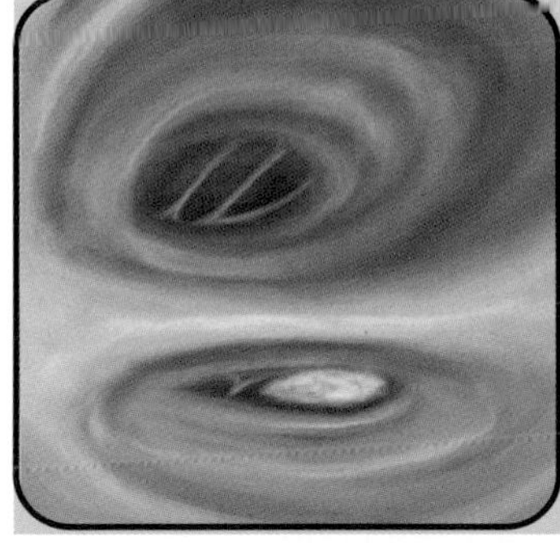
Broncholith

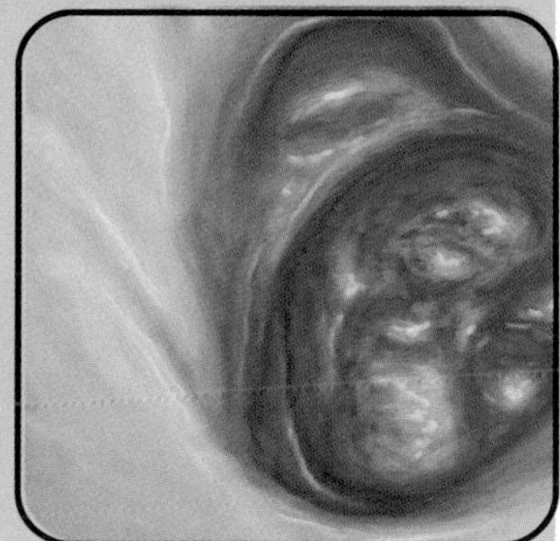
Adenoid cystic carcinoma

Bronchoscopic Views

While the bronchoscope is being passed through the oro- or nasopharynx, the larynx, and the tracheobronchial tree, careful attention should be paid to the mucosa, the size of the lumen, and any difference from expected anatomy. Normal bronchial mucosa is pale pink, but its color varies with the intensity of the light source. The surface follows the contours of tracheal and bronchial walls and becomes paler where it overlies cartilaginous rings. A small amount of mucus and a thin layer of surface lining fluid reflect the light from the bronchoscope. In the trachea and main bronchi, the shape of the lumen is an incomplete circle or arch with a membranous posterior portion; this portion disappears distally as the airways become surrounded first by irregular cartilaginous plates and eventually by concentric muscle and elastic tissue.

Inflammation may be diffuse or localized. The endobronchial changes seen are erythema, increased vascularity, edema, mucosal irregularity, augmented secretion production, and occasionally ulceration. Edema may lead to loss of the cartilaginous prominences, the normal mucosal pattern, and narrowing of bronchial orifices. Excess secretions may be mucoid or purulent and range from thin and watery to thick and viscid. Localized inflammation accompanies carcinomas, tuberculosis, foreign bodies, pneumonia, bronchiectasis, and abscess formation. Healing of endobronchial inflammation may lead to scar formation and permanent stenosis or tracheobronchomalacia or excessive dynamic airways collapse. Newer imaging technologies such as autofluorescence, narrow-band, optical coherence tomography, and confocal microendoscopy each allow visualization of subepithelial changes such as neovascularization. Some of these modalities may allow for visualization of intracellular organelles and provide an "optical biopsy" (i.e., the ability to identify pathology without removing a specimen for external visualization under a microscope).

Extrinsic compression is most commonly caused by malignancy, lymphadenopathy, thyroid goiter, aspirated foreign bodies, and vascular abnormalities. Endobronchial ultrasonography has been shown to be more sensitive than chest computed tomography for differentiating airway compression from invasion. Extrinsic compression from any cause may reduce the airway lumen enough to cause distal atelectasis.

Tissue involved by tumor growth may be firm and fibrous or soft and hypervascular. The mucosa may appear inflamed or pale and yellow. There may be concentric narrowing of the lumen or an irregular mass that at times is polypoid and occludes the bronchus entirely. Engorgement of superficial vessels is common and may result in hemoptysis. The majority of endobronchial tumors are bronchogenic carcinomas, but other neoplasms, such as renal cell, breast, thyroid, colon, and melanoma, can also metastasize to the airway.

Nonmalignant airway obstruction may result from extrinsic disease as listed above or from disease confined to within the airway itself. Inflammatory conditions, including amyloidosis, Wegener granulomatosis, and relapsing polychondritis, may cause significant endoluminal obstruction. Infectious causes of nonmalignant airway obstruction include tuberculosis, fungal disease such as aspergillosis, and papillomatosis caused by human papilloma virus. Granulation tissue resulting from endotracheal or tracheostomy tubes and airway stents is also increasing in prevalence as a form of iatrogenic airway obstruction.

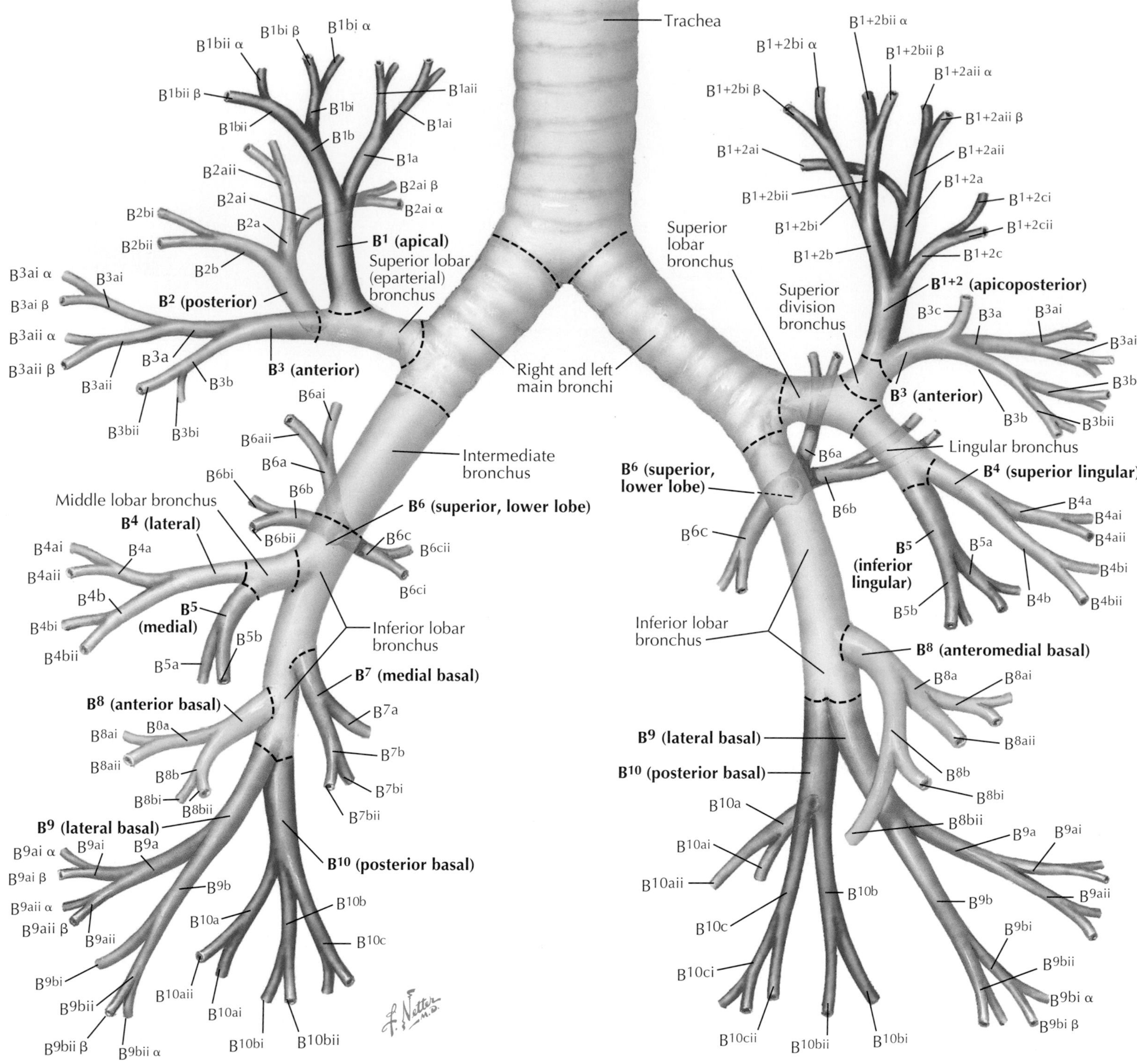

NOMENCLATURE FOR PERIPHERAL BRONCHI

Two nomenclature systems are commonly used to identify the segmental anatomy of the lungs. The one proposed by Boyden uses numerical ordering, and the one proposed by Jackson and Huber names the bronchi. It is recommend that one become familiar with both systems.

There are 10 segments in the right lung and nine in the left (see Plates 1-14 and 1-15). Subdivisions of the bronchial tree correspond to the anatomic segments and are named accordingly. These tertiary bronchi were regarded by Jackson and Huber as the final branches, but the advent of the flexible bronchoscope led Ikeda to introduce additional nomenclature for the fourth, fifth, and sixth divisions because these can now be visualized. A convenient numerical system is used in which segmental bronchi are numbered from 1 to 10 on each side and identified by the capital letter *B* for bronchus. This may be prefixed by a capital letter *R* for right and *L* for left, so that RB^3 identifies the bronchus to the anterior segment of the right upper lobe. The apicoposterior segment of the left upper lobe is LB^{1+2}, and the anteromedial basal segment of the same side becomes LB^8 because each of these paired segments is supplied by a single tertiary bronchus. With rare exceptions, there is no LB^7 designation.

Subsegmental or fourth-order bronchi are indicated by the lower case letter *a* for posterior and *b* for anterior. The letter *c* may also be used when necessary for additional bronchi.

Fifth-order bronchi are designated by the Roman numerals *i* (posterior) and *ii* (anterior). Finally, those at the level of the sixth order of division are characterized by α and β.

Endobronchial variations from the normal anatomy are frequent and are more common in peripheral airways.

Rigid Bronchoscopy

In 1897, Gustav Killian published his success in removing a pork bone from the right mainstem bronchus using a rigid esophagoscope and an external light source. Killian went on to lecture throughout the world, ushering in the era of modern bronchoscopy. Chevalier Jackson perfected the technique of rigid bronchoscopy as we now know it. Much of today's expertise in endoscopy is based on his original methods or modifications of them.

Although the use of the flexible bronchoscope largely replaced the rigid bronchoscope for diagnostic purposes, rigid bronchoscopy remains an indispensable therapeutic tool. The rigid bronchoscope lacks the maneuverability of the flexible bronchoscope, but it is able to provide an airway for oxygenation and ventilation and allows the passage of large-bore suction catheters as well as multiple other tools such as large forceps and lasers. Silicone airway stents can only be placed via a rigid bronchoscope, and the bronchoscope itself can be used to "core out" tumors invading the airway. Because the flexible bronchoscope can be easily passed through the rigid barrel, the two methods of airway visualization should be regarded as complementary.

INSTRUMENTS

The bronchoscope is basically an open steel tube. Some rigid bronchoscopes have a proximal or distal lighting source, but others use an optical telescope. The external diameter of the adult rigid bronchoscope ranges from 9 to 14 mm and is usually 40 cm long. There is a distal beveled end to allow for lifting of the epiglottis and safer insertion through the vocal cords. The diameter of the bronchoscope used depends on the patient's size and degree of airway obstruction. Fenestrations are present at the distal third of the bronchoscope to allow for contralateral lung ventilation when the bronchoscope is inserted into a mainstem bronchus. A variety of instruments such as suction catheters and biopsy forceps should be available for use.

PROCEDURE

Rigid bronchoscopy is generally performed in the operating suite under general anesthesia, which can be delivered via inhalational or total intravenous techniques.

Correct positioning of the head is important to bring the mouth, larynx, and trachea in line with each other. The head is typically extended and sometimes dropped posteriorly to facilitate this alignment. As such, patients with cervical spine instability or ankylosing spondylitis may not be able to be intubated with the rigid bronchoscope. Dentures should be removed, and the upper teeth should be protected, with particular attention to avoid leverage against them.

The bronchoscope is introduced gently with one hand while the other hand keeps the mouth open and maintains head position. The bronchoscope is passed over the base of the tongue, and its tip used to lift the epiglottis anteriorly. The arytenoepiglottic folds, arytenoids, and vocal cords are then visualized. At this point, the bronchoscope is rotated 90 degrees clockwise. The left vocal cord becomes centered in the visual field, and the tip of the bronchoscope is brought between the two cords. With gentle progression and continued clockwise rotation, the bronchoscope will pass into the trachea. At no time should its passage be forced; if there is difficulty, a smaller sized bronchoscope may be needed. Ventilation is then initiated, and inspection of the tracheobronchial tree is continued under direct vision.

To examine the left-sided airways, the head is turned toward the right, and to examine the right-sided airways, the head is turned left. The use of oblique or lateral viewing telescopes is helpful for full visualization of the upper lobes, although this technique has largely been replaced by passing the flexible bronchoscope through the rigid bronchoscope.

Withdrawal of the bronchoscope requires similar care to that used during insertion. If the patient remains anesthetized, an endotracheal tube or laryngeal mask airway can be placed until the effects of anesthesia are reversed.

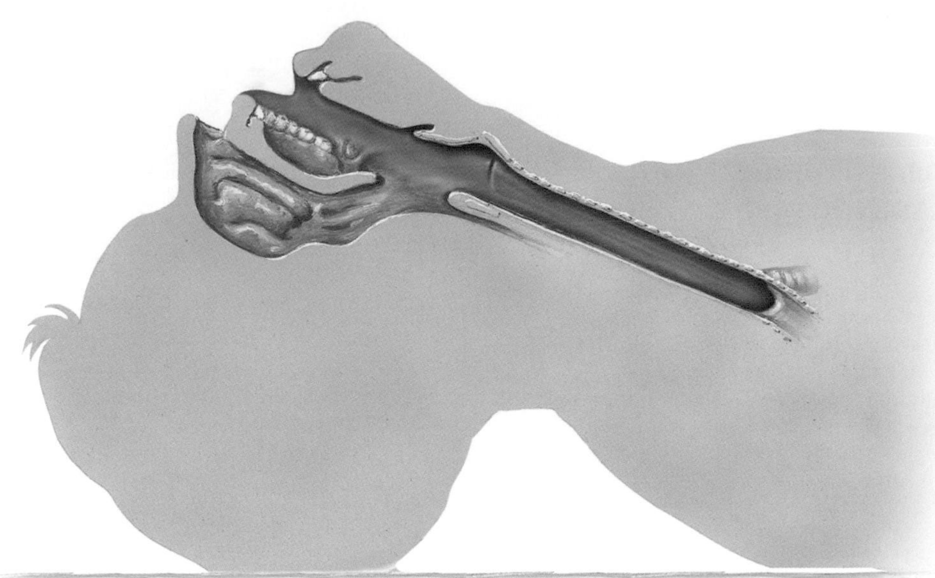

Typical head and neck position for insertion of a rigid bronchoscope used to align mouth, larynx, and trachea

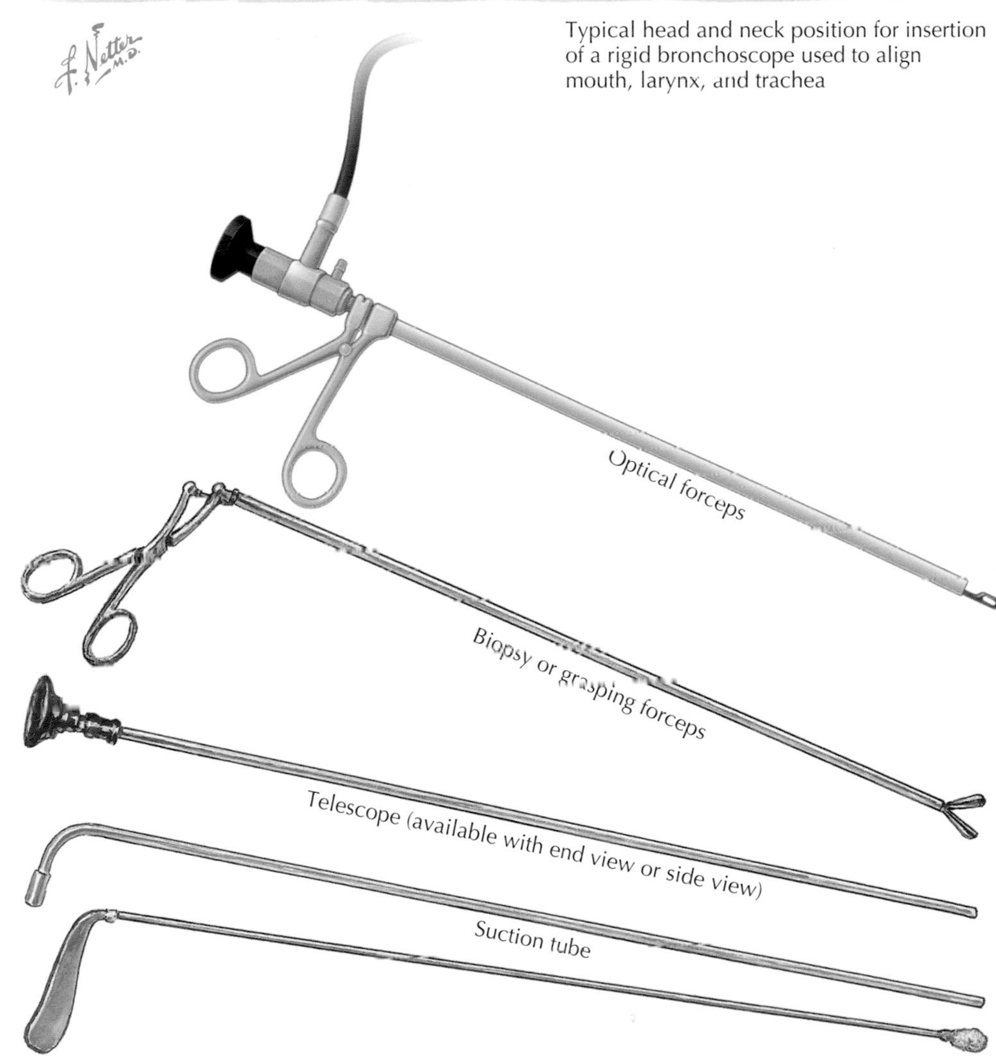

Endobronchial Ultrasonography

Endobronchial ultrasonography (EBUS) has likely had the largest impact on the field of bronchoscopy since the advent of the flexible bronchoscope in 1967. Use of ultrasonography in the airways evolved from endoscopic ultrasonography (EUS). Transducers needed to be made small enough to pass into the airway (or through the working channel of the bronchoscope) without obstructing the airway and to also achieve "coupling" to the airway wall because air is a potent reflector of ultrasound waves.

The first studies investigating EBUS were with a 20-MHz radial probe transducer. This relatively high-frequency probe allows excellent visualization of the layers of the airway wall and has been shown to be more sensitive than chest computed tomography scanning for determining airway invasion versus compression by tumor. Radial-probe EBUS also significantly increased the yield of transbronchial needle aspiration (TBNA). Unfortunately, performing radial-probe EBUS-TBNA is not a real-time sampling technique. The EBUS probe is inserted through the working channel of the bronchoscope, the target lymph nodes are identified, the EBUS probe is withdrawn, and TBNA is performed in the standard fashion.

Radial probe EBUS has also been used to identify peripheral nodules. The diagnostic yield for bronchoscopic sampling of peripheral nodules smaller than 3 cm in size is generally quite poor (25%-70%). Radial probe EBUS has been shown to increase the yield of peripheral nodule sampling, especially when combined with electromagnetic navigation bronchoscopy, up to as high as 90%. The sonographic characteristics of peripheral EBUS have also been shown to correlate with pathologic findings.

More recently, a 7.5-MHz convex-probe EBUS bronchoscope has been developed. The major benefit of this bronchoscope is that it allows real-time visualization of the needle entering the lymph node. Color power Doppler can also be used to identify vascular structures.

Convex-probe EBUS-TBNA has become a technique of choice for the staging of lung cancer. Whereas EBUS-TBNA can reach almost all of the lymph node stations, other procedures such as mediastinoscopy and EUS fine-needle aspiration are more limited. The performance characteristics (sensitivity, specificity, positive and negative predictive values) are nearly equivalent for more invasive procedures such as mediastinoscopy. In many centers, EBUS-TBNA has replaced mediastinoscopy as the initial procedure for the evaluation of mediastinal and hilar lymphadenopathy. It is important to understand, however, that a nondiagnostic EBUS-TBNA procedure is not equivalent to a negative result. Because the false-negative rate for EBUS-TBNA can be as high as 14%, *all* nondiagnostic results from EBUS-TBNA require either appropriate surgical sampling or clinical follow-up.

EBUS-TBNA has also been shown to be extremely useful for the diagnosis of lymphoma and sarcoidosis.

There is a definite skill set that one needs to acquire before performing EBUS-TBNA. A thorough understanding of extrabronchial anatomy, including the location of the various lymph node stations and blood vessels as well their relationship to each other and endobronchial anatomy is essential. One also needs to appreciate the technical differences of the bronchoscope itself. Unlike standard bronchoscopes that have a zero-degree view (i.e., looking straight ahead), the convex-probe EBUS bronchoscope has a 30-degree oblique view. This prevents visualization of the ultrasound probe; however, one needs to appreciate its presence so as to avoid injury to the vocal cords and distal airways. The needle system is also novel, and it is important to review its use with support staff before performing the procedure on a patient. The operator also needs to understand the "knobology" of the ultrasound processor and be able to adjust the depth, contrast, and gain at a minimum.

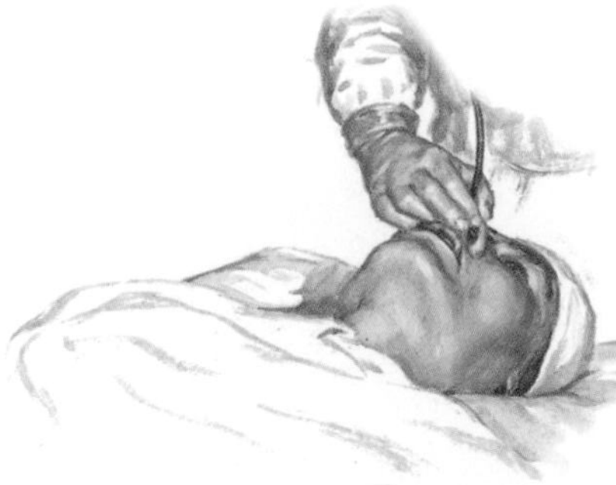

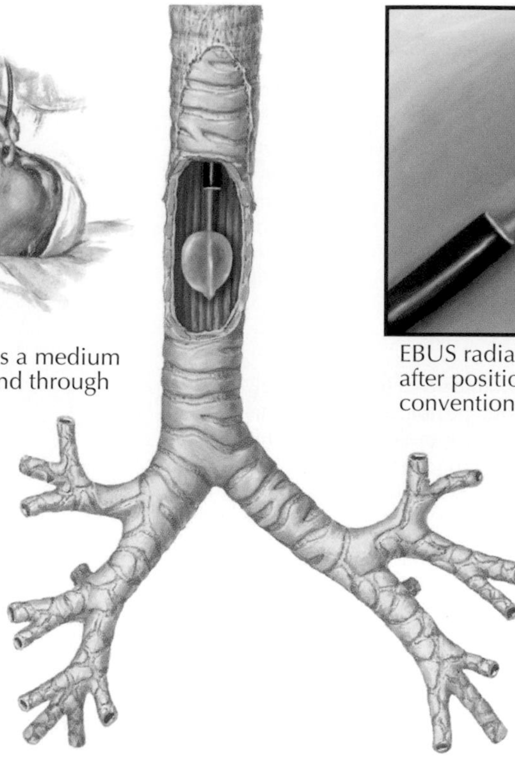

Fluid-filled balloon provides a medium for transmission of ultrasound through to the airway wall

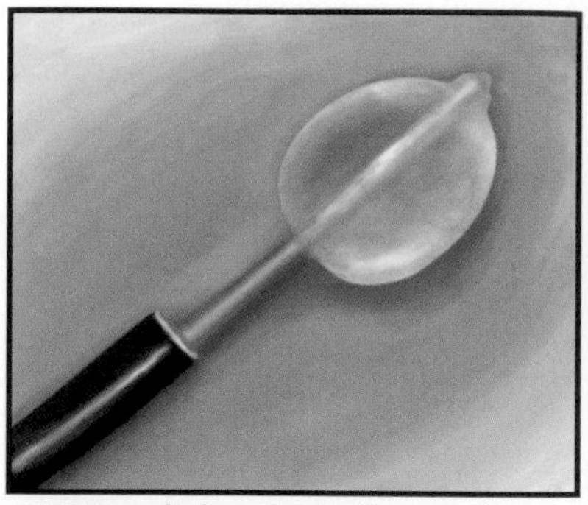

EBUS radial probe balloon inflated after positioning beyond tip of conventional bronchoscope

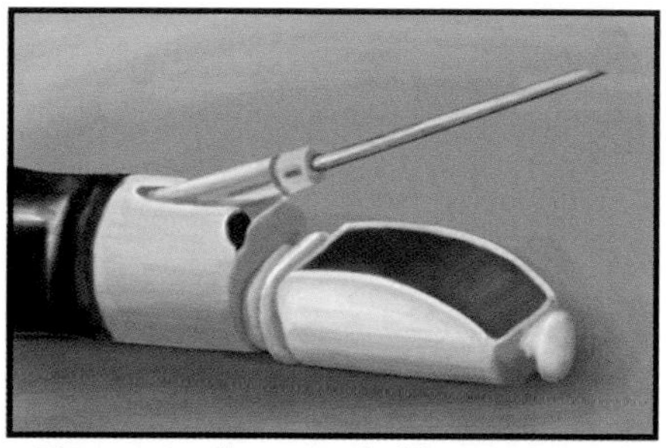

Biopsy needle extended beyond tip of EBUS convex probe bronchoscope

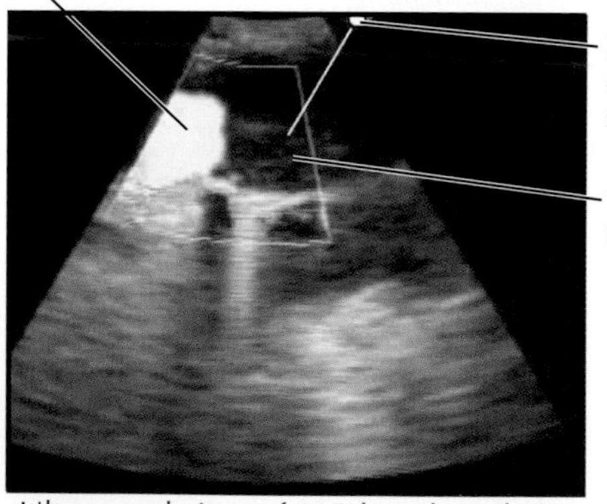

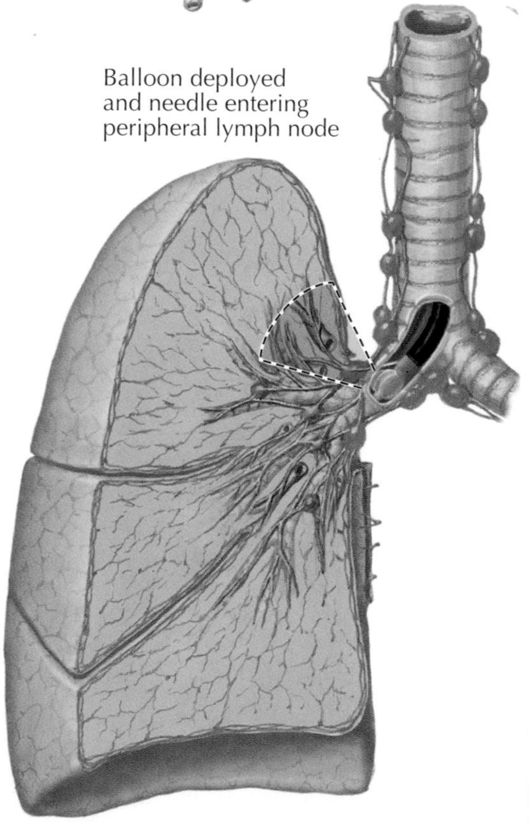

Balloon deployed and needle entering peripheral lymph node

Color power Doppler of right superior pulmonary artery

Needle entrance site

11R lymph node

Ultrasound view of 11R lymph node in relation to right superior pulmonary artery

MEDIASTINOTOMY AND MEDIASTINOSCOPY

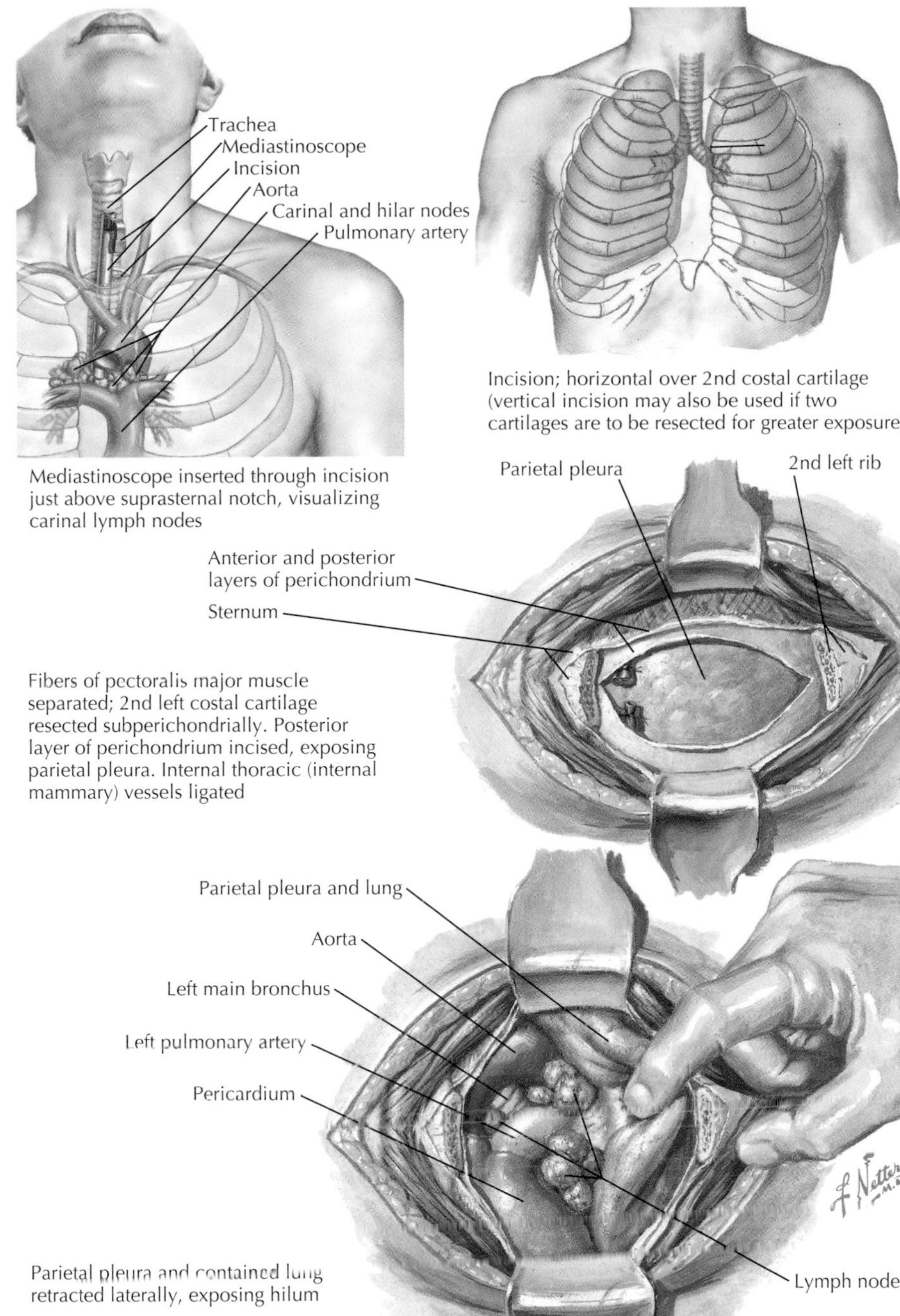

Mediastinoscope inserted through incision just above suprasternal notch, visualizing carinal lymph nodes

Incision; horizontal over 2nd costal cartilage (vertical incision may also be used if two cartilages are to be resected for greater exposure)

Fibers of pectoralis major muscle separated; 2nd left costal cartilage resected subperichondrially. Posterior layer of perichondrium incised, exposing parietal pleura. Internal thoracic (internal mammary) vessels ligated

Parietal pleura and contained lung retracted laterally, exposing hilum

Complete surgical resection is the key curative therapy for early-stage bronchogenic carcinoma. To be effective, resection must be performed under appropriate circumstances; not only must the patient be able to tolerate the required operation but the cancer must also be sufficiently well localized for complete surgical removal. Radical resection in the face of metastases to mediastinal nodes is rarely curative. For this reason, mediastinal nodal staging is essential. Cervical mediastinoscopy and left anterior mediastinotomy remain the gold standard for sampling mediastinal lymph nodes. These procedures may also aid in the diagnosis of lymphoma, sarcoidosis, and other diseases affecting the mediastinum.

STAGING IN THE MANAGEMENT OF LUNG CARCINOMA

For modern thoracic specialists, the selection of patients for lung cancer operations involves a definition and an assessment of certain discriminating factors related to the primary tumor and its lymphatic and hematogenous metastases. In recent years, an effective and meaningful internationally vetted system for staging lung cancer has evolved (see Plate 4-49). Enlarged or hypermetabolic lymph nodes on computed tomography or positron emission tomography scan, respectively, are at risk of harboring metastatic cancer and require acquisition of tissue for definitive pathologic staging.

SURGICAL EVALUATION OF THE REGIONAL LYMPHATIC SYSTEM

Of particular interest is the surgical investigation of the lymphatic drainage of the lung (see Plates 1-30 and 1-31) as it relates to data collection for clinical staging before a pulmonary resection. The lymphatic drainage system provides distinct predictable routes or pathways for the spread of malignancies from each lobe of the lung to the hilum and up the mediastinum to the base of the neck. Usually performed under general anesthesia, a *mediastinoscopy* involves a horizontal suprasternal low cervical skin incision to expose the lower cervical part of the trachea. Through this, central cervical and medially located supraclavicular lymph nodes can be visualized and biopsies performed. The surgeon may also expose and digitally dissect the pretracheal space. Much information can be gleaned through initial palpation of the developed tract. Usually, the presence and location of enlarged lymph nodes, as well as the size, fixation, and relationships to neighboring structures, can best be identified by this means. After the pretracheal tract has been fully developed by preliminary digital exploration, the mediastinoscope is introduced to facilitate direct visualization and biopsy of nodal tissue. Although mediastinoscopy involves some risk of bleeding, information obtained may obviate the need for thoracotomy when resection for potential cure is clearly not feasible.

Debate continues regarding the indications for mediastinoscopy and how to interpret and use the information gained. Most physicians would agree that patients with clearly resectable clinical stage I cancers are unlikely to benefit from the examination. Almost all would concur that contralateral mediastinal lymph node metastases or any metastasis fixed to adjacent structures is not resectable. Less certain is the interpretation of ipsilateral, freely movable, intracapsular nodal metastases that might be included in a radical mediastinal lymph node dissection at the time of thoracotomy and lung resection. Still, current knowledge clearly defines mediastinal lymph nodal metastasis as stage III disease, and despite radical resection, fewer than 10% of patients will experience long-term survival. Most thoracic oncologists view stage III disease as a systemic process requiring combined modality therapy, usually not surgery, to improve survival.

Mediastinoscopy should not be performed in the presence of clinically palpable cervical or scalene lymphadenopathy. Direct surgical biopsy of these nodes can be accomplished at minimal risk, and if malignancy is present, inoperability is confirmed. Biopsy of the scalene nodes should not be carried out on patients with bronchogenic carcinoma when the nodes are not palpable. Furthermore, for a left upper lobe neoplasm, cervical mediastinoscopy is less often definitive in excluding N2 disease and establishing operability than is the case for left lower lobe and right-sided tumors.

For left upper lobe lesions, the left anterior extrapleural *mediastinotomy* developed by Chamberlain has proved most helpful. Ordinarily, anterior mediastinotomy is accomplished through a horizontal incision over the second anterior costal cartilage. The surgeon exposes the mediastinal lymph nodes overlying the left pulmonary artery, phrenic nerve, and subaortic space and can readily perform a biopsy.

Recently, alternative means of sampling mediastinal lymph nodes have been developed. These include video-assisted mediastinoscopic lymphadenectomy (VAMLA) and endobronchial ultrasonography with transbronchial needle aspiration (EBUS-TBNA). VAMLA allows for complete resection and removal of pertinent lymph node stations. Although EBUS-TBNA has been gaining popularity, it has not been found to be as efficacious as mediastinoscopy in routine mediastinal staging.

SECTION 4

DISEASES AND PATHOLOGY

CONGENITAL DEFORMITIES OF THE THORACIC CAGE

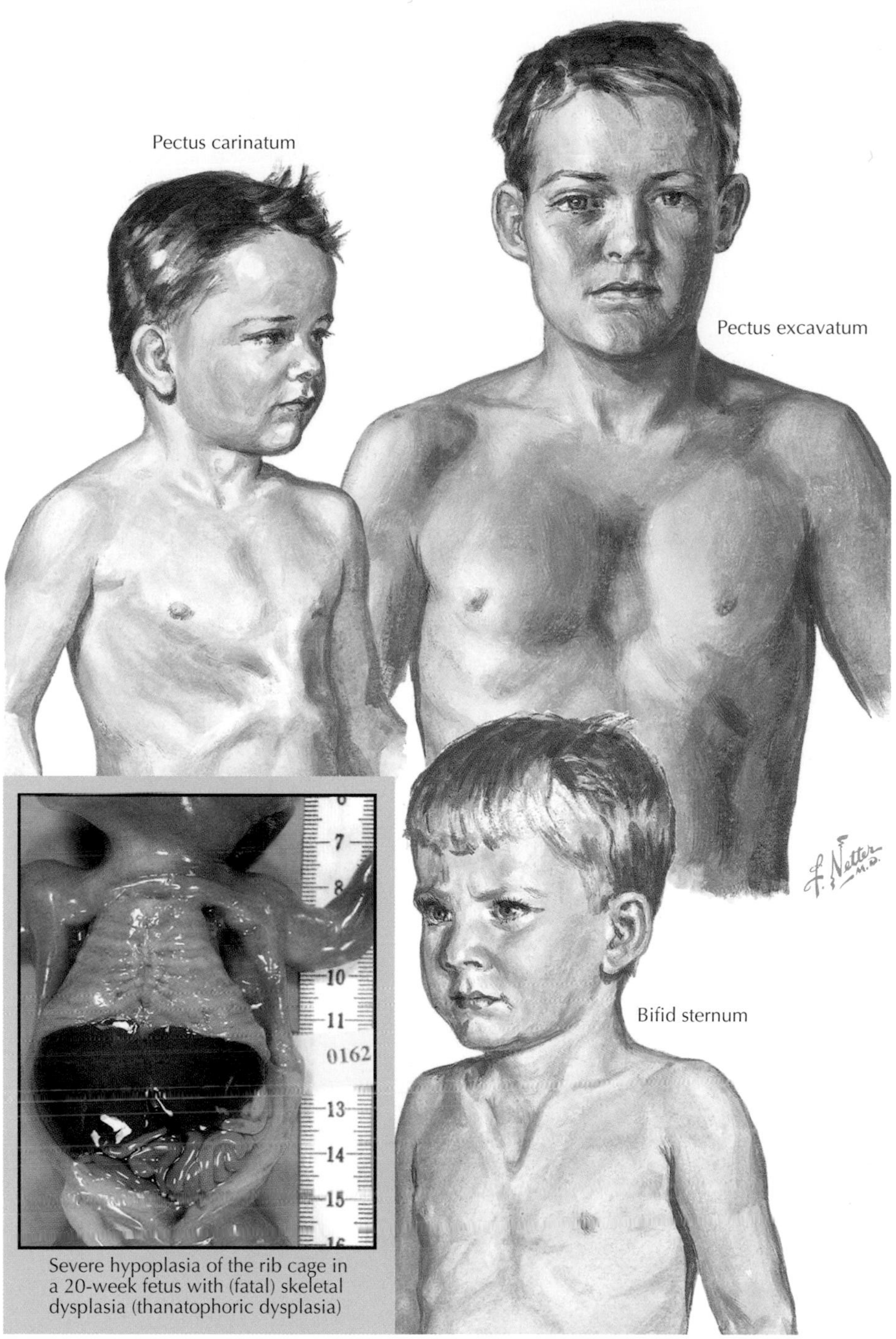

PECTUS EXCAVATUM

Pectus excavatum is also called funnel chest, chonechondrosternon, or trichterbrust. It is a deformity of the anterior chest wall characterized by depression of the lower sternum and adjacent cartilages. The lowest point of the depression is at the junction of the xiphoid process and the body of the sternum. The trait is inherited and may coexist with other musculoskeletal malformations such as clubfoot, syndactyly, and Klippel-Feil syndrome. The cause of funnel chest remains obscure. A short central tendon and muscular imbalance of the diaphragm have been blamed. Most current writers attribute the deformity to unbalanced growth in the costochondral regions.

Symptoms are very uncommon. However, a child with an obvious deformity may experience unfortunate psychological effects. Funnel chest is usually associated with postural disorders such as forward displacement of the neck and shoulders, upper thoracic kyphosis, and a protuberant abdomen. Functional heart murmurs and benign cardiac arrhythmias are frequently seen in these individuals, and the electrocardiogram may show right-axis deviation because of the displacement of the heart. In older patients, there may be an appreciable incidence of chronic bronchitis and bronchiectasis.

Depression of the sternum begins typically at the junction of the manubrium and the gladiolus. The xiphoid process may be bifid, twisted, or displaced to one side. Costal cartilages are angulated internally, beginning with the second or third and extending caudally to involve the remainder. In general, the defect tends to be symmetric, but one side may be more depressed than the other so that the sternum deviates from the middle line. An estimate of the cavitary volume may be obtained by filling the depression with water while the patient lies supine. Standard radiographic films reveal that the heart is displaced toward the left side, and lateral films show the displacement of the body of the sternum posteriorly.

In patients who are symptomatic or who show a significant progression of pectus excavatum, the deformity should be corrected surgically. Because most of the operations are carried out with a cosmetic end in mind, the results are best when surgery is performed between 3 and 7 years of age. Surgical correction consists of excision of the hypertrophied costal cartilages on both sides; osteotomy of the sternum at the junction of the manubrium and body; and then internal fixation by pins or rods, which are removed later. Fixation by a metal strut or wire is required in older patients to prevent recurrence of the deformity, which, in some degree, may occur despite initial overcorrection.

PECTUS CARINATUM

Also known as pigeon breast, chicken breast, or keel breast, this is a protrusion deformity of the anterior chest wall that is unrelated to pectus excavatum and occurs about one-tenth as often. Two principal types are recognized: (1) chondromanubrial, in which the protuberance is maximal at the xiphoid and the gladiolus is directed posteriorly so that a secondary saucerization is evident, and (2) chondrogladiolar, in which the greatest prominence is at or near the gladiolus. The pathogenesis is no better understood than that of pectus excavatum, but the theory of unbalanced or excessive growth of the cartilages makes sense. Although functional cardiac and respiratory difficulties have been observed, the chief reason for surgical correction is cosmetic. If the deformity is minor, no treatment is required. When operation is necessary, the procedure should be tailored to the particular deformity, taking into account the full life circumstances of the patient. When the deformity causes embarrassment, the surgical procedure is aimed at achieving psychological as well as physiologic improvement.

Pectus carinatum

Pectus excavatum

Bifid sternum

Severe hypoplasia of the rib cage in a 20-week fetus with (fatal) skeletal dysplasia (thanatophoric dysplasia)

BIFID STERNUM

Failure of fusion of the sternal bands may occur, creating a defect of the anterior chest wall. Separation of the sternum may be complete or incomplete and may be associated with an ectopia cordis. When the defect is incomplete, surgical correction of the abnormality may be accomplished. If the repair cannot be effected by primary approximation of the sternal segments, a prosthesis or a cartilage autograft may be used.

Other deformities of the chest wall occasionally seen include cervical ribs (with or without compression of the brachial plexus and artery), partial absence of ribs, supernumerary ribs, and thoracic-pelvic-phalangeal dystrophy.

SKELETAL DISORDERS PRESENTING WITH NEONATAL RESPIRATORY DISTRESS

Respiratory distress may result from abnormal lung growth caused by restriction by limited rib growth such as from osteochondrodysplasias (e.g., asphyxiating dystrophy, thanatrophic dwarfism, upper airway obstruction [diastrophic dysplasia]) or abnormal bone, cartilage, or collagen development, leading to a small or abnormal thoracic cage (hypophosphatasia, achondrogenesis, osteogenesis imperfecta).

Kyphoscoliosis

Kyphoscoliosis has long been recognized as a cause of cardiorespiratory failure. Only in recent years, however, has the combination of clinical picture, physiologic measurements, and anatomic observations at autopsy clarified the natural history of the cardiorespiratory disorder.

Unless there is independent lung disease, such as bronchitis or emphysema, only patients with severe spinal deformities are candidates for cardiorespiratory failure. Subjects with mild deformities are consistently asymptomatic. In contrast, those with severe degrees of deformity, particularly if considerable dwarfing has occurred, are often restricted in their activities by dyspnea on exertion. They are most prone to cardiorespiratory failure if an upper respiratory infection should supervene. From the point of view of disability and the likelihood of cardiorespiratory failure, the nature of the deformity (i.e., kyphosis, scoliosis, or both) is unimportant when compared with the severity of the deformity and dwarfing.

One approach to classifying individuals with kyphoscoliosis is on the basis of lung volumes. The more normal the total lung capacity, vital capacity, and tidal volume, the more the subject tends to remain asymptomatic. In those with severe reduction in lung volumes, the stage is set for cor pulmonale.

Estimates of the work of breathing, using pressure-volume loops, show an inordinate work load (and energy expenditure) attributable to the severe limitation of distensibility of the chest wall, which produces markedly reduced compliance. As a consequence of the high cost of breathing, the individual adopts a pattern of rapid, shallow breathing. Although this pattern is economical in terms of the work and energy required, it sacrifices alveolar ventilation for the sake of dead-space ventilation. The resultant alveolar hypoventilation brings about arterial hypoxemia, hypercapnia, and respiratory acidosis by hyperventilating the conducting airways and hypoventilating the alveoli. Thus, whereas individuals with asymptomatic kyphoscoliosis consistently manifest normal arterial blood gases, those with severe kyphoscoliosis often have cyanosis and show not only arterial hypoxemia but also hypercapnia. Between these two extremes are patients who remain breathless on exertion and whose arterial blood gases hover at the brink of important hypoxemia and hypercapnia. They are easily toppled into a state of cardiorespiratory failure by a bout of bronchitis or pneumonia.

In asymptomatic persons, the pulmonary arterial pressure is normal at rest and increases to clinically insignificant levels during exercise. In contrast, the pulmonary arterial pressure in those with severe kyphoscoliosis not only may be high at rest but also increases precipitously during modest exercise. The basis for this pulmonary hypertension is generally twofold: (1) a restricted pulmonary vascular bed caused by the compressing and distorting effects of the deformity on the lungs and on the pulmonary vasculature and (2) the pulmonary pressor effects of hypoxia. These two effects are most marked during exercise because of the increase in pulmonary blood flow into the restricted vascular bed and the pulmonary vasoconstriction elicited by the exercise-induced hypoxemia. The patients show enlargement of the right ventricle at autopsy. During an upper respiratory infection, the pulmonary pressor effects of the arterial hypoxemia may be sufficiently severe to increase pulmonary arterial pressure to very high levels to precipitate right ventricular failure.

In patients in whom chronic alveolar hypoventilation has caused sustained pulmonary hypertension, hypercapnia consistently accompanies arterial hypoxemia. Hypercapnia contributes to pulmonary hypertension by way of the respiratory acidosis that it causes because acidosis acts synergistically with hypoxia in causing pulmonary vasoconstriction. However, hypercapnia exerts its predominant effects on the central nervous system rather than on the heart or circulation. In individuals with kyphoscoliosis who have chronic hypercapnia, there is generally no clinical manifestation of the hypercapnia per se. Ventilatory response to inhaled carbon

Pathology of Kyphoscoliosis

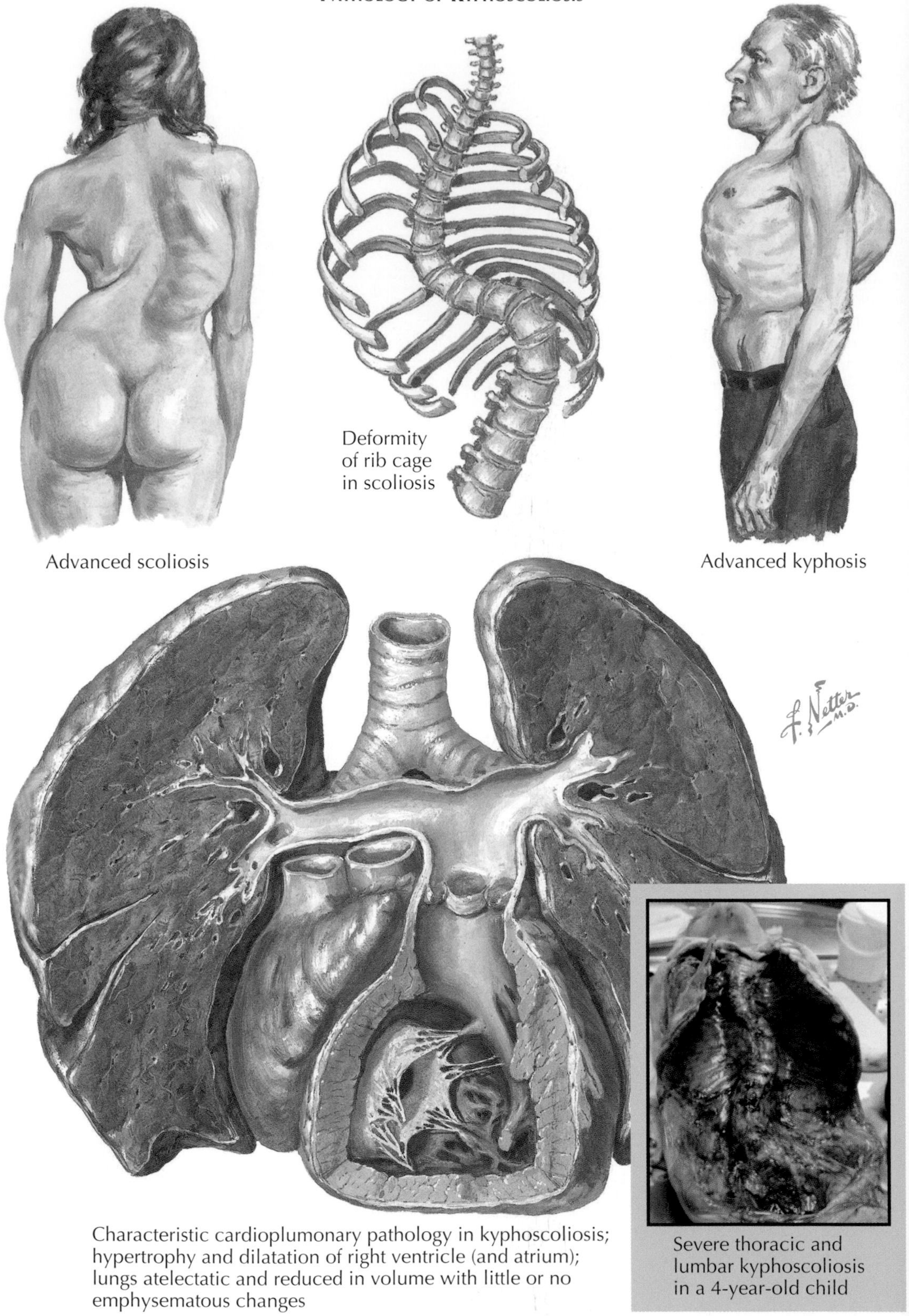

Advanced scoliosis

Deformity of rib cage in scoliosis

Advanced kyphosis

Characteristic cardioplumonary pathology in kyphoscoliosis; hypertrophy and dilatation of right ventricle (and atrium); lungs atelectatic and reduced in volume with little or no emphysematous changes

Severe thoracic and lumbar kyphoscoliosis in a 4-year-old child

KYPHOSCOLIOSIS *(Continued)*

dioxide is depressed compared with that of asymptomatic or individuals with kyphoscoliosis who do not have hypercapnia, reflecting impaired responsiveness to the major chemical stimulus to breathing. As a corollary, greater reliance is placed on the hypoxic drive via the peripheral chemoreceptors. But if a person with kyphoscoliosis develops acute hypercapnia during an upper respiratory infection or exaggerates the preexisting degree of hypercapnia, he or she may manifest personality changes, become unresponsive to conventional stimuli, and lapse into a coma. Accompanying these clinical disorders are cerebral vasodilation, cerebral edema, and an increase in cerebrospinal fluid pressure. The increase in intracranial pressure may be so large as to cause choking of the optic discs, simulating a brain tumor.

All of the disturbances in uncomplicated kyphoscoliosis are greatly exaggerated by intrinsic lung disease. Therefore, smoking and its attendant bronchitis increase the risk of respiratory insufficiency in individuals with kyphoscoliosis. Pneumonia may be disastrous.

From these observations, it is possible to reconstruct the pathogenesis of alveolar hypoventilation and cor pulmonale in individuals with kyphoscoliosis. The sequence begins with severe thoracic deformity, reducing the compliance of the thoracic cage and lung expansion. The work and energy cost of breathing are thus greatly increased. To minimize this work, the patient unconsciously adopts a pattern of rapid, shallow breathing, which results in chronic alveolar hypoventilation. Not only do the small, encased lungs contribute to the increased work of breathing, but they also limit the capacity and distensibility of the pulmonary vascular bed. Pulmonary arterial hypertension is caused by a disproportion between the level of pulmonary blood flow—which is normal for the subject's metabolism—and the restricted vascular bed. After arterial hypoxemia is corrected, polycythemia, hypervolemia, and an increase in cardiac output help to sustain the pulmonary hypertension. The end result of the chronic pulmonary hypertension is enlargement of the right ventricle (cor pulmonale). In this situation, any additional mechanism for pulmonary hypertension, particularly an upper respiratory infection, may precipitate heart failure.

Hypercapnia goes hand in hand with arterial hypoxemia. This is generally well tolerated unless alveolar hypoventilation is acutely intensified, so that carbon dioxide elimination is further impaired. The acute increase in arterial P_{CO_2} may evoke serious derangements in the central nervous system as well as contribute to the pulmonary hypertension and right ventricular failure.

Treatment of cardiorespiratory failure is directed toward reversing the pathogenetic sequence. In this emergency, generally precipitated by an upper respiratory infection, assisted ventilation may be required in conjunction with slightly enriched oxygen mixtures (≤25%-40%) to achieve tolerable levels of blood gases. The ventilatory insensitivity of the chronically hypercapnic patient to an increase in arterial P_{CO_2}, as well as his or her reliance on hypoxic stimulation of the peripheral chemoreceptors for an important part of the ventilatory drive, imposes a need for caution against using excessively high oxygen mixtures. Respiratory depressants are also hazardous because they may cause breathing to stop completely. Antibiotics and supportive measures usually suffice to tide the patient over the crisis brought on by acute respiratory infection. The goal of treatment is to restore the patient to the clinical state that existed before the acute episode. An individual with kyphoscoliosis who was dyspneic on exertion before an acute episode of cardiorespiratory failure can be expected to return to that condition after the crisis has passed. For many patients who have severe kyphoscoliosis, modest arterial hypoxemia and slight hypercapnia may remain. However, it is remarkable how successful adequate therapy can be in restoring the patient to the precrisis state of health.

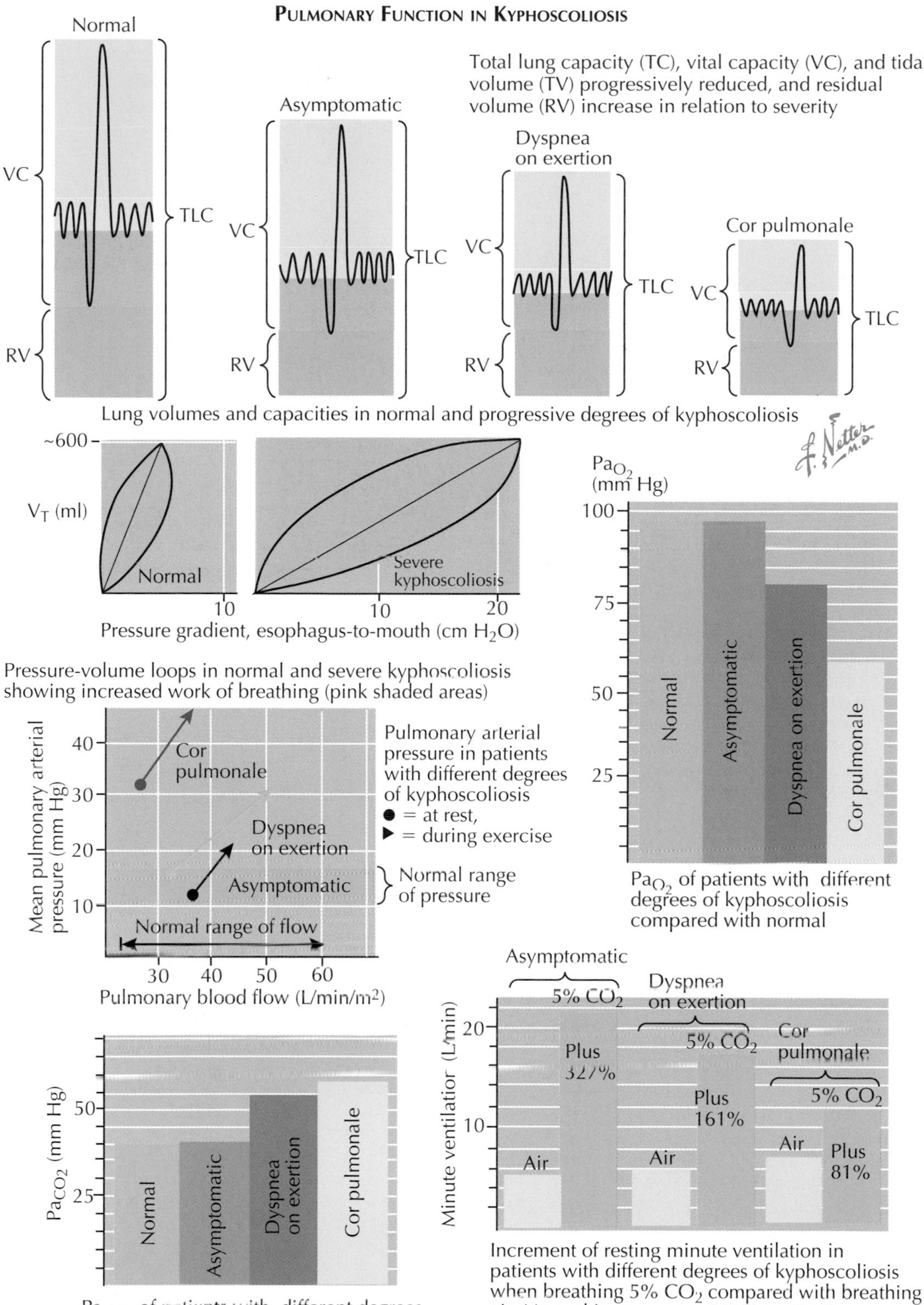

CONGENITAL DIAPHRAGMATIC HERNIA

Left-sided diaphragmatic hernia (Bochdalek) at 24 weeks of gestation

Sites of herniation

Foramen of Morgagni

Esophageal hiatus

A large part or all of diaphragm may be congenitally absent

Original pleuroperitoneal canal (foramen of Bochdalek—the most common site)

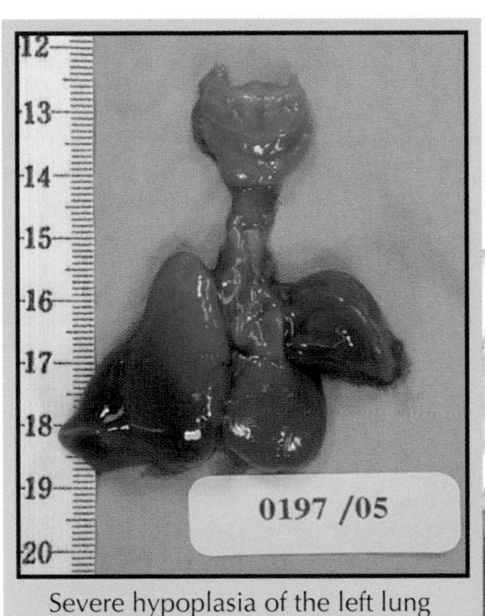

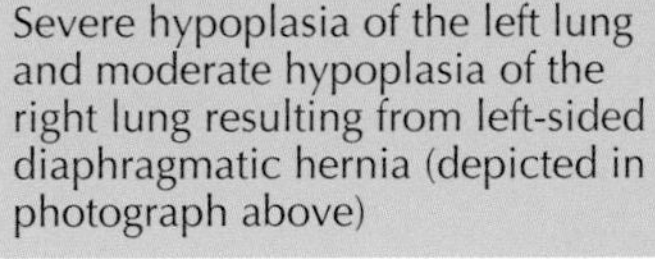

Severe hypoplasia of the left lung and moderate hypoplasia of the right lung resulting from left-sided diaphragmatic hernia (depicted in photograph above)

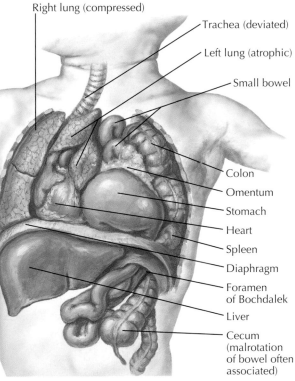

Right lung (compressed)

Trachea (deviated)

Left lung (atrophic)

Small bowel

Colon

Omentum

Stomach

Heart

Spleen

Diaphragm

Foramen of Bochdalek

Liver

Cecum (malrotation of bowel often associated)

F. Netter M.D.

The diaphragm is a septum that separates the thoracic from the abdominal cavity. A domelike structure, it consists of muscular and tendinous elements having their origin in costal, sternal, and lumbar sources. The sternal portions are two flat bands that arise from the posterior aspect of the body of the sternum. Costal elements arise from the lowest six ribs and interdigitate with the transversus abdominalis muscles. The lumbar portions arise from the lateral and medial lumbar costal arches.

True congenital diaphragmatic hernias (CDHs) resulting from defects in embryogenesis are through (1) the hiatus pleuroperitonealis (foramen of Bochdalek) without an enclosing sac, (2) the dome of the diaphragm, (3) the foramen of Morgagni, or (4) a defect caused by the absence of the left half of the diaphragm. The two more common types of CDHs are those through the foramen of Bochdalek and the foramen of Morgagni. Foramen of Bochdalek hernias constitute approximately 90% of diaphragmatic hernias in infants and young children; the left side is involved in 85% of cases, and 5% are bilateral. In left-sided cases, the stomach, portions of the small and large intestines, the spleen, and the upper pole of the kidney may herniate through the defect into the pleural cavity and ascend freely to the apex of the chest. On the involved side, lung growth is compromised, but there may be hypoplasia on the contralateral side because shifting of the mediastinum toward the uninvolved side causes some compression of that lung as well.

The timing of onset and severity of symptoms depend on the degree of pulmonary hypoplasia. In severe cases, the infant presents immediately after birth with severe respiratory distress and is difficult to resuscitate.

The presumptive diagnosis can be made from the occurrence of cyanosis and dyspnea soon after birth in infants in whom the cardiac impulse is abnormally sited. In addition, peristaltic sounds may be heard in the thorax, and at the same time, the abdomen is found to be soft and scaphoid in contour. Nowadays, most infants with CDH will have been diagnosed antenatally by routine ultrasonography in the second or third trimester. Postnatally, a standard chest radiograph will show a shift of the mediastinum and a space-occupying lesion on the affected side (e.g., bowel loops occupying the left hemithorax). The differential diagnosis includes other causes of neonatal respiratory distress such as eventration of the diaphragm, cystic adenomatoid malformation of the lung, mediastinal cystic teratomas, and loculated hydropneumothorax. Hernias that occur on the right side may be confused with segmental collapse or pleural effusion. However, the posterior location of the mass in the lateral projection and the shift of the heart are helpful findings. The diagnosis can be confirmed by ultrasonography, the position of the nasogastric tube, or a barium meal.

Infants who require resuscitation in the labor suite should be intubated; bag and mask resuscitation must be avoided to prevent gaseous distension of the herniated bowel and further respiratory embarrassment. A nasogastric tube attached to low suction should be inserted. Infants with CDH are at increased risk of pneumothorax, and this can affect either lung because they are both hypoplastic. It was previously assumed that infants with CDH required immediate postoperative repair in the hope that removal of the bowel from the thorax and closure of the diaphragmatic defect would lead to improvement in gas exchange through expansion of the lung. Studies have demonstrated that a period of perioperative stabilization reduces mortality and the need for extracorporeal membrane oxygenation. The survival of infants with CDH is approximately 60%, with mortality being caused by pulmonary hypoplasia, pulmonary hypertension, or both. Infants who had a CDH may experience problems at follow-up and reherniation, gastroesophageal reflux, lung function abnormalities, and exercise intolerance even as adolescents. Attempts to repair the hernia in utero have not been promising. Further antenatal interventions have been based on the discovery that obstructing the normal egress of fetal lung fluid enlarges the lungs, reduces the herniated viscera, and accelerates lung growth in experimental models. Temporary occlusion of the trachea has been achieved by external clips and more recently by internal balloon plugs. Appropriately designed randomized trials are required to determine whether such interventions improve long-term outcome.

Congenital defects in the anterior parasternal region (Laney space) may result in the formation of a foramen of Morgagni hernia. These hernias are usually right sided, and most commonly involve the liver and omentum. The hernia must be differentiated from a pericardial cyst. They may be seen as the part of the pentalogy of Cantrell. Anterior hernias are usually asymptomatic in the neonatal period, but when diagnosed coincidentally on a chest radiograph, they should be repaired because strangulation of the abdominal organs may occur.

Tracheoesophageal Fistulas and Tracheal Anomalies

Tracheoesophageal fistula (TOF) and esophageal atresia rarely occur as separate entities, but they are often seen in various combinations: esophageal atresia with upper fistula, lower fistula, and double fistulas. Approximately 10% of infants with esophageal atresia do not have a fistula, but there is a long gap between the esophageal segments. An isolated tracheoesophageal fistula (H or N fistula) can occur without an esophageal atresia. The cause of these congenital anomalies is not well understood. Esophageal atresia is usually sporadic and rarely familial.

Maternal polyhydramnios and a small or absent fetal stomach bubble on antenatal ultrasonography suggest the possibility of esophageal atresia antenatally. Postnatally, the diagnosis can be suspected in a newborn infant who has excessive mucus and cannot handle his or her secretions adequately. Suction provides temporary relief, but the secretions continue to accumulate and overflow, resulting in aspiration and respiratory distress. Feeds are also regurgitated and aspirated. The TOF provides a low-resistance pathway for respiratory gases and gastric distension, and subsequent rupture may further compromise ventilation.

Formerly, the diagnosis was made by using a contrast study with barium or Gastrografin (meglumine diatrizoate); however, there is the danger of aspirating these materials into the lungs. The diagnosis can readily be made by passing a fairly large radiopaque plastic catheter through the nose or mouth into the pouch. When the catheter cannot be advanced into the stomach, the catheter should then be taped in place and put on constant gentle suction. This keeps the pouch free of saliva and minimizes the chances of aspiration pneumonitis. On the chest radiograph, it will be noted that the tip of the catheter is usually opposite T2-T3. If the surgeon prefers a contrast study, no more than 0.5 mL of contrast material should be introduced through the catheter, with the child in the upright position. Radiography will show the typical esophageal obstruction, and the contrast material should then be immediately aspirated.

Initial management is aimed at keeping the airway free of secretions using a 10-Fr double lumen Replogle tube in the proximal pouch on continuous low pressure suction. The ideal surgical procedure consists of disruption of the fistula and an end-to-end anastomosis of the esophagus. If there is a long gap between the esophageal segments, surgery is delayed to allow the pouches to elongate and hypertrophy over a period of up to 3 months. During this time, the infant is fed through a gastrostomy, and the upper pouch is kept clear of secretions.

A. Tracheoesophageal fistula

Most common form (90% to 95%) of tracheoesophageal fistula. Upper segment of esophagus ending in blind pouch; lower segment originating from trachea just above bifurcation. The two segments may be connected by a solid cord

B. Variations of tracheoesophageal fistula and rare anomalies of trachea

Upper segment of esophagus ending in trachea; lower segment of variable length

C. Double fistula

D. Fistula without esophageal atresia

E. Esophageal atresia without fistula

F. Aplasia of trachea (lethal)

Web

Hourglass

G. Stricture of trachea

Inspiration

Expiration

H. Absence of cartilage

I. Deformity of cartilage

To upper lobes

To lower lobes

Left bronchus

Right bronchus

J. Abnormalities of bifurcation

Anomalies and Strictures of the Trachea

Tracheal anomalies are very rare. With stricture of the trachea, there is local obstruction of the passage of air. In the absence of cartilage, the trachea can collapse and therefore obstruct on expiration. With deformity of cartilage, there is obstruction on inspiration and expiration. When abnormal bifurcations are present, the right upper or left upper lobe bronchi (or both) arise independently from the trachea.

Clinically, stenosis may be localized or diffuse. The localized form is caused by a web of the respiratory mucosa or by excessive growth of tracheal cartilage. The diffuse form is caused by a congenital absence of elastic fibrous tissue between the cartilage and its rings in the trachea or by an absence of cartilage. Clinically, obstruction of the trachea causes chronic dyspnea; cyanosis, especially on exercise; and repeated attacks of respiratory tract infection. The diagnosis is established by bronchoscopy and by radiography.

For localized obstruction, surgery is advisable, either dilatation or excision with end-to-end anastomosis. Resection and anastomosis of the trachea can be carried out, including up to six tracheal rings. For generalized stenosis, only supportive therapy is available.

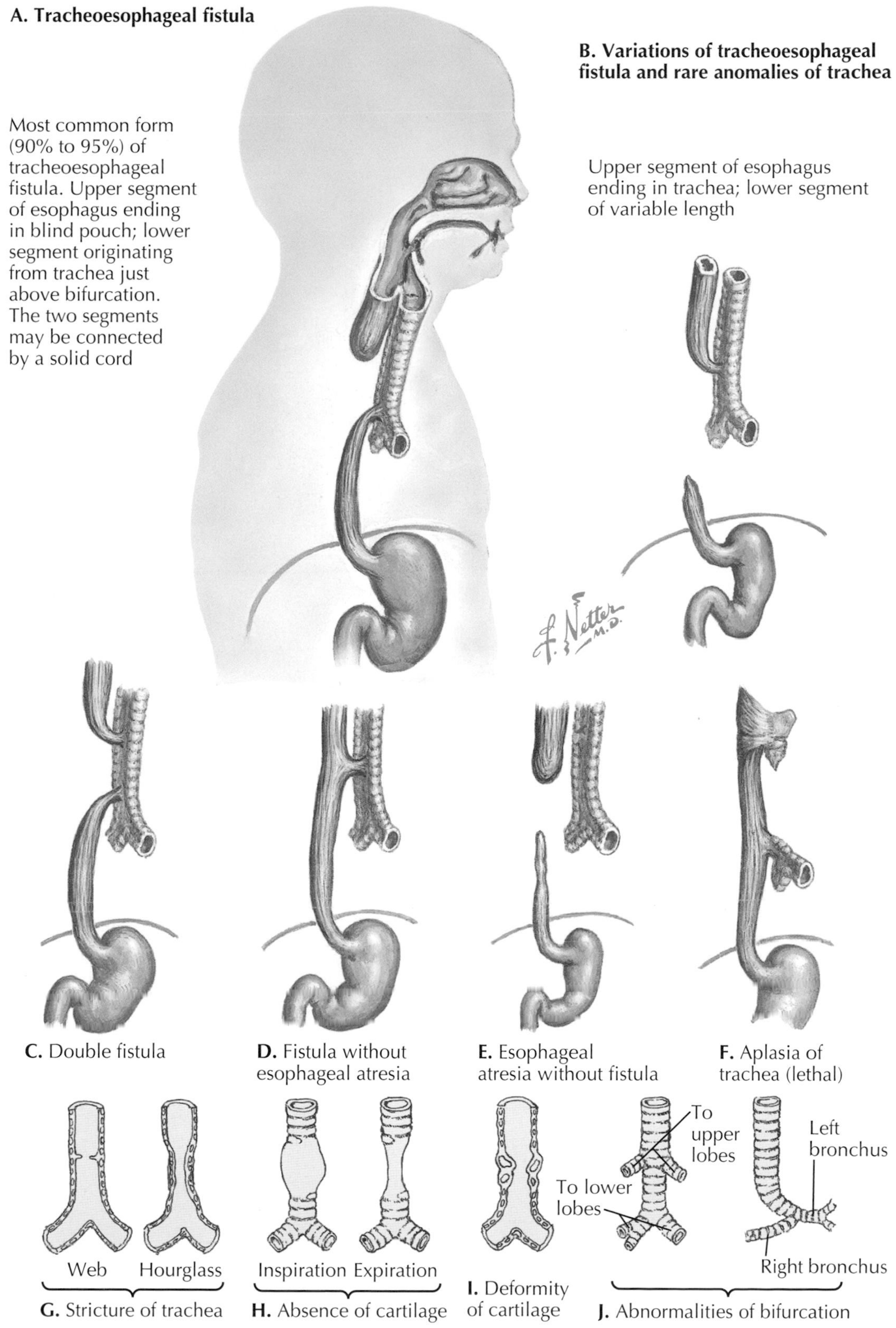

Pulmonary Agenesis, Aplasia, and Hypoplasia

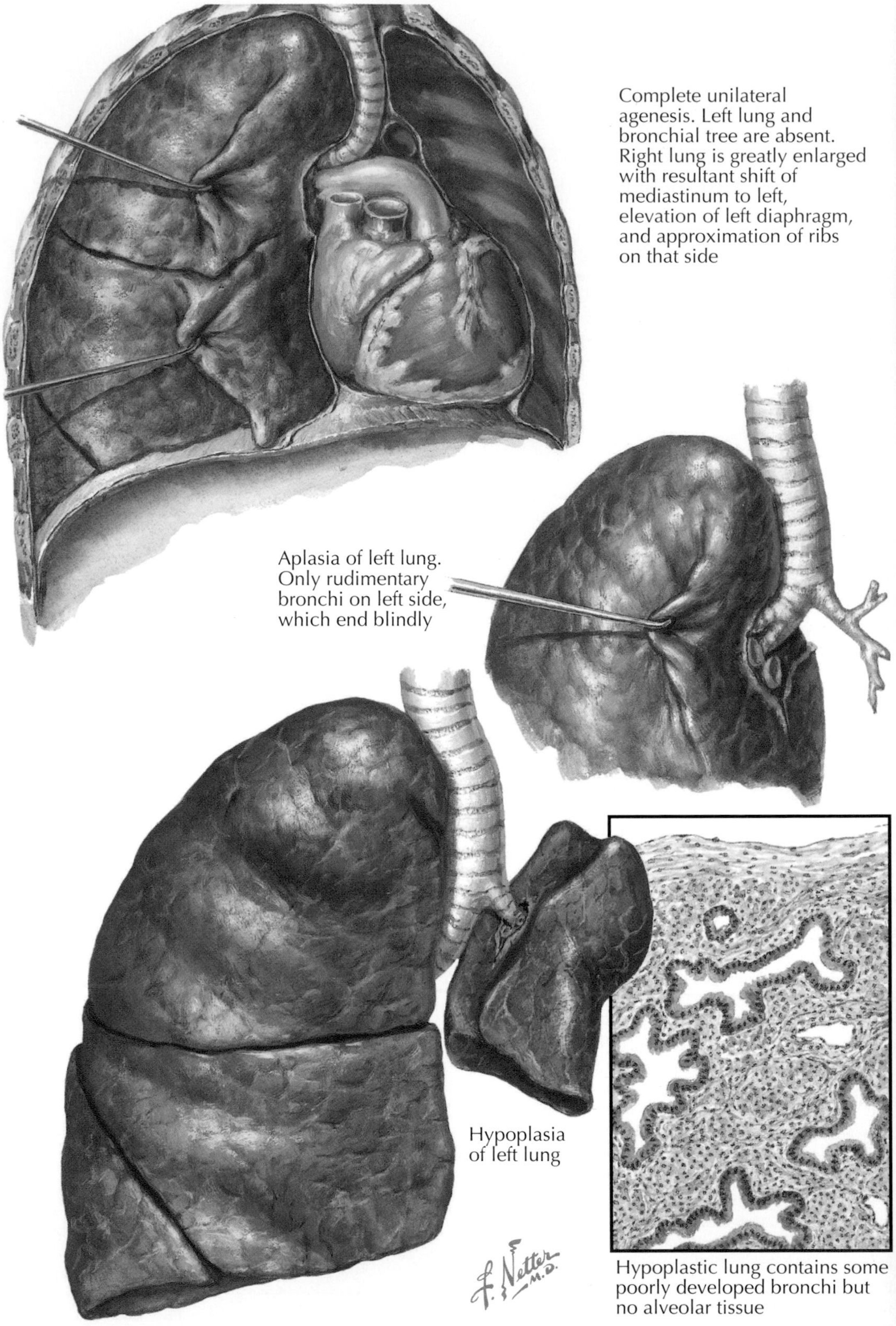

Three different degrees of arrested development of the lungs may occur: (1) *agenesis*, in which there is a complete absence of one lung or both lungs and no trace of bronchial or vascular supply or parenchymal tissue; (2) *aplasia*, in which there is a suppression of all but a rudimentary bronchus ending in a blind pouch and there are no pulmonary vessels and no parenchyma; and (3) *hypoplasia*, in which there is incomplete development of the lung, which is smaller in weight and volume, and there is a reduced number of airways branches, alveoli, arteries, and veins.

The incidence of pulmonary agenesis is low. There is no clear-cut gender predominance; and it does not occur more frequently on one side or the other. Experimental work in rat fetuses has shown that mothers deprived of vitamin A have a greater incidence of pulmonary agenesis in their offspring; however, a similar degree of malnutrition of this type is unlikely to occur in humans. Although absence of the lung is often associated with other congenital defects that terminate life in infancy, many patients with a single lung have lived well into adult life. Sixty percent of patients with agenesis of the lung are found to have other congenital anomalies. The most frequently associated anomalies are patent ductus arteriosus, tetralogy of Fallot, anomalies of the great vessels, and bronchogenic cysts. One normal lung can sustain life because the single lung probably hypertrophies. The condition alone may be asymptomatic, but pulmonary function can more easily be compromised by pneumonia, foreign body, or other insults if there is only one functional lung present. The mortality rate of patients with an absent right lung is 75%, but 25% if the left lung is absent. The difference in mortality rate is caused by the higher frequency of cardiac abnormalities with an absent right lung.

There are many causes of secondary lung hypoplasia, including a reduction in amniotic fluid volume, reduction in intrathoracic space, reduction in fetal breathing movements (neurologic abnormalities or neuromuscular disorders), genetic disorders (trisomy 18 or 21), malnutrition (vitamin A deficiency), maternal smoking, and medications such as glucocorticoid administration.

The finding in cases of agenesis, aplasia, or whole-lung hypoplasia is, as might be expected, total or almost total absence of an aerated lung. The marked loss of volume is indicated by approximation of the ribs, elevation of the ipsilateral hemidiaphragm, and shift of the heart and mediastinum into the unoccupied hemithorax. Because of distension and herniation of the remaining functioning lung tissue across the mediastinum, however, breath sounds may be audible bilaterally, and auscultation alone may not be diagnostic. The diagnosis depends on bronchoscopic and bronchographic determination along with tomography and angiography to demonstrate the absence of the main bronchus on the affected side together with the absence of the pulmonary artery. On histologic study of the hypoplastic lung, a pleural surface can be seen under which there is a small, poorly developed bronchus but no bronchial or alveolar tissue.

Congenital absence of a pulmonary lobe presents similar but less dramatic findings. Physical and radiographic examinations show diminished volume of the affected hemithorax, shift of the heart and mediastinum into the affected side, and ipsilateral elevation of the hemidiaphragm. Bronchography establishes the diagnosis by proving the absence of the bronchus to the missing lobe, and angiography is confirmatory.

Treatment consists in managing intercurrent diseases as they arise. Patients must take precautions to avoid infection, and their prognosis is always guarded because those who survive into adult life have progressively decreased pulmonary function.

Complete unilateral agenesis. Left lung and bronchial tree are absent. Right lung is greatly enlarged with resultant shift of mediastinum to left, elevation of left diaphragm, and approximation of ribs on that side

Aplasia of left lung. Only rudimentary bronchi on left side, which end blindly

Hypoplasia of left lung

Hypoplastic lung contains some poorly developed bronchi but no alveolar tissue

F. Netter M.D.

Congenital Lung Cysts

Congenital lung cysts may be differentiated into three groups—*bronchogenic* cysts that result from abnormal budding and branching of the tracheobronchial tree during its development, *alveolar*, and *combined forms*. Bronchogenic cysts are characterized by respiratory cell mucosa composed of either columnar or cuboidal ciliated cells that line the cavity. They may lie outside the normal lung structure or within it. These cysts do not communicate with the tracheobronchial tree unless they become infected. Bronchogenic cysts must be distinguished from acquired bronchiectasis, which is more common in the dependent portions of the lung; in multiple congenital cysts, the upper lobes are often the site of the disease. The differential diagnosis also includes neurenteric cysts, which are associated with vertebral body anomalies, gastroenteric duplication cysts, congenital lobar emphysema, acquired cysts complicating pulmonary interstitial emphysema, and bronchopulmonary dysplasia.

The cysts are typically located near the carina but may occur in the paratracheal, carinal, hilar, or paraesophageal areas. The location of the cyst is important in determining the clinical presentation. Intrapulmonary cysts with a communication between a cyst and the tracheobronchial tree may incorporate a check valve mechanism, which may result in rapid expansion of the cyst. If they are centrally located, they may produce symptoms (coughing and wheezing, particularly during crying) in the neonatal period because of compression of the trachea or main bronchi. Cysts located in the periphery usually present with infection or hemorrhage later in life or are discovered by chance on a chest radiograph.

Cyst wall lined by cuboidal epithelium of bronchial type

Intrapulmonary cyst communicating with bronchial tree and containing mucus

Cyst wall lined by ciliated columnar epithelium and containing mucous glands and cartilage

Bronchogenic (carinal) cyst of mediastinum compressing esophagus and distorting trachea

Congenital lymphangiectasis

Cystic adenomatous malformation of upper lobe of a lung

Congenital cystic adenomatoid malformation of the lung, type 3. Irregular, small airspaces lined by cuboidal epithelium.

CONGENITAL CYSTIC ADENOMATOID MALFORMATION OF THE LUNG

This lesion consists of a mass of cysts lined by proliferating bronchial and cuboidal epithelium. It is divided into three types: type I, which includes multiple large, thin-walled cysts; type II, which includes multiple, evenly spaced cysts; and type III, which includes a bulky firm mass with small, evenly spaced cysts. The lesion is now frequently diagnosed by antenatal ultrasonography, but some so detected may regress during the third trimester. Approximately 25% of patients are stillborn; they are usually hydropic and have a type III lesion. Fifty percent are born prematurely. Infants may develop respiratory distress immediately after birth, depending on the size of the lesion; other presentations include recurrent infection, hemoptysis, and an incidental finding on the chest radiograph. The lesion may also be premalignant. Infants with life-threatening respiratory distress require surgery in the perinatal period. The treatment of patients with asymptomatic disease is controversial, but intervention in infancy should be considered because of the increased risk of infection, pneumothorax, and malignancy.

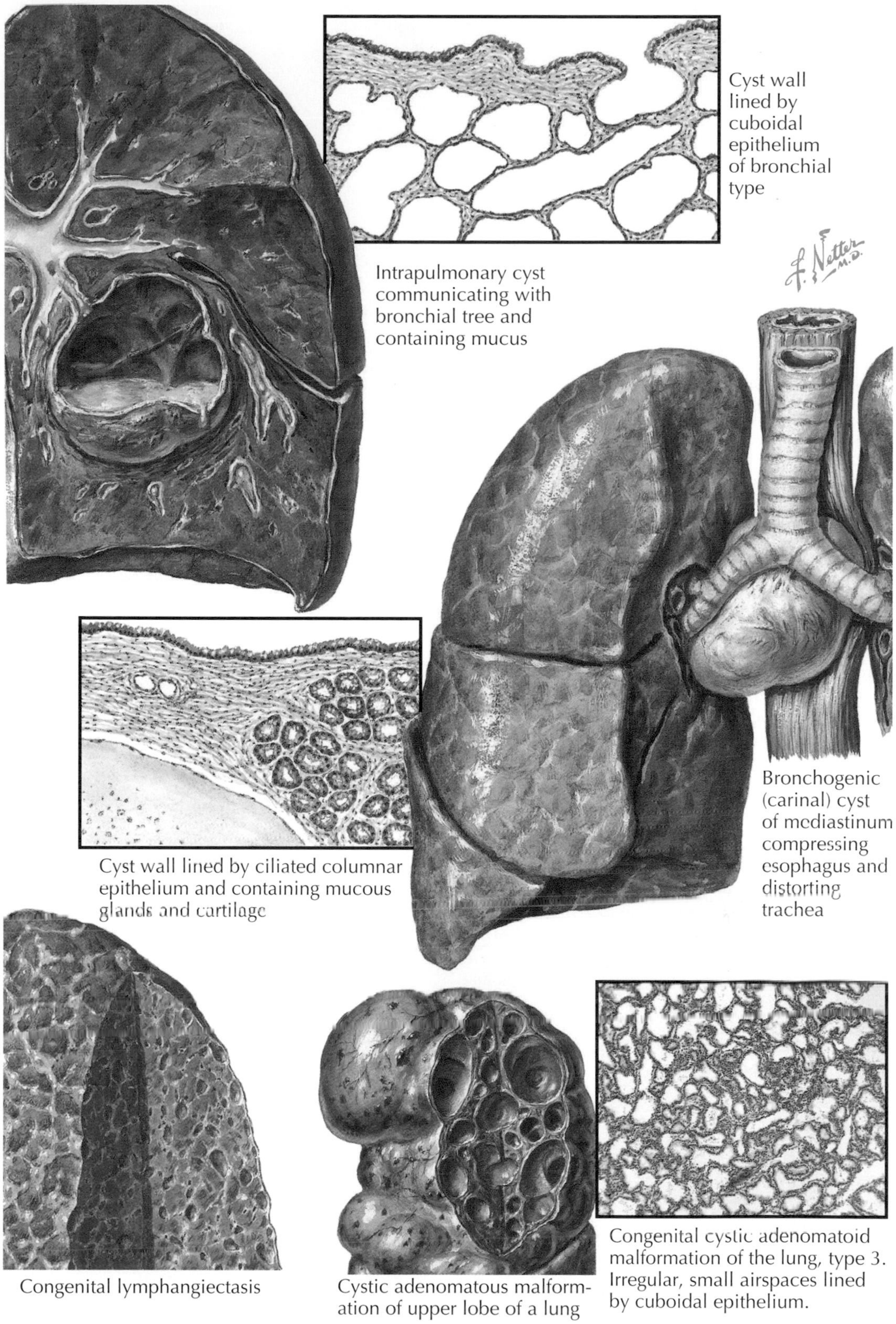

CONGENITAL PULMONARY LYMPHANGIECTASIS

In this condition, there is dilatation of the lymphatic vessels of the lungs and obstruction to their drainage. It may be associated with lymphedema in other portions of the body. Most infants with this problem develop severe respiratory distress at birth, and the majority of them die. Radiologic findings include a ground-glass appearance with fine, diffuse, granular densities representing dilated lymphatics; as with other congenital pulmonary abnormalities, there may be delayed resolution of lung fluid. On examination, the lungs are bulky, with pronounced lobulation, and they contain many thin-walled cystic space–dilated lymphatic vessels.

Pulmonary Sequestration

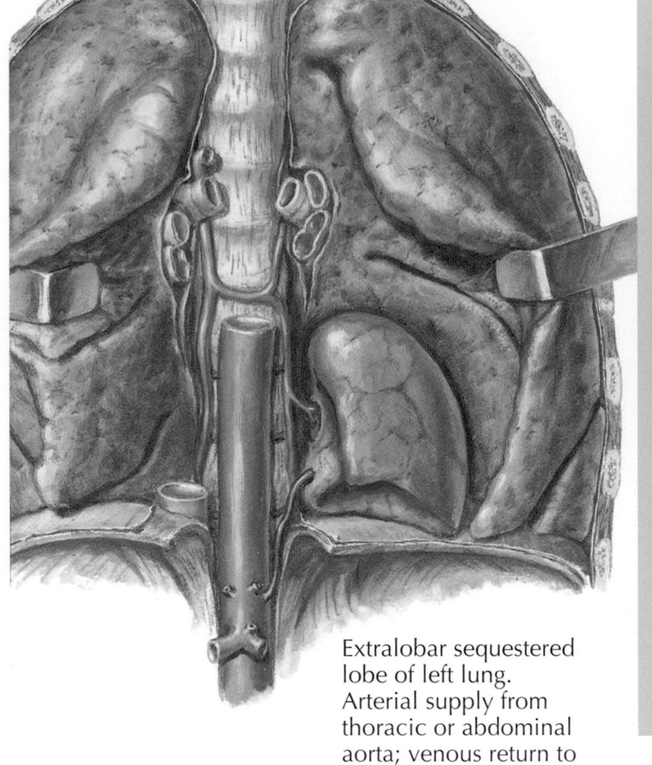

Extralobar sequestered lobe of left lung. Arterial supply from thoracic or abdominal aorta; venous return to hemiazygos vein

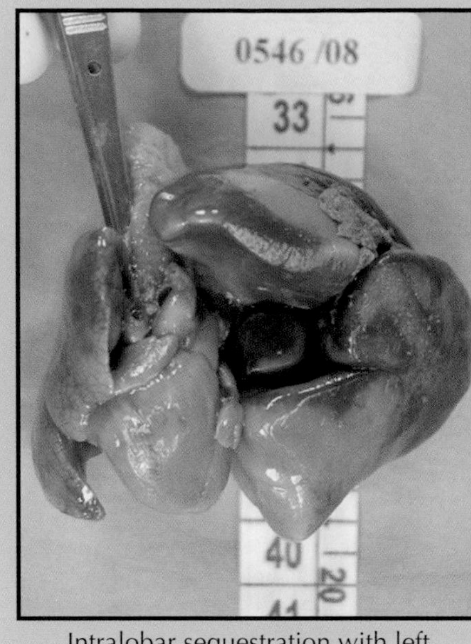

Intralobar sequestration with left lung distorted by large mass and right lung hypoplastic because of compression and mediastinal shift.

Pulmonary sequestration is a congenital malformation in which a mass of pulmonary tissue has no connection either to the parent tracheobronchial tree or the pulmonary vascular tree and receives its blood supply from a systemic artery. The systemic artery usually arises from the aorta either above or below the diaphragm; occasionally from an intercostal artery; or, rarely, from the brachiocephalic (innominate) artery. The sequestered tissue presents itself in two forms: *intralobar* and *extralobar*.

INTRALOBAR SEQUESTRATION

This type comprises a nonfunctioning portion of lung within the visceral pleura of a pulmonary lobe. In the majority of cases, it derives its systemic arterial supply from the descending thoracic aorta or the abdominal aorta. The venous drainage is invariably by way of the pulmonary veins, producing an arterio-arterial communication. Embryologically, it appears to be a failure of the normal pulmonary artery to supply a peripheral portion of the lung; hence, the arterial supply is derived from a persistent ventral branch of the primitive dorsal aorta.

EXTRALOBAR SEQUESTRATION

This malformation may represent a secondary and more caudal development from the primitive foregut that is then sealed off and migrates caudally as the lung grows. Venous drainage is to the systemic circulation, usually the azygos, hemiazygos, or caval veins. Anatomically, it is related to the left hemidiaphragm in more than 90% of cases. It may be situated between the diaphragmatic surface of the lower lobe and the diaphragm or within the substance of the diaphragm.

On pathologic examination, the affected mass is cystic, and the spaces are filled either with mucus or, if infected, with purulent material. The cystic spaces are lined by either columnar or flat cuboidal epithelium.

Only 20% of intralobar sequestrations present in the neonatal period; occasionally, there may be heart failure caused by massive arteriovenous shunting. Extralobar sequestration rarely presents in the neonatal period but may be found incidentally at operation to repair a congenital diaphragmatic hernia. Later presentations include secondary infection, pneumonia, pleural effusion, and empyema. When the sequestered lung becomes infected, it often appears to be a chronic pulmonary abscess accompanied by episodes of fever, chest pain, cough, and bloody mucopurulent sputum.

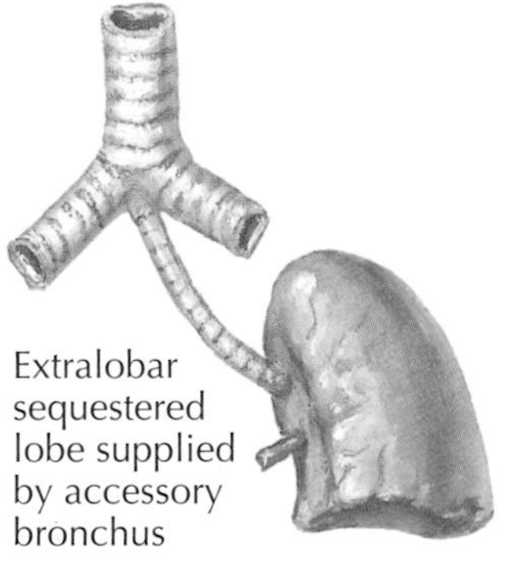

Extralobar sequestered lobe supplied by accessory bronchus

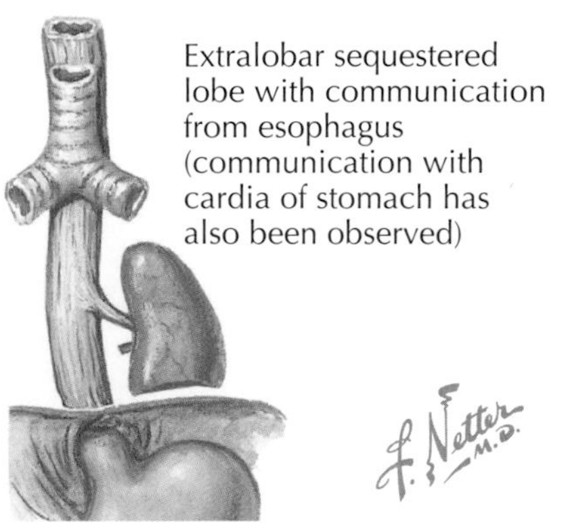

Extralobar sequestered lobe with communication from esophagus (communication with cardia of stomach has also been observed)

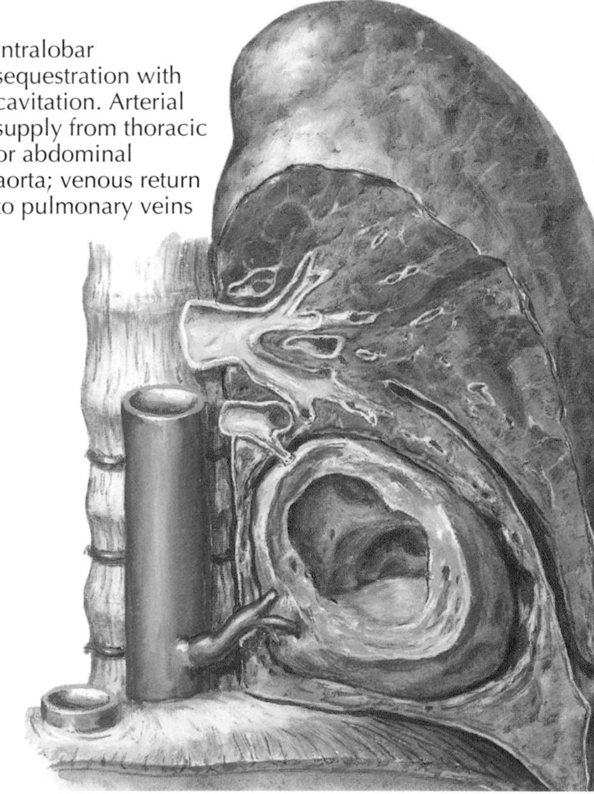

Intralobar sequestration with cavitation. Arterial supply from thoracic or abdominal aorta; venous return to pulmonary veins

On antenatal ultrasonography, the abnormal lung can be seen as an echogenic intrathoracic or intra-abdominal mass. In 50% of cases, there is a pleural effusion, and polyhydramnios is a frequent complication. Postnatally, on radiographic examination the diagnosis should be suspected if there is a dense lesion on the posteromedial part of the left zone of the chest radiograph. Extralobar sequestration is usually seen as a dense triangular lesion close to the diaphragm.

Treatment for either type consists of surgical resection. Because of the threat of secondary infection and hemorrhage, surgery should be recommended even though the patient is asymptomatic at the time. When infection occurs, complete removal is mandatory.

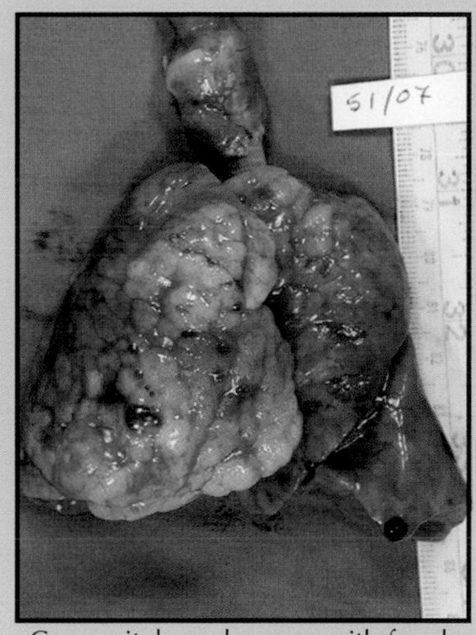

Congenital emphysema with focal, large cysts

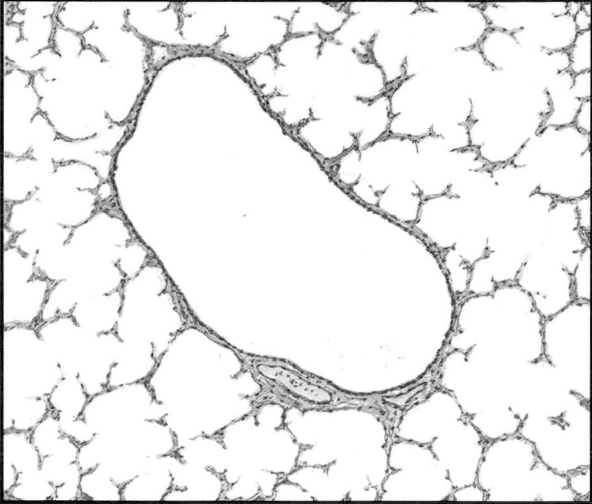
Section showing a fairly large bronchus with almost no cartilage in its wall: a probable cause of emphysema in surrounding lung tissue

Compression of left main bronchus by fibrous ductus arteriosus inserted low on left pulmonary artery. Bullous emphysema of left upper lobe

Ball-valve obstruction of a bronchus by dense mucus and thickened mucosal folds resulting in lobar emphysema

Congenital Lobar Emphysema

This is a rare case of respiratory distress in the neonatal period. The overdistended lobe or lobes cause compression of the remaining normal ipsilateral lung and a marked shift of the mediastinum to the opposite side, so that a ventilatory crisis results with dyspnea, cyanosis, and sometimes circulatory failure.

The pathogenesis of congenital lobar emphysema falls into three categories. In the first group, there are defects in the bronchial cartilage with absent or incomplete rings; the abnormality has also been described in chondroectodermal dysplasia or Ellis-van Creveld syndrome. In the second group, there is an obvious mechanical cause of bronchial obstruction such as a fold of mucous membrane acting as a ball valve, an aberrant artery or fibrous band, tumors, or a tenacious mucous plug. In the third and largest group, no local pathologic lesions other than overdistension of the lobe can be seen, but unrecognized bronchiolitis has been thought to be a possible cause. In each instance, the lobe inflates normally as the bronchus widens during inspiration, but the obstruction to it during expiration results in air trapping and overdistension.

The upper lobes are most commonly involved (80% of cases), particularly on the left side (43% of cases); the right middle lobe (32%) is second in order of frequency. Multilobar bilateral involvement rarely occurs. Differential diagnosis from endobronchial pneumothorax, diaphragmatic hernias, tension cysts, and endobronchial foreign bodies must be made.

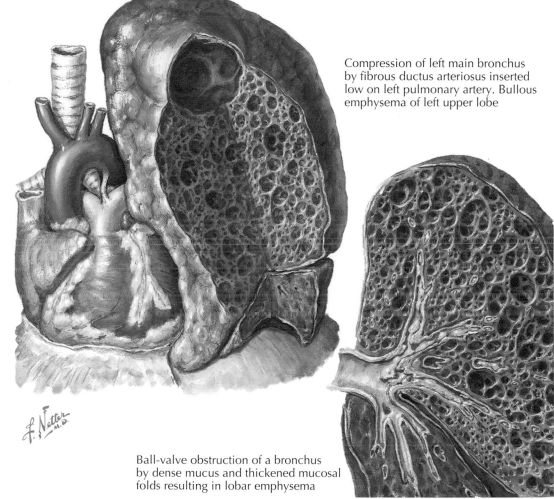

One-third of patients are symptomatic at birth, and approximately half are symptomatic in the first few days after birth. Affected infants may have severe respiratory symptoms and a rapid deterioration, resulting in death. Infants present with increasing dyspnea and recession; cyanosis occurs in 50% of cases and is more obvious on crying. Only 5% of patients are presented after 6 months of age. Physical examination reveals hyperresonance and bulging of the affected hemithorax with a contralateral displacement of the trachea and mediastinum. Hyperlucency of the diseased side is seen on radiography; the ribs are spread farther apart, the diaphragm is lower than normal and flattened, and the uninvolved lobe or lobes may be atelectatic. There is displacement of the mediastinum to the opposite side where the lung appears relatively radiopaque, but the diaphragm is not elevated as seen in atelectasis. In the involved lung, vascular markings may distinguish the abnormality from a pneumothorax.

Lobectomy is indicated for patients who have persistent or progressive respiratory failure, and early lobectomy is required for infants who have significant respiratory distress in the neonatal period. Patients presenting with relatively mild symptoms or diagnosed on chest radiographic examination may be treated conservatively.

Chronic Cough

Neuroanatomy of the cough reflex and common causes of chronic cough

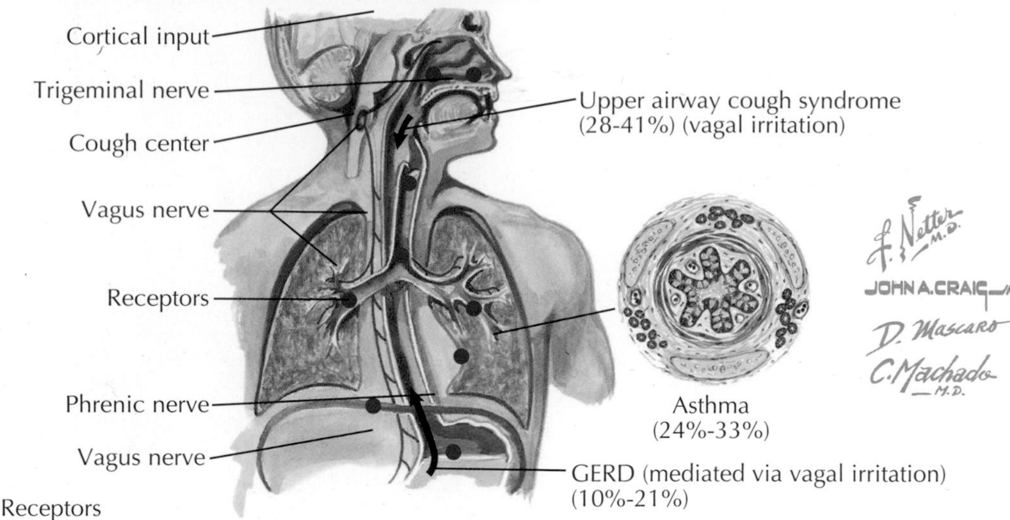

Causes of chronic cough with abnormal chest radiograph

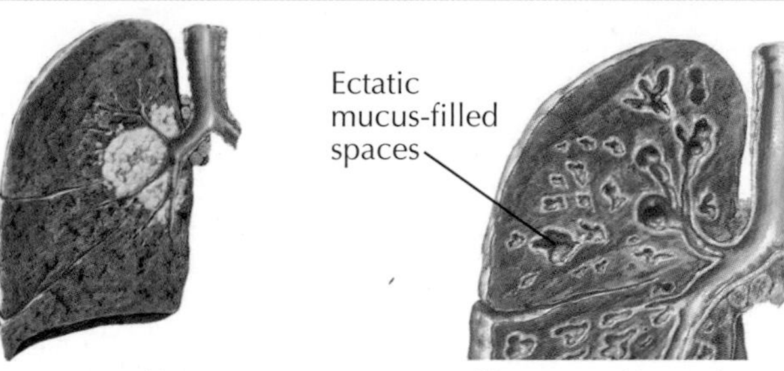

Carcinoma of lung

Cystic fibrosis and bronchiectasis

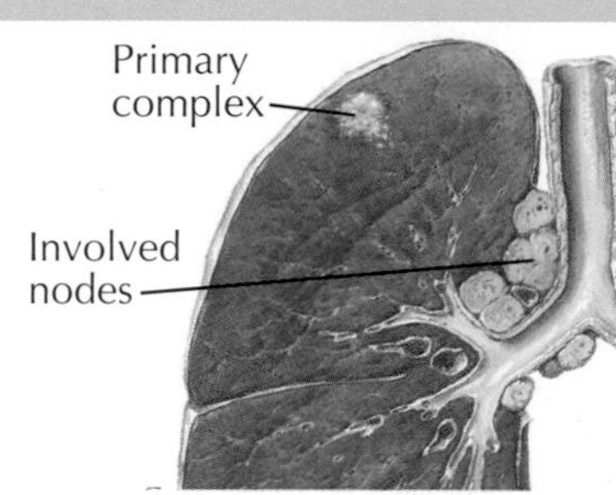

Pulmonary tuberculosis

Causes of acute, subacute, and chronic cough with normal chest radiograph

Acute
- ▶ Upper respiratory tract infections URIs (e.g., the common cold)
- ▶ Bacterial sinusitis
- ▶ *Bordetella pertussis* infection
- ▶ Exacerbations of asthma and bronchitis
- ▶ Allergic rhinitis
- ▶ Environmental irritant rhinitis

Subacute
- ▶ Postinfectious cough (e.g., *Bordetella pertussis* infection)
- ▶ Bacterial sinusitis
- ▶ Exacerbation of asthma, chronic bronchitis; bronchiectasis (x-ray may be abnormal)

Chronic
- ▶ Upper airway cough syndrome caused by a variety of rhinosinus conditions
- ▶ Asthma
- ▶ Nonasthmatic eosinophilic bronchitis
- ▶ GERD
- ▶ Chronic bronchitis
- ▶ Bronchiectasis (x-ray may be abnormal)

Complications of cough

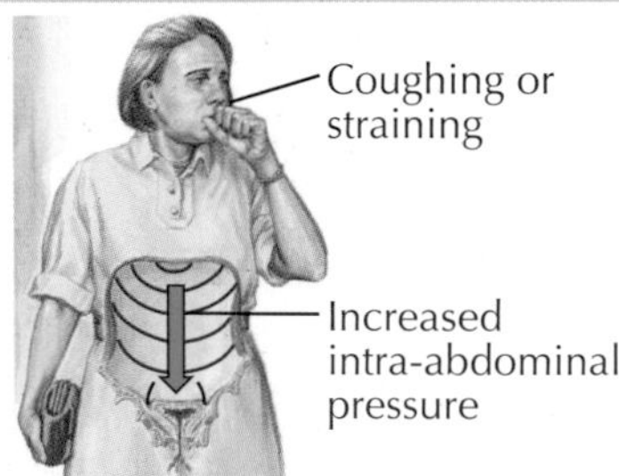

Urinary incontinence

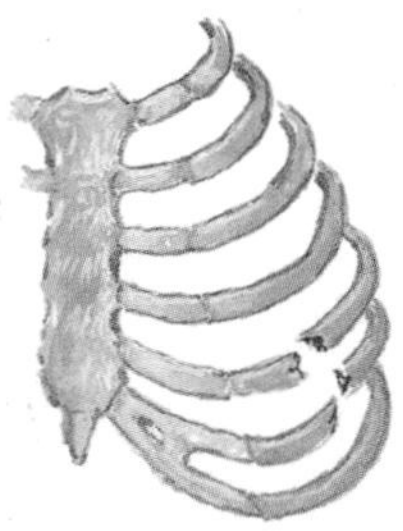

Rib fracture

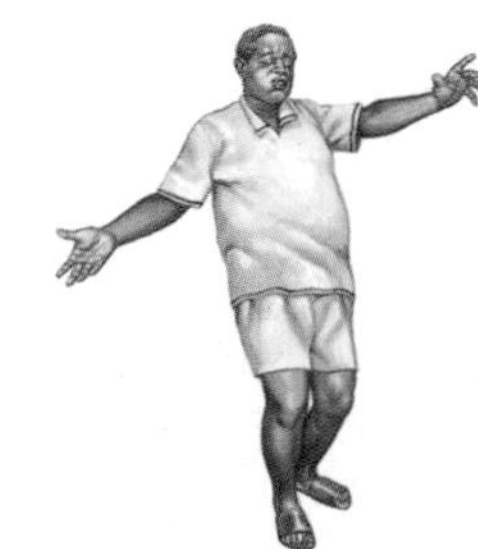

Syncope

Healthy people rarely cough. When they do, it is essentially devoid of any clinical significance. However, when cough is present and persistently troublesome, it can assume great clinical significance. Although cough can become an important factor in spreading infection, this is not the reason why it is one of the most common symptoms for which patients seek medical attention and spend money for medications. They do so because cough adversely affects their quality of life in a variety of ways related to the pressures, velocities, and energy that are generated during vigorous coughing. Although intrathoracic pressures up to 300 mm Hg, expiratory velocities up to 28,000 cm/sec or 500 mph (i.e., 85% of the speed of sound), and intrathoracic energy up to 25 J allow coughing to be an effective means of clearing excessive secretions and foreign material from the lower airways and providing cardiopulmonary resuscitation, these physiologic consequences can lead to physical as well as psychosocial complications. The gamut of complications ranges from cardiovascular, constitutional symptoms, gastrointestinal, genitourinary, musculoskeletal, neurologic, ophthalmologic, psychosocial, quality of life, respiratory, to dermatologic consequences.

Urinary incontinence, rib fractures, syncope, and psychosocial complications such as self-consciousness and the fear of serious disease are particularly bothersome. Coughing-induced urinary incontinence is particularly troublesome in women, especially as they age and in those who have delivered children. Coughing-induced rib fractures may occur in the absence of osteoporosis and typically posterolaterally where the serratus anterior muscle interdigitates with the latissimus dorsi muscle. Syncope caused by coughing can be sudden if the force of the cough causes a concussion wave in the cerebrospinal fluid or more gradual because of hypotension from a decrease in cardiac output.

The modern era of managing cough as a symptom was heralded by the description of a systematic manner of evaluating cough that was based on the putative neuroanatomy of the afferent limb of the cough reflex and the classification of cough based on its duration. Both concepts have been validated (Plate 4-10).

As originally proposed, systematically evaluating the locations of the afferent limb of the cough reflex (i.e., anatomic diagnostic approach) would have the best chance of leading to a correct diagnosis. Although involuntary coughing has traditionally been thought to be solely mediated via the vagus nerve, experimental data suggest that other nerves may also be involved. The anatomic diagnostic approach allowed for the discoveries of extrapulmonary causes of cough such as upper airway cough syndrome caused by a variety of rhinosinus conditions and cough caused by gastroesophageal reflux disease (GERD) without aspiration.

The classification of cough into acute (i.e., <3 weeks), subacute (i.e., 3-8 weeks), and chronic (i.e., >8 weeks) has become one of the most important parts of the workup of cough because it narrows the spectrum of potential diagnostic possibilities (Plate 4-10). The most common causes of acute cough include upper respiratory tract infections (URIs; e.g., the common cold), bacterial sinusitis, *Bordetella pertussis* infection, exacerbations of asthma, chronic bronchitis, allergic rhinitis, and environmental irritant rhinitis. The most common causes of subacute cough include postinfectious cough (e.g., after *B. pertussis* infection); bacterial sinusitis; and exacerbation of preexisting conditions such as asthma, rhinosinus diseases, bronchiectasis, and chronic bronchitis. The most common causes of chronic cough include upper airway cough syndrome caused by a variety of rhinosinus conditions, asthma, nonasthmatic eosinophilic bronchitis, GERD, chronic bronchitis, and bronchiectasis.

When the clinician systematically follows a validated diagnostic protocol and prescribes specific treatment in adequate doses directed against the presumptive cause(s) of cough, cough will improve or disappear in the great majority of cases. At least 20% of the time, chronic cough is caused by multiple conditions that simultaneously contribute. The causes of cough can only be determined when it responds to specific treatment.

COMMON LARYNGEAL LESIONS

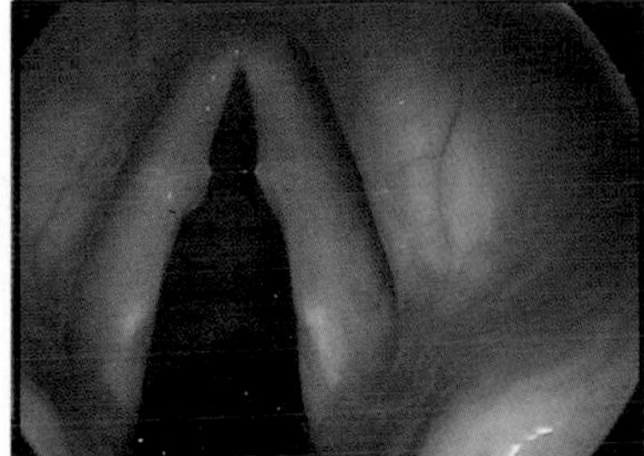
Bilateral vocal cord nodules

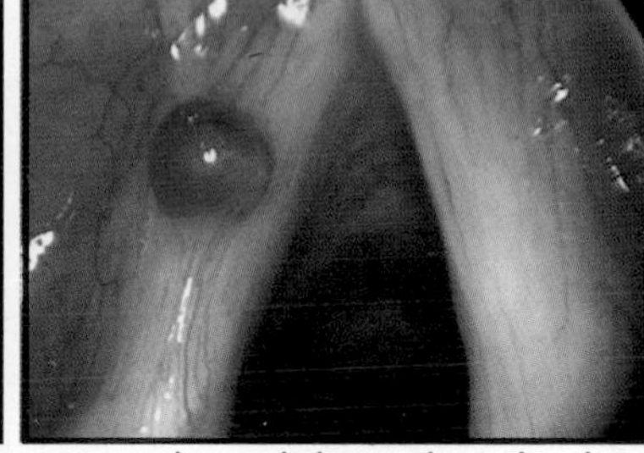
Hemorrhagic left vocal cord polyp

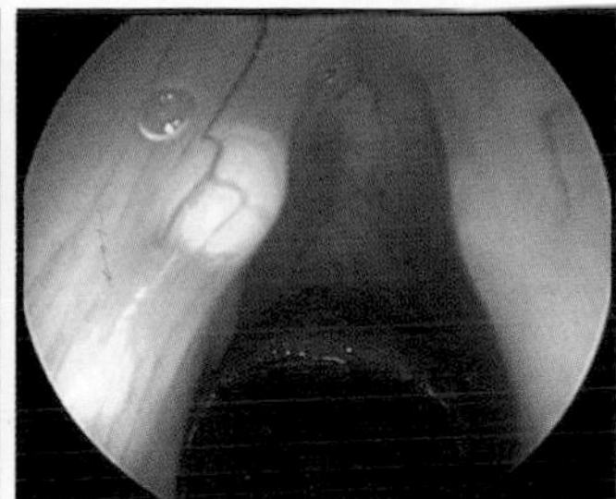
Left vocal cord cyst

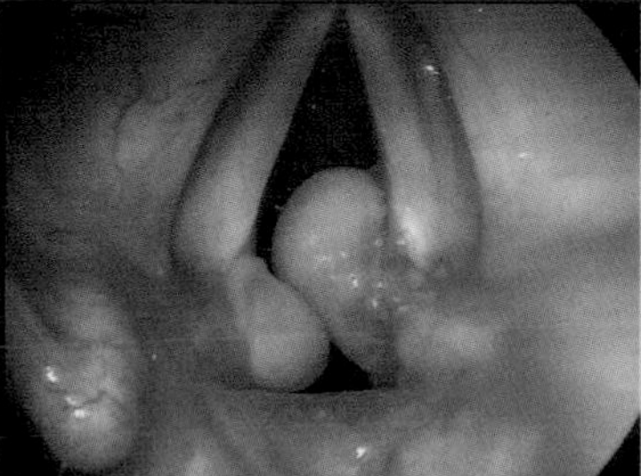
Bilateral laryngeal granulomas after endotracheal intubation. These often regress spontaneously

Etiology. In adults, endotracheal tube impinges on vocal processes of arytenoid cartilages, causing erosion by pressure and movement of tube during mechanical-assisted ventilation, leading to granuloma formation

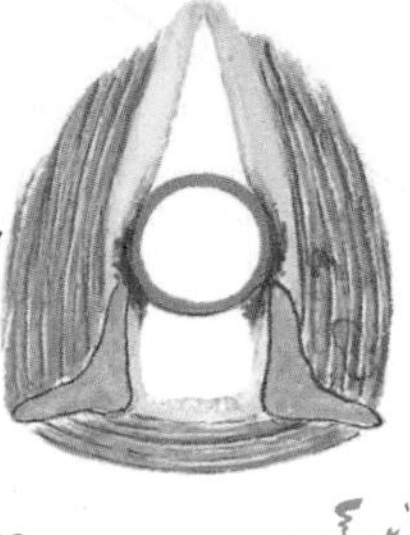

In children, because of smaller larynx, tube lies in interarytenoid space, and subglottic granuloma may result

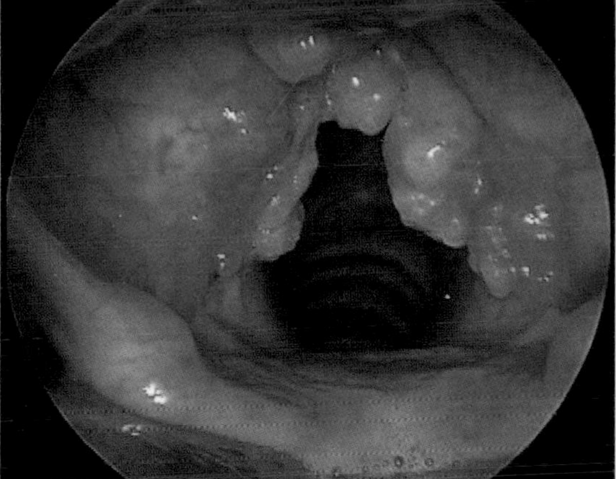
Recurrent respiratory papillomatosis of the larynx

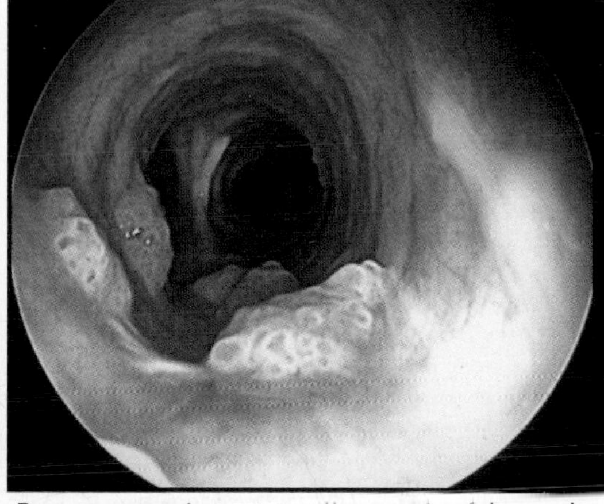
Recurrent respiratory papillomatosis of the trachea

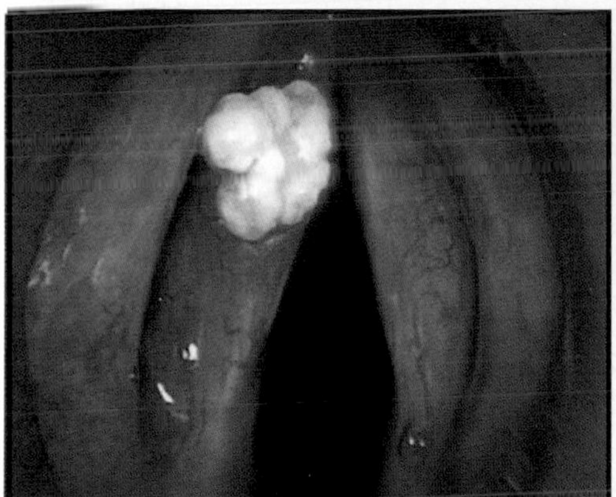
Verrucous carcinoma of the left true vocal cord

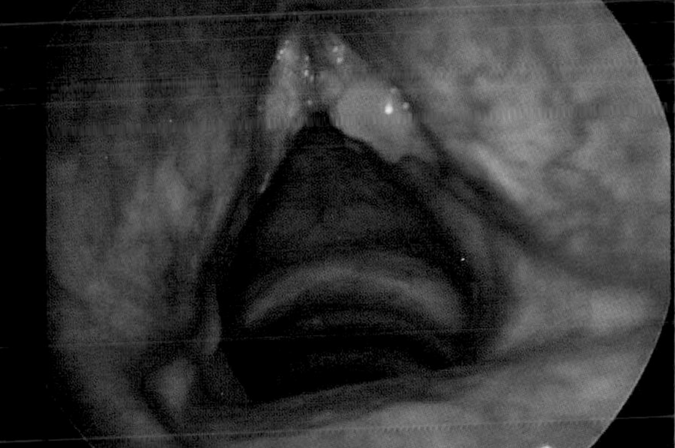
Squamous cell carcinoma of the anterior true vocal cords

Vocal cord nodules, polyps, and cysts are common causes of hoarseness in people with high voice demands, such as teachers, singers, and young children. Excessive or abusive voice use causes repetitive trauma and inflammation within the superficial layer of the lamina propria (Reinke space), leading to the formation of subepithelial lesions affecting the anterior true vocal cord. Mass effect from these lesions impairs vocal cord vibration and disrupts air flow between the vocal cords during phonation, leading to hoarseness. Treatment requires a multifaceted approach, including elimination of vocally abusive behaviors; optimization of laryngeal hygiene; and medical therapy for associated inflammatory conditions such as allergy, infection, and laryngopharyngeal reflux. Surgical excision using modern phonomicrosurgical techniques is indicated for persistent lesions that do not respond to conservative measures.

Laryngeal granulomas are inflammatory lesions arising from the vocal process of the arytenoid cartilage in the posterior larynx. They may be unilateral or bilateral. The most common cause is endotracheal intubation, and the term *intubation granuloma* has been previously used. Pressure from the endotracheal tube causes inflammation and erosion of the thin perichondrium overlying the vocal process of the arytenoid cartilage, leading to granuloma formation. Other common causes include chronic cough or throat clearing, excessive voice use, and laryngopharyngeal reflux. These lesions often regress spontaneously after the localized trauma or underlying inflammatory condition has been addressed. Surgical excision with cold steel or the CO_2 laser is reserved for refractory lesions or large granuloma obstructing the posterior glottic airway.

Recurrent respiratory papillomatosis (RRP) is a disease of viral origin characterized by multiple exophytic lesions of the aerodigestive tract in both children and adults. Laryngeal involvement is common, leading to progressive hoarseness and airway compromise. Extralaryngeal spread to the trachea and lungs is less common but is associated with increased morbidity and potential mortality. Onset of RRP may occur during either childhood or adulthood, with a bimodal age distribution demonstrating the first peak in children younger than 5 years of age and the second peak between 20 and 30 years of age. Juvenile-onset RRP is more common and is the most aggressive form of the disease. It is acquired through vertical transmission of human papilloma virus from an infected mother in utero or during childbirth. Although benign, these lesions are a source of significant morbidity because of their location within the upper and lower airways, the frequency with which they recur despite aggressive medical and surgical treatment, and the potential for malignant degeneration over time.

Squamous cell carcinoma is the most common malignancy of the larynx. These cancers range from well-differentiated, low-grade tumors such as verrucous carcinoma, which can be treated with surgical excision alone and carries an excellent prognosis, to poorly differentiated, high-grade carcinomas, which have a poor prognosis despite aggressive, multimodality treatment. The location of the tumor also has important implications. Glottic cancers, which arise from the true vocal cords, are often diagnosed at an early stage because even small lesions cause symptomatic hoarseness. They also have a relatively low rate of metastasis to regional lymphatics or distant sites. In contrast, supraglottic cancers, which arise from the epiglottis or false vocal cords, are often diagnosed at a more advanced stage when the tumor is large enough to cause symptomatic dysphagia or airway obstruction. Supraglottic cancers have a high rate of regional lymph node involvement and are more likely to metastasize to the lungs or other distant sites. Subglottic cancers are rare but carry a relatively poor prognosis. Prolonged smoking and alcohol consumption are the most important risk factors for laryngeal cancer, with a synergistic effect when combined.

LARYNGEAL AND TRACHEAL STENOSIS

The unique anatomy and delicate tissues of the larynx and trachea predispose these sites to scarring and stenosis in response to injury. Some of the more common causes include prolonged endotracheal intubation, long-term tracheostomy, bacterial or viral infection, systemic inflammatory conditions, neoplasia, and trauma. In many cases, the stenosis is a relatively late sequela of the initial pathologic process and may not be recognized until it progresses to the point of symptomatic airway compromise (stridor or dyspnea) or impaired laryngeal function (hoarseness).

Laryngeal stenosis may occur at any level within the larynx. Supraglottic and glottic stenosis are usually a result of external trauma or prolonged intubation but are also seen with caustic ingestions, inhalation burns, and postsurgical scarring. Subglottic stenosis is the most common form of laryngeal stenosis. Prolonged endotracheal intubation can damage the thin inner perichondrium of the cricoid cartilage, leading to circumferential scarring and cicatrix formation. Long-term tracheostomy tubes can also cause subglottic stenosis as a result of superior migration of the tube and ensuing destruction of the cricoid ring. Other common causes of subglottic stenosis include laryngopharyngeal reflux, Wegener granulomatosis, and a congenital form seen in young children. When a specific cause cannot be identified, the term *idiopathic subglottic stenosis* (ISS) is used. It is likely that many cases of ISS are caused, at least in part, by unrecognized laryngopharyngeal reflux or autoimmune disorders.

Tracheal stenosis is a potentially devastating sequelae of prolonged endotracheal intubation and tracheostomy in patients with respiratory failure requiring cuffed tubes for mechanical ventilation. In the anterior and lateral tracheal walls, the vertical blood vessels that course between the mucosa and the cartilage rings may be readily compressed by a distending cuff or balloon. Decreased blood supply leads to perichondritis, avascular necrosis, and fragmentation of the tracheal cartilage. The resultant stricture often has a triangular configuration on transverse section because of anterior weakening of the cartilaginous arch with lateral wall collapse. Posteriorly, the membranous trachea is more pliable, and the vascular supply is less likely to be compressed. Thus, in about 50% of cases of postintubation or posttracheostomy balloon stenosis, the posterior tracheal wall is spared.

The characteristics and extent of tracheal stenosis can be demonstrated radiographically with traditional tomography in the frontal and lateral projections or with computed tomography (CT) images in the coronal and sagittal planes. The stenotic segment may be narrow and weblike, involving only one tracheal ring, or it may be longer, involving two to five tracheal rings with tapering margins. If the affected segment is thin or pliable, obstruction may only occur with inspiration or expiration (tracheomalacia), depending on whether the affected segment is extrathoracic (neck) or intrathoracic (thorax), respectively. Tracheomalacia may result in greater functional impairment than is apparent radiographically. If dynamic collapse is suspected, flow-volume loops demonstrating reduced inspiratory or expiratory flow or fiberoptic bronchoscopy demonstrating inspiratory or expiratory collapse may be useful diagnostic tools. In some cases, multiple stenoses may occur, especially after the use of tubes of different lengths or tubes with double cuffs.

Postintubation and posttracheostomy balloon stenosis remains a serious problem despite the advent of low-pressure cuffs and increased vigilance in the clinical care setting. It has been recommended that the cuff be deflated at intervals to avoid an excessively prolonged compression of the tracheal mucosa. The problem with this method is that the cuff may not empty completely, and if it is reinflated with the minimal fixed volume of air recommended for filling, overinflation may occur. Proper cuff pressures are best achieved by inflating under auscultatory control until there is no leakage of air with positive-pressure ventilation. If stenosis develops despite these measures, surgery in the form of endoscopic laser incision and dilatation or tracheal resection with anastomosis may be necessary.

Tracheal stenosis

Blood supply of upper trachea

Inferior thyroid artery

Tracheoesophageal branches from inferior thyroid arteries send circumferential vessels to intercartilaginous spaces, with vertical ascending and descending branches beneath mucosa

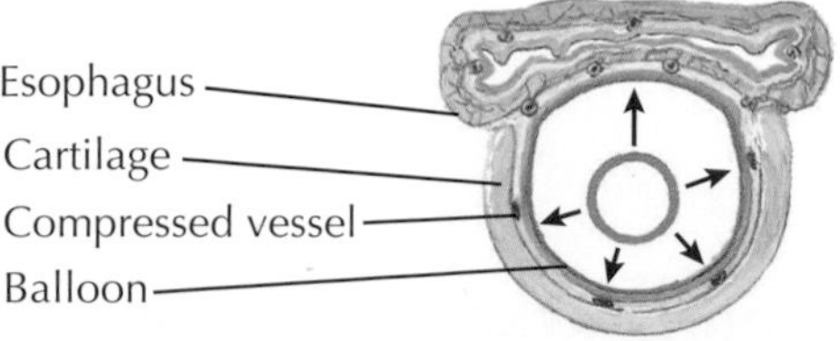

Vertical submucosal vessels may be readily compressed against cartilage rings of anterior and lateral tracheal walls by a distended endotracheal balloon, with resultant erosion followed by avascular ulceration and perichondritis, collapse, and stenosis. Posterior fibromuscular wall, however, is yielding, and vascular compression is therefore less likely here, so that this wall is often spared

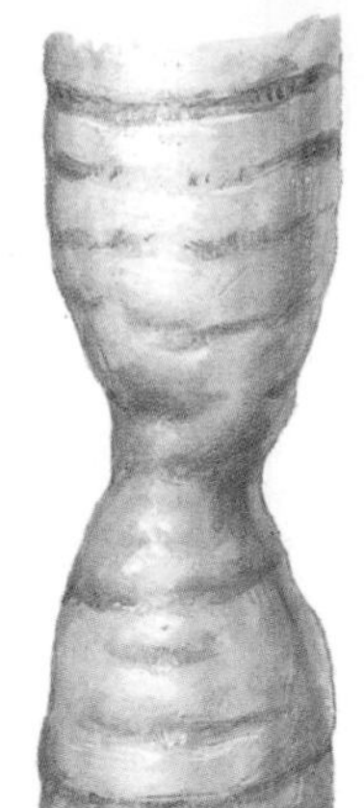

Section through excised specimen viewed from above, showing fragmentation of cartilage and complete concentric stenosis with ulcerations

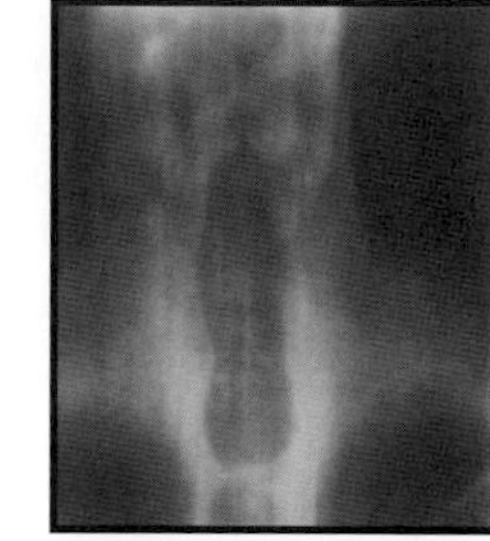

"Weblike" tracheal stenosis

Hourglass constriction of trachea; cartilage rings obscured by perichondritis, so that serial transverse cuts may be required to determine limits of normal tissue

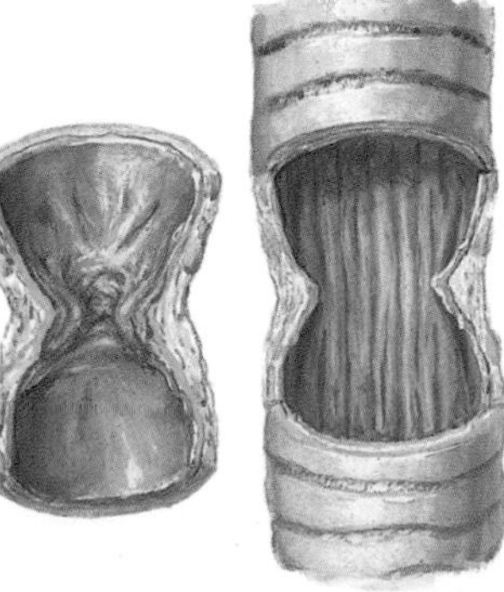

Stenosis involving only anterior and lateral cartilaginous walls; posterior fibromuscular wall intact

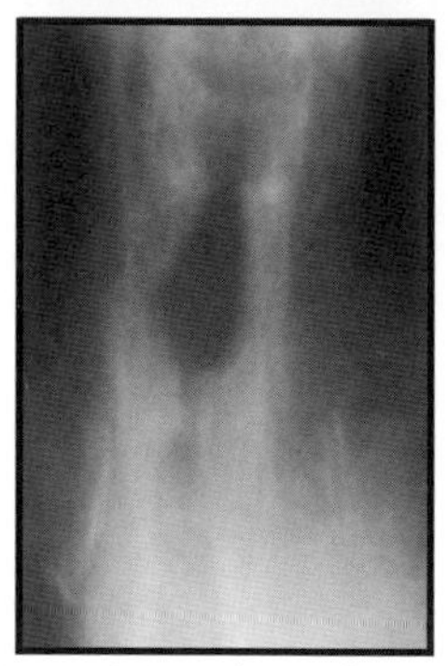

Stenosis involving longer segment of trachea

Subglottic stenosis

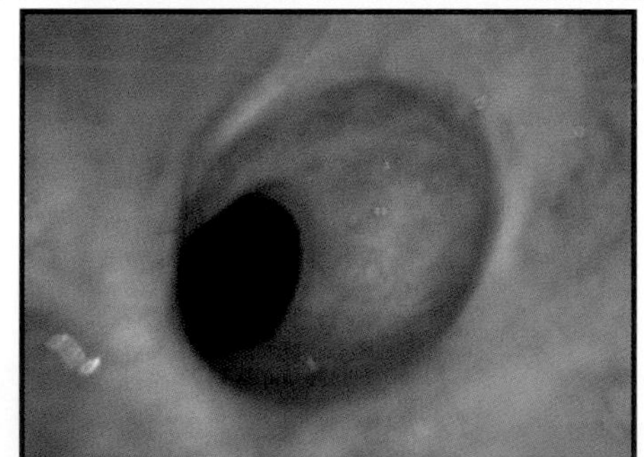

Endoscopic photograph of subglottic stenosis showing circumferential narrowing or cicatrix formation at the level of the cricoid ring

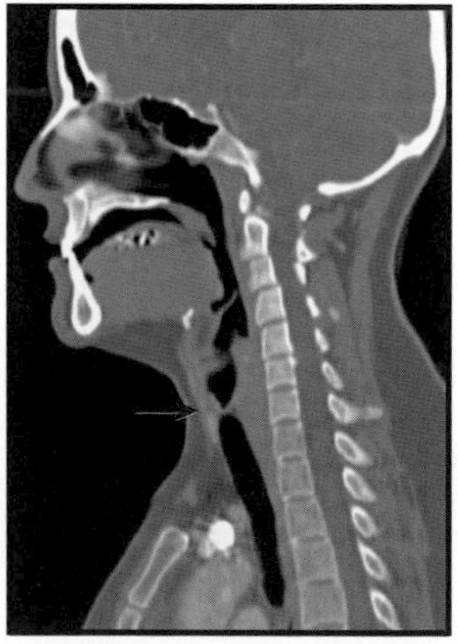

Sagittal CT scan image of subglottic stenosis (marked by red arrow)

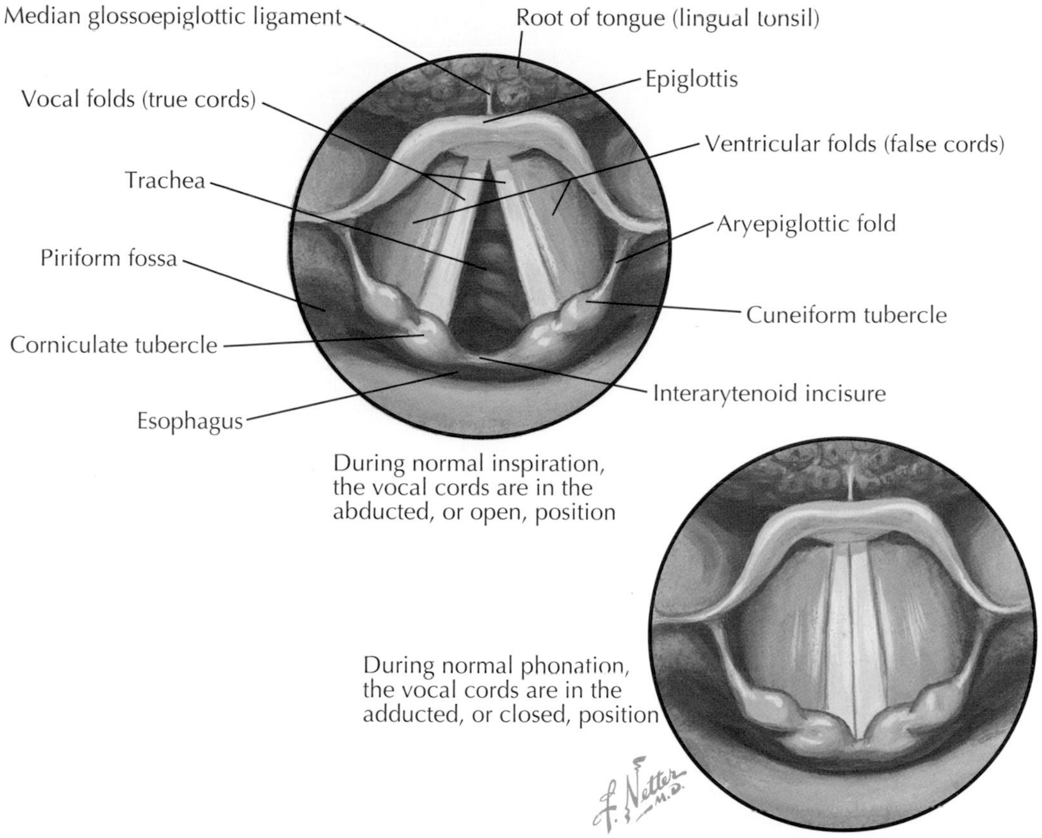

Vocal Cord Dysfunction

Vocal cord dysfunction (VCD), also known as paradoxical vocal cord motion (PVCM), is a relatively poorly understood laryngeal disorder manifest by inappropriate adduction, or closing, of the vocal cords during inspiration. This is in contrast to the normal respiratory cycle, in which the vocal cords are abducted, or open, during inspiration and only begin to adduct toward the end of exhalation or with the onset of phonation. Physiologically, partial adduction of the vocal cords at the end of the expiratory phase maintains alveolar patency by generating positive end-expiratory pressure. Full adduction of the vocal cords occurs normally during phonation. As air expelled from the lungs encounters a closed glottis, subglottic air pressure increases, which in turn provides the force necessary to vibrate the vocal cords and produce voice. In contrast, paradoxical adduction of the vocal cords during inspiration in patients with VCD results in acute, intermittent episodes of functional airway obstruction.

The most common symptoms of VCD are inspiratory stridor, dyspnea, hoarseness, throat tightening, and cough. Unfortunately, these symptoms are relatively nonspecific and may mimic other conditions such as asthma, epiglottitis, angioedema, or anaphylaxis. Many patients with VCD will have been treated aggressively for presumed asthma without improvement. In contrast to asthma, the airway obstruction in VCD occurs with inspiration rather than expiration, and laryngeal stridor should not be mistaken for bronchial wheezing. Pulmonary function testing can help exclude asthma and support a diagnosis of VCD, with attenuation of the inspiratory flow rate on flow-volume loops. It is common to have both asthma and VCD, in which case methacholine challenge testing is often helpful.

A diagnosis of VCD can be further substantiated with transnasal flexible fiberoptic laryngoscopy. As with pulmonary function testing, this should be done while the patient is symptomatic. Because of the episodic nature of VCD, it may be necessary to first challenge the patient with exercise, sustained vocal tasks, or other known triggers to elicit an acute exacerbation. Flexible laryngoscopy demonstrates a structurally normal larynx with paradoxical adduction of the vocal cords during inspiration. This is more pronounced when breathing in through the mouth rather than the nose, which provides a stronger neural stimulus for vocal cord abduction. Adduction of the anterior two-thirds of the vocal cords with a diamond-shaped posterior glottic gap is most commonly described, although additional findings of false vocal cord adduction and anterior to posterior supraglottic constriction have been reported.

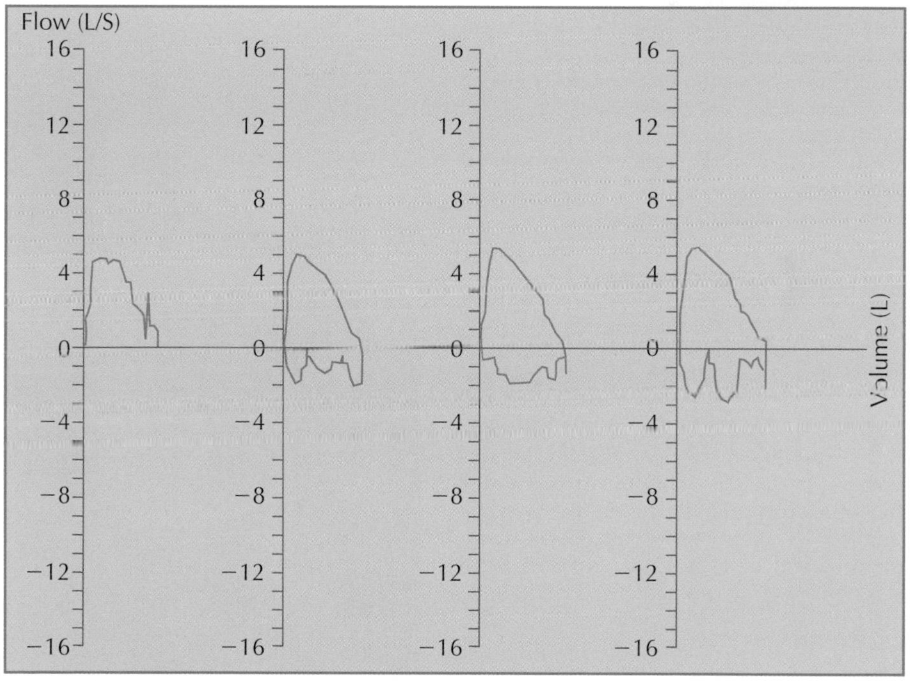

The cause of VCD is poorly understood. Because of the lack of clear organic pathology and the high incidence of underlying psychiatric conditions in these patients, VCD has historically been considered a psychogenic disorder, as evidenced by such antiquated terms as *Munchausen's stridor* and *factitious asthma*. Although VCD may be a manifestation of a somatization or conversion disorder in some patients, nonpsychogenic causes must also be considered. Brainstem compression, upper or lower motor neuron injury, and movement disorders have been associated with VCD. Laryngeal hyperresponsiveness secondary to laryngopharyngeal reflux (LPR) has also been implicated as a potential causative factor in VCD. A diagnosis of LPR is supported by findings of posterior laryngeal erythema, interarytenoid mucosal pachydermy, and posterior pharyngeal cobblestoning on flexible laryngoscopy.

The treatment of VCD involves a multifaceted approach, with identification and elimination of potential irritants or triggers, medical therapy for underlying psychogenic or pathologic conditions, and intensive behavioral therapy with an experienced speech-language pathologist focusing on laryngeal relaxation and diaphragmatic breathing techniques. If necessary, severe attacks may be managed acutely with anxiolytics, heliox, or continuous positive airway pressure ventilation. Most patients with VCD improve with proper treatment and time.

During normal inspiration, the vocal cords are in the abducted, or open, position

During normal phonation, the vocal cords are in the adducted, or closed, position

Flow-volume loops in a patient with known vocal cord dysfunction demonstrate truncated inspiratory flow rates with a characteristic "saw-tooth" pattern corresponding to inappropriate adduction, or closing, of the vocal cords during inspiration

ALLERGIC ASTHMA: CLINICAL FEATURES

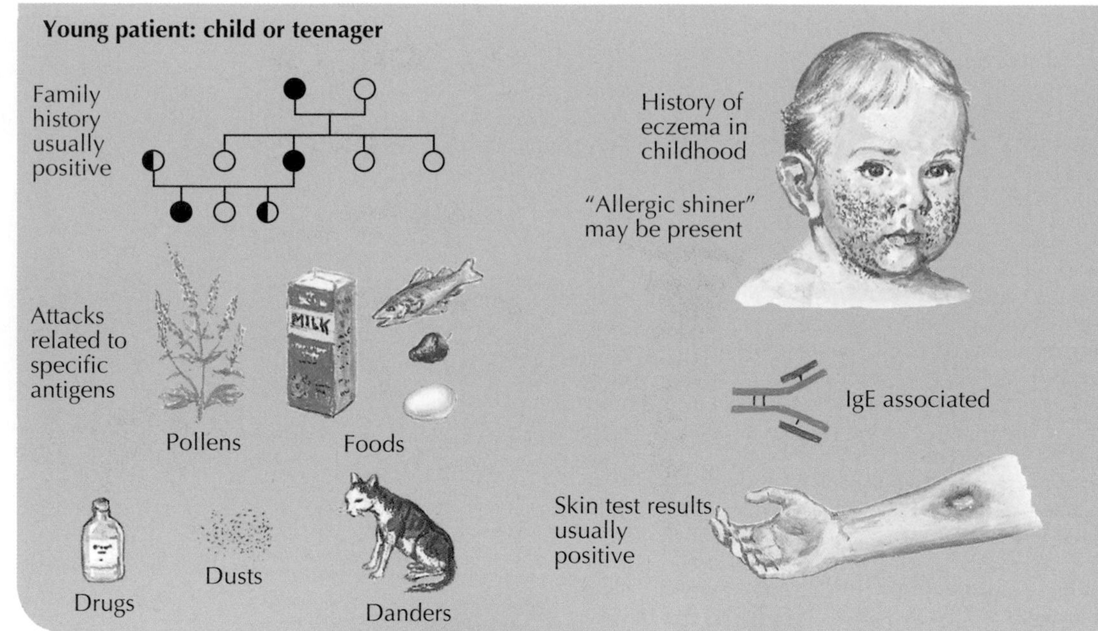

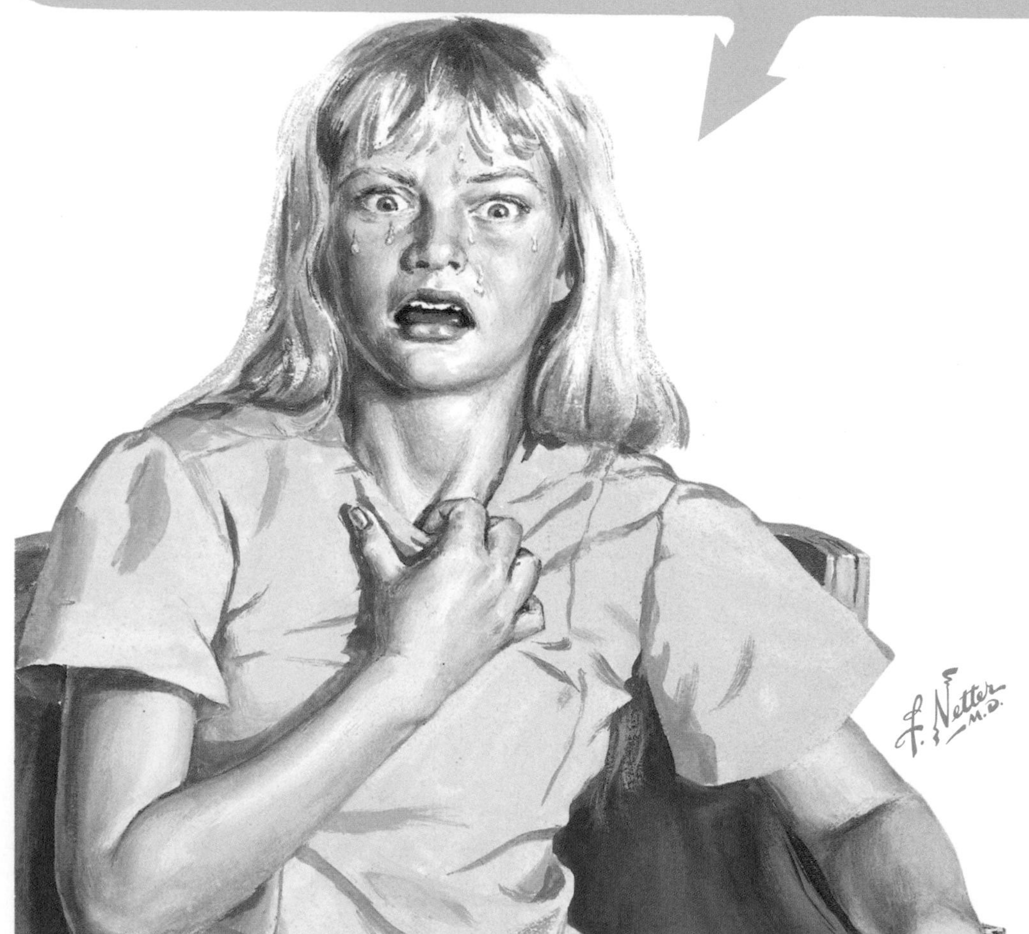

BRONCHIAL ASTHMA

Asthma affects between 5% and 15% of the population in most countries where this has been evaluated. Asthma is a clinical syndrome characterized by variable airflow obstruction, increased responsiveness of the airway to constriction induced by nonspecific inhaled stimuli (airway hyperresponsiveness), and cellular inflammation. Asthmatic symptoms are characteristically episodic and consist of dyspnea, wheezing, cough, and chest tightness caused by airflow obstruction because of airway smooth muscle constriction, airway wall edema, airway inflammation, and hypersecretion by mucous glands. A major feature of the airflow obstruction of asthma is that it is partially or fully reversible either spontaneously or as a result of treatment.

CLINICAL FORMS OF BRONCHIAL ASTHMA

Asthma is a syndrome because, although the clinical presentation is often quite characteristic, its etiologic factors vary. Previous descriptors of asthma included the terms *extrinsic asthma*, implying that an external stimulus was responsible for causing the disease, and *intrinsic asthma*, in which no obvious external cause could be identified. It is now recognized that likely all asthma is initiated by some external stimulus, the most commonly identified of which are environmental allergens.

Allergic Asthma

Allergic asthma most often affects children and young adults (Plate 4-14). A personal history of other allergic manifestations (atopy), such as allergic rhinitis, conjunctivitis, or eczema is common, as is a family history of atopy. Atopy is identified by positive dermal responses to environmental and occupational allergens and elevated serum immunoglobulin E (IgE) levels.

Nonallergic Asthma

Nonallergic asthma is usually identified in patients who develop asthma symptoms as adults (see Plate 4-15). The symptoms may develop after a respiratory tract infection, and occasionally infective agents such as *Chlamydia pneumoniae* or *Mycoplasma* spp. are implicated. Occupational sensitizers are other important causes of nonallergic asthma, and a detailed occupational history is a critical component of the evaluation of the patient. Nonallergic asthma is also commonly associated with comorbidities such as chronic sinusitis, obesity, or gastroesophageal reflux.

INDUCERS AND INCITERS OF ASTHMA

An important distinction needs to be made between stimuli that are inducers of asthma (cause the disease), such as environmental allergens and occupational sensitizers, and inciters of asthma, which are stimuli that cause exacerbations or transient symptoms (see Plate 4-16).

Respiratory Viral Infections

Viral infections are important inducers of asthma and have been associated with a number of important clinical consequences in people with asthma, including

Bronchial Asthma *(Continued)*

the development of wheezing-associated illnesses in infants and small children; the development of asthma in the first decade of life; causing acute asthma exacerbations (particularly rhinovirus); and inducing changes in airway physiology, including increasing airway responsiveness.

Environmental Allergens

Allergens are known to both induce asthma and be inciters of asthma symptoms. Indeed, some people with asthma only experience seasonal symptoms when they are exposed to allergens. Patients with allergen sensitivity can experience acute bronchoconstriction within 10 to 15 minutes after allergen inhalation, which usually resolves with 2 hours (the early asthmatic response); however, the bronchoconstriction can recur between 3 to 6 hours later (the late asthmatic response), which develops more slowly and is characterized by severe bronchoconstriction and dyspnea. The late response occurs because of progressively increasing influx of inflammatory cells, particularly basophils and eosinophils, into the airways. The bronchoconstriction usually resolves within 24 hours, but patients are left with increased airway responsiveness, which may persist for more than 1 week.

Occupational Sensitizing Agents

Occupational asthma is a common cause of adult-onset asthma. More than 200 agents have been identified in the workplace, including allergens such as animal dander, wheat flour, psyllium, and enzymes, which cause airway narrowing through IgE-mediated responses, and chemicals (often small molecular weight, e.g., toluene diisocyanate), which cause asthma through non–IgE-mediated mechanisms. Work-related exposures and inhalation accidents are a significant risk for new-onset asthma. When occupational chemical sensitizers are inhaled by a sensitized subject in the laboratory, an early asthmatic response can often be elicited, similar to that induced by allergen. This can be followed by a late asthmatic response. The airway inflammatory responses caused by occupational sensitizers do not appear to differ substantially from other causes of asthma, such as environmental allergens.

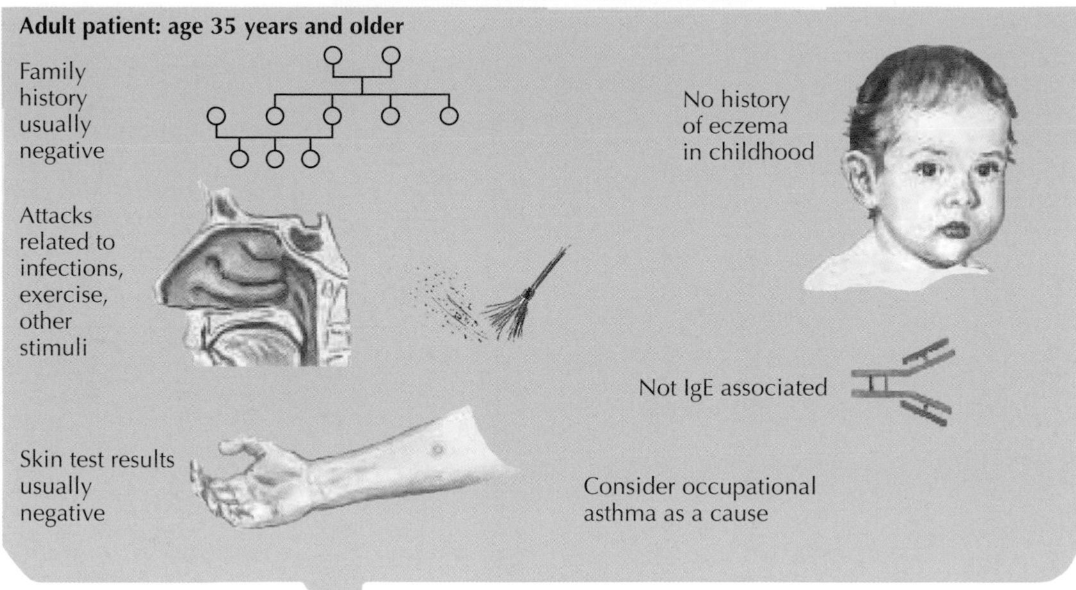

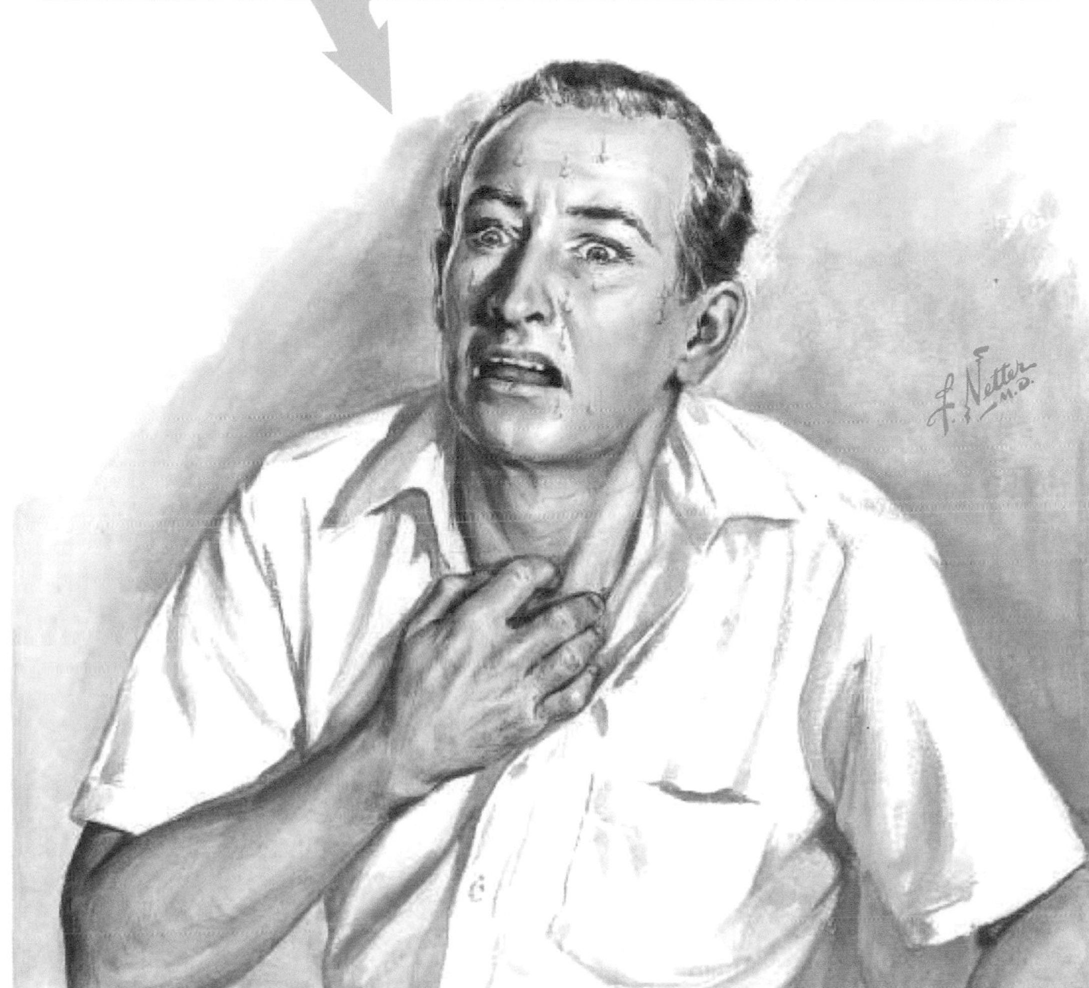

Exercise

Exercise is a very commonly experienced asthma inciter. Bronchoconstriction occurs after exercise, becoming maximal 10 to 20 minutes after the end of exertion, and generally resolves within 1 hour. Bronchoconstriction very rarely occurs during exercise. Bronchoconstriction is caused by the cooling and drying of the airways because the large volumes of air inhaled during exercise are conditioned to body temperature and are fully saturated. Similar symptoms can be experienced by people with asthma who inhale very cold, dry air. Exercise-induced bronchoconstriction can usually be prevented by pretreatment with inhaled β_2-agonists 5 to 10 minutes before exercise.

Atmospheric Pollutants

A variety of atmospheric pollutants are asthma inciters. These include nitrogen dioxide (NO_2), sulfur dioxide

Common Precipitating Factors in Etiology of Bronchial Asthma

Inducers of asthma

Infections

Common cold or other viral infections

Sinusitis

Bronchitis or bronchiolitis

Inhalant allergens

Pollens: weeds, grasses, trees

House dusts

Feathers

Animal danders

Furniture stuffing

Fungal spores

Inducers of asthma symptoms

Irritant inhalants

Paint

Gasoline

Tobacco smoke

Industrial chemicals

Fumes

Cold air

Air pollutants

Trigger mechanisms

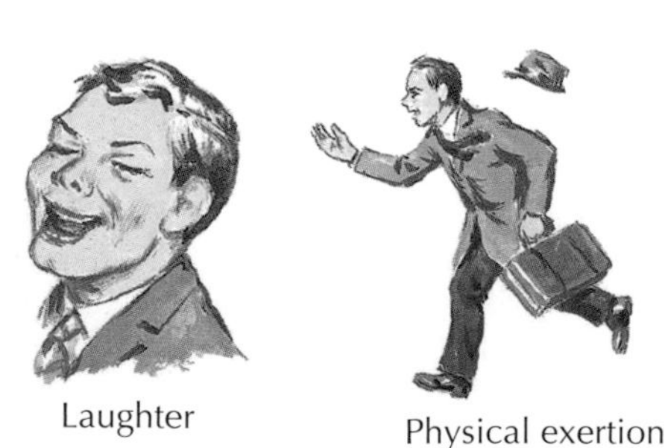

Laughter

Physical exertion

Psychological stress

Drugs

Various drugs

Aspirin

Bronchial Asthma *(Continued)*

(SO_2), ozone, and inhaled particles smaller than 10 μm in diameter (PM_{10}). Other environmental irritants that can incite asthma symptoms include strong smells, such as perfume, car exhaust fumes, and secondhand tobacco smoke.

Aspirin Sensitivity

A triad of aspirin sensitivity, asthma, and nasal polyposis (Samter triad) has been recognized in approximately 5% of individuals with asthma (although nasal polyposis is not invariably present in asthmatics with aspirin sensitivity). Symptoms of asthma develop within 20 minutes of ingestion of aspirin, which may be very severe and occasionally life threatening. This sensitivity exists to all drugs that are cyclo-oxygenase (COX-1) inhibitors and sometimes also to tartrazine. Acetaminophen and COX-2 inhibitors appear to be safe to use in most aspirin-sensitive individuals with asthma.

CLINICAL PRESENTATION

Symptoms and Clinical Findings

Symptoms and signs of asthma range from mild, discrete episodes of shortness of breath, wheezing, and cough, which are very intermittent, usually after exposure to an asthma trigger, followed by significant remission, to continuous, chronic symptoms that wax and wane in severity. For any patient, symptoms may be mild, moderate, or severe at any given time, and even patients with mild, intermittent asthma can have severe life-threatening exacerbations. An asthmatic exacerbation can be a terrifying experience, especially for patients who are aware of its potentially progressive nature.

Symptoms of an asthmatic exacerbation most often develop gradually but occasionally can be sudden in onset. Most often asthma exacerbations are preceded by viral upper respiratory tract infections. Many patients complain of a sensation of retrosternal chest tightness. Expiratory and often inspiratory wheezing is audible and is associated with variable degrees of dyspnea. Cough is likely to be present and may be productive of purulent sputum.

In severe asthma exacerbations, the patient prefers to sit upright; visible nasal alar flaring and use of the accessory respiratory muscles reflect the increased work of breathing. Anxiety and apprehension generally relate to the intensity of the exacerbation. Tachypnea may be the result of fear, airway obstruction, or changes in blood and tissue gas tensions or pH. Hypertension and tachycardia both reflect increased catecholamine output, although a pulse rate greater than 110 to 130 beats/min may indicate significant hypoxemia (PaO_2 <60 mm Hg) and the seriousness of the episode. Pulsus paradoxus (≥10 mm Hg) accompanies pulmonary hyperinflation, occurring when the forced expiratory volume in 1 second (FEV_1) is usually below 30% of predicted normal. If severe hypoxemia and hypercapnia with respiratory acidosis occur, the patient is usually cyanotic, fatigued, confused, and agitated. Chest examination reveals a hyperresonant percussion note, a low-lying diaphragm, and other evidence of hyperinflation. Expiration is prolonged. The patient has generalized inspiratory and expiratory wheezing. With low-grade

Variable airflow Obstruction and Airway Hyperresponsiveness

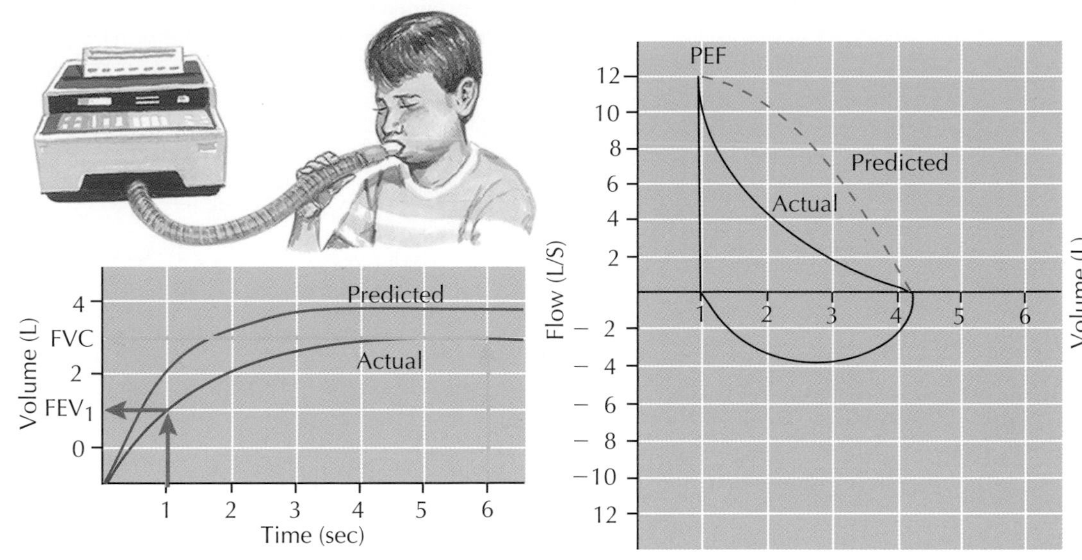

Methacholine and exercise challenges

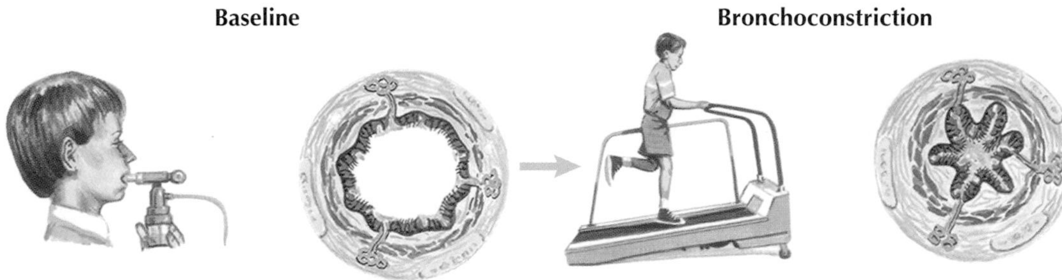

Inhalation of nebulized methacholine at increasing doses. Each dose is followed by spirometry. Fall in FEV$_1$ by ≥20% from baseline at a concentration of ≤8mg/mL is a positive response

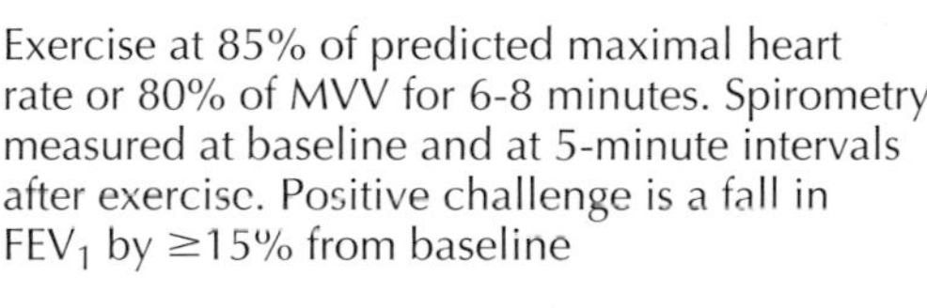
Exercise at 85% of predicted maximal heart rate or 80% of MVV for 6-8 minutes. Spirometry measured at baseline and at 5-minute intervals after exercise. Positive challenge is a fall in FEV$_1$ by ≥15% from baseline

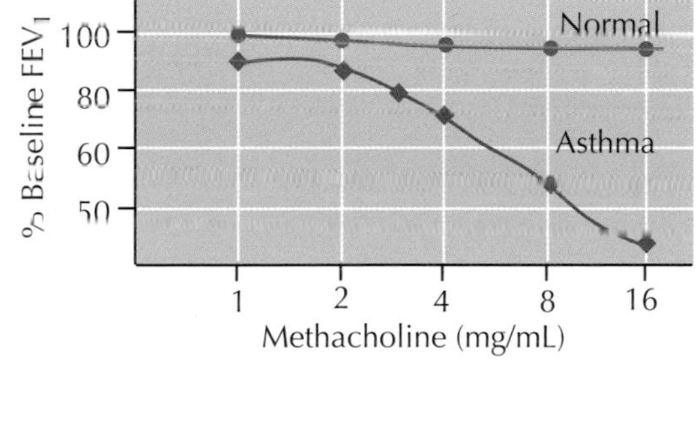

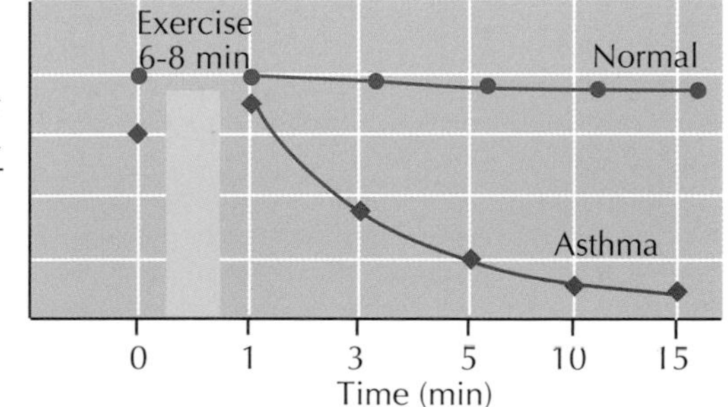

Bronchial Asthma *(Continued)*

obstruction, wheezing may be slight or even absent but may be accentuated by rapid, deep breathing. When airflow is severely reduced, the chest may become paradoxically silent. This ominous finding may be inadvertently induced or worsened by administration of hypnotics, tranquilizers, or sedatives, which depress respiration. At the point where airflow is so decreased that the chest becomes silent, cough becomes ineffective, and ventilatory failure supervenes. This requires immediate and intensive therapy.

DIAGNOSIS OF ASTHMA

Because asthma is a lifelong disease in most patients, it is important to make the correct diagnosis when symptoms first present. Unfortunately, this is sometimes not done, and patients are inappropriately treated. None of the symptoms of asthma are pathognomonic, and the adage "all that wheezes is not asthma" serves as a reminder that wheezing but also cough, chest tightness, and dyspnea are symptoms of other respiratory or cardiac diseases. The diagnosis of asthma must be made by the presence of the characteristic symptoms associated with the presence of variable airflow obstruction or airway hyperresponsiveness to inhaled bronchoconstrictor mediators.

Variable airflow obstruction is best measured using spirometry with a flow-volume loop and demonstrating a reduced FEV$_1$ and ratio of FEV$_1$ to forced vital capacity (FVC), which improves after inhalation of β2-agonists (Plate 4-17). An improvement in FEV$_1$ of more than 12%, with a minimal change of 200 mL, is usually accepted as documentation of reversible airflow obstruction. Some clinics may not have access to spirometry, so variability in peak expired flow (PEF) measurements can also be used for both diagnosis and monitoring asthma. An improvement of more than 20% (or >60 L/min) after inhalation of a β2-agonist or diurnal variation in PEF of more than 20% over 2 weeks of measurements also confirms variable airflow obstruction.

AIRWAY HYPERRESPONSIVENESS

For patients with symptoms consistent with asthma but normal lung function, measurements of airway responsiveness to direct airway challenges (e.g., inhaled methacholine and histamine) or indirect airway challenges (e.g., inhaled mannitol or exercise challenge) may help establish a diagnosis of asthma (Plate 4-17). Measurements of airway responsiveness reflect the "sensitivity" of the airways to factors that can cause asthma symptoms, and the test results are usually expressed as the provocative concentration (or dose) of the agonist causing a given decrease in FEV$_1$. These tests are sensitive for a diagnosis of asthma but have limited specificity. This means that a negative test result can be useful to exclude a diagnosis of persistent asthma in a patient who is not taking inhaled glucocorticosteroid treatment, but a positive test result does not always mean that a patient has asthma. This is because airway hyperresponsiveness has been described in patients with allergic rhinitis and in those with airflow limitation

Sputum in Bronchial Asthma

Unstained smear of asthmatic sputum; schematic (low power)

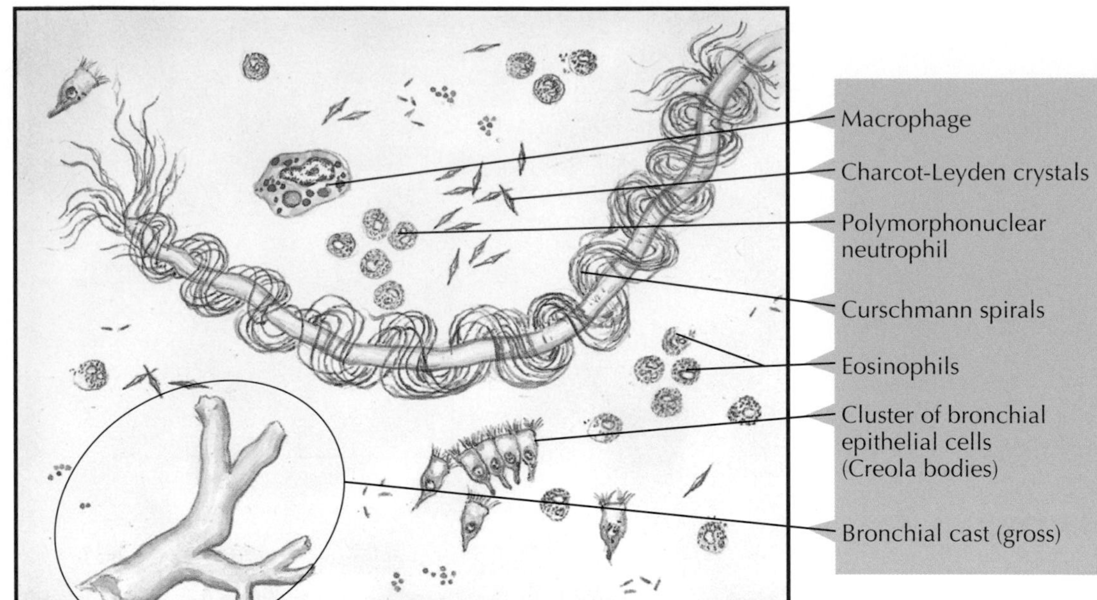

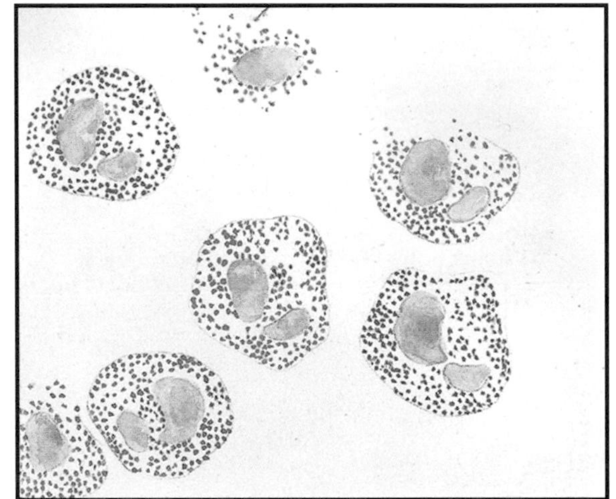

Eosinophils in stained smear

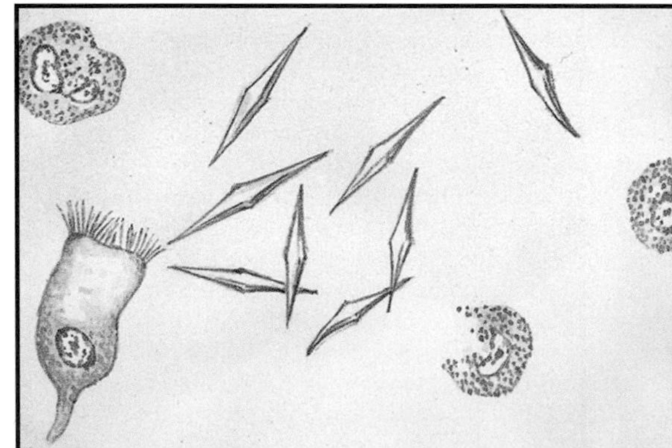

Carcot-Leyden crystals, eosinophils, and epithelial cell under high power

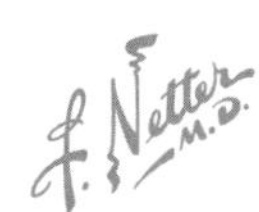

Bronchial Asthma *(Continued)*

caused by conditions other than asthma, such as cystic fibrosis, bronchiectasis, and chronic obstructive pulmonary disease (COPD).

INVESTIGATIONS THAT MAY BE CONSIDERED TO ESTABLISH A DIAGNOSIS

Radiography

The primary value of radiography is to exclude other diseases and to determine whether pneumonia, atelectasis, pneumothorax, pneumomediastinum, or bronchiectasis exists. In mild asthma, the chest radiograph shows no abnormalities. With severe obstruction, however, a characteristic reversible hyperlucency of the lung is evident, with widening of costal interspaces, depressed diaphragms, and increased retrosternal air. In contrast to pulmonary emphysema, in which vascular branching is attenuated and distorted, vascular caliber and distribution in asthma are generally undisturbed.

Focal atelectasis, a complication of asthma, is caused by impaction of mucus. In children, even complete collapse of a lobe may be observed. Atelectatic shadows may be transient as mucus impaction shifts from one lung zone to another. When sputum is mobilized, these patterns resolve.

Radiography is also useful in evaluating coexisting sinusitis. An upper gastrointestinal series may be indicated if gastroesophageal reflux is suspected. A lung ventilation-perfusion scan or computed tomography angiogram may be required if pulmonary emboli are believed to mimic asthma.

Sputum

Spontaneously produced as well as induced sputum can be helpful in confirming the diagnosis of asthma and in deciding treatment requirements (Plate 4-18). Spontaneously produced sputum may be mucoid, purulent, or a mixture of both. Importantly, purulent sputum does not always indicate the presence of a bacterial infection in asthmatic patients.

Thin spiral bronchiolar casts (Curschmann spirals) in sputum, measuring up to several centimeters in length, are strongly indicative of asthma. Ciliated columnar bronchial epithelial cells are frequently found. Creola bodies are clumps of such bronchial epithelial cells with moving cilia and are seen in severe asthma.

In asthma, both sputum eosinophils and neutrophils may be increased or the cellular infiltrate may be predominantly eosinophilic or neutrophilic or occasionally paucigranulocytic. The importance of a sputum eosinophilia is that it indicates inadequate treatment with or poor adherence to inhaled corticosteroids (ICS). Acute exacerbations of asthma are usually associated with an increase in eosinophil or neutrophil cell numbers in sputum.

Skin Prick Tests

It is important to establish the presence of atopy in asthmatic subjects, particularly, whether environmental

SKIN TESTING FOR ALLERGY
Syringe of epinephrine
Tourniquet
Array of commercially available test antigens
A. Scratch test:
1. Single drops of control and suspected antigens applied to volar surface of forearm (or other nonhirsute skin surface)
2. Small prick or scratch made through each droplet; clean stylet used for each
B. Intradermal test: Method more sensitive but more likely to produce systemic reaction
C. Interpretation
Erythema but no wheal
++
Erythema and wheal without pseudopodia
++++
Negative (or control)
Erythema plus 15-mm wheal with pseudopodia
++++

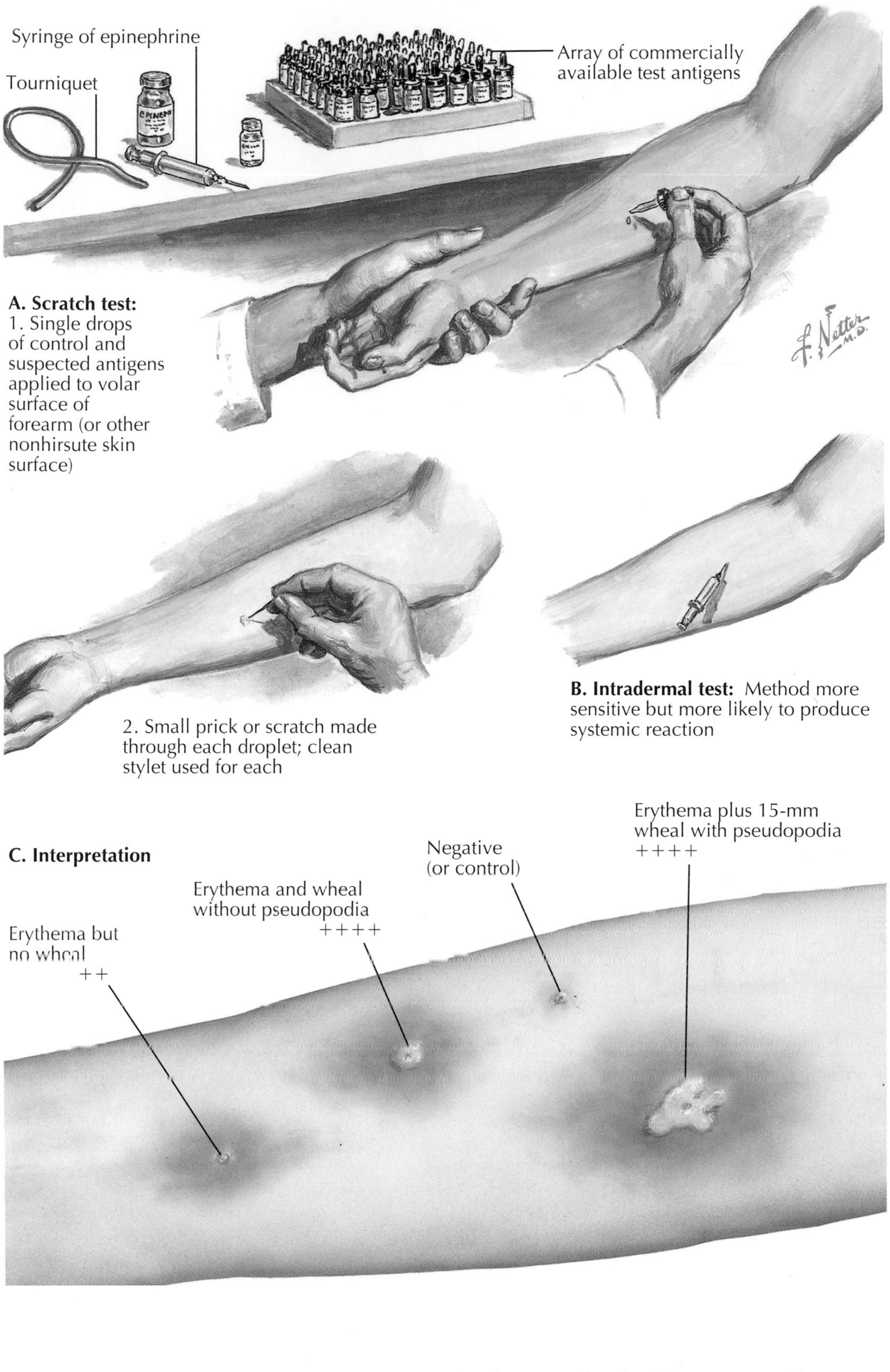

BRONCHIAL ASTHMA *(Continued)*

allergens are important triggers of asthma symptoms. Preferably, skin tests are performed by a skin prick using aqueous extracts of common antigens, such as molds, pollens, fungi, house dusts, feathers, foods, or animal dander technique (Plate 4-19). If skin-sensitizing antibodies to the antigen are present, a wheal-and-flare reaction develops within 15 to 30 minutes; a control test with saline diluent should show little or no reaction.

Optimally, both the history and dermal reactivity will give corresponding results. However, some patients have positive histories but negative skin test results. In other patients, negative histories and positive skin test results indicate immunologic reactivity that is clinically insignificant.

Blood Tests

Blood tests are rarely of value in the diagnosis of asthma, but radioallergosorbent tests (RASTs) are used to identify the presence of allergy to specific allergens. Also, blood eosinophil counts may be increased in asthmatic patients, but they are neither sensitive nor specific for a diagnosis.

Exhaled Nitric Oxide

Elevated levels of exhaled nitric oxide (eNO) may indicate eosinophilic inflammation associated with asthma in the right clinical setting, but the clinical utility of this test is still uncertain.

DIFFERENTIAL DIAGNOSIS

Diseases to be considered in the differential evaluation are depicted in Plate 4-20. In children, diseases that may be misdiagnosed as asthma also include chronic rhinosinusitis, gastroesophageal reflux, cystic fibrosis, bronchopulmonary dysplasia, congenital malformation causing narrowing of the intrathoracic airways, foreign body aspiration, primary ciliary dyskinesia syndrome, immune deficiency, and congenital heart disease. In adult patients, pulmonary disorders, other than those illustrated in Plate 4-20, include cystic fibrosis, pneumoconiosis, and systemic vasculitis involving the lungs.

PHYSIOLOGIC ABNORMALITIES IN ASTHMA

Spirometry and Ventilatory Function in Asthma

In asthma, the prime physiologic disturbance is obstruction to airflow, which is more marked in expiration. This obstruction is variable in severity and in its site of involvement and is, by definition, reversible to some degree. Various combinations of smooth muscle constriction, inflammation, edema, and mucus hypersecretion produce this airflow impediment. In addition, low lung volumes with terminal airspace collapse may compound the airway obstruction. In the larger airways, the rigid cartilaginous rings help maintain patency. In the peripheral airways, however, there is little opposition

Representative Differential Diagnosis of Bronchial Asthma

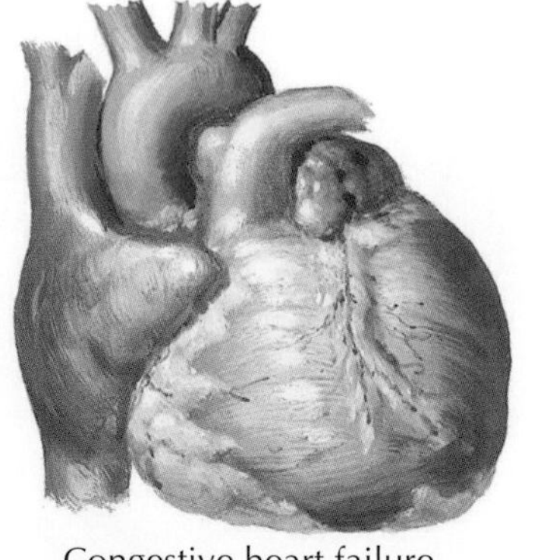
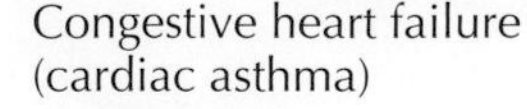
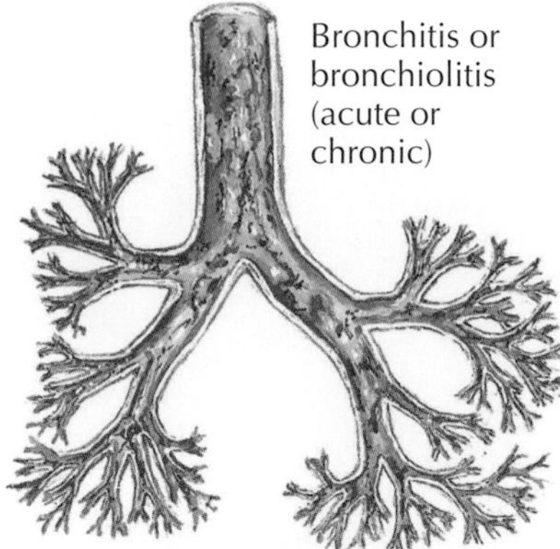
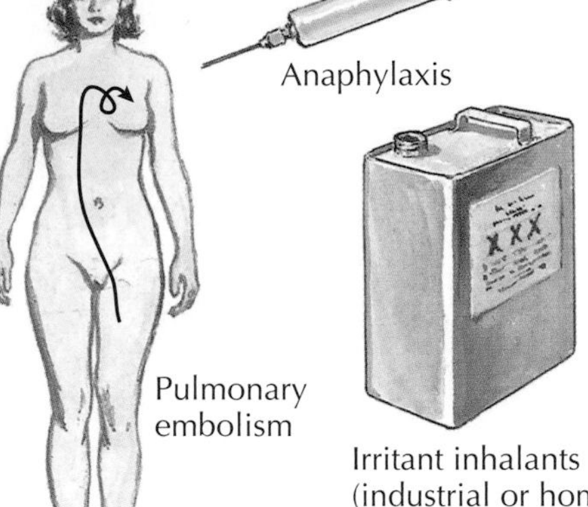
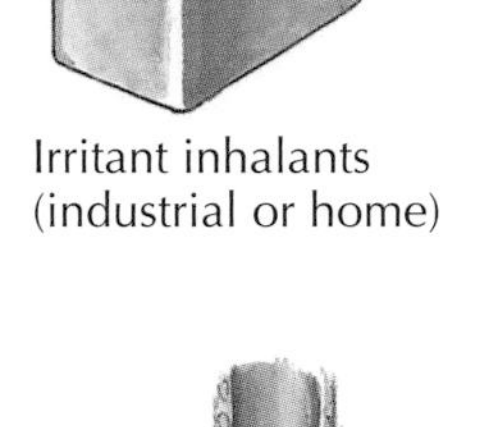
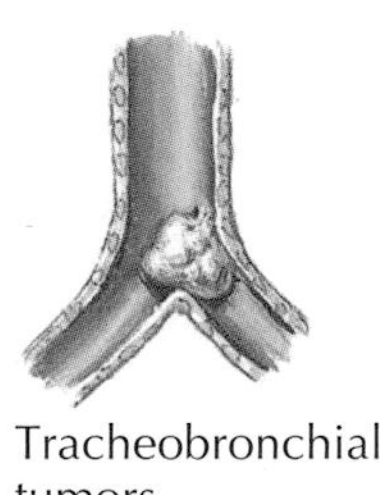
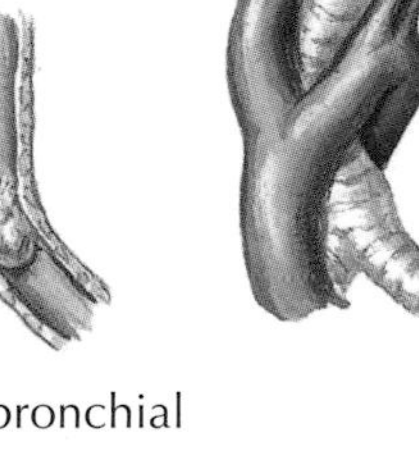
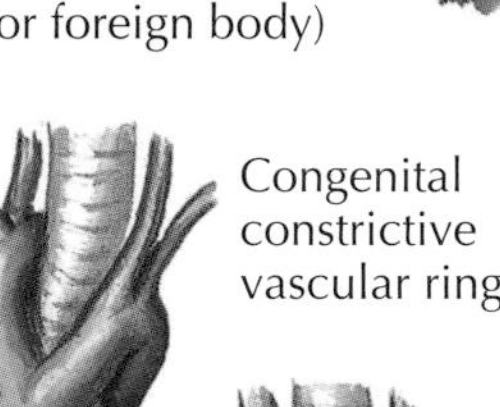
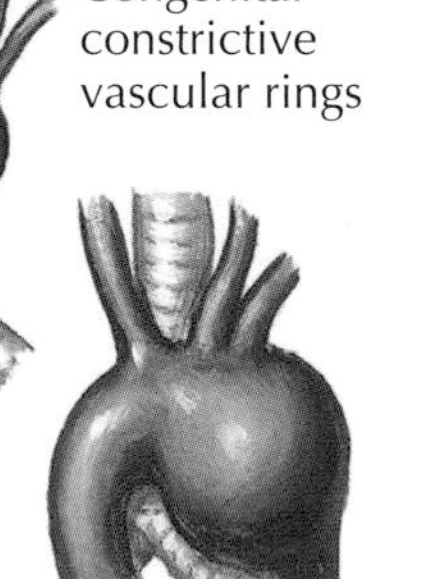
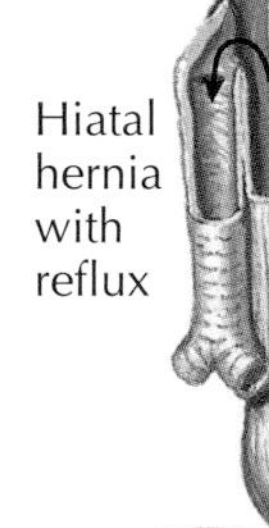
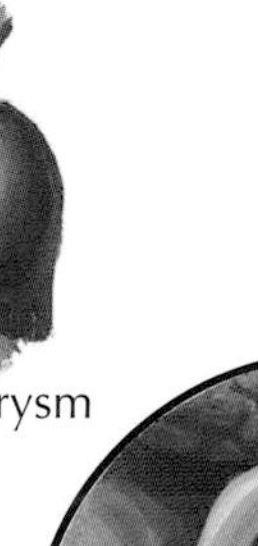
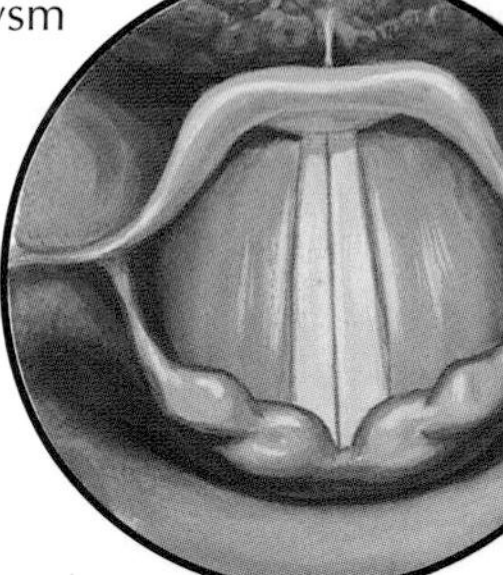
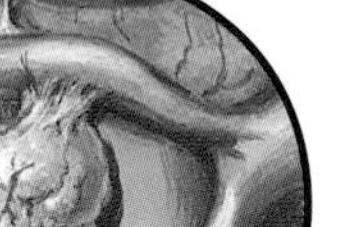
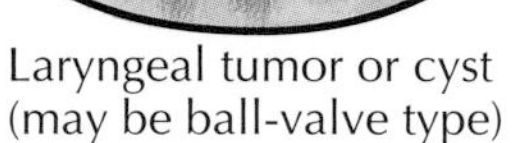

Bronchial Asthma *(Continued)*

to the smooth muscle action because of the paucity of cartilage. Instead, the patency of these airways is influenced by lung volume because they are imbedded in and partially supported by the lung parenchyma.

At the onset of an asthmatic attack, or in mild cases, obstruction is not extensive. As asthma progresses, airways resistance significantly increases. Although inspiratory resistance also increases, the abnormality is more pronounced during expiration because of narrowing or closure of the airways as the lung empties. At this point, further expiratory effort does not produce any increase in expiratory flow rate and may even intensify airway collapse.

Because of these mechanical resistances, the respiratory muscles must produce a greater degree of chest expansion. More important, the elastic recoil of the lungs is insufficient for "passive" expiration. The respiratory muscles, therefore, must now play an active role in expiration. If obstruction is severe, air trapping will occur, with an increase in residual volume (RV) and functional residual capacity (FRC).

Airway obstruction is uneven and results in unequal distribution of gases to alveoli. This and other stimuli result in tachypnea and a consequently shortened respiratory cycle even though the bronchial obstruction requires a lengthened respiratory time for adequate ventilation. These conflicting demands cannot be reconciled while the asthmatic attack continues.

The severity of the obstruction is reflected in the spirometric measurements of expiratory volume and airflow. The FEV_1, FVC, and inspiratory capacity (IC) are all reduced during an acute attack.

The peripheral airways have a proportionately large total cross-sectional area. For this reason, the resistance of the peripheral airways normally accounts for only 20% of the total airway resistance. Thus, extensive obstruction in these smaller airways may go undetected if the physician relies only on clinical findings. The reduction in FVC and FEV_1 shows a good correlation with the decrease in PaO_2, although carbon dioxide retention does not occur until the FEV_1 is about 1 L or 25% of the level predicted.

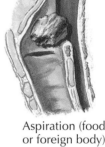

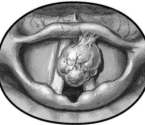

With progressive obstruction, expiration becomes increasingly prolonged. Increases in RV and FRC occur (see Plate 4-39). These volume changes may represent an inherent physiologic response by the patient because breathing at higher lung volumes prevents the closure of terminal airways. The overall effect of these events is alveolar hyperinflation, which tends to further increase the diameter of the airways by exerting a greater lateral force on their walls. This hyperinflation may partially preserve gas exchange. It is disadvantageous because much more work is required, resulting in an increase in O_2 consumption. Moreover, such a state compromises IC and vital capacity (VC). The symptoms of dyspnea and fatigue may also arise in part from this process. Finally, the effectiveness of cough is impaired because the velocity of respiratory airflow is seriously reduced.

As a result of the nonhomogeneous airway obstruction in asthma, the distribution of inspired air to the terminal respiratory units is not uniform throughout the lungs. Alveoli that are hypoventilated because they are supplied by obstructed airways are interspersed with normal or hyperventilated alveoli; hence, the

BLOOD GAS AND PH RELATIONSHIPS

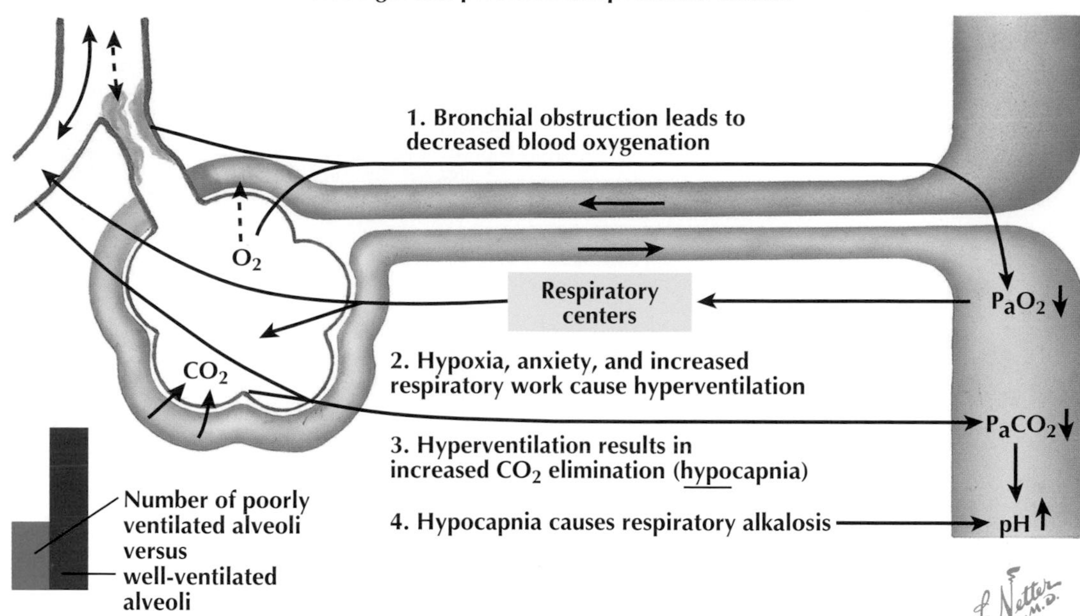

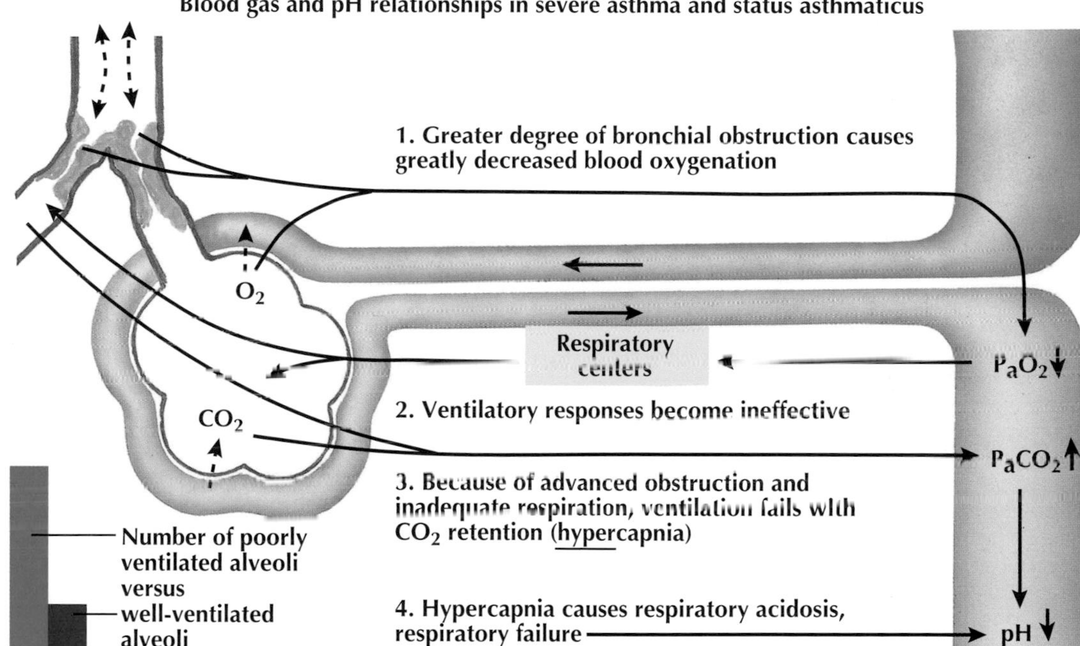

BRONCHIAL ASTHMA *(Continued)*

severity of asthma is directly related to the ratio of poorly ventilated to well-ventilated alveolar groups. Arterial hypoxemia, which is the primary defect in gas exchange in asthma, is caused by this $\dot{V}_A/\dot{Q}_C$ nonhomogeneity (Plate 4-21). As the population of alveolar units with a low $\dot{V}_A/\dot{Q}_C$ ratio increases (because of advancing obstruction), the degree of arterial hypoxemia also intensifies. The $\dot{V}_A/\dot{Q}_C$ disturbance is compounded if some airways are completely obstructed. The right-to-left intrapulmonary shunt effect results in arterial hypoxemia.

Carbon dioxide elimination is not impaired when the number of alveolar-capillary units with normal $\dot{V}_A/\dot{Q}_C$ ratios remains large relative to the number of those with low $\dot{V}_A/\dot{Q}_C$ ratios. As airway obstruction progresses, there are more and more hypoventilated alveoli. Simultaneously, appropriate increases in respiratory work, rate, and depth occur. Such a response initially minimizes the increase in physiologic dead space but eventually becomes limited, and alveolar ventilation finally fails to support the metabolic needs of the body. Carbon dioxide retention now occurs together with increasing hypoxemia. This is a state of ventilatory failure, and it commonly arises when the FEV_1 is less than 25% predicted.

PATHOGENESIS OF ASTHMA

Genetics

Genetic and environmental factors interact in a complex manner to produce both asthma susceptibility and asthma expression. Several genes on chromosome 5q31-33 may be important in the development or progression of the inflammation associated with asthma and atopy, including the cytokines interleukin-3 (IL-3), IL-4, IL-5, IL-9, IL-12, IL-13, and granulocyte-macrophage colony-stimulating factor (GM-CSF). In addition, a number of other genes may play a role in the development of asthma or its pathogenesis, including the corticosteroid receptor and the β2-adrenergic receptor. Chromosome 5q32 contains the gene for the β2-adrenoceptor, which is highly polymorphic, and a number of variants of this gene have been discovered that alter receptor functioning and response to β-agonists.

Other chromosome regions linked to the development of allergy or asthma include chromosome 11q, which contains the gene for the β chain of the high-affinity IgE receptor (FcεRIβ). Chromosome 12 also contains several candidate genes, including interferon-γ (INF-γ), stem cell factor (SCF), IGF-1, and the constitutive form of nitric oxide synthase (cNOS). The *ADAM 33* gene (a disintegrin and metalloproteinase 33) on chromosome 20p13 has been significantly associated with asthma. ADAM proteins are membrane-anchored proteolytic enzymes. The restricted expression of *ADAM 33* to mesenchymal cells and its close association with airways hyperresponsiveness (AHR) suggests it may be operating in airway smooth muscle or in events linked to airway remodeling.

Cellular Inflammation

Persistent airway inflammation is considered the characteristic feature of severe, mild, and even asymptomatic asthma. The characteristic features include infiltration of the airways by inflammatory cells, hypertrophy of the airway smooth muscle, and thickening of the lamina reticularis just below the basement membrane (see Plate 4-22).

An important feature of the airway inflammatory infiltrate in asthma is its multicellular nature, which is mainly composed of eosinophils but also includes neutrophils, lymphocytes, and other cells in varying degrees. Whereas neutrophils, eosinophils, and T

AIRWAY PATHOPHYSIOLOGY IN ASTHMA

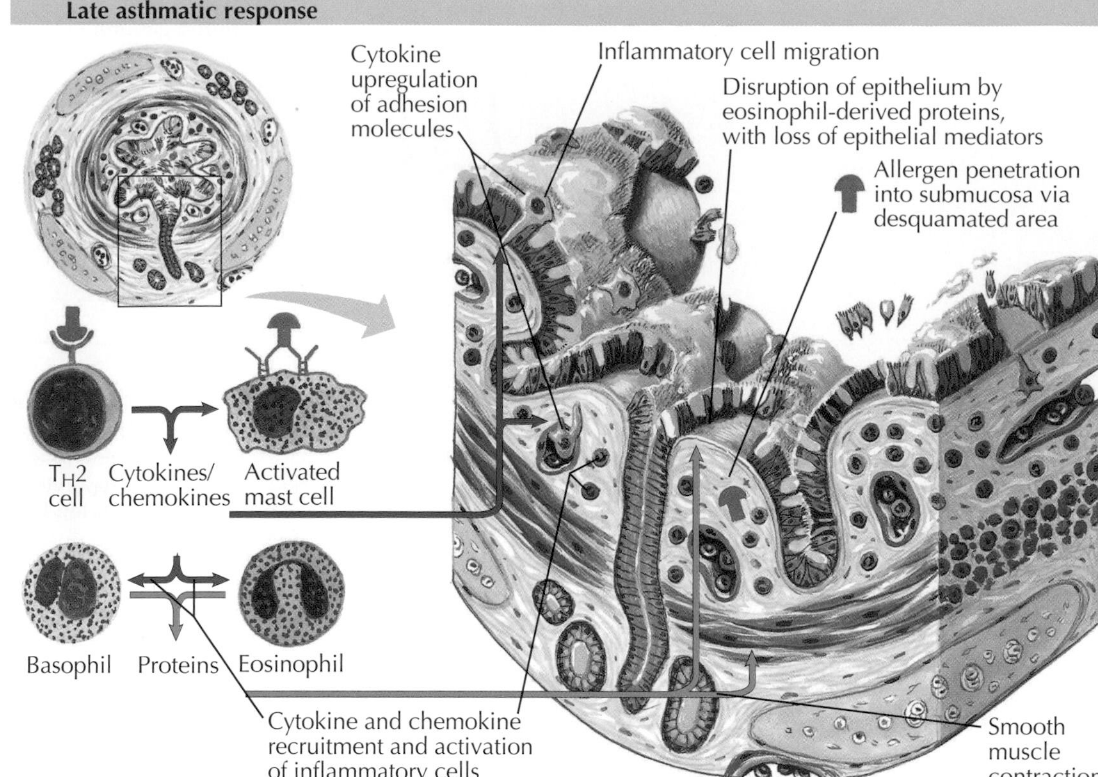

Late asthmatic response characterized by inflammatory changes mediated by cytokines and chemokines, and epithelial disruption mediated by eosinophils and basophils

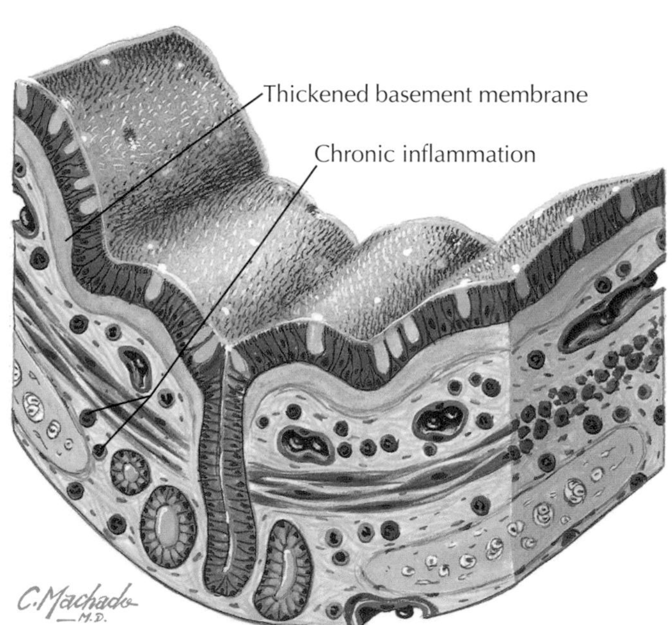

Chronic asthma exhibits chronic low-grade inflammation, which extends beyond the muscularis, where it is less susceptible to inhaled medications. Thickening of basement membrane occurs secondary to inflammation

BRONCHIAL ASTHMA *(Continued)*

lymphocytes are recruited from the circulation, mast cells are resident cells of the airways. Histologic evidence of mast cell degranulation and eosinophil vacuolation reveals that the inflammatory cells are activated. The mucosal mast cells are not increased but show signs of granule secretion in asthmatic patients. Postmortem studies have shown an apparent reduction in the number of mast cells in the asthmatic bronchi as well as in the lung parenchyma, which reflects mast cell degranulation rather than a true reduction in their numbers.

Eosinophils are considered to be the predominant and most characteristic cells in asthma, as observed from both bronchoalveolar lavage (BAL) and bronchial biopsy studies. The bronchial epithelium is infiltrated by eosinophils, which is evident in both large and small airways, with a greater intensity in the proximal airways in acute severe asthma. However, some studies report the virtual absence of eosinophils in severe or fatal asthma, suggesting some heterogeneity in this process. Alveolar macrophages are the most prevalent cells in the human lungs, both in normal subjects and in asthmatic patients and, when activated, secrete a wide array of mediators. Lymphocytes are critical for the development of asthma and are found in the airways of asthmatic subjects in relationship to disease severity. The function and contribution of lymphocytes in asthma are multifactorial and center on their ability to secrete cytokines. Activated T cells are a source of Th2 cytokines (e.g., IL-4, IL-13), which may induce the activated B cell to produce IgE and enhance expression of cellular adhesion molecules, in particular vascular cell adhesion molecule-1 (VCAM-1) and IL-5, which is essential for eosinophil development and survival in tissues.

IMMUNOLOGIC ABNORMALITIES

Allergic asthma and other allergic diseases, such as allergic rhinitis and anaphylaxis, develop as a result of sensitization to environmental allergens and subsequent immunologically mediated responses when the allergens are encountered. These allergic reactions take place in specific target organs, such as the lungs, gastrointestinal tract, or skin. These immune processes leading to allergic reactions represent the disease state referred to clinically as "atopy." The immune sequence consists of the sensitization phase followed by a challenge reaction, which produces the clinical syndrome concerned (see Plate 4-23).

Sensitization to an allergen occurs when the otherwise innocuous allergen is encountered for the first time. Professional antigen-presenting cells (APCs) such as monocytes, macrophages, and immature dendritic cells capture the antigen and degrade it into short immunogenic peptides. Cleaved antigenic fragments are presented to naïve CD4+ T-helper (Th) cells on MHC class II molecules. Depending on a multitude of factors, particularly the cytokine microenvironment, these naïve T-helper cells are subsequently polarized into Th1 or Th2 lymphocytes. Th1 lymphocytes predominantly secrete IL-2, INF-γ, and tumor necrosis factor (TNF)-β to induce a cellular immune response. In contrast, Th2 lymphocytes secrete IL-4, IL-5, IL-9,

Mechanism of Type 1 (Immediate) Hypersensitivity

After sensitization to allergen, T-helper cells are skewed toward a T_H2 cytokine profile, resulting in a humoral immune response (production of IgE) and activation of eosinophils and mast cells and mucus secretion, all of which result in airway inflammation and airway narrowing

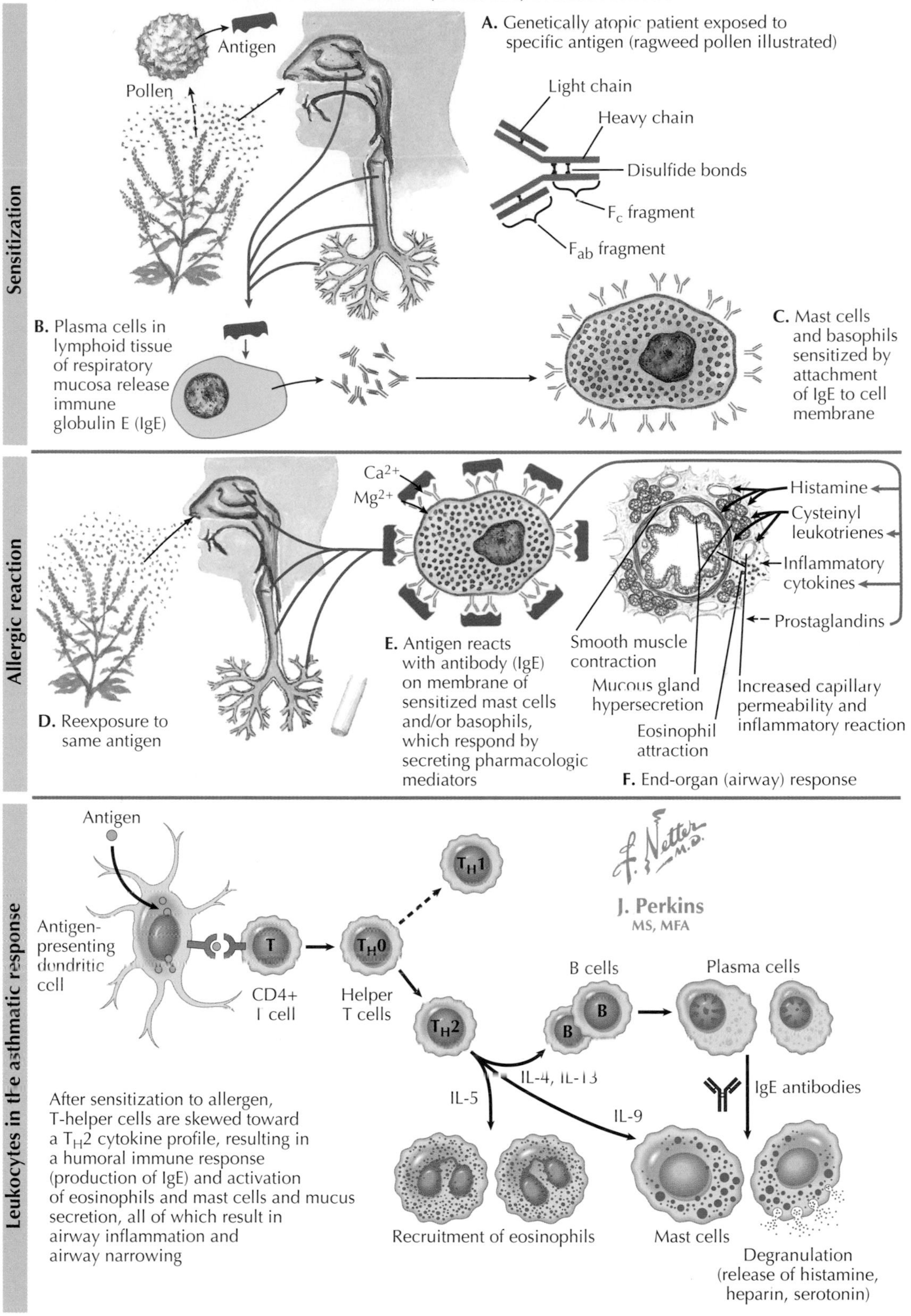

Bronchial Asthma *(Continued)*

and IL-13 cytokines to induce a humoral immune response, particularly the B-cell class switch to allergen-specific immunoglobulin E (IgE) production. In allergic asthma, an imbalance exists between Th1 and Th2 lymphocytes, with a shift in immunity from a Th1 pattern toward a Th2 profile. Accordingly, allergic asthma is often referred to a Th2-mediated disorder, with a persistent Th2-skewed immune response to inhaled allergens (Plate 4-23).

IgE is a γ-l-glycoprotein and is the least abundant antibody in serum, with a concentration of 150 ng/mL compared with 10 mg/mL for IgG in normal individuals. However, IgE concentrations in the circulation may reach more than 10 times the normal level in "atopic" individuals. IgE levels are also increased in patients with parasitic infestations and hyper-IgE syndrome. Increased serum concentration is not necessarily a specific indicator of the extent or severity of allergy in the individual concerned. The IgE molecules attach to the surfaces of the mast cells or other cells such as basophils. The mast cells containing IgE are distributed in the mucosa of the upper and lower respiratory tract and perivascular connective tissues of the lung.

After sensitization to an allergen has occurred, reexposure of the patient to the allergen may result in an acute allergic reaction, also known as an immediate hypersensitivity reaction (Plate 4-23). IgE-sensitized mast cells in contact with the specific antigen secrete preformed and newly synthesized mediators, including histamine, cysteinyl leukotrienes, kinins, prostaglandins and thromboxane, and platelet activating factor. Also, mast cells are sources of proinflammatory cytokines. Each antigen molecule has to bridge at least two of the IgE molecules bound to the surface of the cell. The subsequent airway smooth muscle contraction, vasoconstriction, and hypersecretion of mucus, together with an inflammatory response of increased capillary permeability and cellular infiltration with eosinophils and neutrophils follows, producing asthma symptoms.

Pathologic Changes in Asthma

The initial knowledge of the pathology of asthma came from postmortem studies of fatal asthma or airways of patients with asthma who have died of other causes or who had undergone lung resections. All showed similar, although variably severe, pathologic changes and provided key directives as to the causes and consequences of the inflammatory reactions in the airway (see Plate 4-24).

The characteristic mucus plugs in asthmatic airways can cause airway obstruction, leading to ventilation-perfusion mismatch and contributing to hypoxemia. Mucus plugs are composed of mucus, serum proteins, inflammatory cells, and cellular debris, which include desquamated epithelial cells and macrophages often arranged in a spiral pattern (Curschmann spirals). The excessive mucus production in fatal asthma is attributed to hypertrophy and hyperplasia of the submucosal glands. The mucus also contains increased quantities of nucleic acids, glycoproteins, and albumin, making it more viscous. This altered mucous rheology, coupled

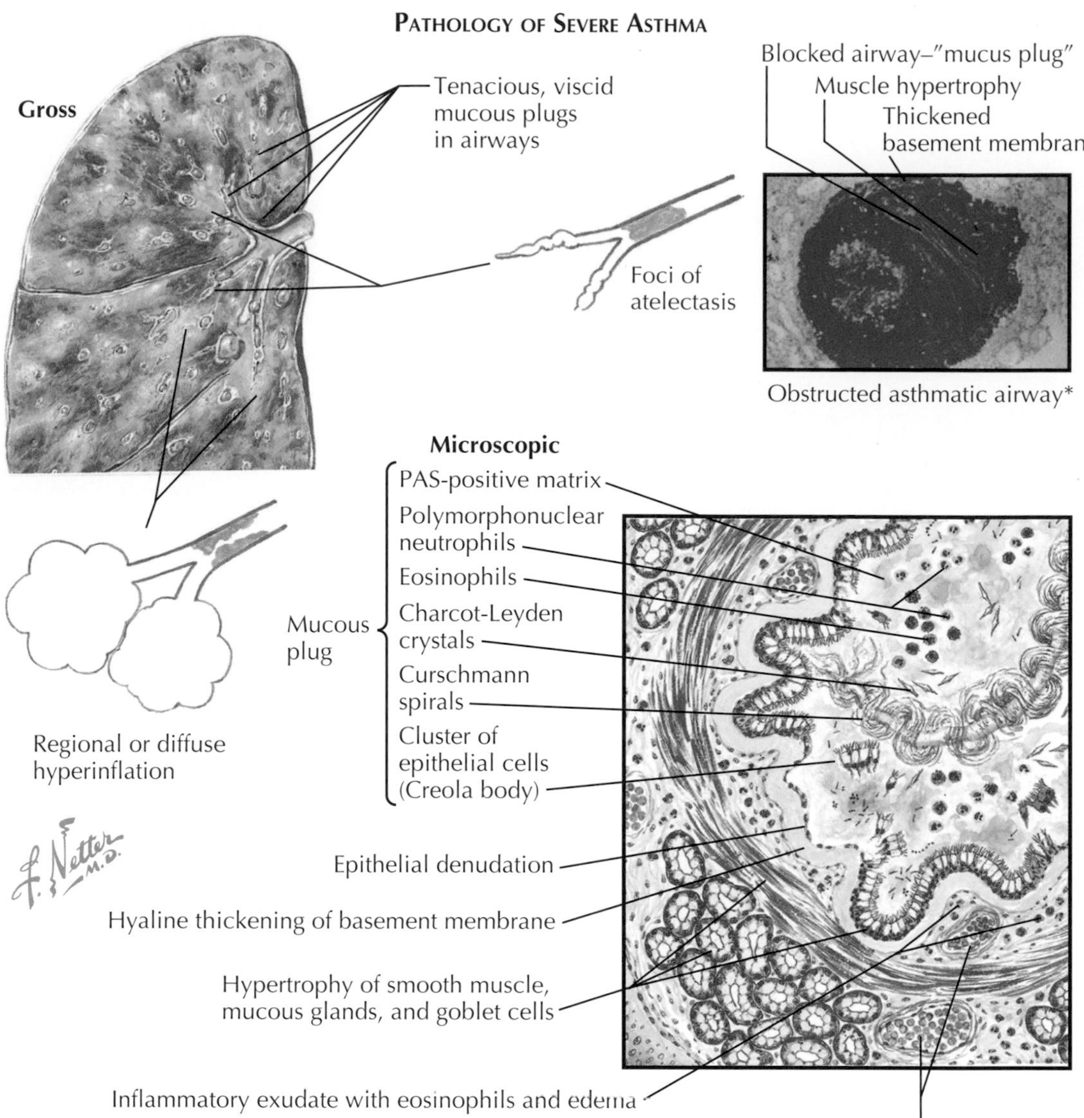

Microscopy of airway

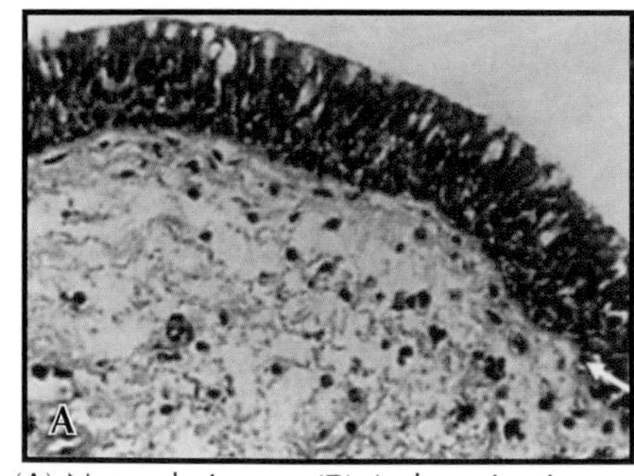

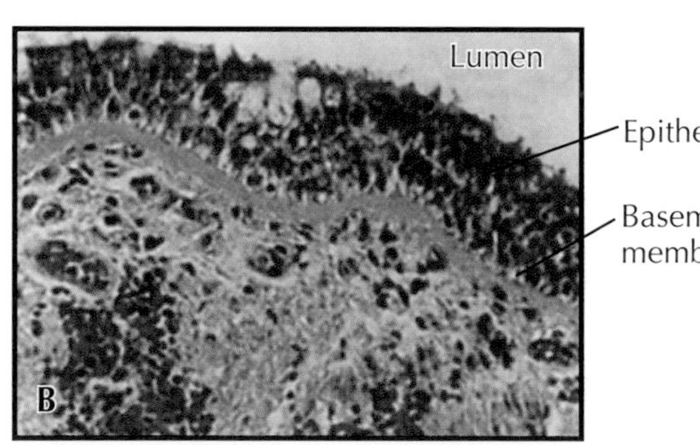

(**A**) Normal airway. (**B**) Asthmatic airway before therapy with high-dose inhaled steroids demonstrating remodeling.

BRONCHIAL ASTHMA *(Continued)*

with the loss of ciliated epithelium, impairs mucociliary clearance.

The airway wall thickness is increased in asthma and is related to disease severity. Compared with nonasthmatic subjects, the airway wall thickness is increased from 50% to 300% in patients with fatal asthma and from 10% to 100% in nonfatal asthma. The greater thickness results from an increase in most tissue compartments, including smooth muscle, epithelium, submucosa, adventitia, and mucosal glands. The inflammatory edema involves the whole airway, particularly the submucosal layer, with marked hypertrophy and hyperplasia of the submucosal glands and goblet cell hyperplasia. Goblet cell hyperplasia and hypertrophy accompany the loss of epithelial cells. There is hyperplasia of the muscularis layer and microvascular vasodilation in the adventitial layers of the airways. Also, morphometric studies have shown that the bronchial lamina propria of asthmatic subjects had a larger number of vessels occupying a larger percentage area than in nonasthmatic subjects and in some circumstances correlated with the severity of disease.

LONG-TERM MANAGEMENT OF ASTHMA

Asthma treatment guidelines have been remarkably consistent in identifying the goals and objectives of asthma treatment. These are to (1) minimize or eliminate asthma symptoms, (2) achieve the best possible lung function, (3) prevent asthma exacerbations, (4) do the above with the fewest possible medications, (5) minimize short- and long-term adverse effects, and (6) educate the patient about the disease and the goals of management. One other important objective should be the prevention of the decline in lung function and the development of fixed airflow obstruction, which occur in some asthmatic patients. In addition to these goals and objectives, each of these documents has described what is meant by the term *asthma control*. This includes the above objectives but also includes minimizing the need for rescue medications, such as inhaled β_2-agonists, to less than daily use; minimizing the variability of flow rates that is characteristic of asthma; and having normal activities of daily living. Achieving this level of asthma control should be an objective from the very first visit of the patient to the treating physician.

The pharmacologic treatment of patients with asthma must only be considered in the context of asthma education and avoidance of inducers of the disease (see Plate 4-25).

Mild Persistent Asthma

Low doses of inhaled corticosteroids (ICS) can often provide ideal asthma control and reduce the risks of severe asthma exacerbations in both children and adults with mild persistent asthma, and they should be the treatment of choice. ICS are the most effective anti-inflammatory medications for asthma treatment. The mechanisms of action of asthma medications are depicted in Plate 4-26. There is no convincing evidence that regular use of combination therapy with ICS and inhaled long-acting β_2-agonists (LABA) provides any

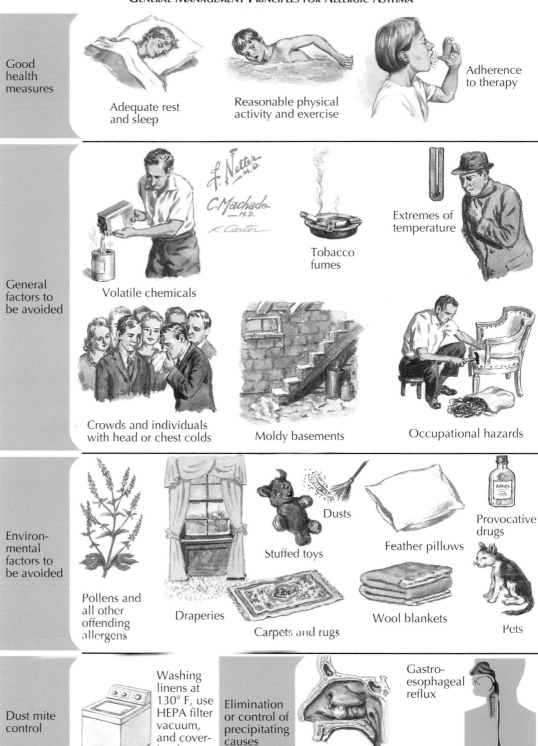

Bronchial Asthma *(Continued)*

additional benefit. Leukotriene receptor antagonists (LTRAs) are another treatment option in this population, but they are also less effective than low-dose ICS. There are considerable inter- and intraindividual differences in responses to any therapy. This is also true for response to treatment with ICS and LTRAs in both adults and in children. Although on average, ICS improve almost all asthma outcomes more than LTRAs some patients may show a greater response to LTRAs. Currently, it is not possible to accurately identify these responders based on their clinical, physiologic, or pharmacogenomic characteristics.

The other issue that needs to be considered when making a decision to start ICS treatment in patients with mild asthma is the potential for side effects. ICS are not metabolized in the lungs, and every molecule of ICS that is administered into the lungs is absorbed into the systemic circulation. All of the studies in patients with mild persistent asthma have used low doses of ICS (maximal doses, 400 μg/d). A wealth of data are available demonstrating the safety of these low doses, even used long term, in adults. However, a significant reduction in growth velocity has been demonstrated with low doses of ICS in children. This is unlikely to have any effect on the final height of these children because the one study that has followed children treated with ICS to final height did not show any detrimental effect even with a moderate daily ICS doses.

Moderate Persistent Asthma

These patients have asthma that is not well controlled on low doses of ICS. Asthma treatment guidelines recommend that combination therapy with ICS and a LABA is the preferred treatment option in these patients. This is because the use of combination treatment of ICS and LABA for moderate persistent asthma has also been demonstrated to improve all indicators of asthma control compared with ICS alone. It is important to note that the evidence of the enhanced benefit of combination therapy with ICS and LABA in moderate persistent asthma exists mainly in adults with asthma. Another recently described treatment approach for the management of patients with moderate asthma is the use of an inhaler containing the combination of the ICS budesonide and the LABA formoterol, both as maintenance and as relief therapy, which has been shown to reduce the risk of severe asthma exacerbations compared with the other approaches studied with an associated reduction in oral corticosteroid use.

Several studies have compared the clinical benefit when LTRAs are added to ICS in patients with moderate persistent asthma in both adults and children. The addition of LTRAs to ICS may modestly improve asthma control compared with ICS alone, but this strategy cannot be recommended as a substitute for increasing the dose of ICS. In addition, LTRAs have been shown to be less effective than LABAs when combined with ICS. Low-dose theophylline has also been evaluated as an add-on therapy to ICS. The magnitude of benefit achieved is less than for LABAs. Another potential treatment option for patients with moderate asthma is omalizumab, which is a

MECHANISMS OF ASTHMA MEDICATIONS

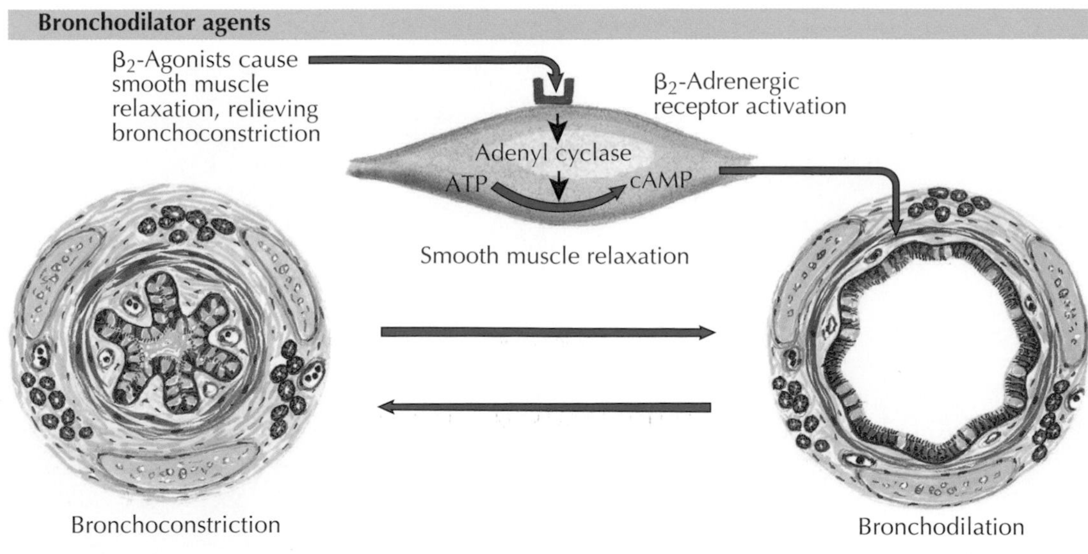

BRONCHIAL ASTHMA *(Continued)*

recombinant humanized monoclonal antibody against IgE. This anti-IgE antibody forms complexes with free IgE, thus blocking the interaction between IgE and effector cells and reducing serum concentrations of free IgE. Compared with placebo in patients on moderate to high doses of ICS, omalizumab reduces asthma exacerbations and enables a small but statistically significant reduction in the dose of ICS. However, this treatment has not been compared with proven additive therapies such as LABAs that are less expensive. Therefore, this therapy is currently recommended in international guidelines for patients with moderate to severe asthma.

Severe Persistent Asthma

Patients with severe asthma are those who do not respond adequately to even high doses of ICS and LABAs. This population disproportionately consumes health care resources related to asthma. Physiologically, these patients often have air trapping, airway collapsibility, and a high degree of AHR. Patients with severe difficult-to-treat asthma are most often adult patients with significant comorbidities, including severe rhinosinusitis, gastroesophageal reflux, obesity, and anxiety disorders. Often this population requires oral corticosteroids in addition to ICS in an effort to achieve asthma control.

TREATMENT OF SEVERE ASTHMA EXACERBATIONS

Episodes of acute severe asthma (asthma exacerbations) are episodes of progressive increase in shortness of breath, cough, wheezing, chest tightness, or some combination and are characterized by airflow obstruction that can be quantified by measurement of PEF or FEV_1. These measurements are more reliable indicators of the severity of airflow limitation than is the degree of symptoms. Severe exacerbations are potentially life threatening, and their treatment requires close supervision. Patients with severe exacerbations should be encouraged to see their physicians promptly or to proceed to the nearest hospital that provides emergency access for patients with acute asthma. Close objective monitoring of the response to therapy is essential.

The primary therapies for severe asthma exacerbations include repetitive administration of rapid-acting inhaled β_2-agonists, 2 to 4 puffs every 20 minutes for the first hour (see Plate 4-27). After the first hour, the dose of β_2-agonists required depends on the severity of the exacerbation and the response of the previously administered inhaled β_2-agonists. A combination of inhaled β_2-agonist with an anticholinergic (ipratropium bromide) may produce better bronchodilation than either drug alone. Oxygen should be administered by nasal cannula or by mask and should be titrated against pulse oximetry to maintain a satisfactory oxygen saturation of 90% or above (≥95% in children).

EMERGENCY DEPARTMENT MANAGEMENT OF ASTHMA

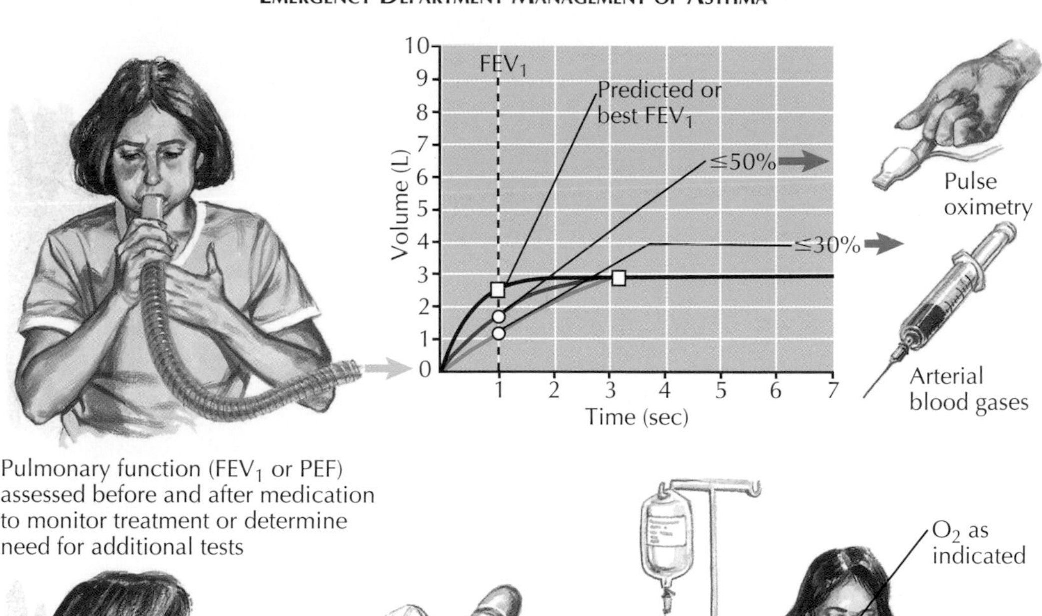

Pulmonary function (FEV$_1$ or PEF) assessed before and after medication to monitor treatment or determine need for additional tests

O$_2$ as indicated

Systemic corticosteroid therapy (oral or parenteral) for all asthma emergencies

JOHN A.CRAIG—AD
C.Machado—M.D.

Patient response to initial therapy better indicator of need for further therapy or hospitalization than severity of exacerbation

Bronchodilator therapy (β_2-agonist) started immediately and maintained intermittently or continuously until pulmonary function within desired limits

1 hour

Discharge criteria

FEV$_1$
Predicted or best FEV$_1$
Posttreatment FEV$_1$ ≥70%
Pretreatment FEV$_1$
Volume (L)
Time (sec)

MANAGEMENT PLAN

Normal physical examination, no symptoms, and FEV$_1$ ≥70% for at least 1 hour since last treatment

Oral corticosteroids, inhaled corticosteroids, long- and short-acting bronchodilators, plus written asthma action plan

BRONCHIAL ASTHMA *(Continued)*

Systemic glucocorticosteroids speed resolution of exacerbations and should be used in all but the mildest exacerbations, especially if the initial rapid-acting inhaled β_2-agonist therapy fails to achieve lasting improvement. Oral glucocorticosteroids are usually as effective as those administered intravenously and are preferred because this route of delivery is less invasive. The aims of treatment are to relieve airflow obstruction and hypoxemia as quickly as possible and to plan the prevention of future relapses. Sedation should be strictly avoided during exacerbations of asthma because of the respiratory depressant effect of anxiolytic and hypnotic drugs.

Patients at high risk of asthma-related death should be encouraged to seek urgent care early in the course of their exacerbations. These patients include those with a previous history of near-fatal asthma requiring intubation and mechanical ventilation, who have had a hospitalization or emergency care visit for asthma in the past year, who are currently using or have recently stopped using oral glucocorticosteroids, who are over-dependent on rapid-acting inhaled β_2-agonists, who have a history of psychiatric disease or psychosocial problems, and who have a history of noncompliance with an asthma medication plan.

The response to treatment may take time, and patients should be closely monitored using clinical as well as objective measurements. The increased treatment should continue until measurements of lung function return to their previous best level or there is a plateau in the response to the inhaled β_2-agonists, at which time a decision to admit or discharge the patient can be made based on these values. Patients who can be safely discharged will have responded within the first 2 hours, at which time decisions regarding patient disposition can be made. Patients with a pretreatment FEV$_1$ or peak expiratory flow (PEF) below 25% percent predicted or those with a posttreatment FEV$_1$ or PEF below 40% percent predicted usually require hospitalization. Patients with posttreatment lung function of 40% to 60% predicted can often be discharged from the emergency setting provided that adequate follow-up is available in the community and their compliance with treatment is assured.

For patients discharged from the emergency department, a minimum of a 7-day course of oral glucocorticosteroids for adults and a shorter course (3-5 days) for children should be prescribed along with continuation of bronchodilator therapy. The bronchodilator can be used on an as-needed basis, based on both symptomatic and objective improvement. Patients should initiate or continue inhaled glucocorticosteroids. The patient's inhaler technique and use of peak flow meter to monitor therapy at home should be reviewed. The factors that precipitated the exacerbation should be identified and strategies for their future avoidance implemented. The patient's response to the exacerbation should be evaluated, and an asthma action plan should be reviewed and written guidance provided.

Chronic Obstructive Pulmonary Disease

Chronic obstructive pulmonary disease (COPD) is a chronic disease that is defined by progressive airflow obstruction that is not completely reversible. COPD is caused by chronic inflammation of the airways and lung parenchyma that develops in response to environmental insults, including cigarette smoke, and manifests clinically with symptoms of cough, dyspnea on exertion, and wheezing. Patients with COPD usually live a number of years with progressive disability and multiple acute exacerbations. Thus, the physician is likely to become involved for many years in the assessment, treatment, and education of a patient with COPD.

SUBTYPES

COPD is a disorder that is characterized by slow emptying of the lung during a forced expiration (see Plate 4-39). In practice, this is measured as the ratio of forced expiratory volume in 1 second (FEV_1) to forced vital capacity (FVC), and the arbitrary definition of airflow obstruction is generally taken to be an FEV_1/FVC ratio lower than 0.70. Because the rate of emptying of the lung decreases with advancing age, many elderly individuals demonstrate airflow obstruction even in the absence of a clinical diagnosis of COPD. The diagnosis of COPD usually describes individuals who have chronic airflow obstruction associated with tobacco smoke or some other environmental insult, although aging of the lung has many features that are similar to those of COPD.

COPD encompasses several clinical subtypes, including chronic bronchitis, emphysema, and some forms of long-standing asthma. *Chronic bronchitis* is defined by cough and sputum production for at least 3 months of the year for more than 2 consecutive years in the absence of other kinds of endobronchial disease such as bronchiectasis. In practice, though, most patients with chronic bronchitis have perennial chronic productive coughs that are dismissed as "smokers' cough." *Emphysema* is defined as enlargement of the distal airspaces as a consequence of destruction of alveolar septa. The resultant loss of elasticity of the lung (i.e., increased distensibility) causes slowing of maximal airflow, hyperinflation, and air trapping that are the pathophysiologic hallmarks of COPD. *Asthma* is defined by completely reversible airflow obstruction and airway hyperresponsiveness. Chronic persistent asthma may lead to irreversible airflow obstruction and a subset of those with asthma smoke and have incompletely reversible airflow obstruction, resulting in a population that meets the definition of COPD. Because most patients have features of more than one subtype and because the treatment approaches are similar, physicians and epidemiologists usually do not distinguish among the various subcategories of COPD. In the future, however, as molecular and imaging methods permit finer distinction of COPD subgroups, it may be possible to more precisely tailor treatments and define prognosis for individual patients.

Interrelationships of Chronic Bronchitis and Emphysema

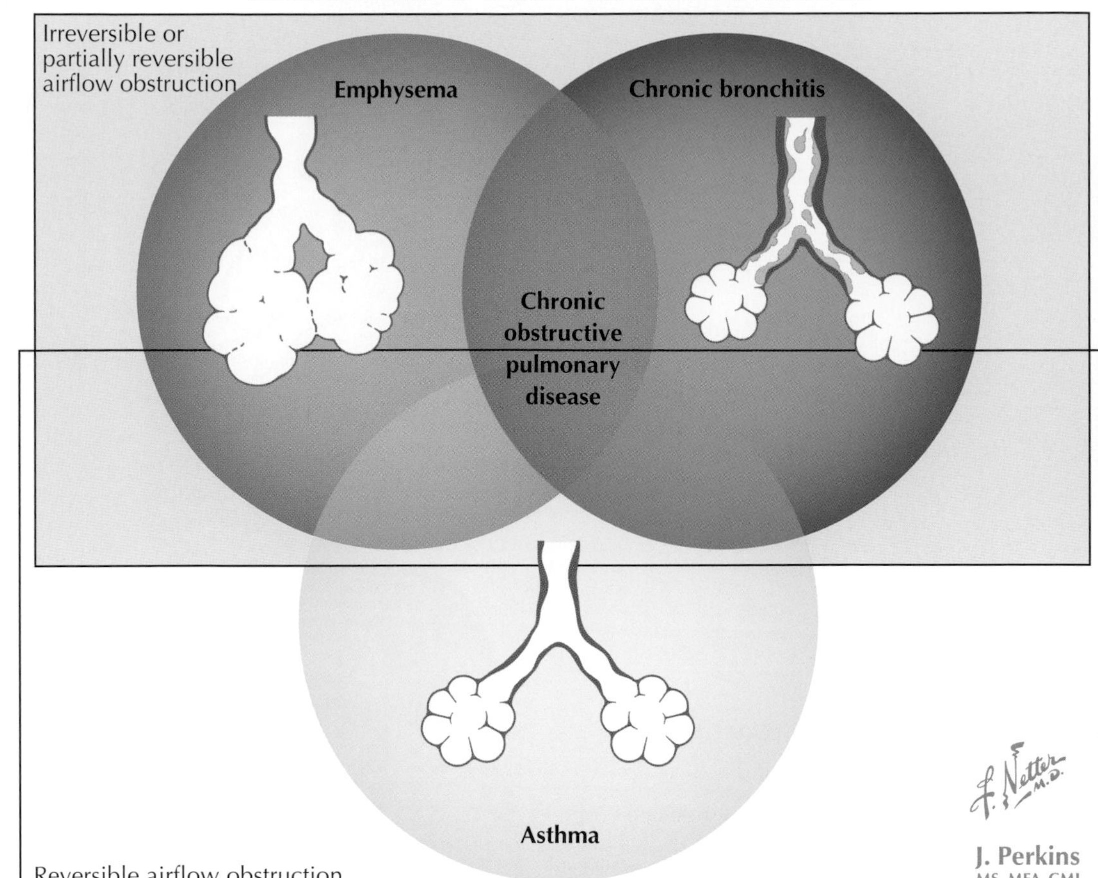

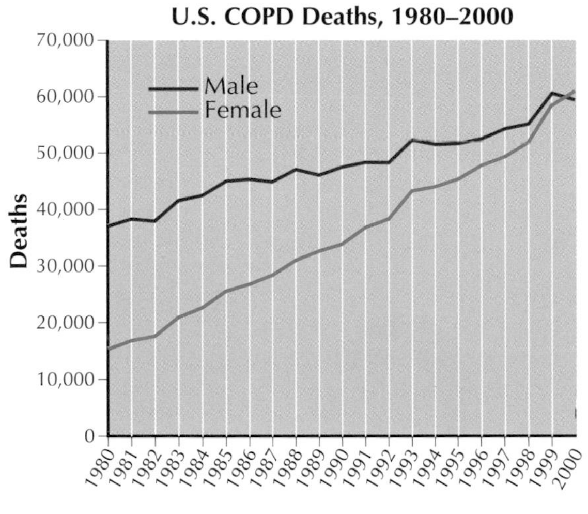

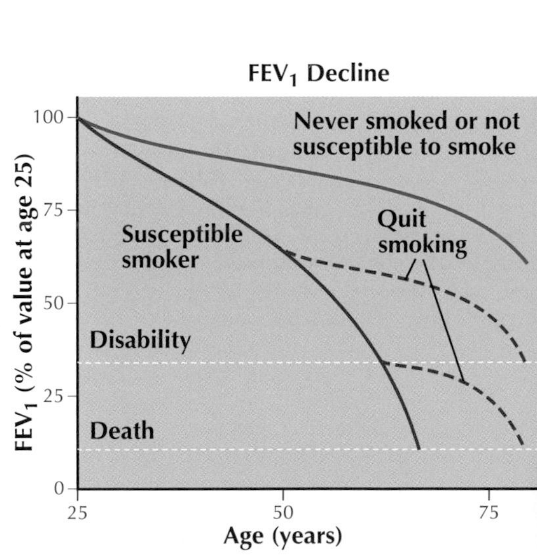

Patients with COPD often seek medical attention after their disease is already severe. Typically, patients have incurred several decades of damage caused by cigarette smoking before they experience dyspnea limiting their functional capacity. Patients may be treated for recurrent lower respiratory tract infections before a diagnosis of COPD is considered. Clinical presentations vary in the severity of the underlying lung disease,

CHRONIC OBSTRUCTIVE PULMONARY DISEASE *(Continued)*

the rate of progression of disease, and the frequency of exacerbations.

EPIDEMIOLOGY

COPD is the fourth leading cause of death in the United States, and mortality related to COPD is projected to increase as cigarette smoking increases in developing countries. COPD is also among the leading causes of chronic medical disability and health care costs in the United States. Morbidity and mortality attributable to COPD have continued to increase, in contrast with other chronic diseases. COPD accounts for a great burden of health care costs, including direct costs of health care and indirect costs related to missed work and caregiver support. Historically, COPD was described as a disease that predominantly affected white men. However, the prevalence of COPD among women and minorities has grown in recent decades as the rate of increase in white men has leveled off. In the United States, morbidity and mortality from COPD in women now exceeds in men, which is largely attributable to increases in the prevalence of cigarette smoking among women. The most rapid increase in COPD mortality is among elderly women. In developing nations, indoor burning of biomass fuel has been an important risk factor for COPD among women. As tobacco use has become more widespread in the developing world, the prevalence of COPD has risen among both men and women (see Plate 4-28).

RISK FACTORS

COPD is caused by a combination of environmental exposures and genetic susceptibility. α_1-Antitrypsin deficiency is the best documented genetic risk factor for COPD and demonstrates the interaction between genetic predisposition and environmental exposures that results in clinical manifestations of COPD. Other genetic associations have been suggested but are not as well substantiated. Inhalational exposures are the major environmental risk factor for COPD, and cigarette smoking is by far the most common risk factor worldwide. Other inhalational exposures include outdoor atmospheric pollution and indoor air pollution from heating and cooking, especially with the use of biomass fuels in developing countries. Occupational exposures and recurrent bronchial infections have also been implicated as pathogenic factors. Socioeconomic status and poor nutrition are other factors that may predispose individuals to developing COPD, and individuals with reduced maximal lung function in early life are more likely to develop COPD later in life.

NATURAL HISTORY

COPD is a heterogeneous disorder with the unifying feature of incompletely reversible airflow obstruction, demonstrated by slow emptying of the lungs during a forced expiration. The natural history of the decline in FEV_1 in patients with COPD was described by Fletcher and Peto (see Plate 4-28). These investigators reported that most cigarette smokers have a relatively normal rate of decline in FEV_1 with aging, but a certain subset of smokers is especially susceptible to cigarette smoke, as demonstrated by an accelerated rate of FEV_1 decline. More recent studies have confirmed that normal

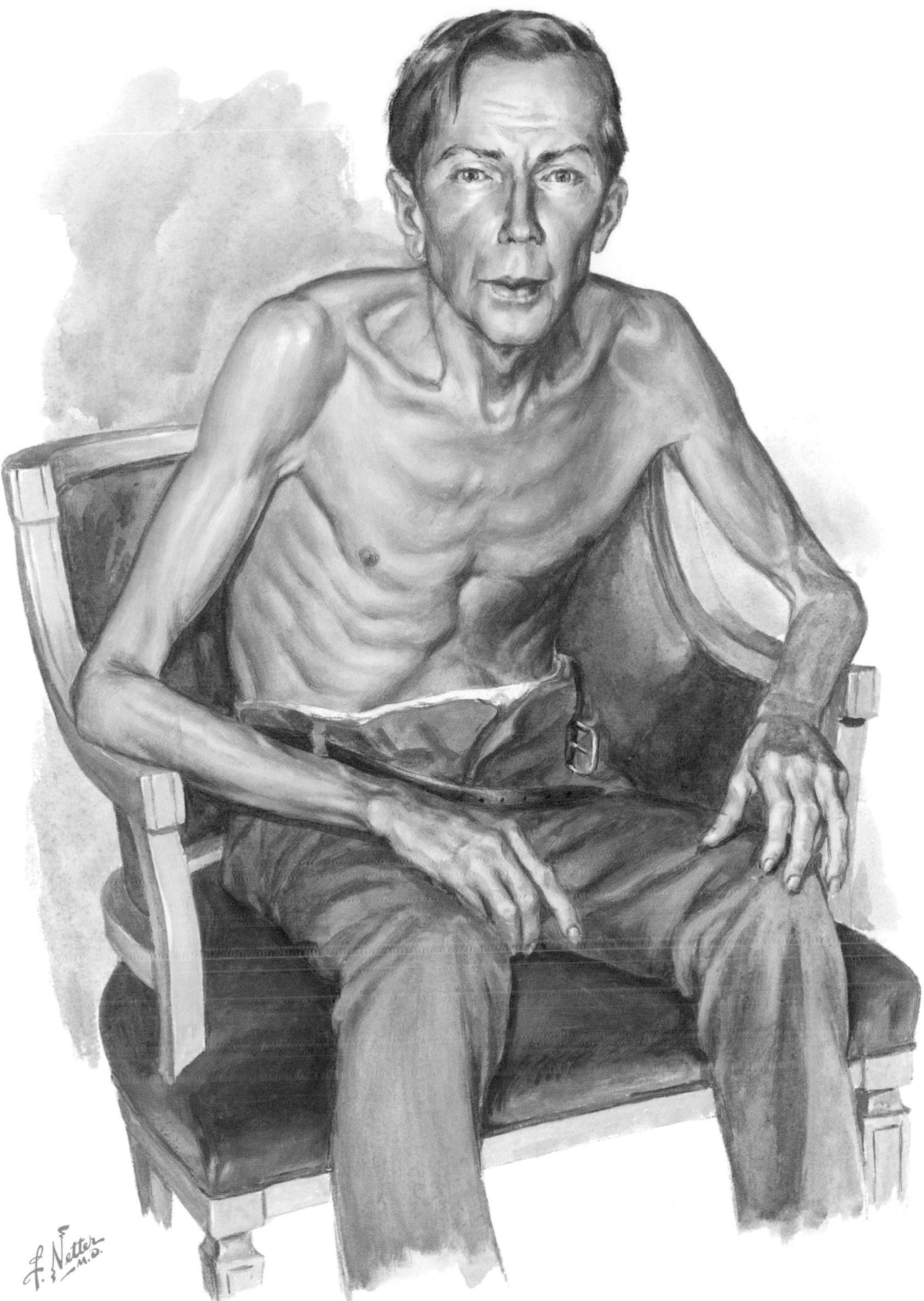

EMPHYSEMA

Chronic Bronchitis

Chronic Obstructive Pulmonary Disease *(Continued)*

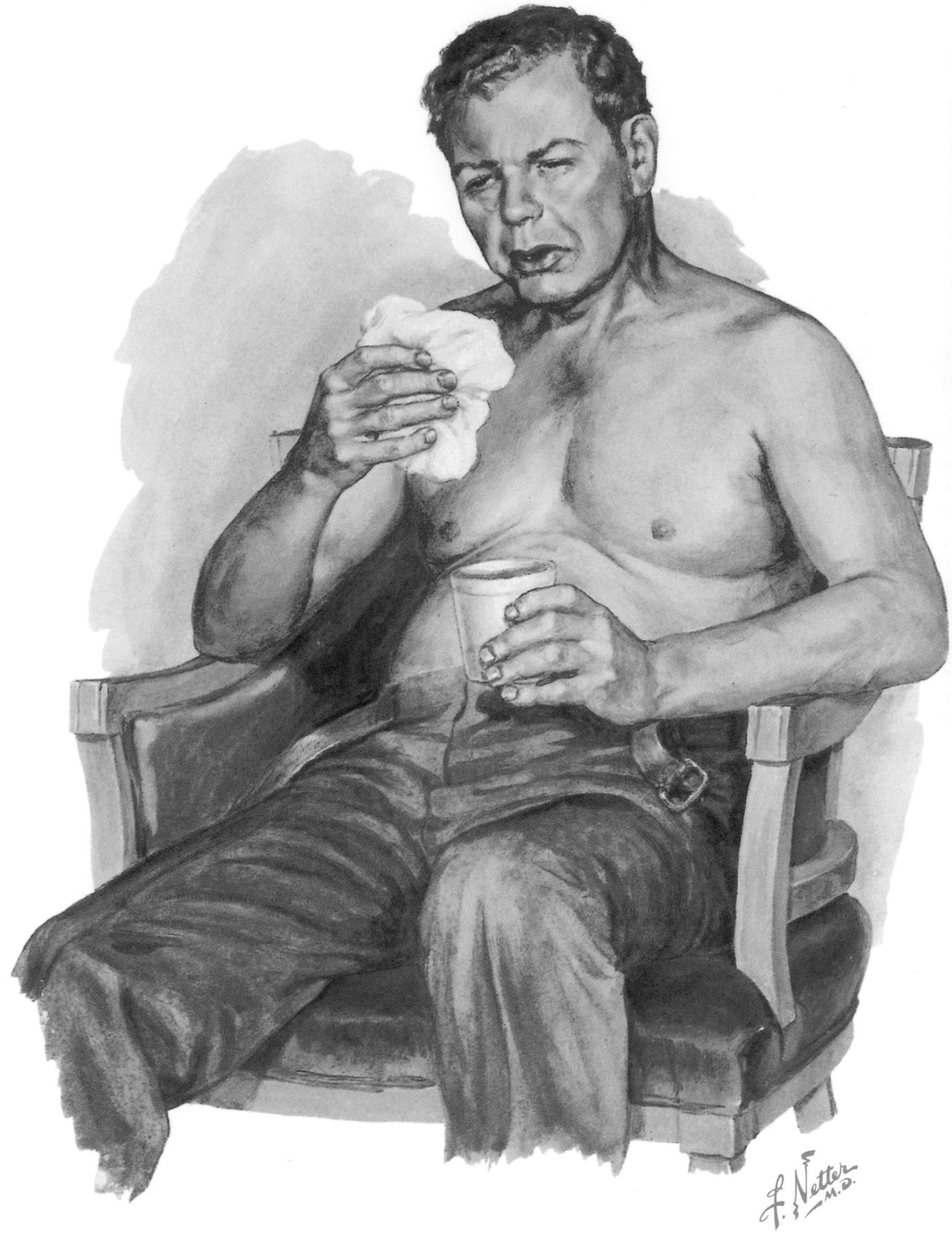

nonsmoking adults lose FEV_1 at a rate of 30 mL per year, a consequence of aging-related loss of elastic recoil of the lung. Studies of patients with COPD show an average annual decline of FEV_1 of 45 to 69 mL per year. Smokers that quit may revert to the normal state of decline (Plate 4-28). Persons who develop COPD may start early adulthood with lower levels of lung function and have increased rates of decline. The decline in lung function is asymptomatic for a period of years, and patients adjust their activities to limit strenuous exercise. In middle age, the onset of an intercurrent respiratory infection, ascent to altitude, or progression of the disease beyond a critical threshold may lead to impairment of routine daily activities or even acute respiratory failure. These events lead the patients with COPD to seek medical attention. Thus, the onset of COPD may appear precipitous even though it is the cumulative result of decades of progression.

CLINICAL FEATURES

COPD is a heterogeneous disease that presents with a spectrum of clinical manifestations. Although end-stage COPD has classically been described as having features typical of emphysema or chronic bronchitis, most patients have features of both (see Plates 4-28 to 4-31). Although COPD represents a spectrum of clinical presentations, the presence of airflow limitation is a unifying feature, and spirometry serves as a diagnostic tool and a means of assessing disease severity (see Plates 4-39 and 4-42). Patients typically have some degree of dyspnea and may also experience cough and wheezing. COPD is progressive, and symptoms and clinical features worsen over time despite available treatments.

PREDOMINANCE OF EMPHYSEMA

The classic representation of a patient with a predominance of emphysema is an asthenic patient with a long history of exertional dyspnea and minimal cough productive of only scant amounts of mucoid sputum (see Plate 4-29). Weight loss is common, and the clinical course is characterized by marked, progressive dyspnea.

On physical examination, the patient appears distressed and is using accessory muscles of respiration, which serve to lift the sternum in an anterior-superior direction with each inspiration. The sternomastoid muscles are well-developed, but the limbs show evidence of muscle atrophy. The patient has tachypnea, with relatively prolonged expiration through pursed lips, or expiration is begun with a grunting sound. Patients who have active grunting expiration may exhibit well-developed, tense abdominal musculature. The hyperinflation of the chest leads to widening of the costal angle of the lower ribcage and elevation of the lateral clavicles. The flattened diaphragm causes the lateral ribcage to move inward with each breath. While sitting, the patient often leans forward, extending the arms to brace him- or herself in the so-called "tripod" position. Patients who brace themselves on their thighs may develop hyperkeratosis of the upper thighs. The neck veins may be distended during expiration, yet they collapse with inspiration. The lower intercostal spaces and sternal notch retract with each inspiration. The percussion note is hyperresonant, and the breath sounds on auscultation are diminished, with faint, high-pitched crackles early in inspiration, and wheezes heard in expiration. The cardiac impulse, if visible, is seen in the subxiphoid regions, and cardiac dullness is either absent or severely narrowed. The cardiac impulse is best palpated in the subxiphoid region. If pulmonary hypertension is present, a murmur of tricuspid insufficiency may be heard in the subxiphoid region.

The minute ventilation is maintained, the arterial Po_2 is often above 60 mm Hg, and the Pco_2 is low to normal. Pulmonary function testing demonstrates an increased total lung capacity (TLC) and residual volume (RV), with a decreased vital capacity. The DL_{CO} (diffusing capacity for carbon monoxide) is decreased, reflecting the destruction of the alveolar septa causing

Chronic Obstructive Pulmonary Disease *(Continued)*

reduction of capillary surface area. When the DL_{CO} decreases below 50% predicted, many patients with emphysema have arterial oxygen desaturation with exercise.

PREDOMINANCE OF CHRONIC BRONCHITIS

Patients with a predominance of chronic bronchitis typically have a history of cough and sputum production for many years along with a history of heavy cigarette smoking (see Plate 4-30). Initially, the cough may be present only in the winter months, and the patient may seek medical attention only during the more severe of his or her repeated attacks of purulent bronchitis. Over the years, the cough becomes continuous, and episodes of illness increase in frequency, duration, and severity. After the patient begins to experience exertional dyspnea, he or she often seeks medical help and is found to have a severe degree of obstruction. Frequently, such patients do not seek out a physician until the onset of acute or chronic respiratory failure. Many of these patients report nocturnal snoring and daytime hypersomnolence and demonstrate sleep apnea syndrome, which may contribute to the clinical manifestations.

Patients with a predominance of bronchitis are often overweight and cyanotic. There is often no apparent distress at rest; the respiratory rate is normal or only slightly increased. Accessory muscle usage is not apparent. The chest percussion note is normally resonant and, on auscultation, one can usually hear coarse rattles and rhonchi, which change in location and intensity after a deep breath and productive cough. Wheezing may be present during resting breathing or may be elicited with a forced expiration.

The minute ventilation is either normal or only slightly increased. Failure to increase minute ventilation in the face of ventilation-perfusion mismatch leads to hypoxemia. Because of impaired chemosensitivity, such patients do not compensate properly and permit hypercapnia to develop with $Paco_2$ levels above 45 mm Hg. The low Pao_2 produces desaturation of hemoglobin, which causes hypoxic pulmonary vasoconstriction and eventually irreversible pulmonary hypertension. Desaturation may lead to visible cyanosis, and hypoxic pulmonary vasoconstriction leads to right-sided heart failure (see Plate 4-32). Because of the chronic systemic inflammatory response that occurs with COPD, these patients often do not have a normal erythrocytic response to hypoxemia, so the serum hemoglobin may be normal, elevated, or even decreased.

Mixed Chronic Bronchitis and Emphysema

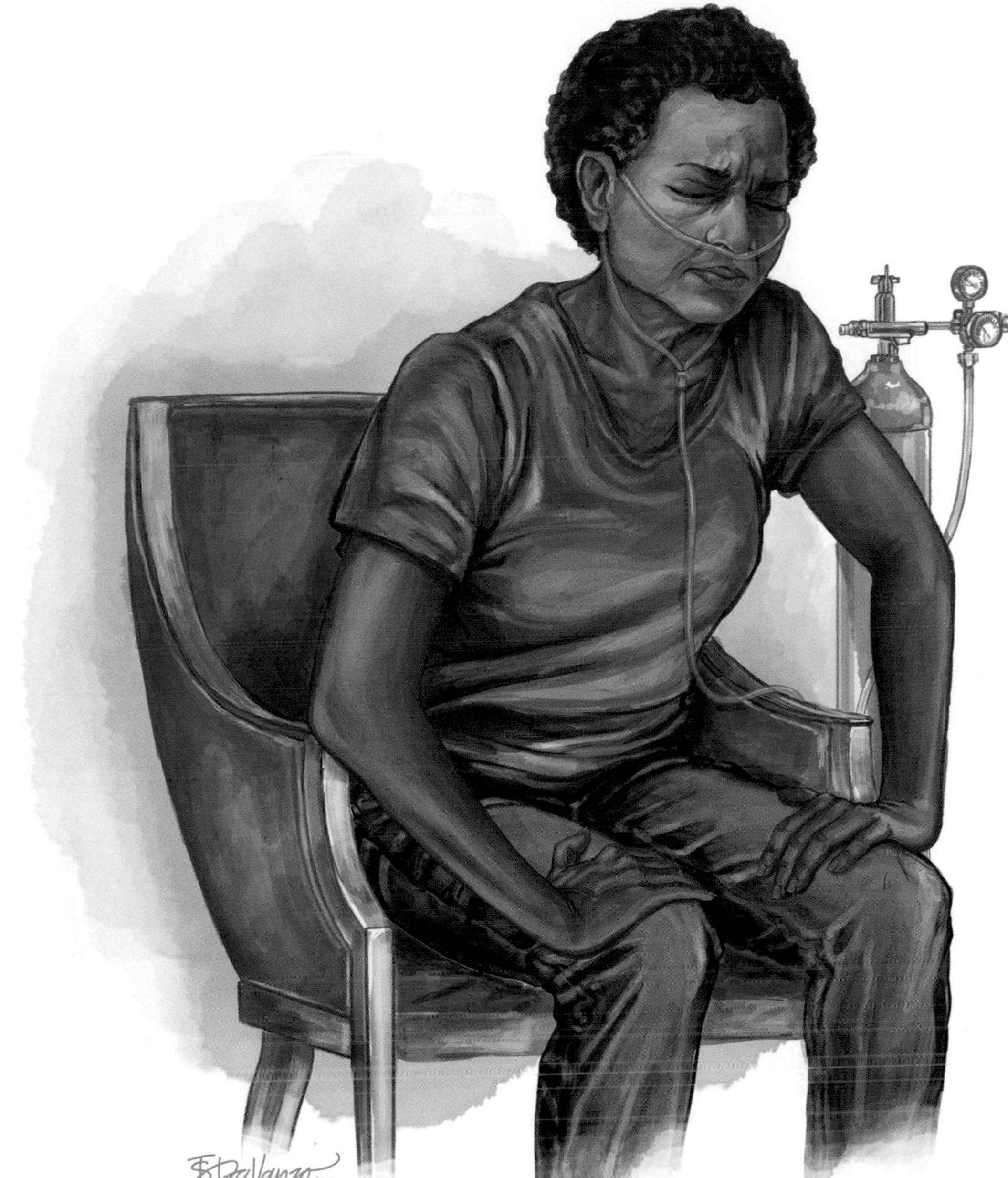

The typical patient with COPD has clinical, physiological, and radiographic features of both chronic bronchitis and emphysema. She may have chronic cough and sputum production, and need accessory muscles and pursed lips to help her breathe. Pulmonary function testing may reveal variable degrees of airflow limitation, hyperinflation, and reduction in the diffusing capacity, and arterial blood gases may show variable decreases in Po_2 and increases in Pco_2. Radiographic imaging often shows components of airway wall thickening, excessive mucus, and emphysema.

The TLC is often normal, and the RV is moderately elevated. The vital capacity (VC) is mildly diminished. Maximal expiratory flow rates are invariably low. Lung elastic recoil properties are normal or only slightly impaired; the DL_{CO} is either normal or minimally decreased.

PATHOLOGY

Large Airways Disease (see Plate 4-33)

Chronic bronchitis is associated with hyperplasia and hypertrophy of the mucus-secreting glands found in the submucosa of the large cartilaginous airways. Because the mass of the submucous glands is approximately 40 times greater than that of the intraepithelial goblet cells, it is thought that these glands produce most airway mucus. The degree of hyperplasia is quantitatively assessed as the ratio of the submucosal gland thickness to the overall thickness of the bronchial wall from the cartilage to the airway lumen. This ratio is known as the *Reid index*. Although the Reid index is often low in the bronchi of patients who do not have symptoms of COPD during life and is frequently high in those with chronic bronchitis, there is sufficient overlap of Reid index values to suggest that a gradual change in the submucous glands may take place. Thus, the sharp distinction of the clinical definition of chronic bronchitis cannot correlate completely with

Chronic Obstructive Pulmonary Disease *(Continued)*

the pathologic changes in large airways. Although patients with chronic mucus hypersecretion with cough and sputum are more prone to respiratory infections and exacerbations of COPD, the presence of cough and sputum are not, by themselves, indicative of a poor prognosis in the absence of airflow obstruction. The magnitude of airflow obstruction is better correlated with the pathologic involvement of the small airways.

Small Airways Disease *(see Plate 4-33)*

COPD is also associated with changes in the small airways, those less than 2 mm and between the fourth and twelfth generation of airway branching in the lungs. The changes in the small airways may occur independently of changes in the larger airways. Changes in the small airways occur across a spectrum and may range from bland intraluminal secretions to a more cellular infiltrate, with polymorphonuclear neutrophils, macrophages, CD4 cells and other lymphocyte subtypes. The presence of lymphoid follicles in the small airways demonstrates increased immune surveillance of the mucosal surface. In addition to cellular inflammation, airway wall thickening, including changes in the epithelium, lamina propria, and adventitia, corresponds to disease progression. The diffuse changes in small airways contribute more to the obstruction and maldistribution of inspired gas than do the abnormalities in large airways. Obstruction of small airways with mucous plugs is associated with increased mortality.

EMPHYSEMA

The several types of emphysema are classified according to patterns of septal destruction and airspace enlargement within terminal respiratory units, or acini (see Plates 4-34 to 4-36). The normal acinus is supplied by a *terminal bronchiole.* The terminal bronchiole undergoes three orders of branching—first into *respiratory bronchioles* with alveolated walls, into *alveolar ducts*, and finally into *alveolar sacs*.

If the septal destruction and dilatation are limited to the central portion of the acinus in the region of the terminal bronchiole and respiratory bronchioles, the disorder is called *centriacinar* or *centrilobular emphysema* (see Plate 4-35). Because of septal destruction, there is free communication between all orders of respiratory bronchioles. Alveolar sacs at the periphery of the acinus lose volume as the central portions enlarge. Although centriacinar emphysema is often considered to be a diffuse disease process, there is considerable variation in severity from acinus to acinus within the same segment or lobe. In general, however, more of the acini are affected in the upper lung zones than in the lower zones. Extensive centriacinar emphysema is most often found in those with histories of heavy smoking and chronic bronchitis.

In contrast to centriacinar emphysema, *panacinar* or *panlobular emphysema* affects the acinus more uniformly with less variability within an individual segment or lobe (see Plate 4-36). There is some tendency for the lower zones to be more severely affected. Panacinar emphysema is the characteristic lesion in α_1-antitrypsin deficiency, although smokers with α_1-antitrypsin deficiency may have centriacinar emphysema as well. Panacinar emphysema to a mild degree is a common finding after the fifth decade of life and may be extensive in elderly nonsmoking patients who have age-related "senile" emphysema. In severe smoking-related chronic obstructive airway disease, both centriacinar and panacinar emphysema are ordinarily found along with chronic bronchitic changes in the airways.

Cor Pulmonale Caused by COPD

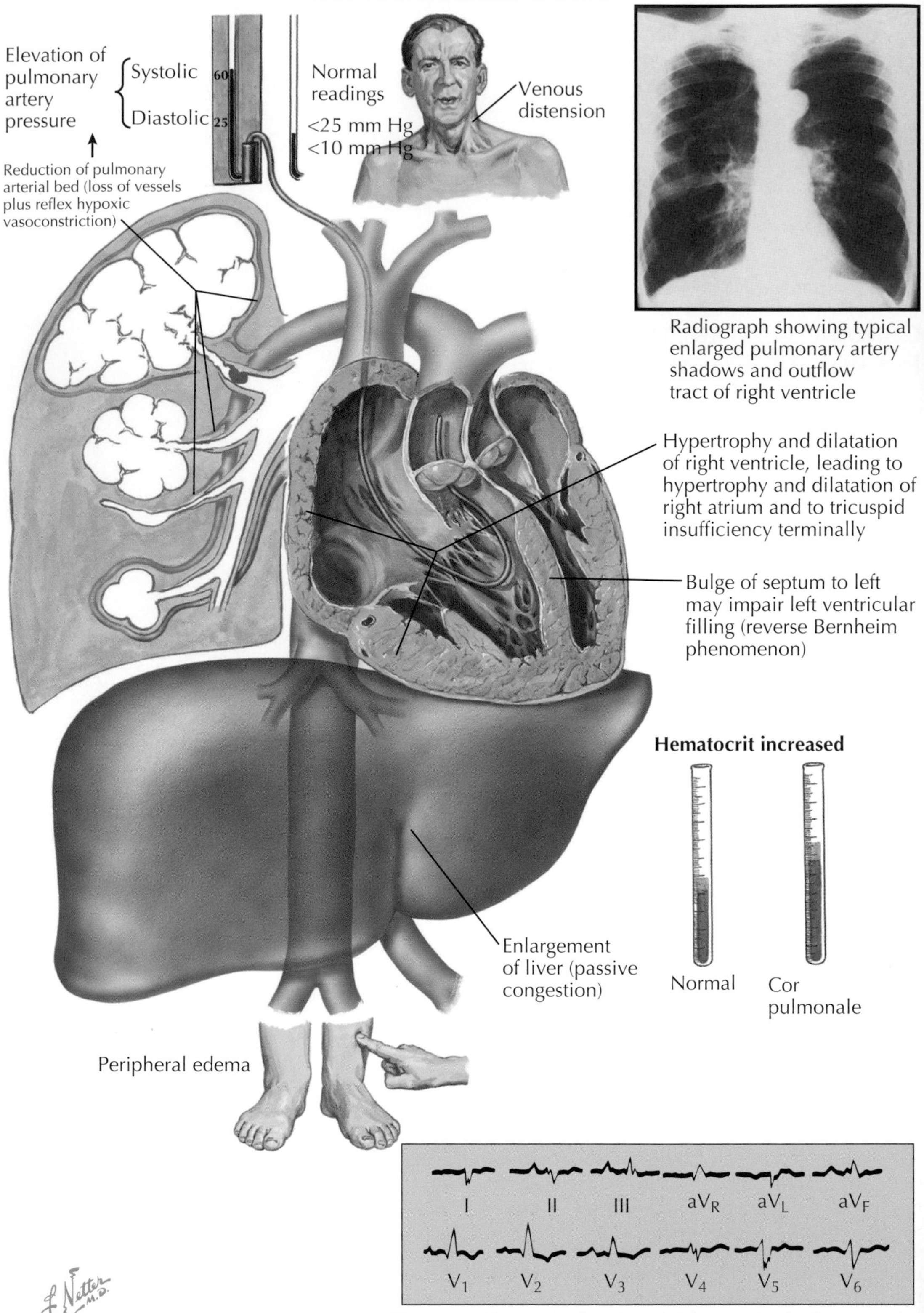

Elevation of pulmonary artery pressure: Systolic 60, Diastolic 25

Normal readings <25 mm Hg, <10 mm Hg

Reduction of pulmonary arterial bed (loss of vessels plus reflex hypoxic vasoconstriction)

Venous distension

Radiograph showing typical enlarged pulmonary artery shadows and outflow tract of right ventricle

Hypertrophy and dilatation of right ventricle, leading to hypertrophy and dilatation of right atrium and to tricuspid insufficiency terminally

Bulge of septum to left may impair left ventricular filling (reverse Bernheim phenomenon)

Hematocrit increased

Normal

Cor pulmonale

Enlargement of liver (passive congestion)

Peripheral edema

I II III aV_R aV_L aV_F

V_1 V_2 V_3 V_4 V_5 V_6

Electrocardiogram indicative of right ventricular hypertrophy

F. Netter M.D.

Chronic Obstructive Pulmonary Disease (*Continued*)

When alveolar wall destruction is restricted to the periphery of the acinus, most often in regions just beneath the visceral pleura, the disorder is designated *paraseptal emphysema*. This form leads to development of subpleural bullae that may result in episodes of spontaneous pneumothorax in otherwise healthy young adults.

PATHOBIOLOGY

COPD is characterized by chronic inflammation in the peripheral airways and the lung parenchyma (see Plates 4-37 and 4-38). The predominant cells are macrophages, CD8+ lymphocytes, and neutrophils. The inflammatory mediators leukotriene B4, tumor necrosis factor-α (TNF-α), and interleukin-8 (IL-8) are increased in the sputum of patients with COPD and may play an important role. An imbalance between proteases and antiproteases is also likely to be important in the pathogenesis of COPD (see Plate 4-38). Macrophages and neutrophils release many different proteases that break down connective tissue, such as elastin, in the lung parenchyma. The proteases may induce direct destruction of lung tissue as well as trigger cascades of intracellular events that lead to apoptotic cell death. Moreover, proteases are potent promoters of mucus cell metaplasia and mucus cell secretion, contributing to chronic bronchitis. Neutrophil elastase, proteinase 3, and cathepsins all produce emphysema in laboratory animals. Neutrophil elastase is inhibited by α_1-antitrypsin and deficiency of this enzyme is the predominant contributor to the emphysema in those with the severe genetic defect. Matrix metalloproteinases (MMPs) from macrophages and neutrophils may also have a key role in inducing emphysema. In the normal state, proteolytic enzymes are counteracted by antiproteases such as α_1-antitrypsin and serum leukocyte proteinase inhibitor (SLIPI). By inducing inflammation, smoking increases release of proteases in the terminal airspaces in patients in whom COPD develops. Moreover, smoking may also inactivate antiproteases via MMP inhibition of α_1-antitrypsin, which itself is an inhibitor of a protease that counteracts the actions of MMPs. By reducing α_1-antitrypsin's inhibition of this protease, known as tissue inhibitor of metalloproteinases (TIMP), the actions of MMPs are enhanced. Smoking also leads to increased reactive oxygen species (ROS), which can promote inflammatory gene transcription by breakdown of the inhibitor of the transcription factor nuclear factor kappa-B (NFκB), known as IN-KB. ROS can also inactivate histone deacetylase (HDAC), leading to increased DNA acetylation and gene transcription. Furthermore, CD8+ cells can promote macrophage production of MMPs through interferon-inducible cytokines, such as inducible protein of 10kD (IP-10), interfection-inducible T-cell alpha chemoattractant (l-TAC), and monokine induced by interferon-gamma (MIG). Thus, an insufficient concentration of antiproteases may result in parenchymal damage.

Oxidative stress may also contribute to the injury characteristic of COPD by oxidation of proteins, cell membranes, and nucleic acids, triggering a cellular stress response that ultimately leads to apoptotic cell death. The inflammation in COPD is not only localized to the lungs but is present on a systemic basis. Patients with COPD have elevated concentrations of C-reactive protein and interleukin-6, even during times of stable symptoms. Weight loss and muscle atrophy in COPD have been associated with increased circulating levels of TNF-α and soluble TNF-α receptors.

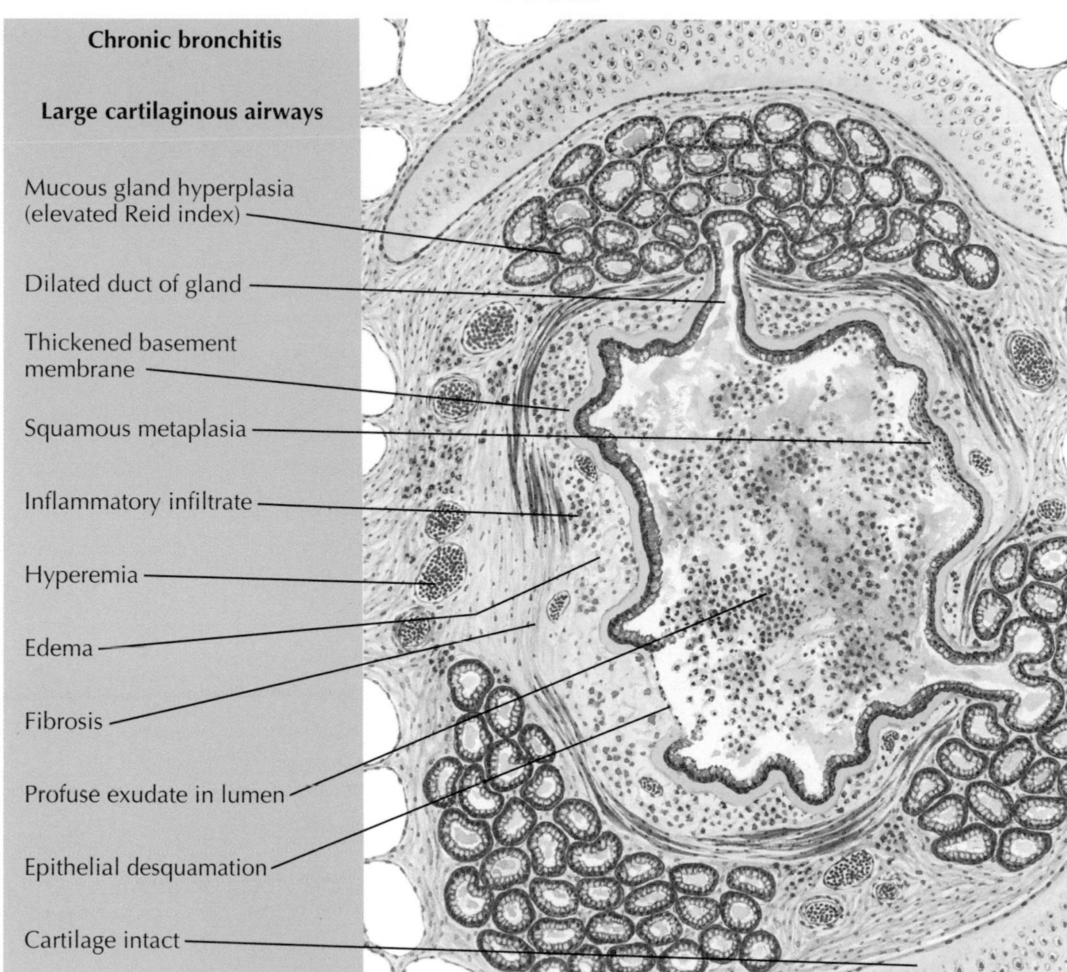

Anatomic Distribution of Emphysema

Normal lung acinus (secondary lobule)

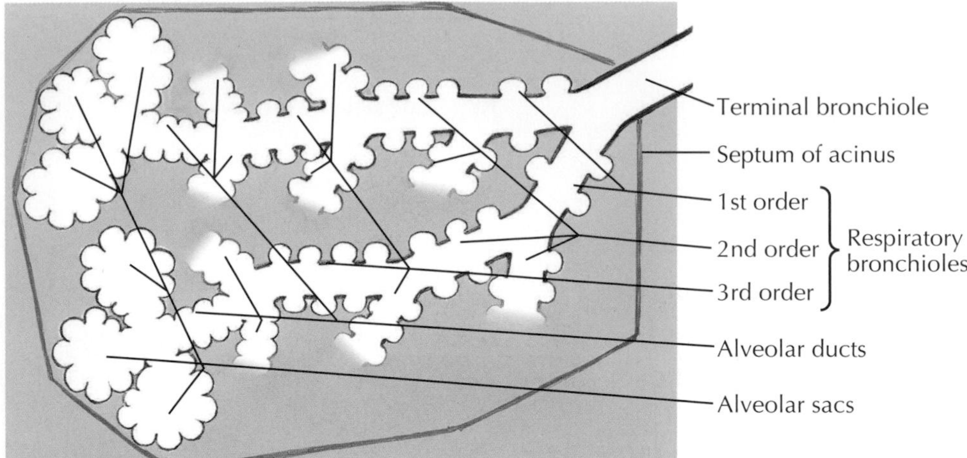
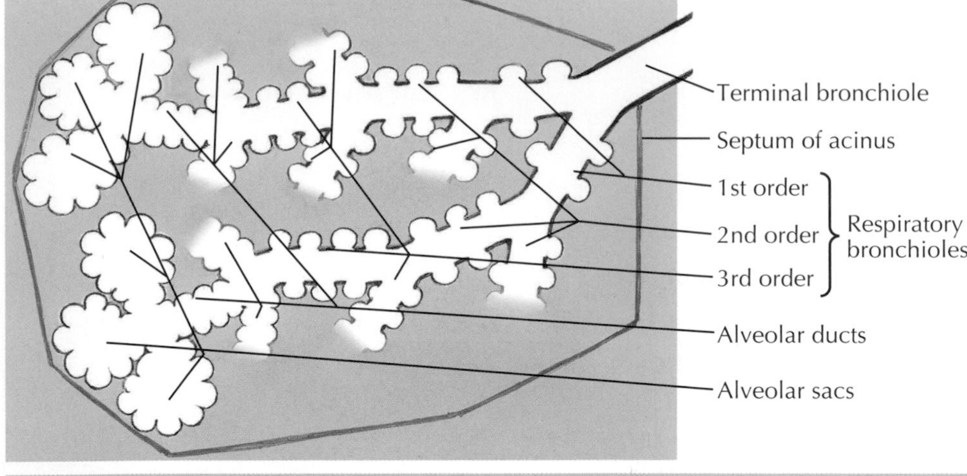

Centriacinar (centrilobular) emphysema

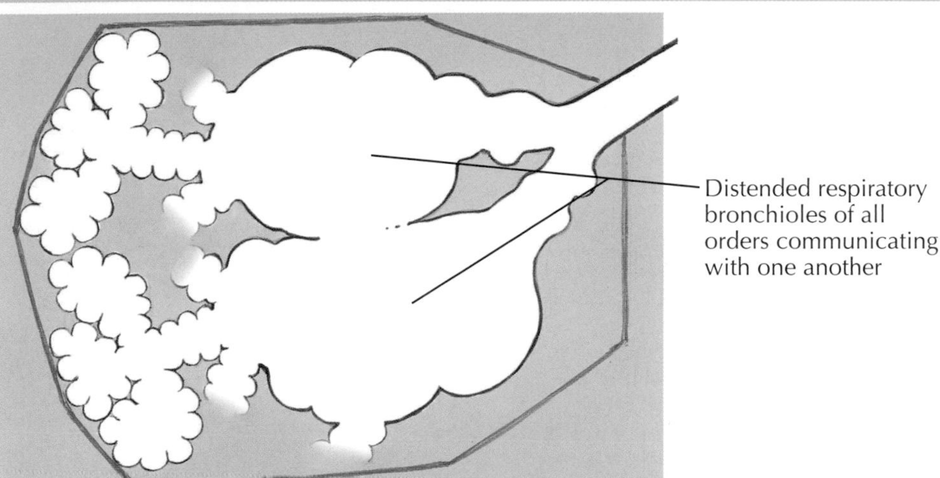

Panacinar (panlobular) emphysema

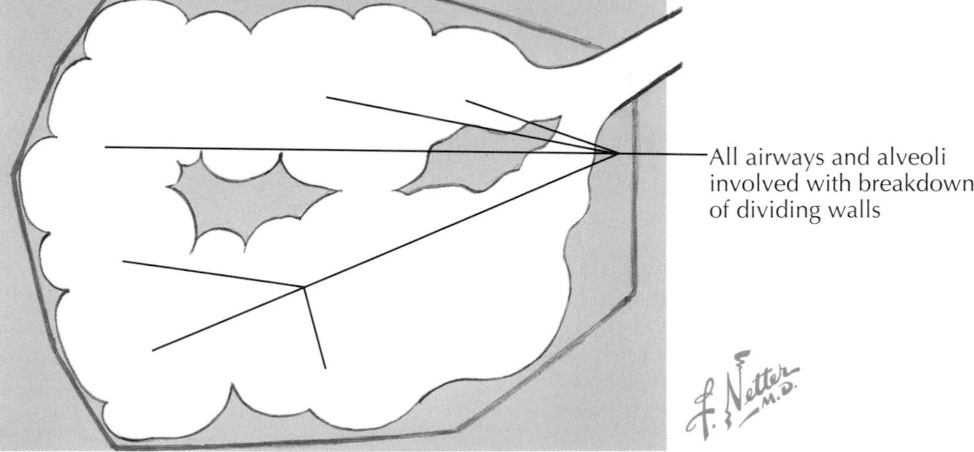

Chronic Obstructive Pulmonary Disease *(Continued)*

The final common pathway of inflammatory cytokines, protease-antiprotease imbalance, and oxidative stress is destruction of alveolar epithelial and capillary endothelial cells by a programmed sequence of cell death, or apoptosis. Because the lung requires replacement of its cellular scaffolding on a continuing basis, any process that leads to an imbalance of cell destruction and cell growth can eventually lead to emphysema. Thus, insufficiency of growth factors is also postulated to contribute to the development of emphysema.

The presence of CD8 cells and airway-associated lymphoid follicles in the lung parenchyma in smokers with COPD has raised the possibility that immunologic processes such as autoimmunity or response to chronic viral infection may also contribute to the pathogenesis of COPD.

α_1-ANTITRYPSIN

Serum levels of α_1-antitrypsin are either deficient or absent in some patients with early onset of emphysema associated with particular genotypes (see Plate 4-38). Most people in the normal population have α_1-antitrypsin levels in excess of 250 mg/100 mL of serum along with two M genes, designated as Pi-type MM. Several genes are associated with alterations in serum α_1-antitrypsin levels, but the most common ones associated with emphysema are the Z and S genes. Individuals who are homozygous ZZ or SS have serum levels of α_1-antitrypsin of less than 50 mg/100 mL and develop severe panacinar emphysema at an early age, particularly if they smoke or are exposed to occupational dusts. The MZ and MS heterozygotes have intermediate levels of serum α_1-antitrypsin. Although smokers with MZ or MS genotypes may have slightly increased decline in FEV_1 if they smoke, the risk of developing COPD is not materially increased beyond other smokers.

α_1-Antitrypsin deficiency is caused by a single amino acid substitution. The Z mutation is caused by a glutamate to lysine mutation at position 342, and the S mutation is caused by a glutamate to valine mutation at position 264. These mutations lead to misfolding of the protein preventing release from the liver, where it is mainly manufactured. The misfolded protein may be destroyed by proteosomal processes, or if it polymerizes, may be stored in the endoplasmic reticulum and not released into the circulation. Excessive liver storage may lead to inflammatory liver disease and cirrhosis, particularly in affected infants and children.

The precise way that antitrypsin deficiency produces emphysema is unclear. In addition to inhibiting trypsin, α_1-antitrypsin effectively inhibits elastase and collagenase, as well as several other enzymes. α_1-Antitrypsin is an acute-phase reactant, and the serum levels increase in association with many inflammatory reactions and with estrogen administration in all except homozygotes. It has been proposed, with some supporting experimental evidence, that the structural integrity of lung elastin and collagen depends on this antiprotease, which protects the lung from proteases released from leukocytes. Proteases released by lysed leukocytes in the alveoli may be uninhibited and consequently free to damage the alveolar walls themselves. Alternative theories suggest that the unopposed protease activity may lead to an ongoing immune-mediated inflammatory response or acceleration of natural programmed cell death.

PATHOPHYSIOLOGY

Whether bronchitis or emphysema predominates, by the time a patient with COPD begins to have

Centriacinar (Centrilobular) Emphysema

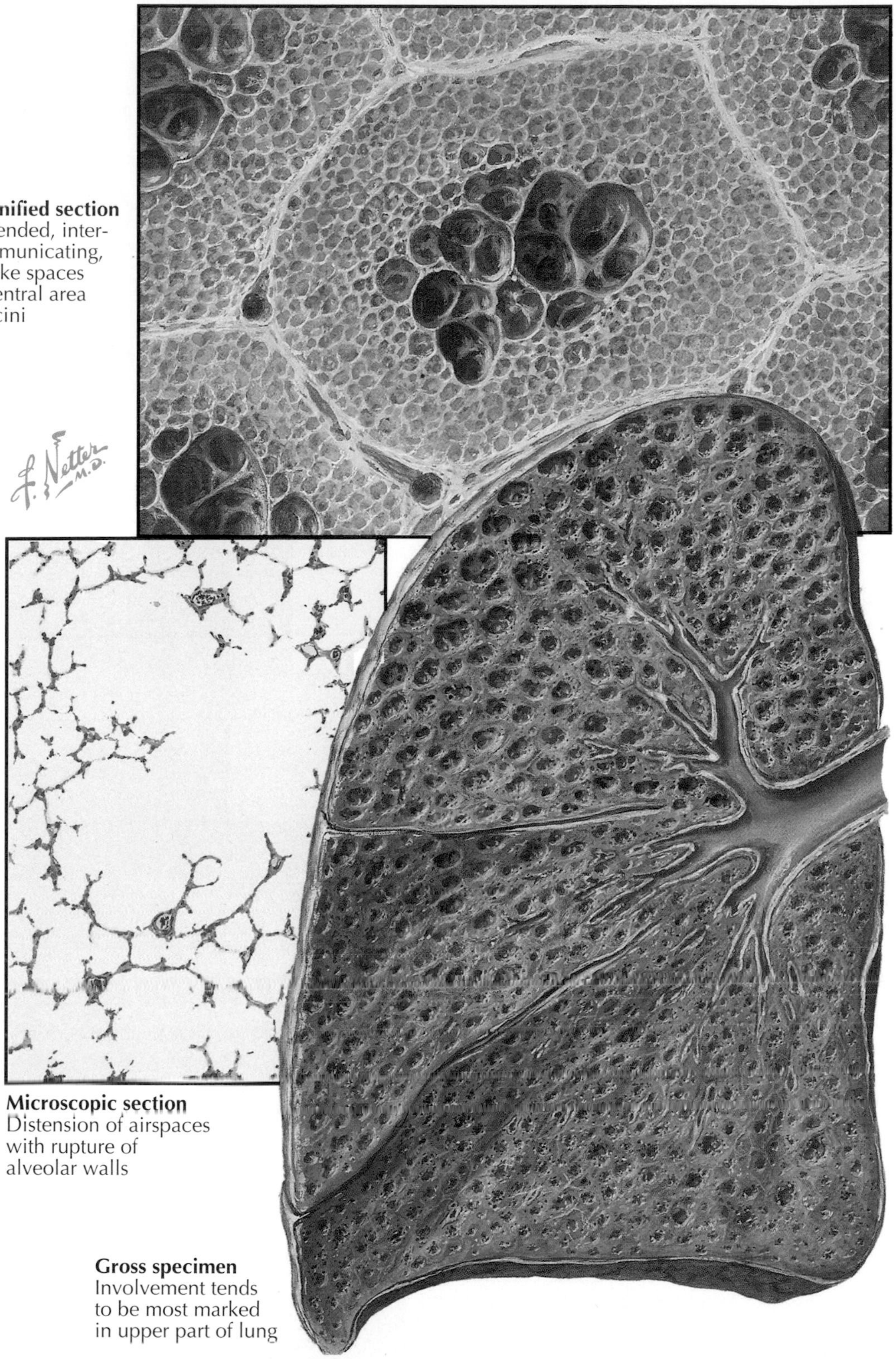

Magnified section Distended, intercommunicating, saclike spaces in central area of acini

Microscopic section Distension of airspaces with rupture of alveolar walls

Gross specimen Involvement tends to be most marked in upper part of lung

Chronic Obstructive Pulmonary Disease *(Continued)*

symptoms, airflow limitation is readily demonstrable as an obstructive ventilatory defect. The most easily measured indexes of obstruction are taken from the volume-time plot of a forced expiratory VC maneuver, classically measured with a spirometer coupled to a rotating drum kymograph. Although volume-measuring spirometers are stable, rugged, and linear instruments, most modern spirometry systems use flow-measuring devices (pneumotachometers) interfaced with a microprocessor that integrates flow over time to produce a time-based record of forced expired volume (see Plate 4-39). The FEV_1 is low both as a percentage of the value predicted for a given gender, age, and height category and as a percentage of the patient's own FVC. Depending on the purpose of the pulmonary function test, an obstructive ventilatory defect is defined either as an FEV1/FVC ratio of less than 70% or less than the 95th percentile for the demographic category.

With COPD, static lung volumes are often abnormal. Plate 4-39 depicts the normal lung volumes and those often found in COPD. The functional residual capacity (FRC) is the lung volume at the end of a quiet exhalation and, in normal subjects, is the volume at which the inward recoil of the lung is equal and opposite to the outward recoil of the *relaxed* chest wall. An elevated FRC in individuals with COPD results from the loss of the static elastic recoil properties of the lung as well as initiation of inspiration before the static balance volume is reached (so-called "dynamic hyperinflation"). TLC is determined by pressures exerted by the diaphragm and muscles of the chest wall in relation to the static elastic recoil properties of both the chest wall and lung. When TLC is elevated in COPD, a significant degree of emphysema is present, although the TLC can also be elevated during acute episodes of asthma. RV is elevated early in the clinical course of COPD and is a sensitive sign of airflow limitation. Early in the course of the disease, elevation of RV is thought to be caused by closure of airways, but late in the disease, emphysematous bullae may also contribute to the elevation in RV. Because the TLC does not increase as much as the RV increases, the VC (i.e., TLC − RV) decreases with advancing COPD.

The measurement of static lung volumes in COPD is subject to some technical issues (see Plate 2-3). Resident gas methods using helium dilution or nitrogen may underestimate the true lung volumes because of incomplete gas mixing or washout in regions with impaired ventilation. Plethysmographic lung volumes that depend on Boyle's law relying on the compressibility of resident gas in the lung are more accurate but are subject to overestimation of the true lung volume if the panting frequency is too rapid to permit equilibration of the mouth and alveolar pressures. Because the difference between the resident gas and plethysmographic measure is caused by regions of lung with little or no ventilation, the difference between the two methods has been called "trapped gas" and used as an indicator of COPD severity (see Section 2).

In addition to the easily demonstrable obstructive abnormalities during forced exhalation, there are significant alterations in the pressure-flow relationships during ordinary breathing in COPD. This contrasts with exhalation in normal subjects who can increase expiratory flow during tidal breathing (see Plate 4-39). Because of the slow emptying of the lung in COPD, the next breath is initiated before the respiratory system can return to the static FRC. This means that the individual breathes at higher lung volumes to maintain adequate expiratory airflow, a condition referred to as *dynamic hyperinflation* (see Plate 4-39). Although breathing at high lung volumes has the advantage of increasing airflow because of the increased lung elastic

Chronic Obstructive Pulmonary Disease *(Continued)*

recoil, it requires an increase in the work of breathing and a decrease in the efficiency of breathing. Increasing respiratory rate accentuates dynamic hyperinflation and can worsen the sensation of dyspnea. Pursed-lip breathing causes patients to slow their respiratory rate and can relieve dyspnea by diminishing dynamic hyperinflation.

The physiologic hallmark of emphysema is a reduction in lung elastic recoil caused by destruction of alveolar septal elements. This causes the pressure-volume curve of the lung to be shifted upward and to the left, resulting in decreased static recoil pressure at a specific lung volume and an increase in the compliance of the lung (see Plates 4-39 and 4-40).

The surface area of the alveolar-capillary membrane is reduced as a consequence of emphysema. This results in decreased transfer of diffusion-limited gases such as carbon monoxide across the alveolar-capillary membrane. This is measured in the pulmonary function laboratory as the DL_{CO}. The DL_{CO} correlates roughly with the magnitude of reduction in maximum elastic recoil of the lung as well as the anatomic extent of emphysema assessed by imaging with computed tomography (CT). In chronic bronchitis, the DL_{CO} may be preserved, and in asthma, the DL_{CO} tends to be elevated.

With the progression of COPD comes progressive exercise limitation. This is caused by the increased work of breathing as ventilation increases with exercise. With increased respiratory rate, patients develop dynamic hyperinflation, a condition in which the end-expiratory lung volume does not return to the static end-expiratory volume of FRC (see Plate 4-40). The hyperinflation that occurs causes an increased work of breathing and exacerbates dyspnea. An indicator of dynamic hyperinflation is the inspiratory capacity (IC), which progressively decreases with increasing ventilation. Measures that reduce dynamic hyperinflation, increasing IC, can improve exercise capacity. These include alterations in breathing pattern, oxygen supplementation, helium inhalation, and use of inhaled bronchodilators, particularly long-acting, and lung volume reduction surgery.

RADIOGRAPHIC APPEARANCE

Chronic Bronchitis

On plain chest radiographs, thickening of bronchial walls is often seen as parallel or tapering shadows, referred to as *tram tracking* or *ring shadows* of airways that are visualized in cross-section. A generalized increase in lung markings at the bases is also frequently seen and is referred to as *dirty lungs*. In patients who have been exposed to occupational dusts, these markings may be accentuated but do not necessarily indicate the presence of pneumoconiosis.

The CT may show airway wall thickening or mucoid impactions in patients with COPD even in the absence of emphysema. The magnitude of these abnormalities, however, does not necessarily correlate with the severity of airflow obstruction or the extent of emphysema, and it remains to be seen whether there are prognostic or therapeutic implications of these findings.

Emphysema

In evaluating plain radiographs, a range of findings can represent emphysema. These include attenuation of the pulmonary vasculature peripherally, irregular radiolucency of lung fields, flattening or inversion of the diaphragm as seen on both posteroanterior (PA) and lateral projections, and an increase in the retrosternal space on the lateral projection. The latter two findings have

Panacinar (Panlobular) Emphysema

Gross section of lung. Dilated, saccular air spaces. In cases of disease caused by α_1-antitrypsin deficiency, lower part of lung tends to be more affected

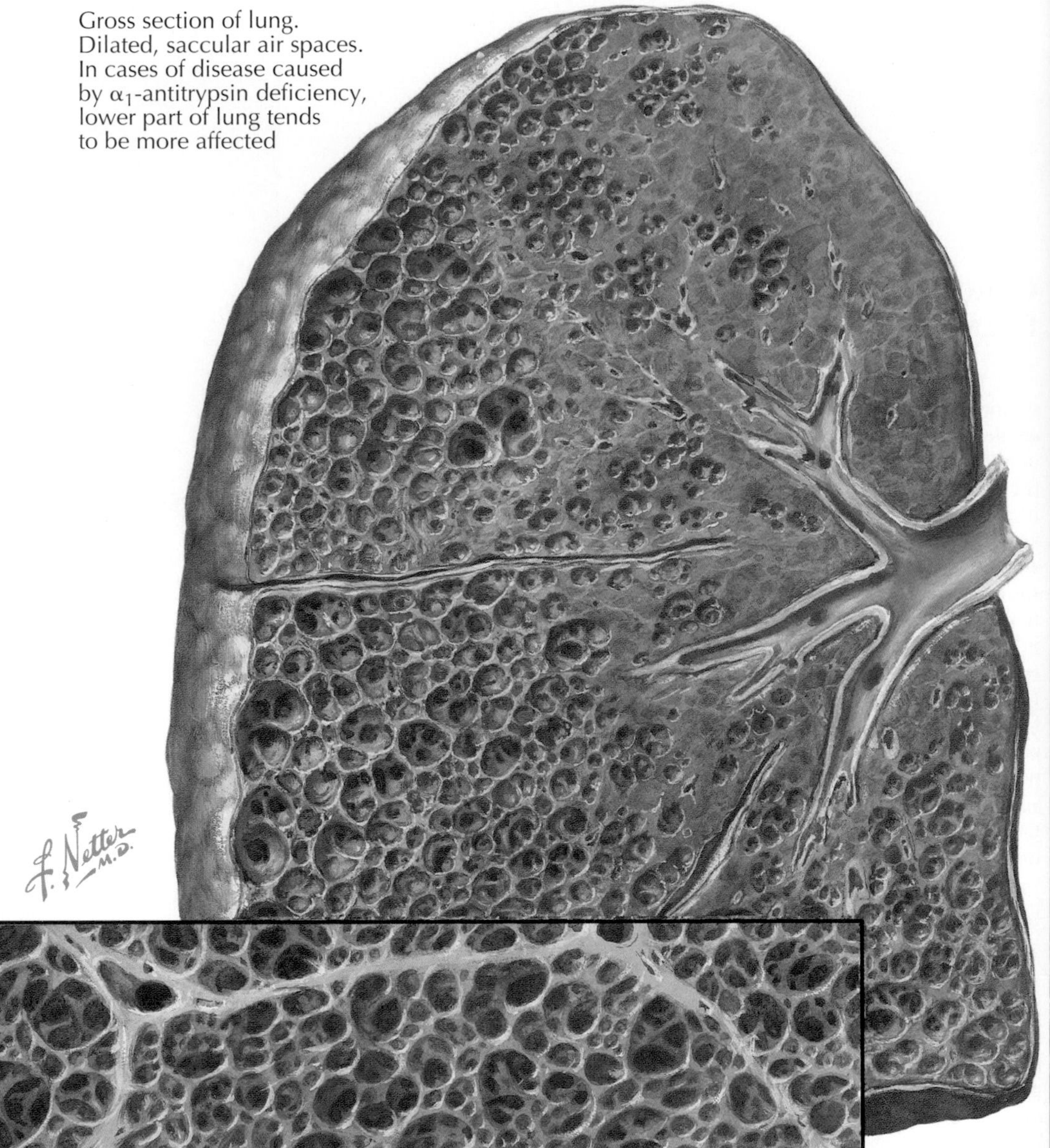

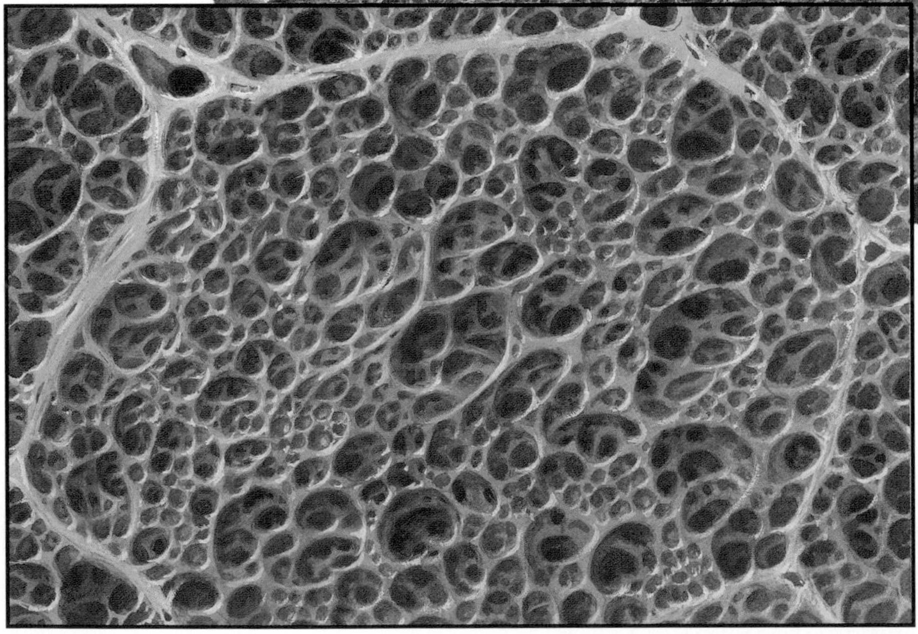

Magnified section. Diffuse involvement of all portions of acini

COPD: Inflammation

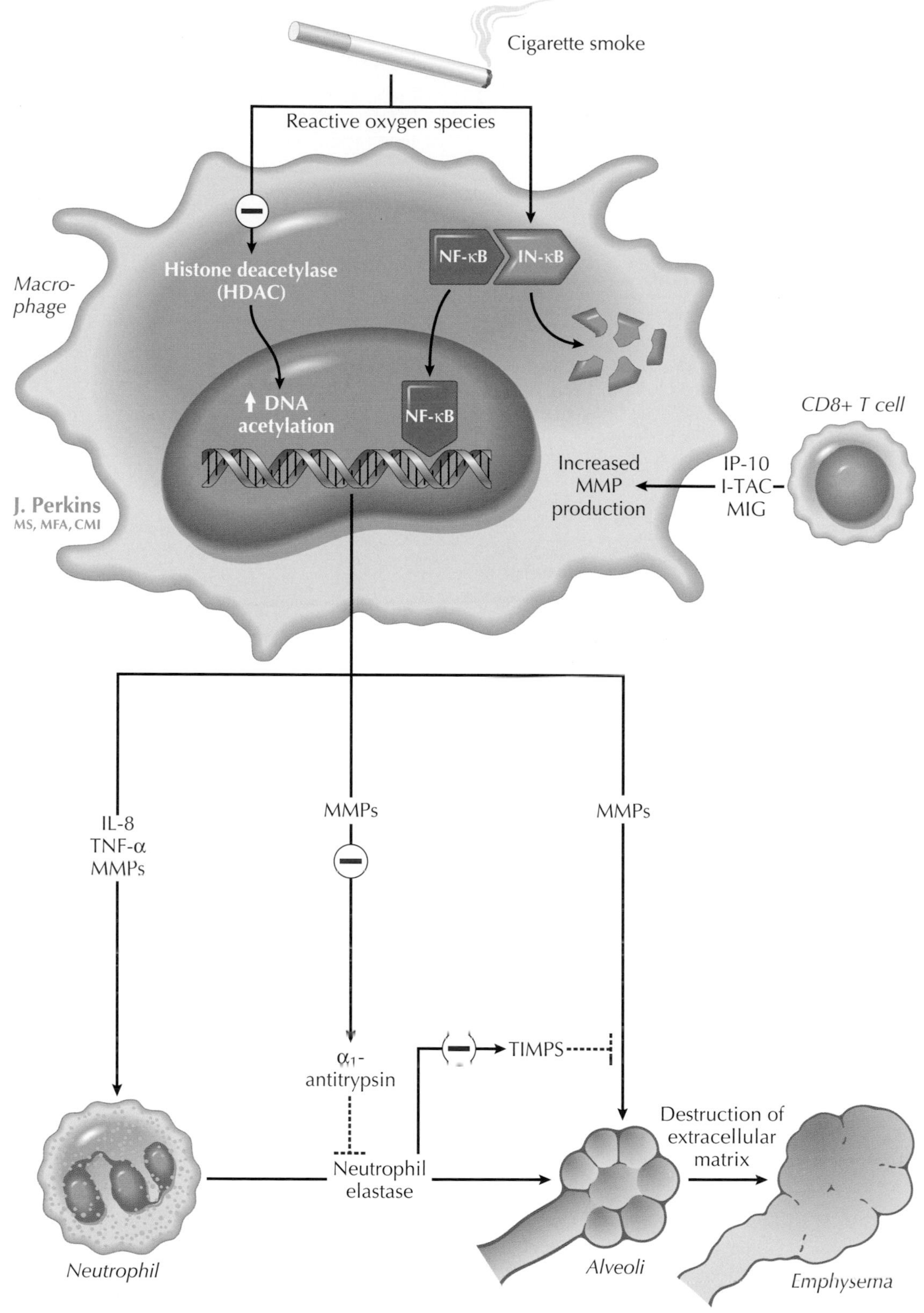

Chronic Obstructive Pulmonary Disease *(Continued)*

correlated best with the severity of emphysema as assessed at subsequent postmortem examination.

High-resolution CT examination of the chest is now considered the best indicator of the extent and distribution of emphysema (see Plate 4-41). Qualitative visual assessments can assess the presence of thin-walled bullae and regions of diminished vascularity. Quantitative assessments use the degree of attenuation of x-rays to estimate the air-tissue ratio as a measure of airspace enlargement. Regions of the lung on thin-section CT scans that approach the radiodensity of air (−1000 Hounsfield units [HU]) are considered to be emphysema. For example, the emphysema index is calculated as the percentage of image voxels in the lung regions that have a density <−950 HU). Other methods rely on the statistical distribution of lung densities, quantifying the severity of emphysema by the lung density at the lowest 15th percentile of voxels.

MANAGEMENT

Patient Education

Educating patients about the chronic nature of their disease and preventive measures is an important, ongoing process that will not be completed in one visit. The health care provider should focus on topics that are most pertinent to the needs of the patient and to the stage of disease. Topics that should be covered include the nature and prognosis of COPD, proper use of inhalers and adherence to medications, role of exercise and pulmonary rehabilitation, nutrition, and use of supplemental oxygen. Providing written materials in addition to office-based education is beneficial. Special counseling is needed for patients with α_1-antitrypsin deficiency and their family members to determine whether genetic testing is necessary or desired. For those with advanced disease, discussions about end-of-life planning and advance directives regarding life support is often welcomed by patients and facilitates communication between the patient and his or her family.

PREVENTIVE MEASURES

Smoking Cessation

Smoking cessation is the single most effective intervention to slow the progression of COPD. and should be a primary goal emphasized by physicians caring for COPD patients. A smoking history should be obtained at each patient encounter. For patients who smoke, a direct, unambiguous, and personalized smoking cessation message should be given by the physician. Assistance with pharmacologic adjuncts and referral to more intensive smoking counseling groups should be offered. A combination of counseling and pharmacotherapy, including nicotine replacement therapy, varenicline, and bupropion, has been shown to be the most effective means of achieving smoking cessation. Guidelines recommend comprehensive tobacco control programs with consistent, clear, and repeated nonsmoking messages that are delivered at every medical encounter.

The Lung Health Study demonstrated the impact of smoking cessation in a landmark trial of more than 5800 smokers with spirometric signs of early COPD who were randomly assigned to smoking intervention plus placebo, smoking intervention plus bronchodilator, or no intervention. Randomization to the smoking cessation intervention was shown to reduce the rate of decline in FEV_1 and to improve mortality, mainly related to cardiovascular disease and lung cancer. Throughout the study, some patients reverted from

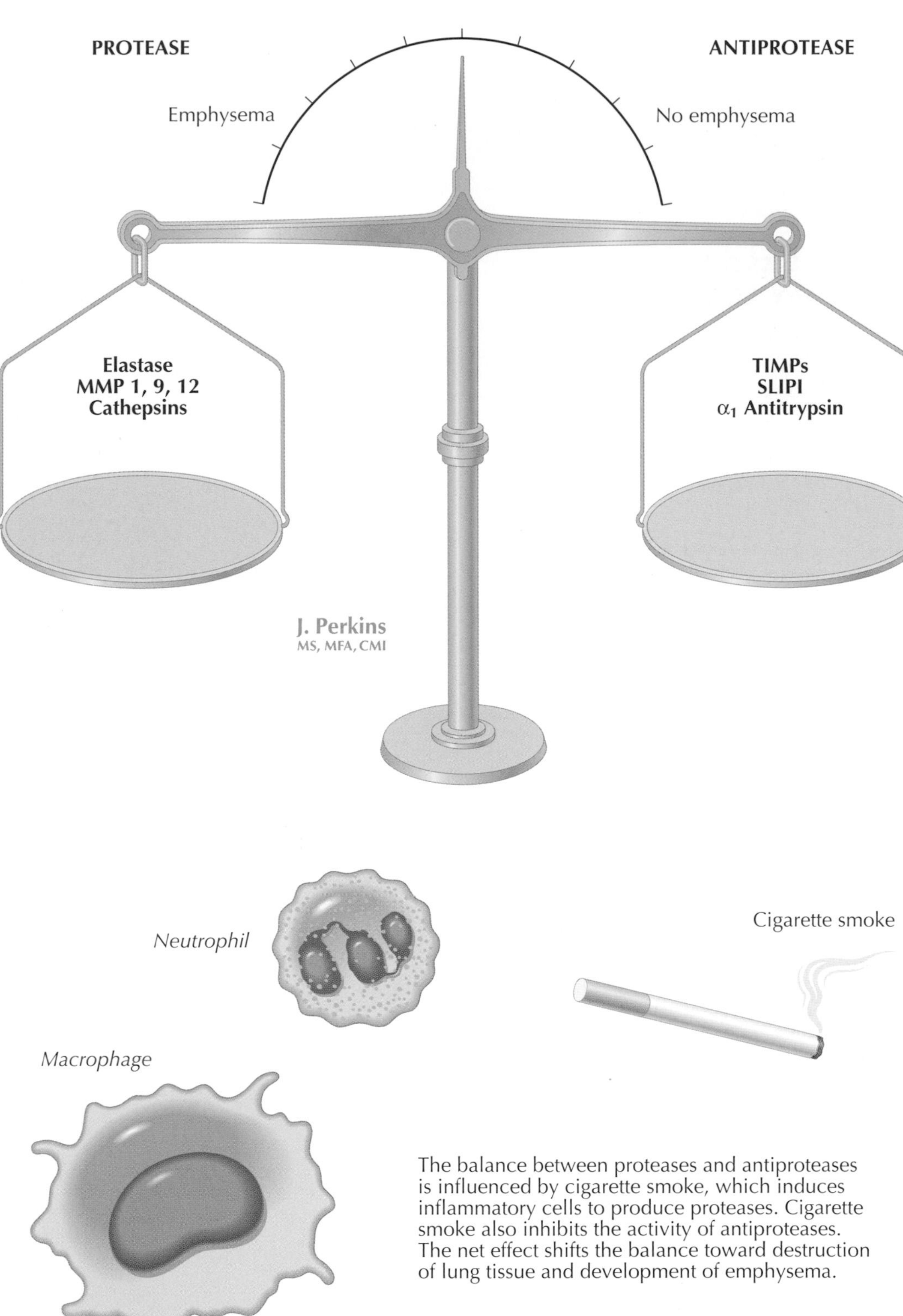

The balance between proteases and antiproteases is influenced by cigarette smoke, which induces inflammatory cells to produce proteases. Cigarette smoke also inhibits the activity of antiproteases. The net effect shifts the balance toward destruction of lung tissue and development of emphysema.

Chronic Obstructive Pulmonary Disease *(Continued)*

being smokers to quitters and vice versa. When patients were followed for 11 years, those who successfully quit smoking had a small initial increase in FEV_1 followed by a slow, normal rate of FEV_1 decline. Quitters who reverted to cigarette smoking showed a more rapid FEV_1 decline than those who were sustained quitters. At 14.5 years, those randomized to the 10-week smoking cessation had a reduced mortality rate compared with those randomized to usual care.

Persons who quit smoking with earlier disease have better outcomes relative to those who continue to smoke than those who quit smoking later in the disease. When the disease is advanced, the inflammatory response persists, and the rate of decline of lung function tends to progress. Because there are many years of asymptomatic decline in lung function, it is possible to diagnose COPD with forced expiratory spirometry before the disease is apparent and to implement aggressive smoking intervention programs. There is no consensus whether it is necessary to screen for COPD among all cigarette smokers, but there is evidence that presentation of a person's FEV_1 in terms of "lung age" does assist in smoking cessation.

Reduce Harmful Environmental Exposures

Reduction of secondhand smoke and other environmental pollutants is important in preventing the progression of COPD. Reducing exposure to indoor and outdoor pollutants requires a combination of public policy to define and uphold air quality standards and steps taken at the individual level to minimize exposure to elevated concentrations of pollutants in the indoor or outdoor environments. Occupational exposures should be ascertained with attention to fumes and dusts, and vigorous measures should be taken to eliminate harmful exposures. Respiratory protective equipment should be worn by COPD patients exposed to heavy dust concentrations. Although there is no level of FEV_1 that absolutely prohibits the use of respiratory protective equipment, some COPD patients will need to change their work environment if they cannot tolerate protective devices.

Minimize Infectious Risks

Although it is not possible to completely eliminate exposure to the many infectious agents, patients should keep away from large crowds and persons with obvious respiratory infections, especially during influenza season. Handwashing or hand sanitization should be emphasized. Patients should be educated about early signs of exacerbations and treated promptly. Some patients may want to keep a prescription or supply of antibiotics or steroids available at home. Pneumococcal vaccination is recommended, although the evidence of its particular efficacy in COPD is lacking. Annual influenza immunization can prevent or attenuate this potentially fatal infection.

Exercise and Rehabilitation

Regular, prudent, self-directed exercise is recommended for all individuals with COPD to prevent the muscle deconditioning that often accompanies the disorder. Individuals should be encouraged to perform at least 20 to 30 minutes of constant low-intensity aerobic exercise such as walking at least three times per week. This is usually feasible even in more severely impaired patients. It is important to instruct patients that they should exercise to a level of dyspnea that is tolerable for the entire exercise period. Supplemental oxygen for exercise is necessary for patients who

Pulmonary Function in Obstructive Disease

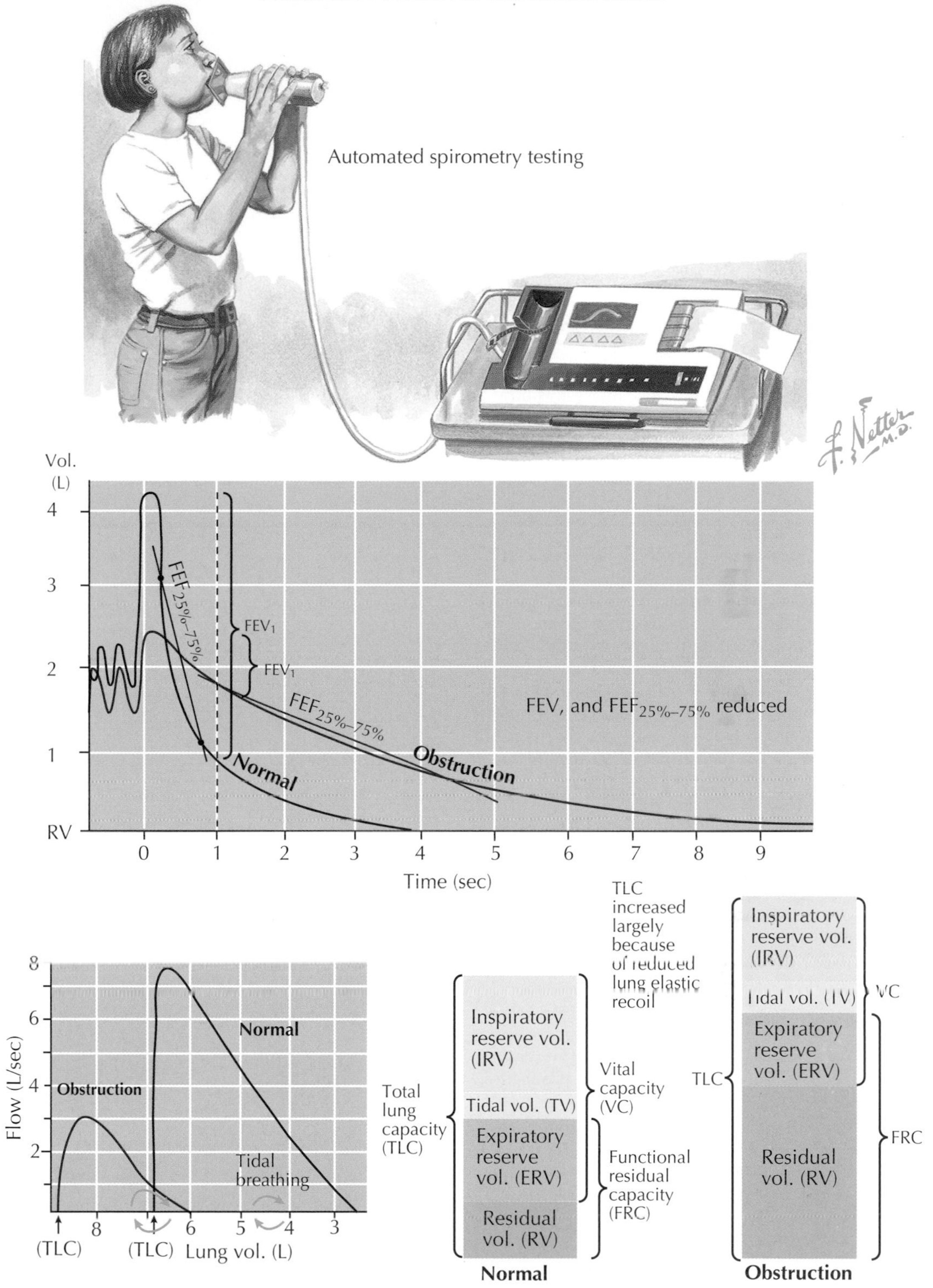

Automated spirometry testing

Maximal expiratory flow-volume curves. TLC may be increased in obstruction but expiratory flow rate decreased. In severe obstruction, tidal breathing may coincide with MEFV curve

Chronic Obstructive Pulmonary Disease *(Continued)*

desaturate with exercise and may benefit some patients without demonstrable oxygen desaturation in terms of exercise capacity and training effect.

Formal rehabilitation programs are established as an effective component of COPD management and should be offered to patients who have substantial limitation in daily activities (see Plate 5-11). The goals of pulmonary rehabilitation are to improve quality of life, reduce symptoms, and increase physical and emotional participation in daily activities. To achieve these goals, pulmonary rehabilitation programs use a multidisciplinary approach, including exercise training, nutrition, education, and psychological support. Smoking cessation programs are often linked to pulmonary rehabilitation programs. Exercise training typically consists of bicycle ergometry or treadmill exercise. Upper extremity weight training is often included as a component of strength training. Practical advice on energy conservation and pacing during activities of daily living can be delivered individually or in group sessions. Proper use of inhalers, oxygen supplementation, and good nutrition are goals of education programs.

Treatment of Stable Chronic Obstructive Pulmonary Disease

The goals of treatment of COPD are to prevent progression and complications of the disease, relieve symptoms, improve exercise capacity, improve quality of life, treat exacerbations, and improve survival. In addition to smoking intervention and treatment of hypoxemia with supplemental oxygen, pharmacologic therapy is available for treatment of patients with COPD. See the section on pharmacology (Plates 5-1 to 5-10) for a more detailed description of many of the drugs discussed below.

The current goals of drug therapy are not only to improve lung function, but also to improve quality of life and exercise capacity and to prevent exacerbations. The recommended approach to drug treatment for COPD is to sequentially add agents using the minimum number of agents and the most convenient dosing schedule, starting with the agents having the greatest benefit, best tolerance, and lowest cost (see Plate 4-42).

Inhaled bronchodilators, including β-agonists and anticholinergic agents, are the foundation of treatment for patients with COPD. They are given on a regular basis to maintain bronchodilation and on an as-needed basis for relief of symptoms. Both β-agonist and anticholinergic classes are available in short-duration (4-6 hour) and long-duration (12-24 hour) forms. Evidence suggests that long-acting agents are more effective than short-acting agents, but the choice of medication should also account for cost considerations and patient preference. Combination of different classes of bronchodilators is often more effective than increasing the dose of a single agent, and combination inhalers can simplify treatment regimens. Individuals with frequent exacerbations or more severe COPD may benefit from a combination inhaler of corticosteroids and long-acting bronchodilator. Long-acting oral theophylline can also be used as adjunctive therapy. Chronic use of systemic corticosteroids should be reserved for individuals with very frequent or life-threatening exacerbations who cannot tolerate their discontinuation.

Replacement therapy with α_1-antitrypsin should be considered for individuals with severe deficiency. Observational studies suggest that individuals with moderate degrees of impairment (FEV_1 35%-65% predicted) seem to benefit most in terms of preservation of lung function and improved survival.

Chronic Obstructive Pulmonary Disease *(Continued)*

Patient education about pharmacotherapy is important to ensure proper use of medications, as well as to enhance adherence. Inhaled agents are administered by metered-dose inhalers or dry powder inhalers or as a nebulized solution. The selection of route of administration is made by cost and convenience of the device because all are similarly effective if used properly. Proper use of inhaled medications is difficult for many patients to learn and retain. Adherence with inhaled medication, particularly when it does not provide immediate symptom relief, is poor. Typically, about half of patients do not take their medication in the dose or quantity prescribed. Reasons for this include a lack of understanding of the role of the medication, failure of the medication to provide meaningful benefit, complexity of the treatment program, and expense of the treatment. Many patients do not want to confide poor adherence to their physician, so it is important for the physician to ascertain this information in a way that does not interfere with the relationship with the patient. If nonadherence is a problem, the treating physician can undertake actions to improve adherence such as simplification of the medication program, education about the benefits of treatment, linking drug use to established habits such as meals or tooth brushing, or prescribing less costly drugs.

Treatment of Exacerbations

COPD exacerbations are characterized by worsening dyspnea, cough, and increased sputum production. There are several formal definitions of a COPD exacerbation, but a useful working definition is that a COPD exacerbation is a worsening of dyspnea, cough, or sputum production that exceeds day-to-day variability and that persists for more than 1 or 2 days. On average, patients with COPD have two to three exacerbations per year, but there is wide variation, and the frequency of exacerbations is only roughly correlated with severity of airflow obstruction. The best predictor of future exacerbations is a history of frequent exacerbations, and these are more common in patients with chronic cough and sputum production. Precipitating events include respiratory and nonrespiratory infections; exposure to respiratory irritants and air pollution; and comorbid conditions such as heart failure, pulmonary embolism, myocardial ischemia, or pneumothorax.

For patients treated at home, increasing the frequency and intensity of inhaled short-acting bronchodilators for several days is effective in mild exacerbations. A nebulizer may be needed for those who have difficulty using inhalers or in those with severe dyspnea. Increasing dyspnea accompanied by a change in the quantity or color of phlegm is usually an indication of bacterial infection and should prompt initiation of antibiotics. A course of corticosteroids, equivalent to 30 to 60 mg of prednisone for 7 to 14 days, will shorten the duration of symptoms for patients with exacerbations managed as outpatients.

For patients admitted to the hospital, intensification of inhaled bronchodilator treatment, systemic corticosteroids, and antibiotics should be administered. Controlled oxygen supplementation should be provided at the lowest level needed to reverse hypoxemia and minimize the induction of hypercapnia. The selection of the oral or intravenous route for antibiotics and corticosteroids is determined by the severity of the illness and the ability of the patient to tolerate oral medication.

Treatment in an intensive care setting should be undertaken for patients with severe life-threatening

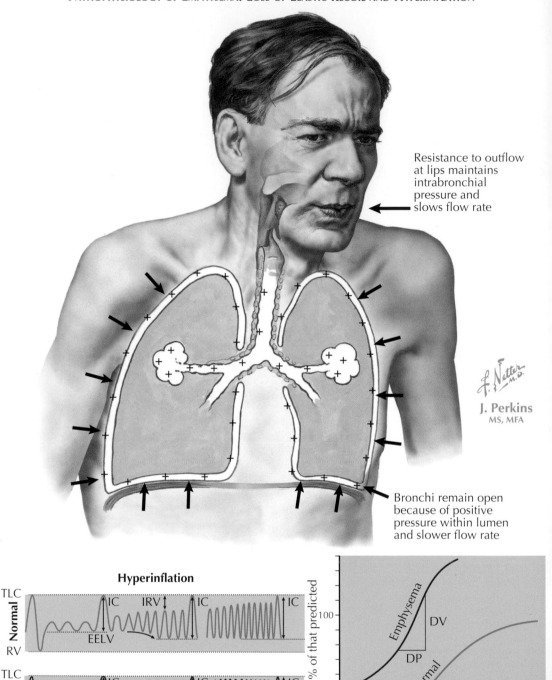

Pathophysiology of Emphysema: Loss of Elastic Recoil and Hyperinflation

Resistance to outflow at lips maintains intrabronchial pressure and slows flow rate

Bronchi remain open because of positive pressure within lumen and slower flow rate

F. Netter M.D.

J. Perkins MS, MFA

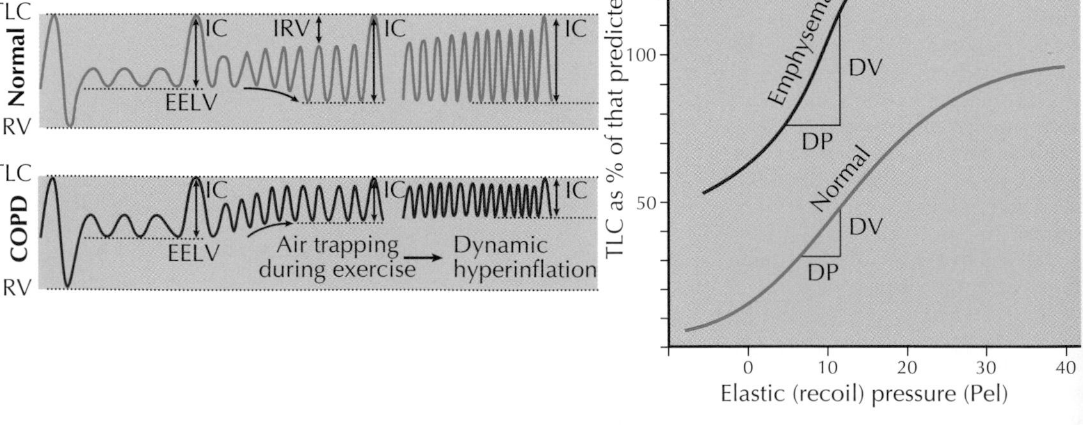

Chronic Obstructive Pulmonary Disease *(Continued)*

exacerbations and those who require more constant attention. For patients with respiratory failure, noninvasive mask ventilation has proven to be an effective strategy to avert endotracheal intubation, shorten the duration of illness, and improve outcomes. When noninvasive mask ventilation is not successful in sustaining ventilation or if the patient is too ill to use the mask, endotracheal intubation and mechanical ventilation are needed to treat respiratory failure. The mechanical ventilator should be set to provide a provide a prolonged duration of expiration to minimize dynamic hyperinflation ("intrinsic positive end-expiratory pressure"), which can lead to dyspnea, ventilator dyscoordination, and barotrauma. Care should be taken not to overventilate the patient and cause alkalemia, which may ultimately impede liberation from the ventilator. Survival after an episode of acute respiratory failure for COPD is about 50% at 2 years after discharge, with about 50% of the patients being readmitted to the hospital within 6 months.

Treatment Complications

Patients with advanced COPD are prone to developing secondary complications of the disease. The goals of treatment are to restore functional status as quickly and as much as possible and to alleviate distress and discomfort.

Pneumothorax

Acute worsening of dyspnea may result from a pneumothorax, which patients with bullous emphysema are prone to have. Treatment involves use of high-concentration oxygen and drainage with a catheter or chest tube connected to a valve or vacuum drainage system. Patients with recurrent, life-threatening, or bilateral pneumothorax are candidates for pleurodesis to prevent recurrence.

Cor Pulmonale

The pulmonary vascular bed normally has an impressive reserve that accommodates large increases in cardiac output with minimal elevations of pulmonary artery pressures (see Plate 4-32). In COPD, there is a decrease in the total cross-sectional area of the pulmonary vascular bed caused by anatomic changes in the arteries; constriction of smooth muscle in response to alveolar hypoxia; and, to the extent that emphysema is present, a loss of pulmonary capillaries. Therefore, the pressures that must be generated by the right ventricle are elevated, and dilatation and hypertrophy of the right ventricle result. Overt right ventricular failure often occurs in association with endobronchial infections, which leads to worsening hypoxemia and hypercapnia. Such episodes are more frequent in patients in whom bronchitis is dominant.

Patients with cor pulmonale are cyanotic and have distended neck veins that do not collapse with inspiration, hepatic engorgement with a tender and enlarged liver, and pitting edema of the extremities. The heart may or may not appear enlarged on a PA chest radiograph, but pulmonary vessels are prominent. Physical examination may disclose a palpable right ventricular heave and an audible early diastolic gallop that is accentuated by inspiration. On occasion, there is dilatation of the tricuspid ring with secondary tricuspid insufficiency; this disappears with effective treatment. The electrocardiogram may show changes of right ventricular hypertrophy. Echocardiographic findings may be inconsistent, especially because of difficulty obtaining

High-Resolution CT Scan of Lungs in COPD

Upper lobe

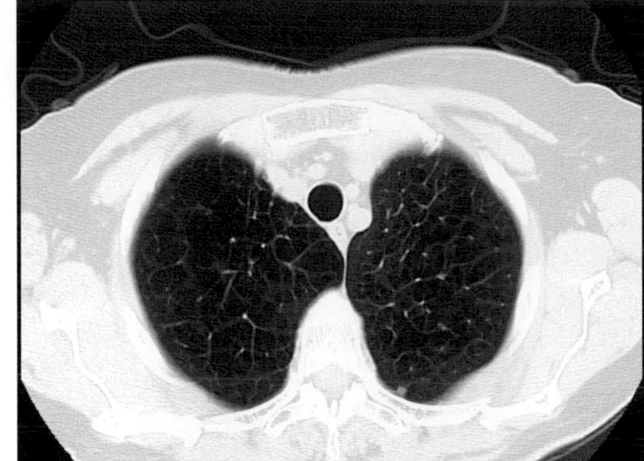

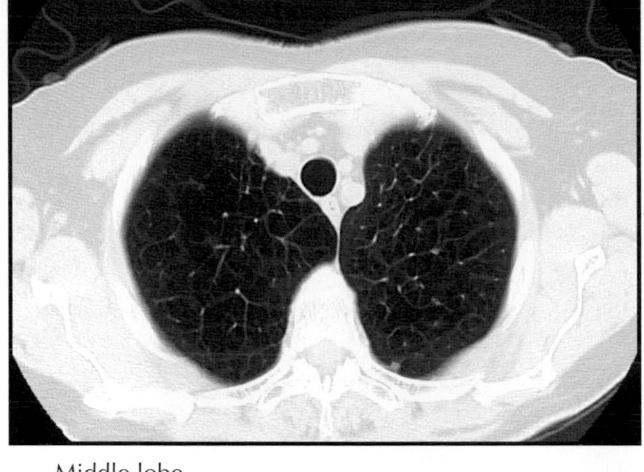

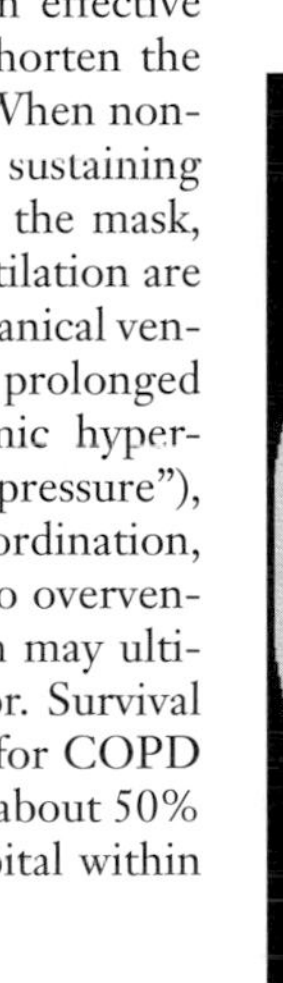

Middle lobe

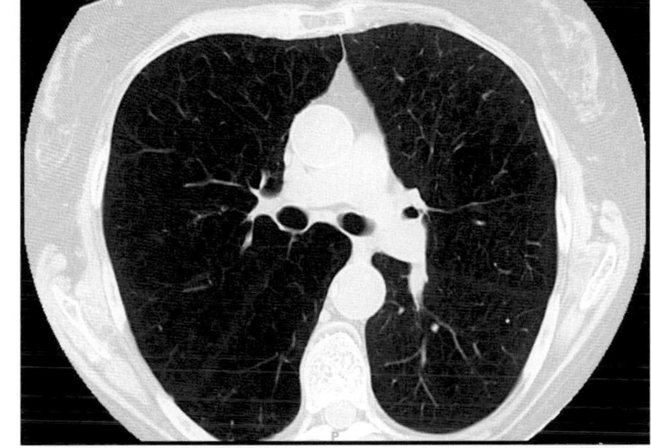

Lower lobe

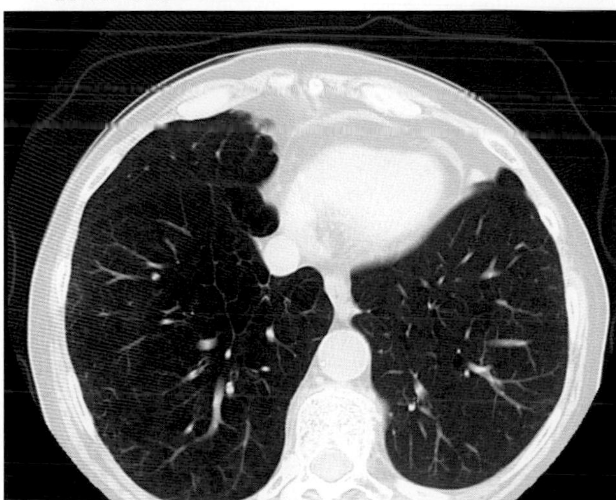

CT scans show severe panacinar emphysema of the upper (above and middle) and lower (below) lobes of the lung

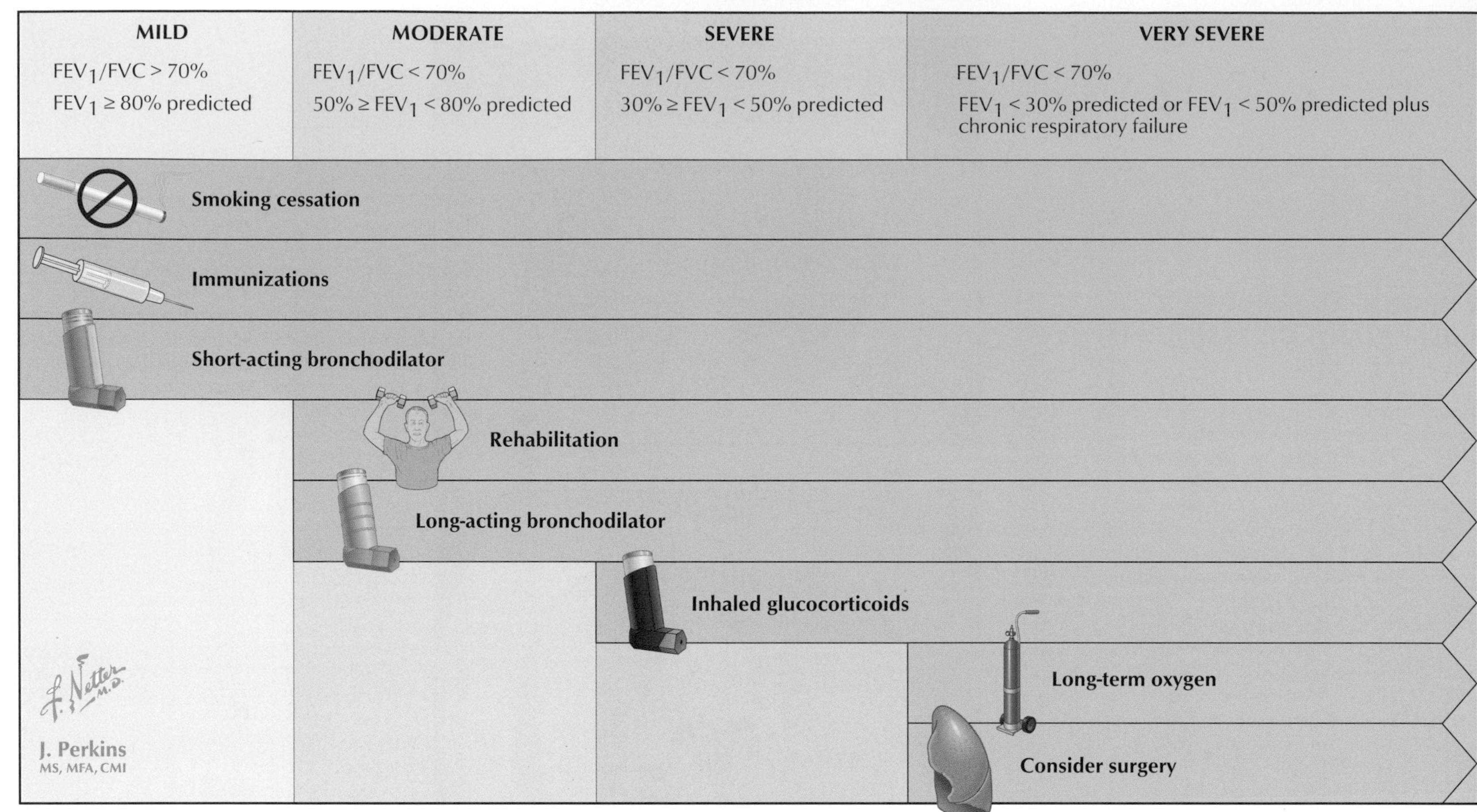

SUMMARY OF COPD TREATMENT GUIDELINES
MILD
FEV1/FVC > 70%
FEV1 ≥ 80% predicted
MODERATE
FEV1/FVC < 70%
50% ≥ FEV1 < 80% predicted
SEVERE
FEV1/FVC < 70%
30% ≥ FEV1 < 50% predicted
VERY SEVERE
FEV1/FVC < 70%
FEV1 < 30% predicted or FEV1 < 50% predicted plus chronic respiratory failure
Smoking cessation
Immunizations
Short-acting bronchodilator
Rehabilitation
Long-acting bronchodilator
Inhaled glucocorticoids
Long-term oxygen
Consider surgery
F. Netter M.D.
J. Perkins
MS, MFA, CMI

CHRONIC OBSTRUCTIVE PULMONARY DISEASE *(Continued)*

good-quality views of the right ventricle because of overlying hyperinflation of the lungs. Thus, in patients suspected to have pulmonary hypertension, a right-sided heart catheterization is the most definitive means of making the diagnosis.

Treatment of hypoxemia is the mainstay of prevention and treatment of cor pulmonale. Supplemental oxygen should be prescribed to maintain adequate oxygen saturations regardless of the development of hypercapnia (see Plates 5-12 to 5-14). The presence of sleep apnea is common in patients with COPD and pulmonary hypertension. Thus, evaluation with a sleep study is often helpful to determine the need for nocturnal oxygen or continuous positive airway pressure (see Plates 4-165 to 4-166). In occasional patients who have severe pulmonary hypertension with minimal COPD, pulmonary thromboembolism should be ruled out. Rarely, pulmonary vasodilators may be used when the magnitude of pulmonary hypertension seems disproportionate to the severity of the COPD and hypoxemia.

SURGICAL TREATMENT

Lung Volume Reduction Surgery (see Plate 5-32)

Lung volume reduction surgery (LVRS) is a surgical procedure that involves stapled resection of 20% to 30% of the lung bilaterally, usually from the apices (see section on LVRS). Although some patients show substantial physiologic and symptomatic improvement after LVRS, many do not. The group of patients that fares best with LVRS is those who have emphysema predominantly in the upper lung zones and who have low exercise capacity despite pulmonary rehabilitation. These patients have improved survival after LVRS and show improved functional status and quality of life. Conversely, patients without upper lobe predominance (i.e., lower lobe emphysema or homogeneous emphysema) and who have adequate exercise capacity after rehabilitation have worse outcomes after LVRS.

Surgical resection of a single large bulla is rarely indicated for treatment of COPD. Isolated giant bullae are usually the result of an expanding congenital cyst. The generally accepted indication for resection of a single large bulla is that it occupies more than one-third of the hemithorax and causes compression of normal lung. Some believe that a preserved DL_{CO} is an indicator of those most likely to improve after bullectomy.

Lung Transplantation (see Plate 5-33)

In younger patients with advanced disease, lung transplantation should be a treatment consideration (see Plate 5-33). Criteria for lung transplantation referral in patients with COPD is an FEV_1 below 25% predicted, severe hypercapnia, or severe pulmonary hypertension in patients younger than age 60 to 65 years. The traditional recommendation is that patients should be referred for transplantation when their life expectancy is less than 2 years because this is the average waiting time on a transplant recipient list. In recent years, the waiting time has lengthened to closer to 4 years, so this may influence physicians to make earlier referrals. Other comorbid conditions, such as poor nutritional status, obesity, chronic mycobacterial infection, or severe osteoporosis, as well as suboptimal psychosocial support, are considered relative contraindications. Current smoking, recent malignant disease, major organ system failure (particularly renal or chronic hepatitis B or C infections) are considered absolute contraindications. Lung transplantation may be either unilateral or bilateral depending on the availability of donor organs and the preference of the transplant surgeon. Generally, younger patients and those with accompanying bronchiectasis are considered more suitable candidates for bilateral lung transplantation.

In the past, COPD has been the most common indication for lung transplantation, accounting for nearly 40% of all lung transplants and about 50% of single lung transplants. This is accounted for by the high prevalence of COPD as well as the better survival rate for patients with COPD than those with other transplant indications while awaiting donor organs. However, current criteria for prioritization of transplant recipients based on diagnosis rather than waiting time alone are likely to diminish the likelihood that COPD patients will receive donor organs. Early survival for patients with COPD after lung transplant is slightly better than that of other diagnostic groups in the first few years. Overall, 30-day survival is 93%, 3-year survival is 61%, and 5-year survival is 45%.

Bronchiectasis

Bronchiectasis is structural damage to conducting airways leading to chronic cough, sputum production, recurrent infective exacerbations, and loss of lung function. Bronchiectasis was first described in 1819 by Laennec as an abnormal dilatation of bronchi and bronchioles caused by a vicious cycle of airway infection and inflammation; this definition still holds true today. Bronchiectasis is being diagnosed with increasing frequency both in the developed and underdeveloped world because of improved diagnostic techniques (high-resolution computed tomography [HRCT] scans) and awareness.

BILATERAL SEVERE BRONCHIECTASIS

Dilated and inflamed airways throughout the lungs, which are filled with pus and retained secretions.

Extensive bronchiectasis in a patient with rheumatoid arthritis

CAUSE

Causes of bronchiectasis may be categorized as an underlying systemic disease or anatomic abnormality, postinfectious or idiopathic. The most common causes differ by age (children vs. adults) and by country.

Systemic Disease

The most important inherited cause of bronchiectasis is cystic fibrosis (CF). CF is reviewed in Plates 4-45 to 4-47; the remainder of this review focuses on non-CF bronchiectasis. Primary ciliary dyskinesia (PCD) is another well-recognized cause of bronchiectasis. PCD is an autosomal recessive, genetically heterogeneous disorder characterized by oto-sino-pulmonary disease caused by abnormal structure and function of cilia. Patients with PCD present with chronic rhinitis, recurrent otitis media and sinusitis, neonatal respiratory distress, chronic cough, and situs inversus (in ~50%). Nasal nitric oxide measurements are a valuable screening tool, with low concentrations seen almost uniformly in patients with PCD. Evaluation of ciliary ultrastructure from a nasal scrape remains the best method of diagnosis. Most PCD patients (~90%) have ultrastructural defects of cilia involving the outer dynein arm (ODA), inner dynein arm (IDA), or both. Genetic diagnosis is becoming increasingly possible. Mutations in DHAI1 and DNAH5 (encoding ODA proteins) are found in about 40% of PCD patients with ODA defects.

α_1-Antitrypsin disease is increasingly recognized as a cause of bronchiectasis. Although emphysema remains the most common pulmonary feature, 27% of patients in one series had clinically important bronchiectasis.

Immune deficiencies may contribute to bronchiectasis, including IgG subclass deficiencies; hypogammaglobulinemia; or, more rarely, chronic granulomatous disease or other causes of abnormal neutrophil adhesion, respiratory burst, and chemotaxis. HIV/AIDS is also a risk factor for bronchiectasis.

Autoimmune or immune-related diseases such as allergic bronchopulmonary aspergillosis (ABPA), collagen vascular diseases (particularly Sjögren syndrome and rheumatoid arthritis) and inflammatory bowel diseases may be associated with bronchiectasis.

Anatomic Abnormality

Patients with chronic obstructive pulmonary disease may have associated bronchiectasis, affecting up to 50% of those with severe but stable disease in one series. Other anatomic lung diseases associated with diffuse bronchiectasis include tracheobronchomegaly (Mounier-Kuhn disease), congenital cartilage deficiency (Williams-Campbell syndrome), and yellow nail syndrome. Obstructive airway lesions, such as endobronchial tumors, granulomatous disease, or foreign bodies, may lead to focal bronchiectasis distal to the obstruction. Other processes, such as unilateral hyperlucent lung (Swyer-James syndrome) and pulmonary sequestration, may also lead to focal bronchiectasis.

Postinfectious Bronchiectasis

The prevalence of postinfectious bronchiectasis plummeted in the developed world with the introduction of antibiotic therapy for lower respiratory infections and routine childhood immunizations. However, it remains the most common cause in the developing world. Although any lower respiratory tract infection can potentially lead to bronchiectasis, infections that place individuals at greatest risk include adenovirus, pertussis, measles, and tuberculosis, as well as *Klebsiella pneumoniae*, *Staphylococcus aureus*, and *Haemophilus influenzae*.

Nontuberculous mycobacteria (NTM), particularly *Mycobacterium avium* complex (MAC), are associated with and may cause nodular bronchiectasis. MAC may present with bronchiectasis, particularly of the lingula and right middle lobe, in immunocompetent individuals without preexisting lung disease. The typical patient is an elderly, thin, white woman. A joint statement on NTM disease by the American Thoracic Society and the Infectious Disease Society of America emphasized the role of NTM in bronchiectasis.

DIAGNOSIS

The diagnosis of bronchiectasis should be considered in individuals presenting with chronic cough and sputum production. Other symptoms may include dyspnea, hemoptysis, and systemic symptoms such as fatigue or malaise. Among adults, bronchiectasis is more common in women than men. Idiopathic bronchiectasis occurs most frequently in middle-aged women who are lifelong nonsmokers. HRCT is the

BRONCHIECTASIS *(Continued)*

gold standard for diagnosis of bronchiectasis. Plain radiography is insufficiently sensitive, and contrast bronchography no longer plays a role. The extent of disease on HRCT has been correlated with functional change and clinical outcomes.

An underlying cause of bronchiectasis is more frequently identified in children than in adults. In two series from the United Kingdom, among 136 children, the cause of bronchiectasis was identified as an immunodeficiency in 34%, aspiration in 18%, PCD in 16%, and idiopathic in 25%. In two adult series from the United Kingdom, idiopathic bronchiectasis was diagnosed in 25% to 47% of individuals.

Examinations to consider in patients with HRCT-diagnosed bronchiectasis may include a sweat chloride test and CF genetic analysis to evaluate for CF, nasal nitric oxide and nasal scrape for PCD, immunodeficiency evaluation (quantitative immunoglobulins with IgG subclasses, antibody response to vaccines with tetanus, *H. influenzae*), barium esophagram for gastroesophageal reflux, α_1-antitrypsin levels, sputum culture, and acid-fast baeilli (AFB). In focal bronchiectasis, evaluation for an airway lesion should be considered.

CLINICAL COURSE

The clinical course of non-CF bronchiectasis is highly variable, depending on the underlying cause and management. Some individuals have daily symptoms, frequent exacerbations, and progressive loss of lung function, but others have minimal daily symptoms and relative preservation of lung function. Factors associated with more rapid decline in lung function include colonization with *Pseudomonas aeruginosa*, more frequent exacerbations, and evidence of systemic inflammation.

MANAGEMENT

There have been few randomized, controlled trials of therapies in individuals with bronchiectasis, partly because of the heterogeneity of the disease. Although the rationale for therapy may be similar in CF and non-CF bronchiectasis, therapies must be tested specifically in this population. For example, because in general, lung function and mortality are less impacted in non-CF bronchiectasis, therapies may be best directed to decreasing exacerbation rates rather than slowing lung function decline. Whereas rhDNase is a mainstay of therapy in CF, it has been demonstrated to have an adverse safety profile in adults with bronchiectasis.

Airway Clearance

Although airway clearance techniques are a mainstay of treatment in non-CF bronchiectasis patients, there are no long-term trials in this population. There is also interest in inhaled hyperosmolar agents such as 7% saline and mannitol to rehydrate airway surface liquid. Mechanical clearance techniques, such as chest physiotherapy and flutter valves, are useful but less proven in non-CF bronchiectasis as important methods of airway clearance.

Antibiotic Therapy

Treatment of exacerbations should be undertaken with antibiotics tailored to the most recent sputum culture. The most common organisms isolated from patients with bronchiectasis include nonenteric gram-negative rods, *S. aureus*, and nontuberculous mycobacteria. About one-third of adults with bronchiectasis are chronically colonized with *P. aeruginosa*. For patients with chronic *P. aeruginosa* colonization, agents include intravenous antibiotics and oral ciprofloxacin. A recent study showed modest microbial benefit but no clinical benefit to the addition of inhaled tobramycin to oral ciprofloxacin for the treatment of acute exacerbations caused by infection with *P. aeruginosa*.

The role of maintenance or prophylactic antibiotics is unclear. Several small pilot studies with agents, including inhaled tobramycin, inhaled colistin, and rotating oral antibiotics, have suggested potential for microbiologic and clinical stability, but longer term studies with more attention to acquisition of resistant organisms are needed.

Antiinflammatory Therapy

Inhaled corticosteroids may reduce airway inflammation and improve clinical outcomes in adults with bronchiectasis, but the long-term safety profile is unclear. In small pilot studies, oral macrolides (erythromycin and azithromycin) may improve lung function and reduce exacerbations, but larger scale trials are needed. Caution must be taken to avoid improper treatment of unrecognized NTM infection, thus causing the emergence of resistant organisms.

Surgery

Surgery may be indicated for resection of areas of focal bronchiectasis that have led to uncontrolled infection or hemoptysis.

LOCALIZED BRONCHIECTASIS

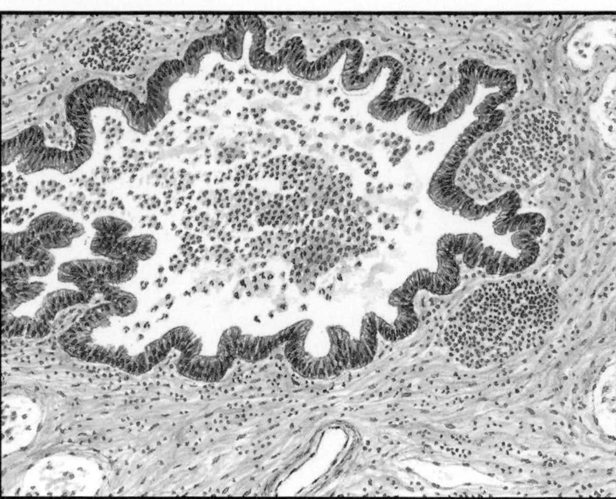

Section through dilated bronchus. Epithelium is hyperplastic and lumen contains cellular exudate. Peribronchial area shows replacement by loose connective tissue with many lymphocytes, both disseminated and aggregated into follicles

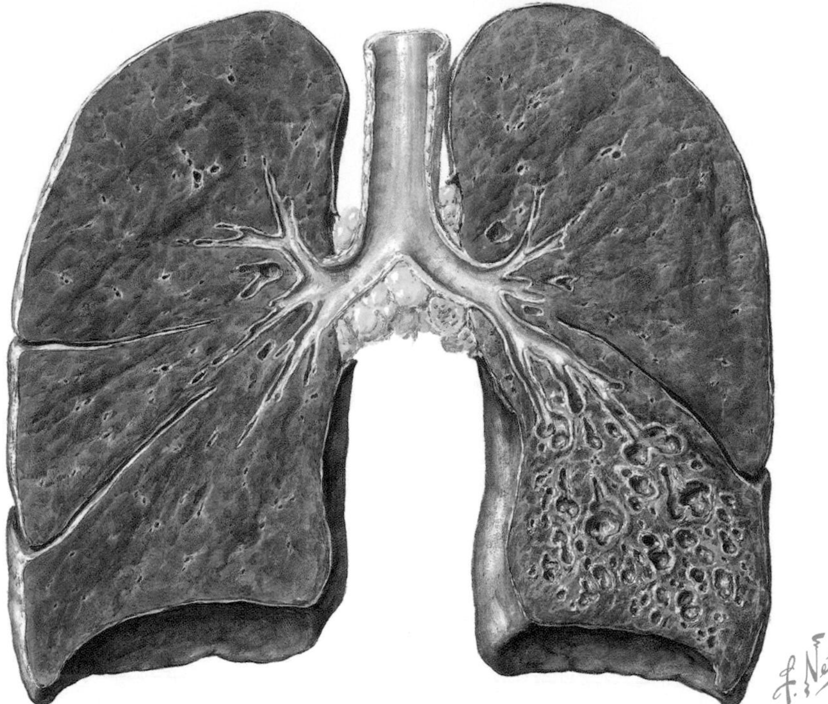

Focal bronchiectasis. Saccular dilatations of bronchi, confined to left lower lobe. Such limited pathology may be amenable to surgery

Cystic Fibrosis

Cystic fibrosis (CF) is the most common autosomal recessive life-shortening disease among whites but also affects all races. There are approximately 30,000 individuals in the United States with diagnosed CF. Progress in the understanding of the underlying genetic defect and pathophysiology and the impact of this knowledge on CF care have been rapid over the past 20 years, resulting in remarkable improvements in quality of life and survival. These gains have converted CF from a respiratory and digestive disease of young children to a complex, multisystem disorder extending into adulthood.

GENETICS

CF is caused by mutations in the CF transmembrane conductance regulator (CFTR), a 230-kb gene on chromosome 7 encoding a chloride channel expressed in epithelial cells in the sweat duct, airway, pancreatic duct, intestine, biliary tree, and vas deferens. More than 1000 mutations in CFTR have been described, although far fewer have been clearly identified as causing disease. These mutations can be grouped into six classes based on their function (Plate 4-45). The level of functional CFTR is important in determining the manifestations of CF, and the broad spectrum of disease related to CFTR dysfunction is increasingly being recognized (Plate 4-45). Attempts to predict the severity of lung disease, the major cause of morbidity and mortality in CF, from the CFTR genotype have been unsuccessful. It is likely that environmental factors and modifier genes play important roles in determining the phenotype of patients with CF.

DIAGNOSIS

Updated guidelines for the diagnosis of CF have recently been published. Although symptoms suggestive of CF include poor weight gain, steatorrhea, rectal prolapse, chronic cough, and recurrent sinusitis, CF is increasingly diagnosed via prenatal or newborn screening. Until the advent of widespread newborn screening for CF, suspicion for CF arose only from the appearance of symptoms or a family history of the disease. But by 2010, newborn screening for CF will be universal throughout the United States, and most individuals will enter the diagnostic algorithm because of a positive newborn screen result. The primary test for establishing the diagnosis of CF remains the sweat chloride test, which is performed by the pilocarpine iontophoresis method. The identification of two CF disease-causing mutations can also establish the diagnosis.

CLINICAL MANIFESTATIONS

Manifestations of CF may include chronic sinusitis, recurrent nasal polyposis, progressive obstructive pulmonary disease, exocrine pancreatic insufficiency,

Pathophysiology and Clinical Manifestations of Cystic Fibrosis

CFTR mutation classes

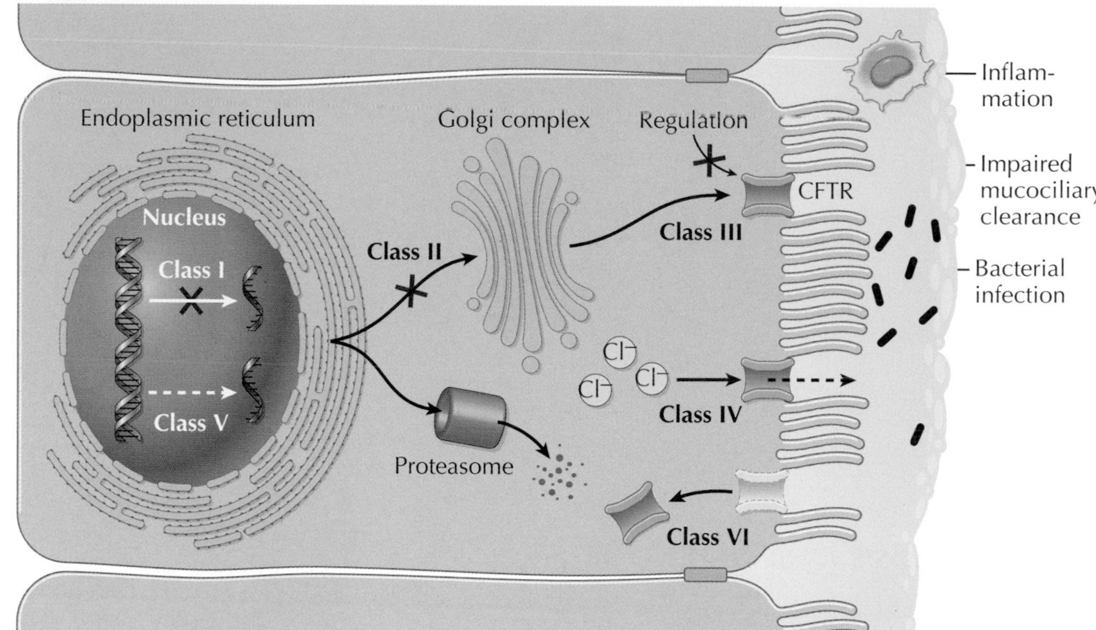

Class I Absent protein synthesis due to defective transcription; **Class II** Defective protein maturation and degradation; **Class III** Defective regulation; **Class IV** Defective chloride conductance; **Class V** Reduced protein synthesis due to reduced transcription; **Class VI** Defective chloride channel stability

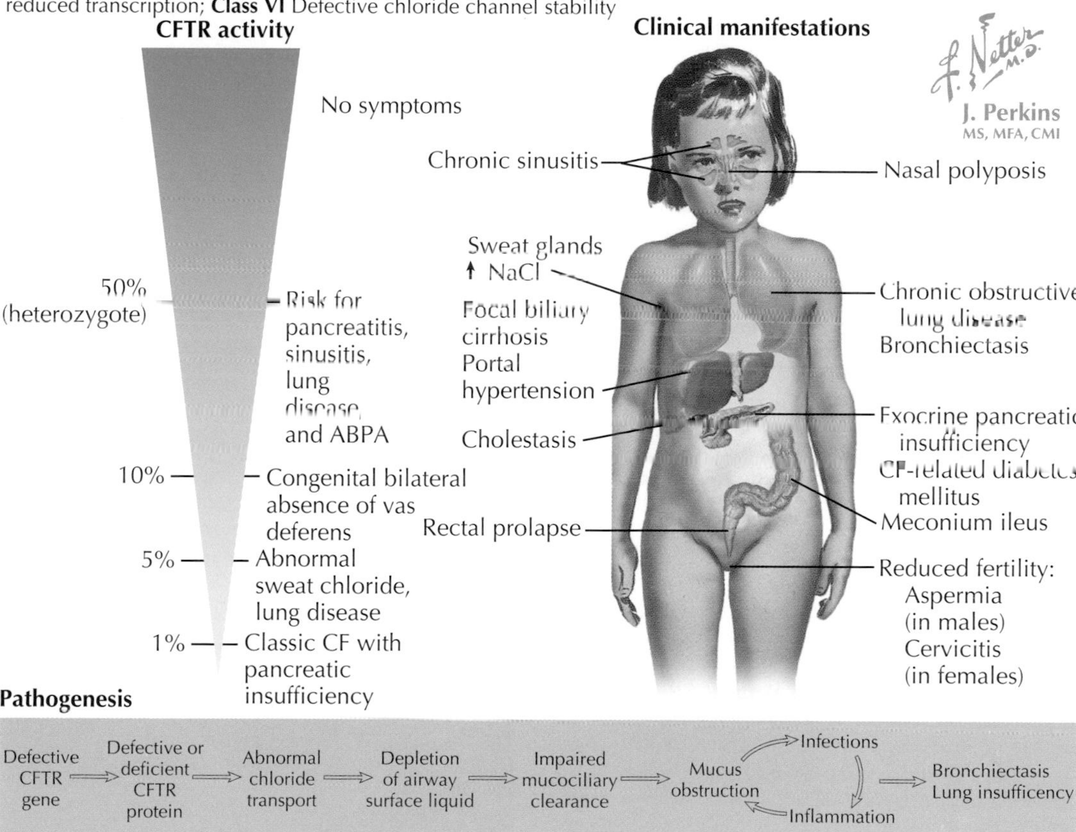

Pathogenesis

Defective CFTR gene ⇒ Defective or deficient CFTR protein ⇒ Abnormal chloride transport ⇒ Depletion of airway surface liquid ⇒ Impaired mucociliary clearance ⇒ Mucus obstruction → Infections → Inflammation → Mucus obstruction ⇒ Bronchiectasis Lung insuffiency

Cystic Fibrosis *(Continued)*

biliary disease, CF-related diabetes, and male infertility. Given the chronic, complex, multisystem nature of the illness, patients with CF should be followed in a specialized CF center, such as those accredited in the United States by the Cystic Fibrosis Foundation.

PULMONARY DISEASE

Lung disease is the primary cause of morbidity and mortality in people with CF. It is characterized by a vicious cycle of endobronchial bacterial infection and a vigorous host neutrophilic inflammatory response, resulting in progressive structural damage (bronchiectasis) and obstructive lung disease (see Plate 4-46). The airways of CF patients become infected with a distinctive spectrum of bacterial pathogens, generally acquired in an age-dependent fashion. Common pathogens at an early age include *Staphylococcus aureus* and *Haemophilus influenzae*. Later, infection with *Pseudomonas aeruginosa* becomes increasingly prevalent. At first, *P. aeruginosa* infection is intermittent and nonmucoid, but it eventually becomes chronic and mucoid in phenotype. Acquisition of *P. aeruginosa*, particularly mucoid strains, is associated with more rapid clinical deterioration.

Respiratory treatments vary by age and disease severity; guidelines have recently been published. These treatments, although dramatically improving pulmonary outcomes over the past 2 decades, also represent the greatest challenge to patients and families. The inhaled therapies and airway clearance can take more than 1 hour each day and can cause financial hardships. Chronic treatments may include airway clearance techniques; mucolytics such as inhaled rhDNase and hypertonic saline; and in patients chronically infected with *P. aeruginosa*, oral macrolides and alternate-month inhaled antibiotics.

Individuals with CF intermittently experience episodes of increased cough, increased sputum production, and decline in lung function, often in conjunction with anorexia and fatigue, termed a *pulmonary exacerbation*. Milder exacerbations are typically treated with oral or inhaled antibiotics coupled with increased airway clearance. Severe exacerbations or those that fail to resolve with outpatient therapy require treatment with intravenous antibiotics, generally in the inpatient setting. In an effort to slow or avoid the decline in lung function associated with chronic *Pseudomonas* infection, first acquisition of *Pseudomonas* spp. is treated with an eradication protocol, which may include oral, inhaled, or intravenous antibiotics, often in combination.

Complications include hemoptysis and pneumothoraces. Bilateral lung transplantation is an option for some CF patients with end-stage lung disease.

GASTROINTESTINAL DISEASE

Approximately 20% of infants with CF present acute intestinal obstruction caused by meconium ileus in the neonatal period. Exocrine pancreatic insufficiency occurs in approximately 90% of individuals affected with CF. Patients with two severe CFTR mutations (class 1, 2, or 3) present with pancreatic insufficiency,

Radiographic and Gross Anatomic Findings of the Lung in Cystic Fibrosis

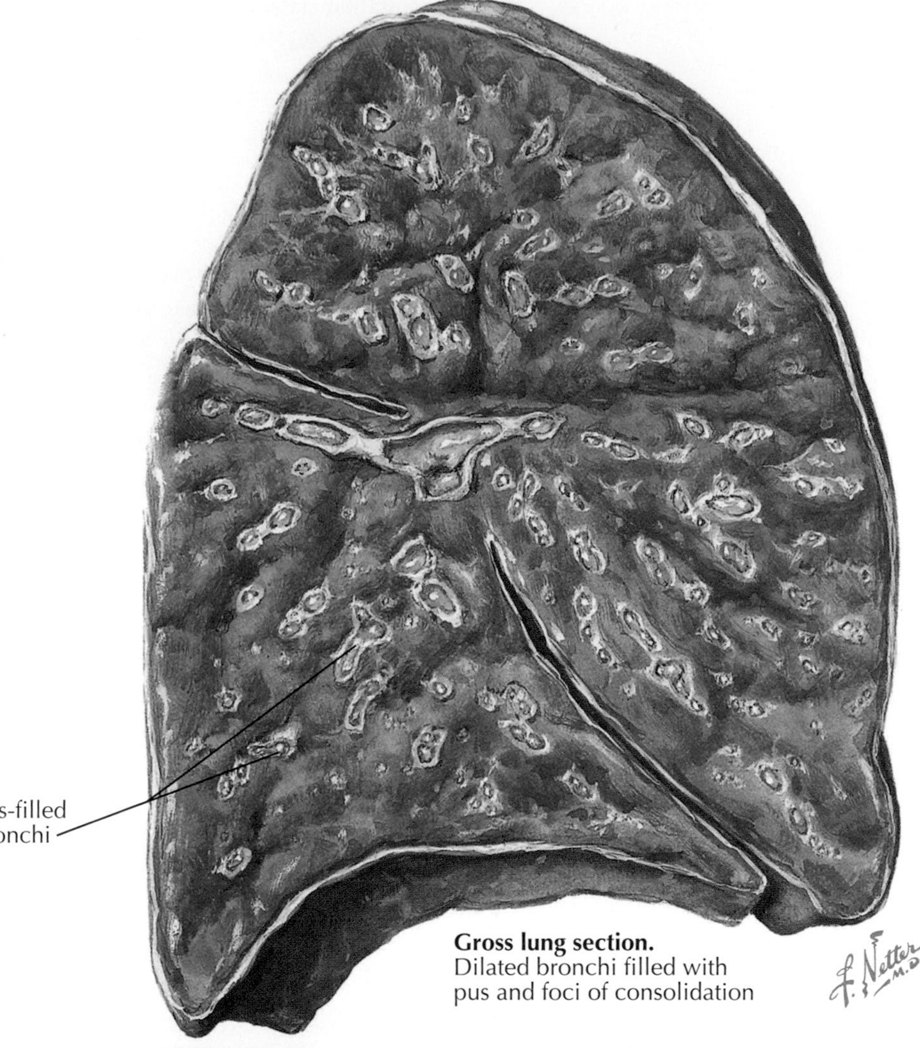

Gross lung section. Dilated bronchi filled with pus and foci of consolidation

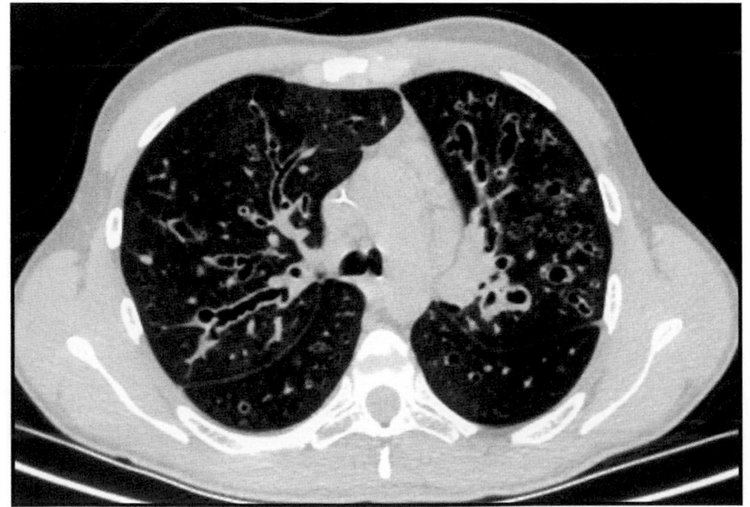

Bilateral, severe bronchiectasis seen on chest CT in a young patient with cystic fibrosis

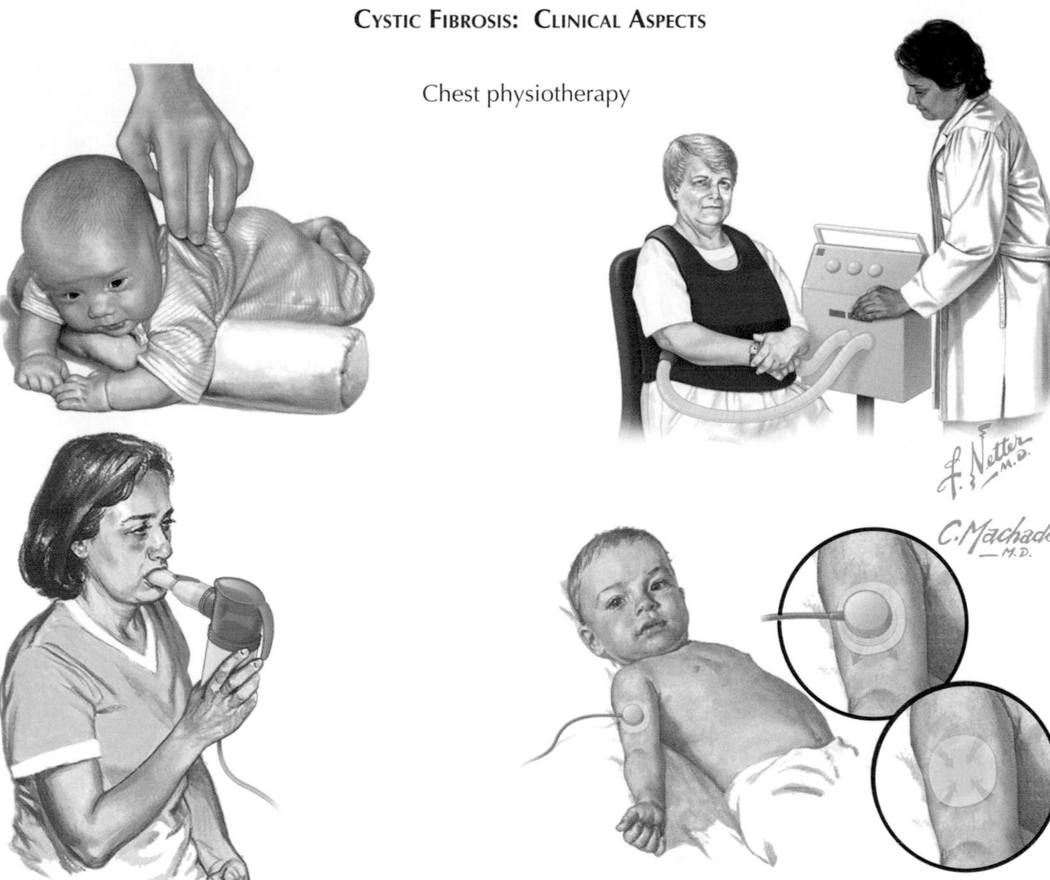

Median predicted survival age, 1986–2008

Median survival age (years): 24, 28, 32, 36, 40

Year: '86 '88 '90 '92 '94 '96 '98 '00 '02 '04 '06 '08

Data from Cystic Fibrosis Foundation, 2009. Annual data report to the center directors. Bethesda, MD: Cystic Fibrosis Foundation 2009.

The median predicted survival is 37.4 years for 2008. This represents the age by which half of the current CF Registry population would be expected to be dead, given the ages of the patients in the Registry and the mortality distribution of the deaths in 2008. The whiskers represent the 95 percent confidence bounds for the survival estimates, indicating that the 2008 median survival is between 35.0 and 40.1.

CYSTIC FIBROSIS *(Continued)*

and those with one or more mild mutations (class 4 or 5) may be pancreatic sufficient. Pancreatic insufficiency places CF patients at risk for fat malabsorption, suboptimal nutrition, and inadequate circulating levels of fat-soluble vitamins. CF patients with pancreatic insufficiency are treated with a high-fat, high-calorie diet and pancreatic enzyme replacement therapy in the form of capsules taken with each meal. Patients with pancreatic sufficiency are at increased risk of acute or chronic pancreatitis.

Some level of liver disease is common in CF patients, with the prevalence increasing with advancing age. Abnormalities may include elevated transaminases, hepatosteatosis, or biliary tract disease. Cholelithiasis is also common. A small number of patients develop frank biliary cirrhosis with portal hypertension. Management of CF liver disease often includes ursodeoxycholic acid.

ENDOCRINE DISEASE

The prevalence of CF-related diabetes also increases with advancing age. The prevalence is 9% at ages 5 to 9 years, increasing to 43% for age older than 30 years. CF-related diabetes is a risk factor for more accelerated decline in lung function and higher mortality. Therefore, routine screening is recommended. Treatment generally involves maintenance of a high-fat, high-calorie diet plus insulin therapy.

Osteopenia is also an increasingly recognized complication of CF. The cause is likely related to poor nutritional status, malabsorption of vitamins K and D, delayed pubertal maturation, steroid exposure, inactivity, and chronic pulmonary inflammation. Routine screening is recommended, and prevention via aggressive nutritional interventions, fat-soluble vitamins, and maximization of pulmonary health is critical.

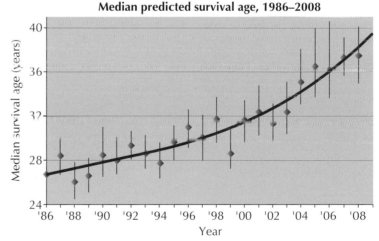

FERTILITY

At least 98% of men with CF are infertile because of absence or atresia of the vas deferens and absent or dilated seminal vesicles. Men with CF can become fathers with artificial insemination procedures. Female reproduction is normal, and an increasing number of women with CF are becoming mothers.

PROGNOSIS

Survival of patients with CF has made continuous, sustained improvements over the past 50 years, with median survival in the United States improving from 8 years in 1969 to more than 37 years today (see Plate 4-47). Female survival has been lower than male, but this "gender gap" appears to be closing. Potential contributors to improved survival include CF center care, aggressive nutritional support, and the introduction of new pulmonary therapies. Major quality improvement initiatives, the widespread uptake of newborn screening, and new therapies aimed at restoring CFTR function and combating chronic inflammation are sure to result in continued improvements in quality of life and survival for individuals with CF.

Lung Cancer Overview

Lung cancer is the most common cause of cancer death in the world, with estimated total deaths of 1.18 million by GLOBOCAN of the International Agency for Research on Cancer (IARC). In the United States, there will be an estimated 222,000 new diagnoses and 157,000 deaths in 2010. Lung cancer is a lethal disease, with only 6% of all new cases surviving 5 years in the United States. The average 5-year survival rate in Europe is 10% and is 8.9% in developing countries. Lung cancer causes more deaths than the four next most common cancers combined (colorectal, breast, prostate, and pancreas). These numbers are staggering, especially because it was a rare disease in the early 1900s.

Cigarette smoking has been identified as the single most common etiologic agent and is estimated to cause 85% to 90% of all cases. Radon is reported to cause 10% of lung cancers. Other etiologic agents are of less frequency and are primarily occupational exposures (e.g., arsenic, asbestos, chromium, nickel, coal, tar). For a complete list of carcinogens to humans, refer to the IARC (http://monographs.iarc.fr). Secondhand smoke increases the risk of lung cancer by 30% or a relative risk of 1.3 versus a never smoker with no secondhand exposure. Lung cancer risk increases with age. Less than 5% of lung cancer occurs before the age of 40 years, and the average age at diagnosis in the United States is 68 years. Family history (genetics) is a risk factor and responsible for a two- to threefold relative risk increase if lung cancer has been diagnosed in a first-degree relative, especially if he or she was at a younger age at diagnosis. The genetic predisposition of lung cancer is a subject of intense research, but to date, a lung cancer gene has not been identified. The gene 15q 24-25 encompasses the nicotinic acetylcholine receptor gene that has a role in nicotine addiction and has been associated with lung cancer risk, but it is currently uncertain if this gene is directly related to lung cancer, independent of nicotine use.

Overwhelming evidence suggests that cigarette smoking is the major cause of lung cancer. The lung cancer epidemic in Western countries parallels the incidence of smoking but lags by about 20 to 30 years. The relative risk among smokers compared with people who have never smoked is 10 to 15 times higher and is dependent on the age of onset of smoking, dose, and duration (pack-years). Stopping smoking has been shown to decrease the relative risk, but the risk does not return to that of someone who has never smoked unless one quits at an early age. Tobacco smoking increases the risk of all major histologic cell types, but the strongest association is with small cell and squamous cell and less strongly with adenocarcinoma. The most common histology in a never smoker is adenocarcinoma.

The frequency of lung cancer in women has risen dramatically in most Western countries over the past 4 to 5 decades. Globally, it is still a male-predominant disease (male : female ratio, 2-3 : 1). However, in the United States, women constitute 45% of all new lung cancer diagnoses. Lung cancer has surpassed breast cancer as the most common cause of cancer death, which occurred in the United States in the mid 1980s. Currently, 72,000 women die of lung cancer versus 40,000 deaths from breast cancer per year. Although there has been some controversy, recent studies have not shown a difference in risk between men and women who have smoked a similar amount. There is no clear evidence of ethnic differences in susceptibility to this disease.

The signs and symptoms of lung cancer are myriad, but the most common are new cough, dyspnea, hemoptysis, chest pain, or weight loss. Paraneoplastic symptoms of lung cancer are discussed later. Symptomatic lung cancer usually results in an abnormal chest radiograph. Approximately 15% to 20% of lung cancers are asymptomatic when they are detected by an incidental chest radiograph or computed tomography scan done for other reasons. Methods of diagnosis include sputum cytology, thoracentesis if pleural fluid is present, bronchoscopy, transthoracic needle aspiration, or needle aspiration and biopsy of distant metastatic sites. In some cases, the diagnosis is made at the time of surgical resection.

The World Health Organization histologic classification of lung tumors is the generally accepted standard. Lung cancer is classified as small cell and non–small cell. Non–small cell lung cancer includes squamous cell, adenocarcinoma, large cell, adenosquamous carcinoma, and sarcomatoid carcinoma. Small cell histology generally has the fastest growth rate, but tumor doubling times can vary tremendously within the same cell type. The slowest growing types have been bronchioloalveolar carcinoma (subtype of adenocarcinoma) and superficial squamous carcinoma (in situ), but again, the variability in growth rate can be enormous.

Classification of Bronchogenic Carcinoma

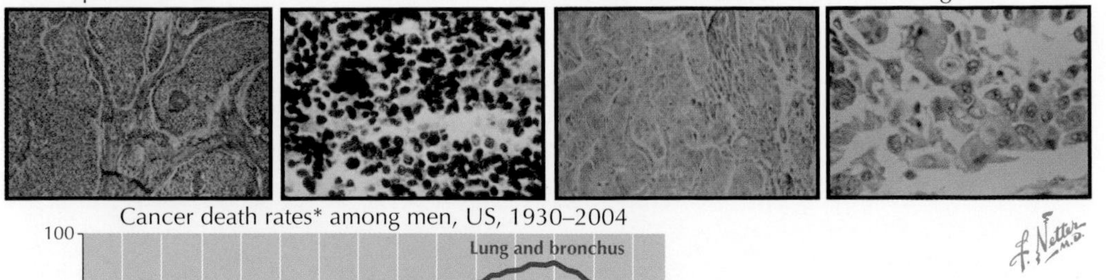

Squamous cell | Small cell | Adenocarcinoma | Large cell

Cancer death rates* among men, US, 1930–2004

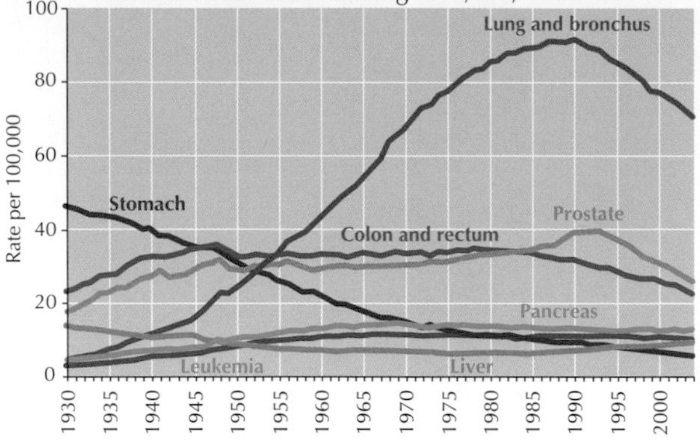

*Age-adjusted to 2000 US standard population.

Source: US Mortality Data 1960–2004, US Mortality Volumes 1930–1959, National Center for Health Statistics, Centers for Disease Control and Prevention, 2006.

Cancer death rates* among women, US, 1930–2004

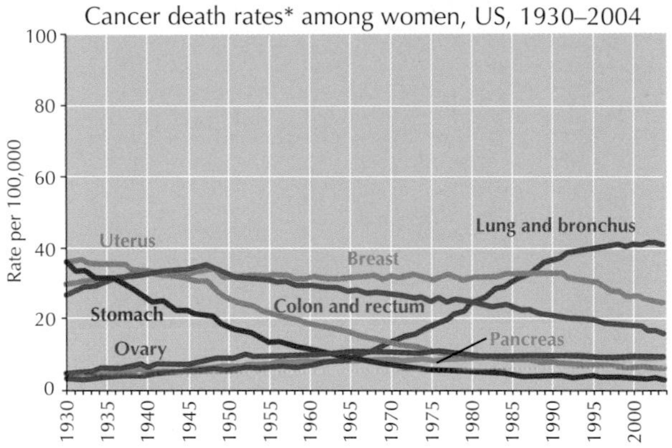

*Age-adjusted to 2000 US standard population.

Source: US Mortality Data 1960–2004, US Mortality Volumes 1930–1959, National Center for Health Statistics, Centers for Disease Control and Prevention, 2006.

Tobacco use in the US, 1900–2004

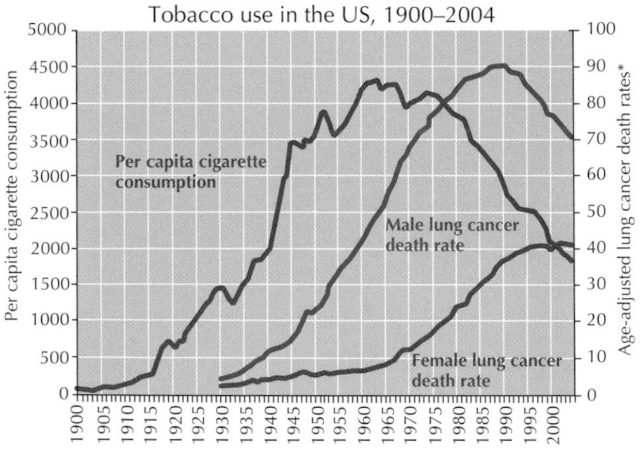

*Age-adjusted to 2000 US standard population.

Source: Death rates: US Mortality Data, 1960–2004, US Mortality Volumes, 1930–1959, National Center for Health Statistics, Centers for Disease Control and Prevention, 2006. Cigarette consumption: US Department of Agriculture, 1900–2004.

Lung Cancer Staging

In 2010, the International Union Against Cancer (UICC) and the American Joint Committee on Cancer (AJCC) published the revised seventh edition of the TNM (tumor, node, metastasis) staging system. This seventh edition was developed on the basis of the International Association for the Study of Lung Cancer (IASLC) and proposed changes to the classification from analysis of more than 67,000 cases of non–small cell lung cancer from around the world. This was the largest data set ever analyzed for the purpose of developing and validating a new staging system. The proposed new TNM staging system has also been validated for small cell carcinoma and bronchial carcinoid tumors. The primary determinant of each T, N, and M descriptor, as well as the overall stage grouping, was based on survival. Detailed algorithms were used to identify unique stages in the simplest way with the least overlap. Stages were internally and externally validated for outcomes across the various databases and geographic regions from which the data were gathered.

There were a number of substantial changes made to the former (sixth) staging system:

- T1 tumors were divided into T1a (tumors ≤2 cm in greatest diameter) and T1b (tumors >2 cm but ≤3 cm in greatest dimension).
- T2 tumors were divided into T2a (tumors >3 cm but ≤5 cm in greatest diameter) and T2b (tumors >5 cm but ≤7 cm in greatest dimension).
- Tumors more than 7 cm in greatest dimension are classified as T3.
- Tumors with additional nodule(s) in the same lobe are classified as T3.
- Tumors with additional nodule(s) in another ipsilateral lobe are classified as T4.
- Pleural dissemination (malignant pleural or pericardial effusions, pleural nodules) is classified as M1a.
- The lymph node classification remained the same, with N1 as intrapulmonary or ipsilateral hilar, N2 as ipsilateral mediastinal or subcarinal, and N3 as contralateral mediastinal or supraclavicular.
- Incorporated proposed changes to T and M (affects T2, T3, T4, and M1 categories).
- Reclassify T2aN1 tumors (≤5 cm) as stage IIA (from IIB).
- Reclassify T2bN0 tumors (>5 cm to 7 cm) as stage IIA (from IB).
- Reclassify T3 (tumor >7 cm) N0M0 as stage IIB (from IB).
- Reclassify T4N0 and T4N1 as stage IIIA (from IIIB).
- Reclassify pleural dissemination (malignant pleural or pericardial effusions, pleural nodules) from T4 to M1a.
- Subclassify M1 by additional nodules in contralateral lung as M1a.
- Subclassify M1 by distant metastases (outside the lung/pleura) as M1b.

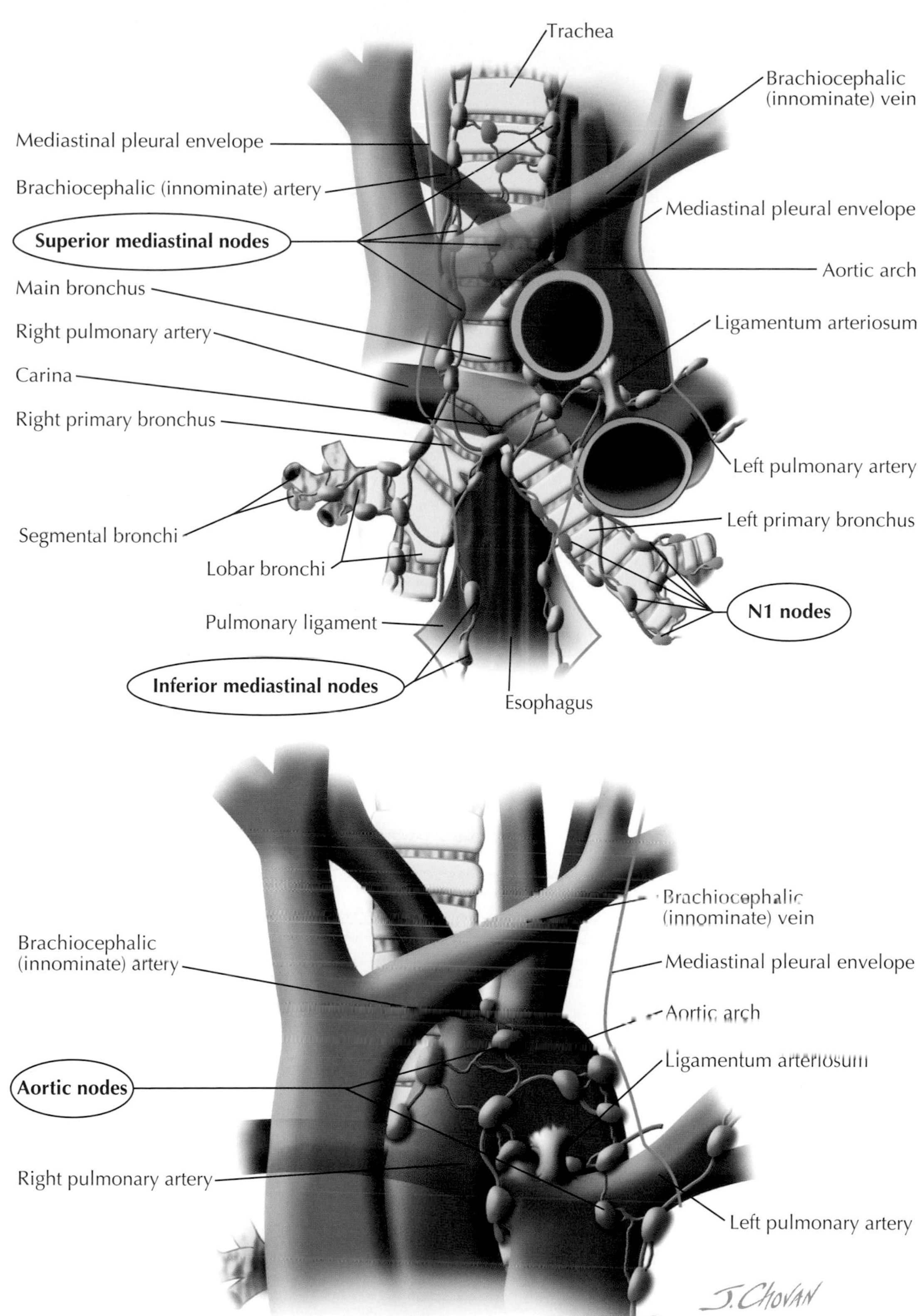

Anatomy of lymph node stations relevant to lung cancer staging. The IASLC proposes grouping the lymph nodes into the zones shown in bold and circled to assist with prognosis.

Because of the addition of new T and M descriptors, the staging definitions have clearly become more complex. However, the new system now provides a more validated system for defining prognosis. In addition, the system also allows common terminology to be used across the world to describe similar patients, which is critical for accurate communication across the medical community and the conduct of worldwide clinical trials. A future goal is the further refinement of the classification system to include the biologic behavior of lung tumors, not just anatomic location, which should promote understanding of tumor biology and provide guidance toward more specific therapies.

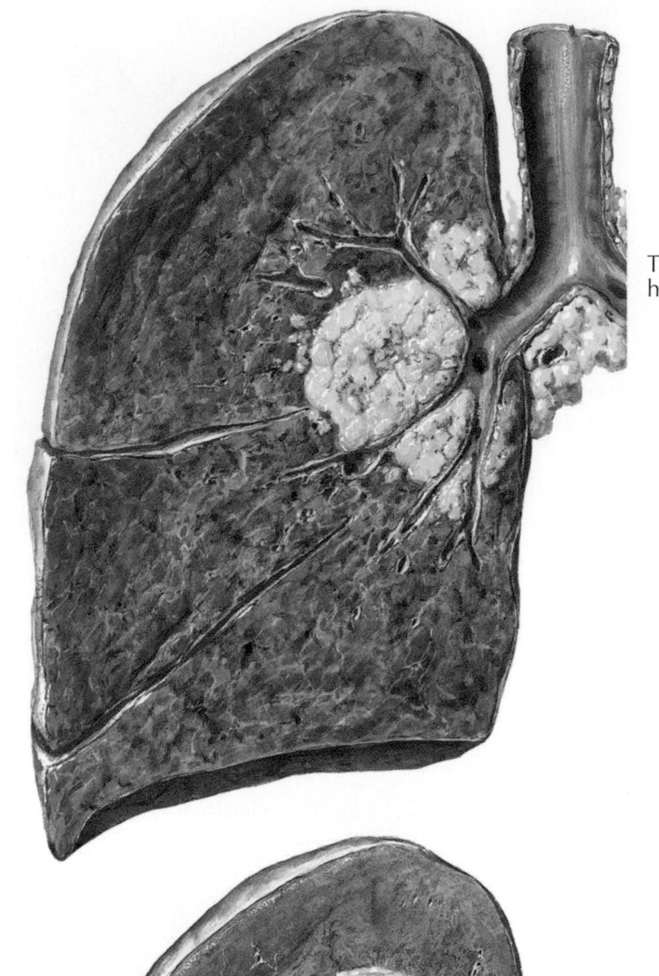

Tumor typically located near hilum, projecting into bronchi

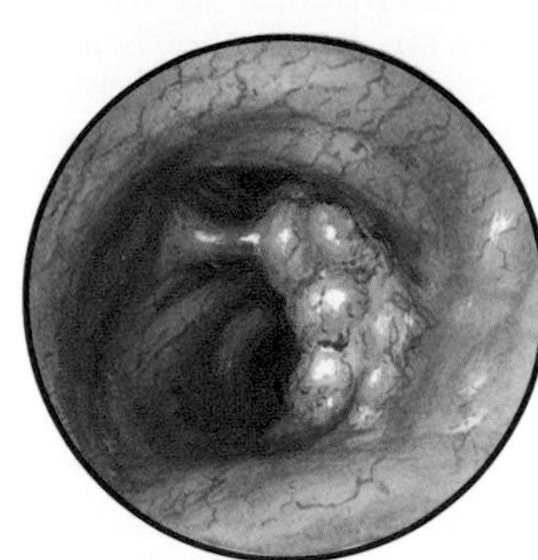

Bronchoscopic view

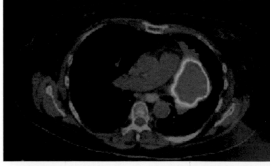

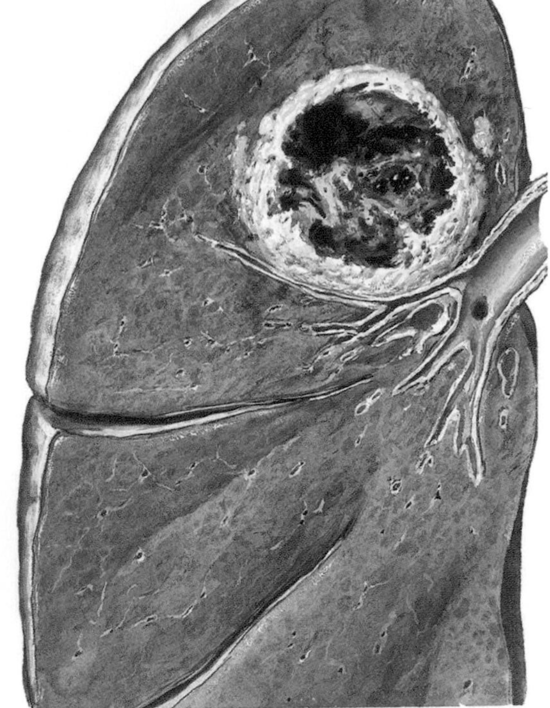

Combined CT/PET image showing a squamous cell carcinoma (*bright area*) of the left lung.

SQUAMOUS CELL CARCINOMA OF THE LUNG

Squamous cell carcinoma (SCC) is defined as a malignant epithelial tumor showing keratinization or intracellular bridges (or both) arising from bronchial epithelium. Previously, SCC, sometimes called *epidermoid carcinoma*, was the most common cell type, but that has changed in the past 1 or 2 decades in the United States, parts of Western Europe, and Japan. Currently, SCCs account for 20% of all lung cancers in the United States (http://seer.cancer.gov). The vast majority of SCC occurs in smokers. Recent Surveillance, Epidemiology and End Results (SEER) data report that SCC accounts for 24% of all cancers in men versus 16% in women. The recent decrease in SCC and increase in adenocarcinoma histology has been attributed to the change in the cigarette, from nonfilter to filter, and the decrease in tar. About 60% to 80% of these cancers arise centrally in mainstem, lobar, or segmental bronchi, but they may present as a peripheral lung lesion.

SCC arises from the bronchial epithelium, and it is thought that the airway abnormality progresses through a series of changes from hyperplasia to dysplasia to carcinoma in situ, which is classified by World Health Organization as preinvasive and a precursor to SCC. Varying degrees of dysplasia have been associated with cumulative genetic alterations, but the critical genetic change(s) before developing frank cancer is still uncertain.

Because of the tendency to occur centrally in the airway, SCC presents more commonly with hemoptysis, new or change in cough, chest pain, or pneumonia caused by bronchial obstruction. The usual radiographic presentation is a central mass or obstructing pneumonia with or without lobar collapse. About 10% to 20% of SCCs present as peripheral lesions. Cavitation may occur in 10% to 15% of all SCCs and is the most common histology associated with cavitation. The cavities are usually thick walled. Cavitation in the lung may also be caused by obstructive pneumonia and abscess formation.

Sputum cytology has the highest diagnostic yield with this cell type because of the predominant central location. Bronchoscopy with brushings and biopsy are diagnostic in more than 90% of SCCs when the cancer is visible endoscopically. The yield for peripheral lesions that are endoscopically negative is significantly less and depends on the size of the tumor. For lesions smaller than 2 cm in diameter, transthoracic needle aspiration has the highest diagnostic yield if a tissue diagnosis is required before surgical resection.

SCC in situ (pre invasive lesion) has an unpredictable course, and the treatment is a topic of current debate. Surgery is the treatment of choice for early-stage disease (stage I or II). Combination chemotherapy and radiotherapy are recommended for good performance score patients with unresectable stage III A or B disease. Stage IV (metastatic disease) is generally treated with systemic chemotherapy, but treatment is noncurative (palliative).

It was previously believed that SCC was more slow-growing than other cell types, but recent analysis of a large international database that controlled for stage of disease does not demonstrate definite survival benefit of SCC versus other non–small cell histologies. In the past, SCCs have been treated the same as all other non–small cell histologies, but recent data show that optimal treatment depends on specific typing.

ADENOCARCINOMA OF THE LUNG

Different histologic types of bronchogenic carcinoma cannot be distinguished by gross specimens or radiography alone. However, a peripherally located tumor <4 cm in diameter is most likely to be adenocarcinoma

Small, peripherally placed tumor

F. Netter M.D.

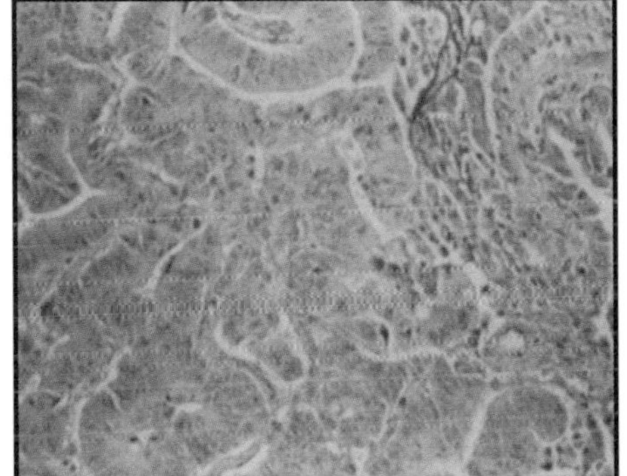

Histology of adenocarcinoma. Tumor cells form glandlike structures with or without mucin secretion

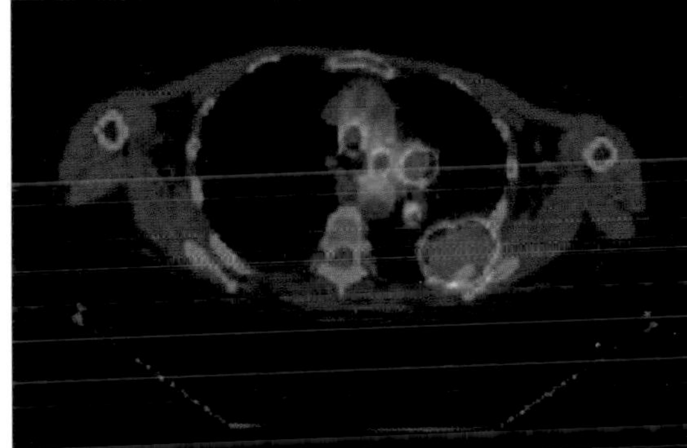

Peripheral adenocarcinoma with mediastinal nodal metastases seen on combined CT and PET imaging (bright areas)

Atypical adenomatous hyperplasia is classified by the World Health Organization (WHO) as a putative precursor of adenocarcinoma (ACA), especially bronchioloalveolar carcinoma (BAC). ACA is defined as a malignant epithelial tumor with glandular differentiation or mucin production. ACA is the most common cell type in the United States and many developed countries. It accounts for 37% of all lung cancers in the Surveillance, Epidemiology and End Results (SEER) database (40% in women; 33% in men; http://seer.cancer.gov). ACA histology is associated with cigarette smoking, but the association is not as strong as it is for squamous cell and small cell carcinoma. ACA is the most common histology of lung cancer in never smokers, especially women.

Bronchioloalveolar cell, also called alveolar cell, is classified by the WHO as a subtype of ACA. BACs are mostly moderate or well-differentiated tumors and grow along preexisting alveolar structures (lepidic growth) without evidence of invasion. If there is evidence of invasion, then the tumor is classified as ACA mixed type. Pure BAC by the current classification is a rare tumor; most are ACA mixed type. It is anticipated that pure BAC will be renamed as *adenocarcinoma in situ* in the new classification.

ACAs are usually peripherally located in the lungs. Because of the peripheral location, more of the patients are asymptomatic, and the lesion is detected on an incidental chest radiograph. Patients may present with a new cough, chest pain, or less commonly hemoptysis. Presenting symptoms caused by distant metastases to the bone, brain, or liver are common with all cell types, especially ACA and large cell carcinoma. Individuals with BAC may present with an asymptomatic solitary pulmonary nodule, pneumonia such as consolidation of the lung, or rarely with a profound bronchorrhea. Bronchorrhea is usually seen in those with extensive bilateral lung involvement.

The most common radiographic presentation is a peripheral lung nodule or mass (mass defined as ≥3 cm) in maximum diameter. It may infrequently present as a central mass and rarely cavitates. ACA is the most common cell type to present with a malignant pleural effusion.

Sputum cytology results are rarely positive. Diagnostic yields with bronchoscopy are less than with squamous cell or small cell carcinoma because of the peripheral location. For lesions that are 2 cm in diameter or larger, the diagnostic yields are approximately 60% to 70%. Transthoracic needle aspirations (TTNAs) are diagnostic in 85% to 90% of all lesions and are the preferred diagnostic test for lesions smaller than 2 cm in diameter. The benefits of TTNA should be balanced against the risk of pneumothorax, especially in patients with chronic obstructive pulmonary disease or emphysema. Thoracentesis and pleural fluid cytology is the preferred diagnostic test in individuals with pleural effusion.

The treatment of choice for patients with stage I, II, or IIIA/B is generally the same as for all non–small cell lung cancers. Patients with stage IV (metastatic) disease have generally been treated with systemic chemotherapy as palliative treatment. In recent years, a number of genetic alterations have been identified in the tumor that are changing the treatment approach. Some ACAs have been identified to have a mutation in the intracellular domain of the epidermal growth factor receptor (EGFR) gene. The predominant mutations include in frame deletions of exon 19 and missense mutation in exon 21. These mutations have been associated with a high response rate to treatment with the EGFR tyrosine kinase inhibitors (TKIs) gefitinib and erlotinib. For reasons that are currently unknown, the frequency of the EGFR tyrosine kinase mutations vary in different ethnic populations. The frequency of mutation in North America and Europe is approximately 15% of all ACA versus 30% of ACA in East Asians. These mutations are almost exclusively limited to the ACA cell type.

Recent reports have documented better survival in individuals when these EGFR mutations are treated initially with EGFR TKIs versus conventional chemotherapy. Other studies have shown that KRAS mutations, which occur in 20% to 30% of patients with ACA, confer resistance to treatment with the EGFR inhibitors. Mutations in KRAS and EGFR are almost always mutually exclusive. It is very likely that future identification of genetic mutations or identification of predominant intracellular pathways of malignant cells will influence the choice of treatment of ACA and other histologies. Most recently a mutation of anaplastic lymphoma kinase (ALK) has been identified in 3% to 5% of ACA, and promising new treatment with the tyrosine kinase inhibitor crizotinib has been reported.

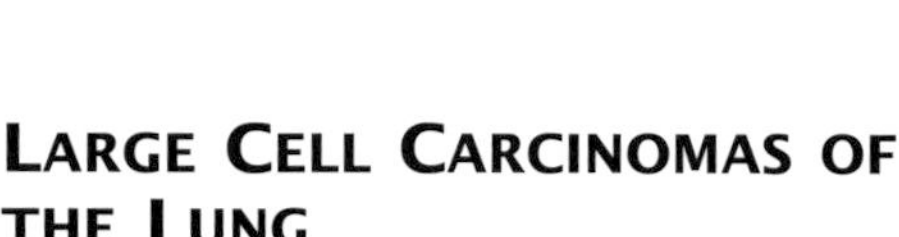

Large Cell Carcinomas of the Lung

Large cell carcinoma is a malignant epithelial undifferentiated neoplasm lacking glandular or squamous differentiation and features of small cell carcinoma. It is a diagnosis of exclusion and includes many poorly differentiated non–small cell carcinomas. Several variants are recognized, including neuroendocrine differentiation (large cell neuroendocrine carcinoma [LCNEC]) and basaloid carcinoma), but it is uncertain if this differentiation is of prognostic or therapeutic importance. Large cell carcinoma and its variants can only be diagnosed reliably on surgical material; cytology samples are not generally sufficient. LCNEC is differentiated from atypical carcinoid tumor by having more mitotic figures, usually 11 or more per 2 mm^2 of viable tumor, and large areas of necrosis are common. Neuroendocrine differentiation is confirmed using immunohistochemical markers such as chromogranin, synaptophysin, or CD56. Patients with LCNEC have a worse prognosis than those with atypical carcinoid tumors. Large cell carcinoma is associated with cigarette smoking. This cell type accounted for 4% of all lung cancers in the Surveillance, Epidemiology and End Results (SEER) database. The SEER database listed the cell type of 24% of all lung cancers as "other non–small cell." These other cancers include non–small cell cancers that pathologists specify as NOS (not otherwise specified). As treatment moves toward specific treatment for specific cell types, it will be important for pathologists to classify the histology as accurately as possible and to decrease the percentages of cases reported as NOS.

The signs and symptoms of this cell type are similar to those of other non–small cell carcinomas. The most common radiographic finding is a large peripheral lung mass. Because of the peripheral location, these cancers may be asymptomatic and detected on an incidental chest radiograph. Because of the rapid growth of this cell type, the radiographic lesion may appear rather suddenly (within a few months) or enlarge rapidly.

Diagnostic procedures are similar to those of other histologic types. Sputum cytology is not generally helpful because of the peripheral location, and bronchoscopic diagnostic yields are similar to those for peripheral adenocarcinomas and squamous cell carcinomas (~60%-70%). Transthoracic needle aspiration is diagnostic in the majority of cases. These cancers are usually aggressive tumors with a strong tendency for early metastases. Nevertheless, surgery is still the treatment of choice for patients with early-stage disease. Currently, there is no convincing evidence that patients with LCNEC should be treated differently than those with any other large cell carcinoma. Patients with stage III and IV disease are treated the same as those with other non–small cell types. Patients with stage III are treated with combined chemotherapy and thoracic radiotherapy. Survival is similar to that of patients with other non–small cell lung cancers, and patients with stage IV are treated with chemotherapy with palliative intent.

Tumors are variable in location

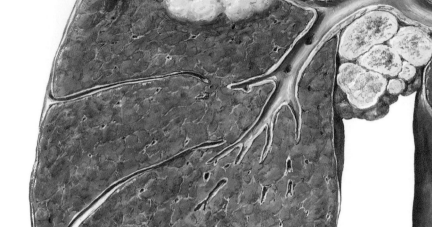

Large cell carcinoma in middle of right upper lobe with extensive involvement of hilar and carinal nodes. Distortion of trachea and widening of carina

Tumor composed of large multinucleated cell without evidence of differentiation toward gland formation or squamous epithelium. These cells produce mucin (stained red). Some tumors may be composed of large clear cells containing glycogen

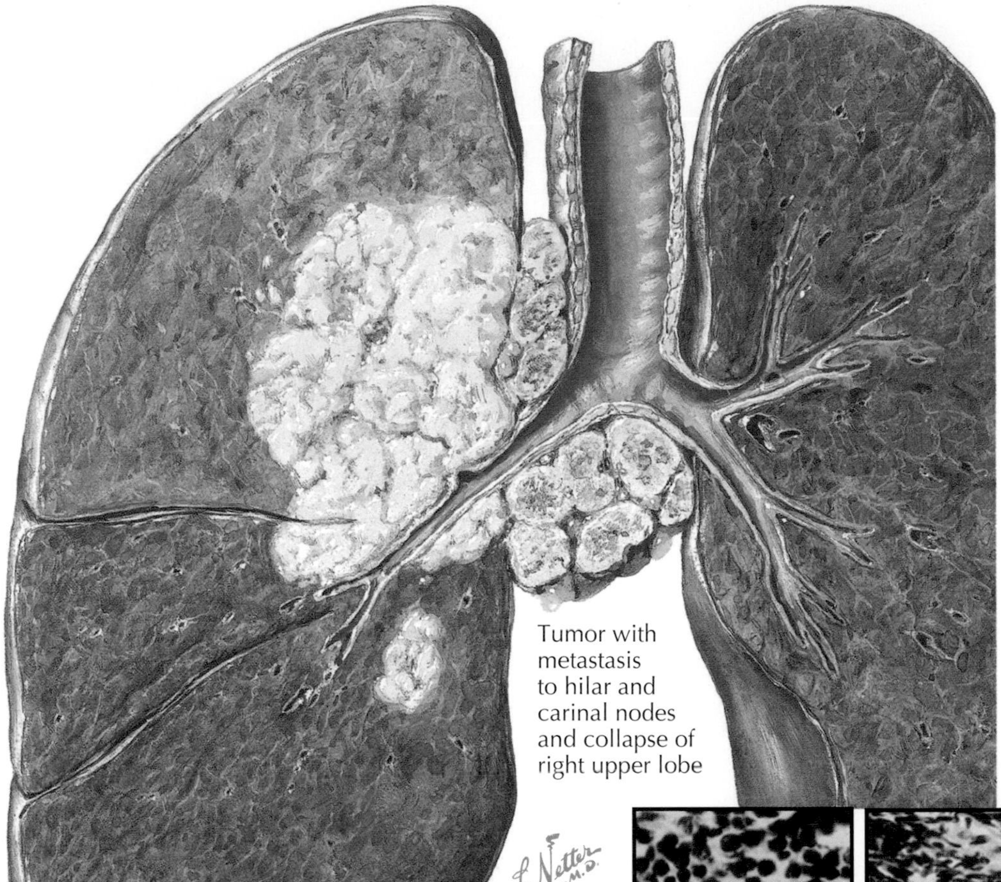

Tumor with metastasis to hilar and carinal nodes and collapse of right upper lobe

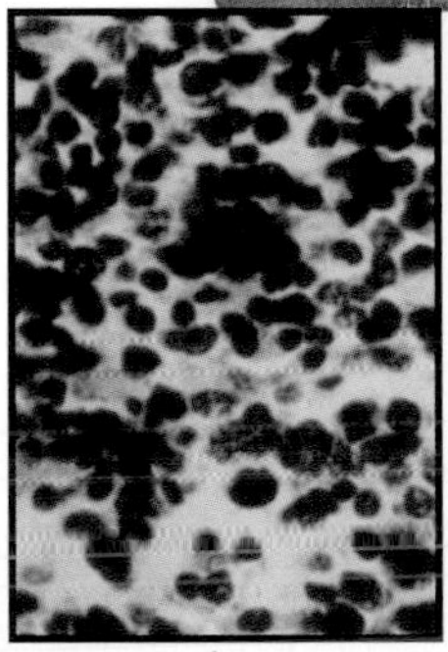

Masses of small cells with hyperchromatic round to oval nuclei and scant cytoplasm

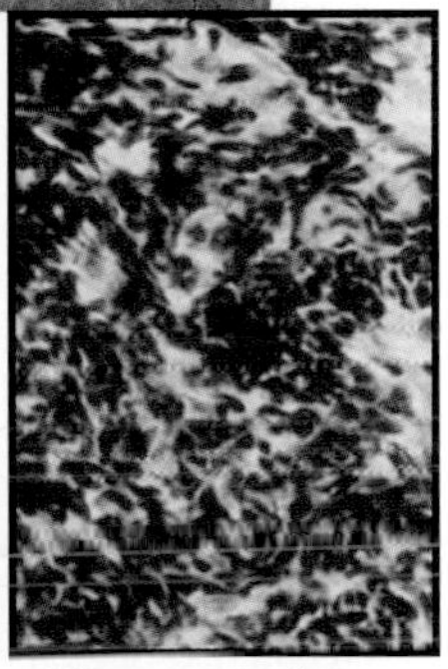

Biopsy specimen. Cells elongated

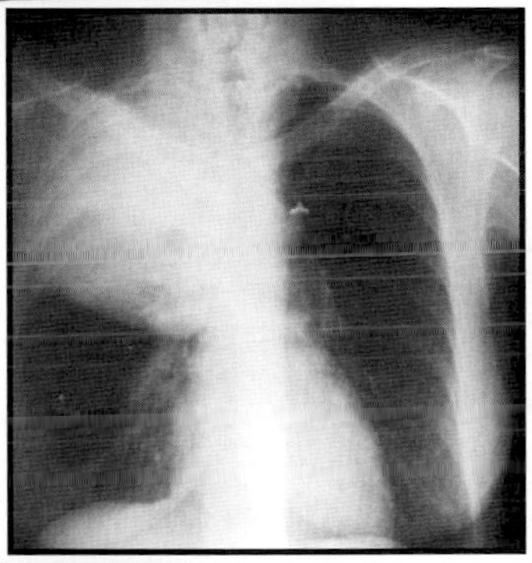

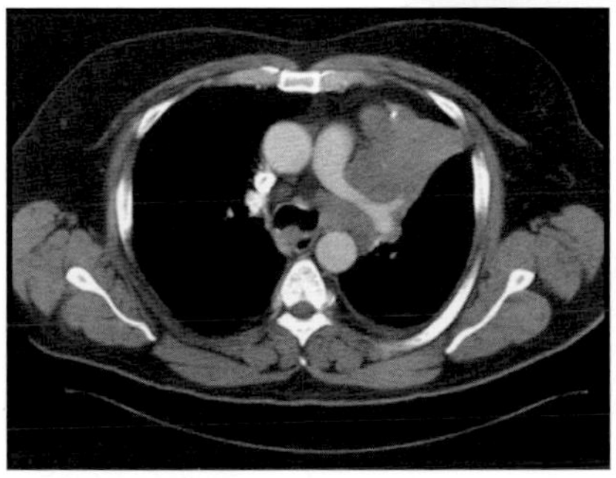

Small cell carcinoma seen by chest CT illustrating extensive hilar involvement and collapse at left upper lobe

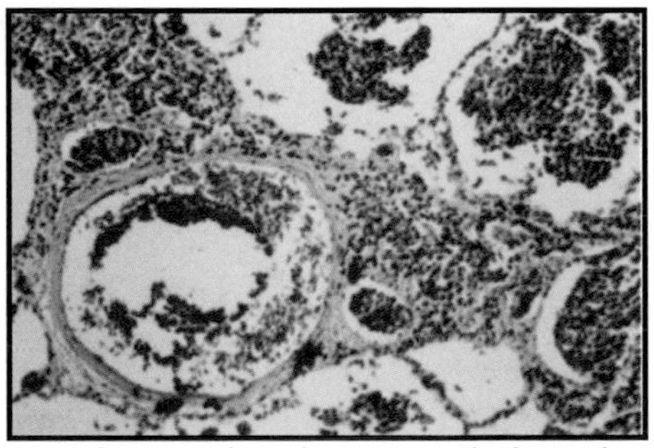

Intrapulmonary lymphatic spread of neoplasm

Small Cell Carcinomas of the Lung

Small cell carcinoma is defined as a malignant epithelial tumor consisting of small cells with scant cytoplasm. If other histologic types of non–small cell carcinoma are also present, then it is classified as *combined small cell carcinoma*. The cells contain neuroendocrine granules, and it is usually considered as a neuroendocrine tumor at the most malignant end of the neuroendocrine spectrum. It usually stains positive for the neuroendocrine markers CD56, chromogranin, and synaptophysin. This cell type has the strongest association with cigarette smoking and rarely occurs in people who have never smoked. Small cell histology accounts for 14% of all lung cancers (13% in men; 15% in women) in the Surveillance, Epidemiology and End Results database (http://seer.cancer.gov). This cell type generally has the fastest growth rate and a tendency to early spread.

Small cell carcinoma is centrally located in the large majority of cases and therefore present with symptoms of cough, hemoptysis, chest pain, or obstructive pneumonia. Because of the tendency for early spread, many individuals present with signs and symptoms of regional or distant metastasis. Mediastinal lymph node spread may result in hoarseness or a change in voice caused by vocal cord paralysis, dysphagia caused by esophageal compression, or superior vena cava syndrome (discussed later). Symptoms caused by brain, bone, or liver metastases may be the first signs of the disease. Small cell carcinoma is the most common cell type associated with paraneoplastic syndromes (discussed later).

Ten percent or fewer of small cell carcinomas present as a peripheral mass or solitary pulmonary nodule. Supraclavicular lymph node metastases may be present and are an easy source for tissue diagnosis. Sputum cytology is rarely positive. Bronchoscopy is the most common method of diagnosis. The tumor is frequently located submucosally, and bronchoscopic biopsies may not yield a diagnosis if deep submucosal samples are not obtained. Pleural fluid cytology may be diagnostic; however, in many cases, the pleural fluid is due to a parapneumonic effusion and not caused by malignant seeding of the pleural space.

Small cell carcinoma is usually staged as limited or extensive stage disease. Limited disease is defined as disease confined to one hemithorax and mediastinal lymph nodes with or without ipsilateral supraclavicular nodes. It is generally disease that can be safely confined within a thoracic radiotherapy field of treatment. Extensive stage is defined as spread of disease beyond the hemithorax with distant metastases. Malignant pleural effusion, cytologically documented, is considered to be extensive stage.

The treatment of limited stage disease is combined concurrent chemotherapy and thoracic radiotherapy in patients with a good performance score and minimal weight loss. Recent cooperative group trials of concurrent treatment have resulted in median survival times of 18 to 20 months and 5-year survival rates of 20% to 25%. For patients with extensive stage disease, the usual treatment is chemotherapy for four to six cycles with a platinum based doublet. The median survival time is 8 to 10 months with 10% or less 2-year survival and virtually no 5-year survivors. Chemotherapy treatment for small cell carcinoma has plateaued with no major advances for the past 2 decades.

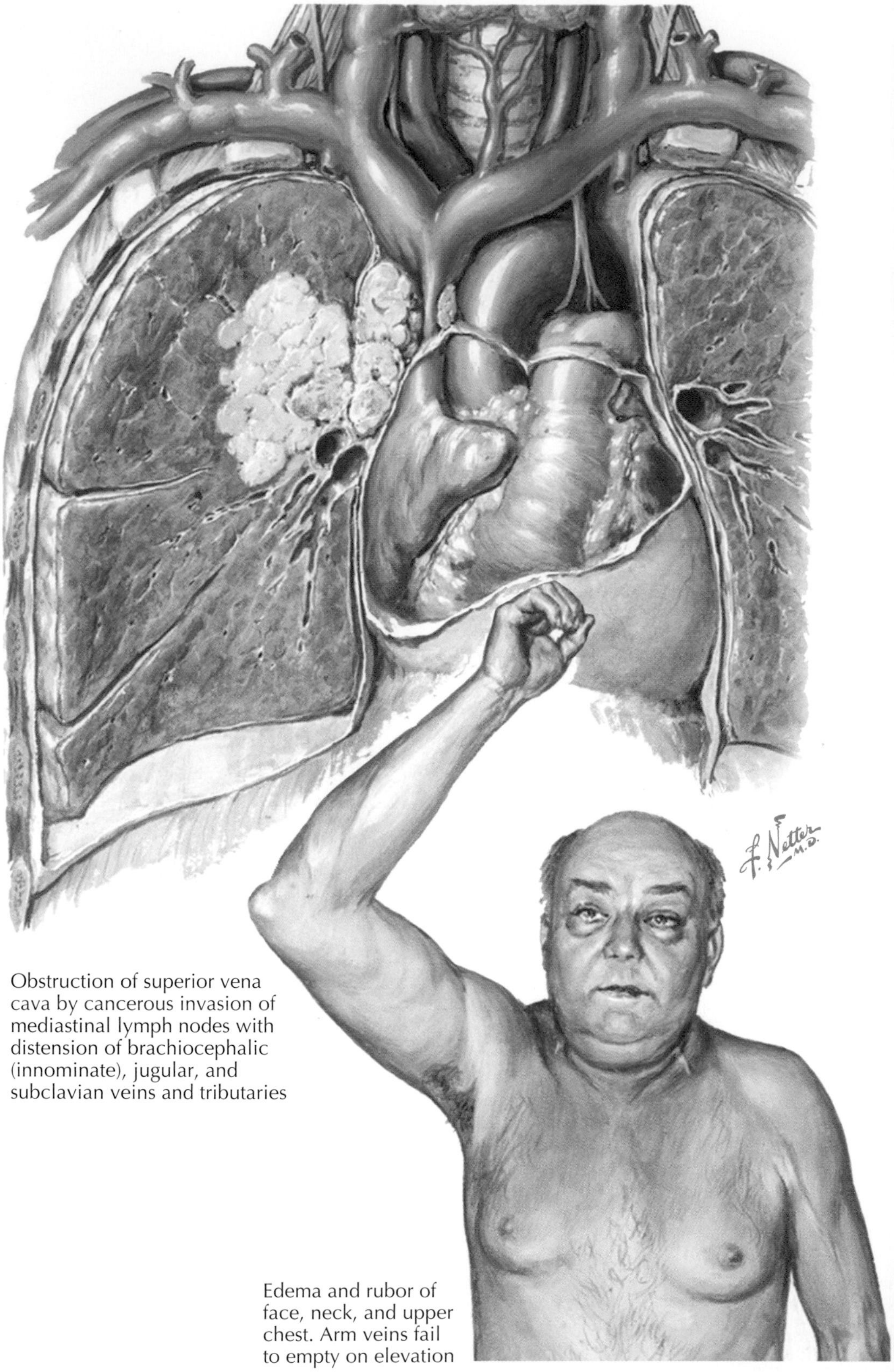

Superior Vena Cava Syndrome

Superior vena cava (SVC) syndrome is caused by extrinsic compression or internal thrombosis of the SVC, which compromises the venous drainage from the head and upper extremities. Lung cancer is responsible for the large majority of SVC syndrome in adults older than age 40 years. Lymphoma is the most common cause in younger individuals. Patients complain of a sensation of fullness in the head, cough, or dyspnea. They may experience lightheadedness, especially when bending over, or have edema and swelling in the head, neck, and arms. Edema of the larynx or pharynx may result in stridor, and cerebral edema may result in headaches or confusion.

Physical findings include dilated neck veins and subcutaneous veins of the chest that persist with the patient in an upright position. Facial edema and a plethoric appearance may be present. Computed tomography chest scans with contrast injected through the arm veins show the mass with narrowing or obstruction of the SVC and the extensive venous collateral circulation of subcutaneous and mediastinal veins. If the SVC syndrome is caused by a benign condition such as fibrosing mediastinitis, then a lung mass will not be identified.

Small cell carcinoma is the classic histology to cause SVC syndrome, but any histologic type may do so. Although SVC syndrome is a serious condition, it is not generally an emergency situation. Accordingly, a tissue diagnosis should be obtained before treatment begins. It is important to know if it is caused by lymphoma, small cell carcinoma, or non–small cell lung cancer before the appropriate treatment is instituted. SVC syndrome may occasionally be caused by other tumors (e.g., breast cancer, germ cell tumor), fibrosing mediastinitis, or an infectious process (rarely). Bronchoscopy has a high diagnostic rate when SVC syndrome is caused by lung cancer. If bronchoscopy results are negative, then mediastinoscopy is the next logical procedure in most cases.

Treatment of patients with SVC syndrome should include stenting of the SVC early on in the process. This treatment quickly relieves the obstruction in more than 90% of cases. Chemotherapy alone as initial treatment is indicated for cases caused by small cell carcinoma or lymphoma, and radiotherapy or combined chemoradiotherapy is used for non–small cell lung cancer. Treatment should rarely be given without a tissue diagnosis. In patients with SVC syndrome caused by lung cancer, the long-term prognosis is related to the histologic type and stage of the disease at the time of initial diagnosis.

Obstruction of superior vena cava by cancerous invasion of mediastinal lymph nodes with distension of brachiocephalic (innominate), jugular, and subclavian veins and tributaries

Edema and rubor of face, neck, and upper chest. Arm veins fail to empty on elevation

PANCOAST TUMOR AND SYNDROME

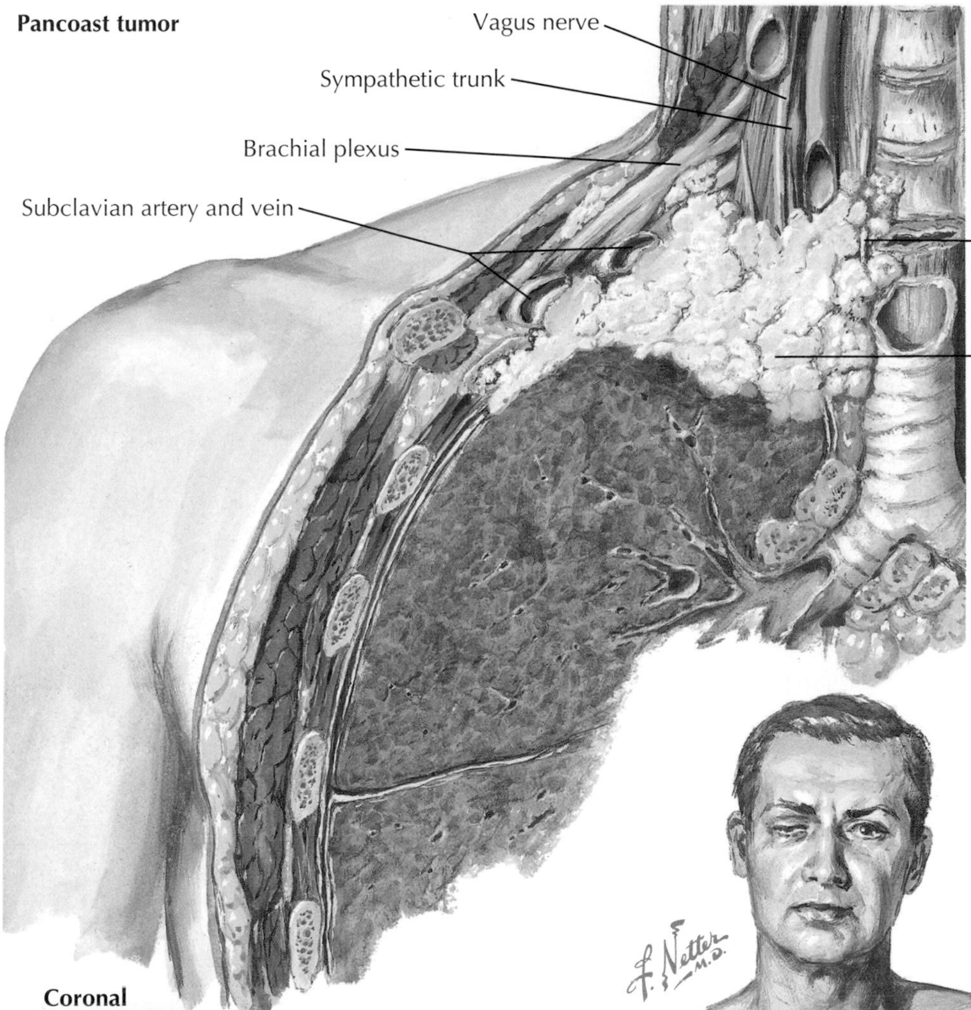

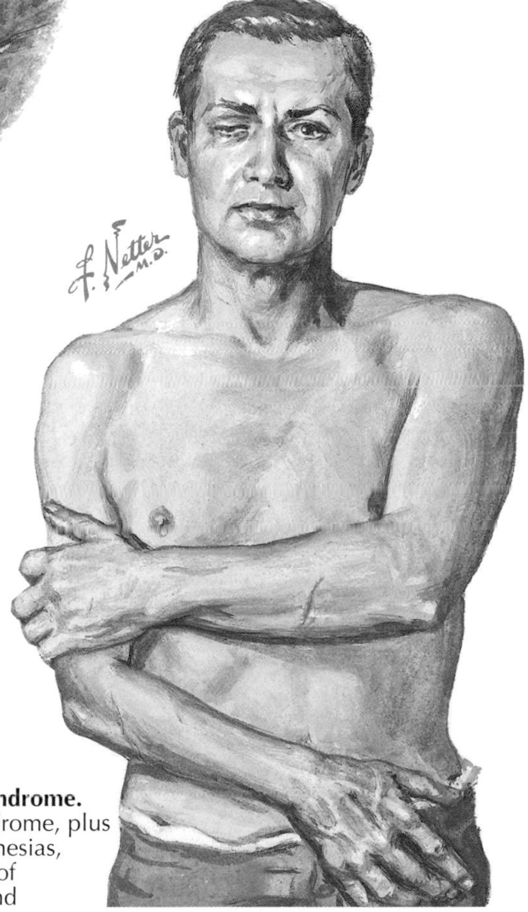

Superior sulcus tumors are located at the apical pleuropulmonary groove adjacent to the subclavian vessels. Superior sulcus tumors received notoriety in reports by Henry Pancoast and are commonly referred to as *Pancoast tumors*. Lung cancer is by far the most common cause of Pancoast and superior sulcus tumors. It is more commonly associated with adenocarcinoma but may be caused by any histologic type. A variety of other rare tumors or infectious diseases have occasionally been reported to cause a Pancoast tumor.

Tumors of the superior sulcus may cause shoulder and arm pain (in the distribution of the C8, T1, and T2 dermatomes), Horner syndrome, and weakness of the muscles of the hand. This complex is referred to as *Pancoast syndrome*. Shoulder pain is the usual presenting symptom and is caused by tumor invasion of the tumor into the chest wall, first and second ribs, vertebral body, and possibly the brachial plexus. Pain may radiate up to the head and neck or to the axilla and arm in the distribution of the ulnar nerve. The cause of the pain is frequently misdiagnosed for months as osteoarthritis or bursitis of the shoulder. Horner syndrome consists of ipsilateral ptosis, miosis, enophthalmos, and anhidrosis of half of the face and head and is caused by involvement of the paravertebral sympathetic chain and the inferior cervical (stellate) ganglion. Contralateral facial sweating and flushing have been reported.

Tumor involvement of the C8 and T1 nerve roots may result in weakness and atrophy of the intrinsic muscles of the hand or pain or paresthesias of the fourth and fifth digits and medial aspect of the arm and forearm. Abnormal sensation or pain in the axilla and medial aspect of the upper arm caused by T2 nerve root involvement may be an early symptom. As these tumors progress, they may invade the intervertebral foramina and cause spinal cord compression and paraplegia. This may especially be a problem for patients with progressive disease who have failed local treatment. Tumors with progressive mediastinal involvement may result in phrenic nerve or laryngeal nerve paralysis.

The classic radiographic finding is that of an apical mass or unilateral apical cap. Occasionally, the abnormality will not be obvious on a chest radiograph; therefore if the diagnosis is suspected, a computed tomography (CT) scan of the chest is required. The CT will demonstrate greater detail and is more likely to elucidate the extent of the tumor locally. Magnetic resonance imaging (MRI) is better at demonstrating brachial plexus involvement and evaluating the spinal canal for tumor extension. MR angiography is better for demonstrating subclavian vessel involvement. Bronchoscopy may be diagnostic for larger tumors, but transthoracic needle aspiration is the most common method of diagnosis of these apical tumors. The usual staging tests include a positron emission computed tomography (PET) scan and MRI of the brain because of the propensity for brain metastases.

The treatment of patients with superior sulcus tumors caused by non–small cell lung cancer with no evidence of mediastinal nodal metastases is initial concurrent chemotherapy and radiotherapy followed by surgical resection 3 to 5 weeks after induction therapy. The 5-year survival with this trimodality treatment is approximately 40%. Patients with documented mediastinal lymph node involvement at initial presentation are treated with definitive chemoradiotherapy alone with somewhat inferior long-term survival. Patients with stage IV or metastatic disease at presentation are treated with palliative radiotherapy and systemic chemotherapy similar to other patients with stage IV disease.

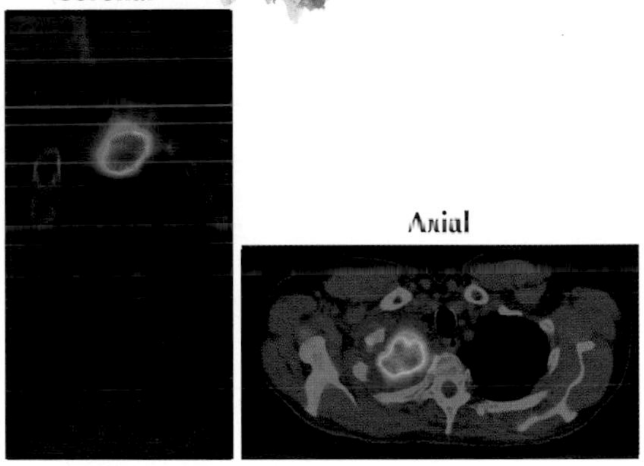

Combined CT/PET images of Pancoast tumor (bright area) seen in coronal and axial views

Pancoast syndrome. Horner syndrome, plus pain, paresthesias, and paresis of arm and hand

Paraneoplastic Manifestations of Lung Cancer

Paraneoplastic effects of tumors are remote effects that are not related to direct invasion, obstruction, or metastases. Paraneoplastic syndromes occur in 10% to 15% of all lung cancers. The following are some of the most common.

The syndrome of inappropriate antidiuretic hormone secretion (SIADH) may be caused by pulmonary infections, central nervous system (CNS) disease or trauma, drugs, or lung tumors. Small cell lung cancer is the most common malignancy to cause SIADH. The tumor secretes ectopic antidiuretic hormone (ADH; vasopressin), which exerts its action on the kidneys and enhances the flow of water from the lumen of the renal collecting ducts to the medullary interstitium with resulting concentration of the urine. Patients present with hyponatremia that is associated with low plasma osmolality and elevated urine sodium and osmolality. To make the diagnosis of SIADH, patients must also have normal renal, adrenal, and thyroid function. The symptoms of hyponatremia may include anorexia, nausea, vomiting, irritability, restlessness, confusion, coma, or seizures. The severity of symptoms is related to the degree of hyponatremia and the rapidity of the decrease in serum sodium. The treatment for mildly symptomatic patients is to restrict fluid intake to 500 to 1000 mL/24 hours. For more severe or life-threatening symptoms, treatment consists of intravenous fluids with normal saline and loop diuretics. For severe symptoms, some experts recommend 300 mL of 3% saline intravenously, but extreme caution must be used because too rapid correction of serum sodium may be associated with central pontine myelinolysis, which is a devastating CNS process that is often fatal. For patients with less severe symptoms from hyponatremia but requiring more than fluid restriction, oral demeclocycline can be used. The onset of action may take from a few hours to a few weeks, and renal function should be monitored. The best treatment for SIADH, if the patient is stable, is to treat the small cell lung cancer with systemic chemotherapy. Regression of the tumor results in normalization of the sodium in most cases.

Cushing syndrome may be related to ectopic production of corticotropin (adrenocorticotropic hormone) or corticotropin-releasing hormone by small cell carcinoma. It has also been reported with bronchial carcinoid tumors or carcinoid tumors of the thymus or pancreas. Small cell lung cancer accounts for 75% of all cases of Cushing syndrome caused by ectopic hormone secretion. Because of the rapid growth of small cell lung cancer, patients are more likely to present with edema, hypertension, and hyperglycemia with or without muscle weakness. This is in contrast to the classic features of Cushing syndrome that include truncal obesity, rounded (moon) facies, buffalo hump (dorsocervical fat pad), and diabetes mellitus. The best screen for Cushing syndrome caused by ectopic hormone secretion is the 24-hour urine free cortisol measurement. Marked elevation of cortisol production and plasma corticotropin levels are highly suggestive of ectopic corticotropin as the cause of Cushing syndrome.

Treatment of patients with ectopic corticotropin production includes metyrapone, aminoglutethimide, mitotane, or ketoconazole given alone or in combination. Ketoconazole is the most commonly used agent. If the patient is stable with no superimposed infection, then systemic chemotherapy is the best treatment for histologically confirmed small cell lung cancer. If the Cushing syndrome is caused by carcinoid tumor, then surgical resection, if possible, is the treatment of choice.

Endocrine Manifestations of Lung Cancer

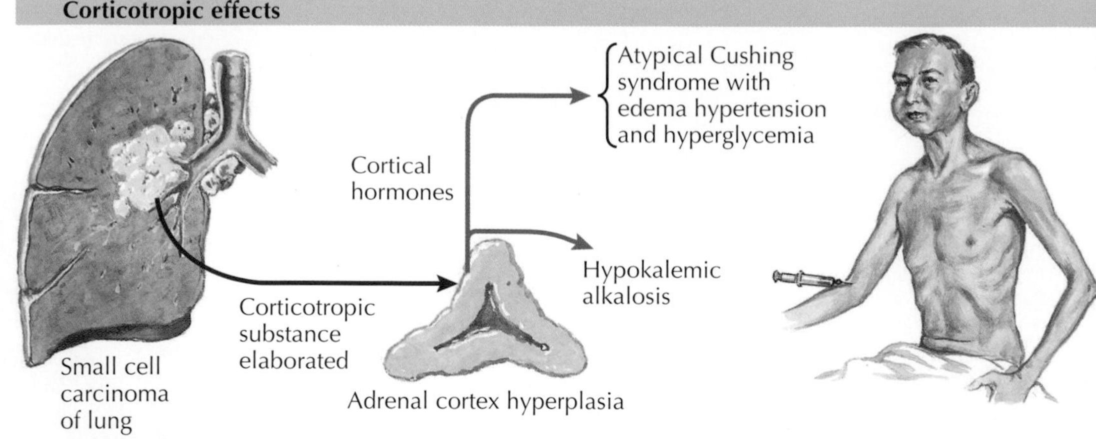

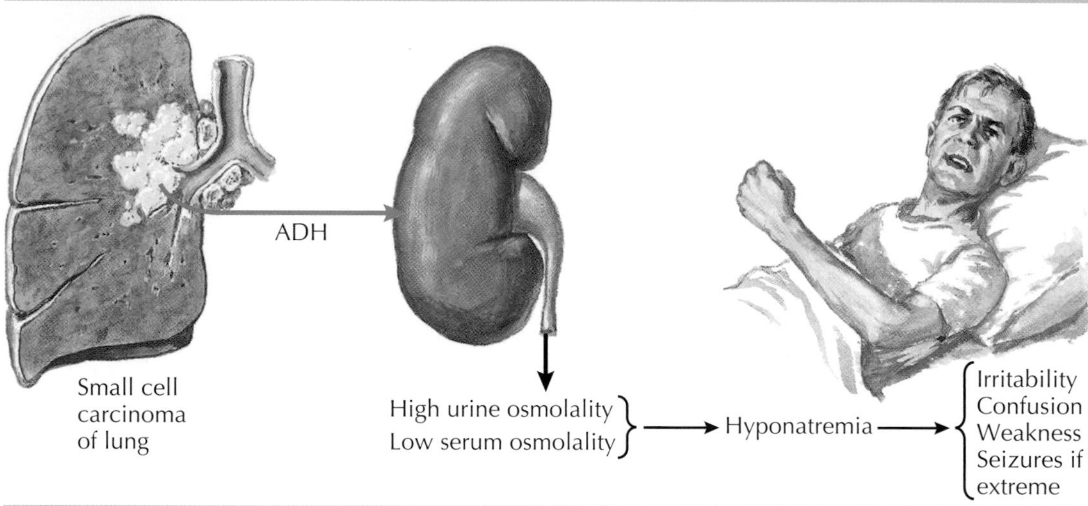

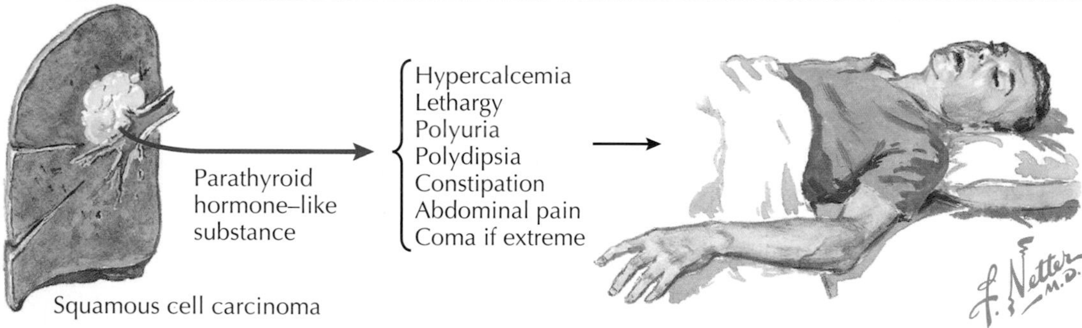

Hypercalcemia in relation to lung cancer may be caused by bone metastases, or less commonly, secretion of parathyroid hormone–related protein (PTHrP) or other cytokines. The most common cancers to cause paraneoplastic hypercalcemia are kidney, lung, breast, myeloma, and lymphoma. For lung cancers, squamous cell carcinoma is the most common cell type associated with hypercalcemia. Symptoms of hypercalcemia include anorexia, nausea, vomiting, constipation, lethargy, polyuria, polydipsia, and dehydration. Confusion and coma are late manifestations. A shortened QT interval on electrocardiography, ventricular arrhythmia, heart block, and asystole may occur. Renal failure and nephrocalcinosis are also possible. Elevated PTHrP levels may be detected in the serum of about half of patients with hypercalcemia of malignancy that is not caused by bony metastasis. Patients with mild elevation of calcium do not require treatment. Treatment is determined by symptoms and includes intravenous fluids to correct dehydration caused by polyuria and vomiting. Intravenous treatment with bisphosphonates inhibits osteoclast activity, and one dose achieves a normal calcium level in 4 to 10 days in most individuals. If rapid partial correction of hypercalcemia is needed, calcitonin will rapidly lower the calcium level by 1 to 2 mg/dL, but the effects are short lived. If the lung cancer is localized, then the treatment of choice, after the patient has been stabilized, is surgical resection. However, the usual situation is that the patient has metastatic disease. For these individuals with hypercalcemia, the average life expectancy, even with treatment, is 1 month.

Paraneoplastic neurologic syndromes (PNSs) are most commonly associated with small cell lung cancer

PARANEOPLASTIC MANIFESTATIONS OF LUNG CANCER *(Continued)*

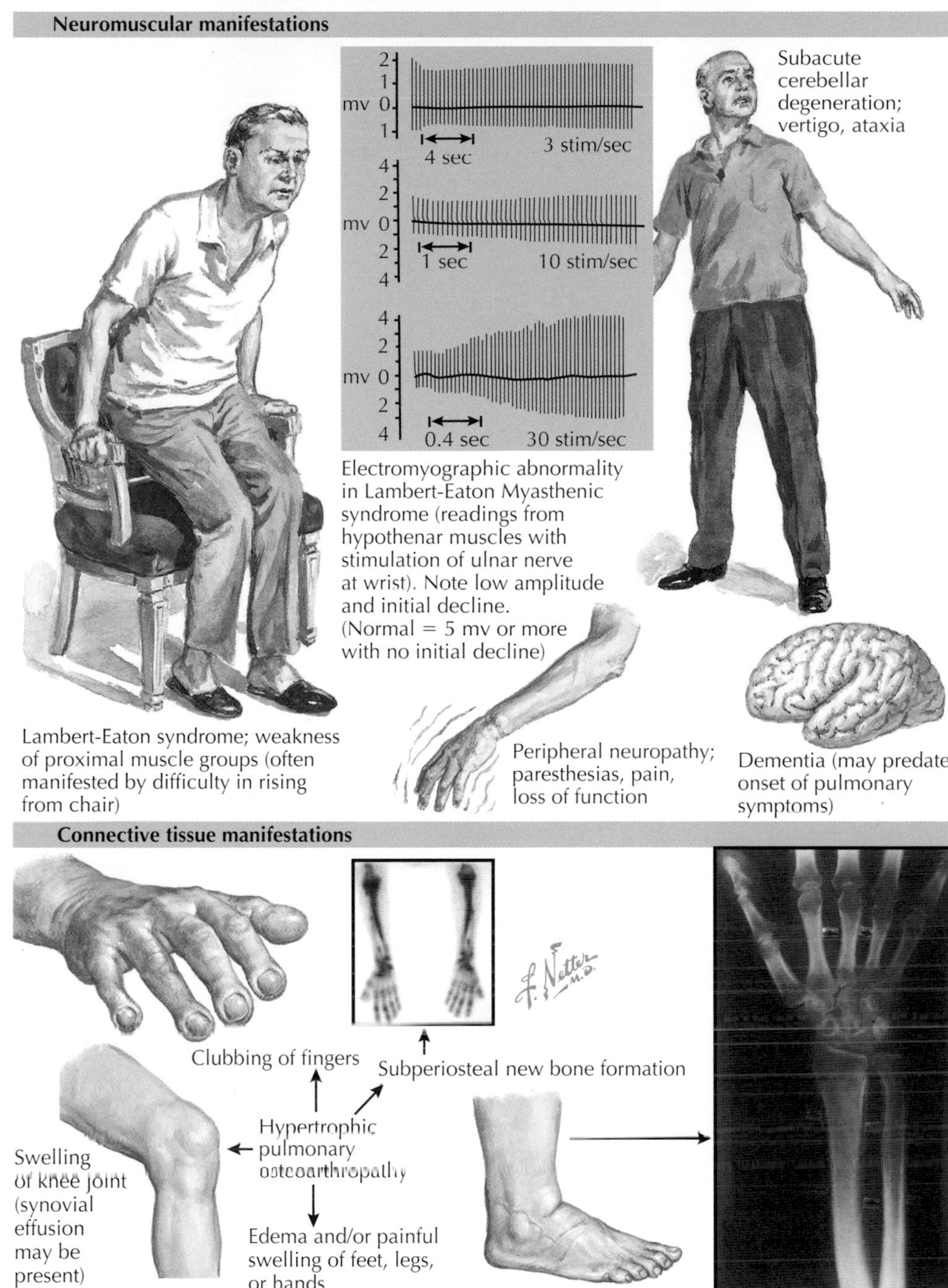

and are quite variable. They include Lambert-Eaton myasthenic syndrome (LEMS), sensory neuropathy, encephalomyelopathy, cerebellar degeneration, autonomic neuropathy, retinal degeneration, and opsoclonus. Limbic encephalitis (dementia with or without seizures) has frequently been observed. The neurologic syndromes may precede the diagnosis of lung cancer by months to years.

PNSs are thought to be immune mediated on the basis of identifying autoantibodies. The antineuronal nuclear antibody (ANNA-1), also known as anti-Hu antibody, has been associated with small cell carcinoma and various neurologic syndromes. ANNA-2 (anti-Ri antibody) and CRMP-5 antibody have also been associated with various PNSs. These antibodies predict the patients' neoplasm but not a specific neurologic syndrome. The ANNA-1 binds to the nucleus of all neurons in the central and peripheral nervous system, including the sensory and autonomic ganglia and myenteric plexus.

Proximal muscle weakness, hyporeflexia, and autonomic dysfunction characterize LEMS. Cranial nerve involvement may be present and does not differentiate LEMS from myasthenia gravis. There is a strong association of LEMS with antibodies against P/Q type presynaptic voltage-gated calcium channels of the peripheral cholinergic nerve terminals. These antibodies have also been identified in 25% of patients with small cell lung cancers with no neurologic syndrome. Myasthenia gravis, in contrast to LEMS, is associated with antiacetylcholine receptor antibodies. Malignancy is identified in approximately 50% of patients with LEMS, and small cell lung cancer is by far the most common type. The diagnosis of LEMS is based on the characteristic electromyographic (EMG) finding that shows a small amplitude of the resting compound muscle action potential and facilitation with rapid, repetitive, and supramaximal nerve stimulation. A single-fiber EMG is optimal for making the diagnosis. Careful radiographic evaluation of the lungs and mediastinum is indicated, especially in current or former smokers who have a suspected PNS. In many cases, the radiographic findings are very subtle. If the patient has a positive paraneoplastic autoantibody blood test result and the computed tomography (CT) chest scan does not reveal an abnormality, then current guidelines recommend that a positron emission computed tomography (PET) scan be performed to look for an occult malignancy. Strong consideration should be given to biopsy of even subtle abnormalities because without diagnosis and treatment the PNS will progress, frequently with devastating consequences.

The best treatment for patients with PNS caused by small cell lung cancer is to treat with chemotherapy with or without thoracic radiotherapy, depending on the stage of disease. LEMS may improve with treatment, but not always. The other PNSs rarely improve with treatment, but the goal is to treat the lung cancer as soon as possible to try to prevent progressive neurologic disease.

Skeletal muscular paraneoplastic syndromes include digital clubbing, hypertrophic pulmonary osteoarthropathy (HPO), and dermatomyositis or polymyositis. Clubbing may involve the fingers and toes and consist of selective enlargement of the connective tissue in the terminal phalanges with loss of the angle between the base of the nail bed and cuticle, rounded nails, and enlarged fingertips. There are nonmalignant causes of clubbing such as pulmonary fibrosis or congenital heart disease. HPO is uncommon in association with lung cancer and is characterized by painful joints that usually involve the ankles, knees, wrists, and elbows and is most often symmetric. Some patients may complain of pain or tenderness along the shins. The pain and arthropathy is caused by a proliferative periostitis that involves the long bones but may involve metacarpal, metatarsal, and phalangeal bones. Clubbing may be present along with HPO. Large cell and adenocarcinoma are the most common types to cause HPO. The cause of HPO is uncertain but is thought to be attributable to a humeral agent. A radiograph of the long bones (tibia and fibula or radius and ulna) may show the characteristic periosteal new bone formation. An isotype bone scan or PET scan typically demonstrates diffuse uptake in the long bones. Symptoms of HPO may resolve with thoracotomy with or without resection of the malignancy. For inoperable patients, treatment with nonsteroidal anti-inflammatory agents is often of benefit. Recently, the use of intravenous bisphosphonates has been reported to alleviate the symptoms of HPO.

There have been reports of the association of lung cancer with dermatomyositis-polymyositis (DM-PM), but the relationship is uncertain. Patients may present with painful muscles and weakness. Blood tests for the muscle enzymes creatine kinase or aldolase will demonstrate elevated levels. An EMG or muscle biopsy is diagnostic. A CT scan of the chest is warranted in a patient with DM-PM who is at high risk for lung cancer. The treatment of patients with malignancy-related DM-PM is the same as for nonmalignancy-related disease plus appropriate treatment of the underlying lung cancer.

Other Neoplasms of the Lung

Uncommon malignant tumors of the lung include bronchial carcinoid and salivary gland tumors of adenoid cystic carcinoma and mucoepidermoid carcinoma. Bronchial carcinoid tumors account for 1% to 2% of all lung malignancies and 20% of all carcinoid tumors. The annual rates in men and women are 0.52 and 0.89, respectively, per 100,000 population. These tumors are characterized by growth patterns that suggest neuroendocrine differentiation. Bronchial carcinoids are classified as typical or atypical. Typical carcinoid tumors are low-grade tumors with fewer than 2 mitoses per 2 mm^2 (10 high-power microscopic fields) and no necrosis. Atypical carcinoids are intermediate-grade neuroendocrine tumors with 2 to 10 mitoses per 2 mm^2 or foci of necrosis. Typical carcinoid tumors are about four times more common than atypical carcinoids. There is no clear relationship to smoking.

Approximately 75% of these tumors arise in the central airways. The usual symptoms are cough, wheeze, hemoptysis, and recurrent pneumonia. One-fourth are peripherally located and are usually asymptomatic or present as an obstructive pneumonia. Five percent may present with an endocrine syndrome such as carcinoid syndrome, Cushing syndrome, or acromegaly.

Centrally located tumors are likely to cause bronchial obstruction with atelectasis, lobar collapse, or pneumonia on chest radiography or computed tomography (CT) scan. Cavitation and pleural effusion, unless related to pneumonia, are rare. The CT scan may show an intraluminal tumor in the central airways. Carcinoid tumors are more commonly smooth bordered but may also be lobulated and are less likely to have irregular borders.

Bronchoscopy is able to visually identify an endobronchial lesion in a majority of cases because 75% are centrally located. The pink to red vascular-appearing mass is typical. Biopsy is frequently diagnostic. Bleeding may be a little more prominent than with non–small cell lung cancer, but serious bleeding complications are uncommon. Sputum cytology and bronchial brushings are usually nondiagnostic. Transthoracic needle biopsy may be diagnostic, but occasionally carcinoid tumor and small cell lung cancer have been confused histologically on small samples from needle biopsy.

The treatment of choice is surgical resection for stage I, II, and IIIA disease (the staging system is same as for non–small cell lung cancer). The 10-year survival with typical carcinoid tumors is 80% to 90%. Survival of those with atypical tumors is significantly less but still approximately 50% at 5 years and depends on the stage of disease at the time of diagnosis. Carcinoid tumors, both typical and atypical, are more chemoresistant and radiotherapy resistant than non–small cell lung cancer. Nevertheless, concurrent chemoradiotherapy is the treatment of choice for patients with unresectable stage IIIA/B disease. Stage IV disease is very chemoresistant, but the somatostatin analog octreotide is effective at controlling the symptoms of carcinoid syndrome (flushing and diarrhea) and may impact survival.

Salivary gland tumors of the tracheobronchial tree are histologically similar to their counterparts in the salivary glands. The two most common airway tumors are adenoid cystic carcinoma (cylindroma) and mucoepidermoid carcinoma; both are less common than carcinoid tumors. There is no clear association of these tumors with smoking. Adenoid cystic carcinoma causes fewer than 1% of all lung tumors, and the vast majority of cases originate intraluminally in the trachea, mainstem, or lobar bronchi. These tumors are typically very slow growing, and the symptoms and presentation are similar to those of centrally located carcinoid tumors. The chest radiograph is frequently normal because of the central endoluminal location of the tumor, but CT usually identifies the tumor. Bronchoscopy is the most common method of diagnosis.

Surgical resection is the treatment of choice, but multiple local recurrences are common before developing distant metastases. The 5- and 10-year survival rates for resected adenoid cystic carcinoma are approximately 70% and 60%, respectively, compared with unresectable disease, in which the 5- and 10-year survival rates are 50% and 30%, respectively.

Mucoepidermoid carcinomas account for fewer than 1% of lung tumors. They form a significant proportion of endobronchial tumors in children. These tumors tend to occur centrally in the tracheobronchial tree. Tumors are divided into low- or high-grade types on the basis of histology. High-grade tumors are rare and have a significantly worse prognosis. The clinical and radiographic presentations of this tumor are similar to those of adenoid cystic carcinomas, and bronchoscopy is the most common method of diagnosis. The treatment of choice is surgical resection. Low-grade tumors metastasize in 5% or fewer of cases. High-grade tumors are treated similarly to non–small cell lung cancer and have a poor prognosis. The overall survival rate for resected mucoepidermoid carcinoma is 80% to 90% at 5 years. Patients with mucoepidermoid carcinoma have better survival than those with adenoid cystic carcinoma.

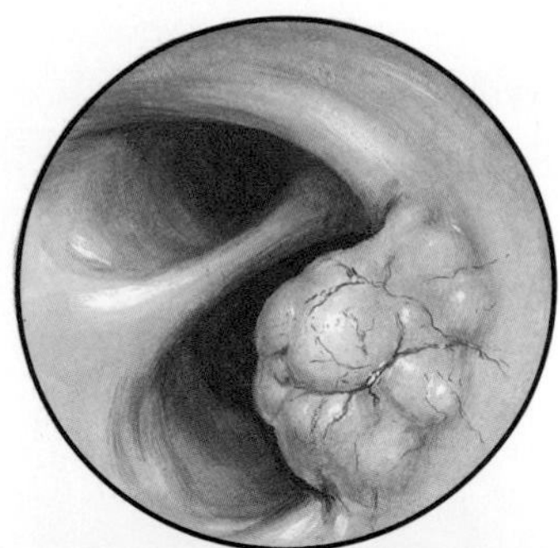
Bronchoscopic view of a primary bronchial tumor

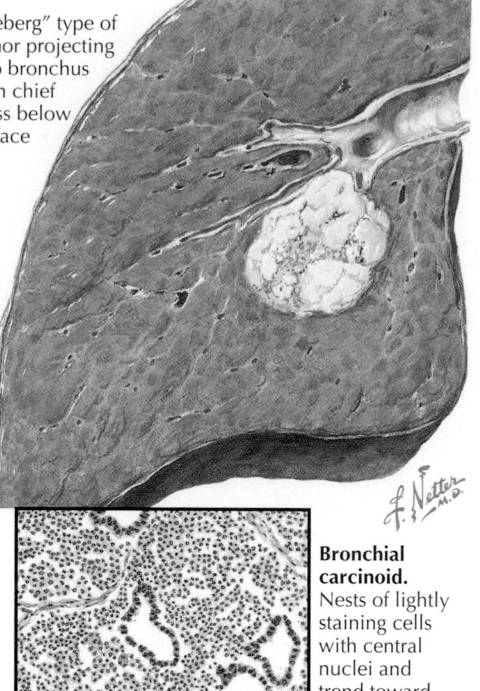

"Iceberg" type of tumor projecting into bronchus with chief mass below surface

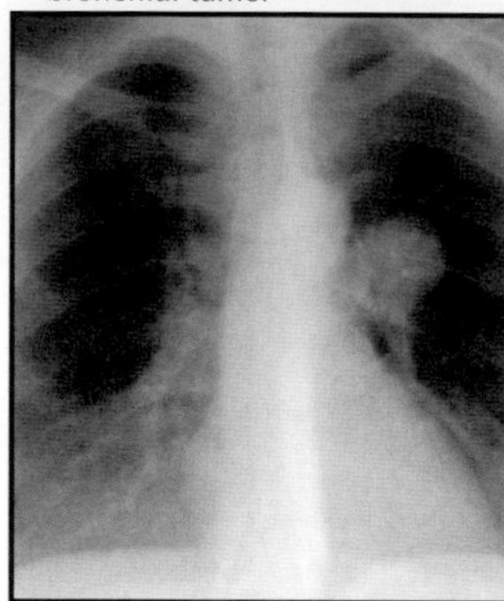
Central carcinoid lesion

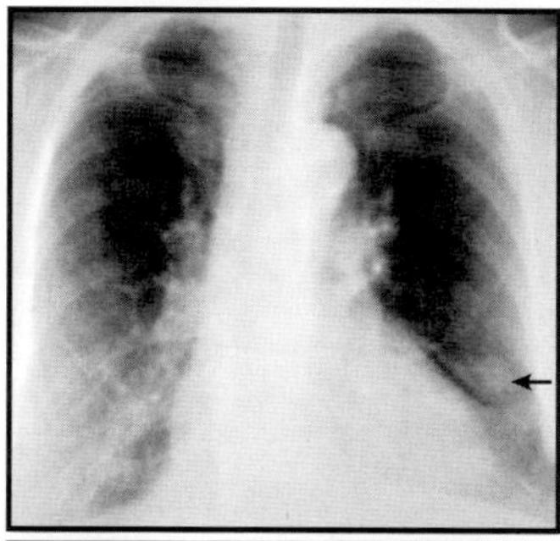
Peripheral carcinoid lesion

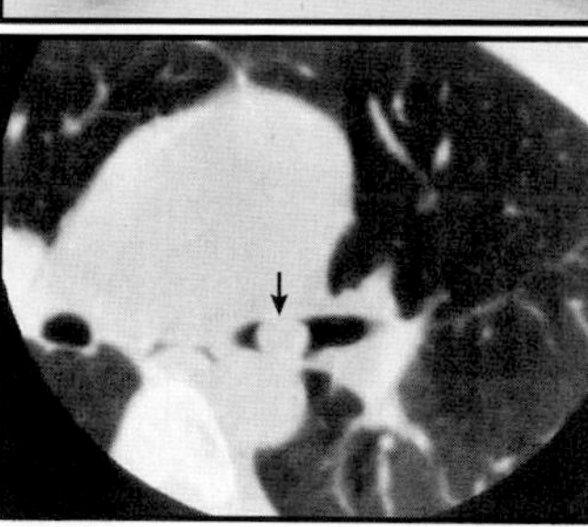
CT of mainstem airway carcinoid lesion

Bronchial carcinoid. Nests of lightly staining cells with central nuclei and trend toward tubule formation

Adenoid cystic carcinoma (cyclindroma). Cylinders of tumor cells with surrounding and central areas of myxomatous tissue

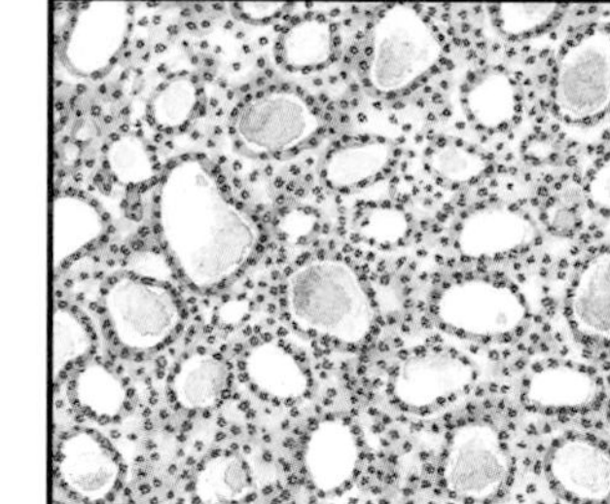
Mucoepidermoid carcinoma. Many glandlike formations (most of which contain mucus) resembling a salivary gland tumor

BENIGN TUMORS OF THE LUNG

Hamartoma

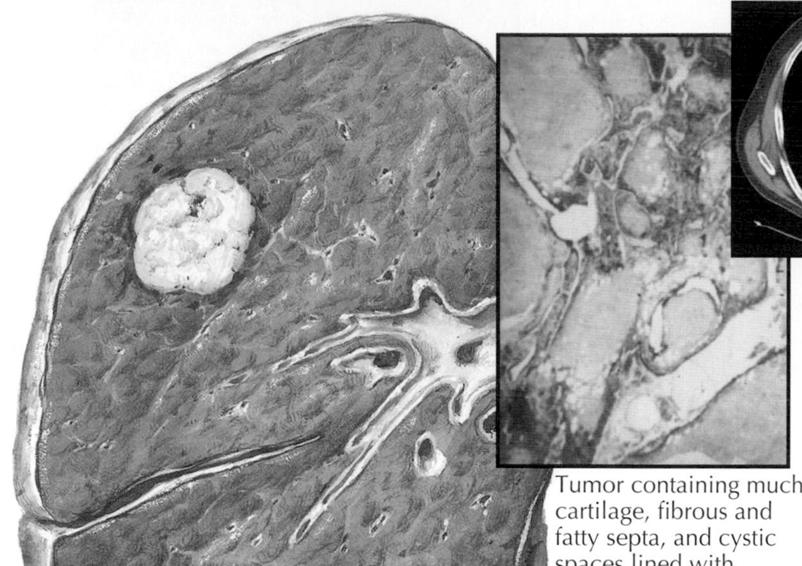

Sharply circumscribed growth with calcified areas

Tumor containing much cartilage, fibrous and fatty septa, and cystic spaces lined with cuboidal epithelium

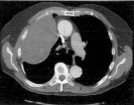

CT scan showing "popcorn" calcification and areas of fat density in a hamartoma in the right lung

Solitary fibrous tumor

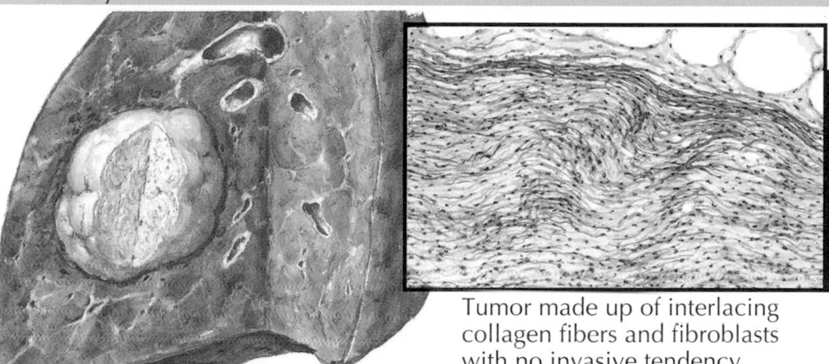

Peripherally located solitary fibrous tumor; these are usually local on the pleural lining.

Tumor made up of interlacing collagen fibers and fibroblasts with no invasive tendency

CT scan of solitary fibrous tumor

Chondroma

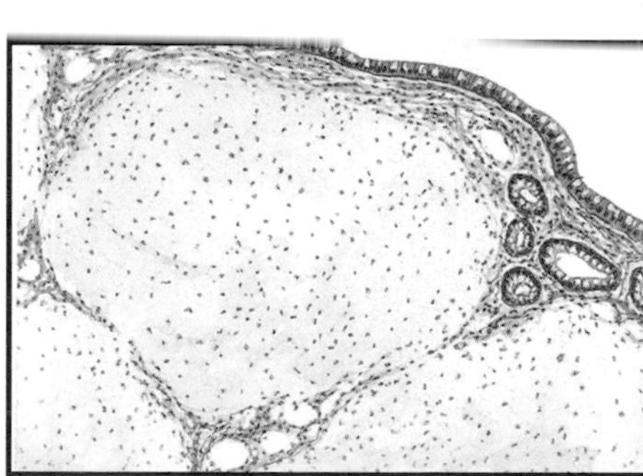

Tumor composed almost entirely of cartilage and covered by bronchial epithelium

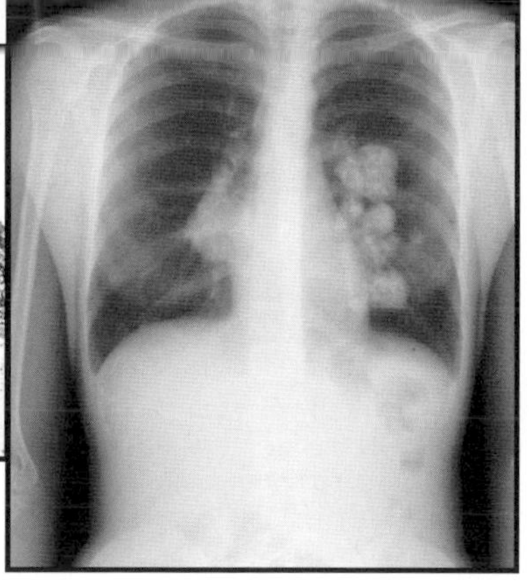

Chest radiograph showing multiple chondroma lesions

Pulmonary granulomas are the most common cause of a benign pulmonary nodule and are a sequela of infection. The next most common benign tumor is hamartoma. It is composed of varying proportions of mesenchymal tissues, including smooth muscle, fat, and connective tissue and cartilage. The incidence in the population is 0.25% with two to four times male predominance. Most hamartomas occur in the periphery of the lung and present as an asymptomatic solitary pulmonary nodule. The edges of the tumor are typically smooth. Approximately 10% may occur endobronchially and may present with symptoms of cough, wheeze, dyspnea, or obstructive pneumonia. The presence of "popcorn" calcification on chest radiography or computed tomography (CT) scan is a classic pattern but is present in only a small percentage of cases. The presence of fat on thin-section CT chest images or fat alternating with areas of calcification is diagnostic of this lesion, but many hamartomas do not have either of these findings. Because of the peripheral location, bronchoscopy is typically nondiagnostic. The positron emission tomography (PET) scan is negative for increased metabolic activity. Because of the indeterminate diagnostic results, many of these tumors are treated with surgical resection, although removal is not necessary for the peripherally located and asymptomatic tumor if it has the diagnostic radiographic appearances discussed above.

Solitary fibrous tumors occur in numerous sites, including the pleura, and may present as a mass in the chest. Previously called *benign localized mesothelioma* (this term is now discouraged), it has no association with asbestos exposure, and 80% to 90% of these lesions are benign and do not spread. It is an uncommon tumor of spindle cell mesenchymal growth thought to be of fibroblastic origin and arises from the visceral pleura most commonly but may also arise in the lung parenchyma or mediastinum. The tumor is usually detected as an asymptomatic nodule or mass on chest radiography. Some patients may present with cough, dyspnea, or chest pain. Rarely, patients may present with hypertrophic pulmonary osteoarthropathy or symptomatic hypoglycemia caused by production of insulin-like growth factor. These latter symptoms are more likely when the tumor is quite large. There are no diagnostic radiographic features, and the PET scan results are usually negative or have a low level of uptake. Bronchoscopy is nondiagnostic because of the pleural origin of these lesions, and transthoracic needle biopsies are unreliable for a definitive diagnosis. The treatment of choice is surgical resection. Local recurrence may occur in 10% to 15% of cases.

Chondromas are a rare tumor of cartilage. They usually occur in female patients with the Carney triad of gastrointestinal stromal tumor, pulmonary chondroma, and paraganglionoma. Pulmonary chondromas are usually asymptomatic unless they are numerous or of large size. Occasionally, they may cause obstructive pneumonia. Radiographically, they are well-circumscribed tumors, usually multiple, and calcified or may have "popcorn" calcification. If the pulmonary tumors are asymptomatic, then there is no reason for treatment. Symptomatic tumors may require surgical resection.

Inflammatory myofibroblastic tumor, previously called *inflammatory pseudotumor* or *plasma cell granuloma*, is composed of a mixture of collagen, inflammatory cells, and the cytologically bland spindle cells showing myofibroblastic differentiation. It occurs in all ages, with an equal gender distribution. It is the most common pulmonary tumor of childhood and may have a significant endobronchial component. Symptoms may include cough, dyspnea, fever, and weight loss. Some patients are asymptomatic. The majority of these tumors are solitary in lung parenchyma but occasionally may involve the chest wall or mediastinum. The mass is usually well circumscribed, lobulated, or smooth, but irregular borders occur in 20%. Calcification may be present, and rarely cavitation has been reported. Complete surgical resection is the treatment of choice with excellent long-term survival of 90% at 5 years in one reported series. Local recurrence may occur with incomplete resections.

Malignant Pleural Mesothelioma

Malignant pleural mesothelioma (MPM) is a tumor arising in the pleura from mesothelial cells. It may also arise in the peritoneal cavity, pericardium, and tunica vaginalis (rarely). Pleural mesothelioma may be restricted to a small area or grow diffusely in a multifocal or continuous manner. The histologic types of MPM are epithelioid, which is the most common; sarcomatoid; and biphasic or mixed. Desmoplastic mesothelioma is considered a subtype of sarcomatoid mesothelioma. Localized malignant mesothelioma presents as a nodular lesion without diffuse pleural spread but is histologically identical to diffuse MPM. Results of immunohistochemical staining with cytokeratin 5/6, calretinin, and Wilms tumor-1 are positive in the vast majority of epithelioid mesothelioma but are less often positive in sarcomatoid mesothelioma. These markers are typically, but not always, negative in adenocarcinoma.

The etiologic agent of MPM is asbestos in a large majority of the cases, but documentation requires a careful exposure history, and the delay between exposure and disease is generally 30 to 50 years. The frequency of MPM increases with increasing asbestos exposure, but there is no documented lower limit or safe threshold level of asbestos exposure. Certain individuals are believed to be genetically more susceptible, but the exact genetics have not been delineated.

The most common presentations are pleural effusion or pain. Dyspnea may be present if the pleural effusion is of significant size. Pain is generally described as a dull ache or pulling sensation in the chest wall. The chest radiograph may show pleural effusion or pleural thickening with or without irregular thickening of the interlobar fissure. Calcified pleural plaques may be present and are a sign of prior asbestos exposure. Computed tomography (CT) of the chest usually demonstrates pleural thickening and nodularity if it is not hidden by the pleural effusion that is present in most cases. Thickening of the intralobar fissure is frequently present. With more extensive involvement, contraction of the involved hemithorax may occur.

The diagnosis can be difficult. Pleural fluid cytology results are positive for malignant cells in one-third of cases, but pathologists have difficulty determining adenocarcinoma involving the pleura versus MPM. Percutaneous or closed pleural biopsy often yields adequate tissue for diagnosis. When these test results are nondiagnostic, then thoracoscopy with biopsy under direct visualization is diagnostic in 90% of cases. The typical description at visualization is that of multiple nodular densities of the pleura. Because of the paucity of cases (~2000-3000 per year in the United States), many pathologists see few cases of MPM. It is therefore very important that biopsy samples be reviewed by a pathologist with particular expertise in mesothelioma.

The treatment of patients with MPM is difficult and somewhat controversial. For those with earlier stage tissue, aggressive trimodality treatment has been advocated by some. This approach includes induction chemotherapy followed by extrapleural pneumonectomy and postoperative hemithoracic radiotherapy. Most patients with MPM are clinically or medically inoperable, and these individuals should be considered for systemic chemotherapy or supportive care only.

The natural history of this disease is that of initial local progression in the pleura (with encasement of the lung), mediastinum, pericardium, and diaphragm. Intraabdominal spread, contralateral pleura, and distant organs occur later in the disease process. The median survival in 9 to 12 months in most nonsurgical series and 16 to 18 months in surgical series with earlier stage patients. Twenty percent or fewer patients survive beyond 2 years, but there are reports of 4- to 5-year survival in selected patients with minimal treatment. Patients generally die of cardiorespiratory failure caused by encasement of the heart and lungs by tumor.

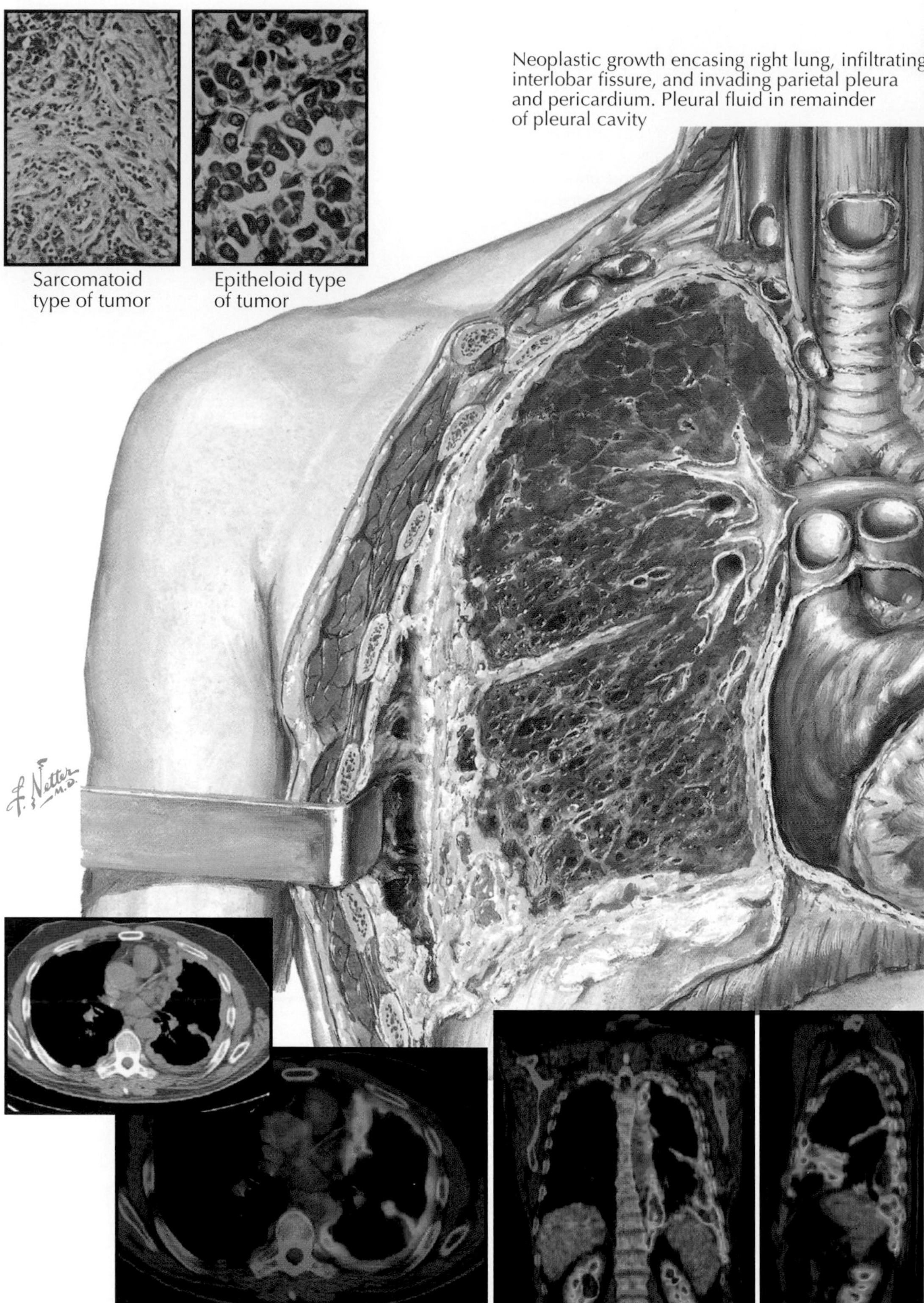

Sarcomatoid type of tumor
Epitheloid type of tumor
Neoplastic growth encasing right lung, infiltrating interlobar fissure, and invading parietal pleura and pericardium. Pleural fluid in remainder of pleural cavity
F. Netter M.D.

Combined CT/PET images showing mesothelioma (bright areas) in axial, coronal, and sagittal views of the lungs

Mediastinal Tumors: Anterior Mediastinum

The mediastinum is the central space in the chest cavity that is bounded by the sternum anteriorly, the pleura of the lungs laterally, the vertebrae posteriorly, the thoracic inlet superiorly, and the diaphragm inferiorly. The mediastinum does not have rigid structures that divide it into compartments, but for anatomic and clinical purposes, it is generally divided into anterior, middle-posterior, and paravertebral compartments. It should be noted that the paravertebral regions do not form part of the mediastinum proper. The anterior mediastinum is defined by an imaginary line drawn along the anterior trachea and posterior cardiac border on a lateral chest radiograph. The most common tumors of the anterior mediastinum are thymoma, lymphoma, germ cell tumors, and thyroid (goiter). Cystic hygroma should also be considered, usually in children.

Tumors of the anterior mediastinum account for 50% of all mediastinal tumors. They may be asymptomatic at diagnosis, or patients may complain of cough, dyspnea, or vague chest discomfort. Thymoma is the most common mediastinal tumor in adults. From 30% to 50% of patients with thymoma also have myasthenia gravis. Of patients diagnosed with myasthenia gravis, approximately 15% have a thymoma. Other syndromes associated with thymoma include hypogammaglobulinemia and pure red blood cell aplasia. A significant percentage of thymomas are malignant and have spread beyond the capsule of the tumor at the time of diagnosis. Surgical resection is the treatment of choice for localized tumors. Unresectable disease confined to the chest is treated with chemotherapy and thoracic radiotherapy. These tumors are generally moderately sensitive to treatment. Survival with early stage and resectable tumors is excellent, but even unresectable malignant thymomas have a 50% 5-year survival rate with treatment. Specific treatment and outcomes are stage and histology dependent.

Lymphomas account for 10% to 20% of all mediastinal tumors and occur in both the anterior and middle mediastinum. Hodgkin disease and diffuse large B-cell lymphoma are the most common types in the anterior mediastinum. Patients may present with local symptoms or systemic symptoms of fever, night sweats, and weight loss. Superior vena cava syndrome may be the presenting symptoms or signs in some cases (see Plate 4-54).

Germ cell tumors may present in the anterior mediastinum. Teratomas are the most common germ cell tumor and are usually benign. Teratomas consist of tissues from more than one germ cell layer. They typically occur in children and young adults. Most are asymptomatic but may cause local symptoms. Radiographically, these tumors are lobular and well circumscribed and may contain calcification or toothlike structures. The computed tomography (CT) scan demonstrates a multiloculated cystic mass that frequently contains fat. Surgical resection is the treatment of choice. Seminomas or nonseminomatous germ cell neoplasms may also occur in the anterior mediastinum. These almost always occur in males, and most are accompanied by elevated blood tumor marker levels of α-fetoprotein (AFP) or β-human chorionic gonadotropin (HCG). These tumors are very responsive to chemotherapy, which is the initial treatment and may be followed by surgical resection of residual disease. The cure rate for seminomas is high, and nonseminomatous germ cell tumors of the mediastinum have an approximate 50% 5-year survival rate.

Intrathoracic goiters are mostly caused by extension from cervical thyroid goiters that can be detected on careful examination of the neck. Patients are usually asymptomatic but may have symptoms related to compression of the trachea or esophagus such as cough, dyspnea, or dysphagia. The vast majority of these tumors are benign. They are located in the anterosuperior mediastinum. The CT demonstrates a lobular, well-defined mass that may have cystic changes or calcifications. Surgical resection is the treatment of choice.

Cystic hygromas (lymphangiomas) are an abnormal collection of lymphatic vessels that dilate and collect lymph. They usually occur in the neck in children but rarely are detected in adults. They are uncommonly isolated to the mediastinum alone. CT may demonstrate a solitary or multiple liquid-filled cysts. If asymptomatic, there is no need to remove them. Other rare tumors of the anterior mediastinum include parathyroid adenomas; pericardial cysts; and mesenchymal neoplasms such as lipomas, liposarcomas, angiosarcomas, and leiomyomas. A foramen of Morgagni hernia of the anterior diaphragm may result in herniation of abdominal contents into the low anterior mediastinum.

Anterior mediastinum

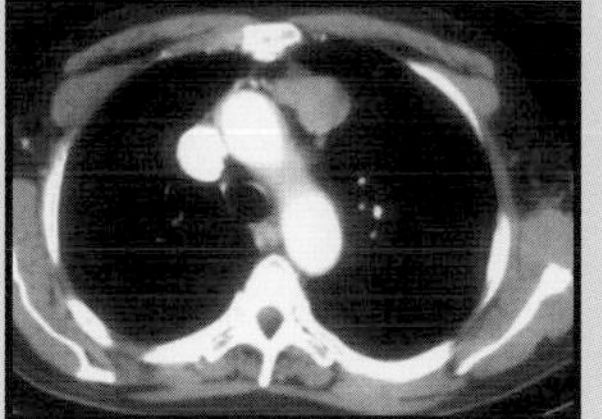

CT scan showing thymoma

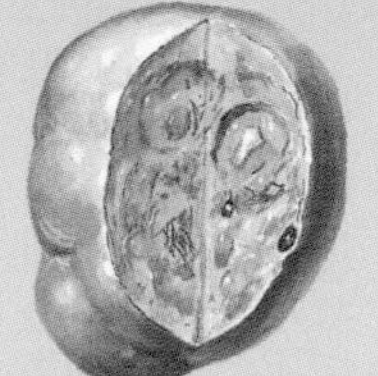

Thymoma

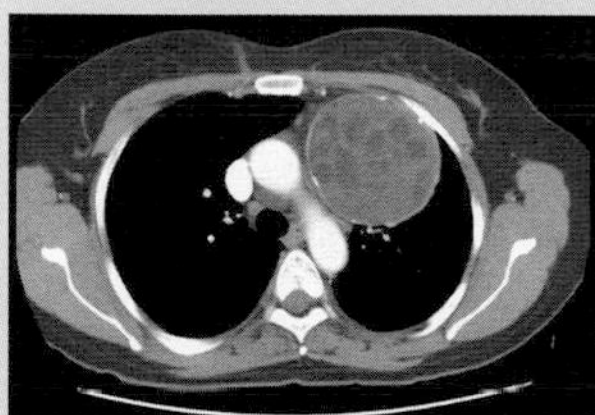

CT scan showing a benign cystic teratoma

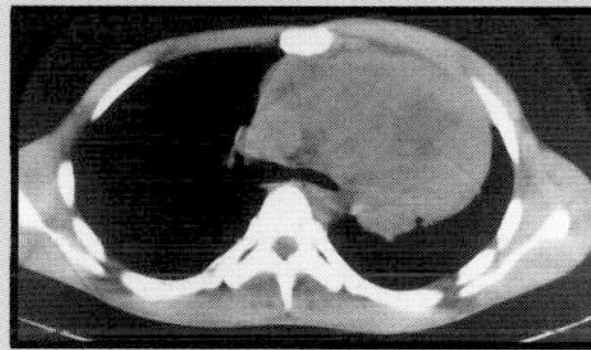

CT scan of diffuse large B-cell lymphoma

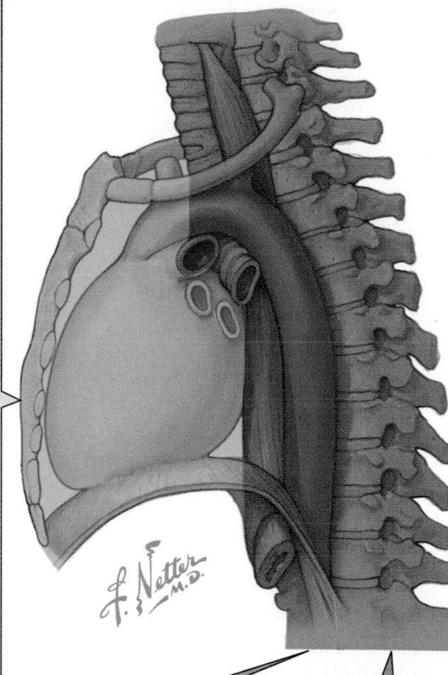

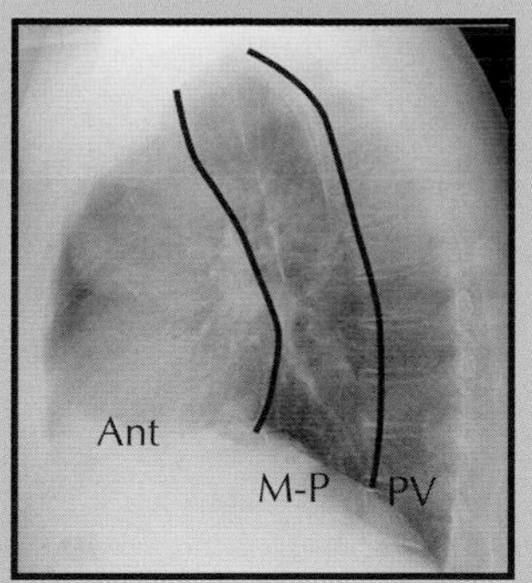

The mediastinum is the central compartment of the thorax that is lined by mediastinal pleura laterally and is continuous from cervical to abdominal structures

The mediastinum is arbitrarily divided into three radiographic compartments on chest radiography. Recall that there are no true mediastinal compartments, so this division is used to localize and categorize disease processes

A line drawn along the anterior aspect of the trachea and the posterior aspect of the heart separates the anterior (*Ant*) from the middle-posterior (*M-P*) mediastinum

A line drawn just posterior to the anterior margin of the thoracic vertebral bodies separates the M-P mediastinum from the paravertebral (PV) region. The paravertebral region is *not* a part of the mediastinum but is included here to help localize and categorize various pathologies

Middle-Posterior and Paravertebral Mediastinum

The middle-posterior mediastinum is the compartment located between the anterior and the paravertebral compartments. The paravertebral compartment is located posterior to an imaginary line drawn just posterior to the anterior margins of the thoracic vertebral bodies. Approximately 10% to 15% of mediastinal tumors occur in the middle-posterior mediastinum. The most common abnormalities are caused by lymph node enlargement from lymphoma, granulomatous disease caused by tuberculosis, fungal infection, or noninfectious conditions of sarcoidosis or silicosis. Metastatic lymphadenopathy may be caused by cancers of the lung, kidney, breast, or gastrointestinal tract. Rare causes of lymphadenopathy are Castleman disease and amyloidosis. Symptoms may be absent or related to the underlying systemic disease process, such as fever and night sweats caused by lymphoma or an infectious process. Some patients may complain of dysphagia caused by compression of the esophagus or vague chest discomfort.

Congenital foregut cysts are a common cause of middle mediastinal lesions. These include bronchogenic cysts, esophageal duplication cysts, and (uncommonly) neurenteric cysts. Bronchogenic cysts are most common and are thought to be caused by an abnormal budding of the foregut during development. Most are located paratracheally or subcarinally. These cysts are lined by respiratory epithelium (pseudostratified, columnar, ciliated). Enteric cysts (esophageal duplication and neurenteric) arise from the dorsal foregut and are usually located in the middle-posterior mediastinum. Enteric cysts are lined by squamous or enteric epithelium. The cyst walls have smooth muscle layers with a myenteric plexus. Esophageal duplication cysts usually adhere to the esophagus. Neurenteric cysts may be associated with the esophagus or cervical or upper thoracic vertebral abnormalities with an attachment or extension into the spine. Most enteric cysts are diagnosed during childhood. Radiographically, these cysts are well-circumscribed, spherical masses. On computed tomography (CT) scan, they are unilocular, homogeneous, and nonenhancing.

Asymptomatic cysts may be observed, but their chance or rate of enlargement is uncertain. Large cysts may compress the airways and lead to pneumonia or dysphagia with esophageal compression. The treatment of choice for patients with symptomatic cysts is surgical resection. Unresected cysts rarely transform into malignant lesions.

Esophageal disorders such as achalasia, benign tumors, diverticula, and carcinoma are common causes of middle-posterior mediastinal lesions. Hiatal hernia is very common and presents as a mass in the inferior middle-posterior mediastinum, usually seen as a retrocardiac mass on routine chest radiography. Barium swallow studies and endoscopy are generally diagnostic.

Vascular lesions may present as a mass in the middle-posterior mediastinum and should always be considered before attempting biopsy. Thoracic aortic aneurysm is the most common of these, but pulmonary artery aneurysm and mediastinal hemangiomas are occasionally encountered. Contrast-enhanced CT chest examinations are generally diagnostic for a vascular aneurysm and likely demonstrate the vascular nature of hemangiomas.

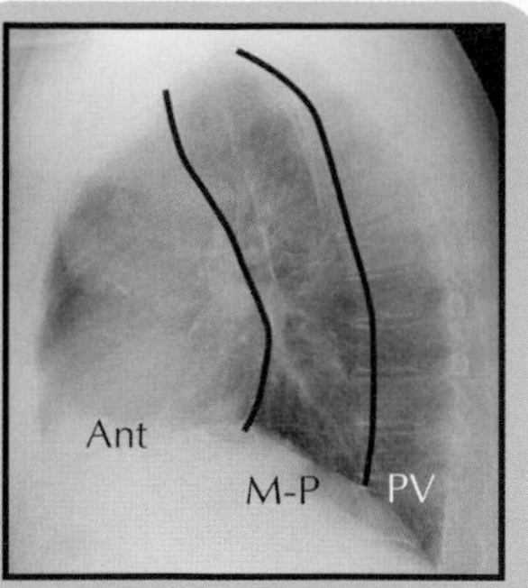

The mediastinum is the central compartment of the thorax that is lined by mediastinal pleura laterally and is continuous from cervical to abdominal structures.

The mediastinum is arbitrarily divided into 3 radiographic compartments on CXR. Recall that there are no true mediastinal compartments so this division is used to localize and categorize disease processes.

A line drawn along the anterior aspect of the trachea and the posterior aspect of the heart separates the anterior (*Ant*) from the middle-posterior (*M-P*) mediastinum.

A line drawn just posterior to the anterior margin of a line drawn just posterior to the anterior margin of the thoracic vertebral bodies separates the M-P mediastinum from the paravertebral (*PV*) region. The paravertebral region is NOT a part of the mediastinum, but is included here to help localize and categorize various pathologies.

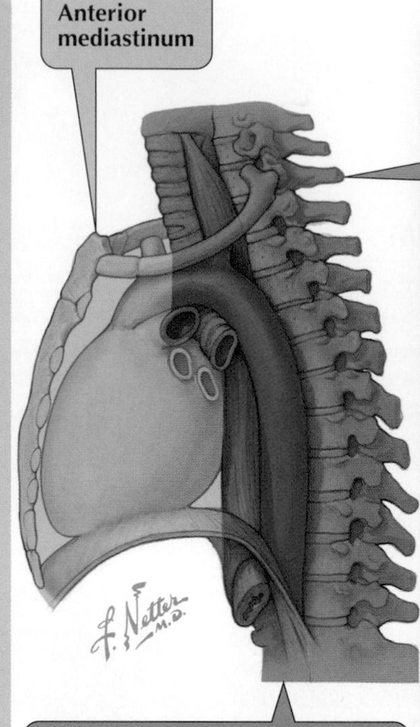

Middle-posterior mediastinum

Vascular aneurysm

Lymph nodes; lympoma, metastitic cancer

Esophageal tumors; achalasia, diverticula

Bronchogenic or esophageal duplication cyst

Paravertebral region

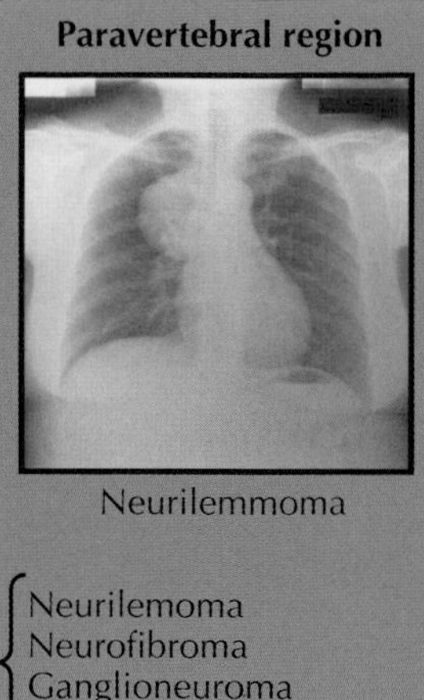

Neurilemmoma

- Neurilemoma
- Neurofibroma
- Ganglioneuroma
- Meningocele

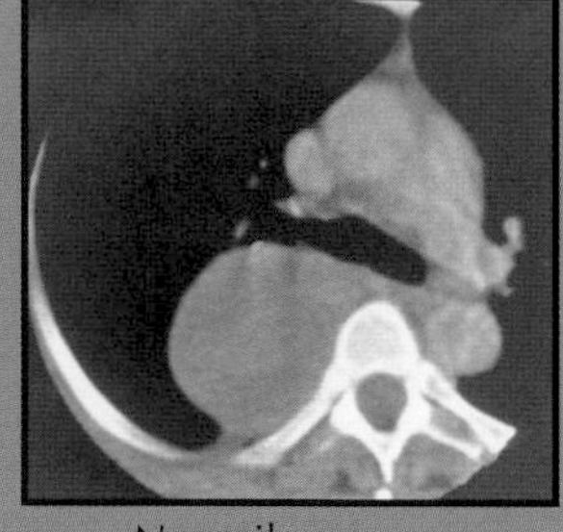

Neuroilemmoma

Tumors of the paravertebral compartment are generally caused by neurogenic neoplasms. Neurogenic tumors account for 20% of adult and 40% of pediatric mediastinal tumors. The large majority of these tumors in adults are benign, but 50% of the neurogenic tumors in children are malignant. Schwannomas (also called *neurilemmomas*) and neurofibromas are the most common neurogenic neoplasms. More than 90% are benign, and a small percentage are multiple. They are slow growing and arise from a spinal nerve root. Neurofibromas often occur in individuals with von Recklinghausen disease (neurofibromatosis). They may have multiple tumors, and malignant transformation is more common with this disease. These tumors are most commonly asymptomatic and detected accidentally. Occasionally, they may result in pain that leads to discovery of the tumor. The malignant form of these neurogenic tumors is classified as a malignant peripheral nerve sheath neoplasm. Radiographically, schwannomas and neurofibromas are well-marginated, spherical, or lobular paravertebral masses. They are usually small and span one to two vertebrae but can grow to a large size. They may cause erosion of the rib or vertebral body, and 10% grow through and enlarge the neuroforamina and expand on either end to give a "dumbbell" shape. For this reason, magnetic resonance imaging of the spine is indicated before surgical resection is attempted. Surgery is the treatment of choice.

Ganglioneuromas are benign neoplasms of the sympathetic ganglia that typically occur in older children or young adults. They may be asymptomatic or symptomatic because of local tumor effects. They are well-demarcated, oblong paravertebral masses that usually span three to five vertebrae. Ganglioneuroblastomas and neuroblastomas are malignant sympathetic ganglia neoplasms that occur in young children.

Pheochromocytomas or paraganglionomas are rare neoplasms of paraganglionic tissue and rarely occur in the mediastinum, usually adjacent to the aorta or pulmonary arteries, but they may present in the posterior mediastinum. A lateral thoracic meningocele is uncommon and may be multiple. Radiographic studies demonstrate the typical cystic structures in the paravertebral foramina location. Asymptomatic lesions do not require treatment.

PULMONARY METASTASES

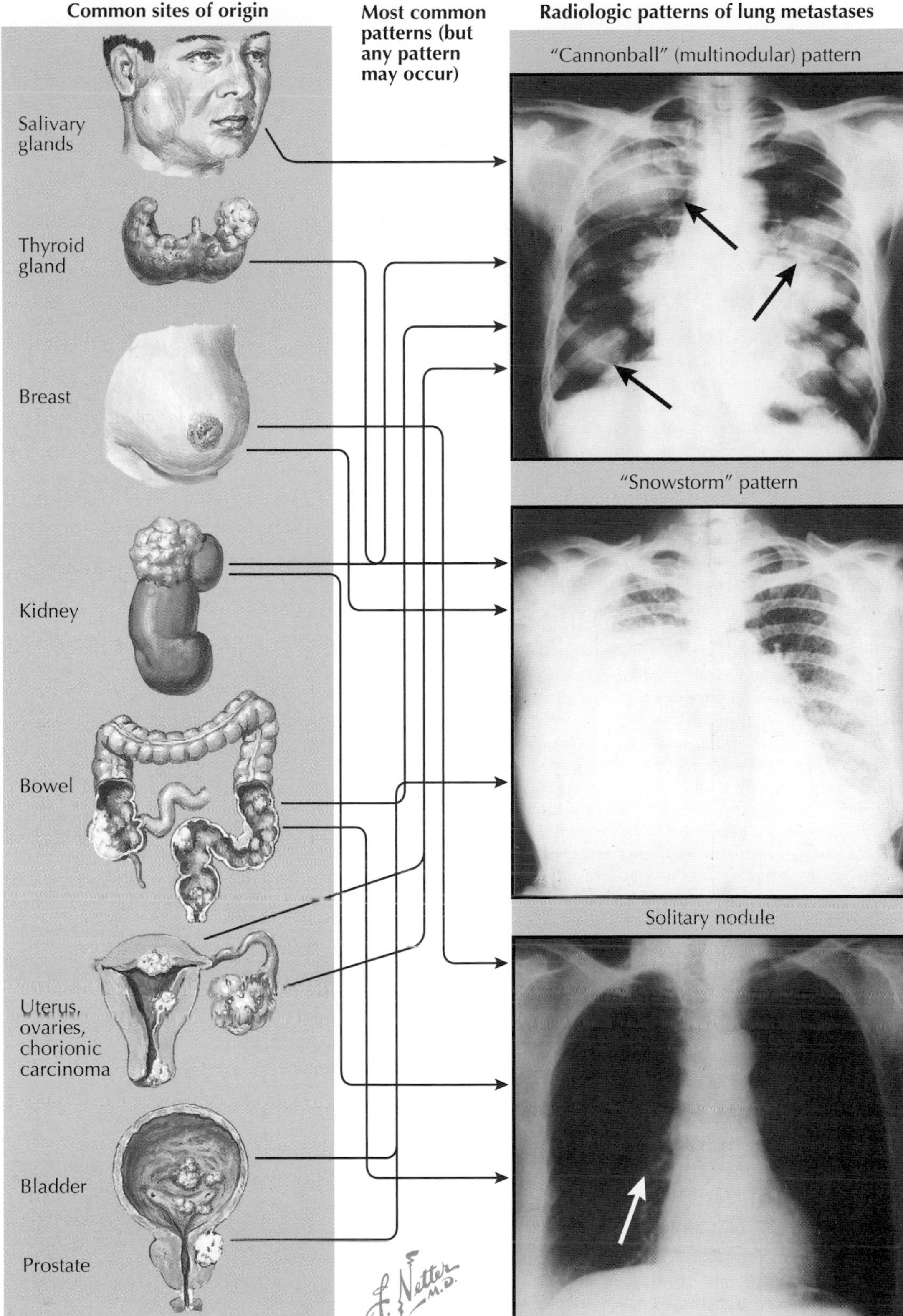

Lung metastasis occurs in one-third to one-half of all patients with a non-lung primary malignancy at the time of death based on autopsy data. Primary malignancies with the greatest tendency to metastasize to the lung are breast, lung, melanoma, osteosarcoma, choriocarcinoma, and germ cell tumors. Most pulmonary metastases are caused by common malignancies that include breast, colorectal, prostate, and renal cell carcinomas. Recent studies have demonstrated a high number of circulatory tumor cells in many different primary cancers. These are believed to lodge in the small pulmonary vessels, proliferate, and ultimately form nodules. Multiple pulmonary nodules are the most common manifestations of pulmonary metastasis. They are frequently spherical and variable in size. Multiple nodules larger than 1 cm in diameter are more likely to be malignant than benign. Larger lesions or "cannonballs" are a classic manifestation. Approximately 90% of individuals with pulmonary metastasis have or had a known primary malignancy. Solitary pulmonary metastasis may occur and in general should be treated as a possible new primary lung cancer if no other metastatic sites are identified and benign disease cannot be confirmed. Surgical resection is the treatment of choice in medically fit individuals.

Cavitation of metastatic nodules occurs in 5% or fewer of cases and is most commonly associated with squamous cell carcinoma of the head and neck, esophagus, and cervix. Sarcomas, especially osteosarcoma, are well known to cavitate. Cavitation has also been observed with adenocarcinoma of colorectal origin and transitional cell carcinoma of the bladder. Pneumothorax occurs with cavitary pulmonary metastasis in the subpleural location because of rupture into the pleural space. Osteosarcoma is the most common metastatic malignancy to cause a spontaneous pneumothorax. A spontaneous pneumothorax in a patient with a history of a sarcoma should raise the question of occult pulmonary metastasis. Calcification of nodules, although generally a sign of benignity, has been observed in metastatic chondrosarcoma and osteosarcoma and very rarely from other primary sites.

Airspace consolidation is most often seen with metastatic adenocarcinoma for gastrointestinal sources. The adenocarcinoma may spread along intact alveolar structures (lepidic growth) and form consolidation with air bronchograms or extensive ground-glass opacities. Sometimes this pattern is confused with primary bronchioloalveolar cell lung cancer.

Lymphangitic pulmonary metastasis is most commonly associated with adenocarcinoma. It is believed to be caused by hematogenous spread of tumor to the periphery of the lung and subsequent lymphangitic spread centrally toward the hilum. By this mechanism, it is most commonly bilateral. Some cases may develop because of hilar tumor involvement with centrifugal spread and account for cases of unilateral lymphangitic spread. The primary malignancies that account for most lymphangitic metastases are the lung, breast, and gastrointestinal tract, especially the stomach. The chest radiograph may reveal increased interstitial markings or demonstrate a sunburst pattern radiating from the hilar area. High-resolution computed tomography is more sensitive at detecting lymphangitic disease than chest radiography. Characteristic findings are a thickened interlobular septum with beading with or without polygonal formations. A thickened subpleural interstitium is also a frequent occurrence.

Patients will usually present with dyspnea with or without cough. The chest radiograph may be normal. Bronchoscopy with bronchoalveolar lavage and transbronchoscopic biopsy will result in a high diagnostic yield. The prognosis of lymphangitic carcinoma is generally poor unless the patient has a chemoresponsive tumor such as breast cancer, lymphoma, or choriocarcinoma.

Overview of Pneumonia

Classification of pneumonia

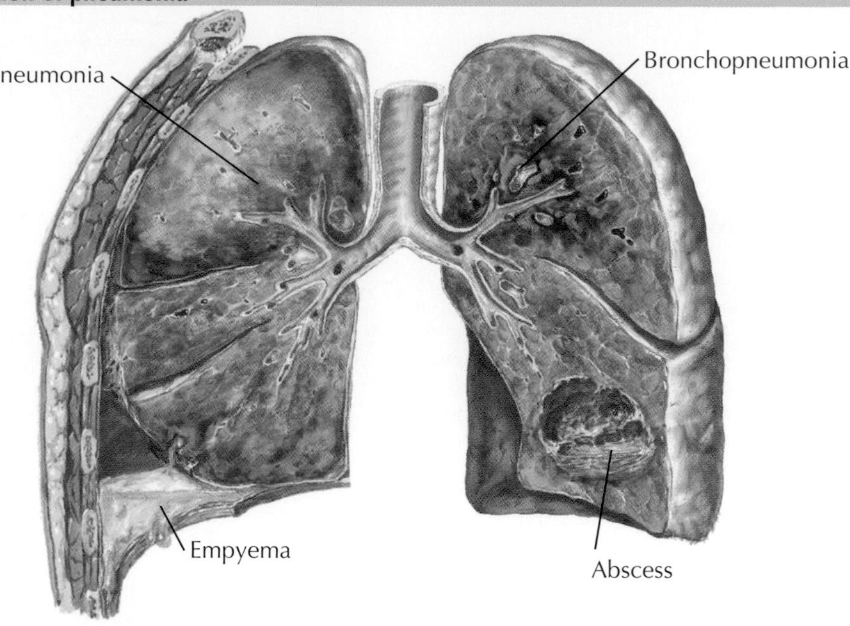

Community acquired pneumonia (CAP)

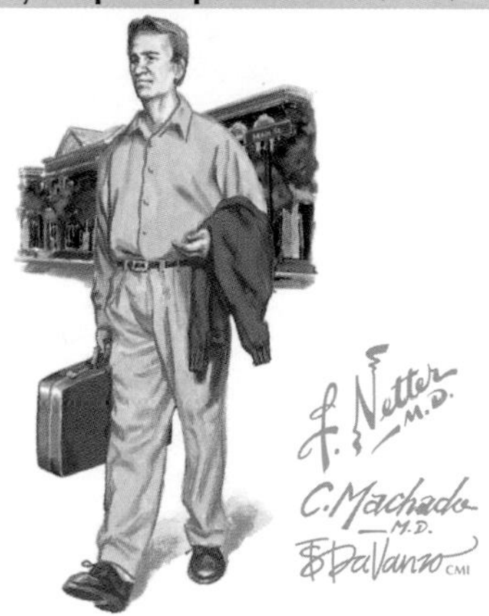

Hospital acquired pneumonia (HAP)

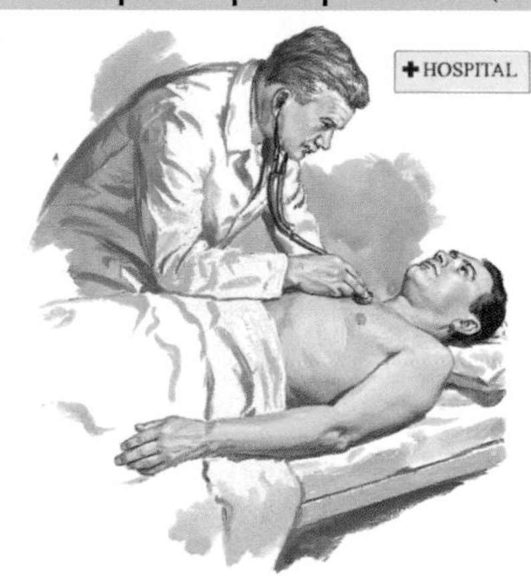

Healthcare-associated pneumonia (HCAP)

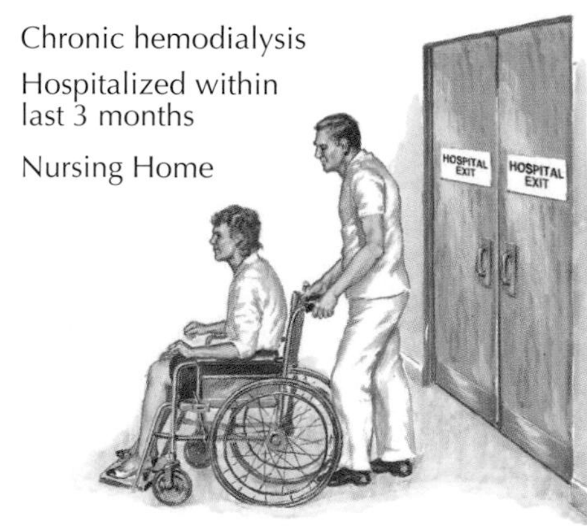

Ventilator-associated pneumonia (VAP)

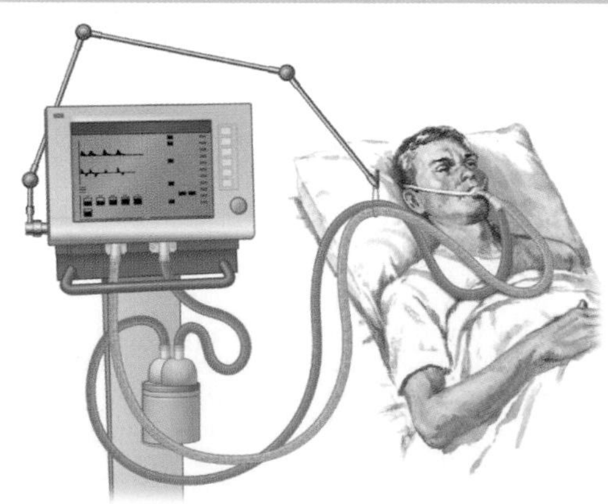

Infections of the lower respiratory tract may involve the airways, lung parenchyma, or pleural space. Pneumonia is an infection of the gas exchanging units of the lung, most commonly caused by bacteria, but occasionally by viruses, fungi, parasites, or other infectious agents. In immunocompetent individuals, pneumonia is characterized by a brisk filling of the alveolar space with inflammatory cells and fluid. If the alveolar infection involves an entire anatomic lobe of the lung, it is termed *lobar pneumonia*, and some episodes may lead to multilobar illness and more severe clinical manifestations. When the alveolar process occurs in a distribution that is patchy and adjacent to bronchi, without filling an entire lobe, it is termed *bronchopneumonia*.

Based on clinical presentation, pneumonias have also been classified as being typical or atypical. The typical pneumonia syndrome is characterized by a sudden onset of high fever, shaking chills, pleuritic chest pain, and productive cough, and it can be expected only if the patient has an intact immune response system and if the infection is caused by a bacterial pathogen such as *Streptococcus pneumoniae*, *Haemophilus influenzae*, *Klebsiella pneumoniae*, *Staphylococcus aureus*, aerobic gram-negative bacilli, or anaerobes. If a patient is infected by one of these organisms but has an impaired immune response, the classic pneumonia symptoms may be absent, as can be the case in elderly and debilitated patients. The atypical pneumonia syndrome, characterized by preceding upper respiratory symptoms, fever without chills, nonproductive cough, headache, myalgias, and mild leukocytosis, is often the result of infection with viruses, *Mycoplasma pneumoniae*, *Chlamydophila pneumoniae*, *Legionella* organisms, and other unusual infectious agents (as in psittacosis and Q fever). In clinical practice, it is often very difficult to use clinical features to predict the microbial cause of pneumonia.

When a parenchymal lung infection leads to breakdown of lung tissue, it may cause tissue necrosis and cavity formation, and this type of infection is termed a *lung abscess*. These infections usually result when a patient aspirates a highly virulent pathogen into the lung in the absence of effective clearance mechanisms; the etiologic agents include *S. aureus*, *K. pneumoniae*, *Escherichia coli*, and *Pseudomonas aeruginosa*. Empyema is an infection of the pleural space characterized by grossly purulent material that is usually caused by extension of parenchymal infection outside the lung; it is caused by anaerobes, gram-negative bacilli, *S. aureus*, and occasionally tuberculosis (TB).

Another classification system that is applied to pneumonia relates to the place of origin of the infection. When the infection occurs in patients who are living in the community, it is termed *community-acquired pneumonia* (CAP), although it is called *nosocomial pneumonia*, or *hospital–acquired pneumonia* (HAP) if it arises in a patient who is already in the hospital. When HAP develops in a patient who has been on mechanical ventilation for at least 48 hours, it is termed *ventilator-associated pneumonia* (VAP). The distinction between CAP and HAP is becoming increasingly blurred because of the complexity of patients who reside out of the hospital. When pneumonia develops in patients who come from a nursing home, in those receiving chronic hemodialysis, and in those admitted to the hospital in the past 3 months, it is termed *health care–associated pneumonia* (HCAP). Because of their contact with the health care environment, these patients may already be colonized with multidrug-resistant organisms when they arrive at the hospital. Thus, the relationship between bacteriology and the place of origin of infection is a reflection of several factors, including the comorbid illnesses present in the patient, their host-defense status, and their environmental exposure to specific pathogens.

Patients who develop pneumonia while receiving immunosuppressive therapy or who have an abnormal immune system are referred to as *compromised hosts*, and the infectious possibilities vary with the localization of the immune defect. In recent years, particularly with the application of immunosuppressive therapy for a variety of illnesses, with the emergence of AIDS, and with an increasing number of institutionalized elderly individuals, TB, fungal, and parasitic lung infections have reemerged as important and common infections.

Pneumococcal Pneumonia

CAUSE

Streptococcus pneumoniae is the most common pathogen for community-acquired pneumonia (CAP) in all patient populations, including those without a cause recognized by routine diagnostic testing. The organism is a gram-positive, lancet-shaped diplococcus, of which there are 84 different serotypes, each with a distinct antigenic polysaccharide capsule. Eighty-five percent of all infections are caused by one of 23 serotypes, which are now included in a vaccine. Infection is most common in the winter and early spring, which may relate to the finding that up to 70% of patients have a preceding viral illness. Patients at risk include elderly individuals; people with asplenia, multiple myeloma, congestive heart failure, or alcoholism; after influenza; and patients with chronic lung disease. Individuals with HIV infection have pneumococcal pneumonia with bacteremia more commonly than those in healthy populations of the same age.

PATHOGENESIS AND PATHOLOGY

The organism spreads from person to person, and asymptomatic colonization of the oropharynx usually precedes the development of parenchymal lung invasion. Pneumonia develops when colonizing organisms are aspirated into a lung that is unable to contain the aspirated inoculum, often because of host defense impairment or because of acquisition of a particularly virulent strain, such as serotypes I and III. Virulence factors exist in the pneumococcus that facilitate its invasion in the lung; these include pneumococcal surface proteins A and C, which promote binding to airway epithelium and interfere with host defense against the bacteria, and pneumolysin, which can promote tissue invasion and interfere with ciliary beating.

The initial response to pneumococcal lung infection is extensive edema formation, which fills the lung and spreads the infection. At this phase, the lung looks grossly purple and is filled with frothy fluid when sectioned. In the next few hours, fibrin and neutrophils enter the alveolar space, and gradually over the next 24 to 48 hours, the bacteria move intracellularly as they are phagocytosed. The lung then becomes firmer and of a liverlike consistency, but with capillary congestion, and there are foci of hemorrhage that lead to a red color and a phase of "red hepatization." As the blood clears over the next 2 or more days, a phase of "gray hepatization" follows. Generally, the lung returns to its normal appearance in 5 to 10 days, but in some instances, fibroblasts enter the lobe, and organization and fibrosis may occur. In most patients, the inflammation initially extends to the pleura and leads to a parapneumonic effusion, but some patients may develop infection of the pleural space, or empyema.

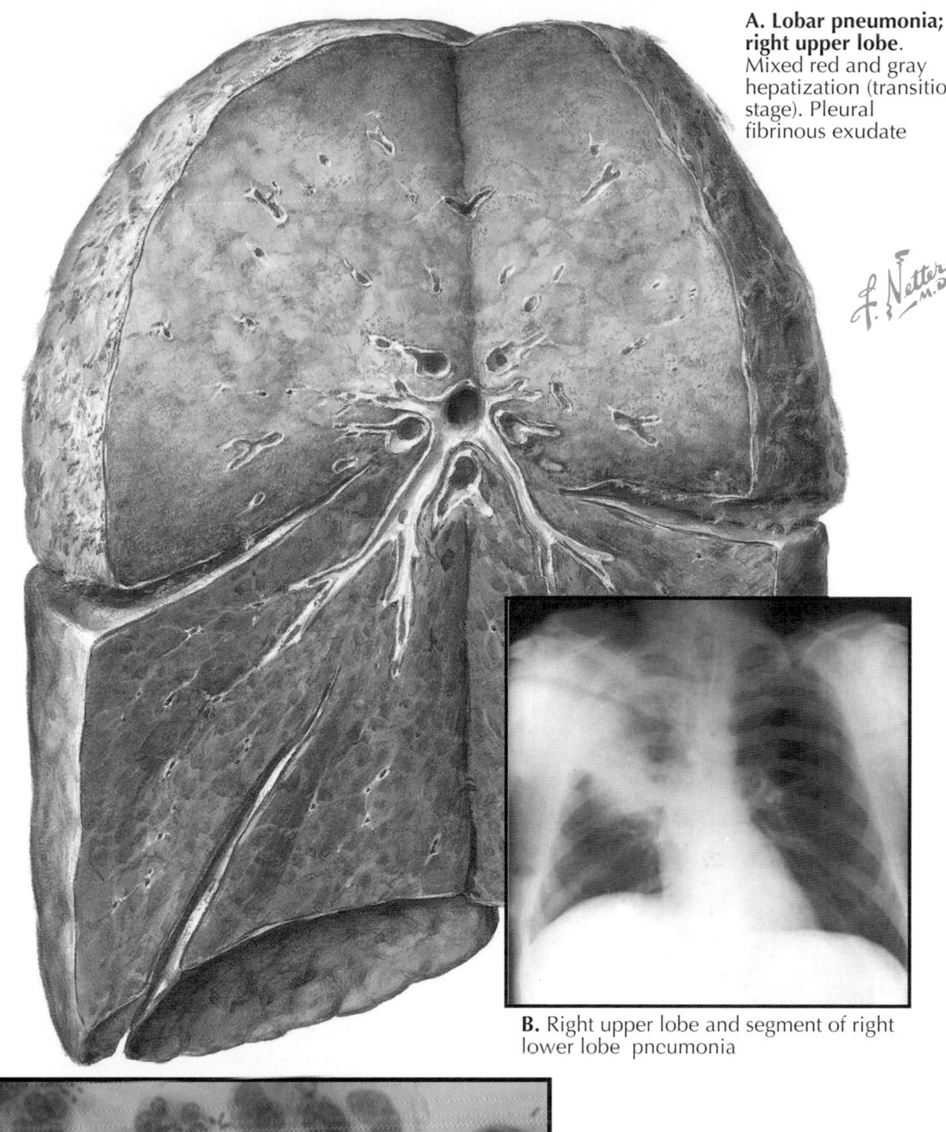

A. Lobar pneumonia; right upper lobe. Mixed red and gray hepatization (transition stage). Pleural fibrinous exudate

B. Right upper lobe and segment of right lower lobe pneumonia

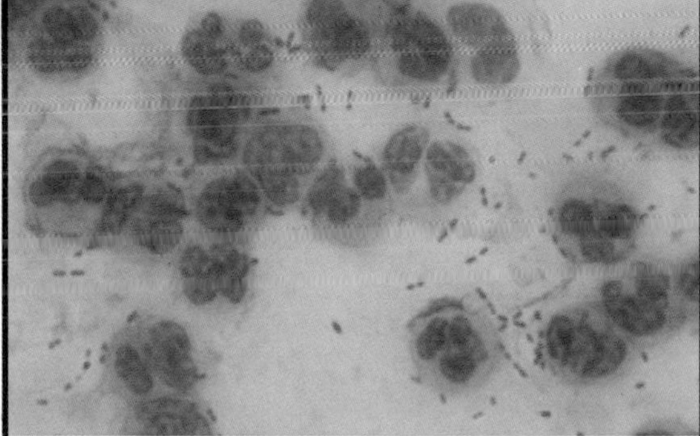

C. Purulent sputum with pneumococci (Gram stain)

CLINICAL FEATURES

A previously healthy individual who develops pneumococcal pneumonia has symptoms of "typical pneumonia" with a sudden onset of high fever, shaking chills, pleuritic chest pain, leukocytosis with a left shift, and purulent (or even blood-tinged, "rusty" colored) sputum. Elderly patients with immune impairment, often caused by the presence of comorbid illness, may not have these classic symptoms and may only have malaise, dyspnea, confusion, and failure to thrive.

The classic radiographic pattern is a lobar consolidation, but bronchopneumonia may also occur. Bacteremia is present in up to 20% of hospitalized patients with this infection, but its presence probably does not lead to increased mortality, although it may be associated with delayed clinical resolution. Extrapulmonary complications, which may lead to a failure to respond to therapy, include meningitis, empyema (which is distinguished from a complicated or uncomplicated parapneumonic effusion by sampling of pleural fluid), arthritis, endocarditis, and brain abscess. In the absence of any of these complications, patients usually show clinical improvement within 24 to 48 hours of the initiation of adequate antibiotic therapy.

The diagnosis of pneumococcal pneumonia can be confirmed by positive blood culture results, but other diagnostic tests include sputum for Gram stain and culture and urinary antigen testing. The value of sputum Gram stain for establishing the diagnosis and for guiding therapy is controversial because the test is not always sensitive or specific, many patients cannot produce a good specimen for evaluation, and the yield of Gram stain is reduced if the patient has been on antibiotic therapy before sampling. When a sputum culture is obtained, it should be interpreted in conjunction with the findings of the Gram stain. Urinary antigen testing for pneumococcus is also commercially available.

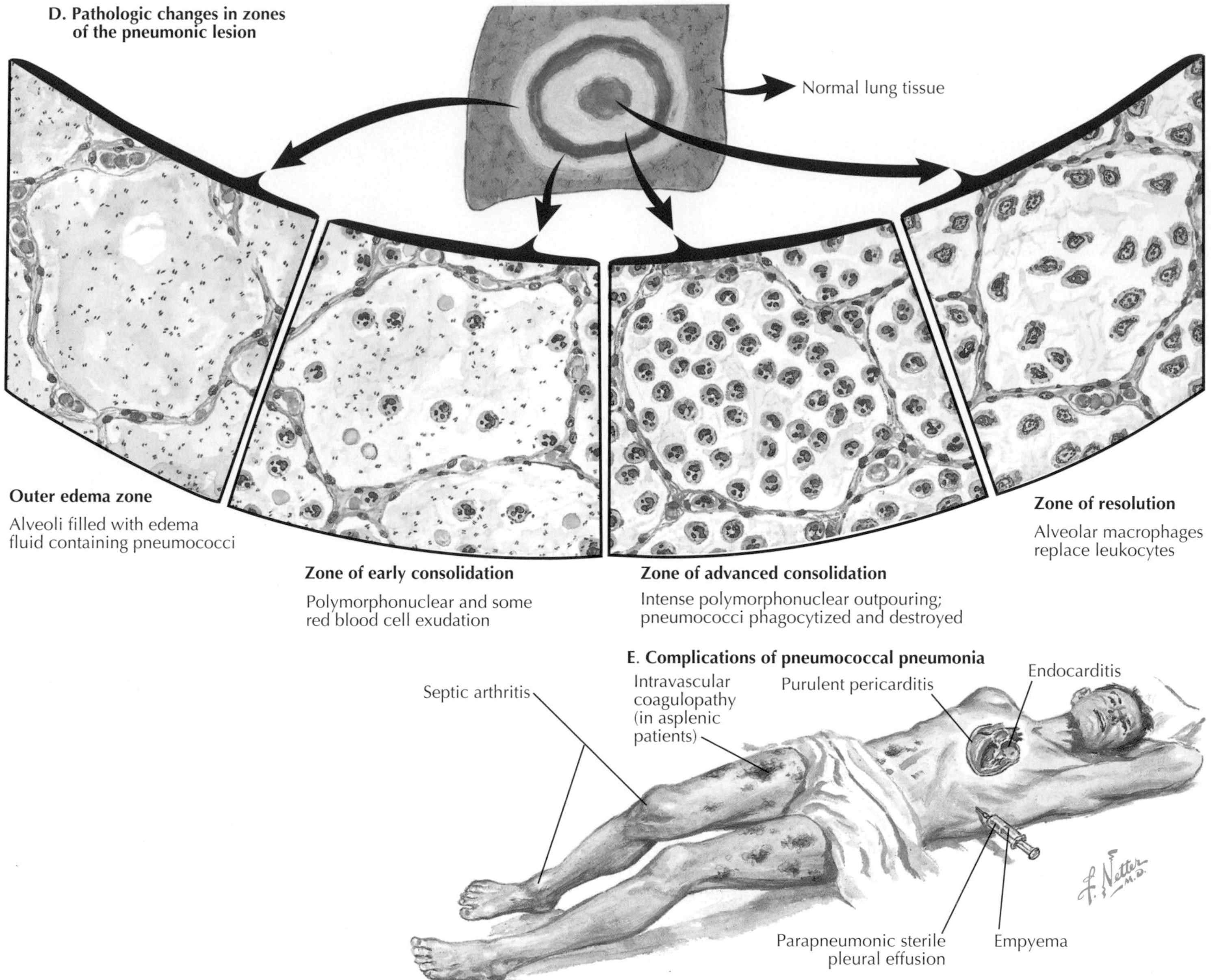

Pneumococcal Pneumonia
(Continued)

THERAPY

Current recommendations are to treat for a minimum of 5 days, provided that the patient is afebrile for 48 to 72 hours and other clinical signs of pneumonia have resolved. Pneumococcal bacteremia may delay the clinical response but does not by itself necessitate prolonged therapy. In recent years, some investigators have measured serum levels of procalcitonin, an acute phase reactant synthesized by the liver in response to bacterial infection, and used serial levels to guide the duration of therapy. Penicillin is the drug of choice, but penicillin resistance has become increasingly common since the mid-1990s, with some level of resistance seen in more than 40% of these organisms in the United States and Europe. Many of these organisms are also resistant to other common antibiotics (macrolides, trimethoprim-sulfamethoxazole, selected cephalosporins, and even the quinolones). The clinical impact of resistance on outcomes such as mortality is uncertain but may lead to an increased risk of death.

PREVENTION

Pneumococcal capsular polysaccharide vaccine may prevent pneumococcal pneumonia and is recommended for those at risk, including those older than age 65 years, those residing in a nursing home or institution, those with splenic dysfunction (splenectomy, sickle cell disease), anyone with a chronic medical illness (e.g., heart or lung disease, diabetes), and those who are immunosuppressed (corticosteroid therapy, chemotherapy). Adults should receive the 23-valent capsular polysaccharide vaccine (PPV), although children are given the 7-valent conjugate vaccine (PCV), which is more immunogenic.

The benefits of the PPV have been confirmed in immunocompetent patients older than age 65 years, and effectiveness has been estimated to be 75%, although it ranges from 65% to 84% in patients with chronic diseases, including diabetes mellitus, coronary artery disease, congestive heart failure, chronic pulmonary disease, and anatomic asplenia. Its effectiveness has not been as well established in immune-deficient populations such as those with sickle cell disease, chronic renal failure, immunoglobulin deficiency, Hodgkin disease, lymphoma, leukemia, and multiple myeloma. A single revaccination is recommended in patients 65 years old or older who initially received the vaccine more than 5 years earlier and were younger than 65 years of age when first vaccinated. If the initial vaccination was given at age 65 years or older, repeat is only indicated (after 5 years) if the patient has anatomic or functional asplenia or has one of the immune-compromising conditions listed above. Although the PCV is recommended for healthy children and has not yet been shown to be effective in adults, it has had benefit for adults who live with vaccinated children, demonstrating a "herd immunity" effect. Recently, some children who have received the 7-valent PCV have developed infection with strains not included in the vaccine, leading to a higher frequency of severe necrotizing pneumonia, especially with serotype 3.

Atypical Pathogen Pneumonia

ATYPICAL PATHOGENS

Originally, the term *atypical* was used to describe the nonclassic clinical features of infection with certain organisms, but today the term has been retained to refer to a group of organisms that includes *Mycoplasma pneumoniae*, *Chlamydophila pneumoniae*, and *Legionella* spp. These organisms cannot be reliably eradicated by β-lactam therapy (penicillins and cephalosporins) but must be treated with a macrolide, tetracycline, or quinolone. The frequency of these organisms as community-acquired pneumonia (CAP) pathogens has varied in studies, but they may be present in up to 60% of CAP episodes because they can serve as copathogens, along with bacteria, in up to 40% of patients. When mixed infection is present, particularly with *C. pneumoniae* and pneumococcus, it may lead to a more complex course than if a single pathogen is present. In patients with more severe forms of CAP, atypical pathogens can be present in almost 25% of all patients, but the responsible organism may vary over time. Although atypical pathogens have been thought to be most common in young and healthy individuals, some population data have shown that they are present in patients of all ages, including elderly people and those in nursing homes.

Studies reporting a high frequency of atypical pathogens have made the diagnosis with serologic testing, which may not be as accurate and specific as culture and antigen identification. The importance of atypical pathogens has also been suggested by a number of studies of inpatients, including those with bacteremic pneumococcal pneumonia, showing a mortality benefit from therapies that include a macrolide or quinolone, agents that would be active against these organisms.

MYCOPLASMA PNEUMONIA

M. pneumoniae is an organism that closely resembles a bacterium, lacks a cell wall, and is surrounded by a three-layered membrane (see Plate 4-67).

Most of the respiratory infections caused by *M. pneumoniae* are minor and in the form of upper respiratory tract illness or bronchitis. Although pneumonia occurs in only 3% to 10% of all *Mycoplasma* infections, this organism is still a common cause of pneumonia, with a slight increase in frequency in the fall and winter. All age groups are affected, and although it is common in those younger than 20 years of age, it is also seen in older adults.

Respiratory infection occurs after the organism is inhaled and then binds via neuraminic acid receptors to the airway epithelium. An inflammatory response with neutrophils, lymphocytes, and macrophages then follows accompanied by the formation of IgM and then IgG antibody. Some of the observed pneumonitis may be mediated by the host response to the organism rather than by direct tissue injury by the organism. Up to 40% of infected individuals have circulating immune complexes.

When pneumonia is present, it is usually characterized by a dry cough, fever, chills, headache, and malaise after a 2- to 3-week incubation period. Chest radiographs show interstitial infiltrates, which are usually unilateral and in the lower lobe but can be bilateral and multilobar, although the patient usually does not appear as ill as suggested by the radiographic picture. Rarely, patients have a severe illness with respiratory failure or a necrotizing pneumonia, but most cases resolve in 7 to 10 days in an uncomplicated fashion. Many patients also have extrapulmonary manifestations such as upper respiratory tract symptoms (present in up to 50% of all affected), including sore throat and earache (with hemorrhagic or bullous myringitis). Pleural effusion is seen in at least 20% of patients, although it may be small. Other manifestations include neurologic illness such as meningoencephalitis, meningitis, transverse myelitis, and cranial nerve palsies. The most common extrapulmonary finding is an IgM autoantibody that is directed against the I antigen on the red blood cell and causes cold agglutination of the erythrocyte. Although up to 75% of patients may have this antibody and a positive Coombs test result, clinically significant autoimmune

Mycoplasmal Pneumonia

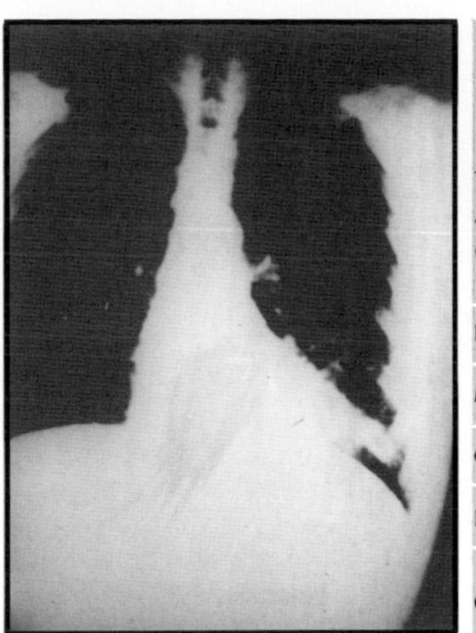

Posteroanterior chest radiograph: patchy perihilar infiltrates chiefly in left lung

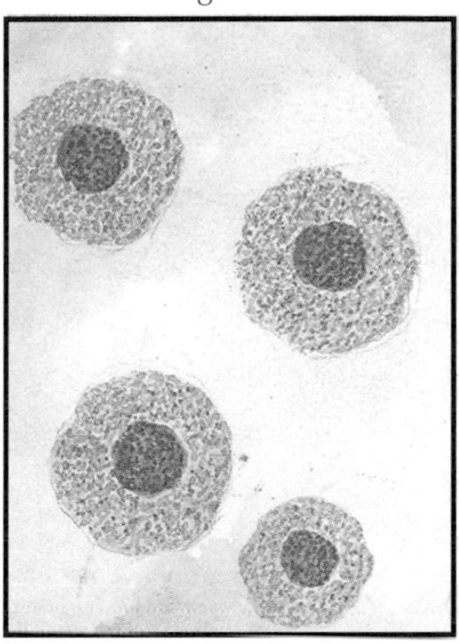

Colonies of *Mycoplasma* spp. growing on agar and stained, showing typical "fried egg" appearance due to penetration of agar by the growth in central area of each colony

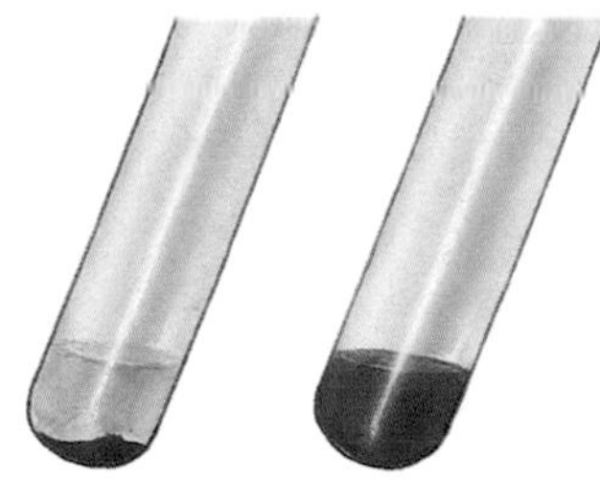

Cold agglutinin test

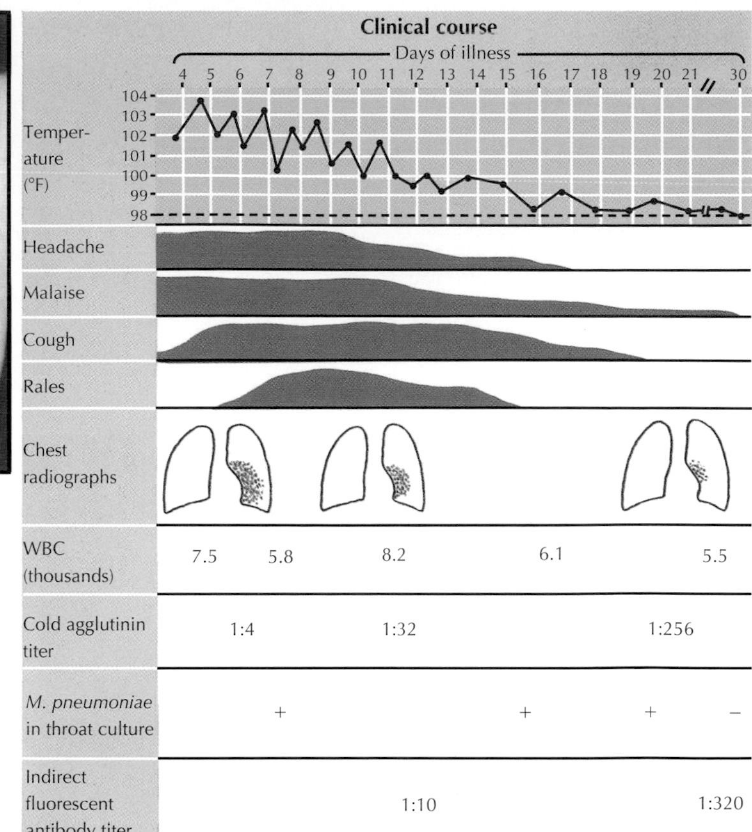

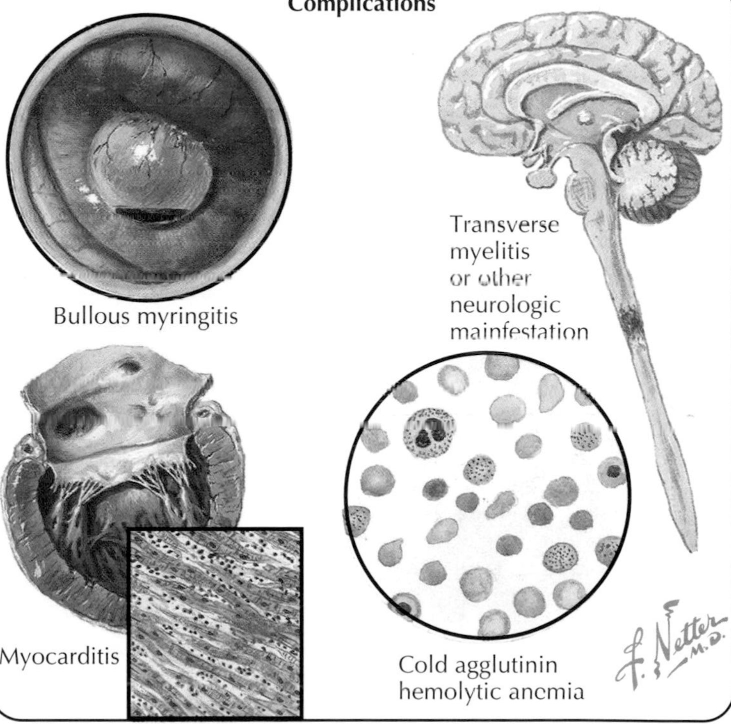

ATYPICAL PATHOGEN PNEUMONIA *(Continued)*

hemolytic anemia is uncommon. Other systemic complications include myocarditis, pericarditis, hepatitis, gastroenteritis, erythema multiforme, arthralgias, pancreatitis, generalized lymphadenopathy, and glomerulonephritis. The extrapulmonary manifestations may follow the respiratory symptoms by as long as 3 weeks.

Diagnosis is suspected by finding a compatible clinical picture and radiograph in a host with pneumonia and possibly extrapulmonary findings. Confirmation can be made by isolating the organism in culture from respiratory tract secretions. Serologic diagnosis is made by documenting a fourfold increase in specific antibody to *M. pneumoniae* by complement fixation test, although a single titer of 1:64 is suggestive of infection. The diagnosis is also suggested by a cold agglutinin titer of 1:64. Testing for IgM antibody has also been used to define infection, and with this methodology, some investigators have found that *M. pneumoniae* can be a copathogen along with bacterial agents in patients with CAP. After the diagnosis has been made, therapy is given for 10 to 14 days with a macrolide, quinolone, or tetracycline, which can reduce the duration and severity of the illness. Radiographic resolution is generally rapid, similar to *Chlamydophila* spp., and more rapid than with *Legionella* spp. or pneumococcal pneumonia.

CHLAMYDOPHILA INFECTIONS

As already mentioned, *C. pneumoniae* can be found in patients of all ages with CAP, as either a primary or coinfecting pathogen and is relatively common (see Plate 4-68). *Chlamydophila* species can also cause a less common form of pneumonia, termed psittacosis, when a patient is infected by *Chlamydophila psittaci*, an agent transmitted by inhaling infected excrement from avian species; the infectious bird does not need to be ill to transmit disease.

Patients with psittacosis commonly have headache, high fever, splenomegaly and dry cough, all of insidious onset after a 1- to 2-week incubation period. A macular rash similar to that of typhoid fever may also be seen along with relative bradycardia. Other extrapulmonary findings may occur, including hepatitis, encephalitis, hemolytic anemia, and renal failure. Diagnosis is on the basis of a compatible contact history and can be confirmed serologically. Treatment is with a tetracycline (2-3 g/d) for 14 to 21 days.

Although *C. pneumoniae* has been recognized as a common cause of CAP and may be a cause of sporadic pneumonia, it has also led to epidemics of respiratory infection, including pneumonia in patients residing in nursing homes. The disease has no specific features but is commonly seen with laryngitis and pharyngitis. Patients have fever, chills, pleuritic chest pain, headache, and cough and occasionally have respiratory failure. Therapy can be with tetracycline, the newer macrolides, or the fluoroquinolones, but the duration of therapy is uncertain. However, this form of pneumonia tends to resolve more rapidly than other forms of CAP unless it is part of a mixed infection with pneumococcus. More than 85% of patients have complete radiographic resolution by 6 weeks and 100% by 12 weeks.

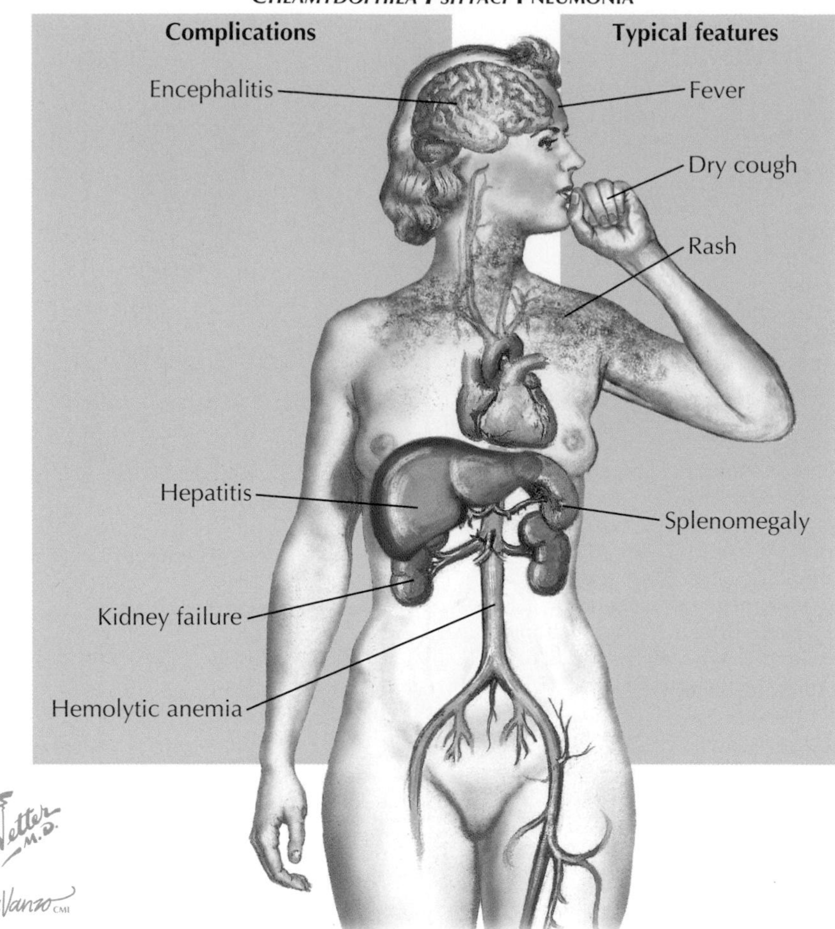

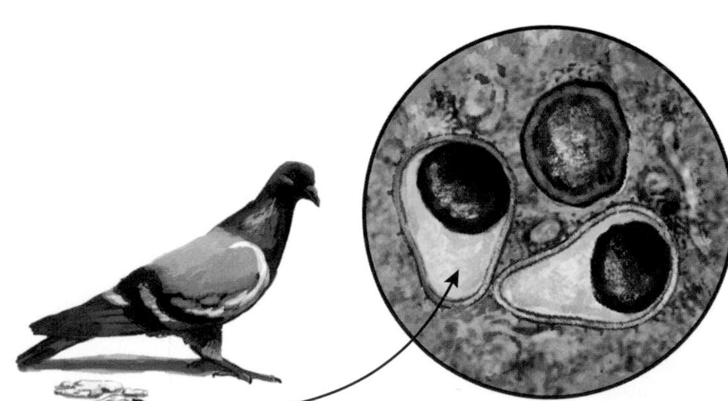

Electron micrograph showing *C. pneumoniae*

Chlamydophila psittaci

LEGIONELLA PNEUMOPHILA

This small, weakly staining, gram-negative bacillus was first characterized after an epidemic in Philadelphia in 1976, which infected primarily the attendees at an American Legion convention (see Plate 4-69). The pathogen is not really new, and after it was identified, evidence was obtained of infection involving this pathogen before 1976. Infection may occur either sporadically or in epidemic form, with the organism being transmitted via the aerosol route from an infected water source such as air conditioning equipment, drinking water, lakes and river banks, water faucets, saunas, and shower heads. Infection is more common in the summer and early fall. When a water system becomes infected in an institution, nosocomial outbreaks may

Atypical Pathogen Pneumonia *(Continued)*

occur, as has been the case in some nursing homes and hospitals.

After the organism enters the lungs, the incubation period is 2 to 10 days. Initially, the organism localizes intracellularly to the alveolar macrophage and multiplies, generating an inflammatory response that involves neutrophils, lymphocytes, and antibody. Because cell-mediated immunity is needed to contain infection, the disease may occur in compromised hosts, particularly hospitalized individuals who are receiving corticosteroids, and may relapse if not treated long enough.

At present, there are more than 46 species of *Legionella* and at least 68 serotypes, but serogroup 1 of *Legionella pneumophila* is the most commonly diagnosed, and it can be identified by a urinary antigen test. The other species that commonly causes human illness is *Legionella micdadei*. In its sporadic form, *Legionella* spp. may account for 7% to 15% of all cases of CAP, being a particular concern in patients with severe forms of illness.

The varying incidence of *Legionella* infection among admitted patients is a reflection of geographic and seasonal variability in infection rates, as well as the extent of diagnostic testing. For a serologic diagnosis, it is necessary to collect both acute and convalescent titers, and this can take at least 8 to 9 weeks. A diagnosis is made if the indirect fluorescent antibody titer increases fourfold to a level of at least 1:64 or if a single convalescent titer is above 1:128; however, the latter finding is not always specific for acute infection. The organism can be recovered in culture of infected secretions grown on charcoal yeast extract agar, but this requires patients to produce sputum, and the results are positive in 10% to 80% of patients. Direct fluorescent antibody staining for the organism in infected secretions is another method of diagnosis. Urinary antigen test is the single most accurate acute diagnostic test for *Legionella* spp. but is specific to serogroup 1 infection only. In recent years, most cases have been diagnosed with urinary antigen, and with reliance on urinary antigen testing the case fatality rate of *Legionella* has fallen, possibly reflecting diagnosis of less severe illness than in the past. In the future, real-time polymerase chain reaction testing on respiratory secretions may become available.

Patients with *Legionella* pneumonia commonly have high fever, chills, headache, myalgias, and leukocytosis. Features that can suggest the diagnosis are the presence of pneumonia with preceding diarrhea and mental confusion, hyponatremia, relative bradycardia, and liver function abnormalities, but this classic *Legionella* syndrome is not usually present. Symptoms are rapidly progressive, and the patient may appear to be quite toxic. The patient may have purulent sputum, pleuritic chest pain, and dyspnea, but the sputum Gram stain generally shows inflammatory cells but no identifiable organisms. The chest radiograph is not specific and may show bronchopneumonia, unilateral or bilateral disease, lobar consolidation, or rounded densities with cavitation. Up to 15% have pleural effusion, but empyema is uncommon. Proteinuria is common, and some patients have developed glomerulonephritis and acute tubular necrosis. Myocarditis and cerebellar dysfunction have been reported as rare complications of *Legionella* pneumonia.

When the diagnosis is suspected, therapy should be with either a macrolide or quinolone, with recent reports showing excellent results with the use of levofloxacin or moxifloxacin. Macrolide therapy has generally been given for 14 to 21 days; quinolones have shown efficacy with shorter durations of therapy. With effective therapy, the decline in fever may be slow, and high spikes in temperature may continue for 1 week after starting appropriate therapy. Radiographic resolution is much slower than for other forms of atypical pathogen pneumonia and nonbacteremic pneumococcal pneumonia. The mortality rate is less than 5% in normal hosts but may be as high as 25% in compromised hosts.

Legionella Pneumonia

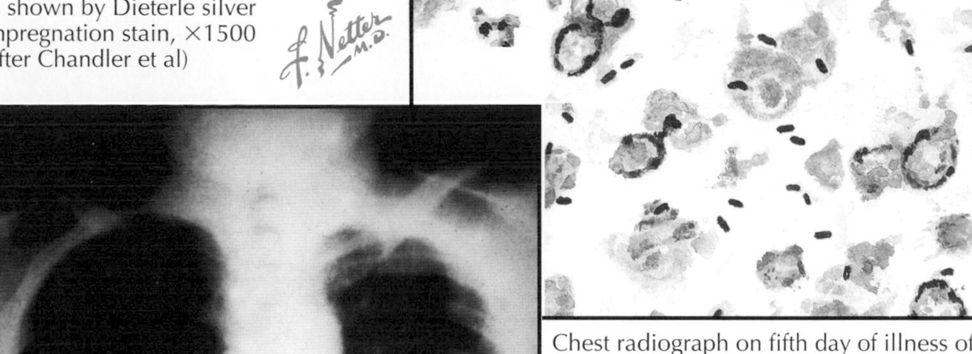

Small, blunt, pleomorphic intracellular and extracellular bacilli in lung of patient with Legionnaires disease as shown by Dieterle silver impregnation stain, ×1500 (after Chandler et al)

Chest radiograph on fifth day of illness of 58-year-old man with serologically confirmed Legionnaires disease. Left lower lobe consolidation the only involvement. Clinical improvement within 2 to 3 days of initiation of treatment with erythromycin. Radiologic changes did not completely disappear for 2 months

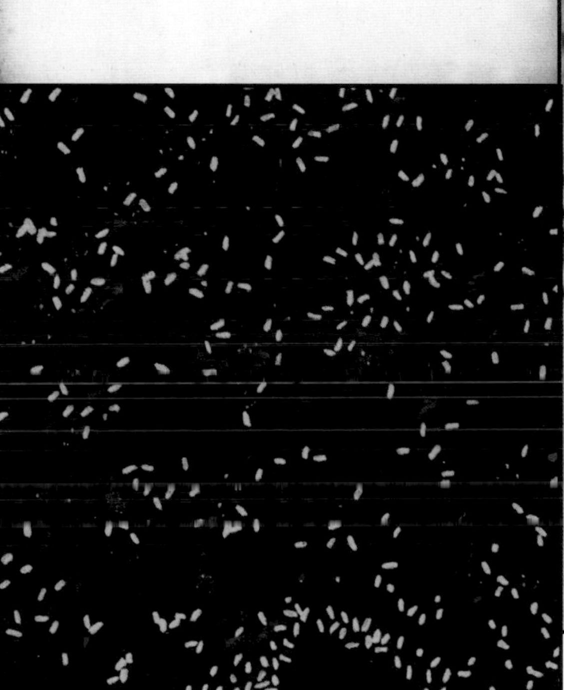

Legionella spp. identified by specific fluorescent antibody stain

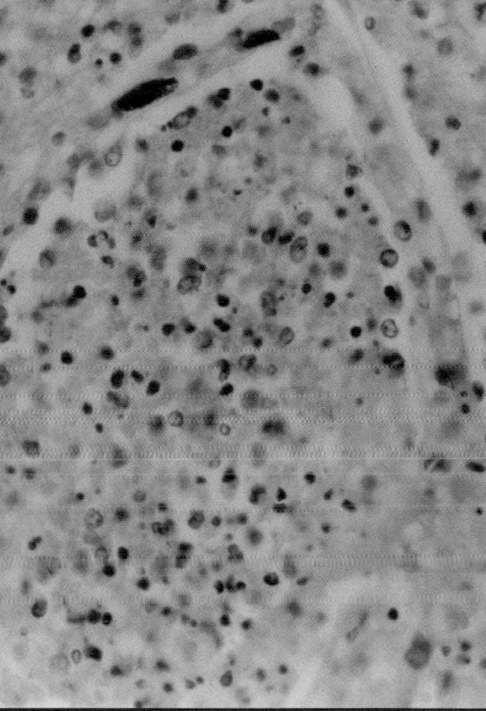

Histologic section of lung (H & E stain) from fatal case of Legionnaires disease. Extensive intraalveolar exudate present containing many large macrophages

STAPHYLOCOCCUS AUREUS PNEUMONIA

Staphylococcus aureus is a necrotizing gram-positive coccus that often appears in a grapelike cluster when stained in tissues and secretions. It can lead to infection at a variety of sites in the body, including the lung, and can be responsible for all forms of pneumonia, including community-acquired pneumonia (CAP), health care–associated pneumonia (HCAP), and nosocomial pneumonia. Although the organism can lead to a deep-seated lung infection, it can also spread hematogenously from the lung to multiple sites throughout the body. Lung involvement may not only be the result of a primary pneumonia but can also be secondary to bacteremia from a variety of sites, including the skin and from right-sided endocarditis. The virulence of this organism is promoted by its ability to acquire from other organisms exogenous genetic material (insertion sequences, transposons, and bacteriophages) that are responsible for tissue invasion and the acquisition of antibiotic resistance. CAP can be caused by antibiotic-sensitive organisms or by methicillin-resistant S. *aureus* (MRSA), the latter being seen in both the community as well as in hospital-acquired infections.

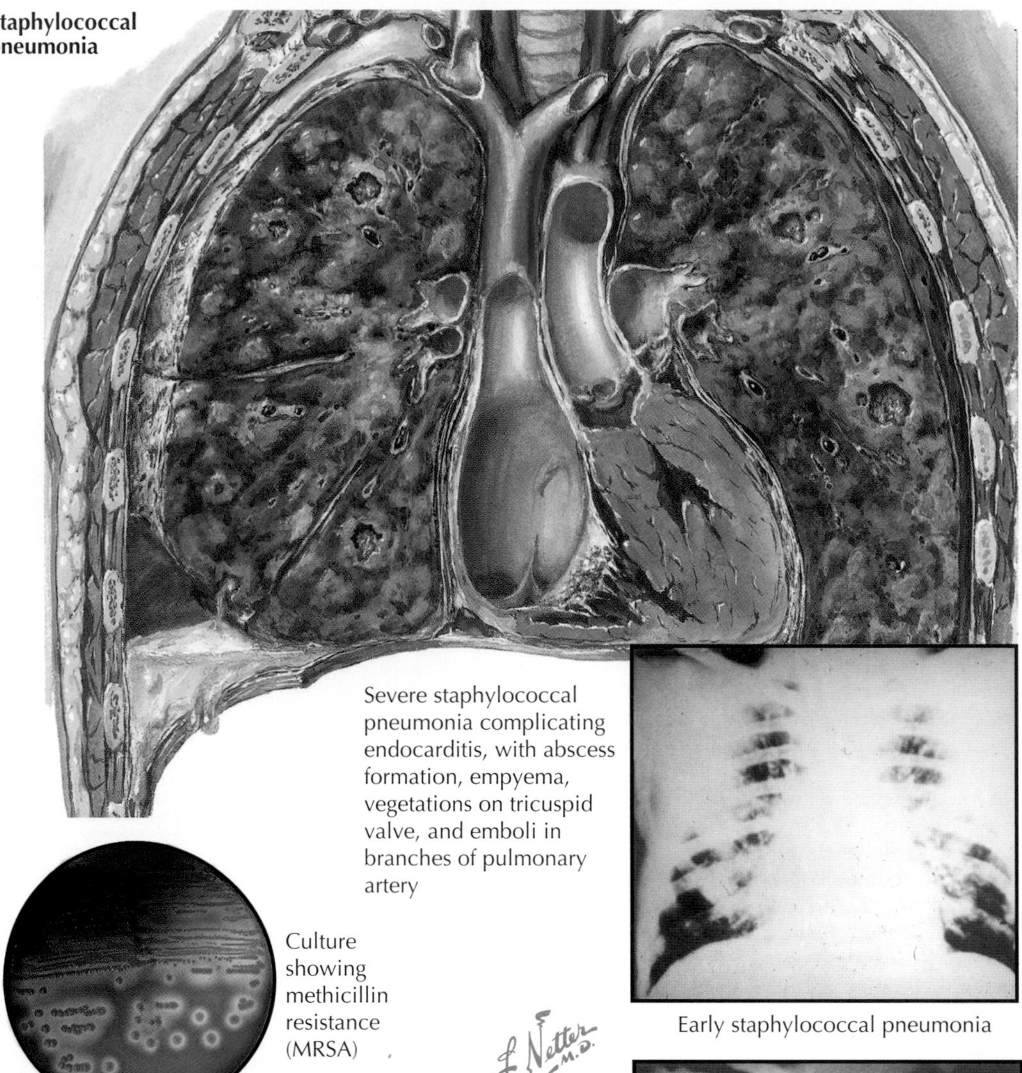

Severe staphylococcal pneumonia complicating endocarditis, with abscess formation, empyema, vegetations on tricuspid valve, and emboli in branches of pulmonary artery

Culture showing methicillin resistance (MRSA)

Early staphylococcal pneumonia

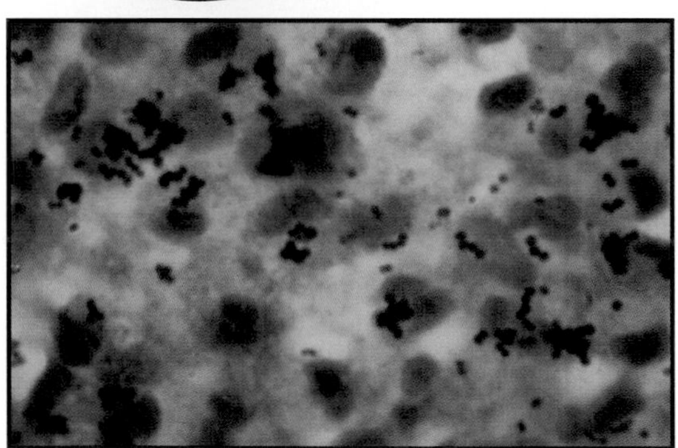

Staphylococci and polymorphonuclear leukocytes in sputum (Gram stain)

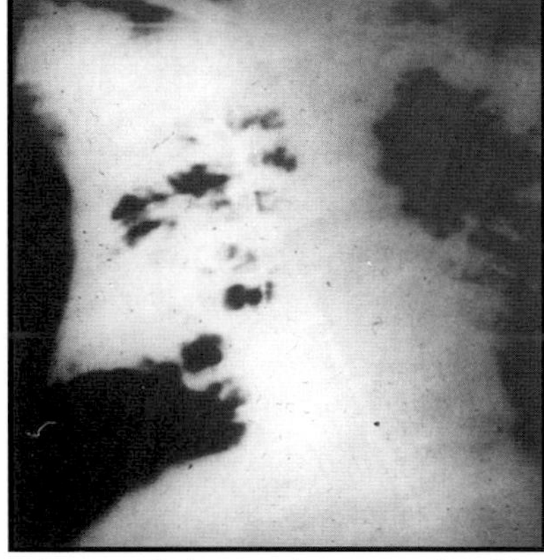

Late staphylococcal pneumonia with abscesses and pneumothorax

EPIDEMIOLOGY

S. aureus is generally not a common cause of CAP but has traditionally been seen in elderly individuals, in those with chronic lung disease (cystic fibrosis and bronchiectasis), and as a cause of bacterial pneumonia complicating influenza. In the past several years, community-acquired strains of methicillin-resistant *S. aureus* (CA-MRSA) have emerged, primarily in skin and soft tissue infections but also as a cause of severe CAP. The frequency of CAP caused by CA-MRSA is still relatively low, but it does occur sporadically, with certain geographic areas having a high frequency, especially during influenza season. CA-MRSA is a clonal disease, emanating from the USA 300 clone of *S. aureus*, and is clinically and bacteriologically different from the strains of MRSA that cause nosocomial pneumonia. CA-MRSA can infect previously healthy individuals, usually as a complication of preceding viral infection, although nosocomial MRSA tends to infect chronically ill and debilitated individuals. CA-MRSA is often a necrotizing infection that may be mediated by a variety of staphylococcal toxins, including the Panton-Valentine leukocidin toxin.

CLINICAL FEATURES

Hematogenous seeding of the lung, leading to staphylococcal pneumonia, can occur in drug addicts with right-sided endocarditis or from septic venous thrombophlebitis (from central venous catheter or jugular vein infection). In patients with primary pulmonary infection, the disease tends to be severe and is often bilateral, multilobar, rapidly progressive, and necrotizing. Patients present with a sudden onset of fever, tachypnea, and cough with purulent sputum, and the condition can progress rapidly to septic shock and respiratory failure. The radiograph may show pleural effusion, cavitary infiltrates, lung abscess, or pneumatoceles (a late sequela of infection). Empyema is a common complication, but extrapulmonary complications include endocarditis and meningitis.

TREATMENT

Therapy for antibiotic-sensitive organisms is with an antistaphylococcal penicillin (e.g., oxacillin or nafcillin) or a first-generation cephalosporin. For MRSA, vancomycin may be used, but linezolid may be a more effective agent because it penetrates better to respiratory sites of infection. Therapy should be continued for 4 to 6 weeks in complicated infections, such as those complicated by bacteremia or distant seeding to extrapulmonary sites. Reinfection can occur, and the mortality rate may exceed 30%. Because the pathogenesis of CA-MRSA pneumonia may be related to bacterial toxin production, therapy may need to involve both an antibacterial agent and an antitoxin-producing agent (e.g., linezolid alone or the combination of vancomycin and clindamycin).

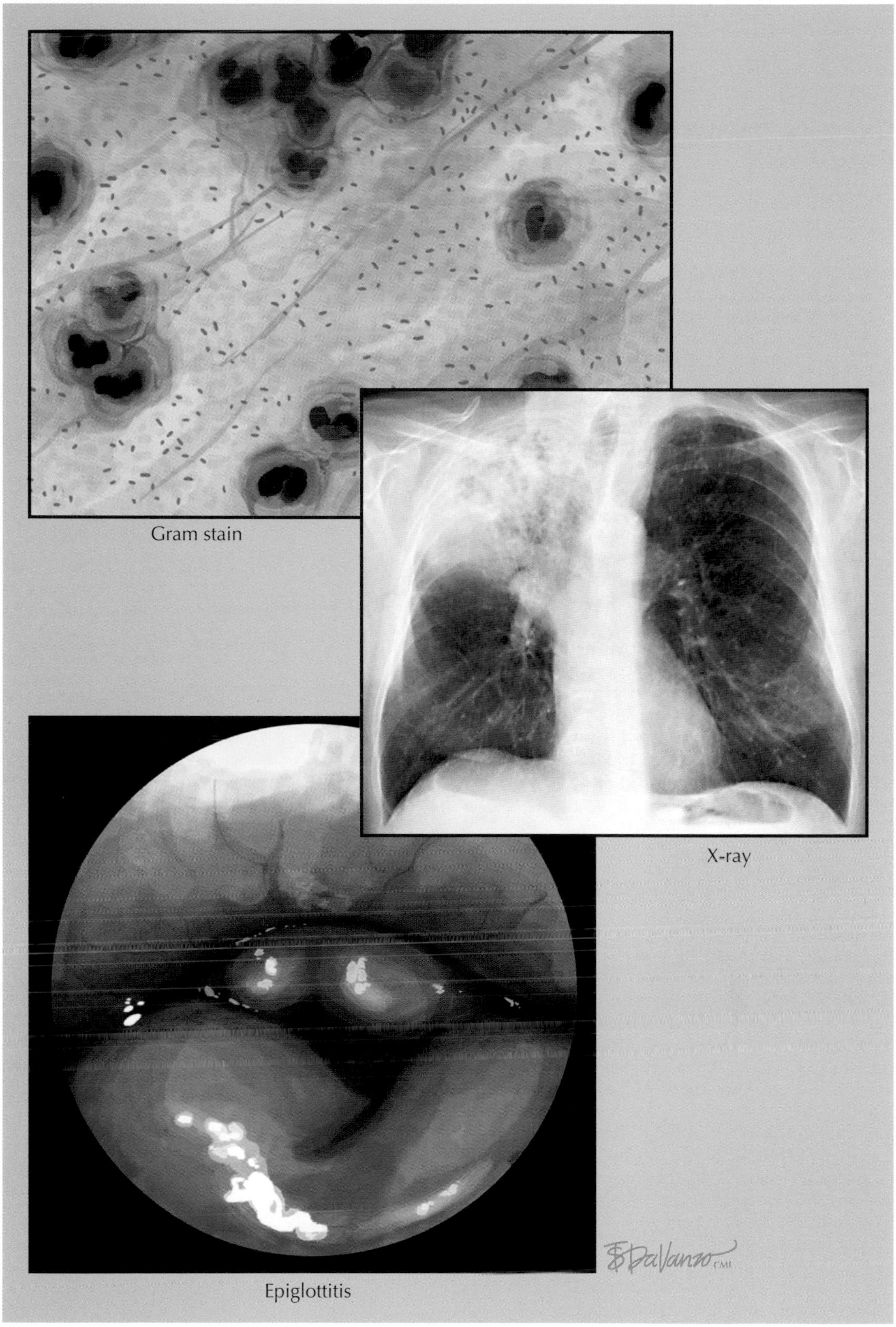

Haemophilus Influenzae Pneumonia

This gram-negative coccobacillary rod can occur in either a typeable, encapsulated form or a nontypeable, unencapsulated form, and either can cause pneumonia. The nontypeable organisms are also a common cause of bronchitis and a frequent colonizer in patients with chronic obstructive pulmonary disease (COPD). The encapsulated organism can be one of seven types, but type B accounts for 95% of all invasive infections. Opsonizing IgG antibody (directed at the capsular polysaccharide PRP and at membrane antigens) is required to phagocytose the encapsulated organisms, and because encapsulated organisms require a more elaborate host response than unencapsulated organisms, they are generally more virulent. However several studies have shown that in adults, particularly those with COPD, infection with unencapsulated bacteria is more common than infection with encapsulated organisms, and that opsonizing antibody is needed to control unencapsulated bacteria as well. Patients who develop pneumonia with these bacteria usually have some impairment in host defense, which may include both humoral immunity and local phagocytic dysfunction, but this organism may occur in patients whose only risk is cigarette smoking.

When pneumonia is present, some patients may develop bacteremia, particularly those with segmental pneumonias rather than those with bronchopneumonia. It has been estimated that 15% of cases are segmental but that up to 70% of these patients have bacteremia, although only 25% of bronchopneumonia cases are bacteremic. The encapsulated type B organism is more common in patients with segmental pneumonia than in those with bronchopneumonia. In patients with COPD, bronchopneumonia is more common than segmental pneumonia.

Patients with segmental pneumonia present with a sudden onset of fever and pleuritic chest pain along with a sore throat. Those with bronchopneumonia have a slightly lower fever, tachypnea, and constitutional symptoms. Multilobar, patchy bronchopneumonia is the most common radiographic pattern, and pleural reaction is also common, being seen in more than 50% of patients with segmental pneumonia and in approximately 20% with bronchopneumonia. Complications may include empyema, lung abscess, meningitis, arthritis, pericarditis, epiglottitis, and otitis media (particularly in children).

Therapy had traditionally been with ampicillin, but now up to 40% of nontypeable *Haemophilus influenzae* isolates and up to 50% of type B organisms are resistant because of bacterial production of β-lactamase enzymes. Currently, effective antibiotics are the third-generation cephalosporins, β-lactam/β-lactamase inhibitor combinations, newer macrolides (azithromycin is more active than clarithromycin), and fluoroquinolones. A conjugate vaccine against type B organisms is available but is not used in adults at risk for pneumonia but rather in children beginning at 2 months of age to prevent invasive infection such as meningitis.

Gram stain

X-ray

Epiglottitis

GRAM-NEGATIVE BACTERIAL PNEUMONIA

Enteric gram-negative bacteria (GNB) are an uncommon cause of CAP but have been reported in up to 10% of patients, particularly those with severe community-acquired pneumonia (CAP) admitted to the intensive care unit. The enteric GNB that have been reported to cause CAP are *Klebsiella pneumoniae*, *Pseudomonas aeruginosa*, *Enterobacter* spp., *Escherichia coli*, *Serratia marcescens*, and *Acinetobacter* spp. (which have been particularly prevalent in Asia and in war veterans from the Persian Gulf region). With the separation of patients with health care–acquired pneumonia (HCAP) from those with CAP, the frequency of GNB CAP may be quite low because many of the risk factors for these organisms place the patient in the HCAP category. Identified risks for GNB in CAP include pulmonary comorbidity (particularly severe chronic obstructive pulmonary disease, those treated with corticosteroids, and patients with bronchiectasis), probable aspiration, prior hospitalization, and prior antibiotics. These last two risk factors often are present in patients with HCAP. Patients who reside in nursing homes may also be commonly infected with these organisms, but these patients would be classified as having HCAP. Patients with GNB CAP have a higher mortality rate than patients with other forms of CAP. These organisms are commonly associated with septic shock and hyponatremia, and patients may have underlying malignancy, cardiovascular disease, and a smoking history. As discussed below, GNB are a common cause of hospital-acquired pneumonia (HAP), particularly ventilator-associated pneumonia (VAP), where they account for the majority of patients with an established etiologic diagnosis. More details about *P. aeruginosa* are provided in the section on HAP.

Klebsiella pneumoniae is an encapsulated gram-negative rod that can also cause both CAP and HAP, as well as lung abscess. It usually is acquired by micro- or macroaspiration from a previously colonized oropharynx. The histologic picture is one of a peripheral zone of edema, with central consolidation. The organism differs from other CAP pathogens because it can often lead to necrotizing pneumonia with cavitary infiltrates and abscess formation. Known as Friedländer pneumonia, after the physician who first observed this illness, patients are predominantly male and usually middle-aged or older, with alcoholism being the most common coexisting condition.

Gram stain of sputum containing *Klebsiella pneumoniae* organisms

Consolidation of right upper lobe with sticky, mucinous exudate on cut surface and in bronchi, which forms characteristic "currant jelly" sputum. Beginning abscess formation. Fibrinopurulent pleuritis

Klebsiella colonies on Endo agar. Growth is slimy and translucent and strings out when drawn up on a loop

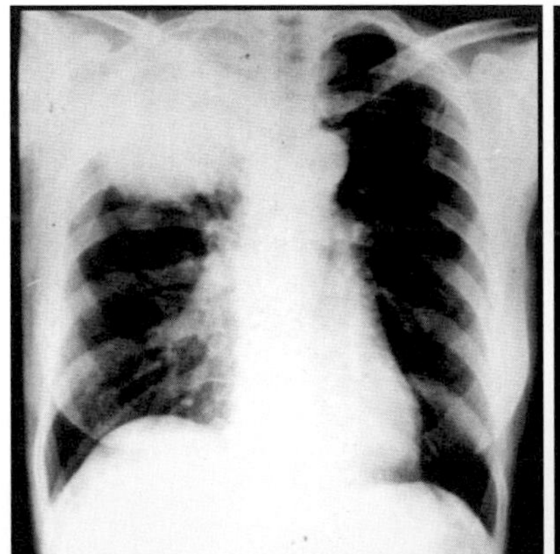
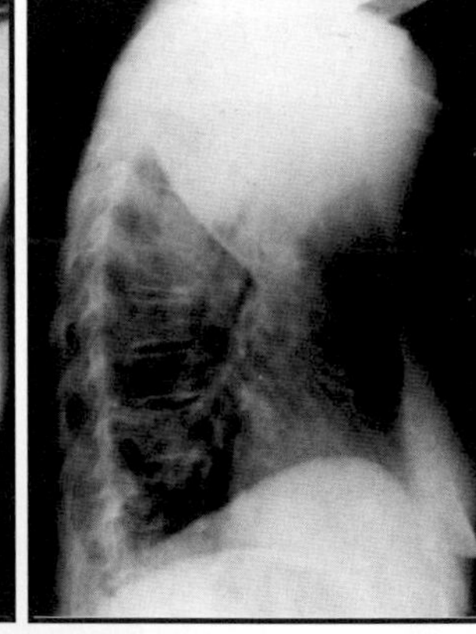

PA and lateral chest films; *Klebsiella pneumoniae*, right upper lobe

When CAP is caused by *K. pneumoniae*, the illness is usually of sudden onset, with productive cough, pleuritic chest pain, rigors, and cardiovascular collapse in a patient who has underlying chronic illness. The cough is usually associated with sputum that is often thick and purulent with blood (reflecting necrosis), or the sputum can be thin with a "currant jelly" appearance. On physical examination, the patient is usually toxic appearing, with high fever and tachycardia, and has findings of lobar consolidation. Although not common or specific, the classic radiographic finding is a bulging upper lobe fissure, usually on the right side, representing lobar consolidation with bulging downward because of the dense infiltrate. Lung abscess and bronchopneumonia may also occur as primary presentations, but lung abscess can complicate pneumonia, as can pericarditis, meningitis, and empyema. The lung abscess syndrome associated with *K. pneumoniae* differs from that seen with anaerobic bacteria. Compared with anaerobic lung abscess, the illness is more acute, sputum is not putrid smelling, multiple cavities are often present, and underlying diabetes is more common.

The diagnosis is made by finding gram-negative rods in a sputum Gram stain and culture in a patient with appropriate risk factors and clinical features. Therapy is usually for 10 to 14 days, depending on clinical response, often with two drugs that are active against the organism, to ensure efficacy and to avoid emerging resistance during therapy. Third-generation cephalosporins should not be used as monotherapy because they can select for the development of resistant organisms with inducible chromosomal β-lactamases. Effective antimicrobial agents include an aminoglycoside, an antipseudomonal penicillin or fourth–generation cephalosporin, aztreonam, a carbapenem, or sometimes a fluoroquinolone. In some hospitals, epidemics of nosocomial infection caused by carbapenemase-producing *K. pneumoniae* have been described; therapy of patients infected with these organisms is challenging and often unsuccessful.

Viral Community-Acquired Pneumonia

The frequency of viruses as a cause of community-acquired pneumonia (CAP) is difficult to estimate because very few patients have routine serologic testing (acute and convalescent titers), some viral pathogens do not have routinely available diagnostic tests, and viral cultures of respiratory tract secretions in the setting of pneumonia are not commonly collected or available. During the fall and early winter in North America, influenza should be considered in all patients with CAP, and it can lead to a primary viral pneumonia or to secondary bacterial pneumonia. One careful study of more than 300 non–immune-compromised CAP patients looked for viral pneumonia by paired serologies and found that 18% had a viral cause, with about half being pure viral infection and the others being mixed with bacterial pneumonia. Influenza (A more than B), parainfluenza, and adenovirus were the most commonly identified viral agents.

Although influenza A and B are the most common causes of viral pneumonia, they can be prevented to a large extent by vaccination. Other viruses also cause severe forms of pneumonia, as evidenced by the recent experience with severe acute respiratory syndrome (SARS), which demonstrated the potential of epidemic, person-to-person spread of a virulent respiratory viral infection. Continued concern about epidemic viral pneumonia remains with the current focus on avian influenza and bioterrorism with agents such as smallpox and Ebola.

ETIOLOGIC VIRAL PATHOGENS

Influenza

This RNA virus can be of either type A, B, or C with the disease from type A being generally more severe and serving as the most important respiratory virus on a global scale with the highest overall morbidity and mortality rates (see Plates 4-73 and 4-74). Influenza B can also cause severe disease, but influenza C is a mild disease that does not have a seasonal occurrence. Influenza A has two major surface glycoprotein antigens, the hemagglutinin (H, with 15 subtypes) and neuraminidase (N, with nine subtypes), which can change yearly (antigenic drift), making previous immunity at least partially ineffective, and thus the disease appears in epidemics annually. Infrequently, major antigenic changes in influenza A occur, and this antigenic shift exposes individuals to a new virus, against which they have no immunity. This has led to worldwide pandemics, with high attack rates and high mortality. Both antigenic drift and waning immunity make this infection a particular threat to those who have underlying chronic cardiac or respiratory illnesses, elderly individuals, people with HIV infection, and pregnant women. The virus has an incubation period of 2 to 4 days and is spread via aerosol or mucosal contact with infected secretions. The yearly epidemics occur in North America in the late fall and extend into the early spring and can be caused by one of three types of influenza—influenza A/H3N2, influenza A/H1N1, and influenza B. Influenza A can coexist with other viral infections, including respiratory syncytial virus (RSV) and parainfluenza virus, particularly in elderly people.

Varicella Zoster

This DNA virus leads to chickenpox, which is primarily a viral exanthema of children, but in adults, the virus can disseminate and lead to viral pneumonia, especially in pregnant women (see Plate 4-75). Adults with chickenpox are more prone to disseminated disease than are children. Most reports have shown that when varicella pneumonia complicates pregnancy, it is usually in the third trimester and that infection occurring at this time is more severe and complicated than if it occurs earlier. The incidence of pulmonary involvement in primary varicella infection in pregnancy ranges from 15% to 30%. When varicella occurs in pregnancy, it not only affects the mother but can also lead to a

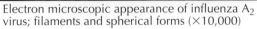

Influenza Virus and its Epidemiology

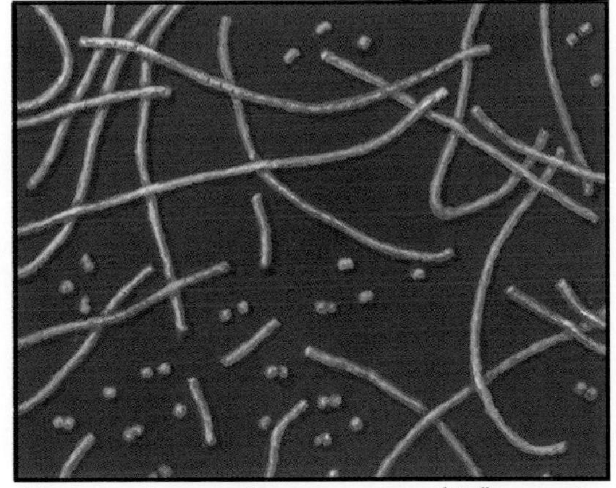

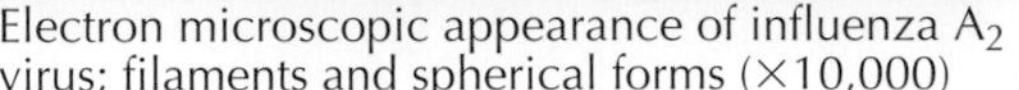

Electron microscopic appearance of influenza A_2 virus; filaments and spherical forms (×10,000)

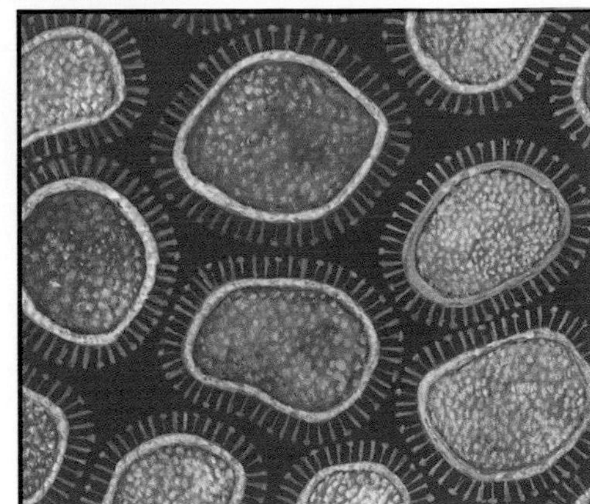

Virus viewed in section at much higher magnification (×300,000)

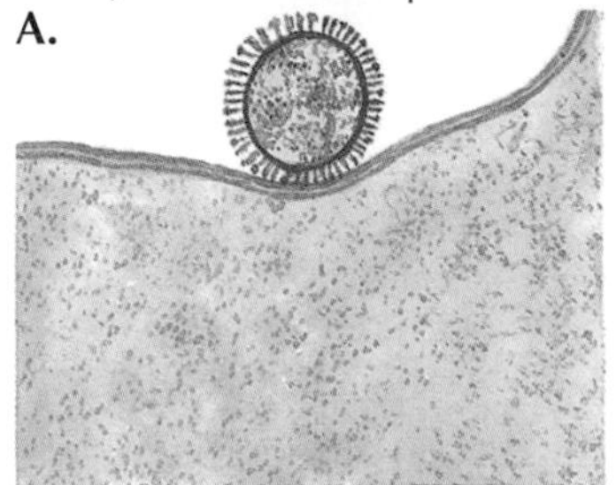

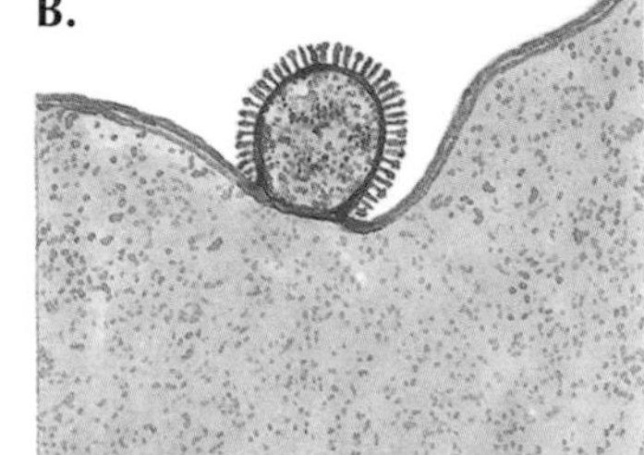

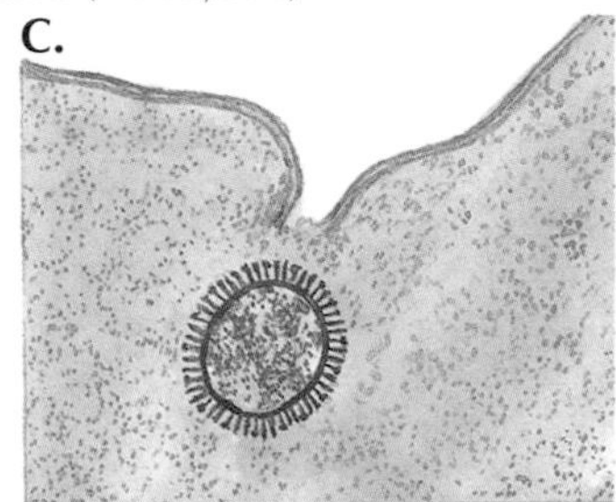

Influenza virus invasion of chorioallantoic membrane cell of chick embryo. **A.** Attachment to cell membrane. **B.** Fusion of viral envelope with cell membrane. **C.** Penetration into cell cytoplasm

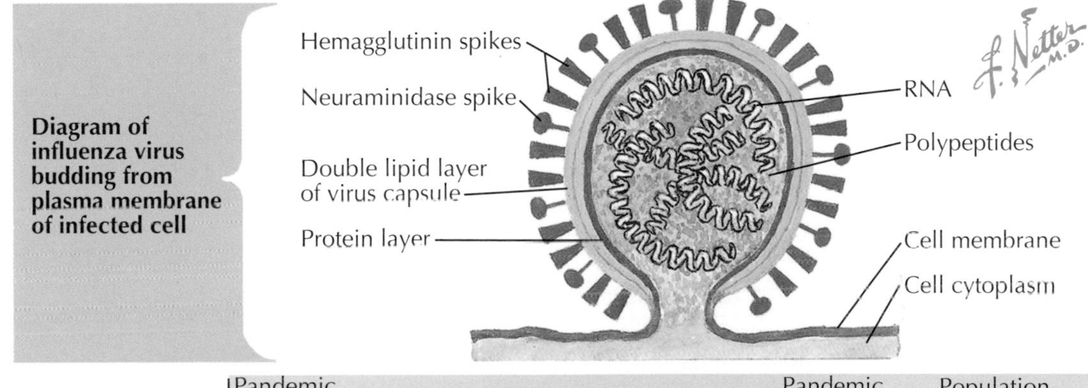

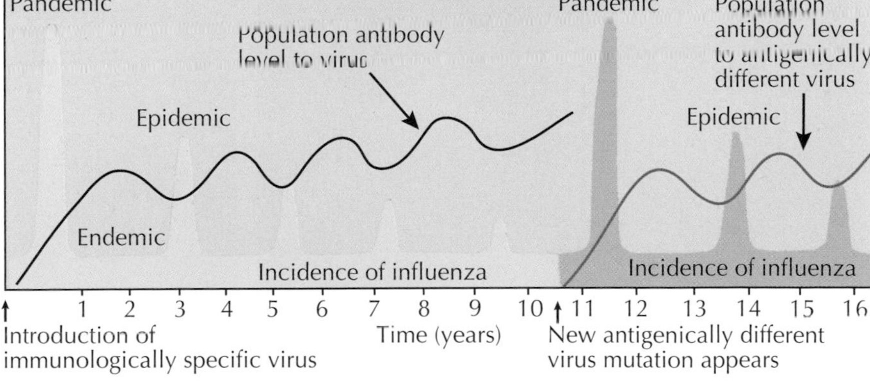

Relationship of influenza incidence to population antibody levels*

*Modified after Kilbourne

INFLUENZA PNEUMONIA

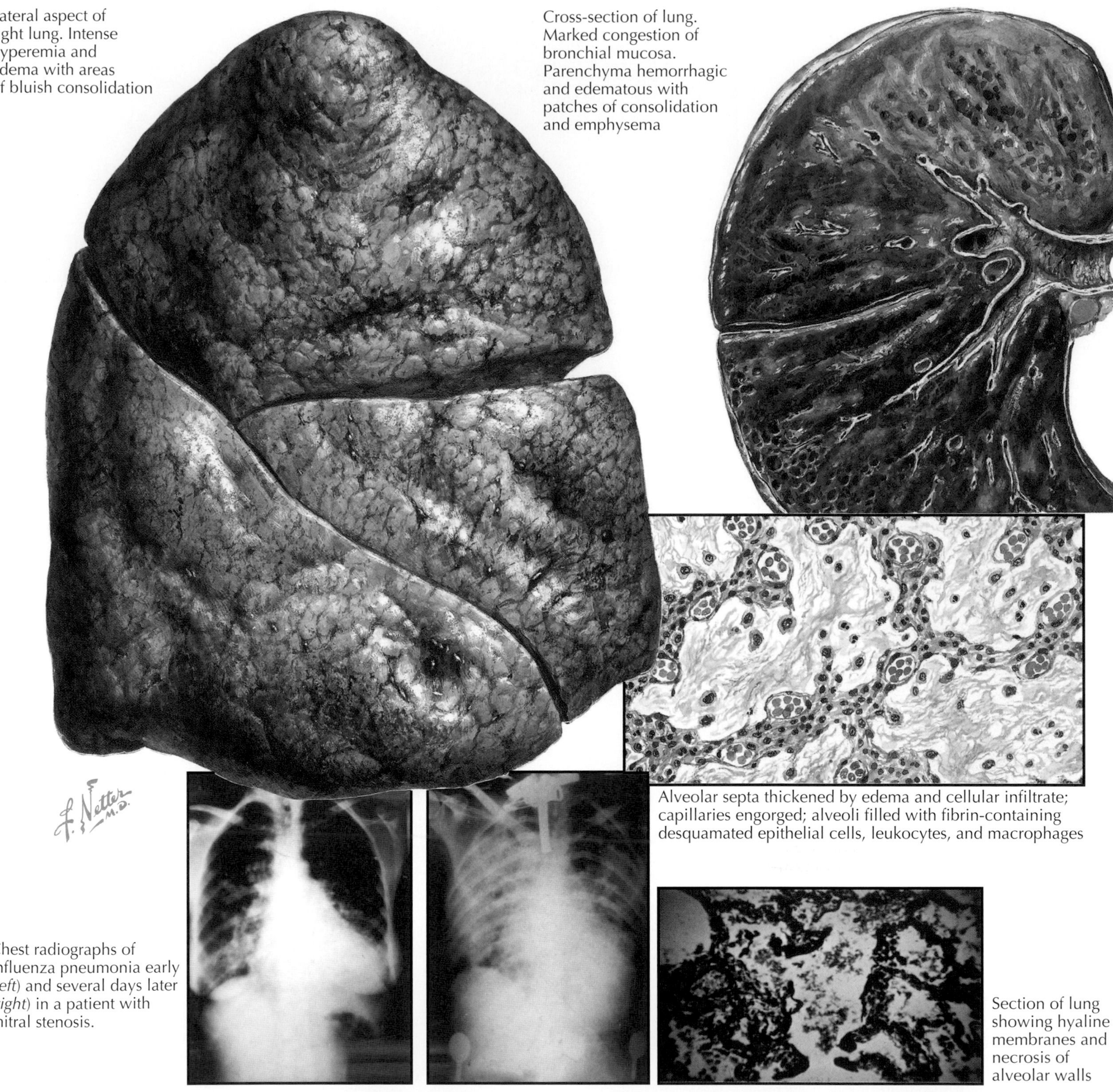

Lateral aspect of right lung. Intense hyperemia and edema with areas of bluish consolidation

Cross-section of lung. Marked congestion of bronchial mucosa. Parenchyma hemorrhagic and edematous with patches of consolidation and emphysema

Alveolar septa thickened by edema and cellular infiltrate; capillaries engorged; alveoli filled with fibrin-containing desquamated epithelial cells, leukocytes, and macrophages

Chest radiographs of influenza pneumonia early (*left*) and several days later (*right*) in a patient with mitral stenosis.

Section of lung showing hyaline membranes and necrosis of alveolar walls

VIRAL COMMUNITY-ACQUIRED PNEUMONIA *(Continued)*

congenital varicella syndrome characterized by limb hypoplasia, skin scarring, central nervous system involvement, and other skeletal lesions. This embryopathy has been reported with infection occurring as late as 26 weeks of gestation.

Cytomegalovirus

By serologic data, up to 60% of adults have been infected with cytomegalovirus (CMV), but it can be a cause of pneumonia in immunosuppressed patients, particularly those with HIV infection, when it reactivates from a latent form of infection (see Plate 4-76). In those with HIV infection, retinitis is the most common form of infection, but pneumonia can also occur.

Other Viral Pathogens

SARS can be a severe type of primary viral pneumonia caused by a coronavirus that often leads to respiratory failure (see Plate 4-77). Other common, important viral pathogens include RSV (bronchiolitis, especially in children), rhinovirus, adenovirus, and parainfluenza viruses (common cold). Unusual causes of viral pneumonia further include Hantavirus (inhalation of rodent excreta, acute respiratory distress syndrome [ARDS],

VIRAL COMMUNITY-ACQUIRED PNEUMONIA *(Continued)*

neutrophilia, thrombocytopenia, elevated hematocrit), measles, and herpes simplex (immunocompromised patients).

Pathogenesis

Viral lower respiratory infections usually involve the tracheobronchial tree or small airways, but primary pneumonia may also occur. The virus first localizes to the respiratory epithelial cells and causes destruction of the cilia and mucosal surface. The resulting loss of mucociliary function may then predispose the patient to a secondary bacterial pneumonia. If the infection reaches the alveoli, there may be hemorrhage, edema, and hyaline membrane formation, and the physiology of ARDS may follow. For example, the main site of infection for influenza virus is the respiratory mucosa, leading to desquamation of the respiratory mucosa with cellular degeneration, edema, and airway inflammation with mononuclear cells. When viral lower respiratory tract involvement only involves the airway, the chest radiograph is normal, but the radiograph can be abnormal if the patient has a primary viral pneumonia, a bacterial superinfection, or a combined viral and bacterial pneumonia.

The status of a patient's immune defenses can dictate the likely infecting viral pathogens. Immunocompromised patients with AIDS, malignancy, and major organ transplantation are often infected by CMV, varicella zoster, and herpes simplex virus. As mentioned with CMV, these patients are usually ill as a result of reactivation of latent infection that was obtained years earlier. Previously healthy adults can be infected with influenza A and B, parainfluenza, adenovirus, the SARS virus, and RSV. Influenza can also develop with a higher frequency and more severe consequences in debilitated and elderly adults. Immune naïve children are most affected by RSV and parainfluenza virus, which can cause both airway and parenchymal lung infections. Children and military recruits develop pneumonia with adenovirus and influenza.

CLINICAL MANIFESTATIONS

Influenza

Primary viral pneumonia caused by influenza may be a severe illness with diffuse infiltrates and extensive parenchymal injury along with severe hypoxemia. This pattern is often seen in those with underlying cardiopulmonary disease, immunosuppression, or pregnancy. However, many patients with primary viral pneumonia get only a mild "atypical" pneumonia with dry cough, fever, and a radiograph that is more severely affected than the patient.

Although up to half of influenza infections are subclinical, when the typical illness occurs, it lasts 3 days and is characterized by sudden onset of fever, chills, severe myalgia, malaise, and headache. As the major symptoms recede, respiratory symptoms dominate, with dry cough and substernal burning, which may persist for several weeks. When viral pneumonia develops, the disease follows the classic 3-day illness without a hiatus and is characterized by cough (dry or productive) and severe dyspnea. The chest radiograph reveals bilateral infiltrates, and mortality is high. Bacterial pneumonic superinfection follows the primary influenza illness with a hiatus of patient improvement for 3 to 4 days before the pneumonia begins. In this setting, pneumonia is usually lobar, and the most common pathogens are pneumococcus, *Haemophilus influenzae*, enteric gram-negative organisms, and *Staphylococcus aureus*. Other respiratory complications include obliterative bronchiolitis, croup, airway hyperreactivity, and exacerbation of chronic bronchitis. Nonrespiratory complications include myocarditis and pericarditis, Guillain–Barré syndrome, seizures, encephalitis, coma, transverse myelitis, toxic shock, and renal failure.

SARS

Clinically, SARS patients present after a 2- to 11-day incubation period with fever, rigors, chills, dry cough, dyspnea, malaise, headache, and frequently pneumonia and ARDS. Laboratory data show not only hypoxemia but also elevated liver function test results. During the

VARICELLA PNEUMONIA

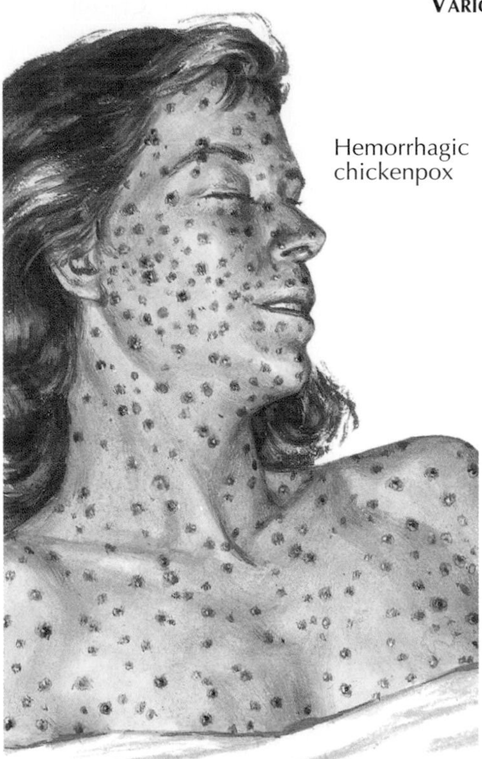

Hemorrhagic chickenpox

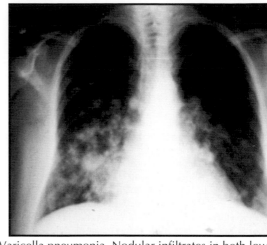

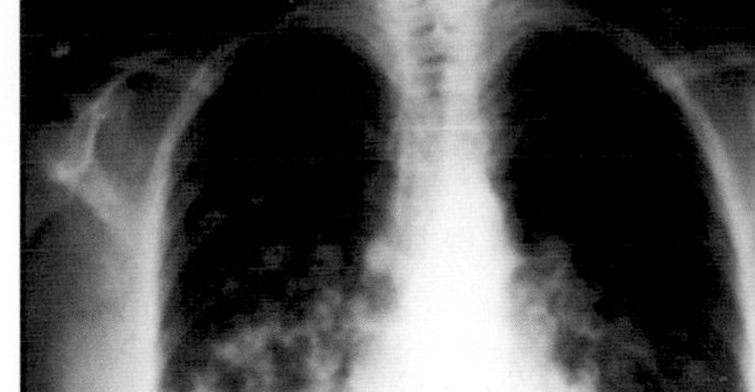

Varicella pneumonia. Nodular infiltrates in both lower lobes, more marked and coalescing on right side

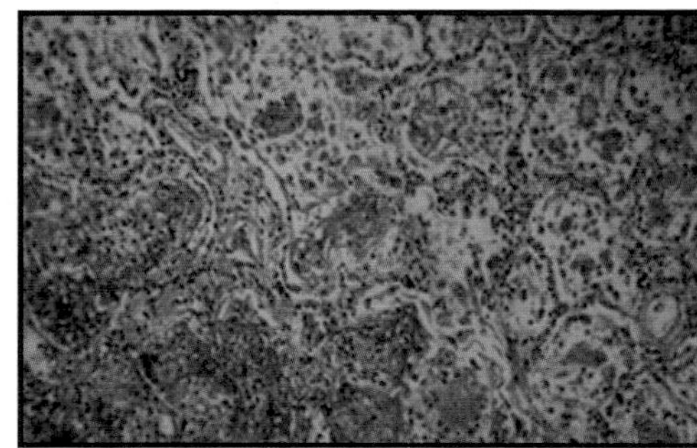

Pulmonary histology, low power. Alveoli filled with fibrin, fluid, and cellular exudate

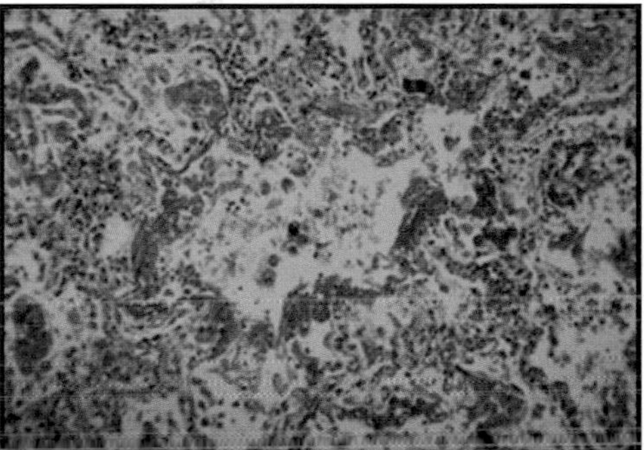

High power: Mononuclear infiltrate in interstitium and fibrin lining alveoli

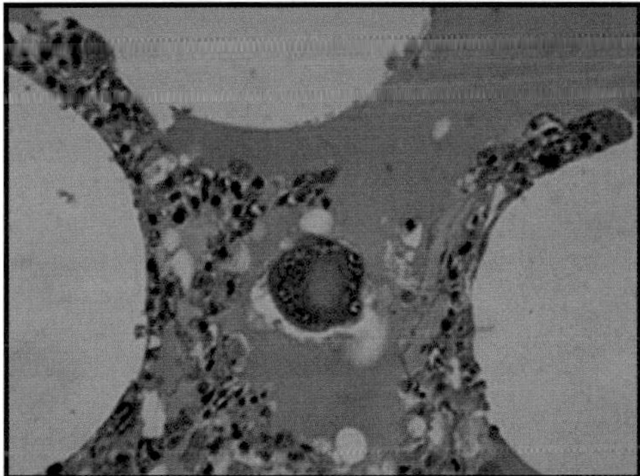

Multinucleated giant cell with much significant alveolar fluid

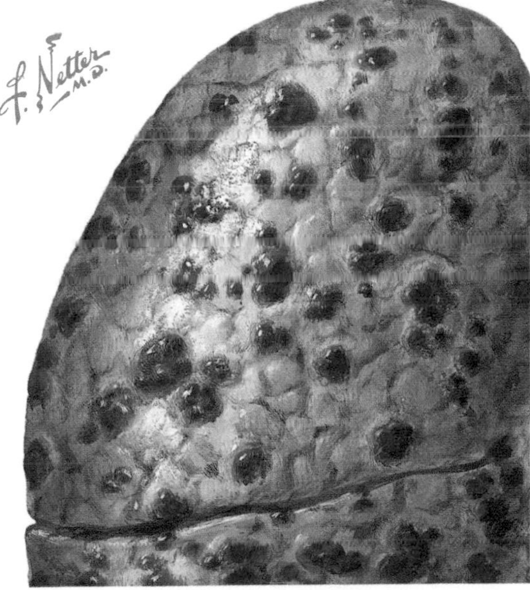

Pleural hemorrhagic pocks

VIRAL COMMUNITY-ACQUIRED PNEUMONIA *(Continued)*

initial epidemic, up to 20% of cases occurred in health care workers, particularly those exposed to aerosols generated by infected patients, as can occur during noninvasive ventilation and during the process of endotracheal intubation. Up to 15% to 20% of infected patients developed respiratory failure, with lung involvement typically starting on day 3 of the hospital stay, but respiratory failure often did not start until day 8. The mortality rate for intensive care unit–admitted SARS patients has been greater than 30%, and when patients died, it was generally from multiple system organ failure and sepsis. There is no specific therapy, but anecdotal reports have suggested a benefit to the use of pulse doses of steroids and ribavirin.

Varicella

Varicella can lead to pneumonia and has an incubation period between 14 and 18 days. Clinically, varicella pneumonia presents 2 to 5 days after the onset of fever, vesicular rash (chickenpox), and malaise and is heralded by the onset of pulmonary symptoms, including cough, dyspnea, pleuritic chest pain, and even hemoptysis. In one series, all patients with varicella pneumonia had oral mucosal ulcerations. The severity of illness may range from asymptomatic radiographic infiltrates to fulminant respiratory failure and acute lung injury (ALI). Typically, chest radiographs reveal interstitial, diffuse miliary or nodular infiltrates that resolve by 14 days unless complicated by ALI and respiratory failure. The severity of infiltrates has been described to peak with the height of the skin eruption. One late sequela of varicella pneumonia is diffuse pulmonary calcification.

Other

The major clinical distinctions between the many viral agents that can cause pneumonia are in the type of host who becomes infected (discussed above) and in the type of extrapulmonary manifestations that accompany the pneumonia. Extrapulmonary signs may suggest a specific viral agent. Rash may be seen with varicella zoster, CMV, measles, and enterovirus infections. Pharyngitis may accompany infection by adenovirus, influenza, and enterovirus. Hepatitis may be seen with CMV and infectious mononucleosis (Epstein-Barr virus). Retinitis is common with CMV, but the pneumonia is not distinctive, with patients having dyspnea, dry cough, and diffuse bilateral lung infiltrates with hypoxemia.

CYTOMEGALOVIRUS PNEUMONIA

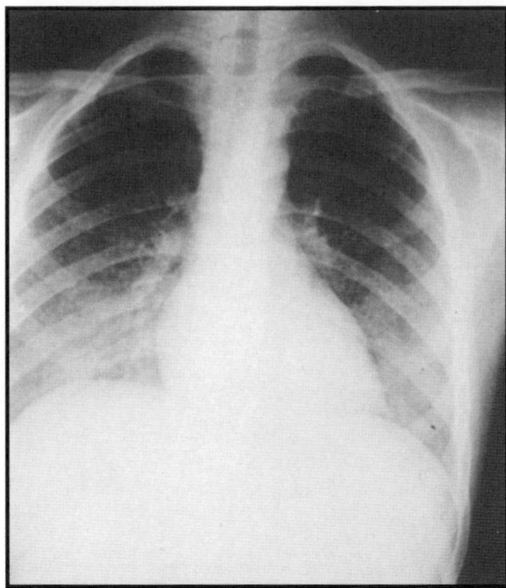

Diffuse densities in both lower lobes

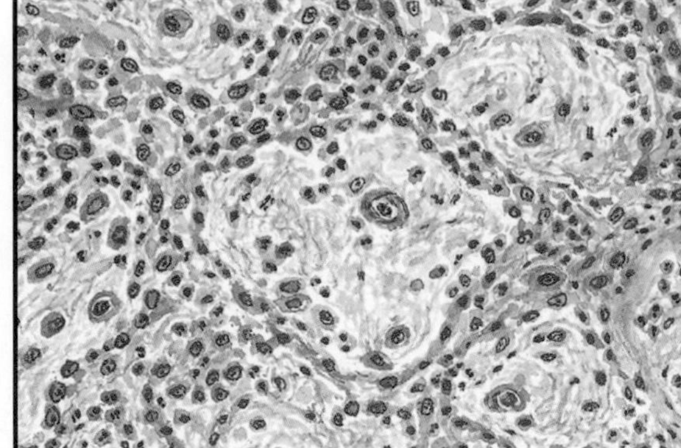

Lung histology in cytomegalovirus pneumonia; cellular and fibrinous exudate in alveoli and in interstitium plus inclusion-bearing cells and epithelial desquamation

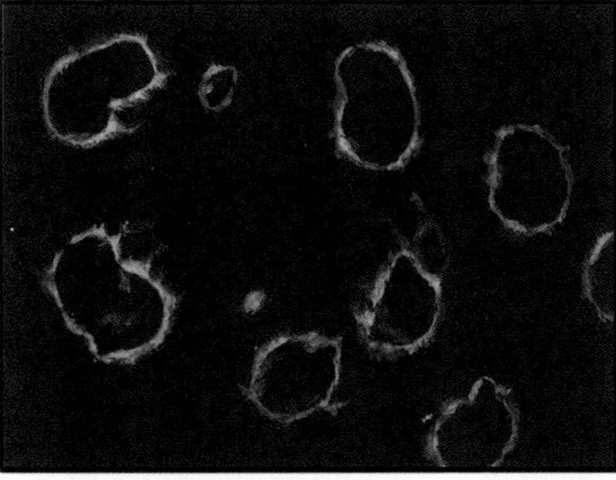

Cells infected with cytomegalovirus stained by immunofluorescent technique

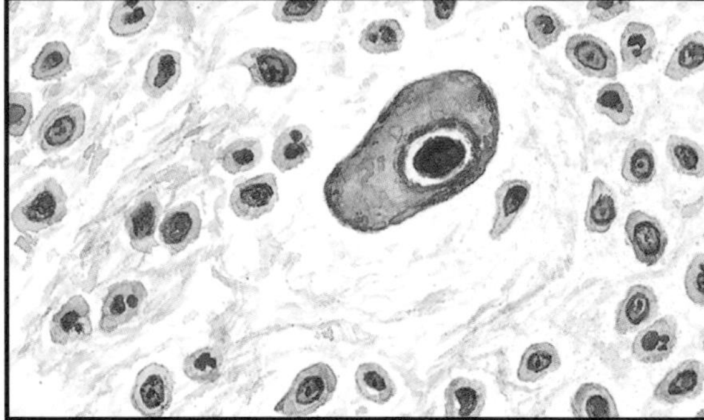

High-magnification view of cell with inclusion body and cytomegaly

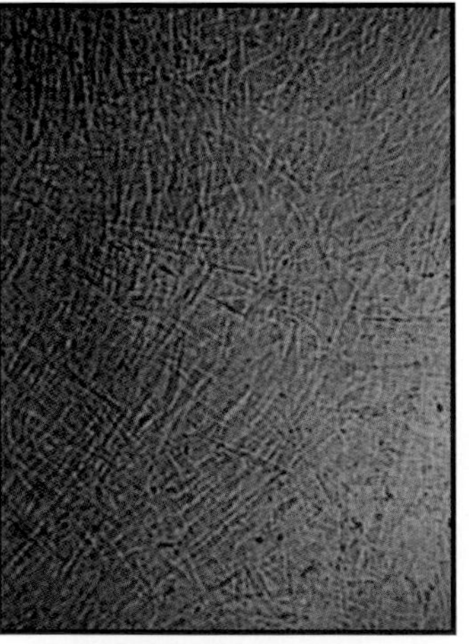

Normal tissue culture (HeLa) cells

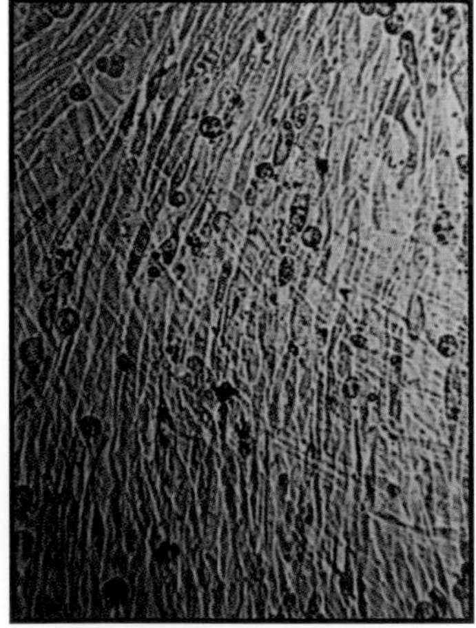

Tissue culture with early rounding of cells due to cytomegalovirus

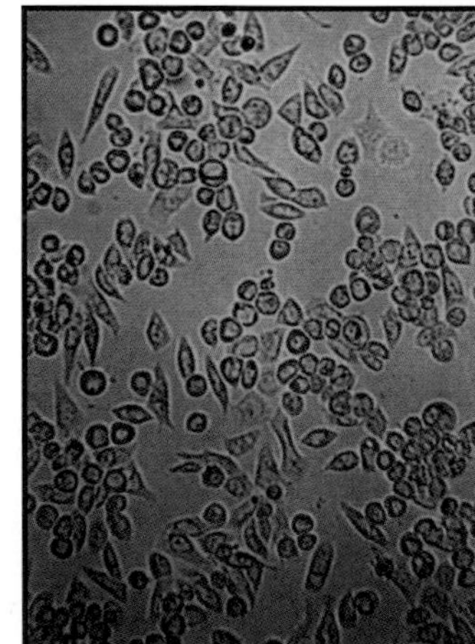

Tissue culture with late cytopathogenic effects due to cytomegalovirus

DIAGNOSIS

The diagnosis of viral illness can be clinical or can be confirmed by specific laboratory methods. Viruses can be isolated with special culture techniques if specimens are properly collected and prepared. Upper airway swabs, sputum, bronchial washes, rectal swabs, and tissue samples should be placed in viral transport media as early in the patient's illness as possible while viral shedding is still prominent. Bronchoscopy serves as the most important method to obtain respiratory tract samples from immune-compromised patients. These respiratory samples can be cultured on certain laboratory cell lines, and viral growth may be detected in 5 to 7 days. More recently, the shell vial culture method has allowed for identification of viruses within 1 to 2 days. In this method, a clinical specimen is centrifuged onto a tissue culture monolayer and then stained with virus-specific antibodies. Viral illness can also be rapidly diagnosed by using immunofluorescence or enzyme-linked immunosorbent assay (ELISA) to test patient samples for viral antigens. Immunofluorescent tests are available for influenza, parainfluenza, RSV, adenovirus, measles, rubella, coronavirus, and herpesvirus. ELISA assays are also available for most of these agents. Serology can be used retrospectively to diagnose a suspected viral infection, but this technique may be difficult if specific viruses are not suspected and sought directly. A new technique that may be valuable is the use of genetic probes to detect specific viral DNA or RNA. Such methodology is now available for CMV, varicella zoster virus, herpes simplex, and adenovirus.

Viral Community-Acquired Pneumonia *(Continued)*

THERAPY

With the current interest and understanding of viral infections, some specific therapy with antiviral agents has become available. Patients with pneumonia from herpes simplex and varicella zoster viruses can be treated with acyclovir. Influenza A can be treated or prevented by the use of amantadine 200 mg/d orally or rimantadine, which acts against the M2 protein of influenza A, or the newer neuraminidase inhibitors oseltamivir and zanamivir (which are also active against influenza B). Amantadine dosing must be reduced with renal insufficiency, and confusion may occur in 3% to 7% of treated individuals. Rimantadine, a derivative of amantadine, is also effective for the therapy of patients with influenza A infection; it can be given once daily because of its long half-life, and it has fewer central nervous system and other side effects than amantadine. The neuraminidase inhibitors can be used during acute infection and reduce the duration of symptoms if given within 36 to 48 hours. Ribavirin aerosol has been used to treat patients with RSV, SARS, and influenza B. Patients with CMV infection have been successfully treated by the acyclovir analog DHPG (ganciclovir), valganciclovir, or foscarnet.

All patients with varicella pneumonia require aggressive therapy with antiviral agents (acyclovir), and multiple investigators have used acyclovir, a DNA polymerase inhibitor, even in pregnant patients, demonstrating its safety in pregnancy and its lack of teratogenicity. Treatment is recommended for 7 days. Some small series have suggested a benefit from adjunctive corticosteroid therapy at modest doses. During pregnancy, women who are exposed to varicella can receive prophylactic varicella immune globulin, which may attenuate the fetal embryopathy if administered within 96 hours of exposure.

Severe Acute Respiratory Syndrome (SARS)

Patient characteristics

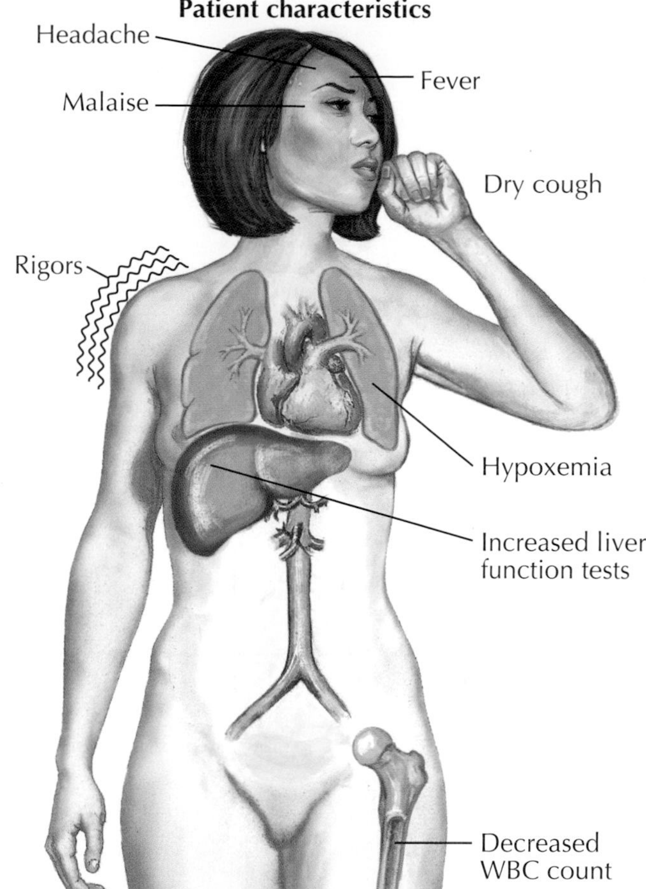

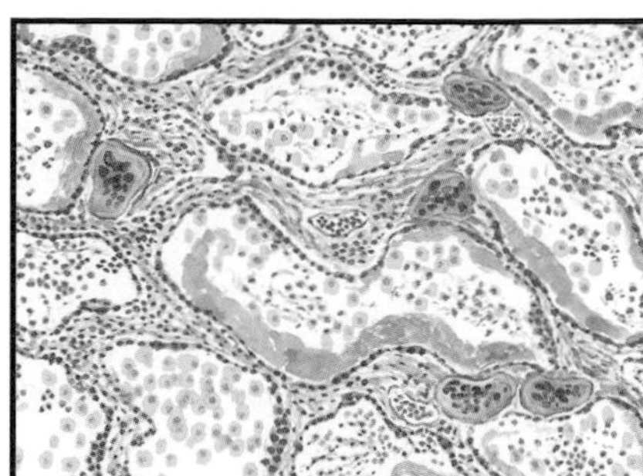

Diffuse alveolar damage, foamy macrophages, and multinucleated syncytial cells

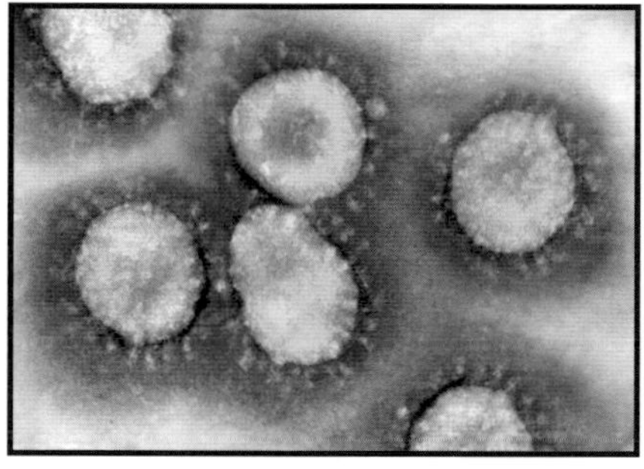

Coronavirus

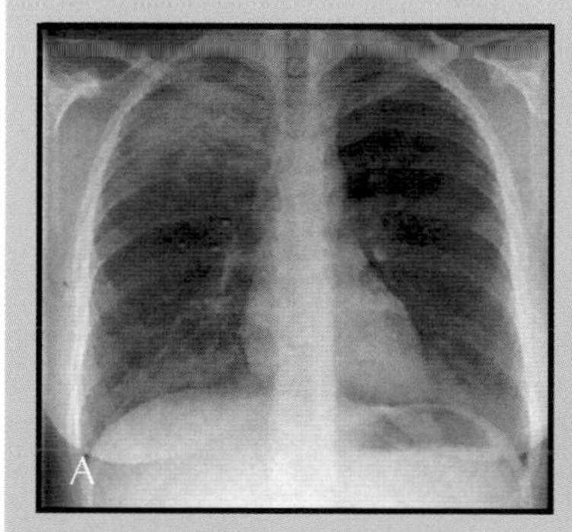

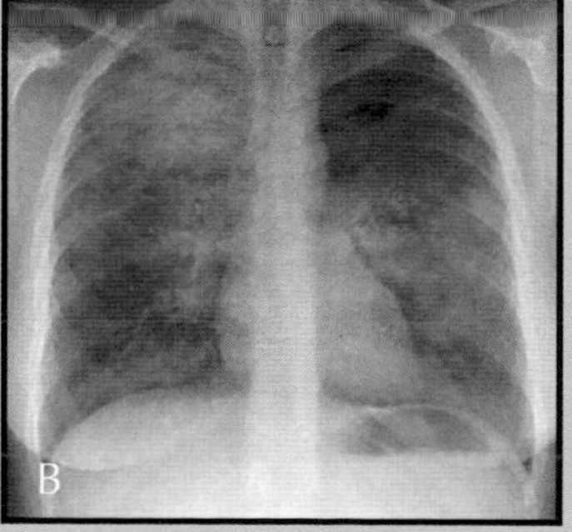

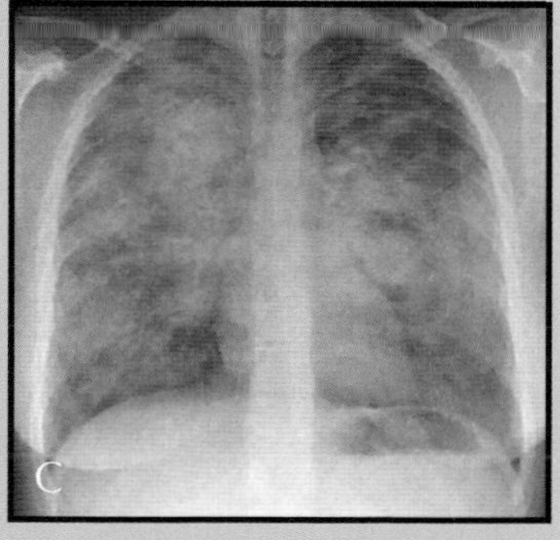

Course of disease

PREVENTION

A vaccine is available for influenza, and immunization should be given to all high-risk patients yearly, with a vaccine prepared against the strains that are anticipated most likely to be epidemic. The vaccine that is generally used is a chemically inactivated vaccine, originally grown on embryonated chicken eggs (and thus cannot be used in egg-allergic patients), and the yearly vaccine is trivalent, with two strains of influenza A (one an H3N2 and the other an H1N1) and one influenza B strain. A live-attenuated vaccine is also available for individuals ages 5 to 49 years. The vaccine includes antigens from influenza A and B, and it has generally been effective, but there is concern for using it in patients with HIV or severe immune suppression because of the live nature of the vaccine.

Parenteral influenza vaccination should be given yearly in the late fall and early winter to high-risk individuals. These include individuals at high risk for complications (people who are older than age 65 years; residents of nursing homes or chronic care facilities; people with chronic heart or lung disease; those with diabetes, renal failure, or immune suppression; women who will be in the second or third trimester during influenza season; and children 6 to 23 months of age) and those who can transmit influenza to high-risk individuals (health care workers, those who work in nursing homes and contact residents, those who give home health care to patients at high risk, and household contacts of high-risk individuals).

If an epidemic of influenza develops in a closed environment (e.g., a nursing home) among nonimmunized patients, antiviral therapy should be given along with vaccination, and antiviral therapy should be continued for 2 weeks until the vaccine takes effect. Either amantadine or the neuraminidase inhibitors can be used in this setting, remembering that amantadine is active only against influenza A but the neuraminidase inhibitors act against both influenza A and B.

LUNG ABSCESS

A lung abscess is a localized (usually >2 cm in diameter), suppurative, and necrotizing infectious process within the pulmonary parenchyma caused by either a respiratory or systemic illness. Most abscesses are primary and result from necrosis in an existing pulmonary process (usually an infectious pneumonia), although necrotization and secondary infection may result from a lung neoplasm. Between 8% and 18% of lung abscesses are associated with neoplasms in all age groups, but in patients older than age 45 years, as many as 30% have an associated cancer. Primary squamous carcinoma of the lung is the most common malignancy associated with abscess formation. An abscess can also result from a systemic process such as a septic vascular embolus (e.g., from right-sided endocarditis) or can be a secondary complication of a pulmonary process such as bronchial emboli (e.g., aspirated foreign bodies) or rupture of an extrapulmonary abscess into the lung (e.g., empyema).

Although any necrotizing pathogen can cause an abscess (such as *Staphylococcus aureus*, *Pseudomonas aeruginosa*, parasites, or mycobacteria), the classic lung abscess is caused by anaerobic bacteria. In the past 40 years, the incidence has declined 10-fold, although the mortality rate has decreased to 5% to 10%, presumably because of improved availability of antibiotics to treat pneumonia.

Sagittal section of lung with abscess (cavity in superior segment of lower lobe containing fluid and surrounded by fibrous tissue and pneumonic patches). Also pleural thickening over abscess

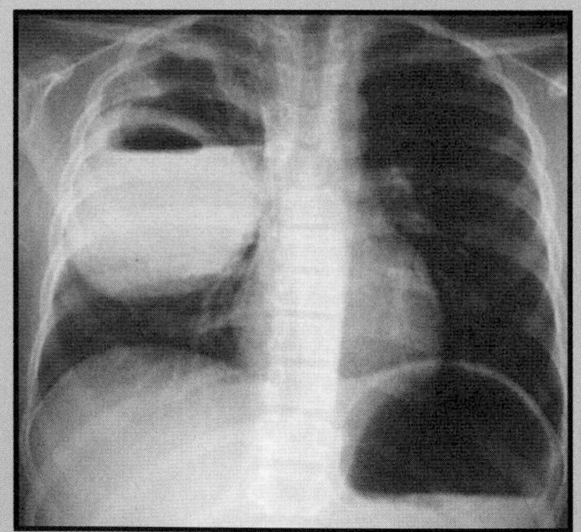

Frontal chest radiograph demonstrating large right upper lobe mass with air-fluid level and thick wall

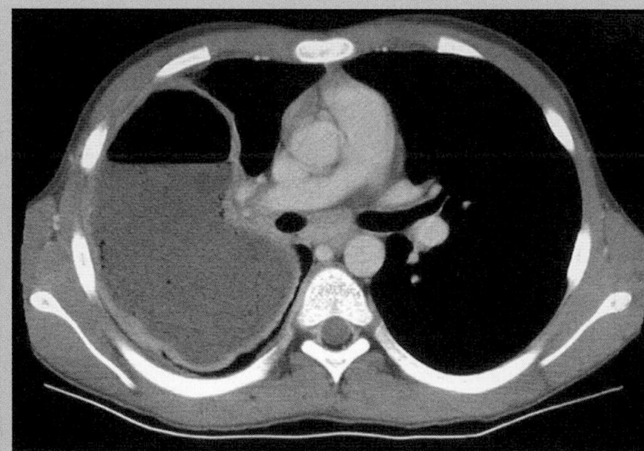

Axial CT image of same lesion, again demonstrating air-fluid level and thick surrounding wall that enhances with contrast as well as pockets of air within mass indicative of necrosis

PATHOGENESIS

Most lung abscesses are caused by a mixed bacterial flora, including anaerobes, up to 90% of the time. Aerobic organisms may be present in up to 50% of patients, but in most cases, they coexist with anaerobes. Typically, an abscess occurs when infected orogingival material is present in a host who has a predisposition to aspirate this material into a lung and who cannot adequately clear the challenge either because of impaired consciousness or because of exposure to a large inoculum (as in massive aspiration). Impaired consciousness can predispose to aspiration, as well as causing impaired clearance, but aspiration can also occur in those with oropharyngeal or esophageal dysfunction. At-risk patients are those with a history of alcoholism, seizure disorders, drug overdose, general anesthesia, protracted vomiting, neurologic disorders (e.g., stroke, myasthenia gravis, amyotrophic lateral sclerosis), esophageal diverticulum, and gastropulmonary fistulas. Aspiration of orogingival material, especially from a patient with poor dental hygiene, is pathogenic, although aspiration of gastric contents may not always lead to infection, especially if the aspirate is only acid, in which case chemical pneumonitis may result.

Based on animal and some human data, the development of a lung abscess occurs 7 to 14 days after aspirating infectious orogingival material into the terminal bronchioles. The location of the abscess is determined by gravity and body position at the time of aspiration, making the most common sites the basal segments of the lower lobes, the superior segment of the lower lobe, and the posterior segments of the upper lobes. In general, the right lung is involved more than the left because of the straight direction of its takeoff from the trachea. (see Plate 4-79). Based on these principles, if an abscess occurs in an edentulous patient (without oral anaerobes) or in a location other than the ones dictated by gravity, there should be suspicion of an endobronchial obstruction, a gastropulmonary fistula, or infection with a non-anaerobic organism (e.g., tuberculosis [TB]).

The most common anaerobic organisms causing lung abscess are *Peptostreptococcus* spp. (an anaerobic gram-positive coccus), *Fusobacterium nucleatum*, *Fusobacterium necrophorum*, *Porphyromonas* spp. (formerly classified in the genus *Bacteroides*), and *Prevotella melaninogenicus* (also formerly classified in the genus *Bacteroides*). Although most necrotizing lung processes are caused by anaerobic organisms, other necrotizing pathogens include *Staphylococcus aureus*, *Escherichia coli*, *Klebsiella pneumoniae*, *Pseudomonas aeruginosa Streptococcus pyogenes*, *Pseudomonas pseudomallei* (melioidosis), *Haemophilus influenzae* (especially type b), *Legionella pneumophila*, *Nocardia asteroides*, *Actinomyces*, and rarely

Lung Abscess *(Continued)*

pneumococcus, parasites (*Paragonimus westermani*, *Entamoeba histolytica*), fungi, and mycobacteria.

CLINICAL FEATURES

An acute lung abscess presents with symptoms of less than 2 weeks' duration and is commonly caused by a virulent aerobic bacterial pathogen, although patients with a chronic lung abscess (symptoms lasting >4-6 weeks) are more likely to have an underlying cancer or an infection with a less virulent anaerobic agent. Most patients with lung abscess have an insidious presentation, with symptoms lasting at least 2 weeks before evaluation. Findings include cough, foul-smelling sputum that forms layers on standing, hemoptysis (in 25% of patients), fever, chills, night sweats, anorexia, pleuritic chest pain (in 60% of patients), weight loss, and clubbing. The presence of foul-smelling or putrid sputum is highly suggestive of anaerobic infection. A history of weight loss is also common, occurring in 60% of patients, with an average loss of between 15 and 20 lb, and this finding further raises the suspicion of malignancy.

DIAGNOSTIC TESTING

Sputum culture may have some value if it shows a specific nonanaerobic pathogen, but because the sample is expectorated through the oropharynx, the finding of anaerobes (which must be specifically sought) is of limited usefulness. Bronchoscopy may be valuable for ruling out endobronchial obstruction and for promoting abscess drainage. If the abscess is associated with an empyema, as is the case 30% of the time, then culture of the pleural fluid may be valuable. Radiography is needed to define the presence of a cavitary lung lesion and typically shows a solitary cavitary lesion measuring 2 to 4 cm in diameter with an air-fluid level. When there is extensive inflammation surrounding the abscess, infection is likely, neoplasms tend to have less surrounding radiographic infiltrate. Lung cavities caused by TB appear different and tend to be thin-walled and without air-fluid levels. Sometimes it is necessary to use a computed tomography (CT) scan to distinguish a lung abscess from an empyema, the latter usually being confined to the pleural space. On the CT scan, whereas a lung abscess usually appears as a thick, irregular-walled cavity with no associated lung compression, an empyema has a thin, smooth wall with compression of the uninvolved lung. When a lung abscess is complicated by a bronchopleural fistula, it may be difficult to distinguish from an empyema. If the radiograph reveals multiple cavitary lesions, it usually suggests a necrotizing pneumonitis caused by a virulent nonanaerobic organism and the possibility of septic pulmonary emboli.

THERAPY

Before the availability of antibiotics, treatment included supportive care, postural drainage with or without bronchoscopy, and surgery. Currently, the mainstay of therapy is antibiotics directed at orogingival anaerobes. The initial antibiotic is usually intravenous penicillin or clindamycin. Although penicillin has historically been the first choice of therapy, recent trials have compared clindamycin with penicillin and found clindamycin to be associated with fewer treatment failures and a shorter time to symptom resolution. Metronidazole is not recommended and has had failure rates above 40%. Therapy is usually for a long duration, and until the pulmonary infiltrates have resolved or until the residual lesion is small and stable and the cavity closed. Many patients require a total of 6 to 8 weeks of antimicrobial therapy. Complications of lung abscess include empyema formation resulting from a bronchopleural fistula, massive hemoptysis, spontaneous rupture into uninvolved lung segments, and nonresolution of the abscess cavity. Although uncommon, these complications often require prolonged medical therapy as well as surgical intervention, either with tube thoracostomy in the case of empyema or lung resection in the case of massive hemoptysis. Surgery for lung abscess is also used in the setting of fulminant infection and in patients who fail medical therapy.

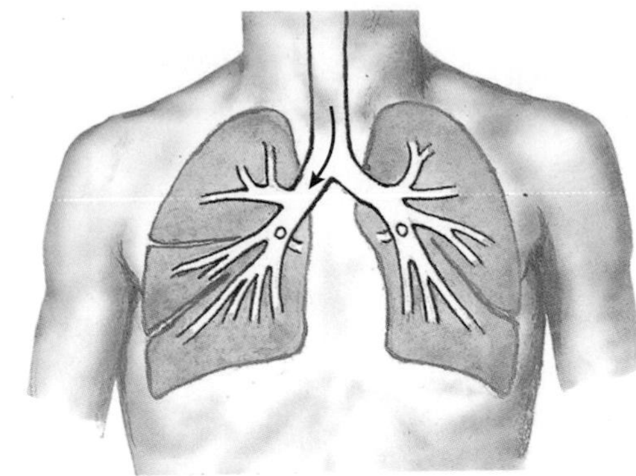

Right main bronchus is more in line with trachea than is the left, so that aspiration is more likely and incidence of abscess is greater on right side

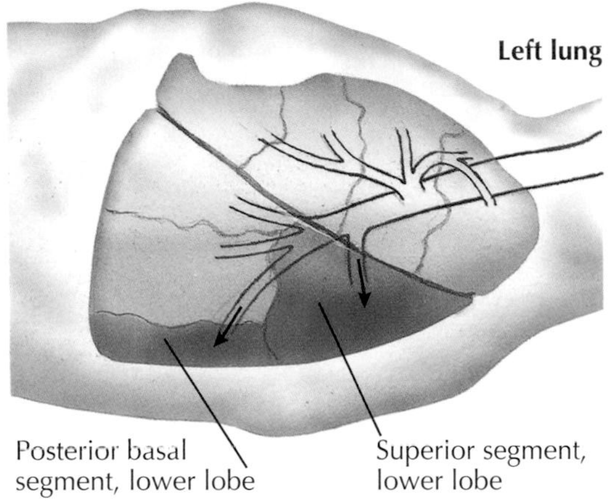

Although left lung is less commonly affected, superior and posterior basal segments are most vulnerable on that side

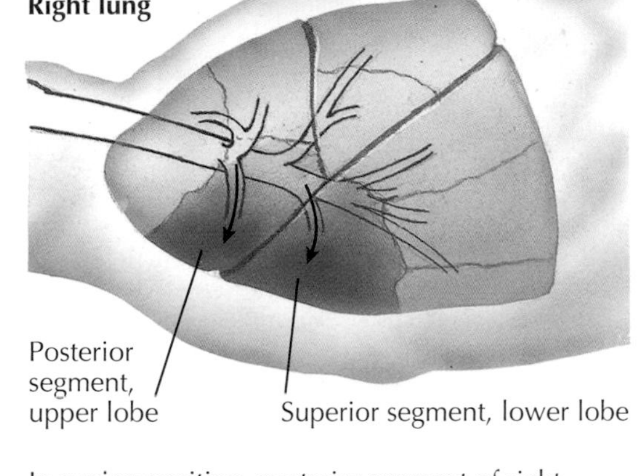

In supine position, posterior segment of right upper lobe and superior segment of lower lobe are most vulnerable to aspirational abscess due to gravitational influences

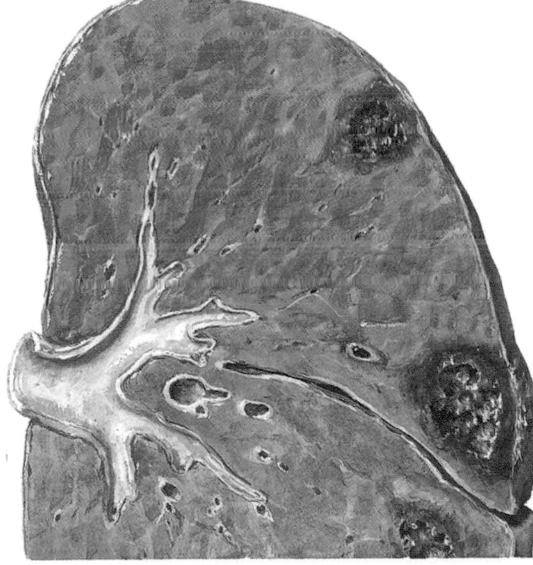

Multiple lung abscesses after septic embolization

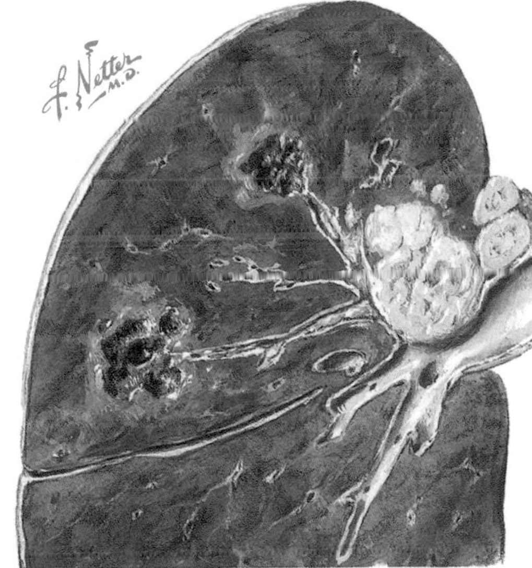

Abscesses distal to bronchial obstruction (in this case by carcinoma)

Overview of Health Care–Associated Pneumonia, Hospital-Acquired Pneumonia, and Ventilator-Associated Pneumonia

HEALTH CARE–ASSOCIATED PNEUMONIA DEFINITIONS AND EPIDEMIOLOGY

Health care–associated pneumonia (HCAP) refers to pneumonia in patients who have had contact with the health care environment before developing pneumonia and thus may be at risk of being colonized and infected with potentially drug-resistant pathogens. This group includes patients who have been in the hospital for at least 2 days in the past 90 days, those coming from a nursing home or extended care facility, those getting hemodialysis or home wound care, and those exposed to a family member harboring drug-resistant pathogens. Because many of these patients are at risk for infection with multidrug-resistant (MDR) gram-negative and gram-positive organisms, these patients do not have CAP, but are now defined as having HCAP. Clinical risk factors for MDR pathogens include severe pneumonia, poor functional status, recent antibiotic therapy (within the past 3 months), recent hospitalization, and immune suppression (including corticosteroid therapy).

It is important to recognize patients with HCAP because some may have a more complex spectrum of etiologic agents than those with community-acquired pneumonia (CAP), including a higher mortality rate, longer length of stay, higher frequency of aspiration, and more frequent receipt of incorrect empiric antibiotic therapy. In this regard, patients with HCAP are similar to those with hospital-acquired pneumonia (HAP).

HOSPITAL-ACQUIRED PNEUMONIA AND VENTILATOR-ASSOCIATED PNEUMONIA DEFINITIONS AND EPIDEMIOLOGY

In critically ill patients, pneumonia is the second most common intensive care unit (ICU)–acquired infection and the one that is most likely to lead to mortality. By definition, HAP occurs after the patient has been in the hospital for at least 48 hours and can occur in patients who are intubated and mechanically ventilated or in those who are not. If the patient has been intubated for at least 48 hours and then develops pneumonia, it is termed ventilator-associated pneumonia (VAP).

HAP occurs with increased frequency in any patient population with impaired immune function (either as a result of serious underlying illness or because of therapy-associated immune dysfunction) and increased exposure of the lower respiratory tract to bacteria (via aspiration with or without an endotracheal tube in place). VAP is present in 20% to 50% of mechanically ventilated patients, depending on the diagnostic criteria that are used and the risk factors in the patient population being considered. The risk of pneumonia increases with the duration of mechanical ventilation. Up to 40% of VAP is early onset (in the first 5 days of hospitalization).

In addition to mechanical ventilation, other risk factors for nosocomial pneumonia include age older than 60 years, malnutrition (serum albumin <2.2 g/dL), acute lung injury (acute respiratory distress syndrome), coma, burns, recent abdominal or thoracic surgery, multiple organ failure, transfusion of more than 4 U of blood, transport from the ICU, prior antibiotic therapy, elevation of gastric pH (by antacids or histamine-type 2 blocking agents), large volume aspiration, use of a nasogastric tube (rather than a tube placed in the jejunum or a tube inserted through the mouth), use of inadequate endotracheal tube cuff pressure (allowing aspiration of oral secretions into the lower respiratory tract), prolonged sedation and paralysis, maintaining patients in the supine position in bed, use of total parenteral nutrition feeding rather than enteral feeding, and repeated reintubation.

The mortality rate for patients with HAP can be as high as 50% to 70% in mechanically ventilated patients. In addition, the odds ratio for mortality in patients who acquire VAP compared with those who do not is nearly twofold, and the presence of VAP can prolong length of stay by at least 6 to 7 days. The greatest contributors to attributable mortality of VAP are use of an inappropriate antibiotic therapy (one that is not active against the identified etiologic pathogens), the presence of certain high-risk drug-resistant organisms (e.g., *Pseudomonas aeruginosa*, *Acinetobacter* spp., or *Staphylococcus aureus*), and the development of illness in a medical (rather than surgical) patient. Other mortality risk factors for HAP include coma on admission, creatinine level above 1.5 mg/dL, transfer from another ward to the ICU, bilateral radiographic abnormalities, age older than 60 years, an ultimately fatal underlying condition, shock, prior antibiotic therapy, pneumonia being a superinfection, multiple system organ failure, and an increasing APACHE (Acute Physiology and Chronic Health Evaluation) score during pneumonia therapy.

CAUSE AND DIAGNOSTIC TESTING

A variety of classification schemes for HAP are available that divide patients into categories based on the likelihood of specific pathogens. If the patient has early-onset infection (within the first 5 days of hospitalization) and no risk factors for MDR pathogens (recent hospitalization, recent antibiotic therapy, the presence of HCAP), then the patient is likely to be infected with a group of "core pathogens." These include nonresistant

Risk Factors of Hospital Acquired Preunionia

Patient-specific risk factors

Advanced age

Chronic underlying disease

Immunosuppression

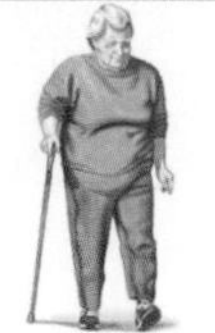

Obesity

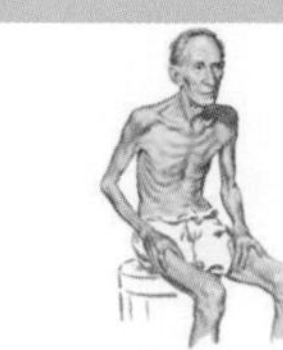

Malnutrition

Altered level of consciousness

Smoking

Alcohol abuse

Drug abuse

Treatment-related risk factors

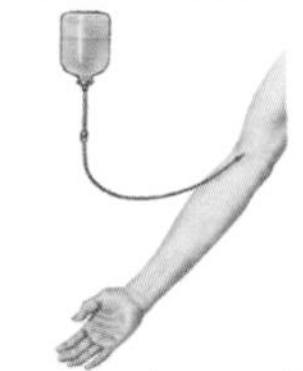

Parenteral nutrition

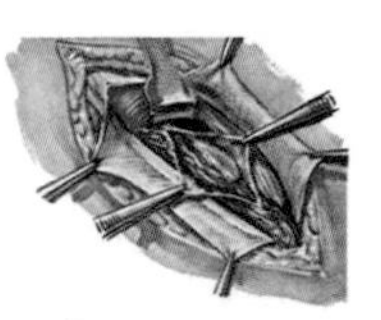

Recent surgery

Recent antibiotic exposure

Risk factors for infection with an antibiotic-resistant organism

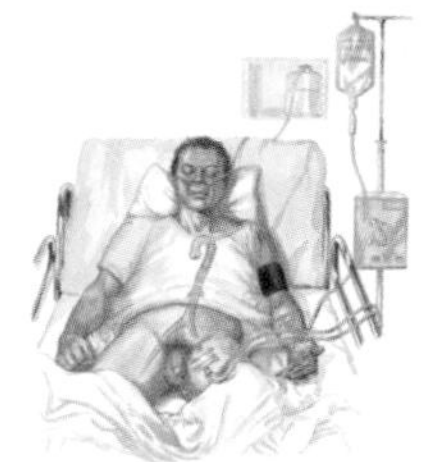

Prolonged hospitalization

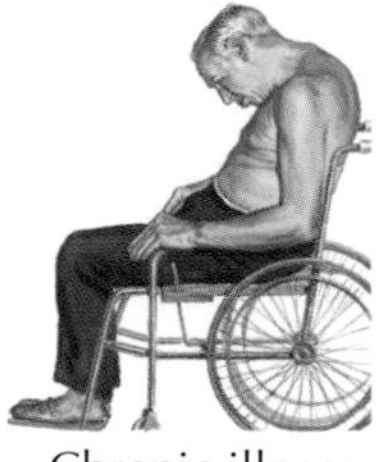

Chronic illness

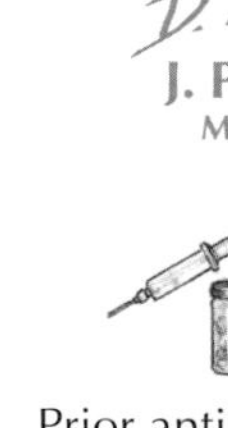

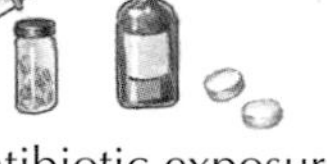

Prior antibiotic exposure

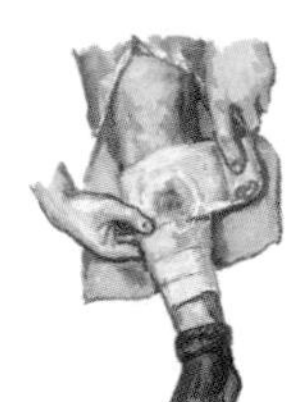

Home infusion therapy or home wound care

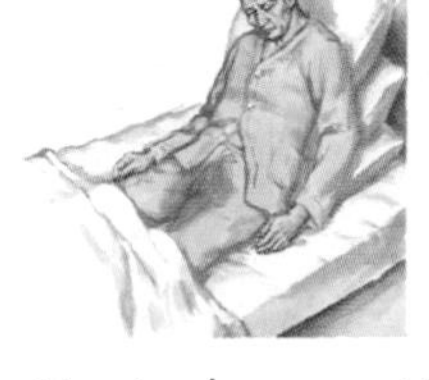

Nursing home resident

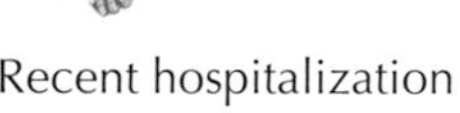

Recent hospitalization

Hemodialysis

Immunosuppression

Overview of Health Care–Associated Pneumonia, Hospital-Acquired Pneumonia, and Ventilator-Associated Pneumonia *(Continued)*

gram-negative organisms (*Escherichia coli*, *Klebsiella* spp., *Enterobacter* spp., *Serratia marcescens*, and *Proteus* spp.), methicillin-sensitive *S. aureus*, and pneumococcus. On the other hand, if the patient has late-onset infection (day 5 or later) or any of the risk factors for MDR pathogens, then in addition to the core pathogens, the patient is also at risk for infection with MDR gram-negative organisms such as *P. aeruginosa*, *Acinetobacter* spp., and extended-spectrum beta-lactamase (ESBL) producers such as *Klebsiella* and *Enterobacter* spp. or MDR gram-positive organisms such as methicillin-resistant *S. aureus* (MRSA).

The diagnosis of HAP, particularly VAP, is controversial because the clinical diagnostic criteria are sensitive but not specific for infection. These include the finding of a new or progressive lung infiltrate plus at least two of the following: temperature below 36.0°C or above 38.3°C, leukocyte count above 10,000/mm^3 or below 5000/mm^3, and purulent sputum. Another common clinical finding in patients with pneumonia is worsening oxygenation. All of these findings are not specific for pneumonia, so they are supplemented by microbiologic testing to define both the presence of pneumonia and the etiologic pathogen. Although some studies have suggested that clinical management can be improved if therapy decisions are guided by quantitative culture data, not all studies have confirmed this finding, and quantitative cultures are not routinely used to establish the diagnosis of HAP and VAP.

Therapy is initially empiric based on the likely etiologic pathogens and is generally done with a single agent if only the core pathogens are expected, although a broad-spectrum multidrug regimen is used if MDR pathogens are likely. After culture data become available, therapy is focused on the organism(s) identified.

Testing for Suspected Hospital-Acquired Pneumonia

Chest radiographs

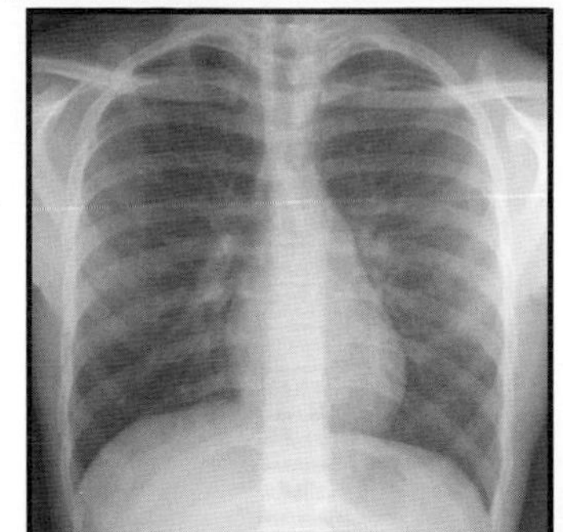

Laboratory evaluations

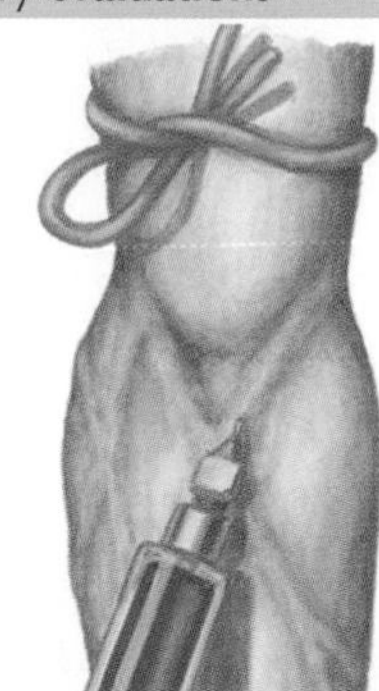

Sputum culture and Gram stain

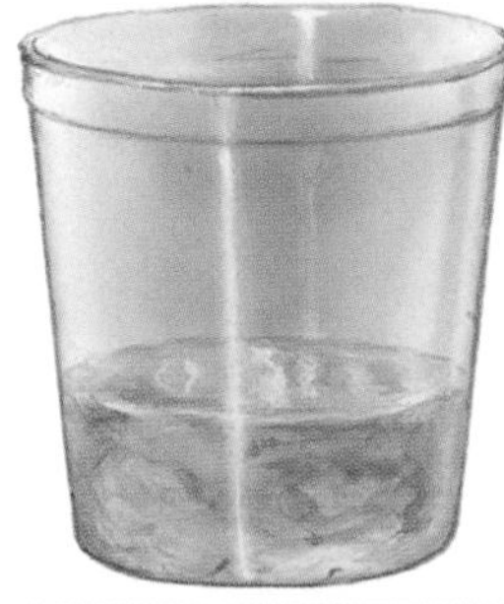

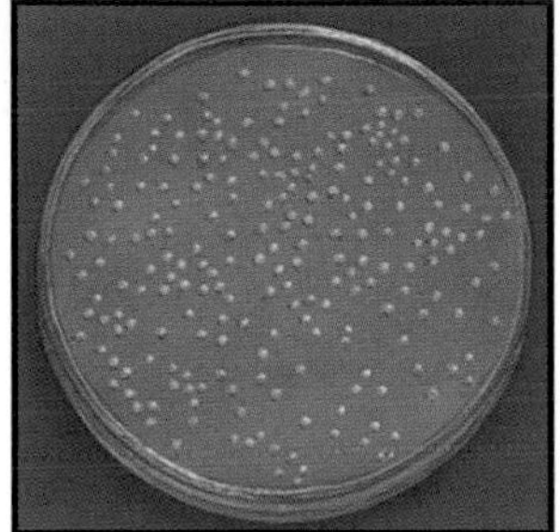

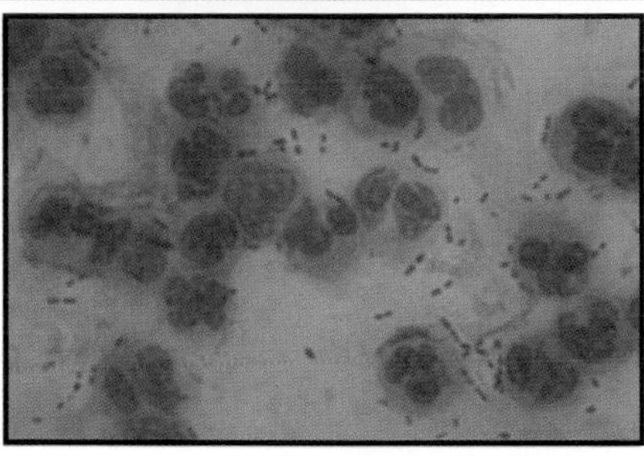

Bronchoscopic evaluation

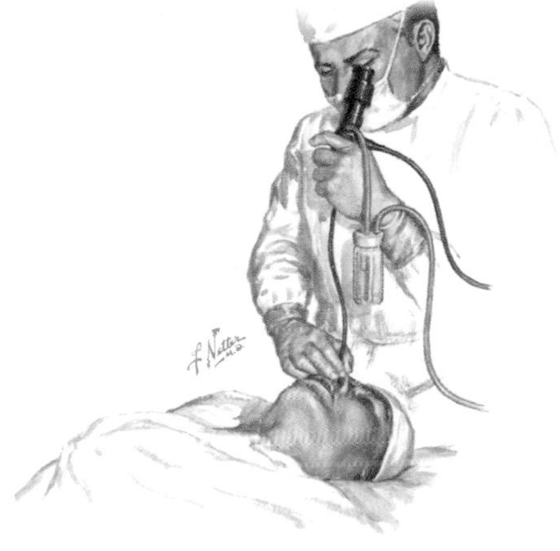

Antibiotic Resistance

When a patient develops HAP or VAP, there is a high likelihood that the etiologic agent will be antibiotic resistant. In fact, in patients with VAP the frequency may exceed 50% if the patient has been in the hospital for at least 7 days and has a history of prior antibiotic use. Drug-resistant organisms are not intrinsically more virulent than sensitive pathogens, but because their presence is often not anticipated, the initial therapy may be incorrect, and this factor contributes to the excess mortality associated with these organisms when they cause VAP.

Multidrug-Resistant Gram-Negative Organisms

Patients with VAP are most commonly infected by gram-negative organisms, including *P. aeruginosa*, *Acinetobacter baumannii*. *K. pneumoniae*, and extended-spectrum β-lactamase (ESBL)–producing Enterobacteriaceae. All of these organisms can be antibiotic resistant, making therapy difficult. *P. aeruginosa* is the most common of these organisms causing VAP, but *A. baumannii* is occurring with increasing frequency, and many hospitals have epidemics of ESBL-producing Enterobacteriaceae and carbapenemase-producing *K. pneumoniae*, making the challenges presented by these bacteria quite daunting.

P. aeruginosa is an especially virulent organism because of its production of destructive exoenzymes and its resistance to a wide range of antibiotics. Patients often have upper respiratory tract (oropharynx) colonization before colonization and infection of the lung, but primary lower respiratory tract colonization can also occur. In the ICU, nosocomial pneumonia is the biggest concern, but this organism can also lead to ventilator-associated tracheobronchitis, an infection in the airway that may later progress to pneumonia. The organism is also involved in chronic airways infections such as bronchiectasis, with or without associated cystic fibrosis. *P. aeruginosa* is such a prevalent nosocomial pathogen because it can grow in virtually any environment, and it produces a wide range of virulence factors that allow it to infect nearly any body site. In addition, the organism can form a biofilm on an endotracheal tube and persist despite antibiotics and host defense mechanisms. When a critical number of bacteria are present, they can coordinate their growth in a biofilm and overcome host defenses through quorum sensing, which is promoted by the release of signaling substances.

Methicillin-Resistant *Staphylococcus Aureus*

This organism has been discussed above as a cause of CAP. The strain of MRSA causing nosocomial pneumonia is different, is more antibiotic-resistant than the community-acquired strain, and is more prone to causing lung infection. Unlike community-acquired MRSA, it is not a clonal disease, and bacterial virulence factors are not as widely present. Important clinical risk factors for MRSA as a nosocomial pneumonia pathogen are acute neurologic illness, hemodialysis, heart disease, and solid organ transplantation. Most pneumonias are not accompanied by bacteremia, but when they are, endocarditis should be assumed to be present, and patients may develop metastatic infection in the brain, bones, and solid organs, and prolonged therapy (4-6 weeks) is needed.

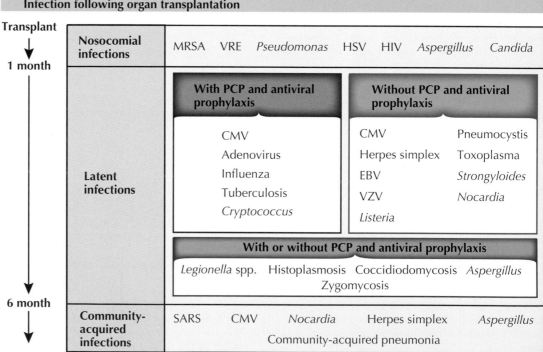

	Splenectomy	Chemotherapy-induced neutropenia	Abnormal T-lymphocyte function
Etiology	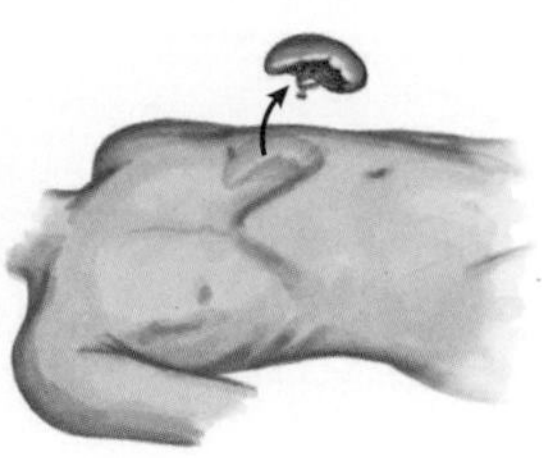	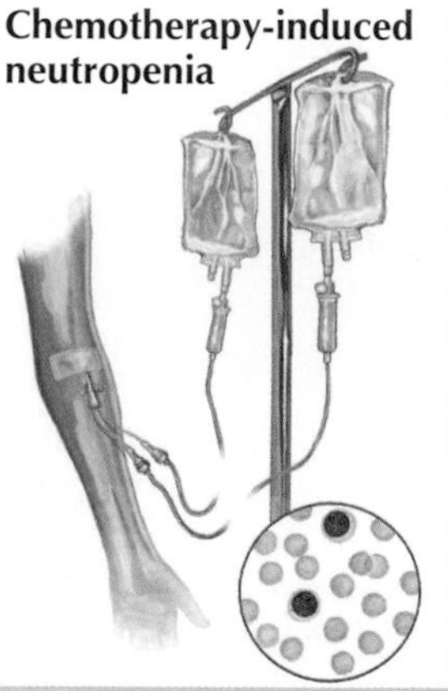	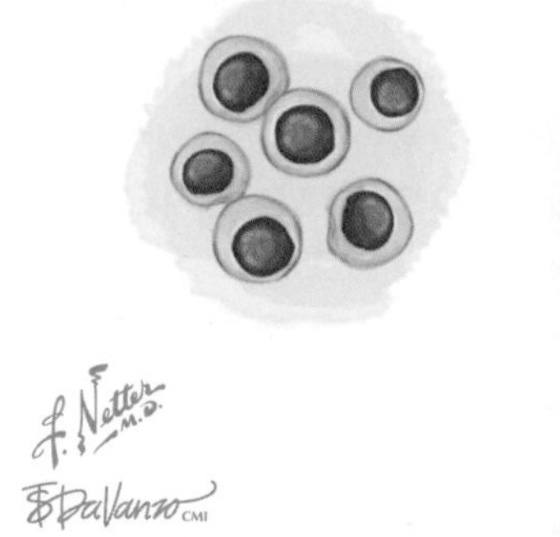
At risk for	Encapsulated bacteria (e.g., pneumococcus, staphylococci, *H. influenzae*, and *N. meningitidis*)	*P. aeruginosa*, other gram-negative bacteria, and *Aspergillus* spp.	Bacteria such as *Listeria monocytogenes*, *Salmonella* spp., *Legionella* spp., *Mycobacterium avium*, or *M. tuberculosis* Fungi such as *Cryptococcus neoformans*, *Histoplasma capsulatum*, *Pneumocystis jirovecii*, or *Coccidioides immitis* Viruses such as cytomegalovirus, herpes simplex Parasites such as *Toxoplasma gondii* or *Cryptosporidium* spp.

Infection following organ transplantation

Time	Infections		
Transplant → 1 month	**Nosocomial infections**	MRSA VRE *Pseudomonas* HSV HIV *Aspergillus* *Candida*	
1 month → 6 month	**Latent infections**	**With PCP and antiviral prophylaxis** CMV Adenovirus Influenza Tuberculosis *Cryptococcus*	**Without PCP and antiviral prophylaxis** CMV, Herpes simplex, EBV, VZV, *Listeria* Pneumocystis, Toxoplasma, *Strongyloides*, *Nocardia*
		With or without PCP and antiviral prophylaxis *Legionella* spp. Histoplasmosis Coccidiodomycosis *Aspergillus* Zygomycosis	
6 month →	**Community-acquired infections**	SARS CMV *Nocardia* Herpes simplex *Aspergillus* Community-acquired pneumonia	

Pneumonia in the Compromised Host

When patients with specific immune impairments related to an underlying primary illness (often malignancy or HIV infection) or arising as a consequence of medical therapy (e.g., chemotherapy- or transplant-related immunosuppression) develop respiratory infections, they are referred to as immunocompromised hosts (ICHs). In recent years, HIV infection has led to a large and important population of ICH patients who may develop pneumonia. In any ICH, a new lung infiltrate may be infectious or noninfectious in origin (e.g., adverse drug reaction, pulmonary hemorrhage, acute lung injury). Because of the broad spectrum of potential pathogens and the seriousness of pneumonia in the ICH, empiric therapy is often supplemented by vigorous efforts at making a specific etiologic diagnosis.

The cause of infection in an ICH is generally dictated by the type of immune impairment (see Plate 4-82). Thus, patients who have had a splenectomy (including those with sickle cell anemia and autosplenectomy) are usually infected by encapsulated bacteria such as pneumococcus, staphylococci, *Haemophilus influenzae*, and *Neisseria meningitides*. Patients with chemotherapy-induced neutropenia may be infected with *Pseudomonas aeruginosa*, other gram-negative bacteria, and *Aspergillus* spp. Patients with abnormal T-lymphocyte function, such as those with certain lymphomas or HIV infection, may be infected by bacteria such as *Listeria monocytogenes*, *Salmonella* spp., *Legionella* spp., *Mycobacterium avium*, or *Mycobacterium tuberculosis;* fungi such as *Cryptococcus neoformans*, *Histoplasma capsulatum*, or *Coccidioides immitis*; viruses such as cytomegalovirus (CMV) and herpes simplex; or parasites such as *Pneumocystis jiroveci*, *Toxoplasma gondii*, or *Cryptosporidium* spp. In HIV-infected patients, the type of infection that develops is directly related to the patient's CD4 lymphocyte count. Those with little immune dysfunction and a CD4 count above 500 per mm^3 usually do not develop opportunistic infection, and their predominant pneumonia is bacterial, especially pneumococcal. Those with counts between 200 and 500 per mm^3 are prone to infection with bacteria and *M. tuberculosis*. As the CD4 count decreases further, the risk of opportunistic infection increases, and patients with a count below 200 per mm^3 are at particular risk for such infections as *P. jiroveci*. With a count below 100 per mm^3, toxoplasmosis is a concern, and below 50 per mm^3, CMV, *M. avium*, and *Cryptococcus* spp. are more likely.

Immunocompromised patients should have a careful clinical examination with attention to the skin, gastrointestinal tract, central nervous system, optic fundi, liver, and lungs. Cough and dyspnea may be present, but respiratory symptoms may be minimal, with fever as the only finding. An etiologic agent can be suggested by certain extrapulmonary findings in conjunction with a specific immune defect. Skin lesions can occur with infection caused by *P. aeruginosa*, *Aspergillus* spp., *M. tuberculosis*, *Nocardia* spp., varicella zoster, herpes simplex, *Cryptococcus* spp., and *Blastomyces* spp. The central nervous system may be affected by *Nocardia* spp., pneumococcus, *H. influenzae*, *P. aeruginosa*, *M. tuberculosis*, *Legionella* spp., *Aspergillus* spp., *Cryptococcus* spp., *Toxoplasma* spp., varicella zoster, and CMV. Liver function abnormalities can be seen with CMV, *Legionella* spp., and *Nocardia* spp. infection; tuberculosis; histoplasmosis; toxoplasmosis; and *Staphylococcus aureus* and *Pseudomonas aeruginosa* infection. Diarrhea may occur with *Legionella* spp., *Cryptosporidium* spp., CMV, or herpes simplex.

After organ transplant, patients can acquire infection that is related to hospitalization, the presence of serious illness, or transplant immunosuppression. Within the first month of transplant, patients' infections are with nosocomial bacterial and *Candida* spp. In the period from 1 to 6 months after transplant, infection is related to immunosuppression and can be with CMV, *P. jiroveci*, fungal agents (molds such as *Aspergillus* spp. and the zygomycoses, and yeasts

Pneumocystis jirovecii pneumonia

Immunosuppression
Steroid therapy
Transplanation
Heart
Bone marrow
Kidney
HIV infection
Leukemia
Lymphoma

Predisposing factors

Pneumonia in the Compromised Host *(Continued)*

such as *Histoplasmosis* spp. and *Coccidioidomycosis* spp.), *L. monocytogenes*, and *Legionella* spp. After 6 months, these same pathogens may cause infection in patients who are heavily immunosuppressed, although chronic viral infection (e.g., CMV) may develop in those less heavily immunosuppressed.

Chest radiography may show specific patterns with certain pathogens. Focal lung lesions may be seen with bacterial, fungal, and mycobacterial illness. Diffuse infiltrates are seen with *P. jiroveci*, CMV, *Legionella* infection, miliary tuberculosis, viral pneumonia, and infection with *Aspergillus* spp. and *Candida* spp. Management usually involves empiric therapy based on risk factors for specific pathogens supplemented by diagnostic procedures (often bronchoscopy or open lung biopsy), especially in nonresponding patients.

Pneumonia with HIV Infection

Patients with HIV infection have impairment of T-cell function but also have humoral immune dysfunction and can be infected with bacteria, fungi, viruses, or parasites. The most common pneumonias in immunosuppressed patients with HIV infection are caused by *P. jiroveci* (see Plate 4-83) and pneumococcus. In early HIV infection with profound immune suppression, *P. jiroveci* is common, but after therapy with antiretroviral agents, bacterial pathogens are more common causes of respiratory infection. *P. jiroveci* can be recognized by methenamine silver stain or by Giemsa stain, usually of lung tissue or bronchoalveolar lavage (BAL) fluid. Most patients probably acquired *P. jiroveci* from environmental sources before the onset of HIV infection, and pneumonia often represents reactivation, but new primary infection and reinfection are also possible. Most patients present with a subacute course of fever, cough, dyspnea, and weight loss. Chest pain, malaise, fatigue, and night sweats may also occur, and some patients are even asymptomatic. Chest radiograph usually shows bilateral diffuse interstitial or alveolar infiltrates. Asymmetric or focal infiltrates may occasionally be seen, as can predominantly upper lobe disease and solitary pulmonary nodules. Less common findings include pneumothorax and pleural effusion. Upper lobe disease and pneumothorax were reported in the past, especially when patients were receiving aerosolized pentamidine for prophylaxis of *P. jiroveci* infection.

The diagnosis of *P. jiroveci* infection is usually made bronchoscopically by BAL or transbronchial biopsy. In addition to a compatible radiograph, other clinical features include leucopenia and lymphopenia, elevated serum lactate dehydrogenase, oral candidiasis, and a widened alveolar-arterial oxygen tension gradient. *P. jiroveci* may coexist with other opportunistic infections such as CMV, toxoplasmosis, or mycobacterial illness. With therapy, improvement is slower in the AIDS patient than in other ICHs with *P. jiroveci* infection. Fever may persist for 7 to 10 days, and overall survival from the infection is as high as 90%. Therapy is begun with intravenous trimethoprim/sulfamethoxazole (15-20 mg/kg/d of trimethoprim and 75-100 mg/kg/d of sulfamethoxazole), but if the patient cannot tolerate this therapy or does not respond, then treatment with alternative agents such as pentamidine (4 mg/kg/d) or atovaquone (750 mg orally three times daily) should be started. Trimetrexate and aerosolized pentamidine have been tried but are generally less effective than standard therapy. Therapy with most regimens is continued for 21 days, and if the illness leads to hypoxemia, with a room-air arterial PO_2 below 70 mm Hg, then corticosteroids should be added to ameliorate the host inflammatory response to the killing of organisms that accompanies therapy. After recovery from pneumonia, patients should receive chemoprophylaxis against recurrent infection, which can be done with oral trimethoprim/sulfamethoxazole or alternative agents.

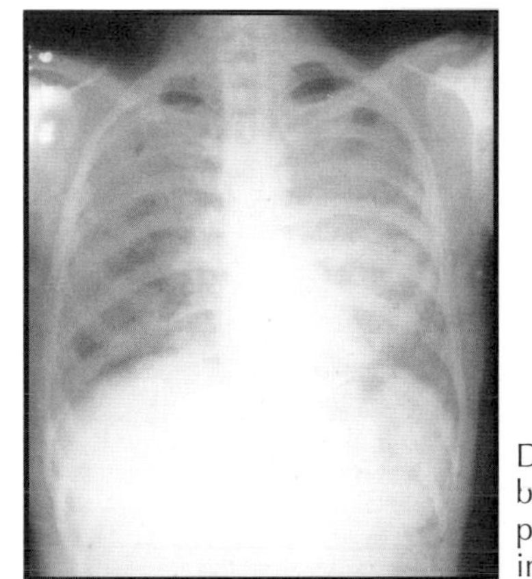

Diffuse bilateral pulmonary infiltrates

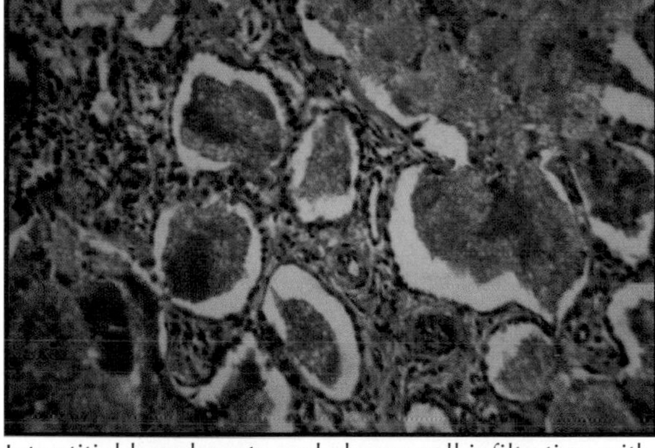

Interstitial lymphocyte and plasma cell infiltration with foamy exudate in alveoli

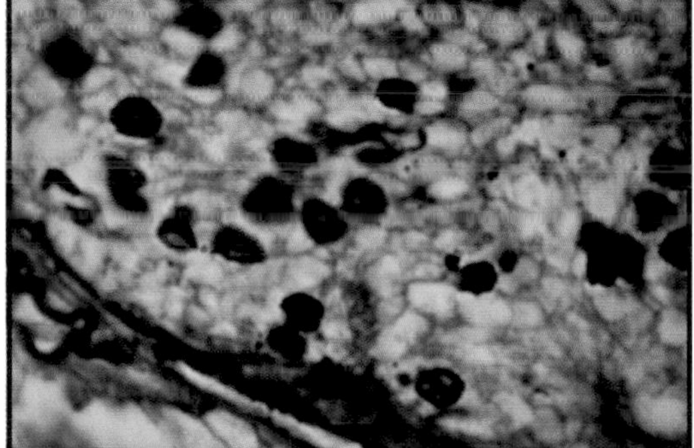

Methenamine $AgNO_3$ stain showing *Pneumocystis* organisims in lung (black spots)

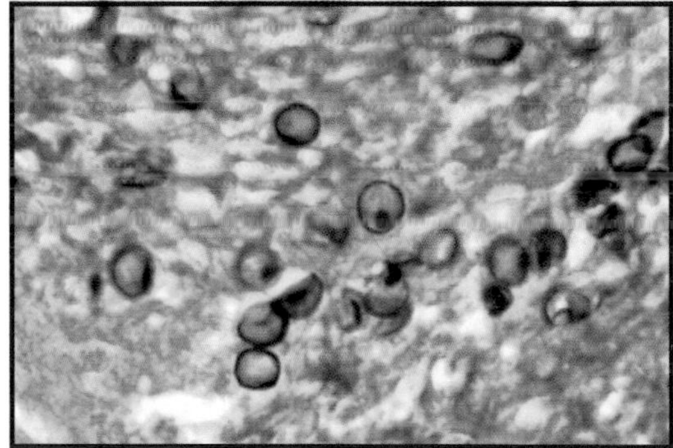

Silver stain of organisms showing cysts

Actinomycosis

Actinomycosis is a chronic suppurative or granulomatous bacterial infection caused by branching, non-spore-forming, gram-positive bacteria belonging to the genus *Actinomyces*. *Actinomyces* spp. are strict or facultative anaerobes. Their cellular morphology is variable, usually diphtheroid or filamentous, although bacillary and coccoid forms may also occur. *Actinomyces* are true bacteria; their filaments are narrower than fungal hyphae; and unlike the latter, they readily fragment into bacillary forms. In addition, *Actinomyces* spp. reproduce by binary fission and not by spore formation or budding as in fungi. They are part of normal oral flora within gingival crevices and tonsillar crypts. Their prevalence is increased with poor oral hygiene, in periodontal pockets, in dental plaques, and on carious teeth.

Actinomycosis is a cosmopolitan, sporadically occurring endogenous infection. Males are 1.5 to 3.0 times more likely to have the disease than females. *Actinomyces israelii* is the usual cause of actinomycosis, although several other species can occasionally cause human disease. Clinical types of actinomycosis and their incidence include cervicofacial (55%), pulmonary (20%), abdominal (20%), and disseminated (5%). A hallmark of actinomycosis is the tendency to spread through anatomic barriers, including fascial planes, and the development of multiple sinus tracts. Cervicofacial infection usually follows tooth extraction or other trauma to the oral mucosa and is characterized by a firm indurated mass in the region of the jaw ("lumpy jaw") that often suppurates and gives rise to multiple cutaneous fistulas. Poor oral hygiene is important as a predisposing factor. Other predisposing conditions include diabetes, immunosuppression, malnutrition, and local tissue damage.

Pulmonary actinomycosis may result directly from a cervicofacial focus or from extension through the diaphragm from an intraabdominal lesion. As a rule, it is secondary to aspiration of the organism from the mouth, and generally the lower lobes are involved. Initial symptoms include mild fever and cough with purulent sputum. With abscess formation, the sputum may become blood streaked. If it is not treated, the infection often spreads to the pleura and through the thoracic wall, causing subsequent empyema, soft tissue abscesses, and multiple draining sinuses. The clinical and radiographic signs of pulmonary actinomycosis are similar to those of nocardiosis, tuberculosis, and other lung disorders.

Abdominal infection most often occurs after appendectomy or bowel perforation, which may be either traumatic or spontaneous. Abdominal actinomycosis is more common in the cecum and appendix, where it is frequently associated with sinus formation. In disseminated actinomycosis, virtually any organ may be involved.

Actinomyces spp. form characteristic sulfur granules in infected tissue but not in vitro. Pus should be placed in a sterile Petri dish and examined with a hand lens against a dark background for these granules. If present, these granules are yellowish white to white firm flecks that vary in size from a barely visible speck to 5 mm in diameter. Under an oil immersion lens, Gram stain of the granules reveals an internal tangle of delicate gram-positive filaments with a rosette of peripheral clubs. Similar granules may be formed by other microorganisms such as *Nocardia brasiliensis*, *Streptomyces* madurae, and *Staphylococcus aureus*. However, these other granules lack the rosette of peripheral clubs.

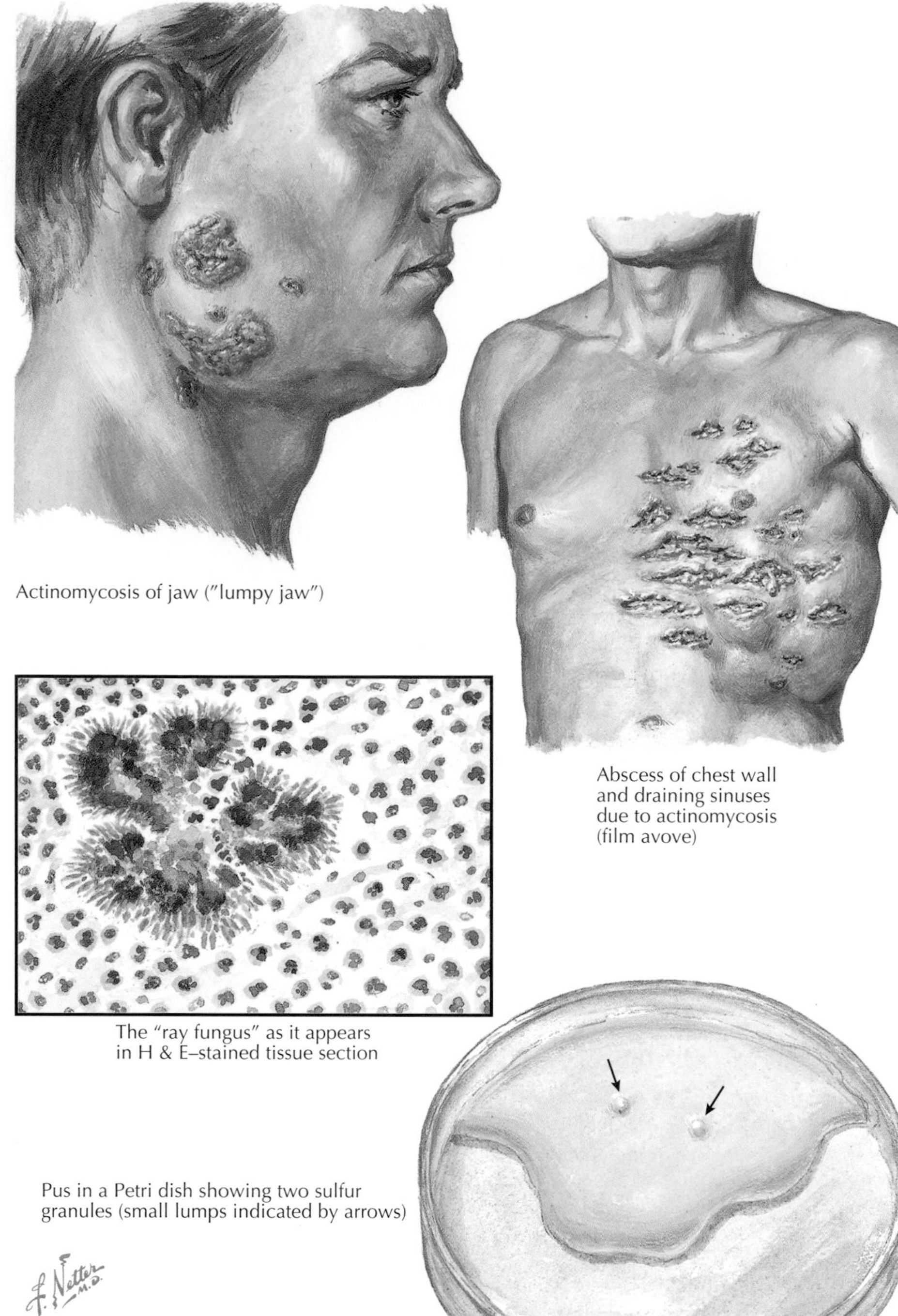

Actinomycosis of jaw ("lumpy jaw")

Abscess of chest wall and draining sinuses due to actinomycosis (film avove)

The "ray fungus" as it appears in H & E–stained tissue section

Pus in a Petri dish showing two sulfur granules (small lumps indicated by arrows)

Diagnosis of actinomycosis is confirmed by culture and occasionally by histopathologic evidence of *Actinomyces* infection. *Actinomyces* spp. are slow-growing, fastidious organisms, which require an enriched medium, anaerobic or microaerophilic conditions, and up to 14 to 21 days for optimal growth. Therefore, the clinical microbiology laboratory should be informed if *Actinomyces* spp. are suspected. *Actinomyces* spp. are almost invariably isolated as part of a polymicrobial flora. However, the significance of these coexisting bacteria in the pathogenesis of actinomycosis is unclear, and these pathogens do not need to be specifically treated with antibiotics.

Treatment

Management of patients with actinomycosis often requires prolonged courses of antibiotics and surgical intervention in complicated cases. High-dose penicillin is the treatment of choice for actinomycosis. For mild infections without significant suppuration or fistulous tracts, oral penicillin V or amoxicillin for 2 to 6 months is recommended. Acceptable alternatives to penicillin include the tetracyclines, erythromycin, and clindamycin. In patients with more severe cervicofacial actinomycosis that requires surgery, intravenous penicillin G for 4 to 6 weeks followed by oral penicillin V for 6 to 12 months is recommended.

In addition to antibiotics, surgical intervention may be required for excision of necrotic tissue or recalcitrant fibrotic lesions and for drainage of extensive abscesses with marsupilation of persisting sinus tracts. Prognosis is excellent with a combined medical-surgical approach. However, recurrences can occur, so prolonged observation of patients after treatment is recommended.

NOCARDIOSIS

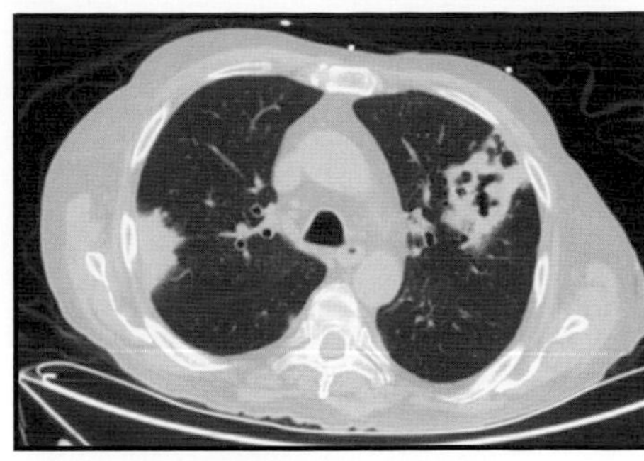

CT at lung windows shows peripheral right upper lobe and left upper lobe mass-like consolidation with cavitation

Multiple necrotic abscesses in right upper lobe covered by extensive pleuritis

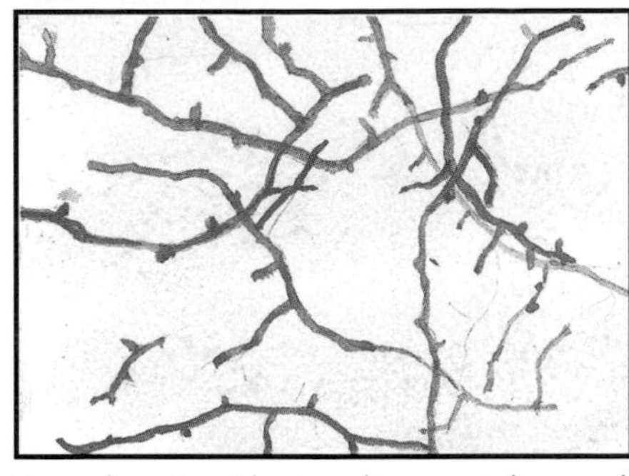

Nocardia asteroides in culture on Sabouraud's glucose agar. The branching filaments do not appear in yeast phase. In sputum or pus, filaments fragment and may be mistaken for tubercle bacilli since they may be acid-fast

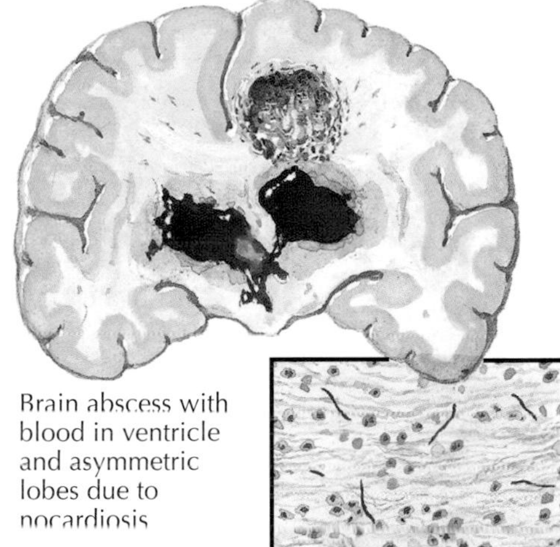

Brain abscess with blood in ventricle and asymmetric lobes due to nocardiosis

Section showing acid-fast organisms in brain tissue

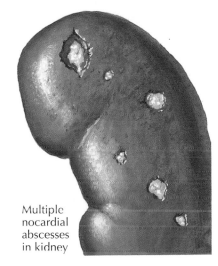

Multiple nocardial abscesses in kidney

Nocardiosis is an uncommon, suppurative, bacterial infection caused by aerobic actinomycetes in the genus *Nocardia*. Although the lungs, skin, and subcutaneous tissues are ordinarily involved, the disease may spread to any other organ, particularly to the central nervous system (CNS). Another characteristic of nocardiosis is its tendency to relapse or progress despite appropriate therapy.

The genus *Nocardia* includes more than 50 species, at least 33 of which cause human disease, most commonly *Nocardia asteroides* complex. *Nocardia* is a gram-positive, nonmotile, nonencapsulated, partially acid-fast, aerobic, highly evolved bacterium with characteristic filamentous branching that fragments into bacillary or coccoid forms. Acid-fastness and growth in aerobic conditions help to distinguish *Nocardia* from *Actinomyces*.

Nocardia spp. occur worldwide and exist in soil, decaying vegetable matter, and aquatic environments as saprophytes. Inhalation is the most common route of infection, although ingestion, direct inoculation, and nosocomial transmission have also been described. Individuals of all ages may be infected, and males contract the disease more frequently, presumably because of occupational exposure. Nocardiosis is usually an opportunistic infection; however, one-third of cases occur in immunocompetent hosts. Immunocompromising illnesses that commonly predispose to nocardiosis include glucocorticoid therapy, malignancy, organ and hematopoietic transplantation, and HIV infection. Less common predispositions include diabetes mellitus, alcoholism, chronic granulomatous disease, pulmonary alveolar proteinosis, tumor necrosis factor-α inhibitor therapy, and tuberculosis.

The location and extent of disease can be used to classify nocardiosis as pulmonary, CNS, cutaneous, and disseminated disease. In the lungs, nocardiosis produces chronic to fulminating disease; in other viscera and skin, it causes chronic suppuration, sinuses, and abscess formation. Hematogenous dissemination can occur to almost any organ.

Presenting symptoms of pulmonary nocardiosis are often similar to those of pneumonia or tuberculosis. Radiographic manifestations include single or multiple nodules (with or without cavitation), lobar consolidation, reticulonodular or interstitial infiltrates, and pleural effusions. Empyema, mediastinitis, pericarditis, and superior vena cava syndrome may occur after contiguous spread.

Nocardial brain abscess may occur in any region of the brain and present clinically with fever, headache, meningismus, seizures, and focal neurologic deficits. CNS nocardiosis may also present as a mass lesion in immunocompetent patients or infrequently as subacute or chronic meningitis.

Manifestations of cutaneous nocardiosis include ulcerations, pyoderma, cellulitis, nodules, and subcutaneous abscesses. Involvement of regional lymphatics and formation of a mycetoma involving subcutaneous tissues and bones with draining sinuses may also occur. Disseminated nocardiosis is defined as two noncontiguous sites of involvement.

Nocardiosis should be suspected in any patient who presents with brain, soft tissue, or cutaneous lesions and a concurrent or recent pulmonary process. Nocardial infection should also be suspected in patients with suppurative pneumonia unresponsive to conventional antimicrobial agents, particularly with immunosuppression. The differential diagnosis primarily includes mycobacterial, fungal, parasitic, and bacterial infections as well as malignancy.

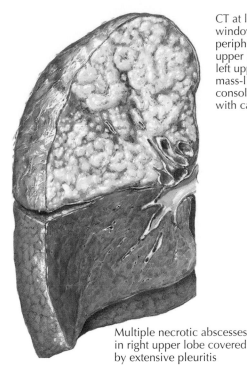

Definitive diagnosis depends on pathogen isolation from clinical specimens. Invasive sampling is often necessary, and the clinical laboratory needs to use specific media and staining procedures. The characteristic appearance on Gram stain and partial acid fastness on direct examination of clinical samples can yield a rapid presumptive diagnosis. *Nocardia* spp. require 5 to 21 days to grow in culture. If possible, isolates of *Nocardia* should be sent to a reference laboratory for precise identification and confirmation of susceptibility testing.

TREATMENT

Nocardia spp. clinical isolates are variably resistant to antibiotics. Monotherapy with an oral agent is appropriate for cutaneous infection in an immunocompetent host. Trimethoprim/sulfamethoxazole is the drug of choice. Empiric coverage with two or three agents is recommended in severe infection (e.g., trimethoprim/sulfamethoxazole in combination with amikacin); with CNS involvement, a third-generation cephalosporin or imipenem should be added. Initial treatment should be administered intravenously for 3 to 6 weeks and until clinical improvement occurs. Therapy should be continued with two oral drugs, such as trimethoprim/sulfamethoxazole, minocycline, or amoxicillin/clavulanate for a total duration of 6 to 12 months. Surgical intervention may be required for brain and large soft tissue abscesses unresponsive to antibiotics, empyema, mediastinal fluid collection, and pericarditis. Prolonged oral maintenance therapy to prevent relapse is required in persistently immunosuppressed patients. The rate for patients with in pulmonary nocardiosis ranges from 14% to 40%. Disseminated disease has a mortality rate of 7% to 44% in immunocompetent and 85% in immunocompromised hosts.

Ulcerating lesion of tongue due to histoplasmosis. Lesion is identical in appearance to carcinoma of tongue

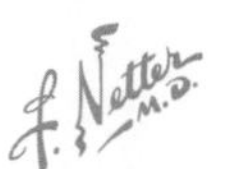

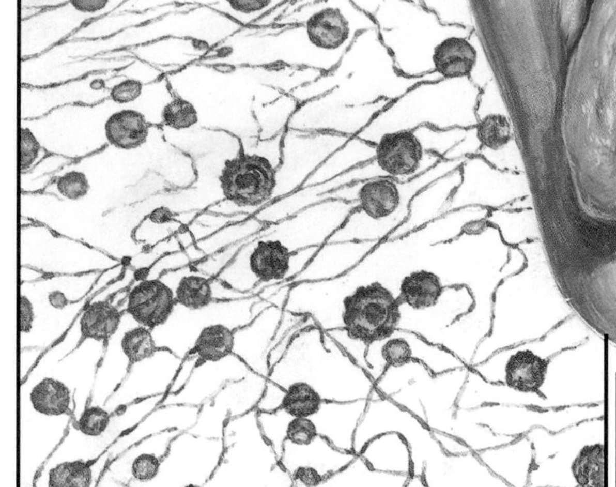

Mycelial or free-living phase of *H. capsulatum* as it exists in nature or in culture

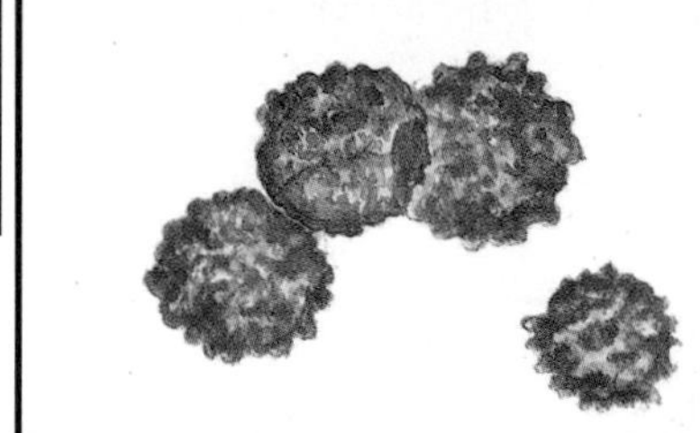

Spores of mycelial phase of *H. capsulatum*. Inhalation of these is source of infection

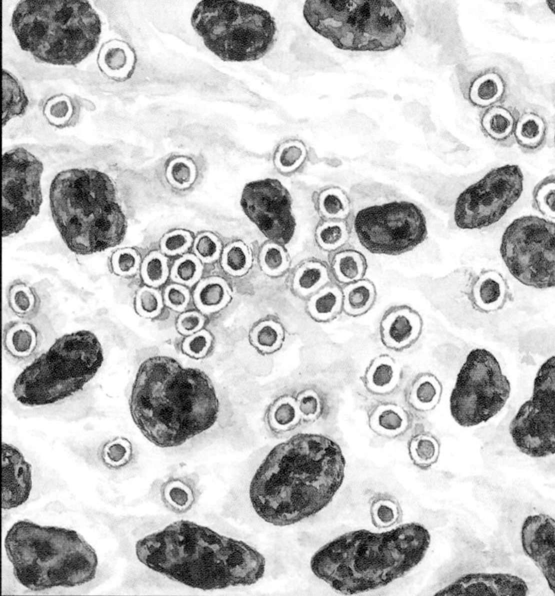

H. capsulatum in tissue

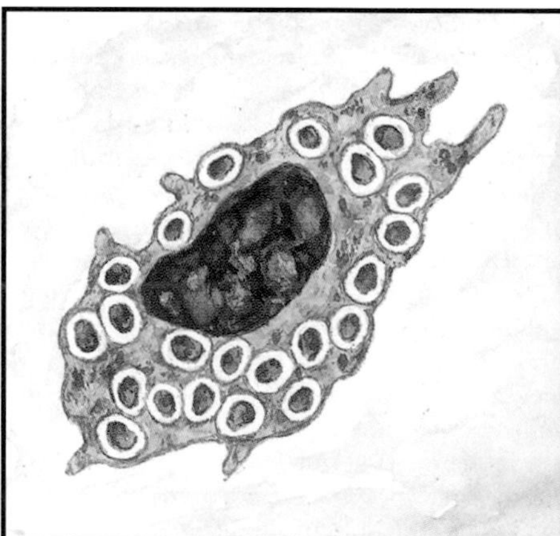

H. capsulatum in a macrophage. In this yeast or tissue phase, organism is not transmissible from person to person

HISTOPLASMOSIS

Histoplasmosis is caused by inhalation of spores of the fungus *Histoplasma capsulatum*. The organism exists widely in nature and is found throughout the United States but is most common in the St. Lawrence and Missouri–Ohio–Mississippi River valleys. It also exists in most of the river valleys throughout the world between the 45th parallel north and the 45th parallel south. Droppings of bats and birds seem to provide in their excreta the essential elements favoring sporulation of the fungus in soil. Therefore, sites commonly associated with exposure to *H. capsulatum* include chicken coops, caves, abandoned buildings, bird roost sites, and wood lots. Activities associated with exposure include excavation, construction, demolition, wood cutting and gathering, and exploring caves. However, in most cases, patients recall no such exposure or only do so when specifically questioned.

Infections with *H. capsulatum* are extremely common; it has been estimated that up to 50 million people in the United States have been infected, and up to 500,000 new infections occur each year. The outcome of acute infection depends on the inoculum size, presence of underlying lung disease, general immune status, and specific immunity to *H. capsulatum*. In more than 95% of cases, the infection is subclinical. In some, the disease may manifest in the form of a flulike syndrome or a mild or severe pneumonia, which is usually self-limited and often undiagnosed. This illness usually presents as a subacute pulmonary infection weeks to months after exposure. Symptoms are usually mild, and radiographs typically show focal infiltrates and mediastinal or hilar lymphadenopathy. Symptoms typically resolve within several weeks, but fatigue and asthenia may persist for months.

With an acute heavy exposure, diffuse reticulonodular or miliary infiltrates are seen, and the infection can progress to respiratory failure or progressive extrapulmonary dissemination. In patients with underlying lung disease, the pulmonary disease can become chronic and progressive and closely simulates cavitary tuberculosis. Chronic disease can also present as broncholithiasis, mediastinal granuloma, and fibrosing mediastinitis. On even rarer occasions, primarily in immunosuppressed patients (e.g., HIV, transplantation, tumor necrosis factor-α inhibitor treatment) or those at extremes of age, *H. capsulatum* may disseminate acutely throughout the body to the bone marrow, skin, liver, spleen, meninges, and alimentary tract. In addition, chronic progressive disseminated histoplasmosis occurs rarely in older immunocompetent adults.

Other pulmonary manifestations of histoplasmosis may include a single small pulmonary density with unilateral hilar lymphadenopathy identical to the Ghon complex; a single nodule or coin lesion, which may

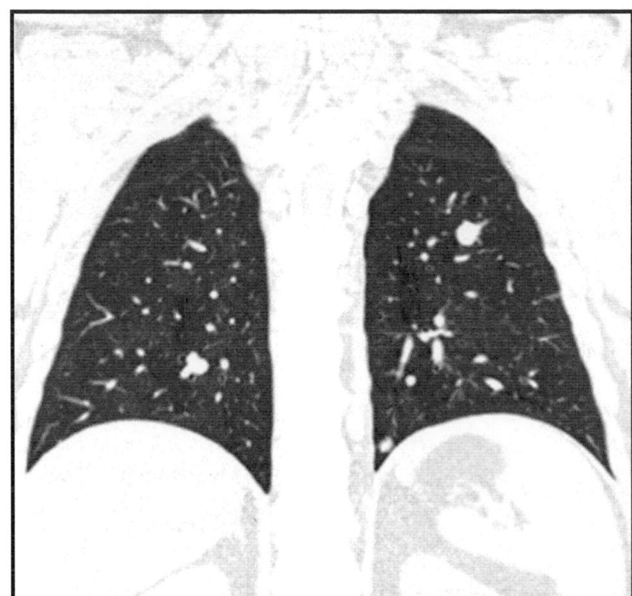

Coronal CT reconstruction at lung windows shows bilateral pulmonary nodules

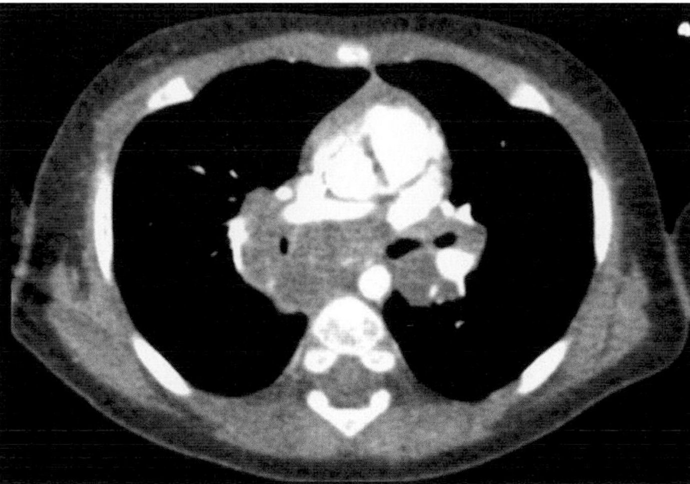

Axial reconstruction from contrast-enhanced CT at the level of the carina shows bulky bilateral hilar and subcarinal lymphadenopathy

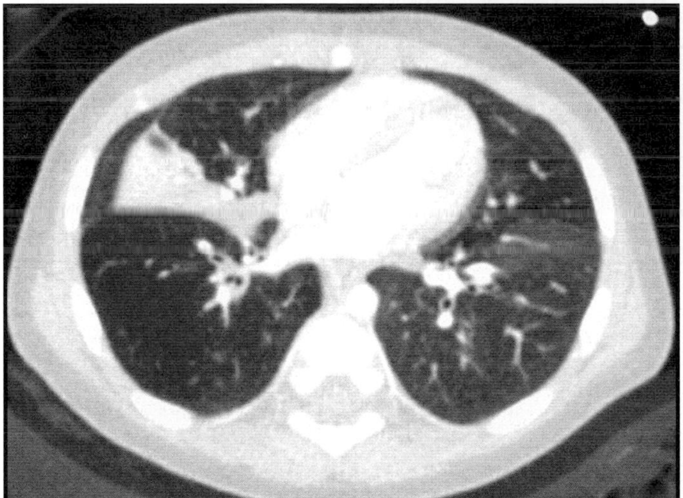

CT scan at lung windows shows atelectasis of the middle lobe likely caused by extrinsic compression of the bronchus by the enlarged nodes

HISTOPLASMOSIS *(Continued)*

simulate a bronchogenic carcinoma; multiple pulmonary nodules simulating metastatic tumor; pleural effusions; mediastinal lymphadenopathy simulating lymphoma; and bilateral hilar adenopathy simulating sarcoidosis.

When the spores from the free-living mycelial phase of *H. capsulatum* gain entry into the body, they convert to the tissue or yeast phase. These appear in tissues and respiratory secretions as intracellular, encapsulated organisms that are ovoid and 3 to 5 μm in diameter that demonstrate narrow-based budding. Accompanying histopathologic findings include granulomas, lymphohistiocytic aggregates, and diffuse mononuclear cell infiltrates.

Diagnosis relies on a combination of histopathology, cultures, antigen detection (in respiratory specimens and urine), and serologic tests (including complement fixation and immunodiffusion). In acute diffuse pulmonary disease, antigen tests and cultures are useful, although serology results are often negative. In acute localized pulmonary disease, serology is often positive, but fungal detection is more difficult. In chronic pulmonary disease, serology and culture results are often positive. Bronchoscopy to obtain adequate respiratory specimens is often required, and on occasion, lymph node or lung biopsy is necessary for diagnosis.

Treatment is indicated for cases of acute pneumonia that are unusually severe, for chronic progressive pulmonary disease, and for disseminated histoplasmosis. Other forms of histoplasmosis require specific treatment only if progression is demonstrated.

TREATMENT

Patients with mild to moderate histoplasmosis are treated with itraconazole, although amphotericin B is indicated for moderately severe and severe infections, especially for initial treatment. Concomitant use of systemic corticosteroids for 1 to 2 weeks is helpful in acute severe disease manifesting as acute respiratory distress syndrome. The duration of antifungal treatment is usually 6 to 12 weeks.

Itraconazole for 18 to 24 months has been successful in the treatment of patients with chronic pulmonary histoplasmosis. After completion of successful treatment, relapse occurs in 10% to 20% of patients over 5 years. Therefore, these patients should be carefully followed during this period. In disseminated disease, severely ill patients should be initially treated with amphotericin B followed by itraconazole for at least 1 year. Less severely ill patients may be treated from the beginning with itraconazole.

COCCIDIOIDOMYCOSIS

Coccidioidomycosis is infection by the dimorphic fungi *Coccidioides immitis* and *Coccidioides posadasii*. *Coccidioides* spp. are endemic to the deserts of the southwestern United States and parts of Mexico and Central and South America. Clinical disease ranges from self-limited pneumonia (valley fever) to disseminated disease, especially in immunosuppressed patients.

Coccidioides spp. grow in the mycelial phase a few inches below the surface of the desert soil. With dry conditions, the mycelia fracture into highly infectious single-cell spores (arthroconidia), 3 to 5 μ in size, that can remain suspended in the air for prolonged periods. On inhalation, an arthroconidium greatly enlarges into a yeastlike spherule, in which endospores evolve. Rupture of mature spherules releases endospores into the infected tissue; each endospore is potentially capable of producing another spherule.

Among persons living in endemic areas, the risk of exposure to *Coccidioides* spp. is approximately 3% per year, with a seasonal pattern, typically highest in dry periods after a rainy season. Infections may also occur in individuals simply passing through an endemic area. Southern Arizona and California account for 90% of the infections seen in the United States. The increase in population in these areas has resulted in increased rates of new infections to 150,000 per year. Infections are subclinical in more than half with only later development of delayed cutaneous hypersensitivity to coccidioidin.

Clinically significant illness can present subacutely, known as valley fever, with respiratory and systemic symptoms often lasting for weeks to months. The most frequent clinical manifestation is community-acquired pneumonia with an incubation period of 1 to 3 weeks. The most common presenting symptoms are chest pain, cough, fever, and fatigue. Arthralgias, erythema nodosum, and erythema multiforme occur occasionally, and hemoptysis suggests the development of cavitary disease.

Chest radiographs may be unremarkable in up to 50% of all patients, even in those with respiratory complaints. Common abnormalities include unilateral or bilateral infiltrates and ipsilateral hilar adenopathy. Less frequently, mediastinal adenopathy and pleural effusion are seen. The primary pneumonitis usually clears spontaneously, leaving a residual nodule or a peripheral thin-walled cavity in about 5% of cases. Dissemination is seen in about 1% of patients to any organ but most commonly skin, bones and joints, and the central nervous system. Risk factors for complicated pulmonary disease and dissemination include defects in cellular immunity, as in HIV infection, organ transplantation, or with high-dose glucocorticoids. Pregnant women, especially during the third trimester, and individuals of African or Philippine descent are at increased risk of dissemination. Diabetes mellitus has been associated with slowly resolving pulmonary infection and residual cavitation.

The diagnosis of coccidioidomycosis is often missed because of the nonspecific clinical presentation and because the diagnosis is not considered. Early specific diagnosis is important because it reduces unnecessary diagnostic testing, inappropriate antibiotic use, and morbidity from progressive pulmonary or disseminated disease. An absolute diagnosis requires isolation of *Coccidioides* spp. in culture from respiratory samples; however, growth may take several days to weeks. The propagation of *Coccidioides* spp. in the clinical laboratory represents a significant health risk to laboratory personnel, who should be notified when a sample with suspected *Coccidioides* spp. is sent for processing. Serologic tests are reliable for the diagnosis of coccidioidomycosis except sometimes early in the disease and in immunocompromised hosts. An immunodiffusion assay that detects serum IgG and IgM antibodies to *Coccidioides* spp. is the most commonly used test, although complement fixation assays are used for testing other body fluids such as cerebrospinal fluid. Most patients lose serologic reactivity within months of an infection, so sustained reactivity indicates residual lesions or active infection. Serial serologic testing is therefore useful to document resolution.

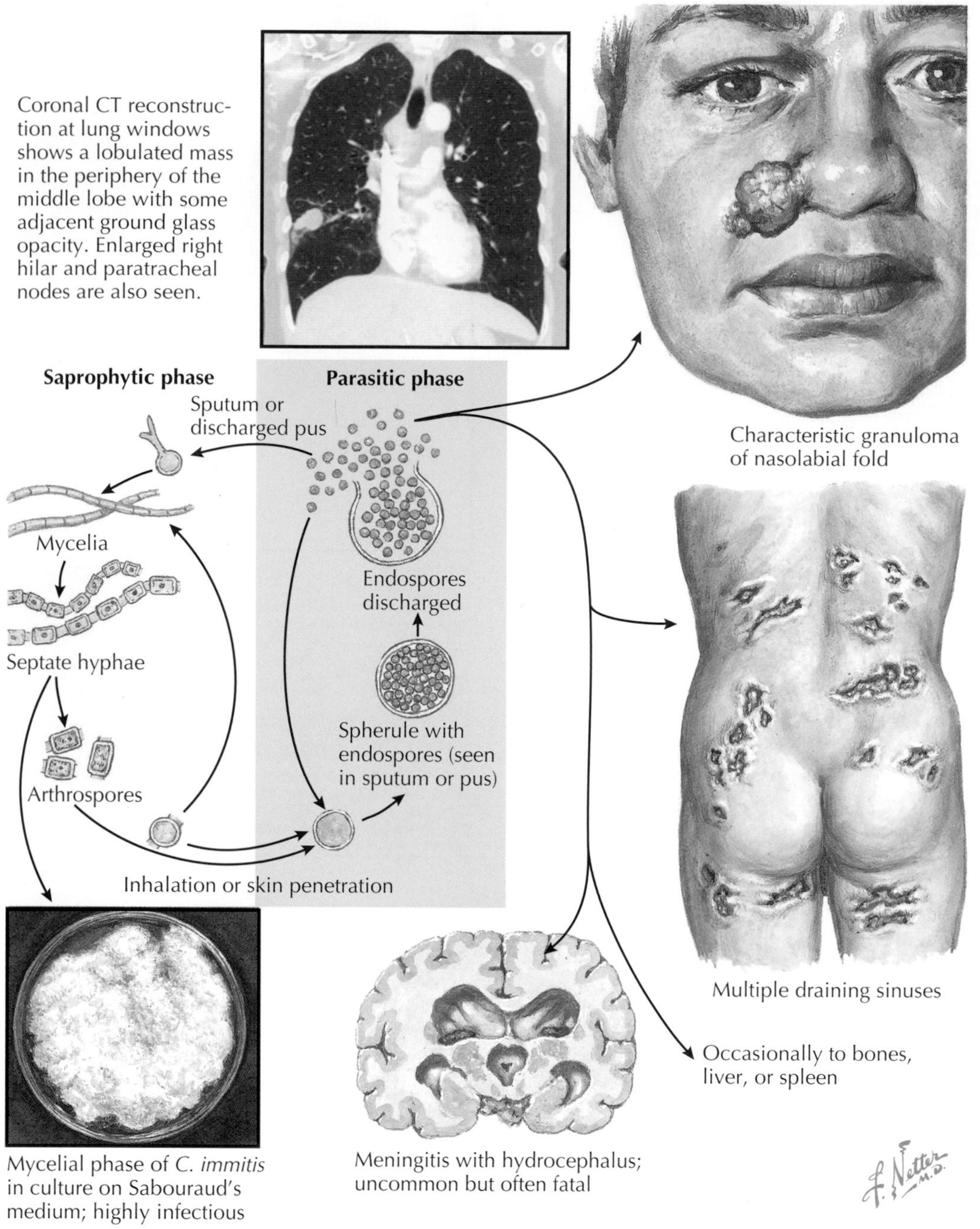

TREATMENT

Most patients with uncomplicated pulmonary coccidioidomycosis resolve their infection without specific antifungal treatment. However, such treatment might benefit some patients, either by shortening the course or by preventing complications. Because of lack of adequate trial data, clinical judgment is used in identifying these patients. Commonly used indicators for treatment include symptoms persisting for more than 2 months, more than 10% loss of body weight, night sweats persisting for more than 3 weeks, inability to work, extensive unilateral or bilateral lung infiltrates, prominent or persistent hilar adenopathy, and complement fixing antibody titers above 1:16. Treatment is also indicated in patients at risk for or manifesting complicated pulmonary or disseminated disease.

Azole therapy with ketoconazole, fluconazole, or itraconazole for 3 to 6 months is the usual regimen. The latter two agents are better tolerated. Posaconazole and voriconazole may have a role in refractory cases. Intravenous amphotericin B is reserved for rapidly progressive cases or with infection at vital sites such as the spine. After discontinuation of treatment, close follow-up is necessary because of a substantial rate of relapse in up to one-third of patients.

Blastomycosis

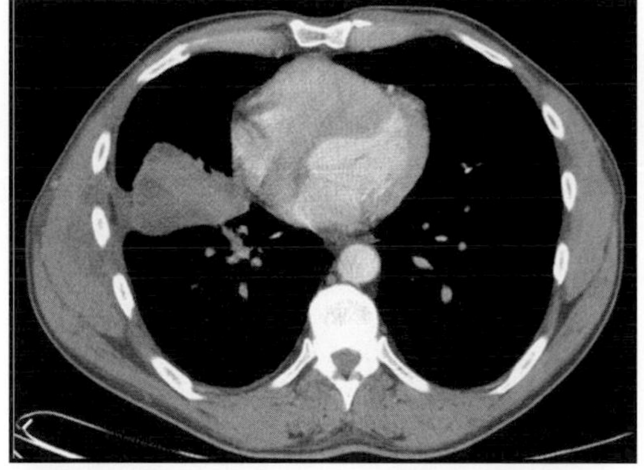

Contrast-enhanced CT scan through the mid-heart shows masslike consolidation in the middle lobe with peripheral necrosis and adjacent pleural thickening

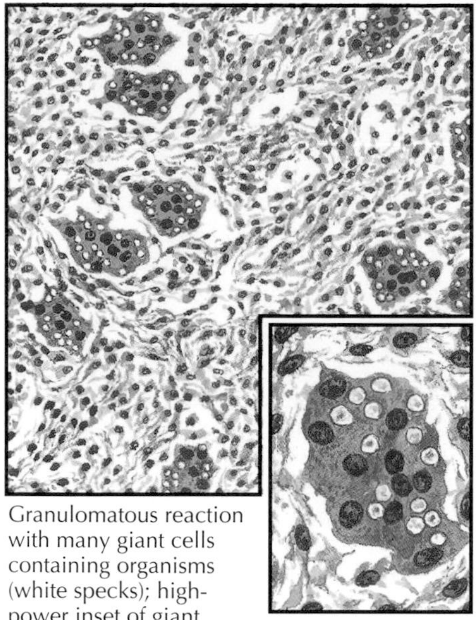

Granulomatous reaction with many giant cells containing organisms (white specks); high-power inset of giant cell with organisms

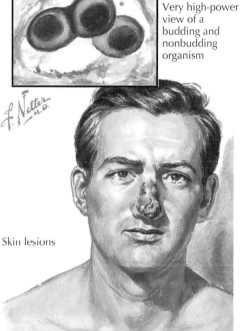

Very high-power view of a budding and nonbudding organism

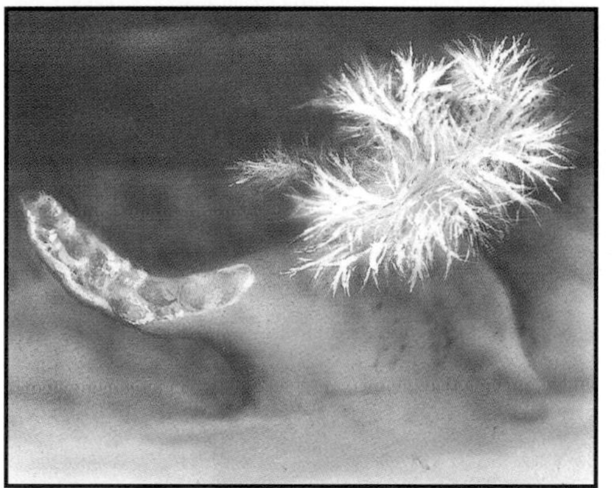

Organism in culture: free-living or infectious phase of *Blastomyces dermatitidis*

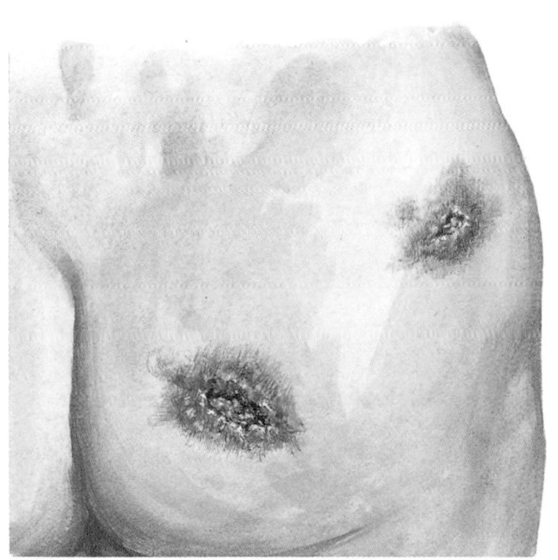

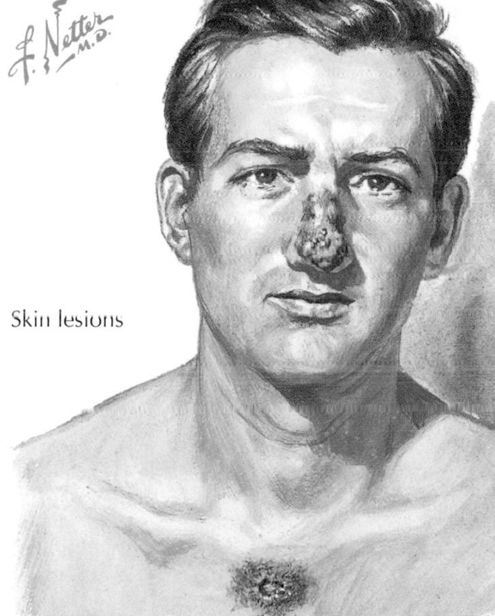

Skin lesions

Blastomycosis is a systemic pyogranulomatous infection primarily involving the lungs that is caused by inhalation of the infective spores of the diphasic fungus *Blastomyces dermatitidis*. The organism exists in soil or on forest vegetation in a mycelial form. When the spores (conidia) from the mycelial growth gain entry into the body, usually by inhalation or rarely by direct inoculation, the organism converts into a yeast form. The yeast phase is found in infected tissue, pus, sputum, or other body exudates and is noninfective. The yeast cells are multinucleate, usually 8 to 15 mm in diameter, and are characterized by a thick refractile cell wall and reproduction is by a single broad-based bud.

The ecologic niche for *Blastomyces* spp. is soil containing decaying vegetation or decomposed wood, with humid conditions fostering its growth. Consequently, a common factor associated with both endemic and epidemic disease is exposure to soil, whether related to work or recreation. Blastomycosis occurs primarily in North America, principally in the Mississippi—Ohio River valleys, the Midwestern states, and in regions bordering the Great Lakes and St. Lawrence River. After North America, blastomycosis has been reported most frequently in Africa, and occasional cases have been identified in Mexico, Central and South America, India, and the Middle East.

In contrast to the conidia, the yeast forms of *B. dermatitidis* are more resistant to phagocytosis and killing by polymorphonuclear leukocytes, monocytes, and alveolar macrophages. Conversion to a yeast form likely contributes to infection and persistence of *Blastomyces* spp., and the capsule and Bad-1, a 120-kd glycoprotein, are major virulence factors expressed in this form.

The major acquired host defense against *B. dermatitidis* is cellular immunity, although humoral (specific antibody)-mediated immunity does not appear to confer resistance to or hasten clinical recovery. A variety of *Blastomyces* antigens are targets of antigen-specific T lymphocytes and lymphokine-activated macrophages after clinical infection.

Blastomycosis can present as a pulmonary disease, multiple organ involvement (disseminated), or less commonly as extrapulmonary disease only. The incidence of the latter two has declined with the availability of effective therapy to about 18% of patients. Blastomyces lung infection can be an asymptomatic or manifest as acute or chronic pneumonia. Hematogenous dissemination frequently occurs; extrapulmonary disease of the skin, bones, and genitourinary system is common, but almost any organ can be infected, including the central nervous system (CNS).

Acute pneumonia with *B. dermatitidis* infection resembles influenza or a bacterial pneumonia. Chronic infection presents as a chronic pneumonia or a potential malignancy. Radiographic manifestations are those of pneumonitis, large and small nodules or masses, cavitation, and diffuse miliary patterns. Lesions may be unilateral or bilateral and involve any or all lobes of the lungs. They may closely simulate a bronchogenic carcinoma in appearance as well as tuberculosis and other pulmonary disorders.

The diagnosis of blastomycosis is made by demonstrating the presence of the causative organism in the patient's sputum, bronchoscopic specimens, urine, other exudates, or body tissue. Direct visualization of the organism in cytologic and histologic specimens can provide a rapid diagnosis. For pulmonary blastomycosis, direct examination of respiratory specimens is 50% to 90% sensitive, and culture yields the diagnosis in 86% to 100% of cases. Serologic tests are unhelpful; however, an antigen detection test for body fluids has promise.

Treatment

Although occasional patients with mild to moderate pulmonary blastomycosis can undergo spontaneous cure, most patients need specific treatment. Both amphotericin B and the azole drugs are active against *B. dermatitidis*. Considerations for treatment include the severity of disease, CNS involvement, and the immune competence of the patient. If severe disease, CNS involvement, or immunosuppression is present, intravenous amphotericin B is recommended, preferably as the lipid formulation, for 1 to 2 weeks or until improvement is observed, followed by oral itraconazole for a total 12-month duration of treatment. In mild to moderate disease in an immunocompetent patient without CNS involvement, therapy can be started with oral itraconazole, and the duration can vary between 6 to 12 months. Other azoles, such as fluconazole (high dose) and voriconazole, can also be used if itraconazole is not tolerated or when the CNS is involved because the latter drug has poor CNS penetration. If the patient does not respond to azole therapy, it should be switched to amphotericin B. Adequately treated patients have low relapse rates of less than 10%.

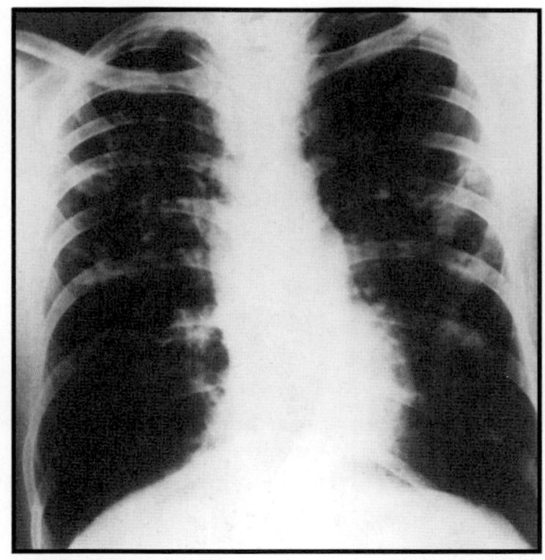

Bilateral pulmonary infiltrates that closely resemble tuberculosis. Pulmonary lesions may range from minimal to very extensive

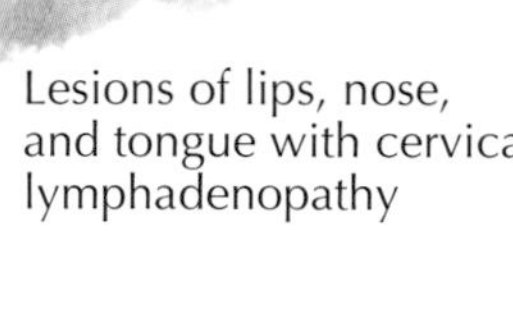

Lesions of lips, nose, and tongue with cervical lymphadenopathy

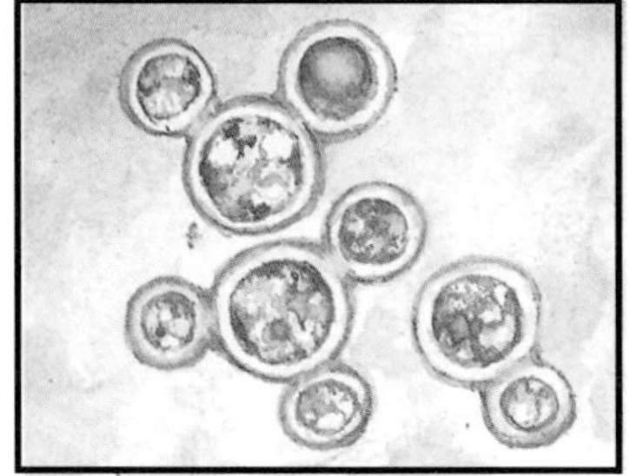

Yeast phase of *P. brasiliensis* in fresh unstained sputum prepared with 10% NaOH, showing double walls with single and multiple budding

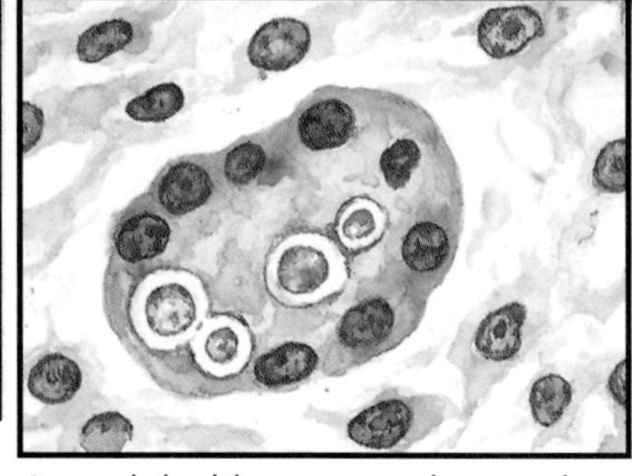

Several double-contoured yeast-phase cells with single buds in a giant cell from skin lesion

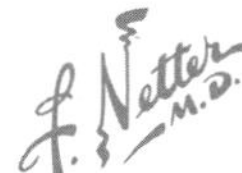

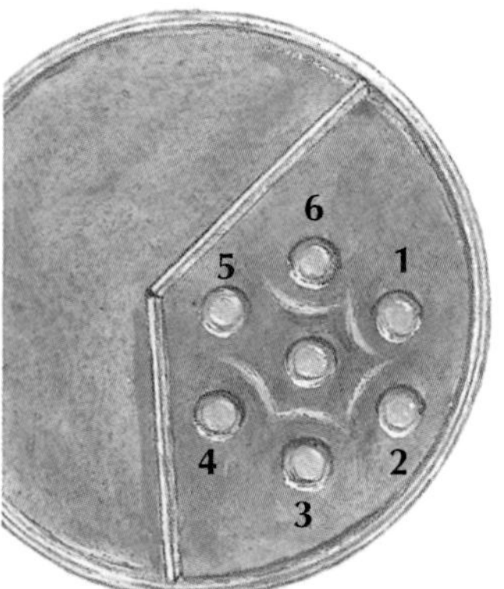

Precipitin test. Antigen in central well, serum from five different patients in peripheral wells showing precipitin bands. Wells 4 and 5 from same patient before and after treatment evidencing response

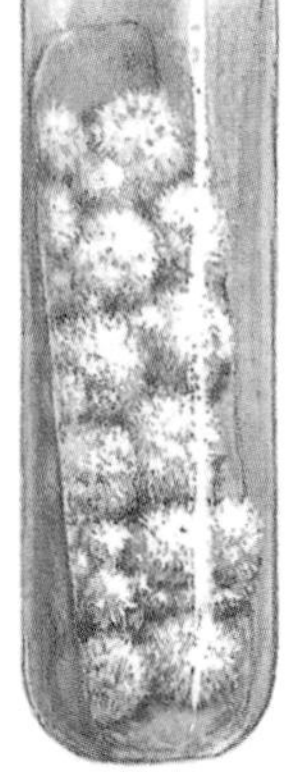

Mycelial colonies of *P. brasiliensis* grown on Sabouraud medium at room temperature. Downy appearance due to filamentous hyphae with intercalate or terminal chlamydospores

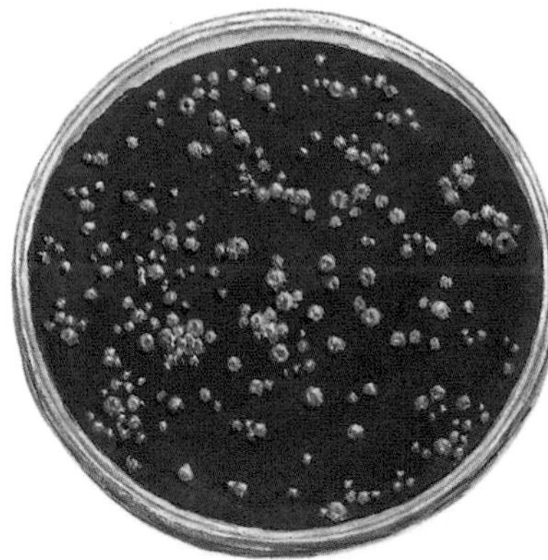

Colonies of yeast form of *P. brasiliensis*, grown on blood agar at 37°C

PARACOCCIDIOIDOMYCOSIS

Paracoccidioidomycosis, formerly known as South American blastomycosis, is caused by inhalation of the spores of a thermally dimorphic fungus, *Paracoccidioides brasiliensis*. The organism lives in soil or on vegetable matter in a mycelial form and can be cultured in this phase on Sabouraud glucose agar at room temperature. After gaining entry into the body, the fungus is transformed into a yeast, which reproduces itself by the formation of multiple buds. However, organisms with single buds are also observed. The yeast form of the fungus can be cultured on blood agar at 37°C but is not infectious.

The disease is limited geographically to Latin America, from Mexico to Argentina, with 80% of the cases occurring in Brazil. Even in an endemic country, the disease is not distributed homogeneously, likely reflecting environmental conditions that favor fungal growth. Because the chronic form of the disease may have a very long incubation period (≥30 years), cases have been detected in former residents of areas where it is endemic after they have lived for years in Europe or the United States. Under these circumstances, the disease has often been confused initially with tuberculosis or other mycoses.

Soil is the likely natural habitat of *P. brasiliensis*, which relates to a high incidence of agricultural or construction exposure in patients with this infection. Children account for less than 10% of the cases with no gender predilection, but in adults, a striking male predominance, as high as 15 : 1, is seen. Smoking appears to be a risk factor for disease in adults.

Clinical presentations of the disease include a chronic "adult" form in the majority, an acute-subacute "juvenile" form in 15% to 20%, and a recently described acute disseminated form in HIV-positive patients. The latter two presentations occur in younger individuals and mainly involve the reticuloendothelial system with little pulmonary manifestations. The chronic form usually occurs in individuals 40 to 60 years of age and is almost always a multifocal disease with predominant pulmonary involvement. Pulmonary symptoms of dyspnea, cough, and sputum are chronic and nonspecific. Often on physical examination, abnormalities are lacking despite significant radiologic findings. Chest radiographs usually show bilateral, symmetric alveolointerstitial or interstitial infiltrates in the lower and central lung zones, sparing the apices, with occasional areas of small cavitations. High-resolution computed tomography scans show a variety of findings, including ground-glass attenuation, nodules, cavitated nodules, interlobular septal thickening, and architectural distortion. After treatment, residual fibrosis is seen in 50% and bullous disease in 25% of patients.

Lesions of the upper airway mucous membranes (oropharyngeal, laryngeal, and nasal) are common in paracoccidioidomycosis. They are painful, hyperemic, and covered with small hemorrhagic dots (mulberry-like) and tend to be progressive and destructive. Draining (submental and cervical) lymph nodes are often enlarged. Dissemination to the skin, bones, adrenal glands, central nervous system, gastrointestinal tract, and gonads may occur with corresponding clinical manifestations.

Definitive diagnosis depends on demonstration of the causative organism by direct visualization in infected tissues as 6- to 40-μm yeast cells with multiple buds or by isolation in culture. Antibody and antigen detection tests are helpful adjuncts to diagnosis and guides to prognosis and therapeutic response.

TREATMENT

The azoles, specifically itraconazole, are the treatment of choice for this infection, with a 95% response rate with a 6-month course. Although sulfonamides, especially trimethoprim/sulfamethoxazole, are effective for paracoccidioidomycosis, these agents must be administered for very long periods (≤3 years), and relapse is frequent. Amphotericin B should be reserved for critically ill patients.

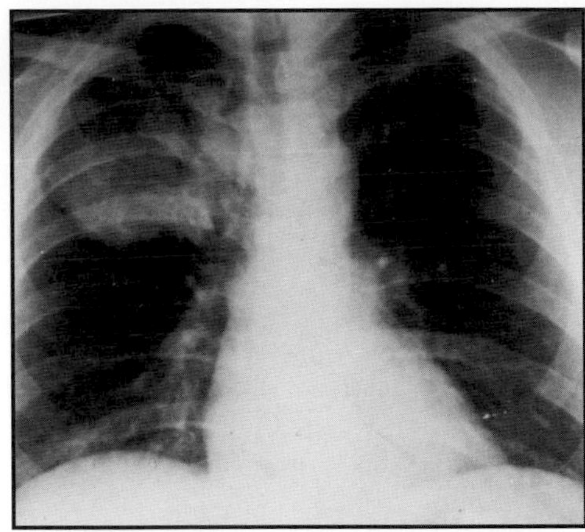

Pulmonary cryptococcosis presenting as a large masslike lesion, easily mistaken for carcinoma

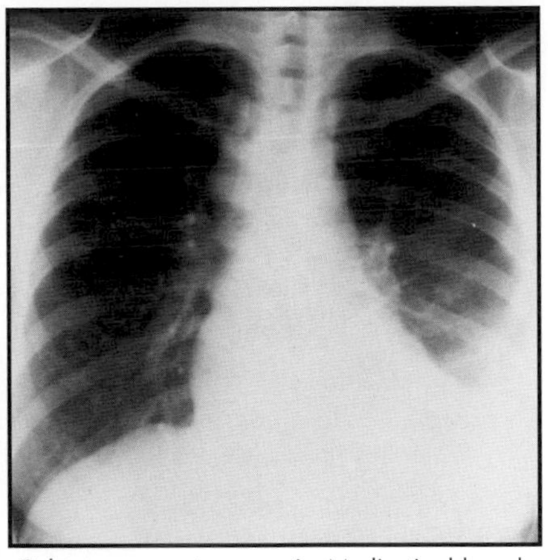

Pulmonary cryptococcosis. Mediastinal lymph nodes enlarged and pleural effusion on left

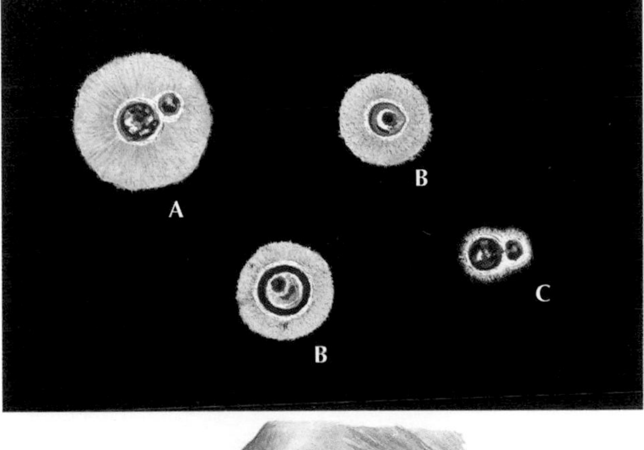

India ink preparation showing *C. neoformans*

A. Budding organism with thick capsule

B. Nonbudding organisms

C. Unencapsulated form (budding)

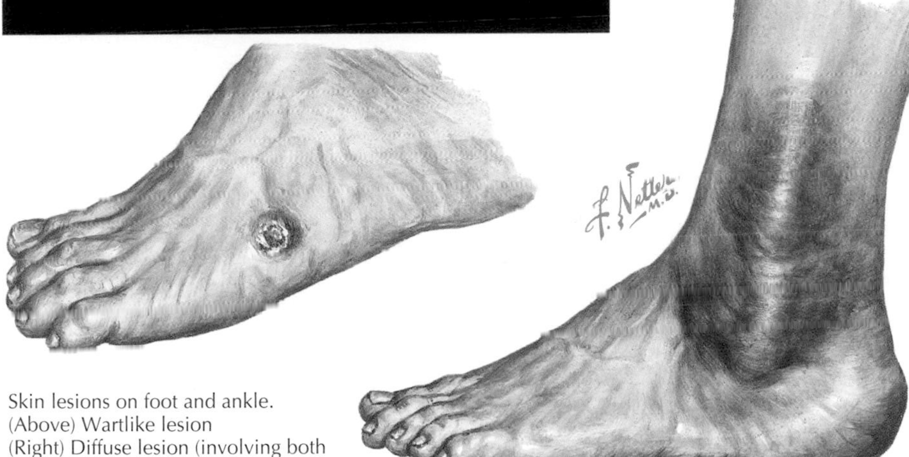

Skin lesions on foot and ankle.
(Above) Wartlike lesion
(Right) Diffuse lesion (involving both medial and lateral aspects of limb)

CRYPTOCOCCOSIS

Cryptococcosis is caused by the closely related, budding, yeastlike fungi *Cryptococcus neoformans* and *Cryptococcus gattii*. *Cryptococcus* is a uniphasic fungus that does not exist in a mycelial form. *Cryptococcus neoformans* has a worldwide distribution in rotting vegetation as well as in soil contaminated by pigeon excreta. However, pigeon exposure does not play an important role in the epidemiology of this infection. It is likely that both humans and pigeons get exposed to this fungus through exposure to rotting vegetation, and the latter act as carriers of the fungus in their gastrointestinal tracts. Most infections in immunocompromised hosts are caused by *C. neoformans*. *C. gattii* has been associated with certain varieties of Eucalyptus trees in Australia and other parts of the world and with other tree varieties in Vancouver Island in Canada. Almost all *C. gattii* infections are seen in immunocompetent hosts.

Cryptococcus spp. probably gain entry into the body through the lungs, by inhalation of the basidiospore form of this fungus. Basidiospores are smaller than the yeast form that facilitates deposition in the alveoli and terminal bronchioles after inhalation. From the lungs, the fungus can disseminate to all organs. Although the lung is the initial site of infection, it is the second most clinically relevant site of infection after the central nervous system (CNS). After inhalation, *C. neoformans* causes a small focal granulomatous pneumonitis; the vast majority of these are clinically and radiographically silent. However, in a manner similar to tuberculosis, these foci of yeasts can persist in a latent stage and cause active infection later if the host immune system becomes compromised.

The thick polysaccharide capsule of *C. neoformans* has antiphagocytic properties and is an important virulence determinant. In the laboratory, the capsule can be visualized as a clear area in a suspension of India ink when examined under a microscope. Another important virulence factor is the enzyme phenol oxidase, which is also unique to *C. neoformans* and can be used for laboratory identification.

Some immunocompetent patients can have symptomatic infection, which may be related to infection with a large inoculum or a virulent strain. These patients usually present with cough, sputum, chest pain, fever, weight loss, and hemoptysis. Chest radiographic findings can vary widely, including solitary or multiple nodules, pneumonic infiltrates, hilar and mediastinal adenopathy, and pleural effusion. Diagnosis is made by visualization of the characteristic encapsulated yeast forms in sputum, bronchoalveolar lavage, or tissue specimens and culture of the organism from these same specimens. Serum cryptococcal antigen is rarely positive and suggests disseminated disease and a need for sampling the cerebrospinal fluid.

Immunocompromised patients represent the majority of cases with cryptococcosis. Reactivation of latent infection is the most likely mechanism of infection, but new infections are also possible. Underlying conditions include HIV infection, malignancies, stem cell and organ transplantation, chronic liver, kidney or lung disease, diabetes, sarcoidosis, sickle cell disease, treatment with systemic corticosteroids, or tumor necrosis factor antagonists. In non–HIV-infected patients, symptoms and radiographs resemble the disease seen in immunocompetent patients, but dyspnea and disseminated disease are more common.

In HIV-infected patents, the pulmonary infection is more acute and severe, and the majority of these patients have CNS involvement. These patients usually have interstitial infiltrates, but alveolar infiltrates, mass lesions, adenopathy, and pleural effusions are also seen. Co-infection with other opportunistic pathogens has been described in HIV-infected patients. Diagnosis relies on microscopy and culture of respiratory secretions or tissue. Serum cryptococcal antigen results are positive in the majority of these patients. CNS involvement should always be assessed in these patients.

TREATMENT

With the exception of immunocompetent asymptomatic patients with a negative serum cryptococcal antigen result, treatment of cryptococcosis is indicated. Asymptomatic patients with positive serum antigen test results should be treated as having mild to moderate disease to prevent symptomatic systemic dissemination. For mild to moderate pulmonary disease in immunocompetent patients, oral fluconazole or itraconazole for 6 to 12 months is indicated. In patients with extensive multiorgan disease or CNS involvement, intravenous amphotericin B and flucytosine is indicated as induction therapy for 2 to 3 weeks followed by oral fluconazole. The same treatment approach is recommended for all immunocompromised patients with cryptococcal infection because the induction therapy is fungicidal. Prognosis is generally good with current treatment of cryptococcosis.

ASPERGILLOSIS

Constantly a part of the natural environment, fungi of the genus *Aspergillus* usually coexist with humans in harmless symbiosis. In special circumstances, however, some species are an opportunistic pathogen in humans. "Aspergillosis" is actually a spectrum of diverse disorders that include illnesses caused by allergy, colonization, or tissue invasion by *Aspergillus* spp., including *Aspergillus fumigatus*, *Aspergillus flavus*, *Aspergillus terreus*, *Aspergillus niger*, *Aspergillus versicolor*, and others.

ALLERGIC BRONCHOPULMONARY ASPERGILLOSIS

Allergic bronchopulmonary aspergillosis (ABPA) is a complex hypersensitivity reaction to bronchial colonization with *Aspergillus* spp. seen in patients with asthma or cystic fibrosis. The clinical picture is of the underlying disease with superimposed recurrent episodes of bronchial obstruction, fever, malaise, expectoration of brownish mucous plugs, peripheral blood eosinophilia, and at times hemoptysis. Major diagnostic criteria for ABPA include a history of asthma or cystic fibrosis, immediate skin test reactivity to *Aspergillus* antigens, precipitating serum antibodies to *A. fumigatus*, serum total IgE concentration greater than 1000 ng/mL, peripheral blood eosinophilia greater than 500/mL, lung infiltrates on chest radiography or chest computed tomography (CT), central bronchiectasis on chest CT, and elevated specific serum IgE and IgG to *A. fumigatus*.

Oral corticosteroids are the mainstay of treatment of acute flares of ABPA. In patients requiring frequent or chronic corticosteroids, itraconazole for 3 to 6 months can reduce the steroid dosage and improve clinical response.

ASPERGILLOMA

Aspergilli often colonize a preexisting lung cavity and form an intracavity aspergilloma or fungus ball. The cavity may be the result of tuberculosis, lung abscess, carcinoma, emphysematous cyst, histoplasmosis, sarcoidosis, bronchiectasis, or other conditions. Colonized cavities are more common in the upper lobes, and radiographic findings are highly characteristic, showing a rounded mass within the dependent portion of the cavity, which is capped with a meniscus of air. The mass moves within the cavity as body position is altered. CT scan and magnetic resonance imaging can be helpful to better define the cavity and presence of parenchymal invasion. The aspergilloma is composed of fungal hyphae, inflammatory cells, fibrin, mucus, and amorphous debris. In most cases, the fungal hyphae do not invade the cavitary wall but apparently produce enough irritation in some cases to cause mild or severe hemorrhage. The finding of a mass within a pulmonary cavity and the recovery of *Aspergillus* spp. from multiple sputum cultures are strongly supportive of the diagnosis of aspergilloma.

Aspergillomas can be asymptomatic; however, hemoptysis occurs in 75% of patients. If bleeding is severe, frequent, or life endangering, treatment is indicated. Surgical removal of the fungus ball and cavity is the preferred mode of treatment. In inoperable patients, oral azole (itraconazole, voriconazole, or posaconazole) treatment or intracavity amphotericin B instillation can be of value.

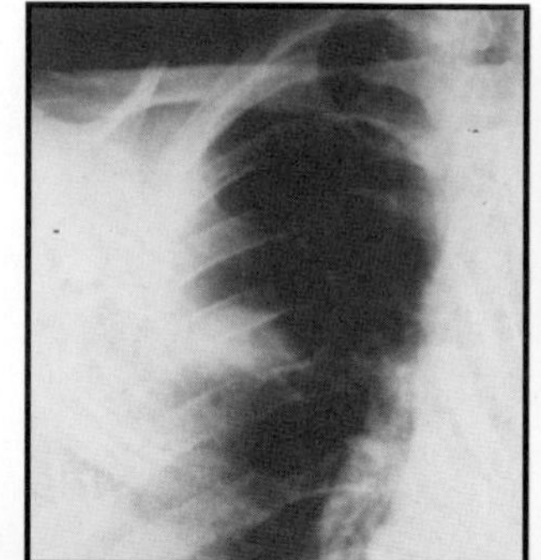

Film showing an asperigilloma within a cavity in right lung

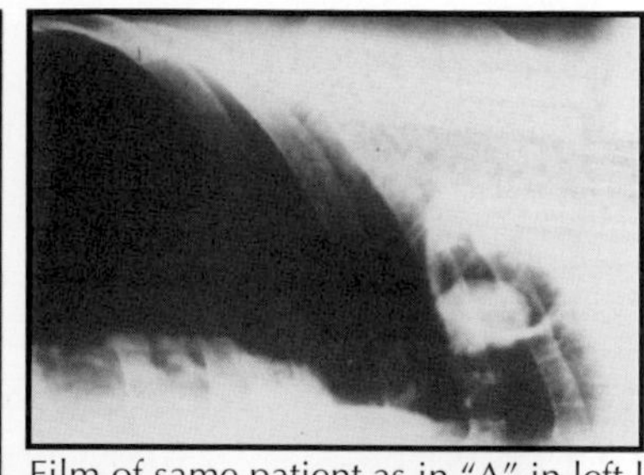

Film of same patient as in "A" in left lateal decubitus positon, demonstrating shift of fungus ball to dependent portion of cavity

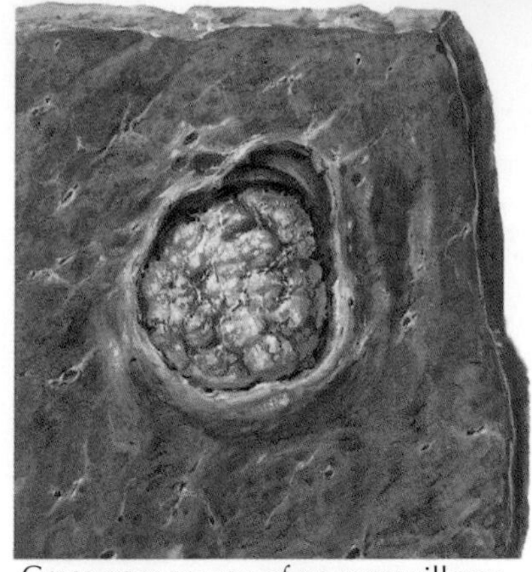

Gross appearance of an aspergilloma in a chronic lung cavity

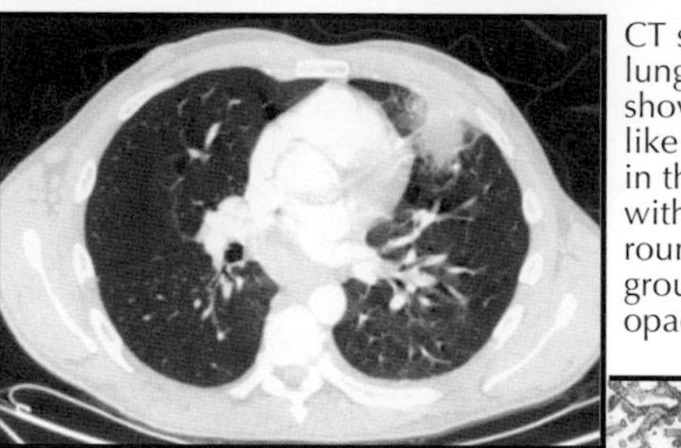

CT scan at lung windows shows mass-like opacity in the lingula with surrounding ground glass opacity

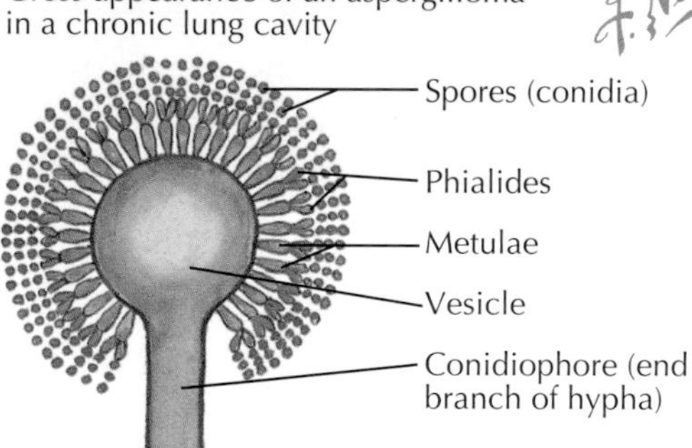

Structure of fruiting form of *Aspergillus niger*. Other species of *Aspergillus* vary in configuration but general structure is similar

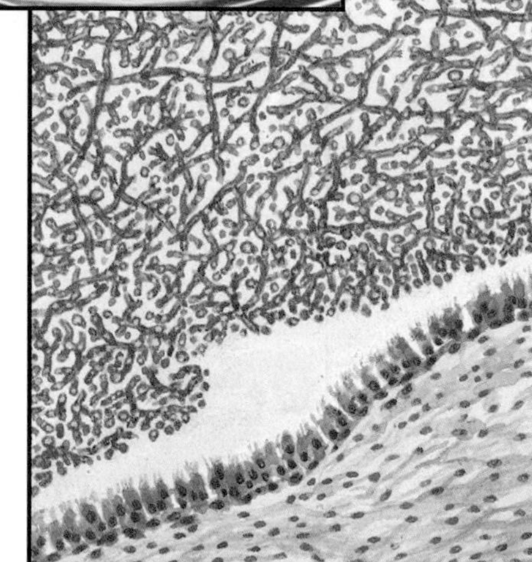

Microscopic structure of an aspergilloma composed of a tangled mass of hyphae within a dilated bronchus. No evidence of tissue invasion

INVASIVE ASPERGILLOSIS

Immunosuppression is as a rule seen in patients with invasive aspergillosis, including prolonged and severe neutropenia, glucocorticoid therapy, hematopoietic stem cell and solid organ transplantation, advanced AIDS, and chronic granulomatous disease. Less frequently, invasive aspergillosis occurs in patients with solid tumors and in those who are only mildly immunosuppressed, such as patients with chronic obstructive pulmonary disease who are taking corticosteroids. From the lungs, which are most often involved, generalized dissemination may take place to any site. The course is usually fulminant.

Invasive aspergillosis is characterized by progression of the infection across tissue planes and vascular invasion with subsequent infarction and tissue necrosis. The major manifestation is fever that is unresponsive to broad-spectrum antibiotics; chest pain, cough, and hemoptysis may also be seen. Chest radiology results can be normal but usually show nodular lesions, patchy infiltrates, or cavitary lesions. On CT imaging, nodules surrounded by a ground-glass appearance, the so-called "halo sign," may be seen; this reflects hemorrhage into the tissue surrounding the area of fungal invasion.

In seriously immunocompromised patients, *Aspergillus* infection may disseminate beyond the respiratory tract and clinically manifest as sepsis. Infection of virtually any organ can occur, but most commonly vascular organs such as the kidney, liver, spleen, and central nervous system are involved.

Diagnosis depends on a combination of clinical judgment with demonstration of the fungus in tissue specimens obtained from the presumed site of infection. Serum *Aspergillus* galactomannan and β-D-glucan assays are useful as diagnostic adjuncts.

Treatment of invasive aspergillosis includes attempts to reverse the underlying immunosuppression and medical and surgical therapy. Voriconazole, an azole, has become the initial therapy of choice for patients with invasive aspergillosis. In patients intolerant of voriconazole, a lipid-based formulation of amphotericin B can be used. For patients who do not respond to these first-line agents, combinations of an echinocandin (e.g., caspofungin) with lipidated amphotericin B or voriconazole can be tried. Surgery can be used to débride necrotic tissue and to remove infected tissue in selected patients.

DISSEMINATION OF TUBERCULOSIS

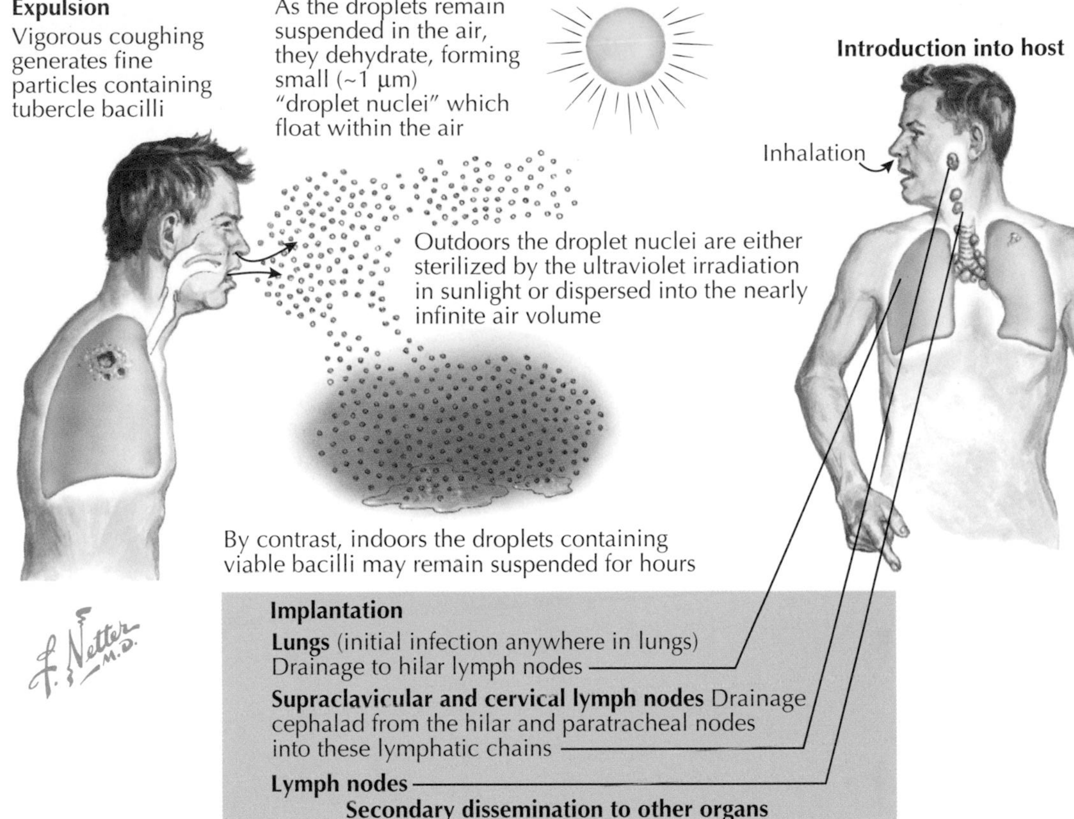

Expulsion
Vigorous coughing generates fine particles containing tubercle bacilli
As the droplets remain suspended in the air, they dehydrate, forming small (~1 µm) "droplet nuclei" which float within the air
Introduction into host
Inhalation
Outdoors the droplet nuclei are either sterilized by the ultraviolet irradiation in sunlight or dispersed into the nearly infinite air volume
By contrast, indoors the droplets containing viable bacilli may remain suspended for hours
Implantation
Lungs (initial infection anywhere in lungs) Drainage to hilar lymph nodes
Supraclavicular and cervical lymph nodes Drainage cephalad from the hilar and paratracheal nodes into these lymphatic chains
Lymph nodes
Secondary dissemination to other organs

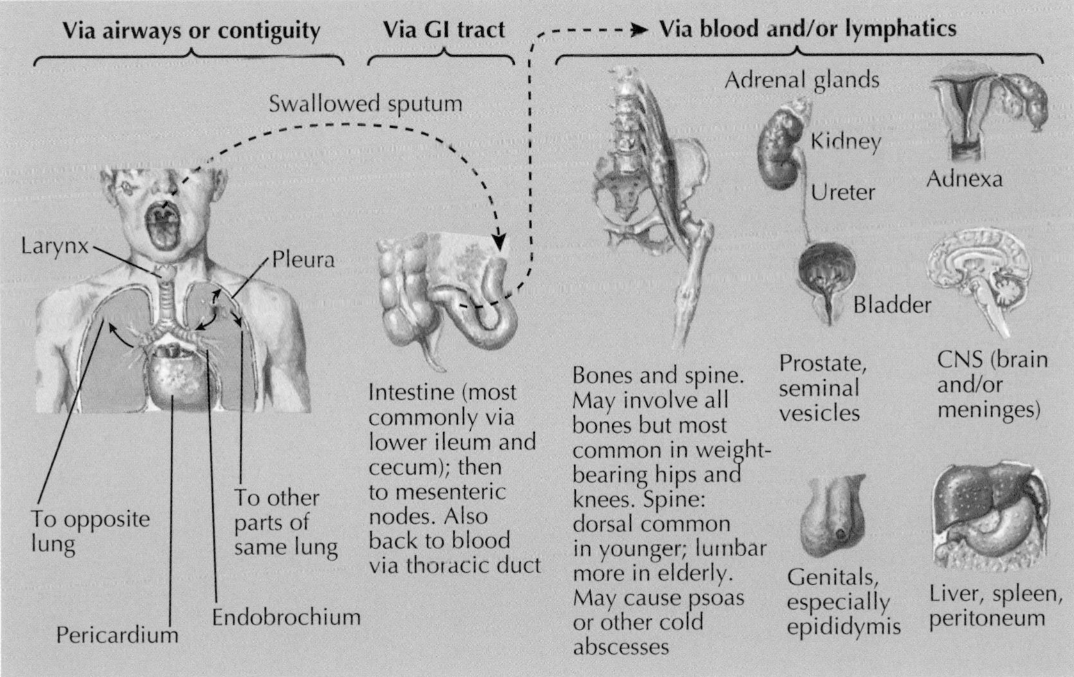

Via airways or contiguity
Via GI tract
Via blood and/or lymphatics
Swallowed sputum
Larynx
Pleura
To opposite lung
To other parts of same lung
Pericardium
Endobrochium
Intestine (most commonly via lower ileum and cecum); then to mesenteric nodes. Also back to blood via thoracic duct
Adrenal glands
Kidney
Ureter
Adnexa
Bladder
Bones and spine. May involve all bones but most common in weight-bearing hips and knees. Spine: dorsal common in younger; lumbar more in elderly. May cause psoas or other cold abscesses
Prostate, seminal vesicles
CNS (brain and/or meninges)
Genitals, especially epididymis
Liver, spleen, peritoneum

TUBERCULOSIS

BACKGROUND

Globally, tuberculosis (TB) remains an immense cause of morbidity and mortality. Approximately one-third of the population, more than 2 billion persons, harbor latent infection with *Mycobacterium tuberculosis*, and 9 million new cases develop annually. Because of delayed diagnosis, lack of access to medications, or nonadherence to prescribed regimens, approximately 1.5 million people die annually of TB.

The progressive appearance of drug-resistant forms of TB has been ominous. Circa 1990, cases of "multidrug resistant tuberculosis" (MDR-TB) were recognized in New York City and Miami, Florida. Strains of TB resistant to the two major drugs, isoniazid (INH) and rifampin (RIF), were associated with hospital-based outbreaks, primarily among persons with AIDS. Similar, highly lethal outbreaks were subsequently recognized around the globe, and by 2007, the World Health Organization estimated that nearly 500,000 new cases of MDR-TB were occurring yearly. More ominously, in 2005 in South Africa, an even more resistant epidemic was noted, extensive drug-resistant TB (XDR-TB). These strains had evolved from MDR-TB and entailed resistance not only to INH and RIF but also to two other major classes of anti-TB drugs, the fluoroquinolones and the second-line injectables such as amikacin, kanamycin, and capreomycin. Cases of XDR-TB have now been reported from 47 nations on all of the continents.

HIV/AIDS has profoundly accelerated case rates and deaths over the past quarter century. The coincidence of TB and AIDS has been most pronounced in sub-Saharan Africa but is increasingly problematic in China, India, Russia, and the former Soviet Republics.

Failure of the TB vaccine, bacillus Calmette-Guérin (BCG), has been a major element of the ongoing epidemic. Although BCG given in infancy does protect against some of the severe forms of childhood TB (meningeal, spinal, or disseminated disease), the vaccine has not curtailed adult pulmonary TB, the vector of ongoing airborne transmission.

In the United States, TB case rates have declined mostly because of the widening use of directly observed therapy (DOT). This practice has increased treatment completion, reduced transmission, and dramatically reduced acquired drug resistance. In 1992 in the United States, when DOT was used in less than 20% of cases, there were nearly 27,000 cases for a rate of 10.4 per 100,000 population, and there were more than 400 MDR-TB cases. By 2007, there were fewer than 14,000 cases, and the rate had fallen to 4.4 per 100K. Notably, 58% of these cases were among foreign-born individuals, the majority of whom brought this infection from their country of origin. Fewer than 100 MDR-TB cases were seen in 2007, mainly among foreign-born individuals who arrived with preformed drug resistance.

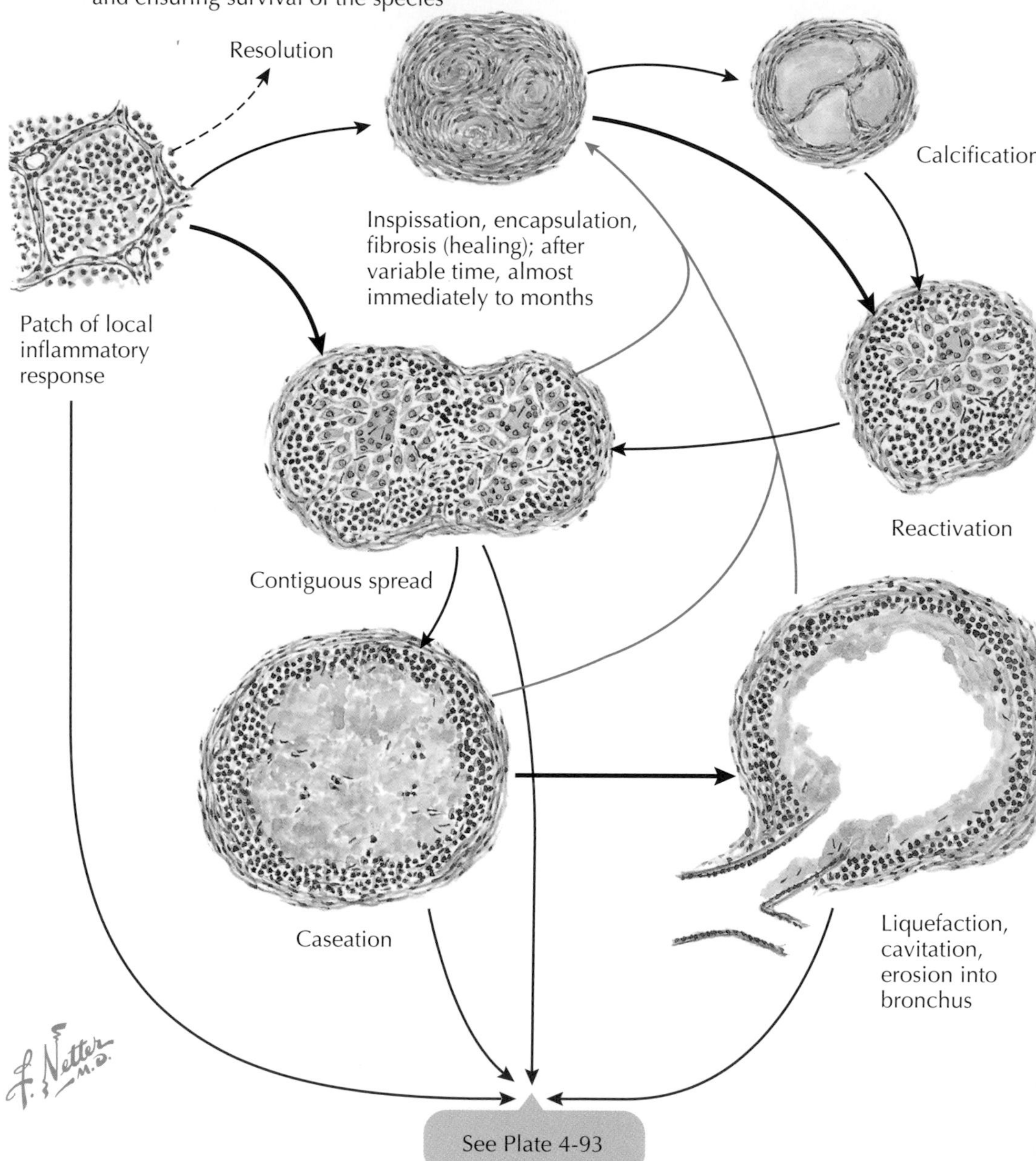
Evolution of Tubercle
Course influenced by:
Inoculum size and strain virulence
Innate and acquired host immunity
Age (infants and elderly most vulnerable), race, cigarette abuse, alcoholism, malnutrition
Pneumoconioses, type I diabetes mellitus, renal failure, HIV/ AIDS
Corticosteroids, cytotoxic agents, organ transplantation (antirejection), TNF-α modifers
From granuloma to cavitation
If confluent regions of granulomatous disease undergo necrosis with resultant formation of a cavity, the tubercle bacilli can enjoy unchecked, exponential replication in the caseum. This allows the hosts to export massive numbers of bacilli in their secretions, infecting others and ensuring survival of the species
Resolution
Calcification
Inspissation, encapsulation, fibrosis (healing); after variable time, almost immediately to months
Patch of local inflammatory response
Reactivation
Contiguous spread
Caseation
Liquefaction, cavitation, erosion into bronchus
See Plate 4-93

TUBERCULOSIS *(Continued)*

TRANSMISSION AND PATHOGENESIS

TB is primarily spread by patients with sputum smear–positive pulmonary disease. Coughing produces small particles, which float in the air and undergo dehydration, forming "droplet nuclei" in the range of 1 μm size. These can reach the alveoli and avoid clearance by the mucociliary escalator of the airways. Transmission occurs exclusively indoors, where these particles are concentrated and protected against ultraviolet irradiation (see Plate 4-93).

After they have been taken up by naïve alveolar macrophages, the bacilli replicate and before inhibitory cellular immunity can limit their growth, there is widespread dissemination (see Plates 4-93 and 4-94). In most instances, host defenses prevail. The infected loci involute, and the only detectable manifestation of the encounter is a reactive tuberculin skin test result. However, in various sites, viable tubercle bacilli may persist for years or decades with the potential to cause "reactivation" TB, either in the lungs or extrapulmonary tissue. Among those with compromised immunity (e.g., very young individuals, people with AIDS, patients on immunosuppressive therapy), however, there may be progressive disseminated disease appearing within a few months of exposure.

Pulmonary disease is the commonest presentation of TB (see Plates 4-95 to 4-98). Among newly infected infants and children, there is a distinctive pattern referred to as *primary TB*. These young patients commonly react to the new infection with exuberant lymphadenopathy in the peribronchial, hilar, or paratracheal nodes, draining the region of the lung where the new infection occurred. The original parenchymal focus may be very small or not visible on routine chest radiographs by this time. Over months or years, this primary lesion may calcify, leaving a "Ghon lesion." Cavitation rarely occurs, and there are very limited numbers of tubercle bacilli in respiratory secretions. Among such patients, many of whom cannot cooperate with sputum collection, gastric aspirates or bronchoscopy may be required to isolate the TB organisms.

The histopathology of tuberculous lesions classically involves granulomas with central caseous ("cheeselike") necrosis. Bacilli, if seen, are typically at the margins of the lymphocyte-macrophage palisades and the necrotic debris. As the disease advances, the lesions erode into the airways, allowing expulsion of the bacilli into the environment. However, the critical component of transmission is the formation of cavities. In the environment of the cavity wall, tubercle bacilli undergo logarithmic extracellular replication. Patients with cavitary disease may shed 10^6 to 10^8 bacilli per milliliter of sputum.

TUBERCULOSIS *(Continued)*

Another aspect of the large population of rapidly multiplying organisms in cavities is the likelihood of spawning drug-resistant mutants. Therapeutically, this places a great premium on the initial intensive phase of treatment (see below).

Pleuritis may occur if the primary parenchymal lesion is close enough to the visceral pleura to induce inflammation of the mesothelial surface. In some cases, there is typical sharp chest pain, but in others, an asymptomatic effusion is observed. The pleural effusion may be accessed by aspiration; classically, it is a lymphocyte-rich exudate. Acid-fast bacilli are rarely seen on stain, and culture results are positive in fewer than half of the cases. Biopsy is the most useful study.

Miliary TB is manifested in the lungs by bilateral fine nodular opacities, predominantly in the dependent zones, where the bacilli have been deposited hematogenously (see Plate 4-98). Disseminated TB is seen among patients with impaired immunity, including those at the extremes of age.

TUBERCULIN SKIN TESTING AND INTERFERON-γ RELEASE ASSAYS

Historically, reactivity to intradermally injected tuberculoprotein has been used in the diagnosis of TB (see Plate 4-99). "Old tuberculin," originally prepared by Koch, was supplanted by purified protein derivative (PPD). The test results were measured by the amount of induration at 48 to 96 hours after placement. However, the tuberculin skin test (TST) was limited by insensitivity and nonspecificity; 15% to 25% of "normal hosts" with TB did not have a significant response to PPD, and prior BCG vaccination or nontuberculous mycobacterial infections may induce significant reactions to PPD.

The primary role of the TST has been identifying latent TB infection (LTBI). Because it has been the only test that defines LTBI, its sensitivity is unknown. However, the lack of specificity has clearly been problematic, particularly among high-risk immigrants who have received BCG.

Recent studies have identified two antigens that are nearly specific to *M. tuberculosis*: culture filtrate protein-10 (CFP-10) and early secretory antigen-6 (ESAT-6). Two new commercial tests have been developed that measure ex vivo production by whole blood of interferon-γ (IFN-γ) on exposure to CFP-10 and ESAT-6 (Quantiferon or T. Spot-TB). Overall, these IFN-γ release assays (IGRAs) appear to be slightly more sensitive and significantly more specific than the TST. Other advantages are that they require only a single encounter, are more objective in interpretation, and do not "boost" reactivity as do serial TSTs. Conversely, the IGRAs are substantially more expensive, technically demanding, and require proximity to a laboratory.

INITIAL (PRIMARY) TUBERCULOUS COMPLEX

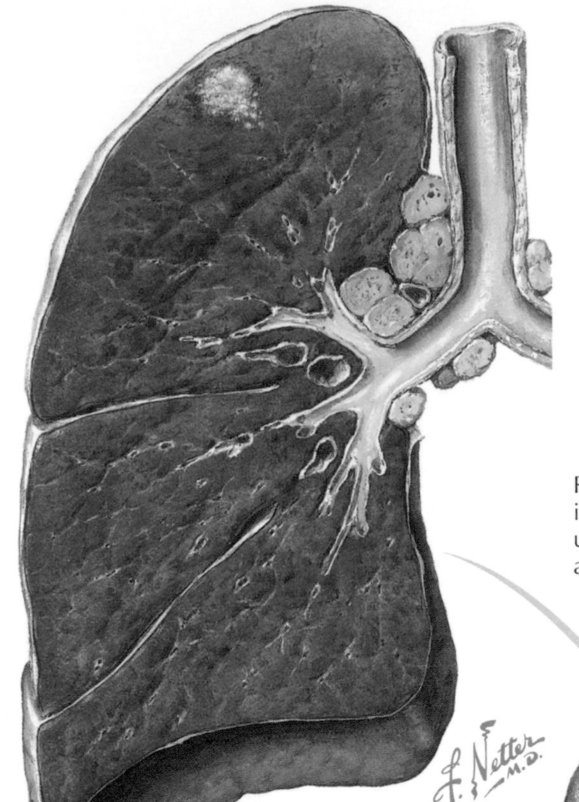

Initial tuberculous infection. Small bronchopneumonic infiltrate in right upper lobe (first infection may be anywhere in lungs) with greatly enlarged hilar and tracheobronchial lymph nodes

Radiograph showing ill-defined shadow of initial infective focus in lateral upper zone of right upper lobe with enlarged lymph nodes in hilar and azygos vein areas in a 6-year-old child

In time, pulmonary focus often heals to a fibrosed, calcified "Ghon lesion," and lymph nodes regress and calcify as shown here

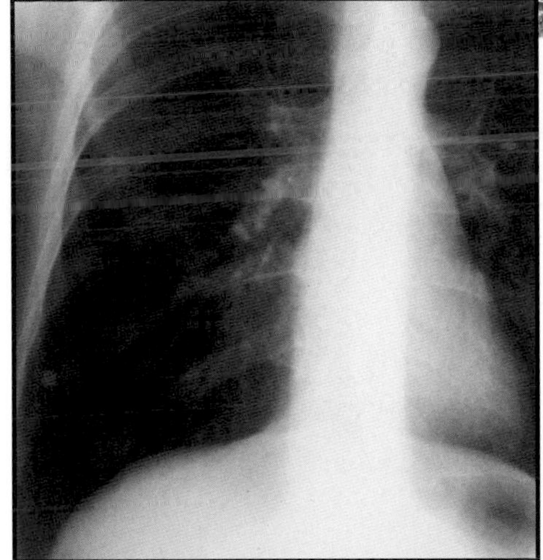

Calcified "Ghon lesion" in lateral portion of right lower lobe

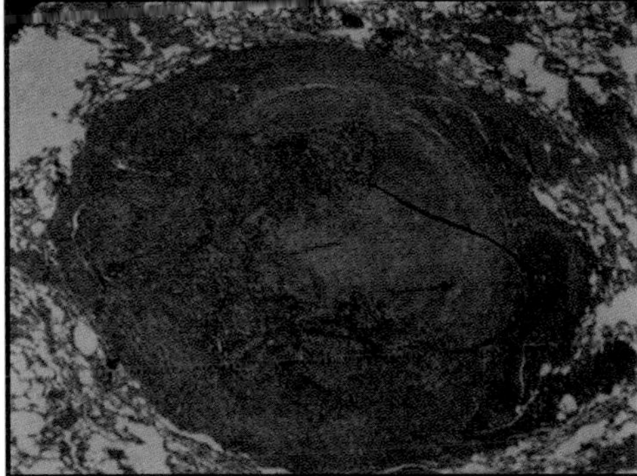

Section of a very inspissated, dried-out focus with fibrous capsule

Progressive Pathology

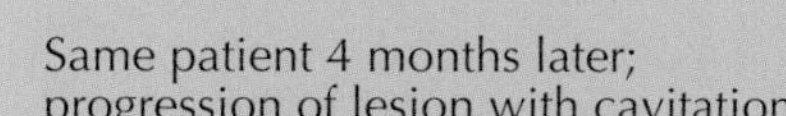

Patch of early active tuberculosis infiltration in right upper lobe
Subtle focus of early disease in right upper lobe
Same patient 4 months later; progression of lesion with cavitation

TUBERCULOSIS *(Continued)*

CHEST RADIOGRAPHY

The routine chest radiograph, posteroanterior (PA) and lateral (LAT) views, has been the traditional test for pulmonary, pleural, and miliary TB. The most common sites for disease area the posterior aspects of the upper lobes and the superior segments of the lower lobes. Common findings include fibronodular stranding extending up from the hilum, retraction cephalad of the pulmonary artery, thickening of the apical pleural cap and (with advanced disease) cavitation. Among HIV-negative "normal" hosts, roughly two-thirds have these typical findings.

Among immunocompromised patients (people with AIDS, those who have undergone organ transplantation, those with renal failure, and recipients of tumor necrosis factor–α [TNF-α] inhibitors), the radiographic presentation may be quite atypical, including lower zone pneumonic infiltrates, prominent lymphadenopathy, huge pleural effusions, and diffuse opacities that begin as tiny, discrete ("millet seed") shadows but may progress to a confluent airspace filling process or acute respiratory distress syndrome.

Computed tomography (CT) scans may reveal important diagnostic findings, including cavities obscured by osseous or soft tissue structures in the apices, grossly enlarged lymphadenopathy with hypodense centers typical of AIDS-TB, or early miliary shadowing not visible on routine chest radiography.

Pleural effusions were typically assessed by performing lateral decubitus views that led the effusions to collect in the dependent zones. Although decubitus views are still popular, ultrasound studies allow for more thorough characterization of the pleural process and increase the yield of aspiration, biopsy, and drainage procedures.

SPUTUM STUDIES

Sputum studies include nucleic acid amplification (NAA) and culture (see Plates 4-100 and 4-101). In much of the world, unprocessed sputum is smeared on a glass slide, stained with the Ziehl-Neelsen or Kinyoun technique, and examined by a technician at high-power magnification under a light microscope. This system is insensitive, identifying fewer than 50% of patients whose sputum would be culture positive in more sophisticated laboratories. This system has been justified by identifying the cases most likely to transmit TB. However, it is diminishingly acceptable given its insensitivity and incapacity for drug susceptibility testing.

In modern laboratories, sputum undergoes decontamination (so the media are not overgrown by microorganisms other than mycobacteria), digestion (to release the mycobacteria from the proteinaceous matrix

EXTENSIVE CAVITARY DISEASE

Large, thick-walled cavities in both upper lobes. Erosion into bronchi has resulted in endobronchial spread to dependent zones. One of the RUL cavities is portrayed as a dilated bronchial artery ("Rasmussen aneurysm"), which may result in massive hemoptysis. There is also typical thickening of the apical pleurae

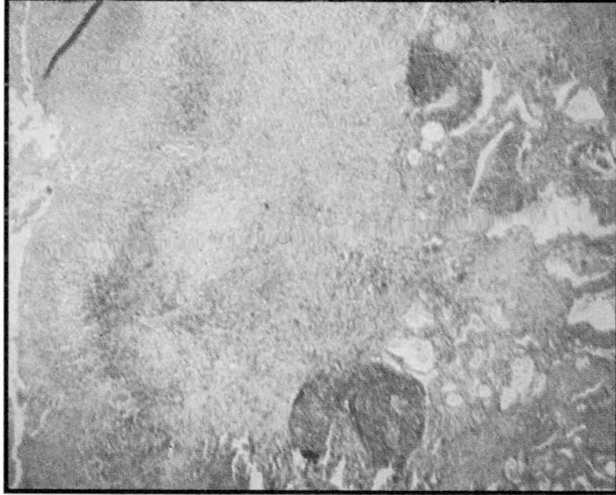

Section through wall of cavity. Cavity is to the left and is bordered by liquefying caseation with degenerating tubercles and collections of lymphoid cells

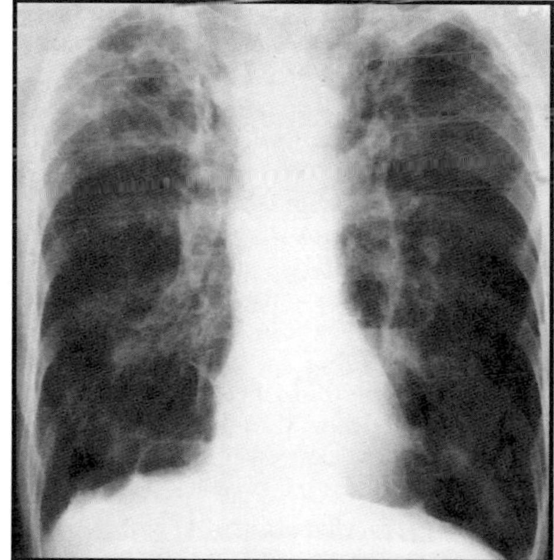

Bilateral advanced fibrocavitary tuberculosis

TUBERCULOSIS *(Continued)*

of the mucus), and concentration (in a centrifuge that is refrigerated so that the heat generated by high-speed centrifugation does not kill too many of the mycobacteria). At the end of this three-step process, the supernatant is decanted, and the pellet is subjected to microscopy, NAA, and culture. Fluorescent microscopy using auramine-O stains the mycobacteria bright yellow on a black background, which allows the reading at 40 × magnification.

NAA may be performed on uncultivated bacilli to establish the species as *M. tuberculosis*. This is particularly valuable in communities with a significant prevalence of pulmonary disease because of nontuberculous mycobacteria (NTM; see below). Early species identification allows optimal selection of the drug regimen (TB or NTM), efficient use of isolation facilities, and appropriate initiation of contact investigation (see below).

Culture remains the central element in the diagnosis of TB. Because microscopy results are positive in only 40% to 60% of cases ultimately proven to be pulmonary TB, culture enhances the sensitivity of sputum study and confirms the species and facilitates drug susceptibility testing.

Solid media such as Löwenstein-Jensen remain in use in many parts of the world. However, such techniques are slow in yielding results, typically requiring 4 to 6 weeks. Liquid media have replaced or supplemented the solid media in many industrialized nations, offering culture results, speciation, and preliminary susceptibility results in 1 to 2 weeks (see below).

Drug susceptibility testing (DST) has become a critical need in the era of epidemic drug resistance. There are a number of variables in DST. Historically, it was common to perform the culture, and when growth was observed and the species confirmed, to take a subculture and perform DST. This "indirect" method required 6 to 8 weeks on average.

DST in the latter 20th century generally used the "proportionality" method. Equal aliquots were put on drug-free clear agar, and "control," and others were placed on agar with various concentrations of the drugs. Then the number of colonies on the drug-containing media was compared with the control count.

More recently, techniques using liquid media containing different quantities of the relevant drugs determined the minimum inhibitory concentration (MIC) of the drugs. MIC techniques have either used the cut points derived from the proportionality method (see above) or have calculated presumed efficacy by comparing the maximum concentration (C_{max}) derived from pharmacokinetic studies with the MIC of a given drug.

Miliary Tuberculosis

Innumerable miliary tubercles scattered throughout both lungs and on pleural surface

TUBERCULOSIS *(Continued)*

However, clinical and public health issues have created pressure to identify MDR-TB (or XDR) in a much shorter period because of high rates of mortality among patients with AIDS and continued nosocomial transmission to health care workers and other patients on hospital units.

Two methods have been used to facilitate early recognition of resistance: accelerated microbiologic methods and molecular probes for chromosomal markers of resistance. The microscopic observation of drug susceptibility (MODS) technique uses multiple wells of control and drug-containing media. The wells are examined regularly for the presence of corded bacilli. This technique has been reported to yield results in as little as 7 to 10 days for multiple drugs.

By contrast, techniques to probe for chromosomal mutations known to be associated with resistance appear to be faster and simpler. Although the mutations related to resistance for many TB drugs are known, the one most reliable and clinically meaningful is that for rifamycin resistance, the RIF polymerase B (*rpo*B) mutation. Because resistance to the rifamycins is the keystone to MDR- or XDR-TB, using this mutation to triage patients appears very attractive.

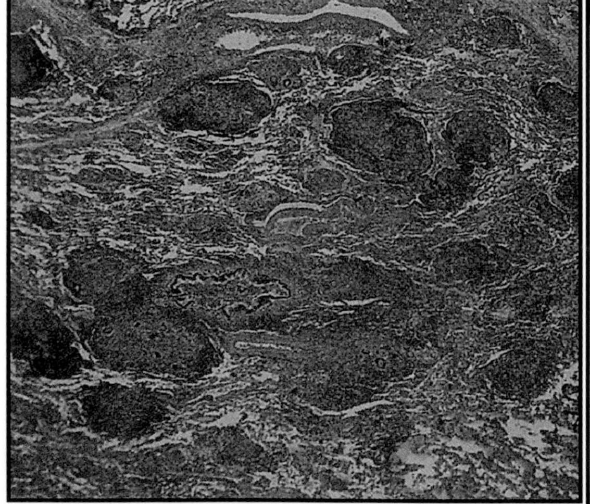

Multiple solitary and conglomerate tubercles composed mostly of epithelioid cells with an occasional giant cell of the Langerhans type and surrounded by numerous lymphoid cells

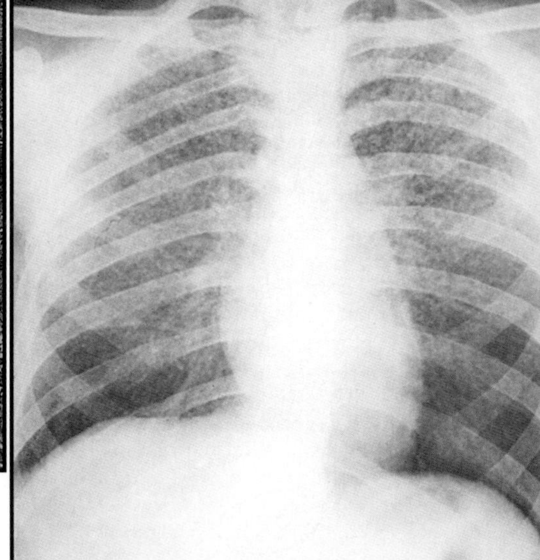

TREATMENT OF TUBERCULOSIS

Modern regimens use four drugs: RIF, INH, pyrazinamide (PZA), and ethambutol (EMB). The current standard duration is 6 months. The RIF, INH, PZA, and EMB are given for the first 2 months, and the RIF and INH are given for the last 4 months. Current guidelines, however, indicate that if the sputum culture taken after the first 2 months is positive, the RIF and INH should be extended to a total of 9 months to lessen the risk of relapse.

Because nonadherence or noncompliance with the prescribed regimen was shown to be associated with delayed conversion to sputum negativity, higher rates of failure or relapse and—most importantly—acquired drug resistance, directly observed therapy (DOT) has become the normative practice in the United States.

Under the typical DOT program, at the time of diagnosis, patients are served notice that they must make themselves regularly available for supervised treatment or will face confinement. Patients cannot be compelled to take medications, but if they are recalcitrant, they can be placed under enforced isolation.

To facilitate supervised therapy, intermittent (less than daily) regimens may be used. One model, based on studies from Hong Kong, used thrice-weekly treatment throughout. Another, first used in Denver, begins with 2 weeks of four drugs daily, switches to 6 weeks of four drugs twice weekly, and concludes with 18 weeks of RIF-INH twice weekly. Of note, the twice-weekly schedule has been found inadequate in the setting of

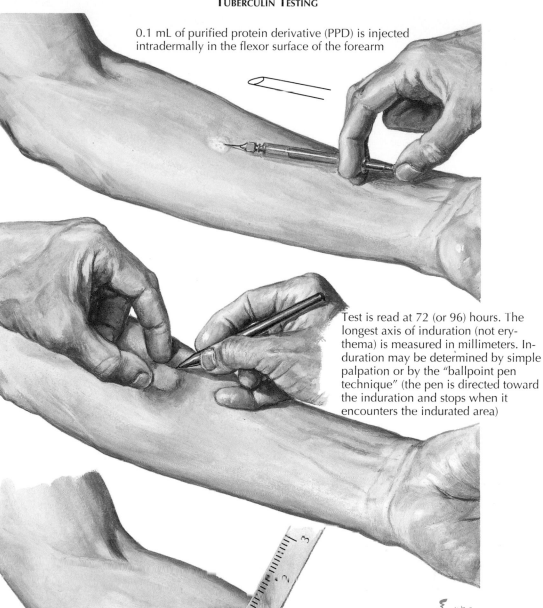

Tuberculin Testing

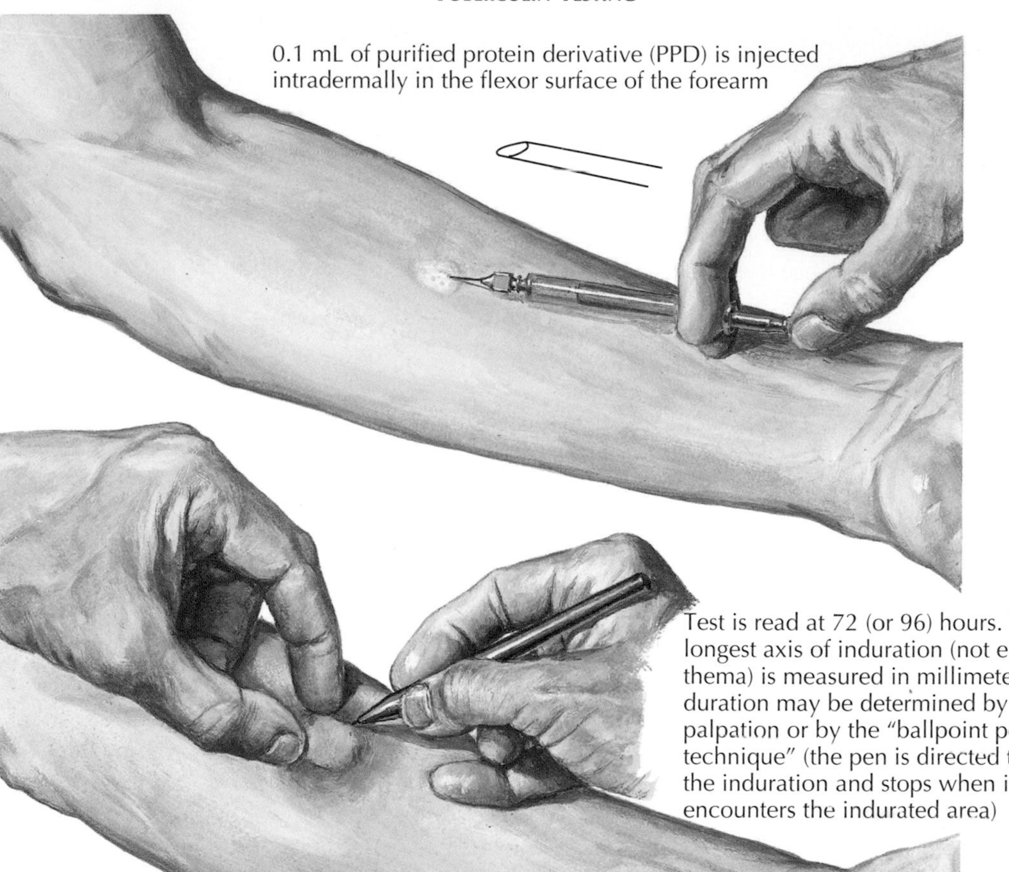

0.1 mL of purified protein derivative (PPD) is injected intradermally in the flexor surface of the forearm
Test is read at 72 (or 96) hours. The longest axis of induration (not erythema) is measured in millimeters. Induration may be determined by simple palpation or by the "ballpoint pen technique" (the pen is directed toward the induration and stops when it encounters the indurated area)
cm
1
2
3
F. Netter M.D.
Diameter of marked indurated area measured in transverse plane. Reactions over 9 mm in diameter are regarded as positive; those 5 to 9 mm are questionable, and the test may be repeated after 7 or more days to obtain a booster effect. Less than 5 mm of induration is regarded as negative

Tuberculosis *(Continued)*

AIDS; either thrice-weekly or daily (five times per week) is indicated.

MDR-TB or XDR-TB

As already noted, MDR (resistance at least to RIF and INH) and XDR [(resistance at least to RIF, INH, one of fluoroquinolone agents, and one of the second-line injectables [amikacin, kanamycin, or capreomycin]) are threatening global TB control.

TB drug resistance is based on chromosomal mutations, not transferable resistance factors. The mutations are not induced by therapy; rather, failure to take an adequate number of drugs in correct dosages allows the resistant mutation to escape and by selection become the dominant strain. Drug-resistant epidemics are amplified by making drugs available without the infrastructure to ensure reliable therapy. After "primary" resistance is established in a patient, he or she can transmit the resistant strain to others (i.e., "transmitted" or "secondary" resistance).

Treatment of patients with highly resistant TB is challenging because the second-line drugs (SLDs) are less efficacious, more toxic, and more expensive than the first-line drugs. Plus the duration of therapy required to cure increases from 6 months to 24 months.

Historically, drug-resistant TB was observed to be less readily transmissible and less virulent (likely to progress to active disease) among contacts. However, over the past 20 years, Beijing strains have tended to replace the older European strains, and these organisms have been shown to be readily transmissible and highly virulent.

Optimal management of drug-resistant cases entails access to in vitro susceptibility testing, including SLDs, experience with the clinical nuances of SLDs and—ideally—access to resectional surgery. Among the agents used are the injectables (streptomycin, amikacin, kanamycin, or capreomycin), the fluoroquinolones (cipro-, levo-, or moxifloxacin), cycloserine, ethionamide, para-aminosalicylic acid (PAS), clofazimine, linezolid, clarithromycin, and amoxicillin/clavulanate. Comprehensive discussions of the treatment of highly resistant TB are beyond the scope of this chapter.

Treatment of Latent Tuberculosis Infection

As noted above, reactivation of latent foci or infection—typically acquired months, years, or even decades earlier—is the commonest pathway in the pathogenesis of TB. Recognizing this pattern, the United States Public Health Service conducted a series of trials to determine whether giving INH to those with latent TB would reduce their risk of developing active disease. Briefly, these placebo-controlled trials, which involved roughly 72,000 diverse subjects, showed approximately 60% to 70% protection. In the group followed longest,

Sputum Examination

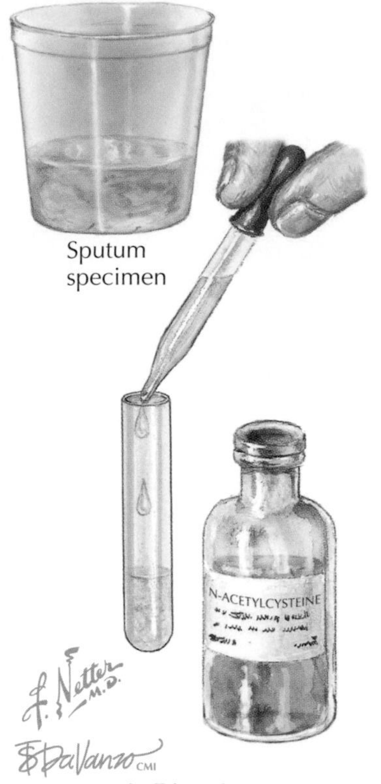

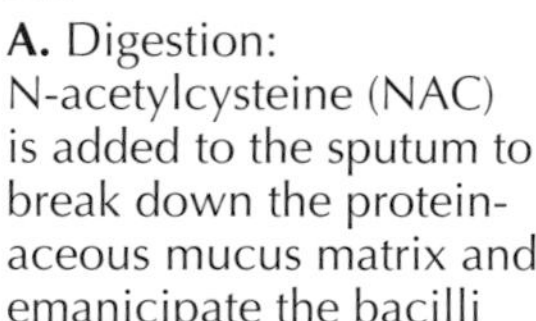

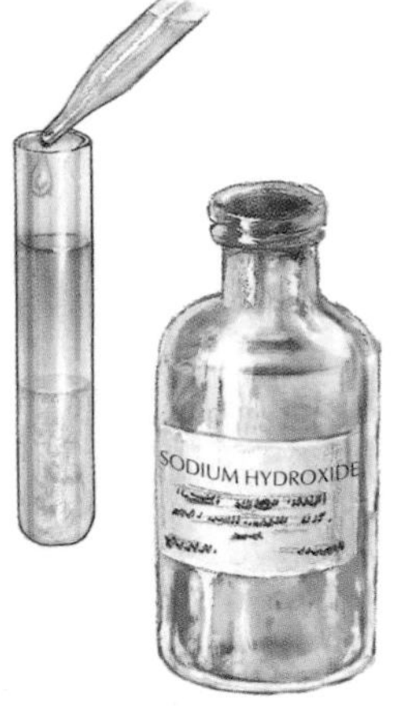

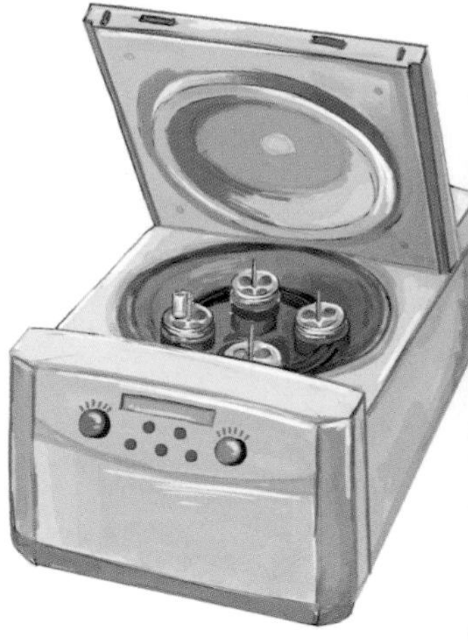

A. Digestion: N-acetylcysteine (NAC) is added to the sputum to break down the proteinaceous mucus matrix and emanicipate the bacilli

B. Decontamination: Dilute sodium hydroxide (NaOH) is added to kill other bacteria in the sputum so they do not overgrow the mycobacteria in culture

C. Concentration: The sputum goes through high-speed centrifugation to concentrate the bacilli for staining and culturing. The centrifuge is refrigerated to keep the heat from killing the bacilli

D. The concentrated pellet is then deployed for staining/microscopy, culture, and, if available, molecular probes for speciation and mutations associated with drug-resistance

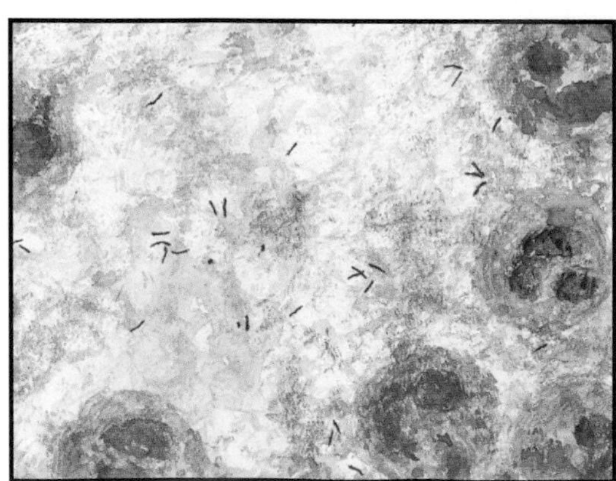

E. Slide of sputum stained with carbol-fuchsin (Ziehl-Neelsen method), viewed under oil immersion, showing acid-fast bacilli (*M. tuberculosis*) as bright red rods

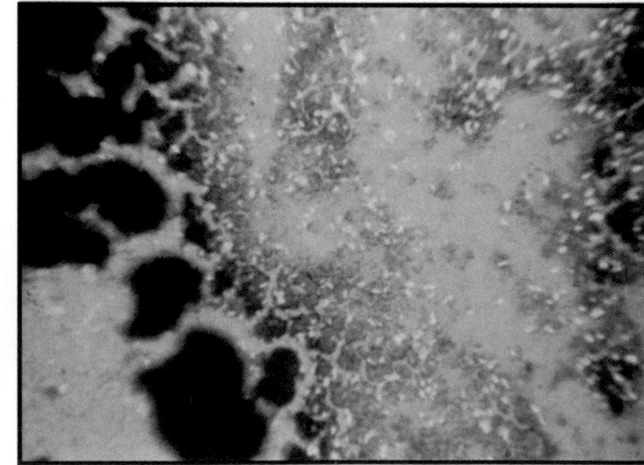

F. *M. tuberculosis* stained with auramine O, which causes acid-fast bacilli to flouresce (×200)

TUBERCULOSIS *(Continued)*

Alaskan villagers, the protection extended over 19 years. Because BCG vaccination would substantially confound the utility of the TST, the sole means of identifying latent infection, vaccination has not been used in the United States.

In the United States, treatment of latent TB infection (TLTI) focuses on identifying individuals or groups historically at high risk for TB and, based on reactivity to the TST or IGRA, administering "preventive therapy": (1) contacts to cases of communicable TB who may be presumed to have been recently infected; (2) those with HIV infection or AIDS; (3) health care workers with recent conversion of their TST or IGRA; (4) immigrants from high-risk regions; (5) individuals with radiographic abnormalities consistent with healed TB; and (6) other immunocompromised subjects, including those with chronic renal failure, organ transplantation, recipients of tumor necrosis factor α inhibitors, or other agents (including high-dose steroids or cytotoxic agents).

The current guidelines from the American Thoracic Society (ATS) and Centers for Disease Control and Prevention (CDC) offer three TLTI regimens: (1) INH for 9 months (first choice), (2) INH for 6 months (acceptable), or (c) RIF for 4 months. The 9-month INH regimen is rated highest by evidence-based analysis; 6 months of treatment is deemed acceptable. The 4 months of RIF option is a reflection of the efficacy of RIF in accelerated sterilization in the treatment of active disease and its superior activity in the murine model. TLTI with INH or RIF substantially lessens the number of viable bacilli in those with latent infection and thereby prevents (or delays) reactivation.

The side effects and toxicity of INH include rare but serious hepatitis. Roughly 10% to 20% of those started on INH will have modest, asymptomatic elevations in their hepatic transaminase values, more common with increased age. A total of 1% to 3% of those receiving INH may develop symptomatic hepatitis, which requires discontinuation. Lethal liver failure occurs with continued use of INH in the setting of worsening liver chemistries and symptoms. Current ATS and CDC guidelines indicate that symptom surveillance is generally sufficient to prevent serious liver damage.

RIF is less likely to cause serious hepatitis and does not have the central nervous system effects (e.g., lethargy, decreased concentration) experienced by some patients taking INH. The major issue with RIF is the potential for drug interactions with a variety of agents, including antiretroviral (ARV) agents, oral contraceptives, warfarin, and a variety of other meds (see the *Physicians' Desk Reference*). It should not be used in people with HIV/AIDS because of the risk of acquired monoresistance.

For contacts with MDR-TB cases, there is no unanimity for TLTI. A 6-month course of a fluoroquinolone (levofloxacin or moxifloxacin) may be appropriate. There are no practical options for TLTI in contacts with XDR-TB.

SPUTUM CULTURE

Concentration and decontamination

Equal amounts of 4% NaOH plus 0.5% *N*-acetyl-L-cysteine added to sputum, shaken for 1 minute, and incubated at room temperature for 15 to 20 minutes. This kills most contaminants but also kills some *M. tuberculosis*

Specimen centrifuged for 15 minutes and supernatant decanted

Sediment diluted with 0.5 mL of water or albumin, neutralized with phosphate buffer (pH 6.8), then spread over plates or slants of medium

M. tuberculosis on slant of Löwenstein-Jensen opaque, egg-containing medium. Colonies nonpigmented or buff colored and rough

M. kansasi colonies on Löwenstein-Jensen medium. Orange pigmentation appears only after exposure to light

M. tuberculosis colonies on 7-H-11 oleic acid agar translucent medium, which allows earlier reading. *M. tuberculosis* as well as other pathogenic mycobacteria appear in about 2 weeks and are read weekly for total of 8 weeks

Drug susceptibility testing
(for selected patients)

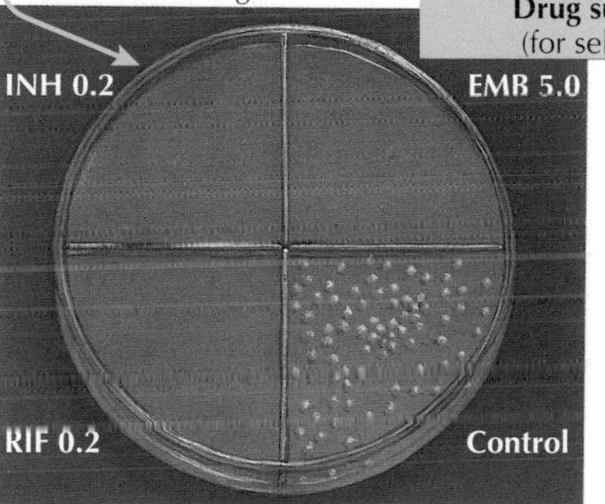

Direct. Medium in each of 3 quadrants contains a different drug; 4th is control. Diluted sediment is spread evenly over all; 3 or 4 plates required as each drug is tested in 2 or 3 concentrations. INH 0.2 and 1.0; EMB 5.0, 10.0, and 15.0; RIF 0.2, 0.5, and 1.0; and SM 2.0 and 10.0 mg are most frequently tested

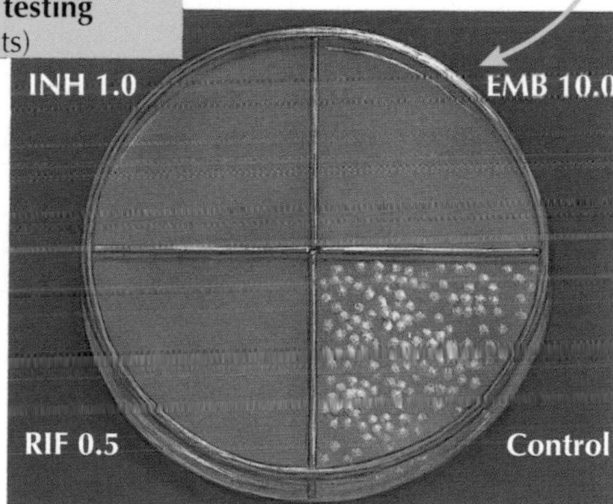

Indirect. Organisms are first cultured, and then measured aliquots of culture are spead over quadrants containing different drugs in varying concentrations as well as control

EMB = ethambutol, INH = isoniazid, RIF = rifampin, SM = streptomycin

TUBERCULOSIS *(Continued)*

Treating Tuberculosis in Persons with AIDS

There are four unique aspects of managing TB in persons with AIDS:

1. The clinical presentation may be atypical, including chest radiography. In the absence of cavitation (rare in AIDS), sputum smears are less readily smear positive. Diagnosis may be established by unusual modalities such as blood culture, lymph node biopsy, and culture or bone marrow biopsy and culture.
2. In persons with AIDS with advanced malnutrition and infectious enteritis, there may be suboptimal TB drug absorption; pharmacokinetic studies may be helpful.
3. There may be significant drug interaction between the rifamycins and the ARV agents. In general, RIF has such a profound effect in accelerating the elimination of the ARVs that they cannot be used together. Instead, rifabutin, which has about 30% of the effect on the cytochrome P450 system, should be used. (See the CDC's website for updates on TB therapy and ARVs.)
4. When ARV therapy is begun and the CD_4 lymphocyte population increases, there may be an amplified immune response to the TB. This immune reconstitution inflammatory syndrome (IRIS) may result in organ-specific flares or exaggerated constitutional symptoms. Recent experience indicates that despite this risk, ARV be begun within 2 to 3 weeks of commencing TB therapy. If serious problems arise, corticosteroids may ameliorate the IRIS.

PREVENTING NOSOCOMIAL TRANSMISSION OF TUBERCULOSIS

The MDR-TB epidemic was highly instructive regarding institutional safety. In retrospect, health care authorities had confused the early bactericidal effects of modern regimens with adequate infection control measures. With drug-susceptible TB, the number of viable bacilli in the sputum falls by two to three logs in the first week of treatment; additionally, the patients' cough frequency decreases abruptly. By contrast, with MDR-TB, the bacillary population and cough do not diminish under standard therapy. In the New York City MDR-TB outbreak in the early 1990s, molecular epidemiology showed that 80% of the cases were nosocomially transmitted.

This recognition led to several protective measures: (1) placing all suspected cases in negative-pressure isolation rooms, (2) establishing six or more air changes per hour in these rooms, (3) having all health care workers potentially exposed to wear fit-tested N95 respirators, and (4) using ultraviolet germicidal irradiation in patient rooms.

These measures appear to have significantly reduced the risk of nosocomial transmission. Nonetheless, health care workers are still required to have annual testing, either TSTs or IGRAs.

NONTUBERCULOUS MYCOBACTERIAL LUNG DISEASE

Throughout the 20th century, cases of pulmonary disease caused by mycobacteria other than *Mycobacterium tuberculosis* were described. Prominent among the "atypical" species have been *Mycobacterium avium*, *Mycobacterium intracellulare*, and *Mycobacterium kansasii*. Unlike *M. tuberculosis* (which has no common reservoir other than infected humans and is spread exclusively by human-to-human aerosols), the nontuberculous mycobacterial (NTM) lung diseases are found widely distributed in water and soil and appear to be acquired from these environmental sources.

The clinical and radiographic features of NTM disease are distinctive. Among the traditional male patients, the illness is mindful of classic TB: upper lobe fibronodular-cavity disease associated with productive cough, hemoptysis, fever, sweats, and weight loss. By contrast, the prototypic female case primarily involves bronchiectasis and centrilobular nodules associated with productive cough and malaise.

Runyon classification of environmental mycobacteria		
Group	**Features**	**Typical pathogens**
I. Photochromogens	Slow-growing; change from cream-colored in dark to yellow-orange in light	M kansasii M marinum
II. Scotochromogens	Slow-growing; pigmented	M scrofulaceum M gordonae M szulgai
III. Nonchromogens	Always cream colored	M avium M intracellulare M xenopi M malmoense
IV. Rapid growers	Visible growth in 3–7 days	M abcessus M chelonae M fortuitum

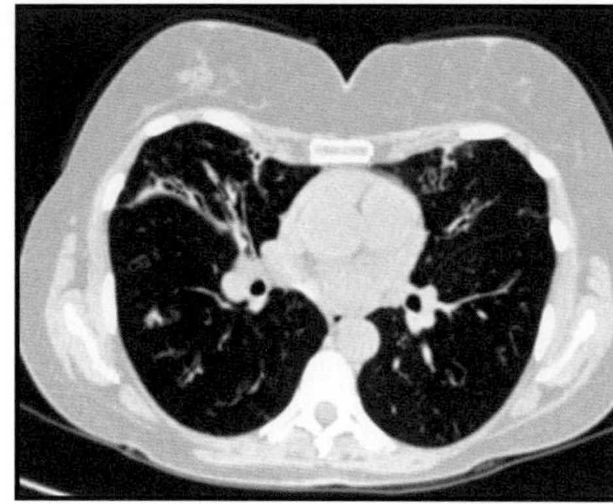

Patient with MAI with bronchiectasis, especially involving right middle lobe and lingua.

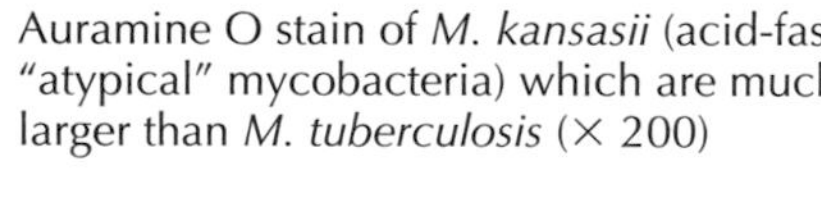

Auramine O stain of *M. kansasii* (acid-fast "atypical" mycobacteria) which are much larger than *M. tuberculosis* (× 200)

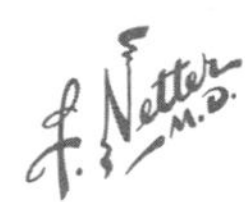

EPIDEMIOLOGY

Unlike tuberculosis (TB), for which there are carefully compiled annual data, there is less reliable information on the prevalence and distribution of NTM lung disease. A major issue is that not all patients whose sputum yields an NTM on culture have true "disease," and, in fact, 50% to 80% of patients with positive NTM cultures may actually be "contaminated" by these environmental microbes.

However, many U.S. clinicians believe that they are seeing more cases, especially among women. In Canada, although the incidence of pulmonary NTM is roughly 60% that of TB, the prevalence of NTM lung disease over the next decade is estimated to become substantially greater than that of TB. This is because of many factors—more than 80% of TB cases are treated and cured within 9 months, the observed incidence of TB is decreasing, cure rates for NTM lung disease are probably in the range of 50% to 60%, and treatment failure or relapses are common. Hence, an accumulation of NTM patients in Canada and the United States over time is expected.

Additional emphasis should be placed on the fact that most TB patients started on therapy rapidly become and remain asymptomatic. By contrast, many NTM patients with bronchiectasis have protracted symptoms and, even if the NTM is cured or suppressed, they experience intercurrent infections, commonly with gram-negative bacilli such as *Pseudomonas aeruginosa*.

NONTUBERCULOUS MYCOBACTERIAL SPECIES

In virtually all recent surveys, the bulk of disease is associated with *M. avium* or *M. intracellulare*. Although distinct species, these organisms are so similar that they are referred to as *M. avium* complex (MAC) or MAI. *M. kansasii* has been a prominent pathogen in the south-central United States but seems relatively less common in recent experience. Rapidly growing mycobacteria (group IV in the Runyon system) are being seen with increasing frequency; *Mycobacterium abscessus* is much more common than *Mycobacterium chelonae*. Other NTM that seem to vary in prevalence regionally include *Mycobacterium xenopi*, *Mycobacterium simiae*, *Mycobacterium malmoense*, and *Mycobacterium szulgai*.

DIAGNOSTIC CRITERIA

Given the potential for contamination, the American Thoracic Society (ATS) has established criteria for clinical relevance, which include typical symptoms, suitable radiographic findings (cavities, bronchiectasis, scattered nodular opacities) and two or more positive sputum cultures or one positive bronchial aspirate or wash. The clinical significance is enhanced if it is one of the more common pathogens. *Mycobacterium gordonae*, by contrast, is almost universally a contaminant.

Distinctive Morphotype

Two of the most intriguing aspects of the cases among women are the physical-anatomic features and racial distribution. Unlike TB, which is more common among persons of color in the United States, the preponderance of NTM disease is seen among whites and, less frequently, Asians. There is a notable paucity among African American individuals. The prototypical patient is variable tall and slender; subtle scoliosis is common, and many patients have narrowed anteroposterior distance or pectus excavatum. Mitral valve prolapse is found with higher than normal frequency. Although the disease can involve any region of the lungs, bronchiectasis and volume loss of the right-middle lobe or lingula are strikingly prominent.

TREATMENT

Antimicrobial therapy is delineated in the 2007 ATS guidelines. For the slowly growing species (*M. kansasii*, MAC, *M. xenopi*, and so on), regimens composed of clarithromycin (or azithromycin), RIF, and EMB are usually used. An injectable agent such as amikacin may be added initially for more extensive disease.

However, for the more common rapidly growing mycobacterial species such as *M. abscessus* and *M. chelonae*, an intravenous regimen such as imipenem or cefoxitin and either amikacin or tobramycin appears more efficacious.

For infections caused by the slowly growing mycobacterial species, therapy usually entails 12 to 18 months of continuous therapy with the objective of cure. However, the rapidly growing mycobacteria are prone to recur, and the strategy includes several months of intensive suppressive treatment with the anticipation of retreatment.

Overview of Inhalation Diseases

The inhalation of dusts and noxious gases into the lung may result in little damage or reaction if the agents have low biological activity or the exposure is minimal, but the results can be devastating injury, inflammation, or fibrosis if the agent is potent and carried by high dose or prolonged exposure. Virtually any fume, particle, or fiber that can be inhaled might cause a response in the lung if the material is in any way biologically active and the dose and exposure are sufficient.

Exposures to inorganic mineral dusts (e.g., silica, asbestos, coal, mixed silicates) result in chronic lung diseases characterized by fibrosis and distortion of tissue that produce progressive respiratory impairment. These diseases generally progress slowly over time, often taking decades from first exposure to clinical symptoms. The extent of disease depends on the interaction between the intensity of exposure (airborne particle load), the duration of exposure (cumulative dose), and the time since exposure began. The key to control of these diseases is prevention by reducing the levels of airborne dust in the workplace.

Many lung diseases caused by inhalation exposure to organic or metal particulates are the result of a specific immune response. Hypersensitivity pneumonitis (prototype, farmer's lung disease), chronic beryllium disease, cobalt pneumoconiosis (hard metal disease), and others only appear after sensitization and the development of highly immunospecific cell-mediated and humoral immune responses. In contrast to the pneumoconioses caused by inorganic dusts and fibers, these diseases usually do not require a high level of exposure to trigger them. After being sensitized, individuals may respond intensely to very low ambient levels of the offending agent and may become symptom free if exposure can be avoided. There is great variation among individuals, and only a minority of those exposed may develop disease. In some instances (e.g., beryllium), the disease may progress for years after the exposure ends. Brief episodes of disease caused by immune responses to inhaled materials may clear and leave no permanent lung damage, but repeated episodes or prolonged exposure may result in end-stage fibrosis and severe respiratory impairment.

Toxic gases and fumes, smoke from fires, and volatile chemicals used in industrial processes can cause injury to the lung when they are inhaled. In most instances, these reactions are acute, occurring within seconds to 48 hours of inhalation. If the injury is mild, complete resolution without permanent impairment can be expected; if the injury is more severe, then repair may be incomplete and may involve scarring. The speed and extent of injury from inhaled gases depends on the biologic reactivity of the chemical and its solubility in the water-based mucus that lines the lung. For example, whereas highly soluble compounds, such as hydrochloric acid (HCl), dissolve readily in mucus and cause injury primarily to the upper airway and larger bronchial airways, relatively less soluble compounds, such as nitrogen dioxide (NO_2), produce damage primarily at the level of the alveoli and small airways. Intense exposure to highly irritating fumes (e.g., chlorine gas, smoke) may cause an instant response in the larynx, producing glottic closure and limiting more distal damage at the expense of respiration.

Specific syndromes with both respiratory and systemic symptoms can occur after inhalation exposures.

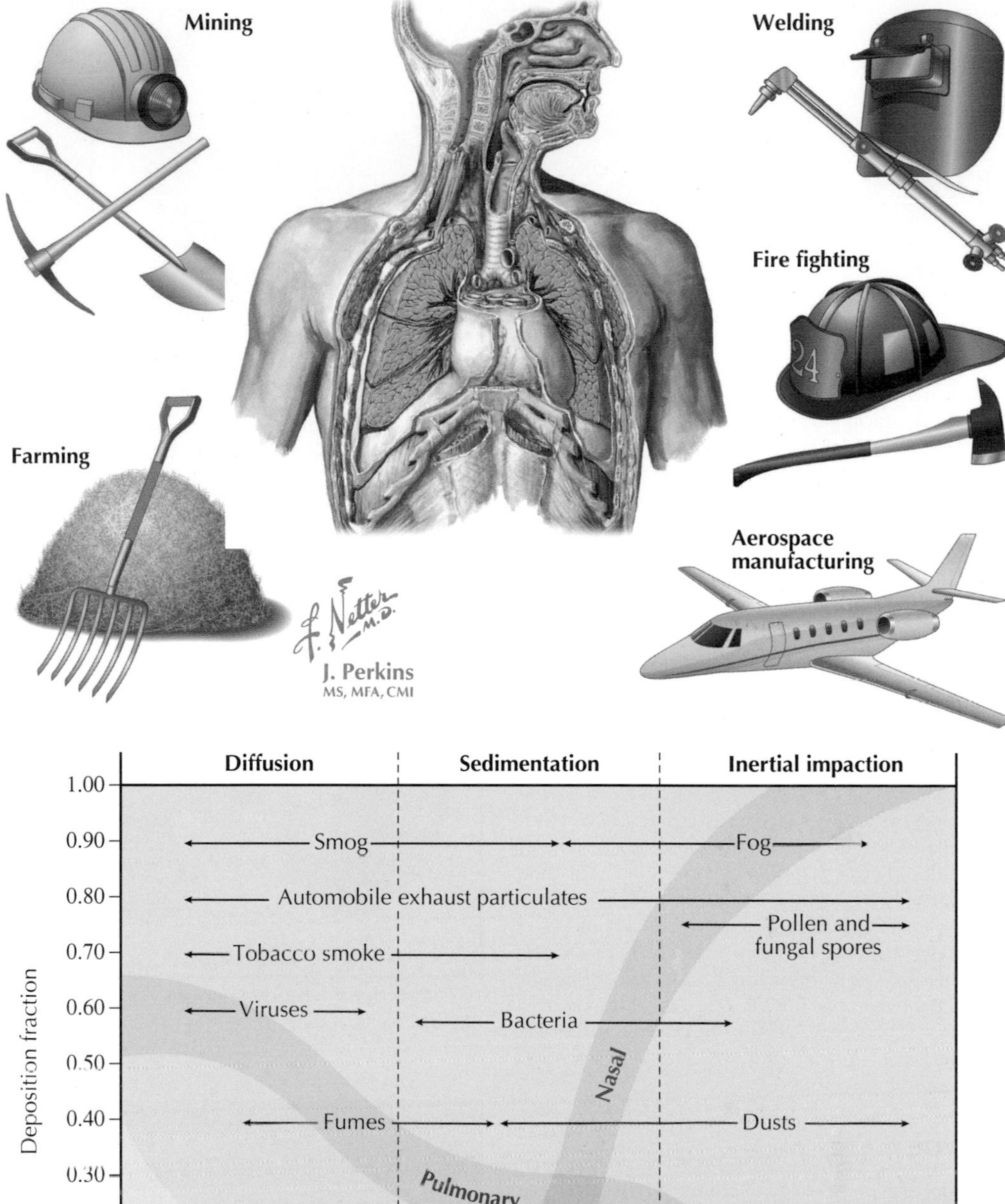

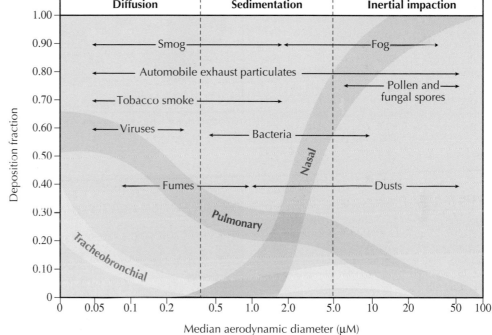

Distribution of common inhaled particles and fumes illustrating their relative deposition in the lung based on size and mechanism of deposition

Metal fume fever is seen in welders and other workers who heat zinc, copper, and other metals to high temperatures, generating fumes and small respirable particles. Symptoms of metal fume fever occur 4 to 8 hours after exposure and consist of an influenza-like illness with fever to 40°C, chills, headache, cough, sore throat, shortness of breath, nausea, muscle aches, and malaise. The illness is self-limited and usually clears within 24 to 48 hours of its onset. It is believed to be caused by both the direct irritation of the respiratory tract and the absorption of the metal into the systemic circulation. Organic dust toxic syndrome (ODTS) is a form of inhalation fever that results from exposure to aerosolized endotoxin (bacterial cell wall products), glucans (fungal cell wall products), and related compounds. A flulike illness develops 4 to 8 hours after exposure, with fever, muscle aches, malaise, cough, shortness of breath, and sometimes wheezing. Exposures can occur in a wide variety of settings, such as swine confinement facilities, sewage treatment plants, cotton processing gins, grain storage silos, and grain milling facilities. In patients with metal fume fever, ODTS, and other inhalation fevers, tolerance may occur if exposure is frequent, with loss of tolerance after an exposure holiday. Daily exposure may cause chronic bronchitis.

SILICOSIS

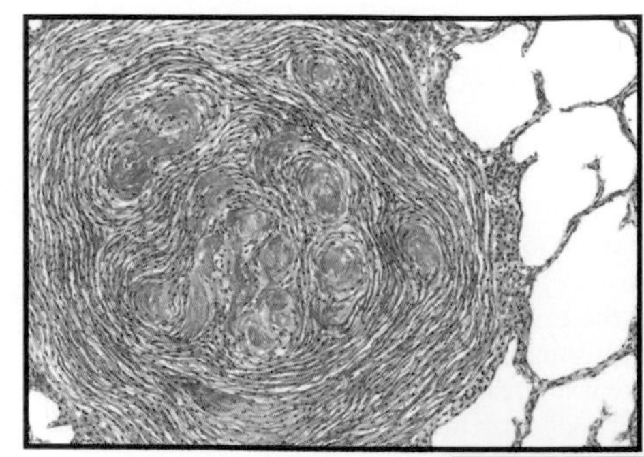

Silicotic nodule with accumulations of mononuclear cells and concentric ("onionskin") whorls of collagen fibrils

Simple silicosis with numerous small nodules in a predominantly upper- and mid-lung zone distribution

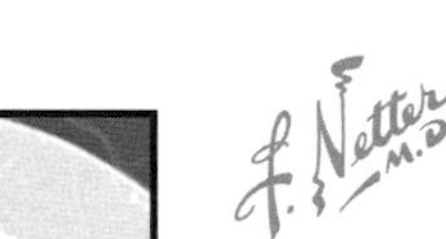

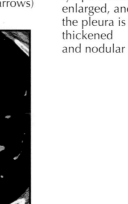

Chest radiograph from a granite worker with simple silicosis and numerous upper lung zone opacities; calcification is evident in the enlarged hilar lymph nodes and some of the opacities

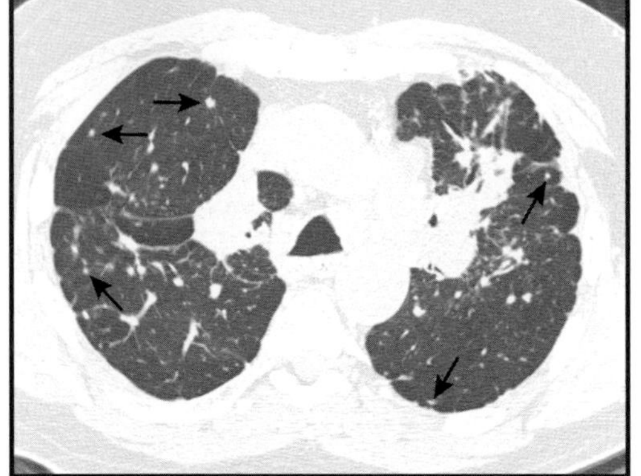

CT scan (lung windows, upper zone) from a foundry worker shows central conglomerate masses and numerous small nodules (arrows)

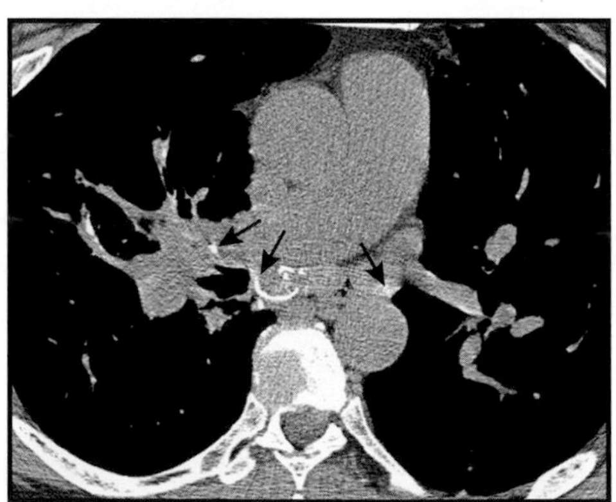

CT scan (mediastinal windows, lower zone) shows a curved rim of eggshell calcification in a subcarinal lymph node and flecks of calcium on hilar nodes

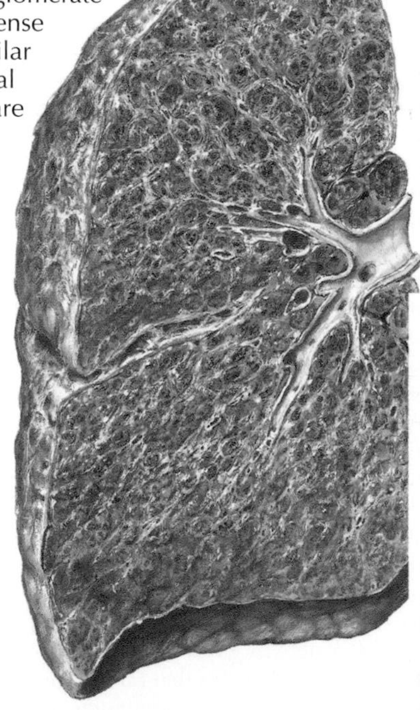

Complicated silicosis, or "progressive massive fibrosis," with coalescence of nodules into large conglomerate masses with dense fibrosis. The hilar and mediastinal lymph nodes are enlarged, and the pleura is thickened and nodular

Silicosis is a chronic diffuse fibronodular interstitial lung disease caused by the inhalation of crystalline particles of silica (silicon dioxide [SiO_2]). The particles must be of respirable size (0.2-10 μm aerodynamic diameter) to reach the distal airspaces of the lung. The biologic activity of silica is attributable to silanol groups and other chemically reactive species on the crystal surface, not to its physical shape or sharp edges. The mineral must be in crystalline form because glass (amorphous noncrystalline silica) is essentially nontoxic in crushed, powdered, or fibrous form. The mineral silica is abundant in nature as either pure quartz or mixed in igneous rock with other minerals; whereas beach sand is pure quartz, granite contains 10% to 15% crystalline free silica. Exposure to respirable silica must be substantial and prolonged to cause clinically significant lung disease.

Silicosis usually presents as a chronic diffuse lung disease with numerous small nodules with an upper lung zone predominance, and it evolves slowly over years or decades. This form is labeled *chronic simple silicosis*. It may progress to more extensive disease with coalescence of the nodules into conglomerate masses with surrounding fibrosis and traction emphysema. The more advanced stage may be referred to as *progressive massive fibrosis* (PMF). Extremely high levels of exposure can cause an acute and usually fatal form of silicosis accompanied by an outpouring of alveolar surfactant lipids and proteinaceous debris, a rare condition known as *acute silicosis* or *silicoproteinosis*. An intermediate form termed *accelerated silicosis* may develop in 2 to 5 years if exposure is intense.

PATHOLOGY

The pathology of silicosis features a characteristic lesion, the silicotic nodule, found in lung tissue and draining lymph modes. This lesion begins as a small collection of macrophages (many containing phagocytosed dust particles), lymphocytes, and fibroblasts; this early lesion is usually located near respiratory bronchioles. Whorls of type I collagen and other matrix proteins accumulate in the center as the nodules enlarge, with an outer rim of mononuclear cells and proliferating fibroblasts. Neutrophils and eosinophils are not abundant. The nodules coalesce gradually, and the fibrotic process extends to infiltrate the surrounding tissue. Finally, dystrophic calcification may be found within the larger conglomerate masses and in the hilar and mediastinal lymph nodes. The silica mineral particles are usually abundant within these lesions and can be visualized by polarized light microscopy or by elemental analysis with scanning electron microscopy and energy dispersive spectrometry.

CLINICAL FEATURES

Patients with silicosis experience gradually progressive shortness of breath with exertion and cough, sometimes with clear or white sputum. Physical examination may be normal, or high-pitched end-inspiratory crackles (rales) may be heard over the mid-lung areas. Digital clubbing is very uncommon in silicosis. Signs of cor pulmonale (accentuated second heart sound, peripheral edema) may be late manifestations of advanced disease. The chest radiograph early in silicosis shows small, rounded opacities with a mid- and upper-zone predominance (International Labour Organization classification p/q opacities, profusion 1/1-2/1). More advanced silicosis includes more widespread opacities with some coalescence, enlarged hilar and mediastinal lymph nodes, and peripheral "egg-shell" calcification of these nodes. Extensive pleural thickening or pleural calcifications are not seen, although some of the nodules may originate at subpleural sites. High-resolution (thin section) computed tomography (CT) is helpful in revealing this pattern and may show more extensive disease than would be suspected from the plain frontal chest radiograph. The radiographic features of silicosis may be much more striking than either the patient's

Silicotuberculosis

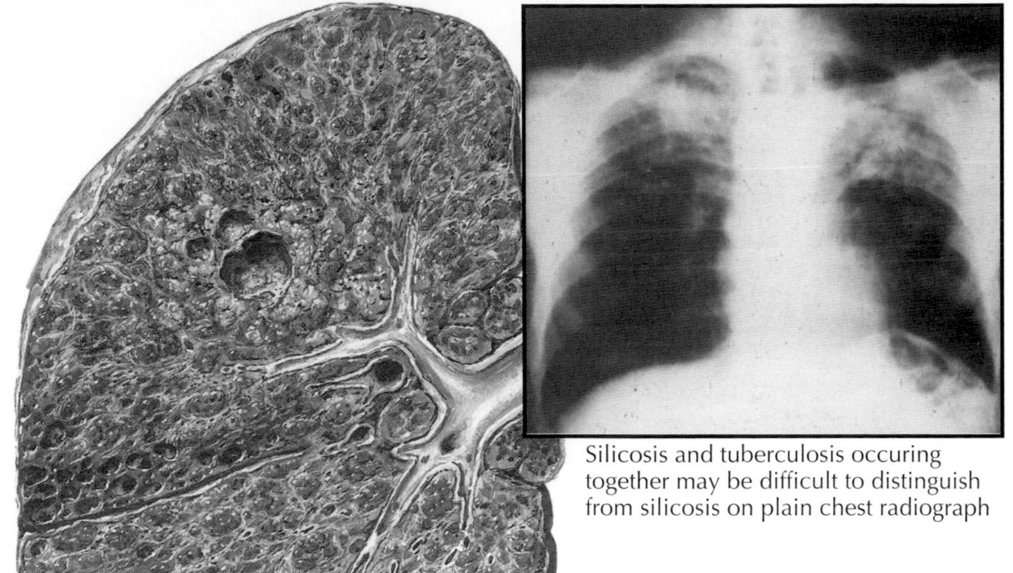

Silicosis and tuberculosis occuring together may be difficult to distinguish from silicosis on plain chest radiograph

Tuberculosis with cavitation superimposed on silicosis

Rheumatoid pneumoconiosis (Caplan syndrome)

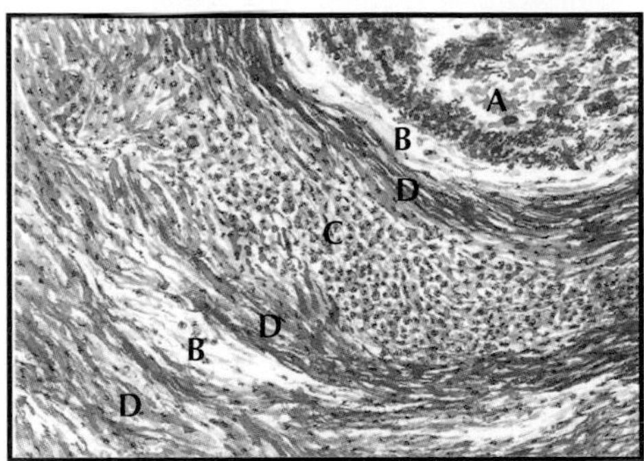

Section through margin of Caplan nodule: (**A**) necrotic central area, (**B**) separation clefts, (**C**) zone of inflammatory cells and fibroblasts, (**D**) rim of collagen

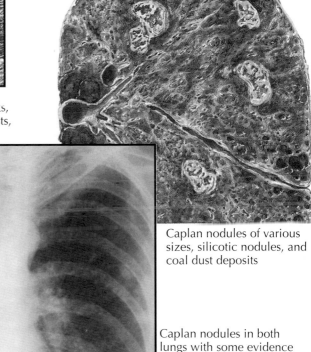

Caplan nodules of various sizes, silicotic nodules, and coal dust deposits

Caplan nodules in both lungs with some evidence of diffuse fibrosis

SILICOSIS *(Continued)*

complaints or the pulmonary function abnormalities. Pulmonary function tests show a pattern of mixed restrictive and obstructive physiology, commonly with oxygen desaturation with exertion. There is no effective treatment for silicosis; it must be prevented by industrial hygiene measures. Chronic silicosis must be managed with supportive care, such as oxygen therapy and treatment of intercurrent infections.

WORKPLACE EXPOSURE

Workers may be exposed to respirable silica dust in a variety of industrial settings where the use of power machinery generates numerous fine particles. A common theme involves drilling where the work takes place in a confined space that may be poorly ventilated, such as through silica-containing rock to extract minerals (mining) or stone (quarrying) or drilling to create passageways (tunneling). Crafting stone for monuments, tombstones, or sculpture can generate substantial airborne dust. Silica sand is used to create abrasives, sandpaper, and grinding and polishing materials. Abrasive blasting using sand for grit or nonsiliceous abrasive blasted against silica-bearing stone also can cause silicosis. Sharpening tools (scissors grinding) or cleaning sand-cast foundry parts with silica-containing abrasives can produce substantial exposures.

Silicosis caused by mining, quarrying, tool grinding, and similar activities can usually be reduced to safe levels by vigilant industrial hygiene measures (air extraction, spraying water on cutting surfaces, abrasive blasting in isolation booths, respiratory protective devices, independent clean air sources). Workers involved in the production of abrasives, glass sand, and particularly silica flour (finely divided silica powder) may experience significant exposure and develop silicosis. Silica flour is used widely as an additive, absorbent, bulking agent or an abrasive in many products such as paints, plastics, toothpastes, and detergents. Control measures and regulation and surveillance of exposures to silica are the major reason for the decline in the number of cases and deaths caused by silicosis in the United States and other industrialized nations over the past 70 years. Silicosis is still common in developing nations where extractive industries are growing and power equipment is being used more widely, but worker protection and industrial hygiene remain limited. The United States Occupational Safety & Health Administration (OSHA) and the Mine Safety Administration (MSA) have established a Permissible Exposure Limit (PEL) for an 8-hour time-weighted average (TWA) for crystalline quartz of less than 0.10 mg/m^3; levels between 0.05 mg/m^3 and 0.10 mg/m^3 are specified by most nations.

SILICOTUBERCULOSIS

Patients with silicosis appear to be particularly susceptible to a chronic indolent form of pulmonary tuberculosis. Diagnosis may be difficult because of the silicotic radiographic changes. Complete eradication of tubercle bacilli is thought to be very difficult, and lifelong antituberculous drug therapy is usually recommended.

CAPLAN NODULES

When silicosis or coal workers pneumoconiosis occurs in a patient who also has rheumatoid arthritis, necrobiotic nodules (rheumatoid nodules) may develop in the lung, a condition known as Caplan syndrome. The lesions are typically large (>1.0 cm), round, and well-defined. These "Caplan nodules" often grow much more quickly than typical silicotic nodules and may undergo central necrosis or cavitation; they may also disappear spontaneously. The Caplan nodules are of little clinical consequence in their own right but may raise great concern about the possibility of tuberculosis caused by the cavitation or lung cancer resulting from their rapid growth.

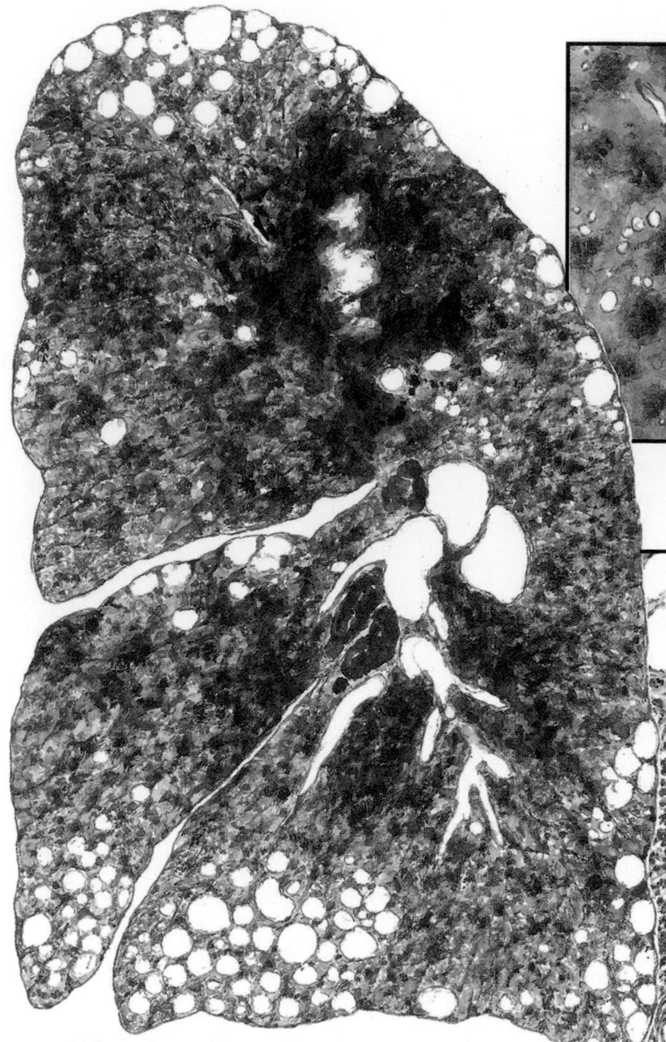

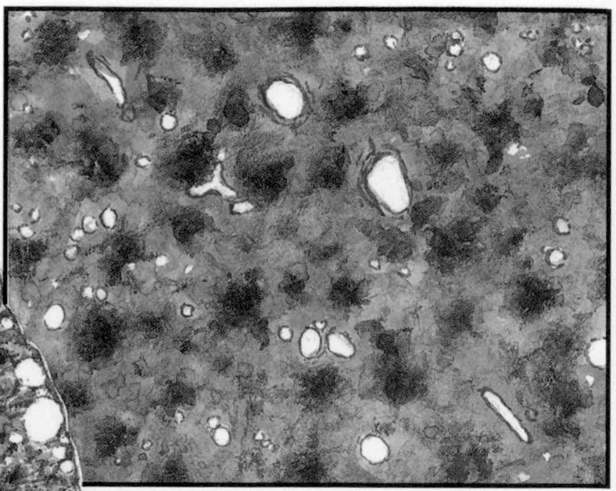

Coal Worker's Pneumoconiosis

Coal worker's pneumoconiosis (CWP) results from the inhalation of respirable coal dust that first settles within the alveoli and later accumulates near the respiratory bronchioles. There, coal macules form with limited scarring, leading to disease of the respiratory bronchioles and focal emphysema. As with most lung diseases caused by the accumulation of indigestible mineral particles or fibers in the lung, CWP develops slowly over decades and requires high levels of exposure. The disease is limited to miners of hard coal, particularly underground tunnel workers, and to those who process or handle coal where large amounts of dust are produced by crushing or bulk moving machines.

CWP was common in the United States and Europe during the late nineteenth through mid-twentieth centuries when coal was used widely for industrial and domestic fuel, mechanized mining techniques generated large amounts of respirable particles, and dust control measures were not used. Coal is elemental carbon, often mixed with small amounts of siliceous minerals. In tunnel mines, it may be necessary to drill and blast through granite or other stone with a high fraction of crystalline silica to follow and extract the coal seam. Occupational safety regulations led to wet cutting techniques, improved ventilation, and robotic mine face equipment that reduced airborne dust and decreased the number of miners needed at the cutting face. Clinically significant CWP has become much less common in industrialized nations but is still a major health problem in developing countries.

Workers with early or limited CWP evidence a pattern on plain chest radiograph of diffuse small nodular opacities 1 to 10 mm in diameter and may have no clinical symptoms or pulmonary dysfunction. A small minority of workers develop progressive disease with coalescence of the small nodules into large opacities surrounded by bands of dense fibrosis and emphysema, usually with upper lobe predominance. This advanced disease is considered complicated pneumoconiosis or *progressive massive fibrosis* (PMF). It is associated with restriction of the vital capacity, overdistension of the residual volume, and often significant airflow limitation as well (a mixed disorder). The diffusing capacity may be reduced early in the course of disease, but hypoxemia is a late consequence. Cough and shortness of breath with exertion become worse as CWP progresses.

The clinical manifestations of CWP appear to be attributable to a combination of factors. High levels of coal mine dust exposure cause "industrial bronchitis" during (and shortly after) exposure, with cough and the expectoration of black sputum but with no pulmonary function effects or only mild airflow obstruction. Pure carbon may have little impact on the function of the lung, although large amounts of black pigment may be stored in prominent dust macules and lymphoid tissues. Silica mixed with carbon or inhaled independently during drilling can cause concomitant silicosis. Most importantly, many miners smoke tobacco and thus emphysema or chronic obstructive pulmonary disease (COPD) synergize with the effects of coal dust. There is no treatment for CWP directly, but complicating diseases such as bronchitis, COPD, rheumatoid arthritis, tuberculosis, and secondary infections can be given specific or symptomatic treatment. Tobacco smoking prevention or cessation is critical.

Magnified detail of lung section shows coal dust macules or nodules

Whole-lung thin section shows central "progressive massive fibrosis" with black carbon deposits, numerous smaller nodules, and emphysematous changes

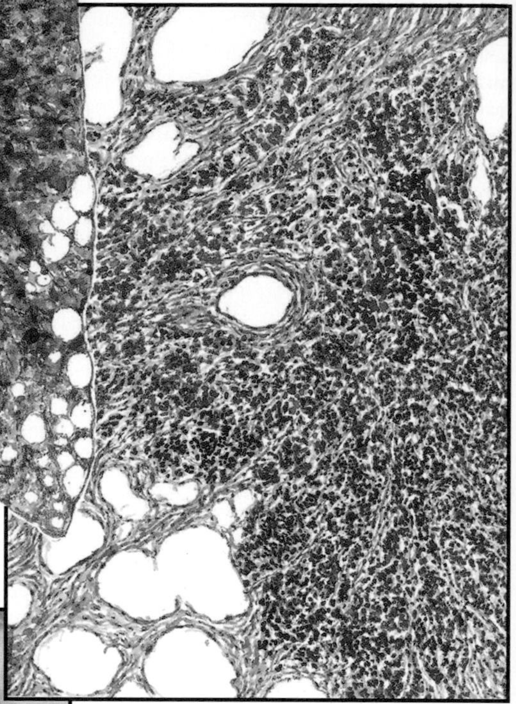

A microscopic section through a coal nodule shows large amounts of black coal dust with interspersed collagen and fibrosis. The nodule surrounds a pulmonary arteriole

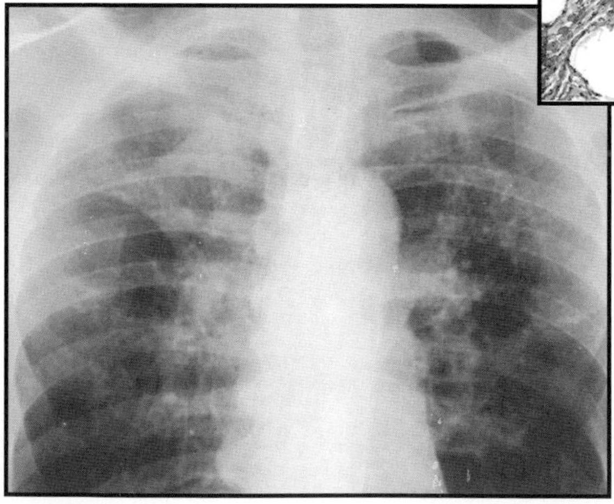

F. Netter M.D.

Chest radiograph of a retired coal miner showing massive upper lobe lesions, sometimes referred to as "angel wings," and numerous small nodules

Asbestosis and Asbestos-Related Diseases

Asbestos causes diffuse pulmonary fibrosis (asbestosis), areas of pleural thickening that may calcify (plaques), and benign exudative pleural effusions. Asbestos exposure is associated with increased risk for bronchogenic carcinoma in tobacco smokers and for malignant pleural and peritoneal mesothelioma. The asbestos-related diseases are caused almost exclusively by occupational exposures, but asbestos also represents a significant risk for mesothelioma for the general population and for workers who contact the material through their jobs.

Asbestos is valuable for its great durability and its thermal insulating properties. Asbestos is an abundant crystalline magnesium silicate that occurs in pure natural deposits as a densely packed fiber. The natural fiber can be crafted into sheets of insulating material, mixed as insulation slurry for spraying or direct application on to walls or pipes, mixed with concrete cement to strengthen it, woven into cloth with great fire-resistant properties, or manufactured into many other products in which durability and resistance to friction are important. After a period of wide use in diverse applications throughout the world during the middle of the twentieth century, the use of asbestos has been largely eliminated in the industrialized nations because of the health hazards from exposure; however, it is still mined, milled, and used widely in many developing countries.

The crystal structure of asbestos is in the form of long, thin fibers. Asbestos is divided into two mineral groups: the serpentine and the amphibole. Chrysotile (serpentine) asbestos is a very long, white, curly fiber that was used extensively for insulation and cloth. The amphibole asbestos types *amosite* (brown asbestos) and *crocidolite* (blue asbestos) have shorter, straight fibers and are particularly valued for their durability.

Exposure to asbestos occurs primarily through breathing airborne fibers into the lungs, and inhaled asbestos is clearly harmful if the dose is sufficient. Workers in all phases of asbestos production and installation experienced very high levels of exposure until the 1960s or 1970s because the health hazards were not recognized or were not publicized. Measures to control airborne fiber levels and then to reduce or eliminate the use of asbestos were implemented during the 1970s and 1980s. Levels of asbestos exposure sufficient to cause all types of asbestos-related diseases were experienced by asbestos miners and millers and by workers manufacturing asbestos cement, insulation products, paper, brake pads, friction products, and similar materials. Commercial ship builders constructing new or renovated vessels during and after World War II experienced very high levels of asbestos exposure. Insulation workers, steam boiler makers, plumbers, and others in the construction trades were exposed to asbestos as they applied the material to walls, ceilings, pipes, and many other surfaces that needed heat protection. Installed asbestos can still represent a health hazard to workers who are employed in these buildings or who maintain, renovate, or demolish them. All of the diseases caused by asbestos have very long delay periods (latency, lag time) between the exposure and the clinical illness, and no acute or short-term toxic effects of asbestos are known.

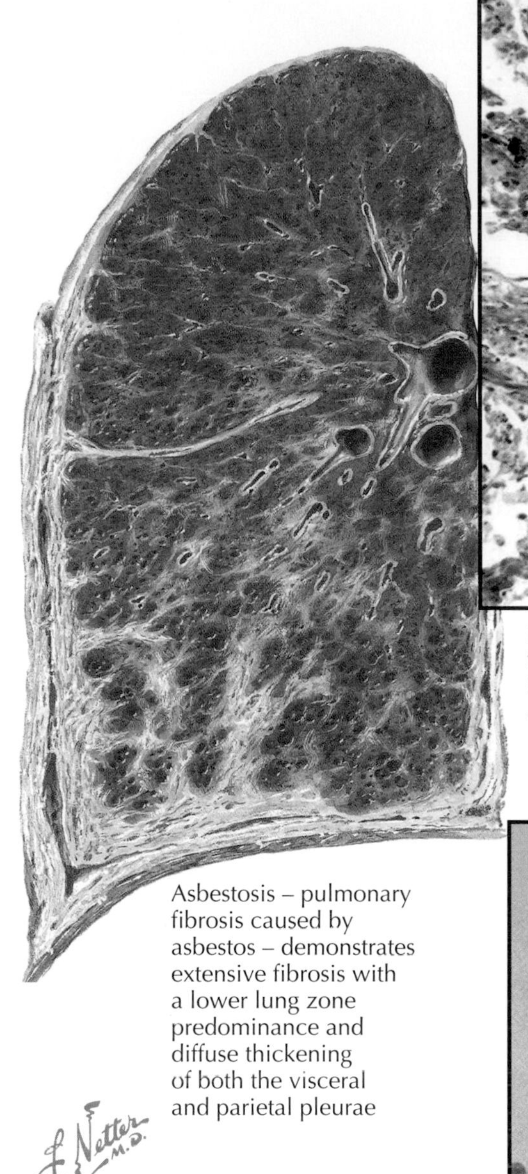

Lung tissue section shows asbestosis, with interstitial fibrosis and dust collections near small airways. Several asbestos fibers and "ferruginous bodies" can be seen (yellow arrows)

Asbestosis – pulmonary fibrosis caused by asbestos – demonstrates extensive fibrosis with a lower lung zone predominance and diffuse thickening of both the visceral and parietal pleurae

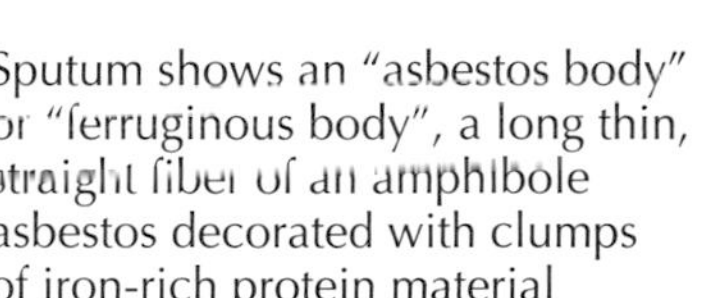

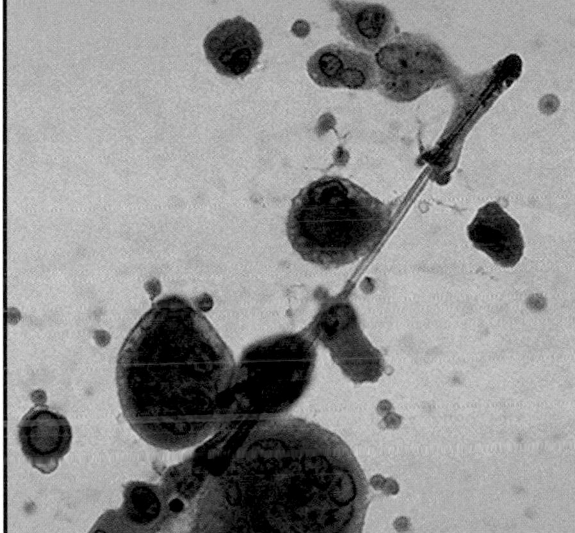

Sputum shows an "asbestos body" or "ferruginous body", a long thin, straight fiber of an amphibole asbestos decorated with clumps of iron-rich protein material

ASBESTOSIS

High levels of exposure to asbestos cause diffuse pulmonary fibrosis known as *asbestosis*. The clinical, radiographic, and pathologic features of asbestosis are nearly identical to those of idiopathic pulmonary fibrosis (IPF; cryptogenic fibrosing alveolitis). The symptoms are slowly progressive shortness of breath on exertion and a dry cough. Physical findings include high-pitched end-inspiratory crackles (dry rales) at the lung bases and digital clubbing in about half of the patients. Pulmonary function tests show a restrictive physiology with hypoxemia that worsens on exertion. The findings on chest radiograph are small irregular opacities at the periphery of the lung with a lower lung zone predominance. High-resolution computed tomography (HRCT) scans show thickening of subpleural septal and interlobular lines, curvilinear lines, and nonseptal linear opacities. Honeycomb cystic changes and traction bronchiectasis become apparent with more advanced disease.

The lung pathology of asbestosis is similar or identical to that of IPF and features the changes characterized as "usual interstitial pneumonitis," but the key distinguishing feature is the presence of abundant asbestos fibers or asbestos bodies. If the fibers are amphibole asbestos, many may become coated with protein and iron to become "asbestos bodies" or "ferruginous bodies," golden-red refractile fibers with beads or cylinders of protein. If the fibers are chrysotile, then few if any asbestos bodies form. The asbestos bodies can be stained blue with iron stains and are visible by light microscopy; smaller or uncoated fibers can be found by transmission electron microscopy.

Asbestosis (pulmonary fibrosis caused by asbestos) develops only after very high levels of exposure and

ASBESTOSIS AND ASBESTOS-RELATED DISEASES *(Continued)*

only appears decades (10-50 years) after exposure began and often after the exposure ended. Thus, workers with abnormal chest radiographs who have had only recent or brief exposure to asbestos are very unlikely to have asbestosis. The diagnosis of asbestosis rests on an appropriate asbestos exposure history, a suitable time interval between exposure and disease, basilar crackles on chest examination, and compatible radiographic changes. Lung tissue biopsy is usually not needed unless the exposure history is uncertain. There is no treatment for asbestosis other than supportive care. The prevalence of pulmonary fibrosis caused by asbestos has increased progressively but may have peaked in developed countries where asbestos use has been curtailed or banned for 25 years. It is expected that current exposure levels in the industrialized countries will be far below the threshold needed to cause pulmonary fibrosis.

BENIGN ASBESTOS-RELATED PLEURAL DISEASE

Asbestos causes several manifestations of disease in the pleural space surrounding the lung. All are believed to be related to the transport of fibers from the epithelial and interstitial spaces through the centrifugal lymphatics to the visceral pleura and across the pleural space to the parietal pleura. The most common clinical manifestation of asbestos exposure is *pleural plaques.* These lesions are benign fibrous deposits in and beneath the parietal pleura, most commonly on the lower costal and diaphragmatic surfaces of the chest. Pleural plaques seen in profile on the plain chest radiograph appear as dense linear thickening of the pleural surface several millimeters deep and several centimeters long. Pleural plaques may show dystrophic calcification that appears in profile as thin dense lines along the pleural surface. HRCT scanning demonstrates plaques easily, and areas of thickening or calcifications can often be found when the plain chest radiograph is normal. The plaques may appear 20 to 50 years after initial asbestos exposure and gradually increase in size and extent of calcification. Plaques require less exposure than asbestosis or other pleural manifestations. Pleural plaques alone cause no significant symptoms and little or no pulmonary function impairment; they require no treatment. Bilateral lower lung zone calcified pleural plaques are virtually pathognomonic of asbestos exposure and thus may serve as confirmation of a significant occupational exposure history.

Moderate asbestos exposure is associated with an exudative or serosanguineous *benign pleural effusion* in a small fraction of workers. This manifestation of asbestos-related pleural disease may be seen relatively early after exposure and often occurs before plaques or fibrosis is apparent. The main issue with a benign asbestos-related pleural effusion is usually the concern that it may represent a mesothelioma; extensive testing may be needed to prove that it does not. Rarely, asbestos can cause diffuse pleural thickening that leads to clinically significant restrictive lung disease. Areas of pleural thickening can lead to entrapment of the subadjacent lung tissue to cause a site of "rounded atelectasis."

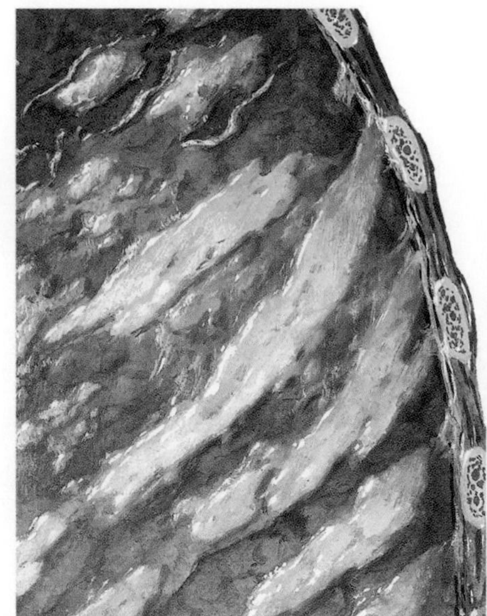

Pleural plaques on the parietal pleurae of the chest wall

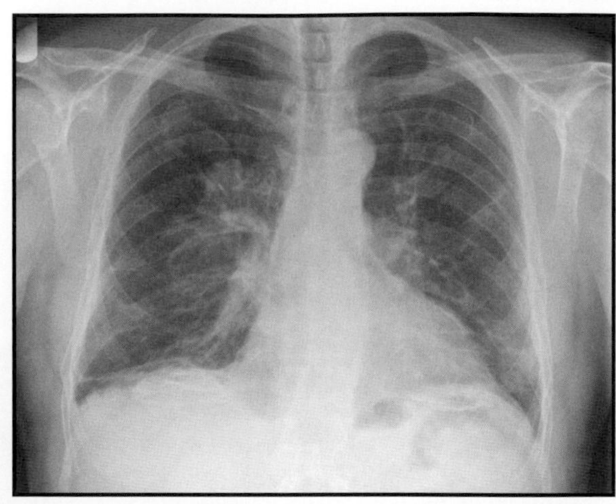

Chest radiograph of an asbestos worker shows diffuse small irregular peripheral opacities in a lower zone distribution (asbestosis) and extensive calcified pleural plaques seen en face (left upper and right lower chest) and as linear densities along the diaphragm

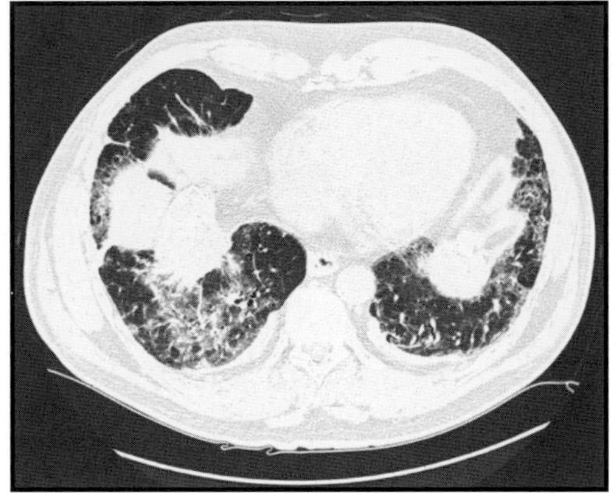

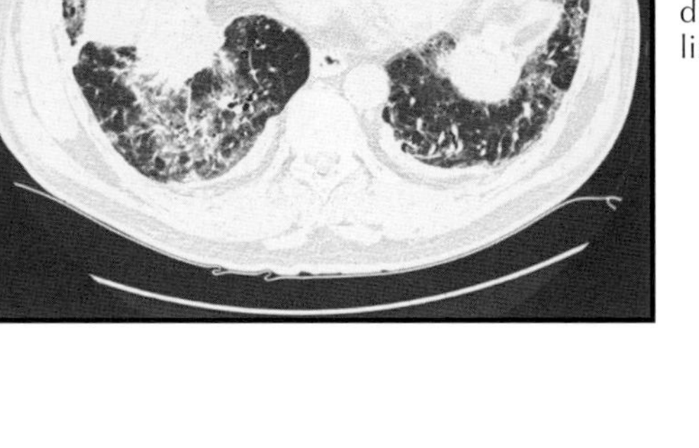

Chest CT scan (lung windows) at the diaphragm shows peripheral subpleural linear opacities of asbestosis

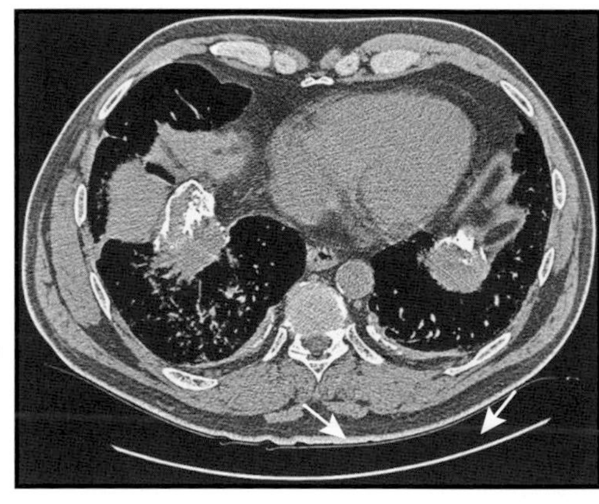

Chest CT scan (mediastinal windows) at the diaphragm shows plates and linear bands of calcification (arrows) on the parietal pleura of the diaphragm and chest wall

ASBESTOS-RELATED MALIGNANCY

Exposure to asbestos is associated with increased risks for two types of malignancy: mesothelioma in nonsmokers and smokers and bronchogenic carcinoma in smokers. The frequency of both cancer types increases with higher asbestos exposure levels, and both may be seen at doses that do not cause asbestosis or benign pleural disease. Malignant mesothelioma of the pleura or the peritoneum is a locally aggressive and invasive mesothelial cancer that occurs very rarely in the general population (fewer than one case per 100,000 per year) but is found with greatly increased frequency among individuals exposed to asbestos. The risk appears to be greater for exposure to crocidolite than to chrysotile. Patients with localized mesothelioma may sometimes respond to aggressive surgery or to chemotherapy, but for most patients, the median survival time remains short (8-14 months from diagnosis), and the mortality rate is high. The prevalence of mesothelioma has risen dramatically in the past 20 years and may now be reaching a peak that will decline in parallel with reduced asbestos use and exposure.

Workers who received substantial asbestos exposure and who smoked tobacco are at greatly increased risk of developing bronchogenic carcinoma compared with smokers who did not have asbestos exposure. Individuals who never smoked tobacco but had moderate to heavy asbestos exposure appear to be at slightly increased relative risk (1.5- to 2.5-fold) of developing lung cancer compared with nonexposed nonsmokers, but the absolute risk is still low. The clinical presentation, radiographic features, anatomic location, frequency of pathologic categories, and treatment of lung cancer with asbestos exposure appear to be similar to those for the general population.

BERYLLIUM

Beryllium (Be) is a metal whose strength, light weight, and other properties make it particularly well suited for aerospace, defense, nuclear, electronic, and other forefront technology applications. Lung diseases caused by beryllium were first publicized in the early 1940s among beryllium-oxide extraction workers in Ohio and fluorescent lamp manufacturing workers in Massachusetts. Both acute chemical pneumonitis and chronic beryllium disease (CBD) resembling sarcoidosis ("Salem sarcoid" in lamp workers) were observed. Industrial hygiene measures limited the high exposures that caused acute pneumonitis, but the continuing effects of very low-dose exposure after sensitization were more difficult to control. Beryllium is mined in the United States, China, Kazakhstan, Russia, and other countries. The ore is processed on site to beryllium hydroxide and then converted into beryllium metal, oxide, and alloys.

Beryllium salts and metal can sensitize susceptible individuals to cause a chronic granulomatous lung disease—berylliosis—that closely resembles sarcoidosis. The disease occurs almost exclusively among workers involved in beryllium extraction and production of beryllium alloy products. Sensitizing exposure does not occur after the metal has been integrated into finished products. Beryllium lung disease may serve as a paradigm for diseases in which the mechanism involves the combination of a genetically determined immunologically susceptible population with exposure to a unique specific antigen.

CHRONIC BERYLLIUM DISEASE

CBD, or berylliosis, usually begins with the gradual onset of shortness of breath and dry cough. As the disease worsens, systemic symptoms of easy fatigue, weakness, anorexia, and weight loss may be seen. Severe pulmonary involvement can produce dyspnea at rest, hypoxemia, and cor pulmonale with edema. The radiographic features resemble sarcoidosis with small reticulonodular opacities in a diffuse or patchy distribution and obscuration of peripheral vasculature by adjacent ground-glass opacities; bullae, lung distortion, or pleural thickening are uncommon. Symmetric bilateral hilar lymph node enlargement is usually moderate rather than massive and is found in fewer than 50% of cases. Progressive coalescence of opacities in an upper or mid-lung distribution can be seen as the disease advances. Pulmonary function tests show a restrictive impairment, diminished gas transfer (DL_{CO} [diffusing capacity for carbon monoxide]), and hypoxemia at rest that often worsens on exertion; a high proportion of patients with CBD also evidence airflow obstruction.

The pathology of CBD shows epithelioid cell nonnecrotizing granulomas in the lung parenchyma, the hilar and mediastinal lymph nodes, and less commonly in the skin and other organs. The lesions show macrophage-derived multinucleated epithelioid giant cells surrounded by smaller macrophage or monocytes and both T and B lymphocytes. Schaumann bodies are common. Fibroblasts and collagen infiltrate the centers of the granulomas as the disease progresses. Beryllium usually cannot be detected within these lesions. Other organ systems beyond the thorax can be involved in CBD, such as the skin, liver, spleen, peripheral lymph nodes, and bone marrow. Clinicians and pathologists agree that sarcoidosis and CBD cannot be distinguished reliably for individual cases.

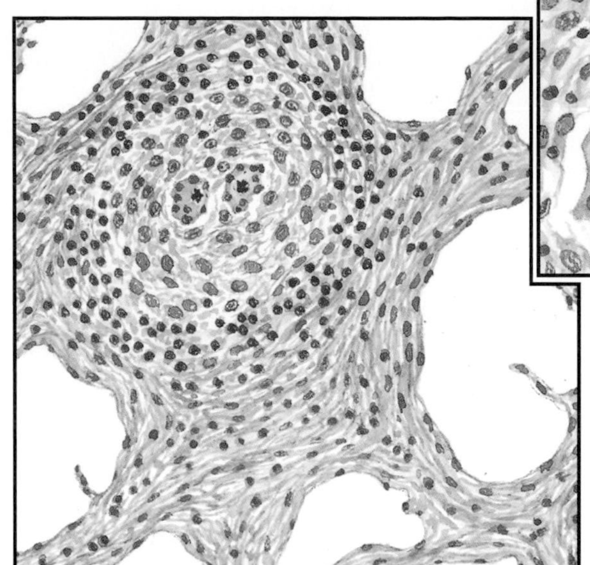

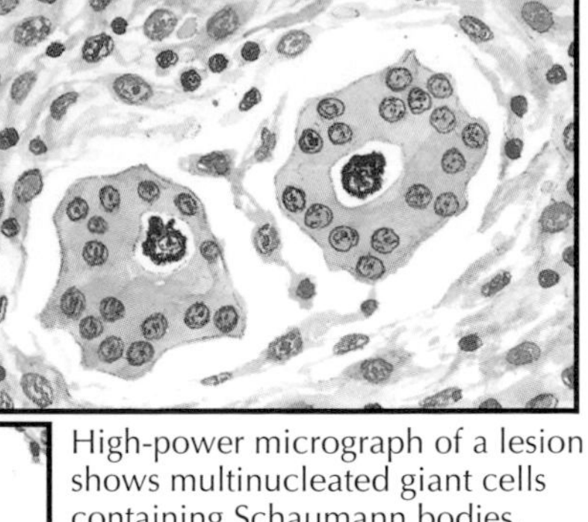

High-power micrograph of a lesion shows multinucleated giant cells containing Schaumann bodies.

Lung tissue shows a granuloma with interstitial fibrosis resembling sarcoidosis. There are central epithelioid histiocytes and multinucleated giant cells with a surrounding cuff of lymphocytes. Skin may show similar lesions.

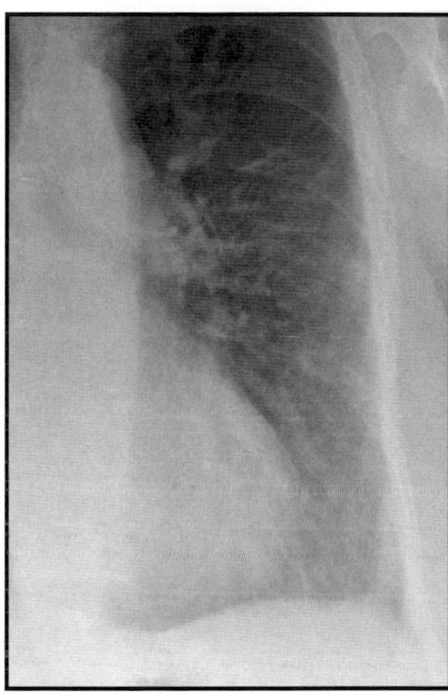

Chest X-ray from a beryllium worker exposed from aircraft parts manufacturing shows hilar adenopathy and patchy reticulonodular opacities.

PATHOGENESIS

The pathogenesis of CBD is driven by the accumulation of beryllium-specific CD4+ Th1-cells at disease sites. Genetic factors appear to determine the efficacy of presentation of beryllium to T cells, the T-cell response, and the cytokine production that influences the subsequent immune inflammatory response. Lung and peripheral blood CD4+ T lymphocytes from sensitized individuals respond to beryllium in vitro by proliferating vigorously (i.e., the beryllium lymphocyte proliferation test). Sensitization alone is not sufficient to produce clinically evident lung disease because many exposed workers develop sensitization without progression to disease. Lymphocyte immune sensitivity to beryllium is found in 1% to 16% of exposed workers, but only half of the sensitized workers evidence lung granulomas.

DIAGNOSIS

The diagnosis of CBD requires a compatible clinical picture, an appropriate environmental exposure history, and the demonstration of cell-mediated immunity (lymphocyte sensitivity in vitro) to beryllium antigen. Clinical evidence of disease with noncaseating granulomas in tissue pathology is essential because not all exposed or sensitized workers develop disease. A clinical syndrome alone is not sufficient because sarcoidosis can present identical features and is much more common. Workers suspected of CBD can be referred to one of several national research centers that offer consultation and specialized testing.

THERAPY

The therapy for berylliosis is similar to the treatment for sarcoidosis but must include strict avoidance of beryllium exposure. Patients with very mild or early disease may require no treatment if avoidance of further antigen exposure is successful. Most patients can be managed with relatively low doses of oral corticosteroids. Higher doses of steroids and cytotoxic or steroid-sparing alternatives (methotrexate, azathioprine, cyclophosphamide) are required by more patients with more severe disease.

Pneumoconiosis Caused by Various Minerals and Mixed Dusts

Numerous minerals and metals that are mined, milled, quarried, carved, or used in industrial processes can cause lung disease if particles or fumes are inhaled. In many instances, the materials are relatively inert. Large amounts of the mineral can accumulate in the lung to create an impressive dust burden on pathologic examination (iron) or a striking chest radiograph (barium) but few symptoms and little pulmonary dysfunction. In some instances, metal fumes (cadmium) or particles (cobalt) can cause acute lung injury or trigger an immune response.

Kaolin pneumoconiosis.
Whole-lung cross-section shows whorled fibrous masses and smaller nodules. Inset microscopic section shows alveoli filled with dust-ladened macrophages containing kaolin (aluminum silicate) clay particles. There is mild interstitial thickening and fibrosis

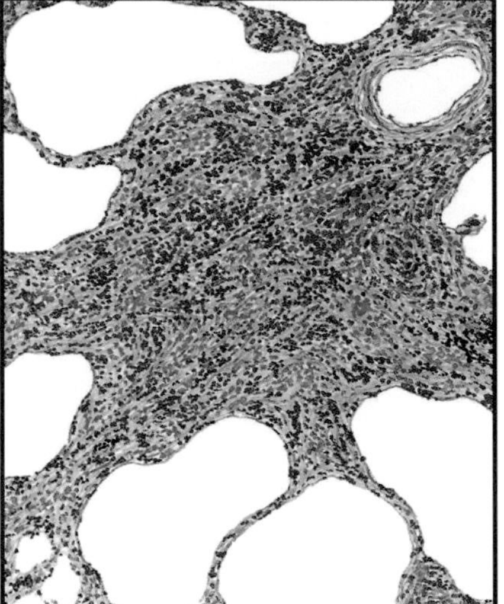

Mixed dust pneumoconiosis. Microscopic section shows fibrosis surrounding deposits of carbon, iron oxide, and silica. These lesions may be found in welders, oxyacetylene torch cutters, sandblasters, and others

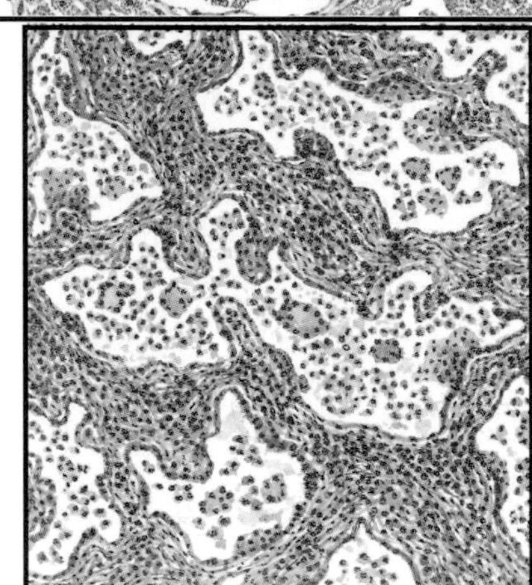

Hard metal disease (cobalt pneumoconiosis). Giant cell interstitial pneumonitis is caused by the immune inflammatory response to cobalt used as a sintering agent for fusing tungsten and carborundum (tungsten carbide) or diamond dust in abrasives

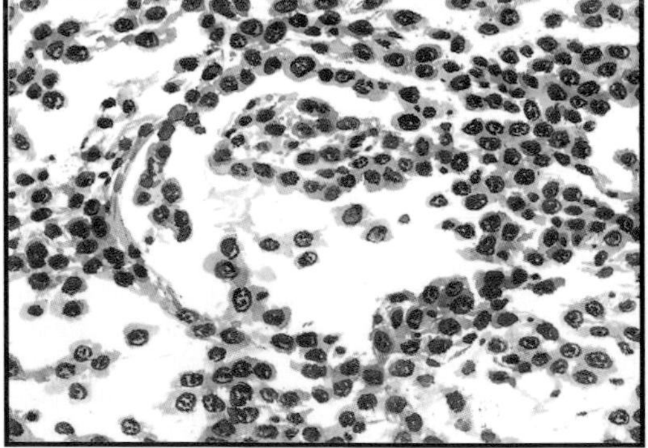

Cadmium injury: The acute effects of cadmium inhalation are seen as injury and metaplasia of the alveolar epithelium

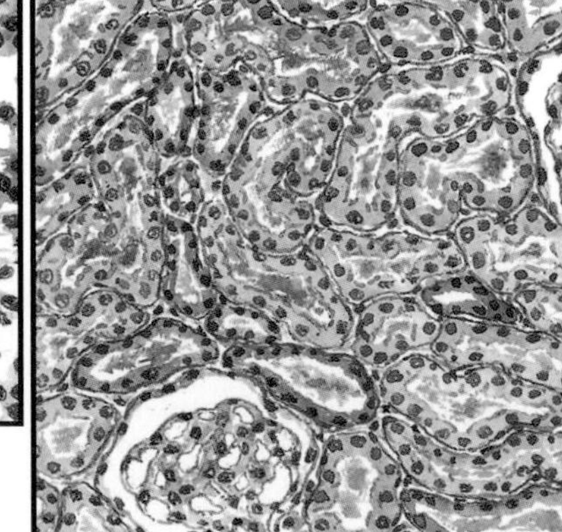

Cadmium injury. Renal effects of chronic cadmium poisoning appear as PAS-positive material clogging the tubules

KAOLIN

China clay (kaolin, aluminum silicate) is mined from surface quarries and crushed to a fine powder. Kaolin is used widely as an absorbent, as an additive to thicken paints and other products, and to manufacture porcelain ceramics. Workers exposed to high levels of kaolin dust may accumulate large amounts of the mineral in their lungs and may develop a mild pneumoconiosis that resembles silicosis.

MIXED-DUST PNEUMOCONIOSIS

Mixtures of various minerals comprise most naturally occurring stone. When stone or earth is excavated, blasted, crushed, or crafted, the airborne dust contains a mixture of crystalline and amorphous minerals that reflect the source. If dust exposure is intense or prolonged, these minerals accumulate in the lungs of exposed workers and may be evident either as a "storage disease" or as overt pulmonary fibrosis. The extent of lung disease depends primarily on the fraction of crystalline free silica present in the mixed dust and the pathogenicity of other silicates (e.g., aluminum silicates, magnesium silicates).

COBALT PNEUMOCONIOSIS (HARD METAL DISEASE)

Cobalt exposure is associated with interstitial lung disease and occupational asthma. These diseases occur only in occupational settings, and there is no indication that cobalt metal or cobalt compounds constitute a health risk for the general population. The interstitial lung disease develops only when the exposure to cobalt occurs in association with tungsten carbide (known as "hard metal") or with diamond dust. This specific pneumoconiosis is known as "hard metal disease." Only a small fraction of exposed workers develop the disease, and the mechanisms appear to be immunologic sensitization rather than (or in addition to) direct lung injury. The clinical features of cobalt pneumoconiosis are variable and include a subacute form with rapidly progressive cough, fever, and shortness of breath as well as a more chronic form with gradually progressive respiratory impairment. Chest radiograph patterns vary from patchy infiltrates to diffuse small nodular infiltrates or reticulonodular opacities. The pathology of cobalt pneumoconiosis is distinctive, and the hallmark features are bizarre giant cells in association with a pattern resembling "usual interstitial pneumonitis" or "desquamative interstitial pneumonitis." A picture similar to that of hypersensitivity pneumonitis can be seen in the subacute form.

The adverse responses to cobalt in the lung appear to be primarily immunologic but may also involve direct injury or toxicity. Cobalt can be detected in the urine of exposed workers. Cobalt may or may not be detected in lung biopsy specimens of patients with cobalt pneumoconiosis. Cobalt can cause asthma and contact dermatitis associated with IgE antibodies and possibly T-cell–mediated responses against cobalt. The granulomatous "giant cell interstitial pneumonitis" characteristic of hard metal disease includes abundant

Pneumoconiosis Caused by Various Minerals and Mixed Dusts *(Continued)*

lymphocytes and macrophages, particularly in the earlier or subacute form.

Cobalt metal is used to sinter, cement, or fuse dissimilar materials when the mixture is heated together. In this application, cobalt is used widely to create "hard metal" coatings on steel tools and parts and abrasives in which tungsten carbide particles or diamond-cobalt particles are applied to disks or wheels for grinding tools. Workers who produce tools or parts coated with hard metal for durability and workers manufacturing tungsten carbide or diamond abrasives are at risk for developing cobalt pneumoconiosis. Individuals who later use these abrasives or who sharpen tools with tungsten carbide tips are also at risk.

CADMIUM

Cadmium is an element that occurs as a soft bluish-white metal, usually refined as a byproduct of smelting other metals such as zinc. It is used for pigment (cadmium yellow), batteries, and other chemical applications. The use of cadmium is sharply limited by its high toxicity and carcinogenicity. Workers can inhale cadmium from the smelting and refining of metals, from the air in plants that make cadmium products, or when soldering or welding metal that contains cadmium. Acute exposure to cadmium fumes may cause flulike symptoms, including chills, fever, and muscle aches. More severe exposures can cause tracheobronchitis, pneumonitis, and pulmonary edema. Symptoms of inflammation may start hours after the exposure and include cough, dryness and irritation of the nose and throat, headache, dizziness, weakness, fever, chills, and chest pain. Inhaling cadmium-laden dust quickly leads to respiratory tract and kidney injuries that can be fatal.

FULLER EARTH

"Fuller earth" (magnesium oxide, calcium montmorillonite, attapulgite, calcium bentonite) is fine clay used to absorb oils from wool, friction pads, and other materials. Exposure during the mining or milling of Fuller earth may cause the accumulation of large amounts of the clay in the lungs. The mineral may be contaminated with silica, calcite, dolomite, or other materials. The lung disease is likely caused by quartz and other silicates that contaminate the magnesium oxide.

GRAPHITE

Graphite mineral is pure carbon, a form of highly compressed coal, and is sometimes referred to as meta-anthracite. It is mined from ore deposits and is used for the "lead" in pencils, as a lubricant, and to compose electrodes. Workers exposed to airborne graphite in mining, milling, or manufacturing may accumulate large amounts of the mineral in their lungs. It resides mostly in the macrophages that ingest it and in the regional lymph nodes where they transport it. Although impressive on pathologic examination, it causes little pulmonary dysfunction. Graphite lung disease might be considered a variant of coal worker's pneumoconiosis caused by a very pure form of coal.

SIDEROSIS

Inhalation of iron ore dust (iron oxide) causes accumulation of the brick-red pigment in the macrophages and lymphatic structures of the lung (i.e., pulmonary siderosis). Workers involved in the surface mining of iron ore, crushing and milling for transport, or smelting the ore into elemental iron for steel manufacture may be exposed to iron dust. The pure iron oxide probably causes little lung injury or fibrosis, but substantial amounts of silica and other silicates may be mixed in the iron ore. These fibrogenic contaminants are probably responsible for the lung disease that may result.

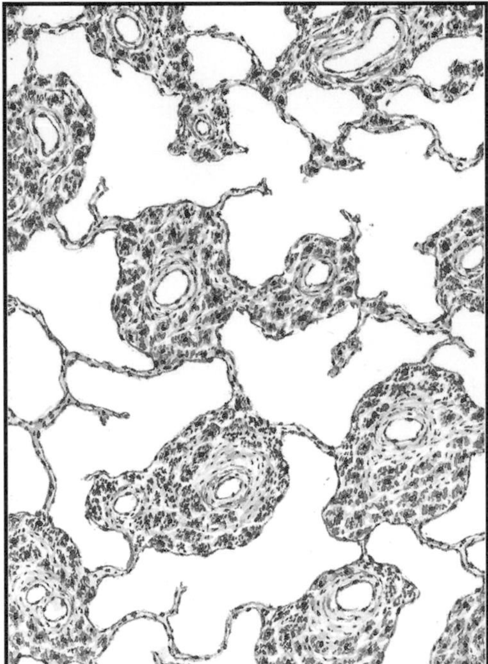

Fuller earth pneumoconiosis. "Fuller earth" (montmorillonite, attapulgite, calcium bentonite) is a fine clay used to absorb grease and oils from wool, friction pads, and other materials. Intense exposure during the mining or milling of Fuller earth may cause lung disease, likely caused by quartz and other silicates that contaminate the magnesium. Perivascular accumulations of macrophages ladened with dust particles are seen in microscopic lung sections

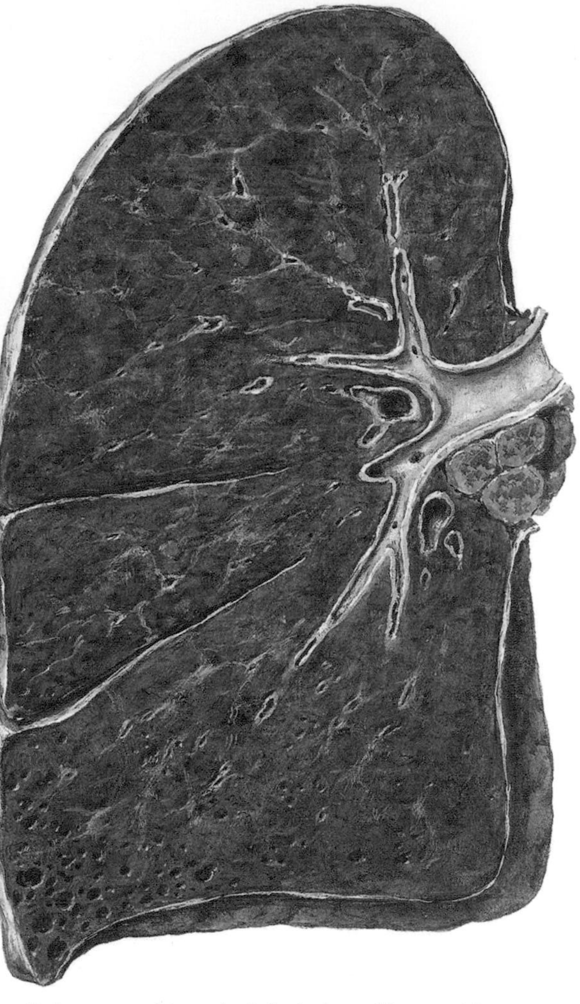

Pulmonary siderosis. Inhalation of iron oxide ore in mining, shipping, and smelting produces accumulation of the dust with brick red pigmentation of the lung. Mild fibrosis with nodules and mild emphysema may result if the ore contains significant silica or silicates

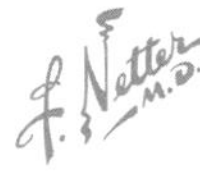

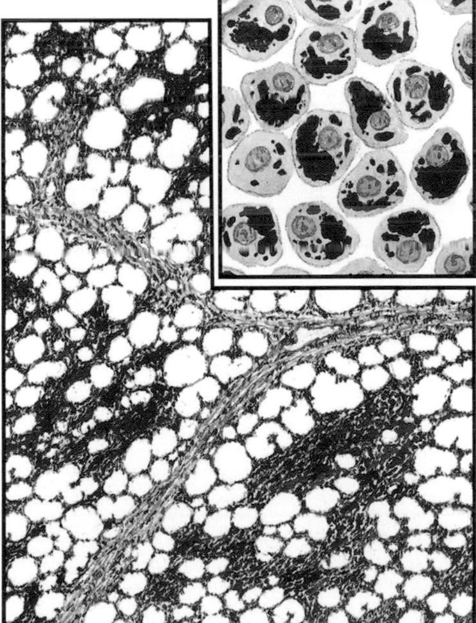

Graphite pneumoconiosis. Black mineral particles pack alveolar macrophages (*inset*) that fill alveoli and coalesce to form dust macules with fibrosis

Hypersensitivity Pneumonitis

Hypersensitivity pneumonitis (HP), or extrinsic allergic alveolitis, is an inflammatory disease caused by immune responses to inhaled antigenic organic particles or fumes. Episodes of acute and subacute HP usually resolve when antigen exposure ceases, although chronic HP may be progressive and irreversible, leading to debilitating fibrotic lung disease. HP can be caused by a wide variety of antigens that result in a common pattern of immune responses and clinical features. Colorful names such as pigeon breeder's disease, bagassosis, and maple bark stripper's lung have been attached to HP when caused by specific occupational exposures, but the patterns of disease and the features of the immune responses appear to be common to all forms.

The classic example of HP is "farmer's lung disease," an illness initially described in dairy farmers who developed episodes of cough, shortness of breath, sometimes fever, and pulmonary infiltrates when exposed to the spores of bacteria that grew in bales of moldy hay. Hay that was wet when baled would support mold growth, and the heat of fermentation would then support growth of thermophilic *Actinomyces* bacteria. As the heated bales dried, the bacteria would convert from replication to the formation of hardy spores of small respirable size and light weight. When cracked open, a cloud of spores would rise from the moldy bale like a puff of smoke and readily be inhaled by the farmer handling it. Because only the occasional bale might be moldy, illness might be intermittent. HP is remarkable for the diversity of occupations and exposures that can cause the disease. Agents include spores from bacteria and molds, amoebae, bird and animal danders, and fragments of plant materials; more than 200 antigens have been identified.

The pathogenesis of HP is based on combined humoral and cell-mediated immune responses. The humoral response is dominated by IgG antibodies that may form immune complexes in vivo and precipitating complexes in vitro in laboratory tests (serum precipitins). The cell-mediated immune response is driven by sensitized T lymphocytes with activated macrophages. Only a small minority of individuals with exposure develop clinical disease, implying a genetically determined immune response capability. A substantial number of exposed individuals may demonstrate serum antibodies but no cell-mediated immune response or clinical illness, indicating that positive laboratory test results for antibodies confirm exposure but are not sufficient to allow diagnosis without other confirmatory evidence.

Three patterns of HP are recognized: (1) an acute form with episodes that occur within 4 to 8 hours of antigen exposure and clear within about 48 hours, (2) a subacute form that last from 48 hours to several months, and (3) a chronic form lasting 4 months or longer. It is believed that occasional, intermittent, intense exposures may favor the acute form (e.g., the rare bale of moldy hay fed in the winter), and continuous or daily exposure may favor the subacute form (e.g., a pet parakeet in the home). With frequent or prolonged exposure, the chronic form of the disease may develop with permanent pulmonary fibrosis.

The clinical features of acute HP include the abrupt onset of flulike symptoms with fever, aches, malaise, cough, and dyspnea within a few hours of known (or unsuspected) exposure. The patient appears ill, and crackles (rales) may be present on lung auscultation. Chest radiographs may reveal infiltrates that lead to an initial diagnosis and treatment of community-acquired pneumonia. Chest computed tomography (CT) scans show scattered ground-glass opacities with small centrilobular nodular opacities. The lung pathology of acute HP features an inflammatory interstitial infiltrate consisting of lymphocytes (predominantly CD8+ T cells), plasma cells, mast cells, and macrophages. Scattered, poorly formed, noncaseating granulomas and

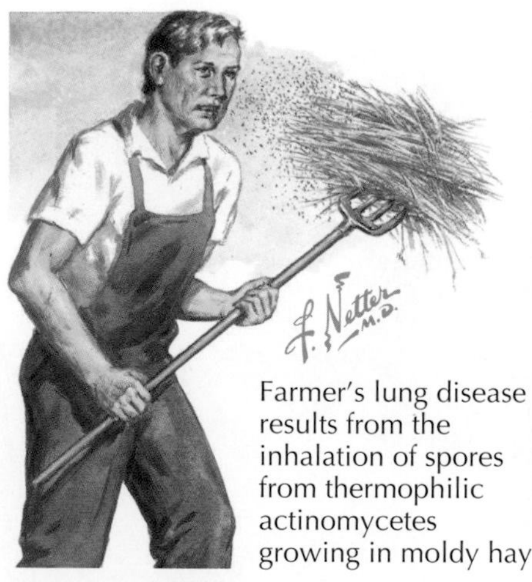

Farmer's lung disease results from the inhalation of spores from thermophilic actinomycetes growing in moldy hay

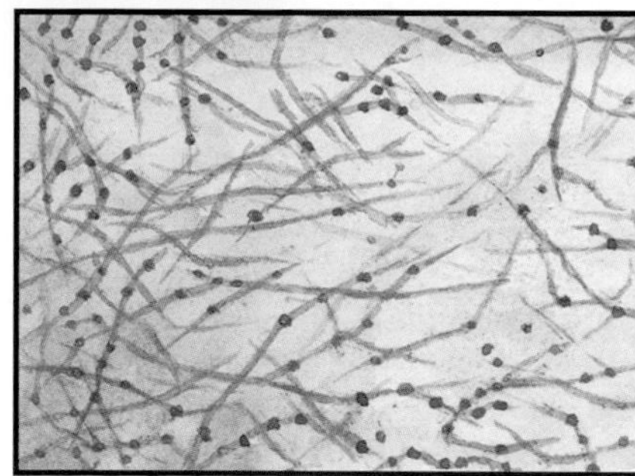

Slide culture of *Saccharopolyspora rectivirgula (formerly Micropolyspora faenae),* a thermophilic actinomycete bacteria that grows in moldy or decomposing organic material and is the cause of farmer's lung, mushroom picker's lung, and other forms of hypersensitivity pneumonitis

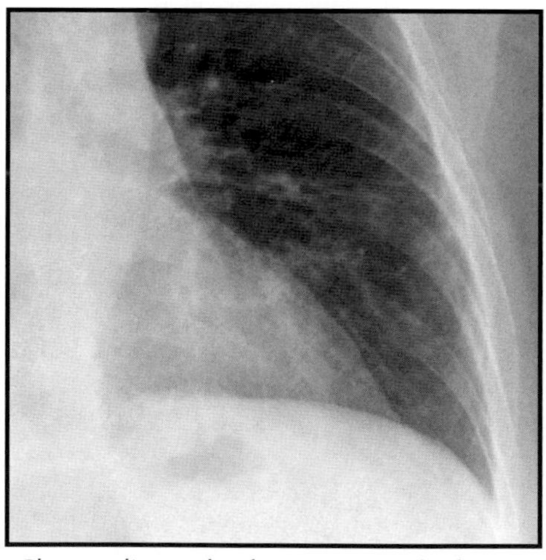

Chest radiograph of a woman with chronic hypersensitivity pneumonitis attributed to household basement mold exposure shows patchy left lower lobe opacities

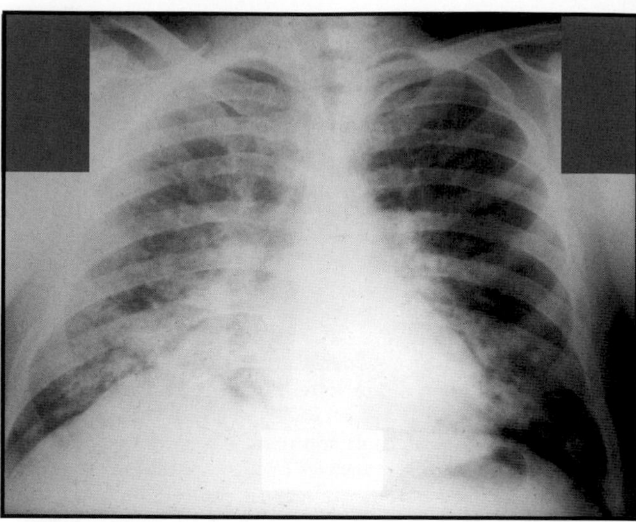

Chest radiograph of a dairy farmer 6 hours after exposure to moldy hay shows bilateral patchy ground-glass opacities. Acute shortness of breath, cough, and fever accompanied the response

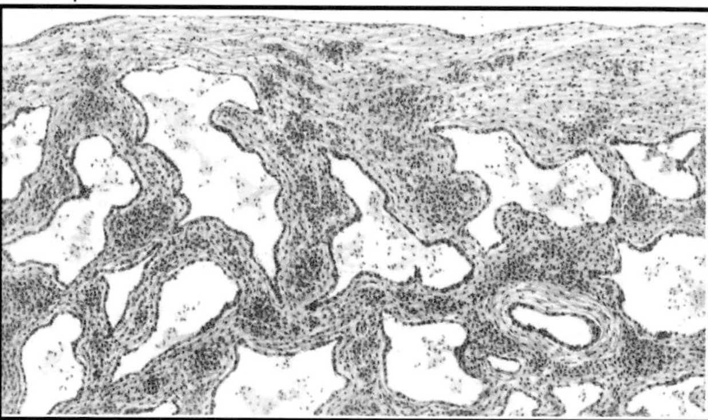

Chronic hypersensitivity pneumonitis shows extensive subpleural and interstitial fibrosis with inflammatory cell infiltrates and loosely formed granuloma-like cell aggregates

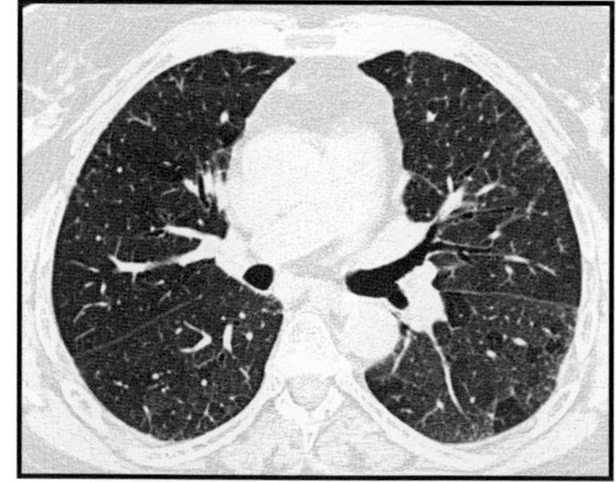

CT scan shows patchy ground-glass opacities, particularly in the left lower lobe, with a mosaic pattern and scattered subpleural linear opacities

Hypersensitivity Pneumonitis
(Continued)

occasional multinucleated giant cells may be seen, particularly adjacent to small airways. Neutrophils may be present, but eosinophils are notably not a prominent part of this immune response. Bronchoalveolar lavage (BAL) reflects the alveolar inflammatory exudate with a very high proportion of lymphocytes (>30%) and usually a predominance of CD8+ cells (in contrast to sarcoidosis, in which CD4+ cells are increased). If the exposure has been limited, the symptoms clear within 48 hours and the radiographs within 4 weeks. Repeated episodes may prompt suspicion for HP rather than infection.

Subacute HP occurs with repeated or continuous exposure to the sensitizing antigen and resembles the acute form with less abrupt onset and fewer systemic symptoms. Cough and dyspnea predominate and may become progressively severe. The chest CT scan may show less ground-glass opacity and centrilobular nodules that are more distinct. Subacute HP exhibits granulomas that may be better formed but with interstitial inflammation away from the granulomas as well. Symptoms and radiographs may clear more slowly when exposure ends, but resolution is usually complete.

Chronic HP may be indolent, progressive, and easily confused with idiopathic pulmonary fibrosis. Symptoms feature dyspnea with exertion and nonproductive cough. Crackles are heard on lung examination, and rarely digital clubbing may be present. The CT scan shows areas of linear and reticular opacities as well as ground glass, and honeycombing may be evident. Chronic HP demonstrates interstitial fibrosis and may sometimes include traction bronchiectasis and honeycomb formation that closely resembles usual interstitial pneumonitis. A predominantly lymphocytic interstitial infiltration and occasional granulomas permit distinction in most cases.

The diagnosis of HP depends on establishing a combination of exposure to a plausible antigen, a compatible clinical syndrome, appropriate radiologic findings, demonstration of an immunologic response to the antigen, and typical lung pathology. BAL with a CD8+ lymphocytosis is confirmatory but not diagnostic. In most cases, all of these dimensions are not needed or available for diagnosis. Historically, most cases of HP were associated with occupational exposures, but hobbies (pet birds), hot tubs, and home environmental exposures now predominate in developed countries. A recent large case series from the United States reported that a specific cause was identified in only 75% of cases despite vigorous attempts; thus, the clinical picture and lung biopsy were needed in the others. Serologic testing offered diagnosis in only 25%. The most common identified causes were avian antigens (34%; parakeets, parrots, pigeons), hot tub lung (21%; *Mycobacterium avium*), and mold (20%; farmer's lung, household exposure).

Removal from exposure to the antigen is the key to the treatment of HP, so correct identification of the antigen is critically important but not successful in many cases. It is very important to establish a diagnosis with confidence because for those with occupational exposures, avoiding the antigen may involve loss of a job or a very costly modification of the workplace. For home or hobby exposures, excluding a beloved pet or a major change in lifestyle may be needed. Systemic corticosteroid therapy is useful in relieving acute symptoms and short-term reversal of lung pathology. Long-term steroid treatment is not recommended because of side effects and uncertain efficacy; fibrosis may continue if exposure does not end. Resolution and a favorable outcome can usually be expected with prompt diagnosis and successful removal from the antigen.

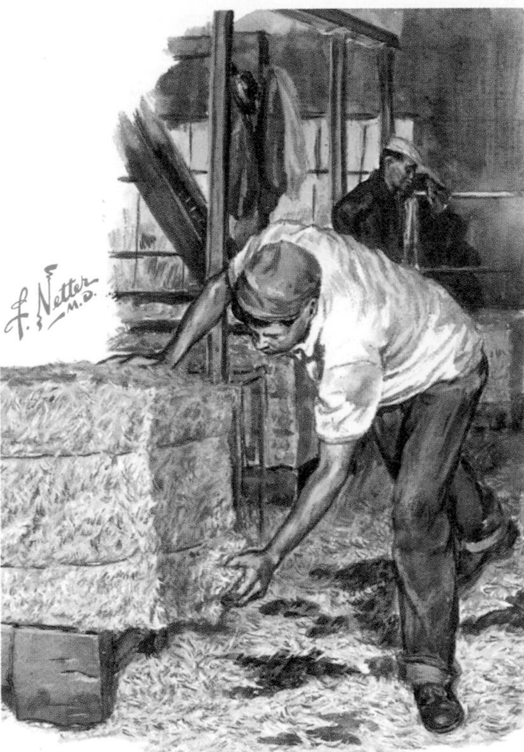

Bagassosis is a form of hypersensitivity pneumonitis caused by inhaling spores from thermophilic organisms that grow in moldy bagasse, the dried leaves and chaff from sugar cane. Bagasse is used to make wall board, paper, and containers or is burned for fuel. It is not the fresh cane material that causes the disease, but the bacteria, such as *Thermoactinomyces sacchari,* growing in it

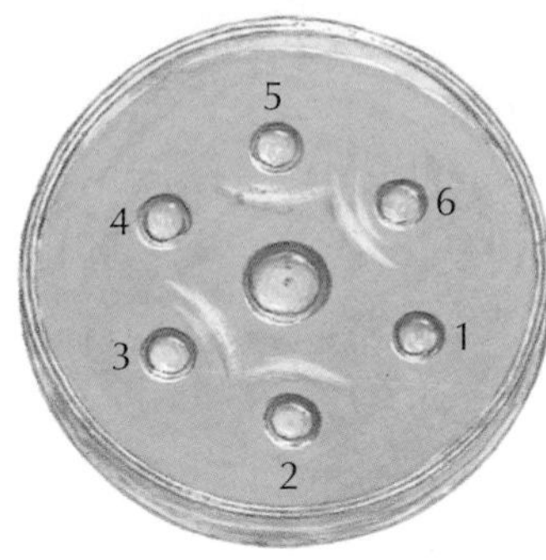

Preciptin reactions in bagassosis: The patient's serum is in the central well, and extracts of bagasse from various sources are in the peripheral wells. Samples 1 and 4 from fresh bagasse show no reactions, but other samples from moldy bagasse show lines of antigen–antibody precipitation

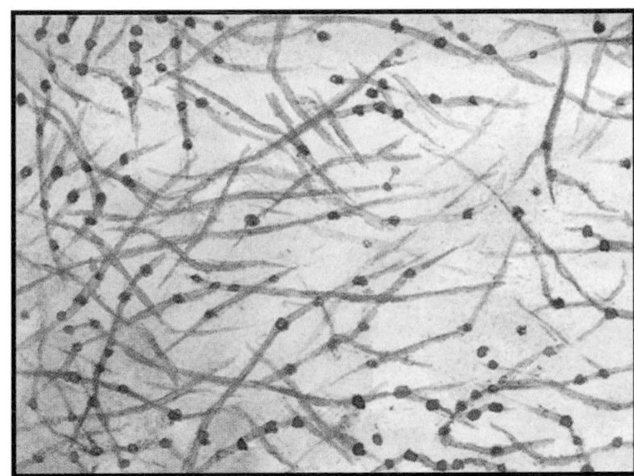

Slide culture of *Thermoactinomyces sacchari*, the principal cause of bagassosis

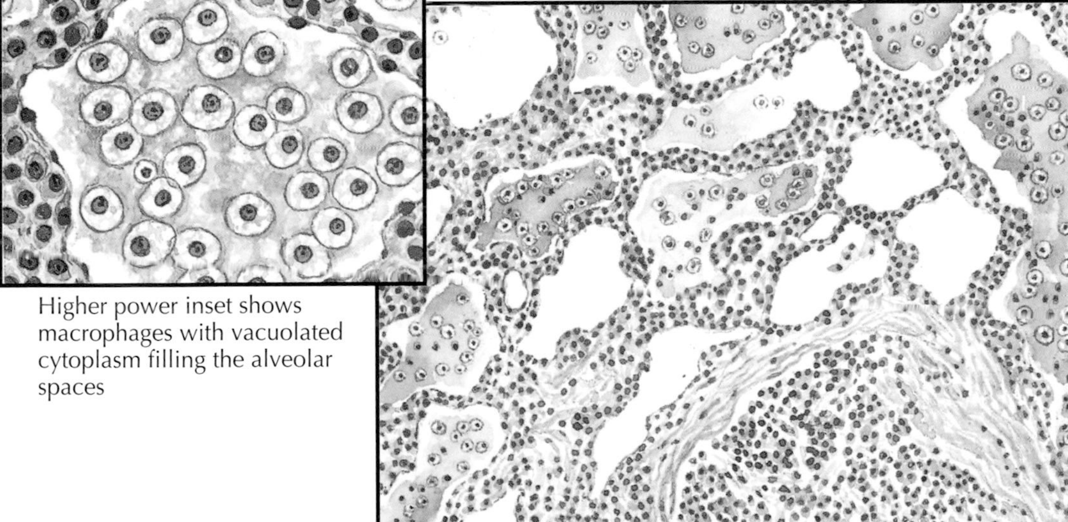

Higher power inset shows macrophages with vacuolated cytoplasm filling the alveolar spaces

In acute bagassosis, the alveolar walls are thickened with an infiltrate of plasma cells and lymphocytes, edema fluid and desquamated alveolar epithelial cells fill the airspaces

Predisposing Factors for Pulmonary Embolism

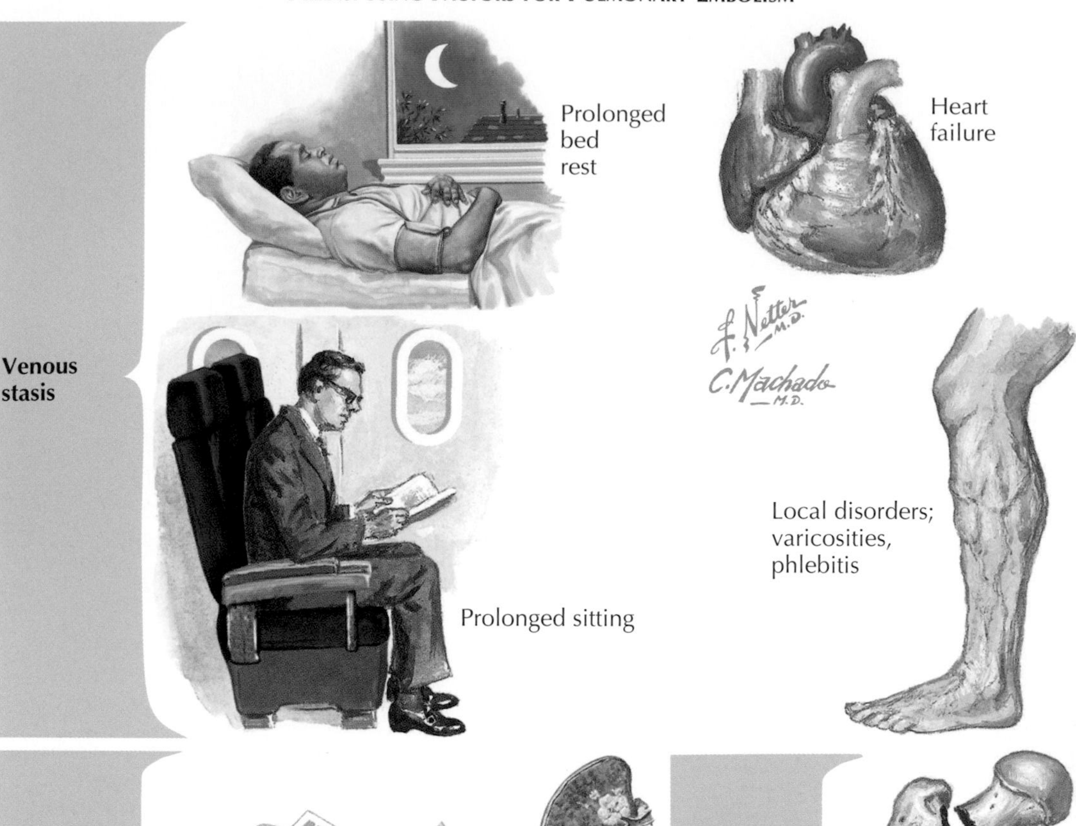

Pulmonary Embolism and Venous Thromboembolism

Pulmonary embolism (PE) and deep venous thrombosis (DVT) are generally considered to be two clinical presentations of venous thromboembolism (VTE). In most cases, PE is a result of embolization of clot from DVT. The diagnosis and management of patients with PE have been addressed in a number of summary articles and guidelines, including guidelines prepared by a Task Force of the European Society of Cardiology.

Risk Factors for Pulmonary Embolism

PE can occur without identifiable predisposing factors, but one or more factors are usually identified, such as age, history of previous DVT, cancer, neurologic disease with paresis, medical disorders associated with prolonged bed rest, thrombophilia, hormone replacement therapy, and oral contraceptive therapy (see Plate 4-114). There may also be associations with obesity, smoking, and systemic hypertension or the metabolic syndrome. Surgery, particularly orthopedic surgery, is associated with an increased risk of PE.

Pathophysiology

The source of clots is generally the deep veins of the legs and pelvis (i.e., a femoral, popliteal, or iliac vein) (see Plate 4-115). Most often, clots in a thigh vein originate as an extension of a clot in a deep calf vein. Superficial thrombophlebitis in the legs or thighs rarely gives rise to emboli but may signal a DVT. The loose propagating thrombus in the deep veins constitutes the hazard of pulmonary embolization. When broken loose, the clot is carried to the lungs through the venous stream and right side of the heart.

Superficial thrombophlebitis, which may be associated with DVT, occurs in fewer than one-third of patients with PE. Signs of DVT in the calf or thigh are difficult to detect until the venous circulation is extensively compromised (see Plates 4-116 and 4-117). When careful examination fails to implicate veins of the extremities, it is usual to suspect thrombosis of less accessible deep veins, particularly the pelvic veins in women who have had complicated obstetric manipulations, pelvic inflammatory disease, or septic abortion associated with suppurative pelvic thrombophlebitis.

Local or systemic disorders that predispose to venous thrombosis in the legs are also potential precursors of pulmonary emboli (see Plate 4-114). Paramount among these is venous stasis. Even in a normal person, a prolonged ride with flexed knees in an automobile or airplane may lead to venous stasis and thrombosis in the legs.

Clinical Manifestations of Leg Vein Thrombosis

Clinical manifestations of thromboses in the leg veins remain an important part of disease recognition and prompt diagnosis (see Plate 4-116).

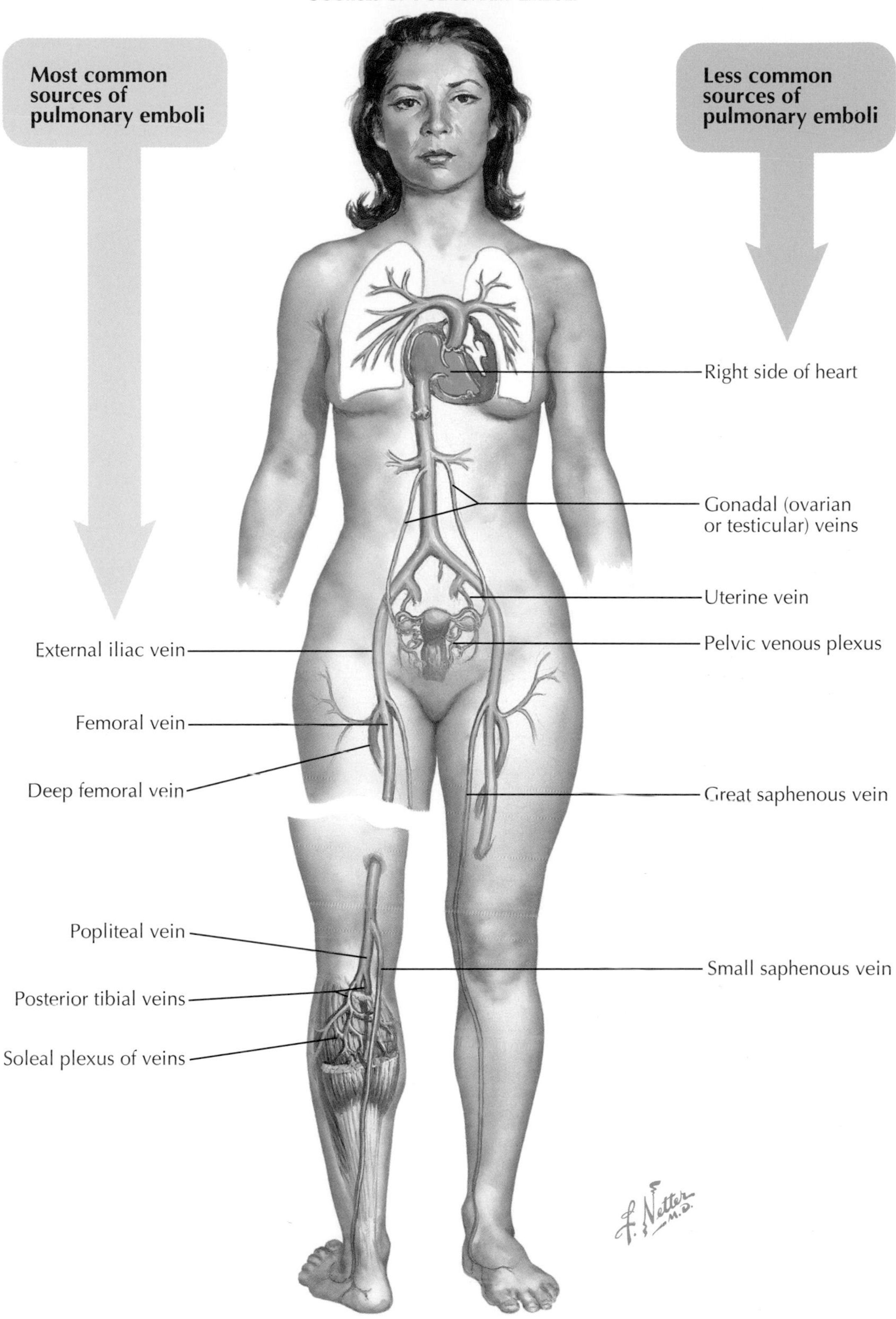

Pulmonary Embolism and Venous Thromboembolism
(Continued)

History

Thrombophlebitis is usually brought to the patient's attention by pain in the muscles of the affected leg. The pain may be diffuse or localized, and the patient usually does not confuse it with joint pain. Patients may notice that the pain is far worse on dependency and, conversely, completely relieved by elevation. There is often swelling of the affected leg and foot; the extremity may be warm locally, and the patient may be febrile.

Certain circumstances are likely to be associated with DVT, and the physician should review these points with the patient. An initial event may be dependency of the leg for several hours. Obesity; chronic illness, particularly carcinoma and most particularly carcinoma of the pancreas; and use of oral contraceptives enhance the possibility of this complication.

Physical Examination

The patient should first be examined in the standing position. The presence of varicose veins should be noted because they increase the patient's susceptibility to thrombophlebitis. Enhancement of the pain by dependency may provide a useful diagnostic clue. The patient is then examined in the recumbent position. A valuable method of detecting unilateral thrombophlebitis is to evaluate the tissue consistency of the affected leg compared with that of the unaffected leg. The examination should be preceded by palpation of the calves for tenderness with the patient's leg slightly flexed. Generalized tenderness of the calf or thigh may be found. In addition, there may be tenderness along the major veins of the calf or thigh and superficial point tenderness of small segments of veins involved with thrombophlebitis. The finding of superficial phlebitis is most important in that the potential for complicating thromboembolism is much less when a segment of vein is tender and a thrombus can be felt but there is little or no tenderness elsewhere. The area of thrombosis may appear red because of inflammation spreading to the skin. Homans sign is difficult to evaluate. The problem is that the tenderness may be bilateral. Elderly people, particularly, experience some pain in their calves with dorsiflexion of their feet.

One of the main techniques for diagnosing and following a patient is that of comparative circumferential measurements of the legs at several levels. The aim is to look for minor amounts of edema that are not readily apparent. A difference of as little as 0.5 cm may be significant. Normally, the patient's dominant leg may be slightly larger than the other leg. This normal increase may be as much as 2 cm at the calf and more in the thigh.

Finally, a serious complication (phlegmasia cerulea dolens) that may arise is the absence of arterial circulation in the affected leg. This represents a medical emergency in that the reflex reduction of arterial circulation, as a relatively infrequent complication of

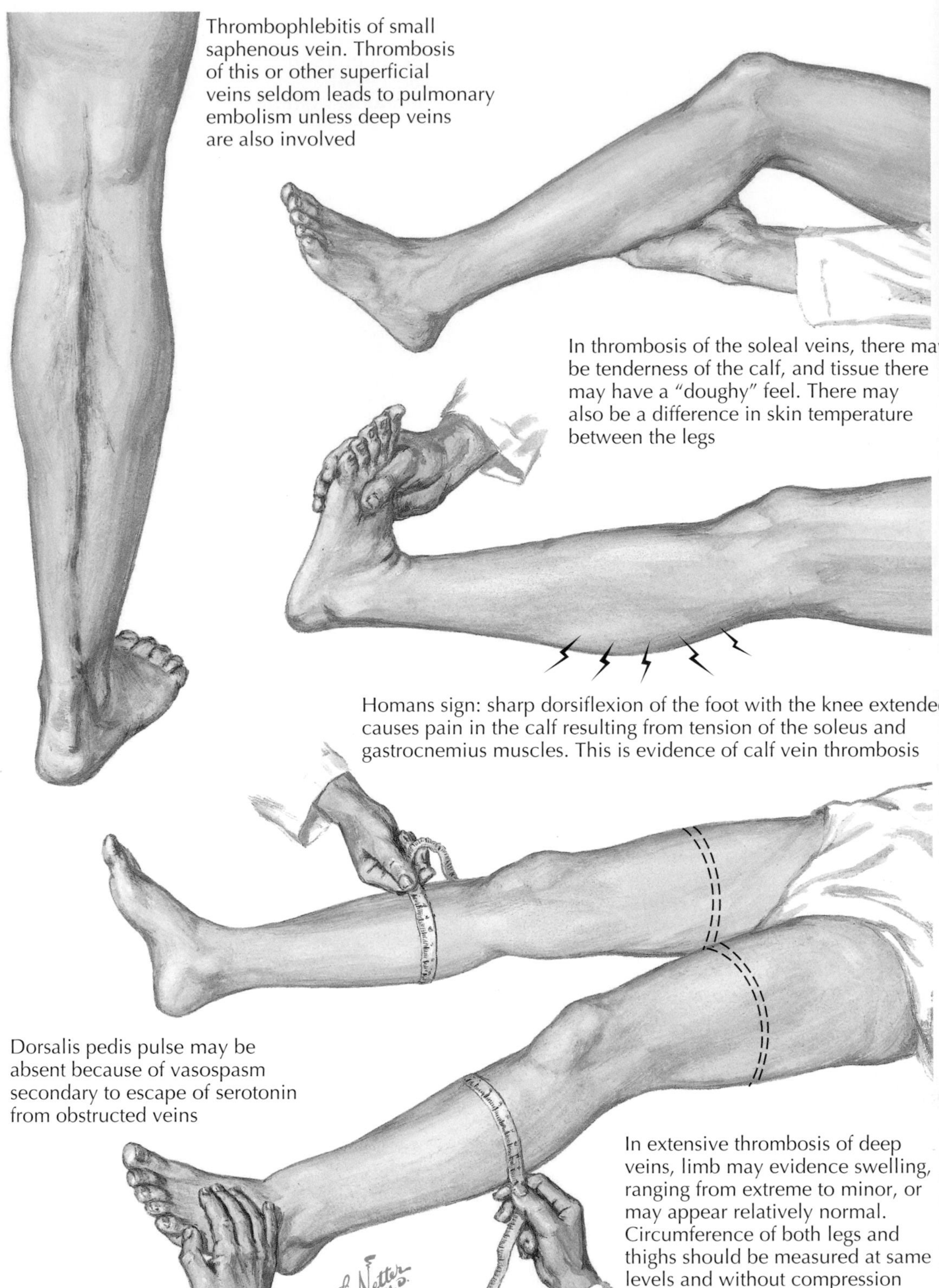
CLINICAL MANIFESTATIONS OF LEG VEIN THROMBOSIS
Thrombophlebitis of small saphenous vein. Thrombosis of this or other superficial veins seldom leads to pulmonary embolism unless deep veins are also involved
In thrombosis of the soleal veins, there may be tenderness of the calf, and tissue there may have a "doughy" feel. There may also be a difference in skin temperature between the legs
Homans sign: sharp dorsiflexion of the foot with the knee extended causes pain in the calf resulting from tension of the soleus and gastrocnemius muscles. This is evidence of calf vein thrombosis
Dorsalis pedis pulse may be absent because of vasospasm secondary to escape of serotonin from obstructed veins
In extensive thrombosis of deep veins, limb may evidence swelling, ranging from extreme to minor, or may appear relatively normal. Circumference of both legs and thighs should be measured at same levels and without compression
F. Netter M.D.

PULMONARY EMBOLISM AND VENOUS THROMBOEMBOLISM

(Continued)

thrombophlebitis, may lead to gangrene of the tissues of the foot. The diagnosis is made by observation of the deepening blue color of the extremity as well as the lack of arterial pulses and coldness of the distal part of the extremity in contrast to the usual warm state in uncomplicated thrombophlebitis.

DIAGNOSIS OF DEEP VENOUS THROMBOSIS (see Plate 4-117)

Ultrasonography

In 90% of cases, PE originates from lower extremity DVT. Lower limb compression venous ultrasonography (CUS) has largely replaced venography for diagnosing DVT. For proximal DVT, CUS has a sensitivity of more than 90% and a specificity of approximately 95%.

Computed Tomography Venography

Computed tomography (CT) venography has been recently advocated as a simple way to diagnose DVT in patients with suspected PE because it can be combined with chest CT angiography in a single procedure using only one intravenous injection of contrast dye. However, it appears as though CT venography increases the overall detection rate only marginally in patients with suspected PE and adds a significant amount of irradiation.

CLINICAL MANIFESTATIONS OF PULMONARY EMBOLISM

The clinical manifestations of pulmonary embolization are generally subtle, unexplained tachypnea and dyspnea; anxiety; vague substernal pressure; and occasionally syncope. In a patient predisposed to PE by bed rest, surgery, or local thrombophlebitis, these symptoms constitute strong evidence for a pulmonary embolus even though the physical examination is unrewarding, the electrocardiogram (ECG) indeterminate, and the chest radiograph normal.

The most common type of PE is one that does not result in infarction (see Plate 4-118). This is because of the protective effect of the dual pulmonary circulation that protects the lung from infarction except in cases of massive embolus or in patients with concomitant left-sided heart failure.

PE resulting in infarction occurs after less than 10% of pulmonary emboli. The evidence for pulmonary infarction is acute onset of pleural pain, hemoptysis, breathlessness, pleural effusion, or pleural friction rub (see Plate 4-119).

A massive embolus that either lodges in the main pulmonary artery or overrides both branches to the point of compromising the bulk of the pulmonary blood flow is a disaster that elicits circulatory collapse and acute cor pulmonale (see Plate 4-120). This form of pulmonary embolization is a dire emergency, but it is difficult to distinguish from an acute myocardial infarction. The chances of detecting it depend on the physician's suspicion that the patient is predisposed to pulmonary embolization. After clinical suspicion has been raised, support for the diagnosis is provided by

Pulmonary Embolism and Venous Thromboembolism

(Continued)

the classic S_1-Q_3 pattern on the ECG. Almost as convincing is a fresh "P pulmonale" pattern, a new right-axis shift, or a new pattern of incomplete right bundle-branch block.

The effect of one or more massive emboli is a reduction in the cross-sectional area of the pulmonary vascular tree and an increase in pulmonary vascular resistance to blood flow. If most of the pulmonary vascular tree is blocked, marked pulmonary hypertension occurs followed by dilatation and even failure of the right ventricle. In patients with previously normal lungs, the severity of these changes correlates closely on a lung scan with the extent of perfusion defects. Whether the total hemodynamic effect is attributable to the restricted vascular bed or to associated reflex or humoral vasoconstrictor mechanisms is unclear. A decrease in cardiac output and a decrease in systemic blood pressure accompany the right ventricular enlargement. Preexisting cardiac or lung disease aggravates these changes and may precipitate intractable heart failure.

When PE is extensive enough to produce acute right-sided heart failure, it often results in syncope and cardiopulmonary arrest. Profound apprehension, central chest pain, and cardiac dysrhythmias (especially atrial flutter)may also occur, and in many patients, death follows within a few hours of the embolic episode. The physical findings of acute cor pulmonale include tachycardia, an elevated jugular venous pressure with prominent A wave, shock, and cyanosis. Wide splitting of the second heart sound may be present and is often fixed. It disappears with the resolution of the embolus and relief of right ventricular failure. Occasionally, a right ventricular gallop can be heard along with a systolic ejection murmur in the pulmonary area. There may be a palpable lift over the right ventricle and a loud pulmonary closure sound.

Diagnosis of Pulmonary Embolism

Chest Radiography

The radiographic appearance depends on the size and number of emboli, whether they have produced pulmonary infarction, and whether the infarcted area reaches the pleural surface to cause pleuritis and pleural effusion. A massive embolus located at the origin of a major pulmonary artery causes hypoperfusion of the ipsilateral lung manifested by a decrease in vascular markings. An increase in size of a major hilar vessel or an abrupt cutoff, the "knuckle sign," is strong supportive evidence when present. If not distinctly oligemic, areas of the lung often show unduly small vessels. Sometimes the only indication of a large embolus is an unusually high diaphragm on the affected side or the presence of a pulmonary infiltrate, a consequence of infarction, hemorrhage, or atelectasis. An ipsilateral pleural effusion may also be the only sign of an otherwise unsuspected pulmonary infarction. All of this radiographic evidence takes on a great significance if the individual is predisposed to peripheral or pelvic venous thrombosis and has been identified as a serious candidate for PE. Often nothing abnormal can be seen.

Ultrasound and CT in Diagnosis of Acute Venous Thromboembolism

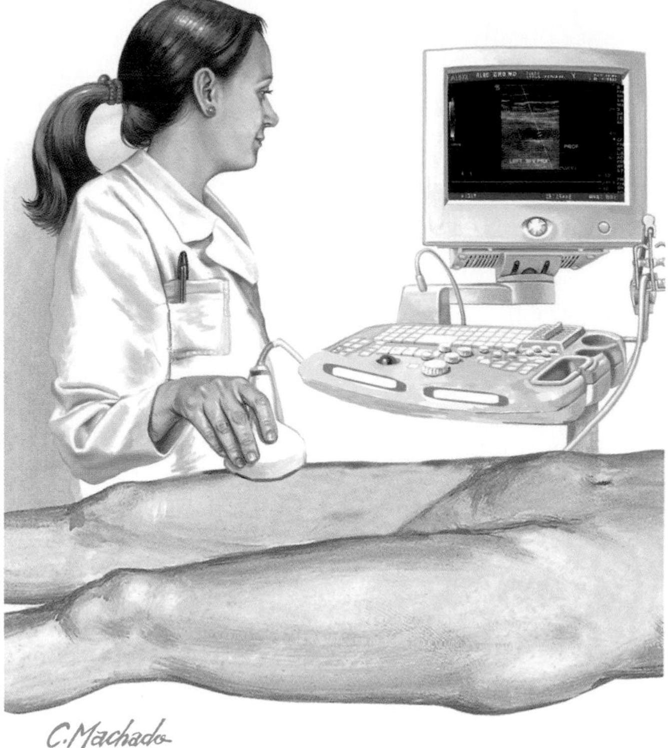

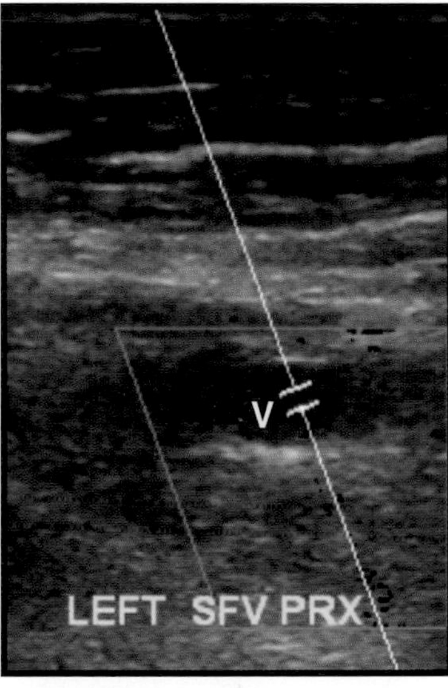

Duplex ultrasound. Notice lack of blood flow (no color or flow wave pattern) in occluded, left superficial femoral vein (*V*).

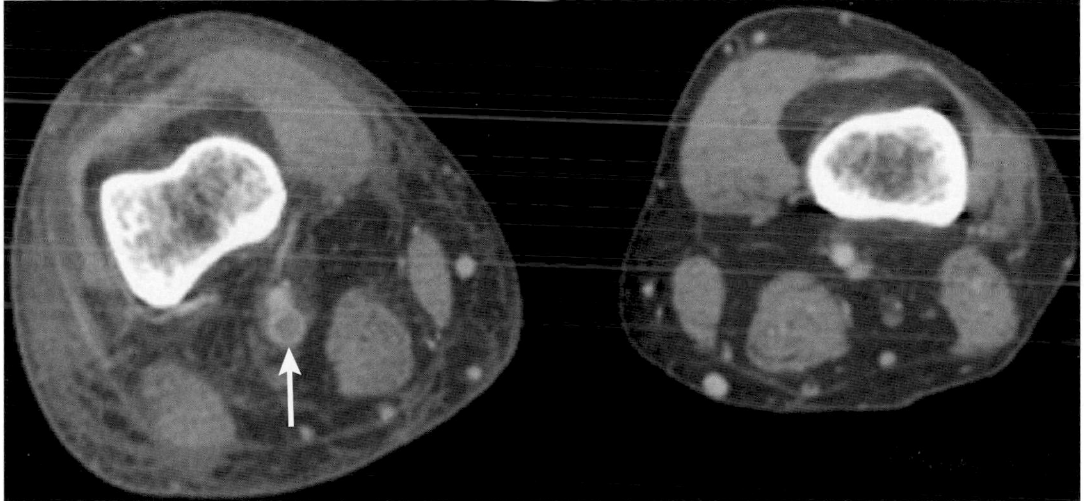

CT venography. CT exam through the legs shows a clot in the right femoral vein (*arrow*). Overall increased size of right thigh compared with left thigh with increased soft tissue swelling and edema is visible

Pulmonary Embolism and Venous Thromboembolism
(Continued)

Embolism of Lesser Degree Without Infarction

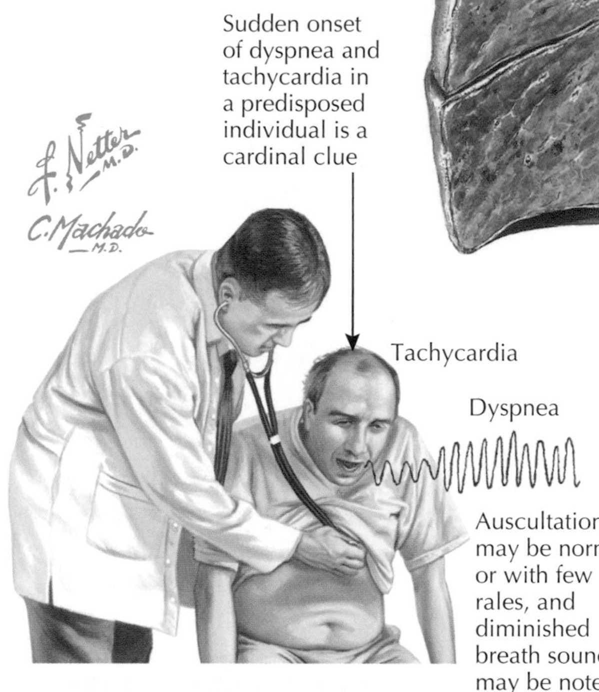
Multiple small emboli of lungs
Sudden onset of dyspnea and tachycardia in a predisposed individual is a cardinal clue
Tachycardia
Dyspnea
Auscultation may be normal or with few rales, and diminished breath sounds may be noted

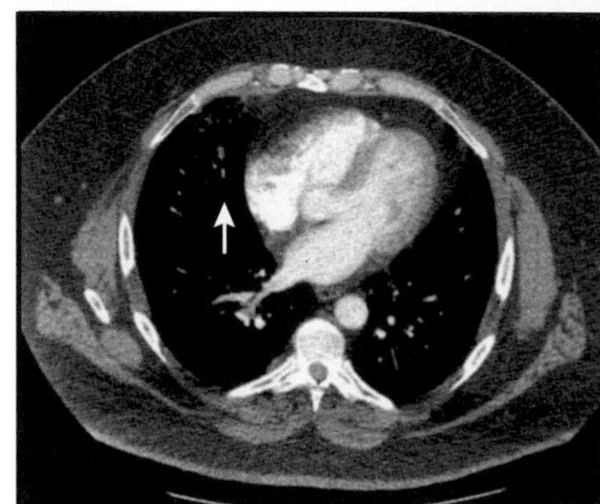

CT shows multiple emboli in right upper lobe pulmonary arteries (*arrow*)

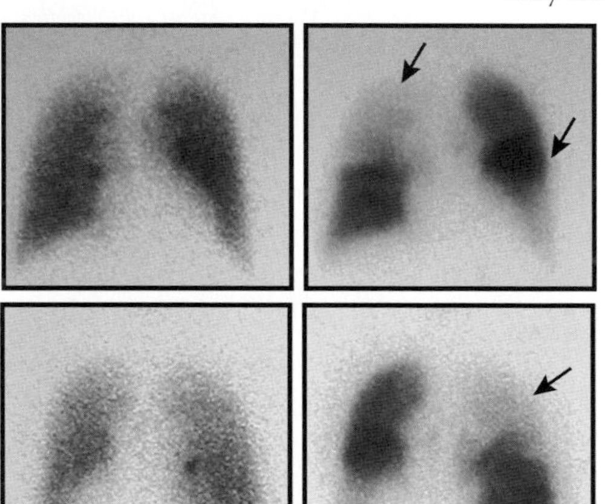

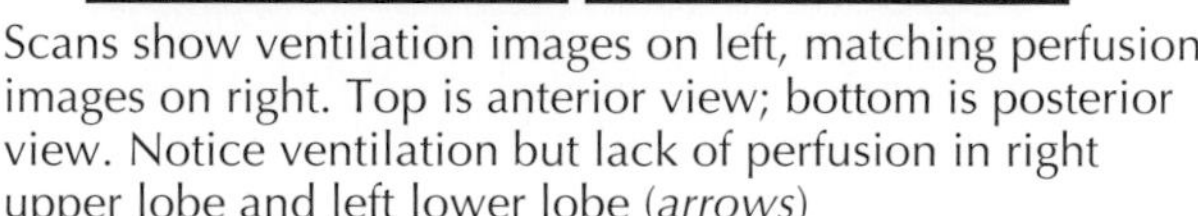

Scans show ventilation images on left, matching perfusion images on right. Top is anterior view; bottom is posterior view. Notice ventilation but lack of perfusion in right upper lobe and left lower lobe (*arrows*)

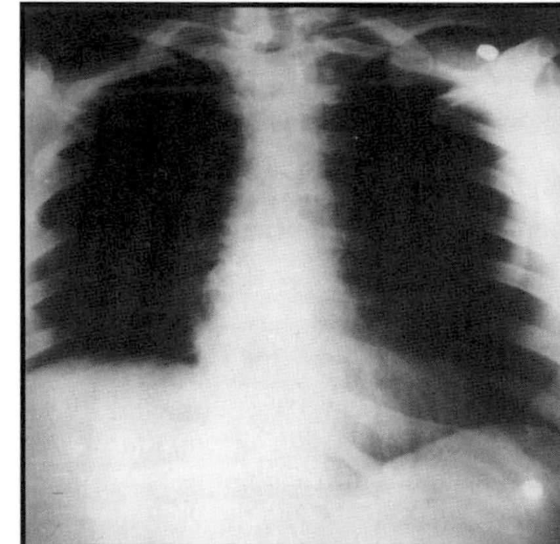

Radiographs are often normal

Arterial Blood Gases

A mainstay in the diagnosis of massive PE is a decrease in arterial oxygen tension, generally in association with reduced arterial carbon dioxide tension. Whereas the arterial hypoxemia is a consequence of ventilation/perfusion (V/Q) abnormalities, the hypocapnia is caused by hyperventilation that is presumed to be reflexly induced by the emboli via the J receptors. Hypoventilated areas probably result from interference with surfactant and resulting atelectasis in small areas of lung.

D-Dimer

Plasma D-dimer levels, a measurement of a degradation product of cross-linked fibrin, are elevated in plasma in the presence of an acute clot caused by simultaneous activation of coagulation and fibrinolysis. A normal D-dimer level makes acute PE or DVT unlikely. The negative predictive value of D-dimer is high. Unfortunately, because of the poor specificity of fibrin for VTE related to the fact that fibrin is produced in a wide variety of conditions, the positive predictive value of D-dimer is low. D-dimer is not useful for confirming PE. When measured by quantitative enzyme-linked immunosorbent assay, D-dimer has a sensitivity of more than 95% and a specificity of about 40%. D-dimer levels can therefore be used to exclude PE in patients with a low or moderate probability of PE.

Ventilation/Perfusion Lung Scan

A lung scan, using a radioisotope as a marker, is often performed to evaluate patients with a suspected diagnosis of PE. Macroaggregated albumin, labeled with iodine 131 or technetium 99, is commonly used for this purpose. The tracer substance is injected intravenously. The radioactive particles, which are on the order of 50 to 100 μm in diameter, are trapped in the microcirculation of the lung. The pattern of distribution of these radioactive particles, detected by an external counter, defines the pattern of pulmonary blood flow. It is helpful to have V/Q scans performed at the same sitting so that areas of inadequate blood flow may be related to ventilation abnormalities. Most specific in reaching a diagnosis is the finding of multiple perfusion defects in normally ventilated lungs.

Lung scans are practical, simple, and safe. They can be repeated as necessary to trace the resolution of defects and to detect fresh emboli. Results are frequently characterized according to criteria established in the North American PIOPED (Prospective Investigation of Pulmonary Embolism Diagnosis) trial into four categories: normal or near-normal, low, intermediate (nondiagnostic), and high probability of PE. A normal perfusion scan virtually excludes PE. A high-probability V/Q scan suggests the diagnosis of PE with a high degree of probability, but further tests may be considered in selected patients with a low clinical suspicion of PE. In other combinations of V/Q scan results and clinical probability, further testing should be performed.

Computed Tomography

Recent studies have supported the value of CT angiography in the diagnosis of acute PE. Multidetector CT

Pulmonary Embolism and Venous Thromboembolism

(Continued)

(MDCT) with high spatial and temporal resolution and quality of arterial opacification allows adequate visualization of the pulmonary arteries to at least the segmental level. MDCT may be adequate for excluding PE in patients without a high clinical probability (suspicion) of PE. Whether patients with negative CT results and a high clinical probability should be further investigated (with compressive ultrasonography of the lower extremities or V/Q scanning or pulmonary angiography) is controversial. A MDCT showing PE at the segmental or more proximal level is considered adequate proof of PE in patients without a low clinical probability.

Pulmonary Angiography

The pulmonary angiographic diagnostic criteria for acute PE were defined many years ago and include direct evidence of a thrombus, either a filling defect or amputation of a pulmonary arterial branch. Pulmonary angiography is, however, invasive and carries some risk. However, when performed by experienced operators, it can be an important confirmatory test.

Echocardiography

The echocardiographic finding of right ventricular dilatation may be useful in risk stratifying patients with suspected high-risk PE presenting with shock or hypotension. A meta-analysis found a more than twofold increased risk of PE-related mortality in patients with echocardiographic signs of right ventricular dysfunction.

Diagnostic Strategies and Algorithms

Pulmonary angiography, the definitive test, is invasive, costly, and carries some risk. Therefore, noninvasive diagnostic approaches are warranted, and various combinations of clinical evaluation and the above-described tests (including D-dimer measurement, lower extremity compressive ultrasonography, V/Q scanning, and CT scanning) have been evaluated to decrease the need for pulmonary angiography. It is important to note that the diagnostic approach to PE may vary according to the local availability of tests. The most appropriate diagnostic strategy should also be determined by the clinical assessment of risk and severity. Various guidelines have been developed that describe diagnostic strategies and algorithms in detail.

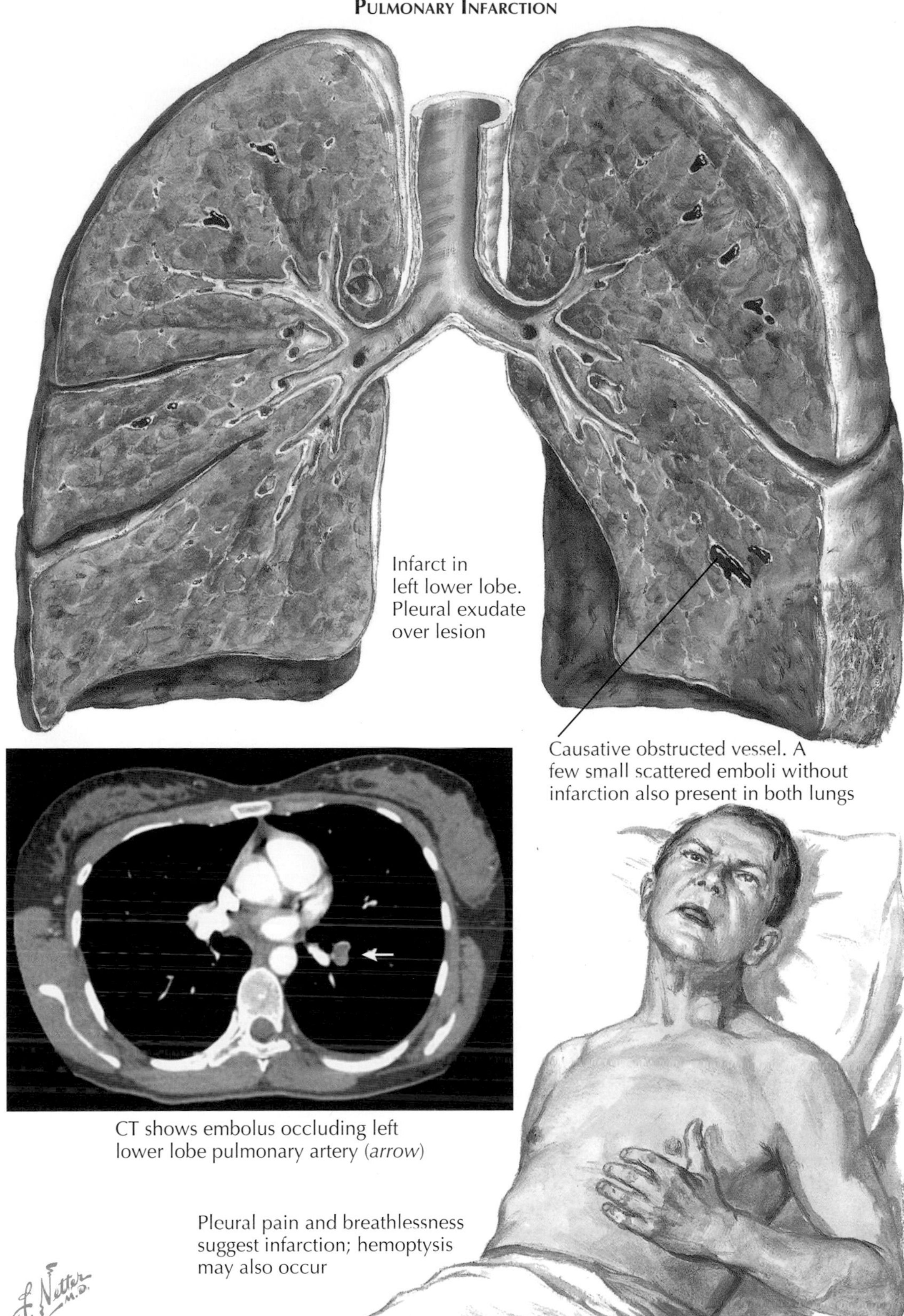
Pulmonary Infarction
Infarct in left lower lobe. Pleural exudate over lesion
Causative obstructed vessel. A few small scattered emboli without infarction also present in both lungs
CT shows embolus occluding left lower lobe pulmonary artery (arrow)
Pleural pain and breathlessness suggest infarction; hemoptysis may also occur
F. Netter M.D.

Prophylaxis and Treatment

Prophylaxis

Prophylaxis of VTE is concerned with the prevention of clot formation in the deep veins of the legs and with the extension of a clot that can break off and travel to the lungs. Because of the morbidity and mortality associated with DVT and PE, appropriate prophylaxis is of paramount importance. Specific guidelines for prophylaxis of VTE have been published by the American College of Chest Physicians (ACCP).

Anticoagulation After Pulmonary Embolism

Anticoagulant therapy plays a critically important role in the management of patients with PE. The objectives

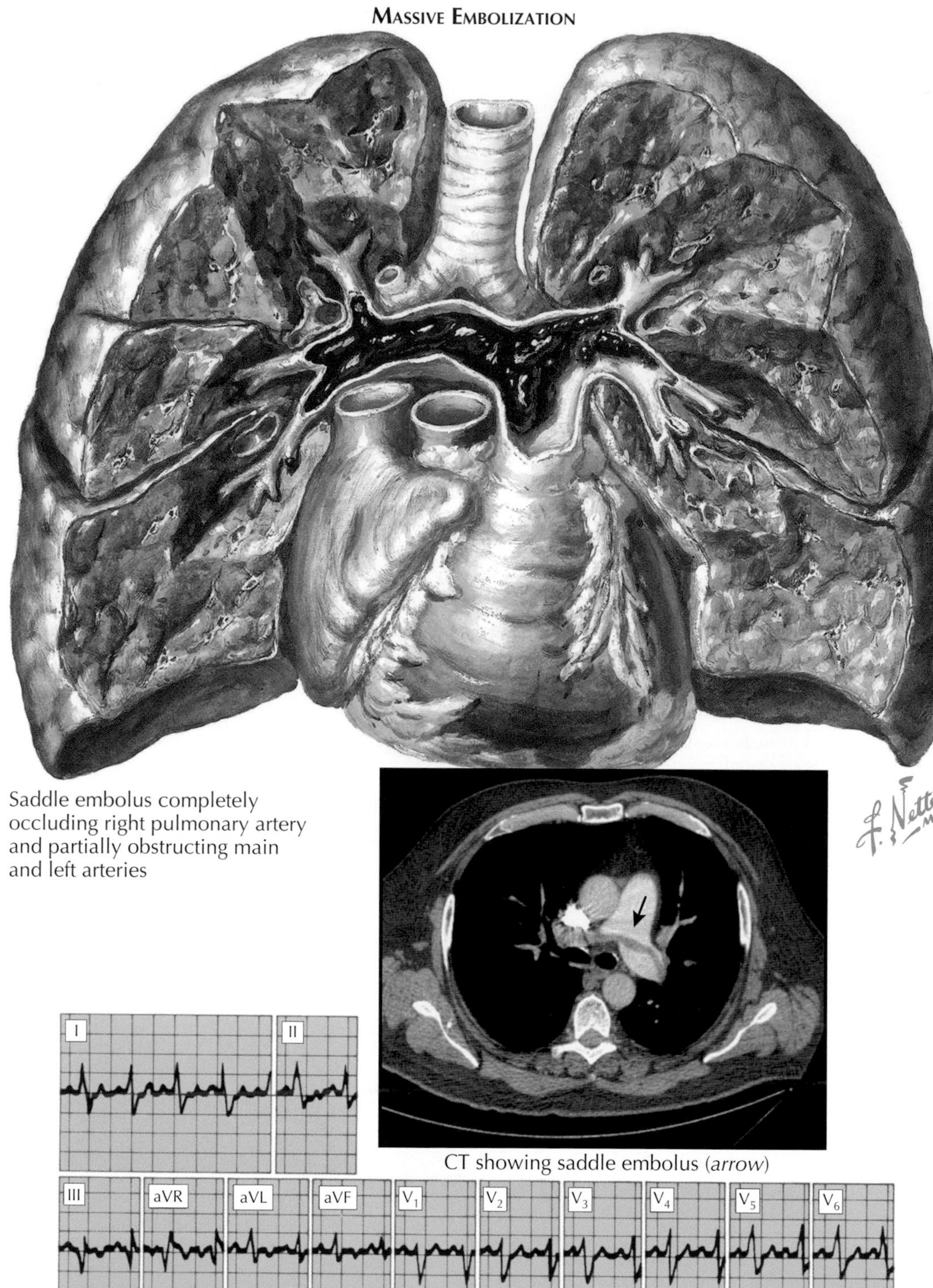

Saddle embolus completely occluding right pulmonary artery and partially obstructing main and left arteries

CT showing saddle embolus (*arrow*)

Characteristic electrocardiographic findings in acute pulmonary embolism. Deep S_1; prominent Q_3 with inversion of T_3; depression of ST segment in lead II (often also in lead I) with staircase ascent of ST_2; T_2 diphasic or inverted; right-axis deviation; tachycardia

Pulmonary Embolism and Venous Thromboembolism
(Continued)

are to prevent death and recurrent events with an acceptable risk of bleeding-related complications. Rapid anticoagulation requires parenteral therapy, such as intravenous unfractionated heparin (UFH), subcutaneous low-molecular-weight heparin, or subcutaneous fondaparinux. Because of the high mortality rate in untreated patients, anticoagulation should be considered in patients with suspected PE while awaiting diagnostic confirmation. Specific guidelines for anticoagulation after PE have been published by the ACCP and are updated regularly. The use of intravenous UFH requires close monitoring of the activated partial thromboplastin time. Treatment with parenteral anticoagulants is usually followed by the use of oral vitamin K antagonists, such as warfarin. Chronic anticoagulation with warfarin requires ongoing monitoring of the prothrombin time or the International Normalized Ratio. Protocols to guide anticoagulant dosing and monitoring and follow-up by a dedicated team of experienced professionals may help to optimize the safety and efficacy of therapy. Drug interactions can be troublesome during warfarin therapy, and each new medication must be examined for its effect in enhancing or diminishing the action of warfarin.

Thrombolysis

Thrombolytic therapy rapidly resolves thromboembolic obstruction and has beneficial effects on hemodynamic parameters. However, the benefits of thrombolysis over anticoagulation with heparin appear to be largely confined to the first few days. Thrombolytic therapy carries a significant risk of bleeding, especially in patients with predisposing conditions or comorbidities. Nevertheless, thrombolytic therapy may be used in patients with high-risk PE presenting with cardiogenic shock or persistent systemic hypotension. Further studies are needed to more precisely define the role of thrombolytic therapy for PE.

Surgical Pulmonary Embolectomy for Acute Pulmonary Embolism

Pulmonary embolectomy may be indicated in patients with high-risk PE in whom thrombolysis is absolutely contraindicated or has failed.

Caval Filters

Inferior vena cava (IVC) filters may be used when there are contraindications to anticoagulation and a high risk of VTE recurrence (see Plate 4-121). They are also often placed in patients with chronic thromboembolic pulmonary hypertension (CTEPH) to provide an additional barrier of protection against recurrent PE. Some filters in use today are retrievable and removable and may be suitable for temporary use.

CHRONIC EFFECTS OF PULMONARY EMBOLISM

Chronic Thromboembolic Pulmonary Hypertension

PEs are occasionally dispatched to the lungs for months to years without clinical evidence of acute embolizations. The patients may present with evidence of severe pulmonary hypertension and often die in right

Mechanical Defenses Against and Chronic Effects of Pulmonary Embolism

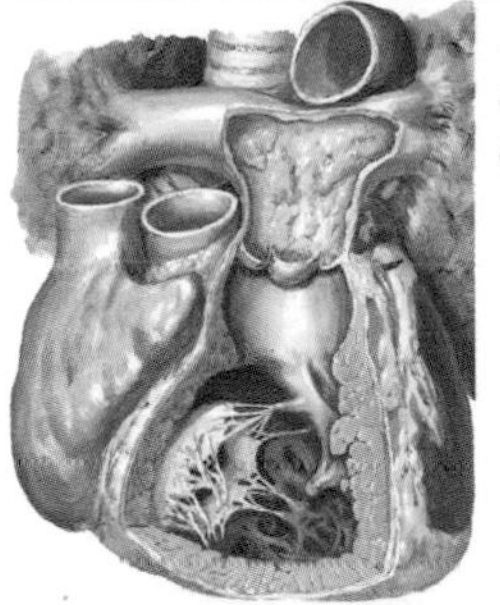

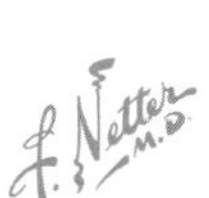

▶Plaque, cords, and web in a lobar pulmonary artery as result of organization of embolus

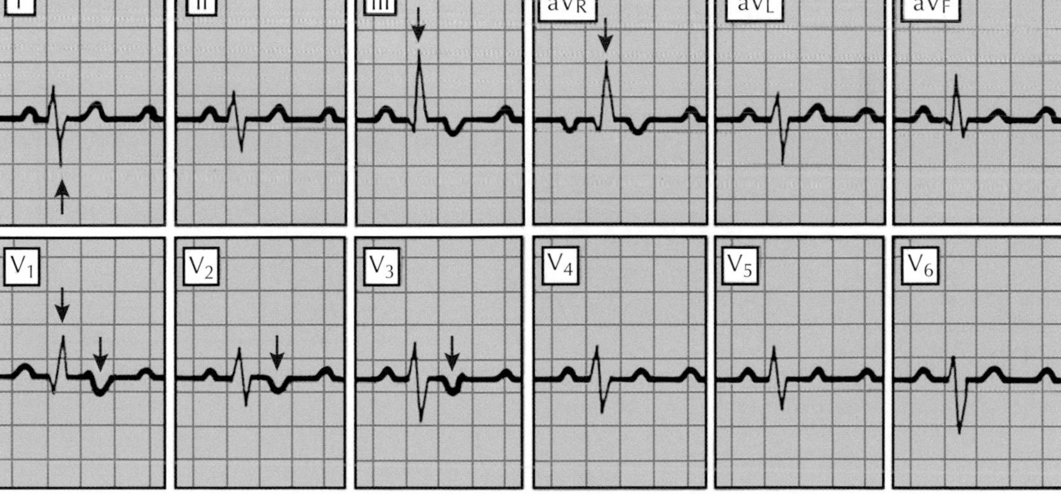

ECG. Deep S_1 and high R_3 indicative of right axis deviation. High R in aV_R and in V_1 plus inverted or diphasic T in V_1 to V_3 evidence of right ventricular hypetrophy

Pulmonary Embolism and Venous Thromboembolism

(Continued)

ventricular failure. The course of patients with multiple pulmonary emboli may be so subtle as to mimic that of patients with idiopathic pulmonary arterial hypertension. CTEPH is a relatively rare complication of pulmonary thromboembolic disease. It is often characterized by progressive dyspnea and hypoxemia and ultimately the development of right-sided heart failure (see Plate 4-121).

In these patients with severe pulmonary hypertension, dyspnea and tachypnea, fatigue and syncopal episodes, or precordial pain during exertion are usually found in some combination. On physical examination, an impulse may be felt over the main pulmonary artery, and there is splitting of the second heart sound with accentuation of the pulmonary component. An ejection click and a systolic or diastolic murmur may be present in the pulmonary valve area. Subsequently, evidence of right ventricular hypertrophy is found, with a prominent A wave in the jugular venous pulse and a right ventricular heave and fourth heart sound. As failure develops, a right ventricular gallop can be heard, and there is evidence of tricuspid valve insufficiency along with the peripheral consequences of an ineffectively functioning right ventricle. Sudden death caused by transient arrhythmias may occur.

Chest radiographs usually show an enlarged heart with right ventricular and right atrial prominence. The main pulmonary artery shadow is increasingly enlarged as hypertension becomes more severe, and the peripheral lung fields are oligemic and lack vascular markings. Evidence of right-axis deviation appears on the ECG, with evidence of right ventricular hypertrophy in the precordial leads. There is usually indication of right atrial enlargement, and when changes are severe, inversion of right precordial T waves. Right-sided heart catheterization and radioisotope lung scans provide definitive evidence of the disease process.

Pulmonary Thromboendarterectomy

Surgical removal of obstructing material related to chronic thromboembolic disease requires a true endarterectomy rather than an embolectomy. The operation is performed on cardiopulmonary bypass, with deep hypothermia and complete circulatory arrest. Selection of appropriate candidates for the operation is extremely important, and criteria include factors such as surgical accessibility and the absence of severe comorbidity. PTE carries substantial risk, but in experienced hands, it may result in dramatic clinical and hemodynamic improvement. Medical therapy for patients with CTEPH is being explored in clinical trials.

Special Situations and Extravascular Sources of Pulmonary Emboli

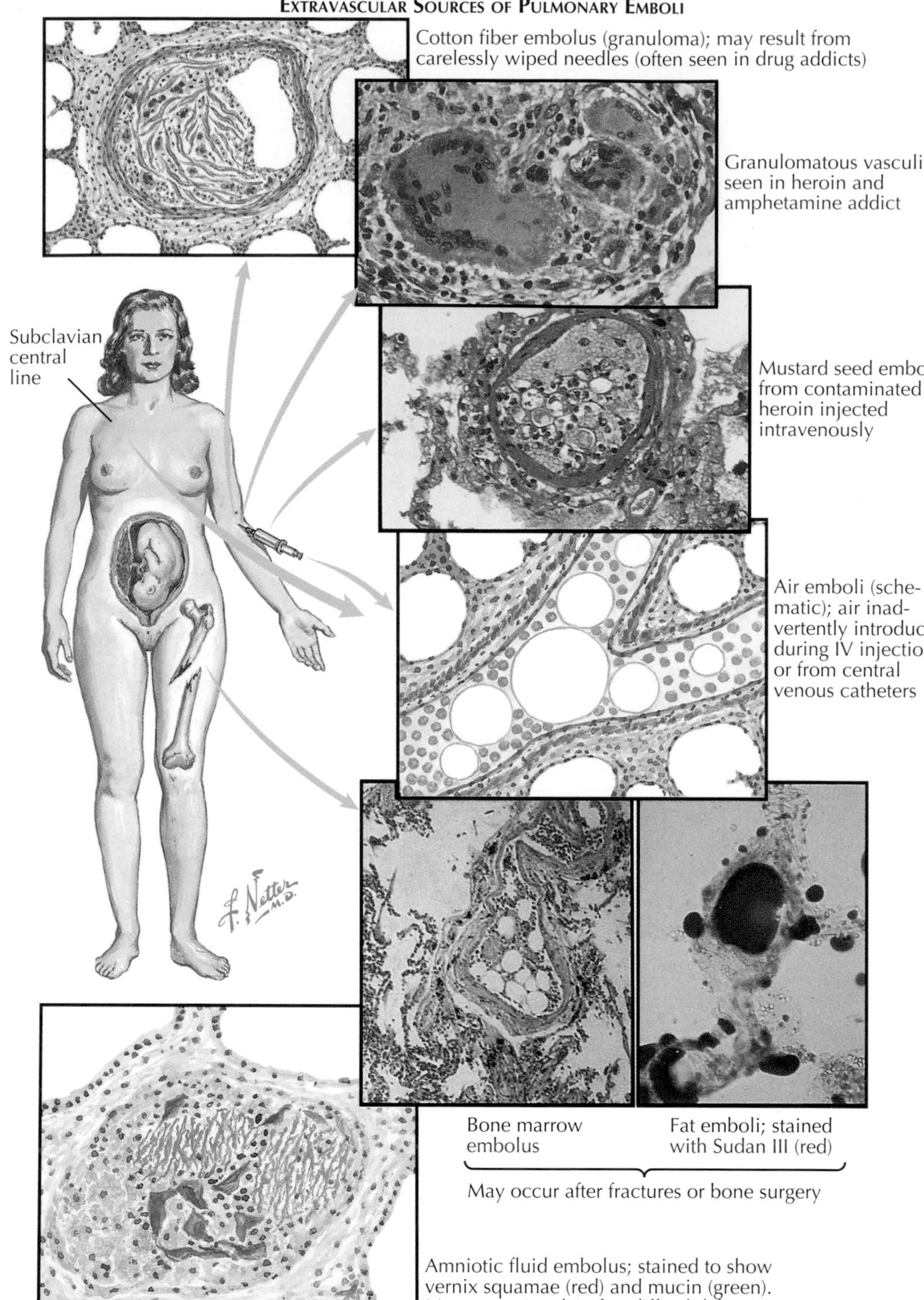

Extravascular Sources of Pulmonary Emboli
Cotton fiber embolus (granuloma); may result from carelessly wiped needles (often seen in drug addicts)
Granulomatous vasculitis seen in heroin and amphetamine addict
Subclavian central line
Mustard seed emboli from contaminated heroin injected intravenously
Air emboli (schematic); air inadvertently introduced during IV injection or from central venous catheters
Bone marrow embolus
Fat emboli; stained with Sudan III (red)
May occur after fractures or bone surgery
Amniotic fluid embolus; stained to show vernix squamae (red) and mucin (green). May occur (rarely) after difficult labor

MALIGNANCY

The risk of thrombosis among cancer patients is substantially higher than in the general population and may be even higher in those receiving chemotherapy. Patients with cancer and venous thromboembolism are more likely to develop recurrent thromboembolic complications and major bleeding during anticoagulant therapy than those without malignancy. Low-molecular-weight heparin (LMWH) may be more effective than warfarin in patients with cancer. LMWH should be considered for the first 3 to 6 months of therapy, and anticoagulant therapy should be continued indefinitely or until cure of the cancer.

PREGNANCY

Pulmonary embolism (PE) is an important potential complication of pregnancy and is associated with substantial risk to the mother. A complete discussion of the diagnosis and management of PE in pregnancy is beyond the scope of this section.

FAT EMBOLISM

The most common cause of fat embolism is trauma to bones, particularly the long bones of the legs. Fat embolism may also be associated with air emboli in decompression sickness (caisson disease). Microscopically, the fat emboli can be demonstrated with fat stains such as Sudan III or IV or oil red O. With these stains, they appear as red-orange droplets, several microns in diameter, filling the small arteries and alveolar capillaries. With routine stains, they appear as optically clear spaces in the vascular lumina. Clinically, fat embolism is often associated with acute respiratory failure (adult respiratory distress syndrome). Cutaneous and conjunctival petechial hemorrhages and embolism of retinal vessels are found in about half the cases.

Bone marrow embolism is also a frequent complication of severe bone trauma or fracture.

AMNIOTIC FLUID EMBOLISM

This relatively rare condition is caused by the massive leakage of amniotic fluid into the uterine veins. The amniotic fluid reaches the uterine venous circulation either as a result of vigorous uterine contraction after rupture of the membranes or through tears or surgical incisions in the myometrium or endocervix. Clinically, the condition is characterized by sudden dyspnea, cyanosis, systemic hypotension, and death during or immediately after delivery. The mechanism of death is not clear because the emboli consist of a suspension of epithelial squamae, lanugo, and cellular debris, usually occluding a few small blood vessels. Death has been attributed to either anaphylactoid reaction to the amniotic fluid or disseminated intravascular coagulation caused by activation of the clotting mechanism by amniotic fluid thromboplastin.

AIR EMBOLISM

Air may be sucked into veins during attempts at abortion, after chest injury as a result of a motor vehicle accident, during the induction of artificial pneumothorax or pneumoperitoneum, placement of central venous catheters, and in a number of other circumstances. The effects of air embolism depend on the amount of air that reaches the circulation and the rapidity of its entry. The volume of air necessary to cause death in humans is usually more than 100 mL. In debilitated persons, a smaller volume of air may be fatal. Death is caused by blockage by an air trap in the outflow tract of the right ventricle, but small air bubbles can be seen in small pulmonary blood vessels.

FOREIGN BODY EMBOLISM

A wide variety of organic or inorganic substances may enter the venous circulation and reach the lungs. This type of embolism has become common in certain groups addicted to narcotic drugs. The drugs are rarely chemically pure and are frequently adulterated with vegetable seeds, talc, and other substances.

As with the other kinds of emboli, the effect of foreign bodies depends to a great extent on the rapidity and extent of embolization. Such particles as fibers or talc are likely to produce an inflammatory response in the wall of small pulmonary arteries, with formation of foreign body granulomas composed of macrophages and multinucleated giant cells. The granuloma may cause partial or total occlusion of the involved blood vessel. If several blood vessels are involved, pulmonary vascular resistance may become elevated and lead to pulmonary hypertension.

Pulmonary Hypertension

CLASSIFICATION

Pulmonary hypertension is an elevation in pulmonary vascular pressure that can be caused by an isolated increase in pulmonary artery pressure or by combined increases in both pulmonary artery and pulmonary venous pressures (see Plate 4-123). Normal pressures in the pulmonary vascular bed are quite low. Pulmonary arterial hypertension (PAH) refers to isolated elevation of pulmonary arterial pressure, hemodynamically defined as a resting mean pulmonary artery pressure above 25 mm Hg with a normal left atrial pressure (<15 mm Hg). PAH that occurs in the absence of a demonstrable cause, formerly known as primary pulmonary hypertension (PPH), may occur sporadically (idiopathic PAH [IPAH]) or as an inherited condition (familial PAH or FPAH). Mutations in the bone morphogenetic protein receptor II (BMPR2) gene occur in 50% of families with a history of FPAH and in nearly 25% of patients thought to have sporadic IPAH. Genetic testing and counseling may be recommended for relatives of patients with FPAH. PAH occurs in association with connective tissue diseases (particularly scleroderma), HIV infection, sickle cell disease, and chronic liver disease (portopulmonary hypertension). The "Venice" classification scheme of pulmonary hypertension is shown in Plate 4-123.

PATHOPHYSIOLOGY OF PULMONARY ARTERIAL HYPERTENSION

Patients with significant PAH rarely undergo lung biopsy because of the surgical and anesthetic risk involved (see Plate 4-124). For this reason, much of the available pathologic information regarding the disease comes from patients with late-stage disease who die or undergo lung transplantation. In these later stages of the disease, IPAH reveals the presence of plexiform arteriopathy. The plexiform lesion is a complex tuft of proliferating intimal cells thought to be of endothelial cell or smooth muscle cell origin. Multiple small channels may remain where there was once an open arterial lumen. This obstructive, proliferative arteriopathy leads to increased resistance to pulmonary blood flow. Some patients with IPAH may demonstrate microscopic in situ thrombosis in the small pulmonary arterioles. Although IPAH is often associated with plexiform arteriopathy, some patients with underlying associated conditions such as scleroderma may demonstrate a more concentric, "onion skin" form of hypertrophy of the pulmonary vascular wall.

Obliteration of the pulmonary vascular lumen leads to an increase in pulmonary vascular resistance, ultimately placing a strain on the right ventricle. If the pulmonary vascular resistance increases slowly, as it often does in patients with PAH occurring in association with congenital heart disease, the right ventricle may adapt over time through hypertrophy, with maintenance of contractility and preservation of cardiac output. A more rapid increase in pulmonary vascular resistance, perhaps in the presence of a genetically determined less adaptive response, may lead to right ventricular dilatation, with a progressive decline in function and ultimately right ventricular failure. Right-sided heart failure is typically manifest clinically by progressive dyspnea on exertion, fatigue, fluid retention, edema, ascites, and signs of venous congestion. The most common cause of death in patients with PAH is right-sided heart failure.

WHO Classification System of Pulmonary Hypertension

1. Pulmonary arterial hypertension (PAH)

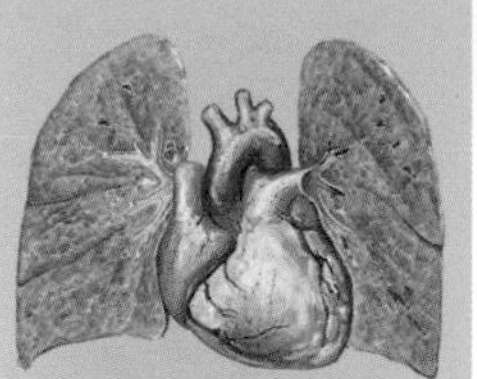

- Idiopathic pulmonary arterial hypertension
- Heritable
- Drug- and toxin-induced
- Persistent PH of newborn
- Associated with:
  - –connective tissue disease
  - –HIV infection
  - –portal hypertension
  - –coronary heart disease
  - –schistosomiasis
  - –chronic hemolytic anemia

1A. Pulmonary venoocclusive disease and pulmonary capillary hemangiomatosis

2. Pulmonary hypertension due to left heart disease

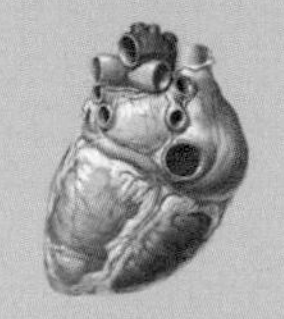

- Systolic dysfunction
- Diastolic dysfunction
- Valvular disease

3. Pulmonary hypertension due to lung diseases and/or hypoxia

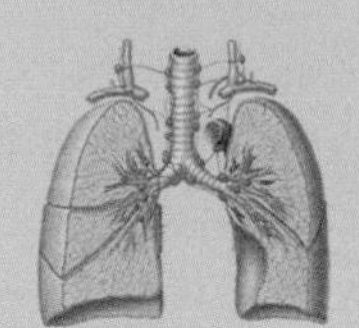

- Chronic obstructive pulmonary disease
- Interstitial lung disease
- Other pulmonary diseases with mixed restrictive and obstructive pattern
- Sleep-disordered breathing
- Alveolar hypoventilation disorders
- Developmental abnormalities

4. Pulmonary hypertension due to chronic thrombotic and/or embolic disease

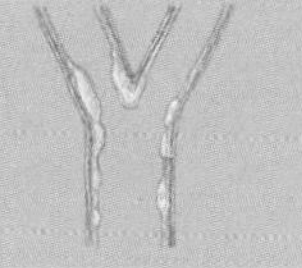

- Chronic thromboembolic pulmonary hypertension

5. Pulmonary hypertension with unclear multifactorial mechanisms

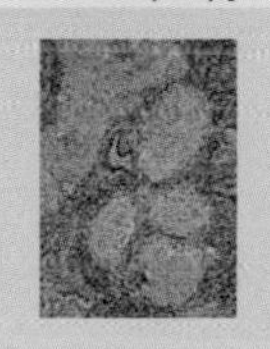

- Hematologic disorders
- Systemic disorders
- Metabolic disorders
- Others

F. Netter M.D.

Simonneau G et al. *J Am Coll Cardiol* 2009;54:S43–S54.

DIAGNOSIS

Screening

Although PAH may be asymptomatic, exertional dyspnea is the most frequently encountered symptom (see Plate 4-125). Accordingly, PAH should be suspected in patients with unexplained dyspnea. Anginal chest pain or syncope is less common and portends a poor prognosis. Peripheral edema or ascites indicates right ventricular failure. The symptoms of PAH are nonspecific and are similar to those occurring in more commonly encountered diseases, such as obstructive lung disease and left-sided heart disease. A family history of pulmonary hypertension may lead to early recognition of clinical disease in other individuals. Pulmonary hypertension occurs more frequently in patients with autoimmune or connective tissue disease, especially scleroderma. Use of amphetamines or cocaine should be explored because these have been implicated in the development of PAH in some users. A history of acute pulmonary embolism requires a careful search for chronic thromboembolic pulmonary hypertension, although this condition may occur in the absence of symptomatic venous thromboembolic disease. Patients with a history of such underlying disorders or exposures who develop unexplained dyspnea should be screened for possible pulmonary hypertension.

The diagnostic strategy uses testing to determine whether PAH is the cause of symptoms and which of its causes is present (see Plate 4-125). A process of screening with less invasive and lower risk tests is followed by specific and confirmatory tests.

The electrocardiogram may provide evidence of pulmonary hypertension, such as right ventricular hypertrophy, right-axis deviation, or right atrial enlargement.

Radiographic signs of pulmonary hypertension include enlarged main and hilar pulmonary arteries (>17 mm) with attenuation of peripheral pulmonary vascular markings ("pruning"). Right ventricular enlargement is evidenced by anterior displacement of the right ventricle into the retrosternal space on the

Pulmonary Hypertension
(Continued)

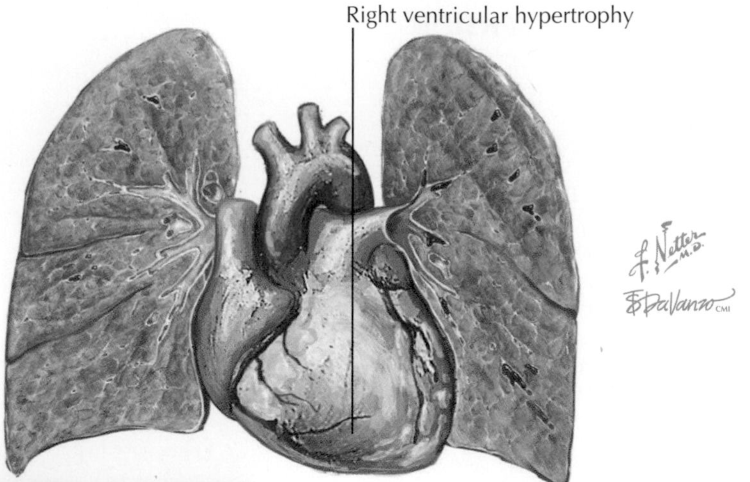

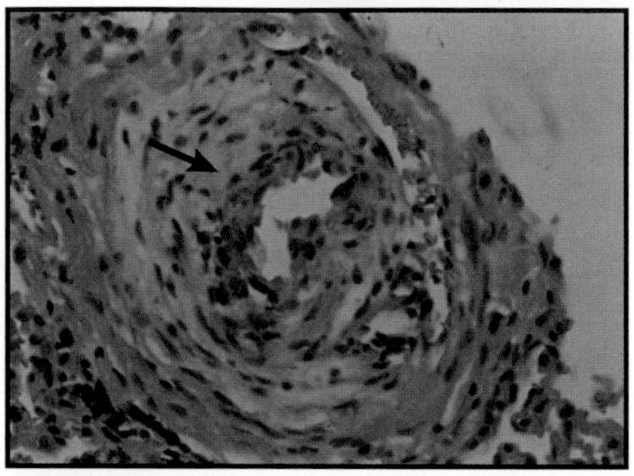

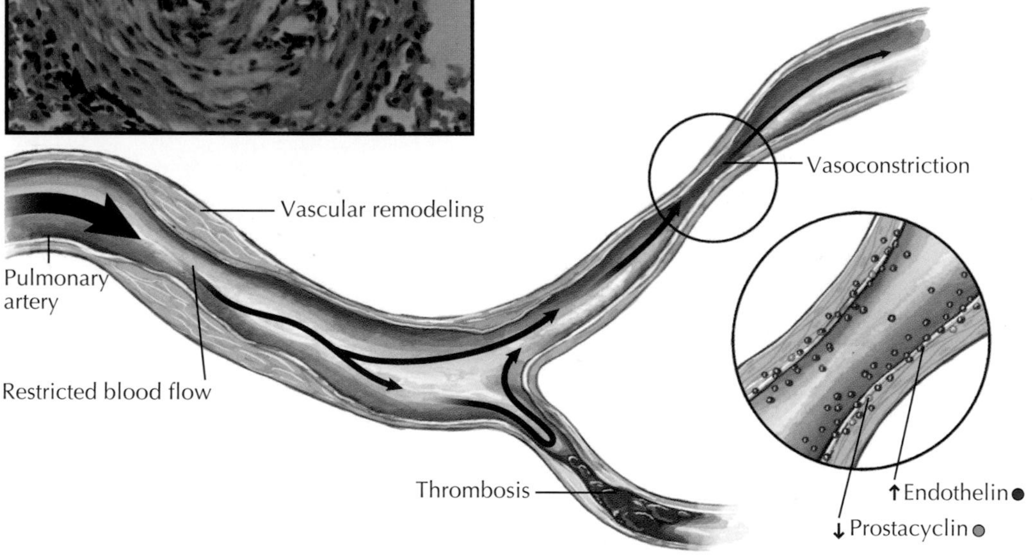

lateral view (see Plate 3-9). The chest radiograph is also useful in demonstrating comorbid or causal conditions, such as pulmonary venous congestion, chronic obstructive pulmonary disease, or interstitial lung disease.

Doppler echocardiography is often the test that suggests a diagnosis of pulmonary hypertension. Echocardiography also provides information about the cause and consequences of pulmonary hypertension. Studies in patients with PAH have reported good correlations between Doppler-derived estimates of pulmonary artery systolic pressure and direct measurements obtained by right-sided heart catheterization. Echocardiography also provides evidence regarding left ventricular systolic and diastolic function and valvular function and morphology that can provide clues to causes of pulmonary hypertension stemming from elevated pulmonary venous pressures. Left atrial enlargement, even in the absence of definite left ventricular dysfunction, should raise the possibility of elevated left-sided filling pressures contributing to pulmonary hypertension.

Cardiac catheterization is ultimately required to confirm the presence of pulmonary hypertension, assess its severity, and guide therapy.

The evaluation of PAH includes assessment for an underlying cause (see Plate 4-125). Pulmonary function testing is a necessary part of the initial evaluation of patients with suspected pulmonary hypertension to exclude or characterize the contribution of underlying airways or parenchymal lung disease. In general, the degree of pulmonary hypertension seen in chronic obstructive lung disease is less severe than in PAH, and the presence and severity of pulmonary hypertension correlate with the degree of airflow obstruction and hypoxemia. Approximately 20% of IPAH patients have a mild restrictive defect. In chronic thromboembolic pulmonary hypertension (CTEPH), a mild to moderate restrictive defect is thought to be caused by parenchymal scarring from prior infarcts. In both conditions, the diffusing capacity for carbon monoxide is often mildly to moderately reduced. Mild to moderate arterial hypoxemia is caused by V/Q mismatch and reduced mixed venous oxygen saturation resulting from low cardiac output. Severe hypoxemia is caused by right-to-left intracardiac or intrapulmonary shunting. In patients with scleroderma, a decreasing diffusing capacity may indicate the development of pulmonary hypertension.

Overnight oximetry may demonstrate oxygen desaturation and might be the first clue to sleep apnea sufficient to contribute to pulmonary hypertension. Nocturnal hypoxemia can occur in patients with IPAH without sleep apnea. Because hypoxemia is a potent pulmonary vasoconstrictor, all patients with unexplained pulmonary hypertension require assessment of both sleep and exercise oxygen saturation.

It is important to screen for autoimmune and connective tissue disease, including physical examination and serologic testing for antinuclear antibodies. However, up to 40% of patients with IPAH have serologic abnormalities, usually an antinuclear antibody in a low titer and nonspecific pattern. Additional serologic studies may be indicated if initial testing suggests an underlying autoimmune disorder.

CTEPH is a potentially curable form of pulmonary hypertension and should be sought in all patients undergoing evaluation for possible pulmonary hypertension. Ventilation/perfusion (V/Q) lung scanning is the preferred test to rule out CTEPH. CTEPH is manifest by at least one segmental-sized or larger perfusion defect, which are typically mismatched and larger than ventilation abnormalities. Patchy, nonsegmental defects are less specific but may be associated with CTEPH. Although a normal perfusion scan essentially excludes surgically accessible chronic thromboembolic disease, scans suggestive of thromboembolic disease may also be seen in other conditions. Pulmonary angiography is the definitive test for diagnosing CTEPH and for determining operability and should be performed in experienced centers when this entity is a consideration.

Computed tomography (CT) scanning may suggest a cause for pulmonary hypertension, such as severe airway or parenchymal lung diseases. A spectrum of abnormalities on CT scan have been described in patients with CTEPH, including right ventricular enlargement, dilated central pulmonary arteries, chronic thromboembolic material within the central pulmonary arteries, increased bronchial artery collateral flow, variability in the size and distribution of pulmonary arteries, parenchymal abnormalities consistent with prior infarcts, and mosaic attenuation of the pulmonary parenchyma.

Open or thoracoscopic lung biopsy entails substantial risk in patients with significant pulmonary hypertension. Because of the low likelihood of altering the clinical diagnosis, routine biopsy is discouraged. Under certain circumstances, histopathologic diagnosis may be needed when vasculitis, granulomatous or interstitial lung disease, pulmonary veno-occlusive disease, or bronchiolitis are suggested on clinical grounds or by radiographic studies.

Plexiform lesion of pulmonary arteriole. Note severe luminal narrowing, with fibrinoid necrosis of vessel wall (arrow).

TREATMENT OF PULMONARY ARTERIAL HYPERTENSION

General Measures

There are few data on which to base recommendations regarding physical activity or cardiopulmonary rehabilitation in PAH (see Plate 4-126). Cautious, graduated

PULMONARY HYPERTENSION
(Continued)

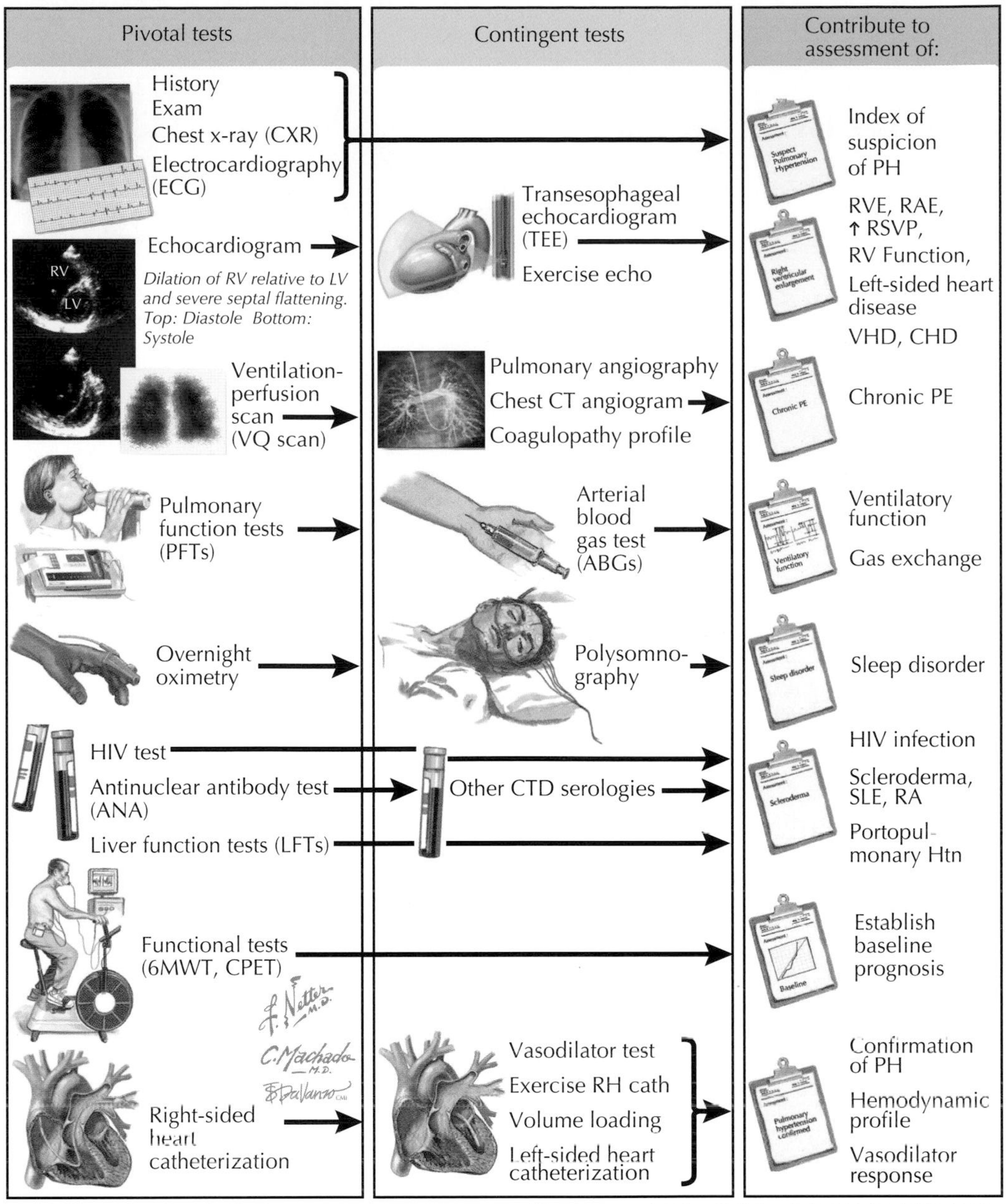

Pivotal tests	Contingent tests	Contribute to assessment of:
History Exam Chest x-ray (CXR) Electrocardiography (ECG)		Index of suspicion of PH
Echocardiogram *Dilation of RV relative to LV and severe septal flattening. Top: Diastole Bottom: Systole*	Transesophageal echocardiogram (TEE) Exercise echo	RVE, RAE, ↑ RSVP, RV Function, Left-sided heart disease VHD, CHD
Ventilation-perfusion scan (VQ scan)	Pulmonary angiography Chest CT angiogram Coagulopathy profile	Chronic PE
Pulmonary function tests (PFTs)	Arterial blood gas test (ABGs)	Ventilatory function Gas exchange
Overnight oximetry	Polysomnography	Sleep disorder
HIV test		HIV infection
Antinuclear antibody test (ANA)	Other CTD serologies	Scleroderma, SLE, RA
Liver function tests (LFTs)		Portopulmonary Htn
Functional tests (6MWT, CPET)		Establish baseline prognosis
Right-sided heart catheterization	Vasodilator test Exercise RH cath Volume loading Left-sided heart catheterization	Confirmation of PH Hemodynamic profile Vasodilator response

F. Netter M.D.
C. Machado M.D.
DalVanzo

McLaughlin, V. V. et al. J Am Coll Cardiol 2009;53:1573-1619.

physical activity is generally encouraged. Heavy physical activity can precipitate syncope. Hot baths or showers are discouraged because resultant peripheral vasodilatation can produce systemic hypotension and syncope. Excessive sodium intake can contribute to fluid retention. Exposure to high altitude (>~6000 ft above sea level) should generally be discouraged because it may produce hypoxic pulmonary vasoconstriction. Supplemental oxygen should be used to maintain oxygen saturations above 91%. Air travel can be problematic for patients with PAH because commercial aircraft are typically pressurized to the equivalent of approximately 8000 feet above sea level. Patients with borderline oxygen saturations at sea level may require 3 to 4 L/min of supplemental oxygen on commercial aircraft, and those already using supplemental oxygen at sea level should increase their oxygen flow rate. Because of the potential adverse effects of respiratory infections, immunization against influenza and pneumococcal pneumonia is recommended.

Pregnancy and Birth Control

The hemodynamic changes occurring in pregnancy impose significant stress in women with PAH, leading to a potential 30% to 50% mortality rate. Although there have been reports of successful treatment of pregnant IPAH patients using chronic intravenous epoprostenol, most experts recommend early termination of the pregnancy. Estrogen-containing contraceptives may increase the risk of venous thromboembolism and are not recommended for women with childbearing potential with PAH. Additionally, the endothelin receptor antagonists bosentan and ambrisentan may decrease the efficacy of hormonal contraception, and dual mechanical barrier contraceptive techniques are recommended in female patients of childbearing age taking these medications.

Concomitant Medications and Surgery

Use of vasoconstricting sinus or cold medications (e.g., pseudoephedrine) or serotonergic medications for migraine headaches may be problematic. Concomitant use of glyburide or cyclosporine with bosentan is contraindicated, and the use of azole-type antifungal agents is discouraged because of potential drug-drug interactions that may increase the risk of hepatotoxicity. Patients taking warfarin should be cautioned regarding potential drug interactions with this medication. Bosentan may decrease International Normalized Ratio (INR) levels slightly in patients taking warfarin.

Invasive procedures and surgery can be associated with an increased risk. Patients with severe PAH are particularly prone to vasovagal events leading to syncope, cardiopulmonary arrest, and death. Cardiac output often depends on the heart rate in this situation, and the bradycardia and systemic vasodilatation accompanying a vasovagal event may result in hypotension. Heart rate should be monitored during invasive procedures, with availability of an anticholinergic agent. Oversedation may lead to ventilatory insufficiency and cause clinical deterioration. Caution should be exercised with laparoscopic procedures in which carbon dioxide is used for abdominal insufflation because absorption can produce hypercarbia, which is a pulmonary vasoconstrictor. The induction of anesthesia and intubation may be problematic because it may induce vasovagal events, hypoxemia, hypercarbia, and shifts in intrathoracic pressure.

Anticoagulation

Anticoagulation of IPAH patients with warfarin is recommended in the absence of contraindications. Although there is little evidence to guide such therapy, current consensus suggests targeting an INR of approximately 1.5 to 2.5. Anticoagulation is controversial for patients with PAH caused by other etiologies, such as scleroderma or congenital heart disease, because of a lack of evidence supporting efficacy, and the increased risk of gastrointestinal bleeding in patients with scleroderma, and hemoptysis congenital heart disease. The relative risks and benefits of anticoagulant therapy should be considered on a case-by-case basis. Patients with documented right-to-left intracardiac shunting caused by an atrial septal defect or patent foramen ovale and a history of transient ischemic attack or embolic stroke should be anticoagulated. Patients receiving treatment with chronic intravenous epoprostenol are generally anticoagulated in the absence of contraindications partly because of the additional risk of catheter-associated thrombosis.

Diuretics

Diuretics are indicated for volume overload or right ventricular failure. Rapid and excessive diuresis may precipitate systemic hypotension and renal insufficiency. Spironolactone, an aldosterone antagonist of benefit in patients with left-sided heart failure, is used by some experts to treat right-sided heart failure.

Digitalis

Although not extensively studied in PAH, digitalis is sometimes used for refractory right ventricular failure. Atrial flutter or other atrial dysrhythmias often complicate late-stage right-sided heart dysfunction, and digoxin may be useful for rate control.

Vasodilator Testing and Calcium Channel Blockers

Patients with IPAH who acutely respond to vasodilators often have improved survival with long-term use of

PULMONARY HYPERTENSION
(Continued)

calcium channel blockers (CCBs) (see Plate 4-126). A variety of short-acting agents have been used to test vasodilator responsiveness, including intravenous epoprostenol or adenosine and inhaled nitric oxide. The most recent consensus definition of a positive acute vasodilator response in PAH is decrease of at least 10 mm Hg in mean pulmonary artery pressure to less than or equal to 40 mm Hg with an increased or unchanged cardiac output. Most experts believe that true vasoreactivity is uncommon, occurring in 10% of patients with IPAH and rarely in those with other forms of PAH. Vasoreactivity testing should be performed in experienced centers. Only patients demonstrating a significant response to the acute administration of a short-acting vasodilator should be considered candidates for treatment with CCBs; treatment should be monitored closely because maintenance of response is not universal. Long-acting nifedipine or diltiazem or amlodipine is suggested. Agents with negative inotropic effect, such as verapamil, should be avoided.

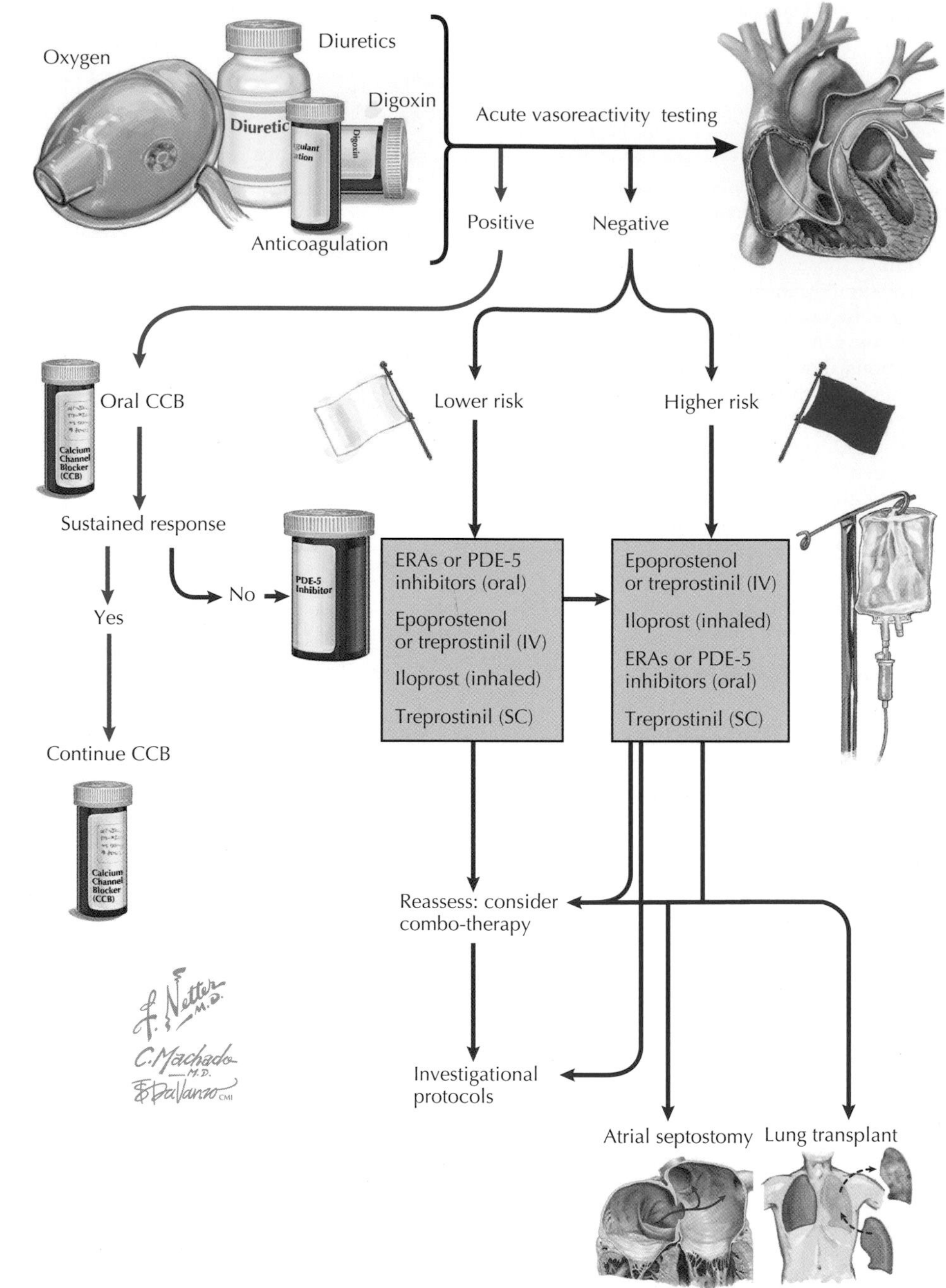

McLaughlin, V. V. et al. J Am Coll Cardiol 2009;53:1573-1619.

Prostanoids

Prostacyclin is a metabolite of arachidonic acid that is produced in vascular endothelium. It is a potent vasodilator, affecting both the pulmonary and systemic circulations, and has antiplatelet aggregatory effects. A relative deficiency of endogenous prostacyclin may contribute to the pathogenesis of PAH. In IPAH, continuously intravenously infused epoprostenol improved exercise capacity, assessed by the 6-minute walk distance (6MWD), cardiopulmonary hemodynamics, and survival compared with conventional therapy (oral vasodilators, anticoagulation). A similar study showed epoprostenol improved exercise capacity and hemodynamics in patients with PAH caused by the scleroderma spectrum of disease. Epoprostenol therapy is complicated by the need for continuous intravenous infusion. Because of its short half-life, the risk of rebound worsening with interruption of the infusion, and its irritant effects on peripheral veins, epoprostenol should be administered through an indwelling central venous catheter. Common side effects include headache, flushing, jaw pain, diarrhea, nausea, a blotchy erythematous rash, and musculoskeletal pain. Serious complications include catheter-related sepsis and thrombosis. Although epoprostenol is approved by the Food and Drug Administration for functional class III to IV patients with IPAH and PAH caused by scleroderma, it is generally reserved for patients with advanced disease refractory to oral therapies.

Other options for prostanoid therapy include subcutaneous or inhaled treprostinil, which has a longer half-life than epoprostenol, and inhaled iloprost, which must be inhaled six to nine times daily. Both drugs have demonstrated improved exercise capacity, functional class, and hemodynamics.

Endothelin Receptor Antagonists

Endothelin-1 (ET-1) is a vasoconstrictor and smooth muscle mitogen that may contribute to increased vascular tone and proliferation in PAH. Two endothelin receptor isoforms, ET_A and ET_B, have been identified. Controversy exists as to whether it is preferable to block both the ET_A and ET_B receptors or to selectively target the ET_A receptor. It has been argued that selective ET_A receptor antagonism may be beneficial for the treatment of patients with PAH because of maintenance of the vasodilator and clearance functions of ET_B receptors. A dual ET_A/ET_B receptor antagonist, bosentan, and a relatively selective ET_A receptor antagonist, ambrisentan, have been approved for use in patients with PAH and moderate to severe heart failure.

Phosphodiesterase-5 Inhibitors

Sildenafil is a highly specific phosphodiesterase-5 inhibitor approved for male erectile dysfunction. Sildenafil reduces pulmonary artery pressure and increases 6MWD and confers additional benefit to background therapy with epoprostenol in patients with PAH. Sildenafil, and the longer acting tadalafil, are approved in the United States for the treatment of PAH.

INTERVENTIONAL AND SURGICAL THERAPIES

Atrial septostomy involves the creation of a right-to left interatrial shunt to decompress the failing pressure/volume-overloaded right side of the heart. Where advanced medical therapies are available, atrial septostomy is seen as a largely palliative procedure or as a stabilizing bridge to lung transplantation. In areas lacking access to advanced medical therapies, atrial septostomy may be an option. Patient selection, timing, and appropriate sizing of the septostomy are critical to optimizing outcomes. Lung transplantation is particularly challenging in patients with PAH and is often reserved for those who are deteriorating despite the best available medical therapy. Survival in patients undergoing lung transplantation is approximately 66% to 75% at 1 year. Most centers prefer bilateral lung transplantation for patients with PAH.

PULMONARY EDEMA

Gas exchange occurs at the delicate interface between air and blood consisting of the alveolar epithelium and capillary endothelium. Flooding of the interstitium and alveoli with fluid and solutes from the pulmonary microvascular space disrupts this interface and is an important cause of dyspnea, hypoxemia, and respiratory failure. The pathophysiologic mechanisms that cause pulmonary edema differ among the conditions that can lead to this problem. Understanding these mechanisms provides a rationale for management (see Plate 4-127).

NORMAL PHYSIOLOGY

The familiar Starling relationship applies to the pulmonary microvasculature as it does in other capillary beds and estimates the net fluid flux (Q) across the capillary membrane from the microvascular space (mv) into the perimicrovascular interstitial fluid (if). The important variables are the total surface area of the microvasculature (S), the vascular permeability per unit surface area (L), and the net hydrostatic pressures across this membrane (Pmv – Pif), offset partially by the plasma colloid oncotic pressure within the microvasculature as opposed to the somewhat lower colloid osmotic pressure in the interstitium (Πmv – Πif). The difference in osmotic pressures across the pulmonary capillaries is less than in other capillary beds, and low albumin states alone do not cause pulmonary edema.

$$\text{Net fluid flux} = \text{Permeability}\ (\Delta\text{Hydrostatic pressures} - \Delta\text{Oncotic Pressures})$$

$$Q = (S * L)[(Pmv - Pif) - (\Pi mv - \Pi if)]$$

In the normal lung, the tight junctions of the alveolar epithelium prevent fluid from entering the alveoli, so that the fluid transudate enters the perimicrovascular interstitial space and then drains proximally through the pulmonary lymphatics into the venous system. The two most common perturbations that overwhelm this homeostasis are an elevation in capillary hydrostatic pressure and an increase in the permeability of the microvasculature (see Plate 4-128).

CARDIOGENIC PULMONARY EDEMA

Pulmonary edema from increased hydrostatic pressures is almost always caused by increased left atrial filling pressures from cardiac dysfunction or volume overload and is termed *cardiogenic pulmonary edema*. Common clinical situations are acute coronary syndromes, systolic or diastolic heart failure, valvular heart disease, and volume overload from acute or chronic renal failure. Because the permeability of the capillaries to proteins is preserved, the fluid in the alveoli is low in protein. Management is focused on reducing the filling pressures with diuresis and afterload reduction, as well as specific therapies for the underlying disorder (e.g., coronary revascularization, valvular surgery, renal replacement therapy).

NONCARDIOGENIC PULMONARY EDEMA

Pulmonary edema may occur even with normal hydrostatic pressures if there is an increase in the permeability of the endothelial and epithelial membranes. As both proteins and fluids leak through these altered membranes, the amount of protein in the edema fluid is elevated. The most frequent cause of noncardiogenic pulmonary edema is acute lung injury (ALI) initiated by inhaled or ingested toxins or by inflammatory mediators released in response to pulmonary or systemic insults. ALI and adult respiratory distress syndrome (ARDS) are most frequently associated with pneumonia, aspiration of gastric contents, sepsis syndromes, pancreatitis, major trauma, and multiple blood transfusions.

The management of patients with ALI and ARDS is definitive treatment of the underlying disorder and supportive care during resolution of the lung injury. Despite the severity of the lung injury, most patients with ARDS do not die from respiratory failure but instead from the underlying illness or from complications of the complex supportive care. Ventilatory strategies for patients with ARDS now use low tidal volumes (6 mL/kg ideal body weight) so as not to damage the remaining aerated alveoli with excessive distending pressures or volumes. Noncardiogenic pulmonary edema can also be worsened by an increase in hydrostatic pressures from sepsis-associated cardiac dysfunction or overly aggressive volume resuscitation.

PULMONARY EDEMA: PATHWAY OF NORMAL PULMONARY FLUID RESORPTION

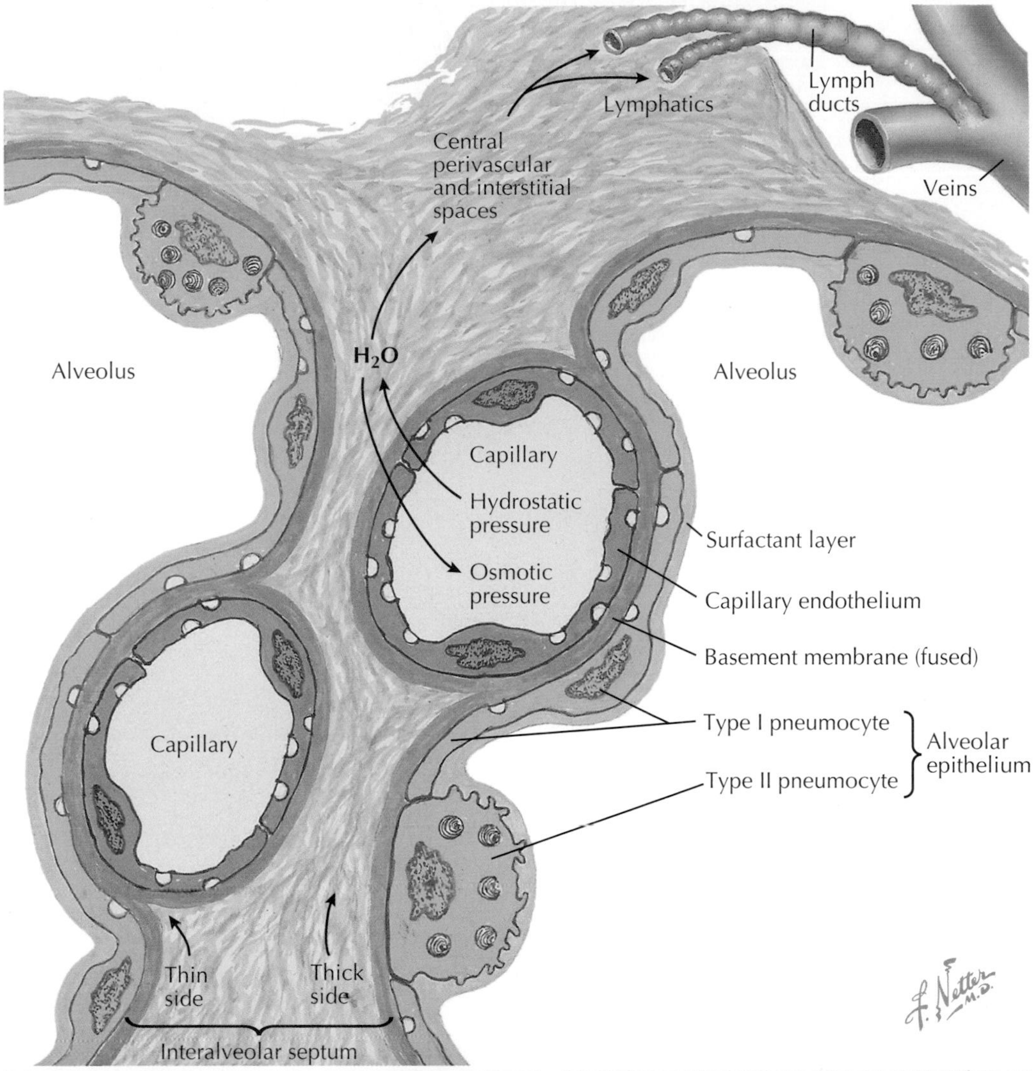

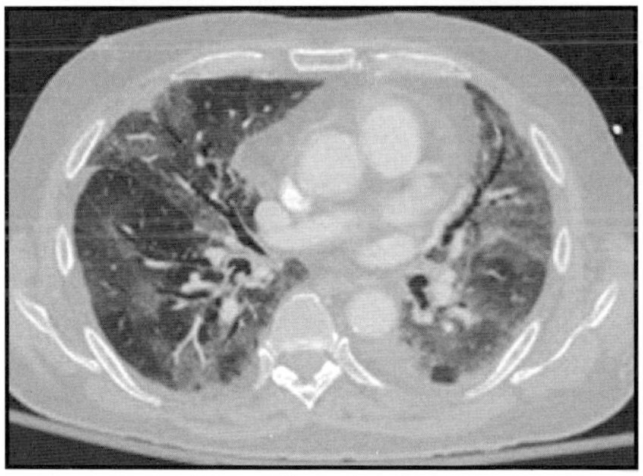

Noncardiogenic edema

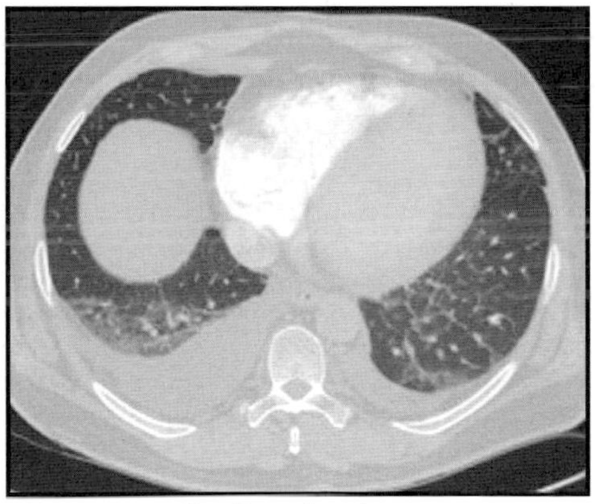

Cardiogenic edema

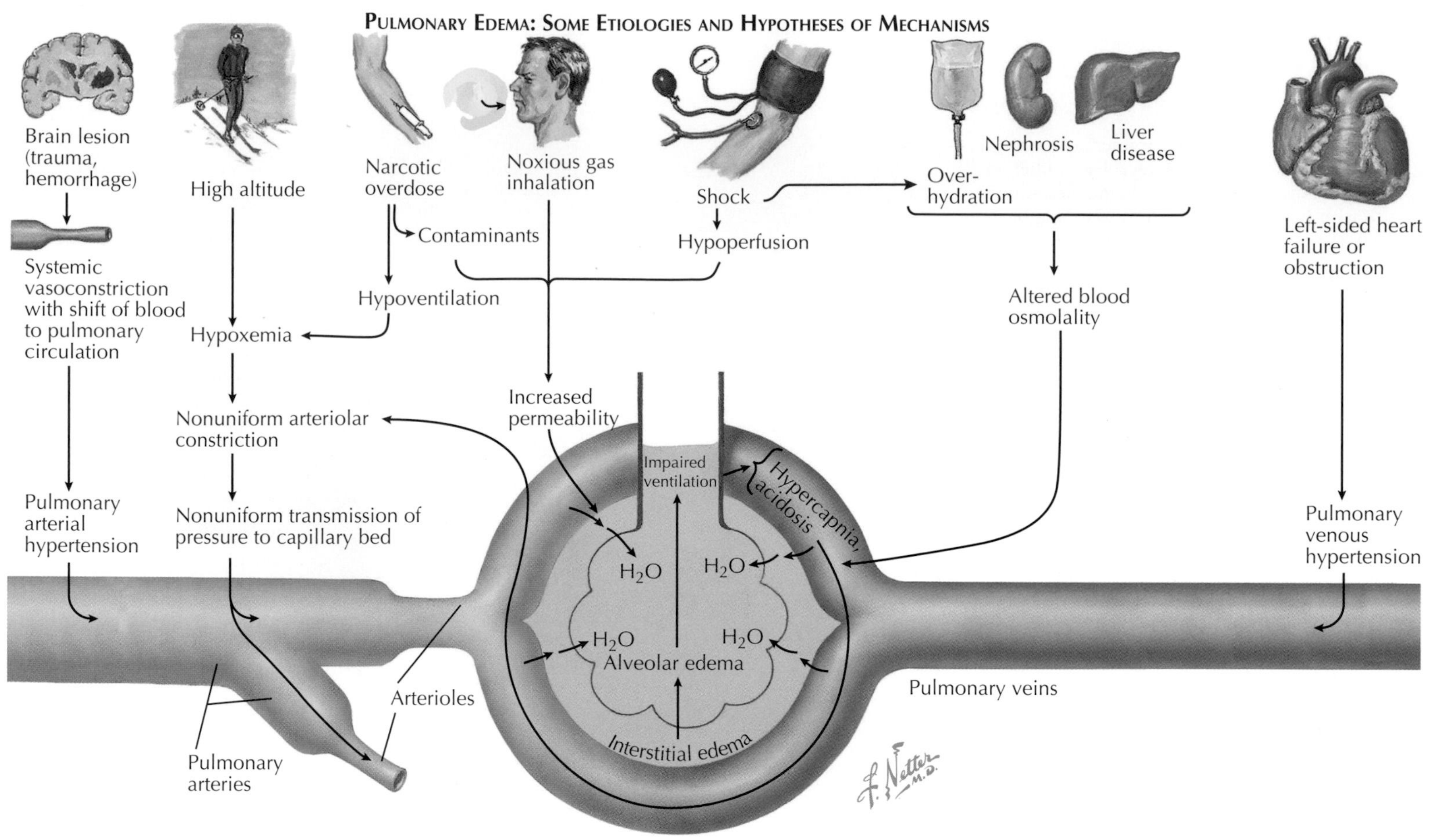

Pulmonary Edema *(Continued)*

SPECIFIC CLINICAL CAUSES OF NONCARDIOGENIC PULMONARY EDEMA

High-altitude pulmonary edema usually occurs in individuals ascending to altitudes above 3000 m (~9000 ft) above sea level even if they are athletically fit. Current evidence suggests that some individuals have accentuated pulmonary vasoconstriction in response to hypoxemia, perhaps from impaired nitric oxide production or exaggerated sympathetic responses, causing high pulmonary artery pressures that tear or fracture the pulmonary capillaries. This can be fatal unless managed promptly with supplemental oxygen and prompt descent to lower altitudes.

Neurogenic pulmonary edema may occur within minutes to hours in patients with acute central nervous system injury, usually in the form of seizures, intracerebral or subarachnoid hemorrhage, or head trauma. The exact pathophysiology is unknown but may involve an abrupt increase in pulmonary venoconstriction from sympathetic stimulation with subsequent elevations in capillary hydrostatic pressures, pulmonary microvascular injury, or both. With supportive care and management of the underlying neurologic insult, the edema usually resolves within 48 to 72 hours.

Certain drug ingestions can cause pulmonary edema, including opiates (heroin and methadone), oral or intravenous β-agonists used to manage preterm labor, and salicylates. Again, the exact mechanisms are not completely understood but may involve a combination of increased pulmonary capillary pressures and altered vascular permeability. The pulmonary edema from salicylate overdose can be exacerbated by standard overdose management with volume resuscitation and alkalinization with intravenous sodium bicarbonate.

EVALUATION OF PATIENTS WITH PULMONARY EDEMA

Patients with pulmonary edema present with the acute onset of dyspnea, tachypnea, and hypoxemia with radiographic studies showing bilateral alveolar infiltrates and increased interstitial markings. The history and clinical context often suggest the cause of the pulmonary edema. Symptoms consistent with an acute coronary syndrome strongly suggest cardiogenic edema, although pulmonary edema in the setting of pneumonia, an acute abdomen, or aspiration points toward ALI. Patients with seizures or intracerebral hemorrhage may have neurogenic pulmonary edema but could also have had gastric aspiration during periods of altered consciousness. Older cardiac patients often are at risk for sepsis syndromes. Thus, although the clinical history is essential, it is not always definitive as to whether the edema is cardiogenic, noncardiogenic, or a combination of both.

The physical examination may suggest cardiac disease, but findings of an S3 gallop or murmurs from valvular disorders may be difficult to hear in the noisy emergency department or intensive care unit environment. Lung examination findings of inspiratory crackles are similar in both forms of pulmonary edema. Peripheral edema is not specific for cardiac disease. Ancillary studies are obviously important. The electrocardiogram may show evidence of ischemia. Laboratory tests assess for evidence of infection, pancreatitis, or drug ingestions. Plasma levels of brain natriuretic peptide (BNP) are elevated when cardiac chambers are distended from congestive heart failure or volume overload. Low BNP levels (<100 pg/mL) strongly support a noncardiogenic cause of pulmonary edema. High levels (>500 pg/mL) suggest a cardiac cause, but intermediate levels are generally not helpful. Direct hemodynamic estimates of the left atrial pressures are possible with placement of a pulmonary artery catheter, but this is an invasive procedure with known complications. Use of these catheters has not been associated with improved patient outcomes.

Imaging of the chest with plain radiographs and computed tomography scans suggests cardiogenic edema if there are pleural effusions, an enlarged cardiac silhouette, widened central vascular structures, septal lines, and peribronchial cuffing. Absence of these features and patchy, peripheral infiltrates suggest noncardiogenic edema. Bedside transthoracic cardiac echocardiography can be a quick and noninvasive way to evaluate for impaired systolic function or valvular disease, but it is less sensitive for diastolic dysfunction.

The systematic approach to pulmonary edema uses history, physical exam, laboratory evaluation, and imaging. Echocardiography and, if needed, invasive hemodynamic monitoring are used in patients in whom the cause of the edema is still not certain.

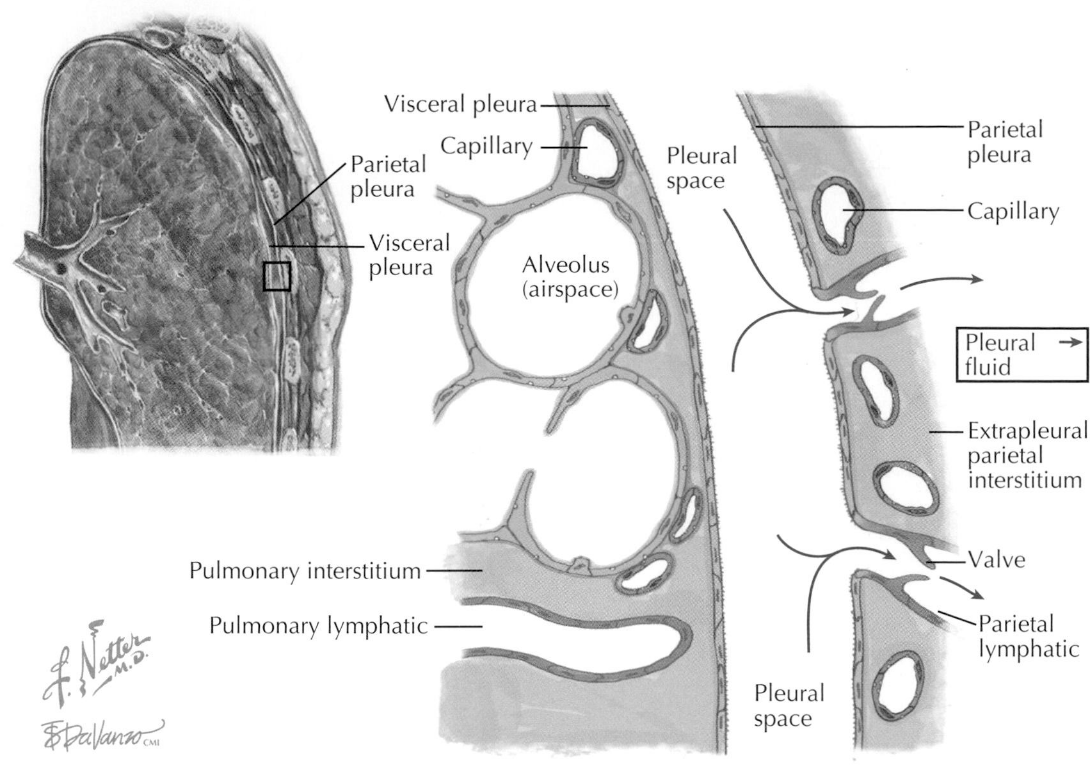

Pathophysiology of Pleural Fluid Accumulation

The pleural space is the potential space between the visceral and parietal pleura. Normally, it contains 7 to 16 mL of hypotonic fluid, which acts to lubricate the membranes to allow near-frictionless movement of the two pleural surfaces against each other during breathing. A large number of disease processes may result in abnormal accumulation of fluid in the pleural space.

Fluid and plasma protein movement across biologic membranes is governed by the revised Starling law describing water flux (Jv) between two compartments:

$$Jv = Kf[(PH1 - PH2) - \sigma(\pi1 - \pi2)]$$

where Kf is the filtration coefficient, PH is hydraulic pressure, π is colloidosmotic pressure, and σ is the solute reflection coefficient of the membrane.

Based mainly on animal studies, pleural fluid is filtered at the parietal level from systemic microvessels into the pleural space. Some contribution from visceral parietal filtration may also be present. Pleural fluid drains primarily via the parietal pleural lymphatics. Fluid drainage can increase markedly to maintain constant pleural fluid volume, approaching approximately 700 mL/d in humans. However, when formation exceeds drainage, pleural fluid accumulation occurs. Plain chest radiography can identify as little as 50 mL of accumulated pleural fluid when examining a lateral view, revealed by blunting of the posterior costophrenic angle. Usually at least 200 mL of fluid is required to be detected by blunting of the lateral costophrenic angles in the posteroanterior view. Chest ultrasonography can detect as little as 5 mL of fluid, and computed tomography is even more sensitive.

Typically, one of four major mechanisms results in excessive pleural fluid formation: elevated hydrostatic pressure (PH), decreased oncotic pressure (π), decreased lymphatic drainage caused by mechanical obstruction, or increased extravasation (Kf) through inflamed pleural membranes. The first two mechanisms typically result in fluid classified as transudative, and the latter two mechanisms usually result in exudative fluid. Transudates and exudates are defined by the ratio of pleural fluid-to-serum levels of protein and lactate dehydrogenase (LDH) with a protein ratio of above 0.50 or LDH ratio (compared with the upper limit of normal serum LDH) of above 0.67 defining an exudate.

Whereas transudates imply normal pleura and can usually be diagnosed based on other clinical characteristics, exudates often require further testing. These tests on the fluid include appearance, character, odor, color, cell count, microbiology, cytology, and biochemical tests (e.g., pH, glucose, amylase, triglycerides). In some cases, pleural biopsy may be required to diagnose the cause of an exudative pleural effusion.

Causes of pleural effusion

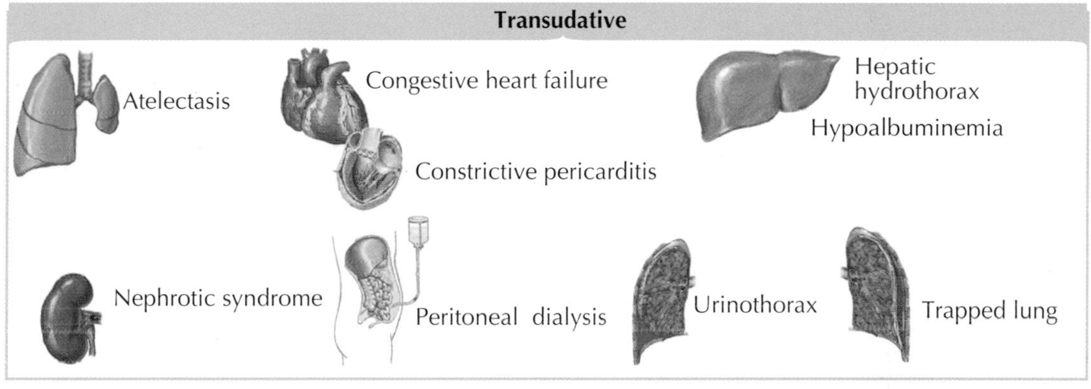

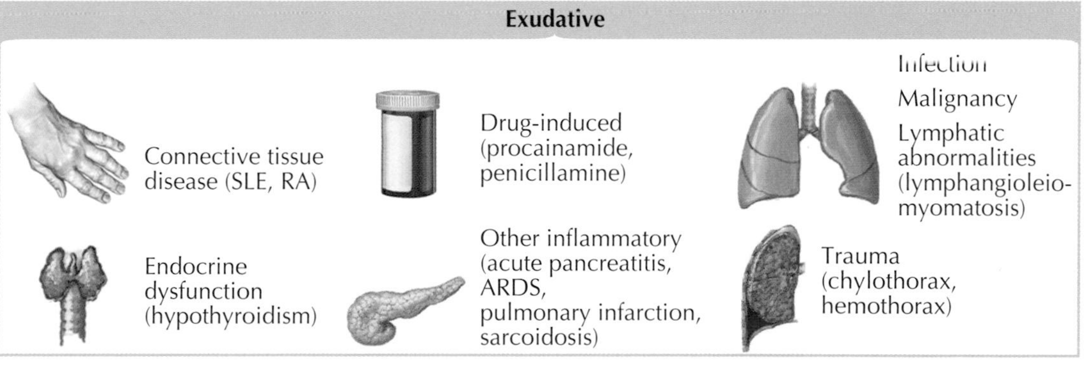

Pulmonary venous hypertension

Increased left atrial pressure

Left heart failure

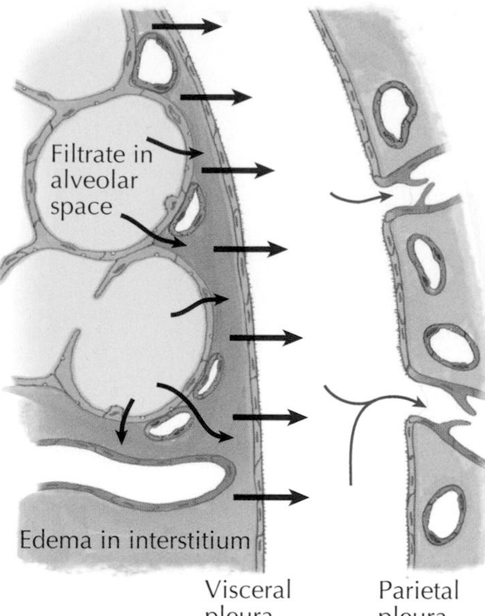

Pleural Effusion In Heart Disease

Pleural effusions commonly occur in patients with congestive heart failure (CHF). The effusions are a sequela of pulmonary venous hypertension and not the result of isolated systemic venous hypertension unless there is associated ascitic fluid with transdiaphragmatic movement into the pleural space. With systolic or diastolic left-sided heart failure, pulmonary venous pressure increases, causing fluid to move into the lung interstitium; the increased interstitial–pleural pressure gradient promotes the movement of fluid between mesothelial cells into the pleural space. If pleural fluid formation exceeds removal through the parietal pleural lymphatics, a pleural effusion will develop.

Pleural effusion from heart disease can also be caused by constrictive pericarditis, which is defined by marked fibrous thickening of the pericardium causing chronic cardiac compression. Causes of constrictive pericarditis include tuberculosis, cardiac surgery, connective tissue disease, radiation therapy, malignancies, and other infections (including viruses). Constrictive pericarditis results in limited ventricular diastolic filling. End-diastolic ventricular pressures and mean atrial pressures increase to virtually equal levels.

Patients with CHF present with the typical manifestations of orthopnea, paroxysmal nocturnal dyspnea, and dyspnea on exertion. Chest radiographs show evidence of pulmonary venous hypertension; extravascular lung water; and bilateral pleural effusions, with the right effusion typically being greater. A unilateral left pleural effusion in the patient with heart disease should suggest an alternate diagnosis.

Constrictive pericarditis is more common in men whose chief complaints include fatigue, dyspnea, weight gain, abdominal discomfort, and peripheral edema. The usual physical findings are sinus tachycardia, distant heart sounds, and prominent cervical neck veins that do not decrease with inspiration (Kussmaul sign). Chest radiographs reveal bilateral effusions with a normal heart size. In contrast to CHF, constrictive pericarditis results in ascites before the appearance of peripheral edema. A pulsus paradoxus is observed in most patients. The diagnosis is confirmed by right-sided and left-sided heart catheterization demonstrating equalization of diastolic pressures.

Pleural effusion in CHF is the classic transudate. The total nucleated cell count is generally less than 500/μL with a predominance of lymphocytes and mesothelial cells. The pH typically ranges from 7.45 to 7.55, and the glucose concentration is similar to the serum concentration. However, it is important to note that diuretic therapy may elevate both the protein and lactate dehydrogenase ratios into the exudative range in approximately 10% of patients. Use of the serum–pleural fluid albumin gradient (serum minus pleural fluid) helps determine whether the effusion is caused solely by CHF. If the albumin gradient is ≥1.2 g/dL, it is highly likely that the effusion is a transudate. Pleural fluid findings in patients with constrictive pericarditis are similar to those of CHF but may be exudative with effusive constriction from inflammatory pericarditis.

Management of patients with CHF is directed at decreasing pulmonary venous hypertension with diuretics, afterload reduction, digitalis, and salt restriction. Treatment of patients with constrictive pericarditis includes pericardiectomy.

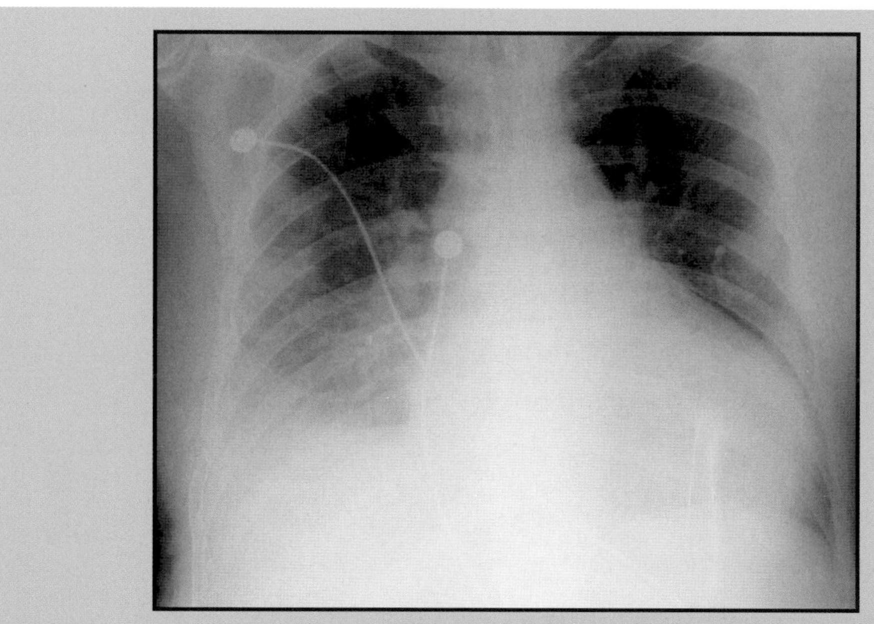

67-year-old man with ischemic cardiomyopathy with cardiomegaly, bilateral effusions, and pulmonary venous hypertension

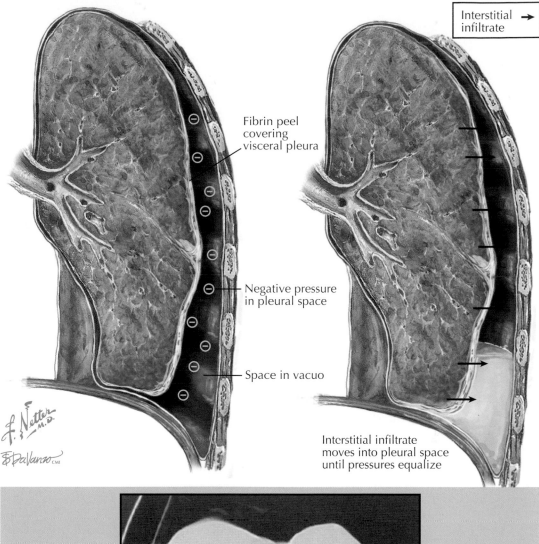

Interstitial infiltrate →

Fibrin peel covering visceral pleura

Negative pressure in pleural space

Space in vacuo

Interstitial infiltrate moves into pleural space until pressures equalize

Unexpandable Lung

An unexpandable lung may result from visceral pleural restriction, an endobronchial lesion, or chronic atelectasis. The most common causes of visceral pleural restriction are malignancy and infection; others include inflammatory pleurisy, such as rheumatoid disease, and coronary artery bypass graft (CABG) surgery.

There are two distinct phases of the unexpandable lung caused by visceral pleural restriction: (1) the early phase, called *lung entrapment*, and (2) the late phase, termed *trapped lung*. Lung entrapment caused by malignancy is associated with two pathophysiologic mechanisms responsible for pleural fluid formation: (1) malignant involvement of the pleura, promoting capillary leak and impaired pleural lymphatic drainage, and (2) visceral pleural restriction from the tumor burden, resulting in hydrostatic imbalance. A trapped lung from remote infection results in pleural fluid formation only from the unexpandable lung and hydrostatic forces.

Patients with a trapped lung may present either with exertional dyspnea if the extent of unexpandable lung is large or with a small, persistent effusion discovered on routine chest radiography if the visceral pleural restriction is small. When a portion of the pleura is restricted and the adjacent lung cannot occupy the resultant space, fluid fills the space in vacuo along a pressure gradient.

A therapeutic thoracentesis will cause a rapid and significant decrease in pleural pressure that can be documented by manometry, resulting in anterior chest pain without relief of dyspnea. The diagnosis of trapped lung can be further substantiated by allowing air entry through an open stopcock into the pleural space with rapid cessation of the chest pain. A chest computed tomography (CT) scan will confirm a "visceral pleural peel," which is typically smaller than 3 mm in thickness and not likely to be detected when not outlined by air.

The character of the pleural fluid will be determined by the stage of the unexpandable lung. With a parapneumonic effusion causing lung entrapment, the fluid will be exudative by protein and lactate dehydrogenase criteria with neutrophil predominance. When the inflammatory or infectious process has resolved, the sole cause of the effusion will be an imbalance in hydrostatic pressures and thus a transudate. However, because lung entrapment and trapped lung represent a continuum of the same disease process, the timing of thoracentesis is critical in revealing whether the fluid is exudative (early) or transudative (later). Although most patients with inflammatory lung entrapment have resolution, others develop a pleural peel and trapped lung. Therefore, the classic pleural effusion from trapped lung is a serous transudate with a low number of mononuclear cells.

In an asymptomatic patient with a small, trapped lung, reassurance is all that is necessary. With a large, symptomatic trapped lung and restrictive physiology, the underlying lung should be examined by CT scan. If the underlying lung is normal, decortication can be recommended in the appropriate circumstance.

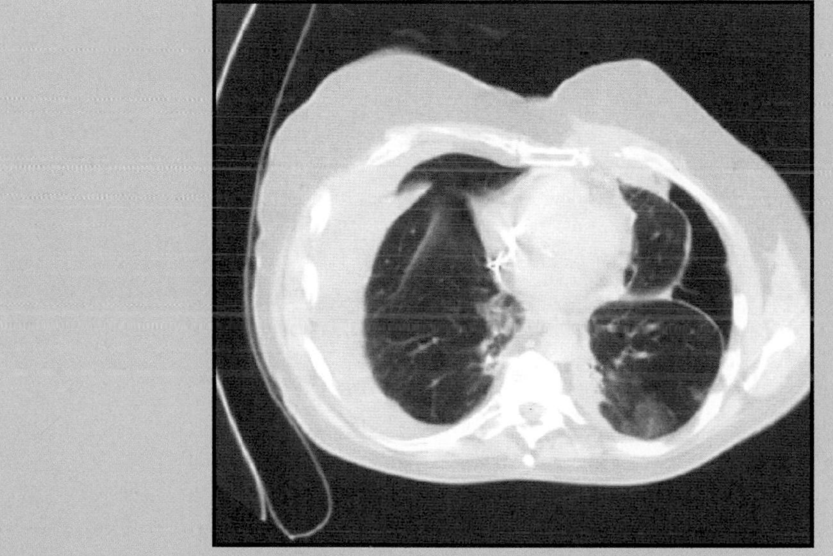

53-year-old woman with complicated parapneumonic effusion and trapped lung on left due to thick visceral pleural peel.

Parapneumonic Effusion

A parapneumonic effusion is defined as pleural fluid that develops from pneumonia. Parapneumonic effusion is the most common cause of an exudative effusion. A practical, clinical classification of a parapneumonic effusion is as follows: (1) an uncomplicated parapneumonic effusion resolves with antibiotic therapy alone without pleural space sequelae; (2) a complicated parapneumonic effusion requires pleural space drainage to resolve pleural sepsis and prevent progression to an empyema; and (3) empyema is the end-stage of a parapneumonic effusion. Empyema is defined by its appearance, which is an opaque, whitish-yellow, viscous fluid (pus) that is generated from serum coagulation proteins, cellular debris, and fibrin deposition.

An empyema develops primarily because of delayed patient presentation and less often from inappropriate clinical management. Early antibiotic treatment prevents progression of the pneumonia, the development of a parapneumonic effusion, and the progression to an empyema. Risk factors for empyema include extremes of age, debilitation, male gender, pneumonia requiring hospitalization, and comorbidities (e.g., bronchiectasis, chronic obstructive pulmonary disease, rheumatoid arthritis, alcoholism, diabetes, gastroesophageal reflux disease).

Pleural fluid analysis allows the clinician to stage the parapneumonic effusion and to guide initial management, with complicated effusions tending to be more cloudy, with pH below 7.20, glucose level below 40 mg/dL, lactate dehydrogenase (LDH) level above 1000 U/L, and neutrophils above 25,000 cells per microliter. Early and appropriate antibiotic treatment prevents the development of a parapneumonic effusion and its progression. A parapneumonic effusion is one of the few clinical situations in which a diagnostic thoracentesis should be performed as soon as possible. There should be timely escalation of treatment if the parapneumonic effusion progresses with continued pleural sepsis. Early pleural space drainage with a small-bore catheter promoting expansion of the lung prevents the development of a complicated parapneumonic effusion and empyema in the majority of patients. Clinical features that suggest the need for surgical drainage include prolonged pneumonia symptoms, comorbid disease, failure to respond to antibiotic therapy, and the presence of anaerobic organisms. Chest radiographic findings that suggest the need for pleural space drainage include an effusion larger than 50% of the hemithorax, loculation, or an air-fluid level. Stranding or septation noted on ultrasonography suggests the need for pleural space drainage; and marked pleural enhancement, pleural thickening, and the split pleura sign on contrast chest computed tomography indicate the need for pleural space drainage. Aspiration of pus is a clear indication for drainage; however, a positive Gram stain or culture, pH below 7.20, glucose level below 40 mg/dL or LDH level above 1000 IU/L all support the need for pleural space drainage. If pleural sepsis persists, video-assisted thoracoscopic surgery is usually successful in resolving the infection and promoting lung expansion.

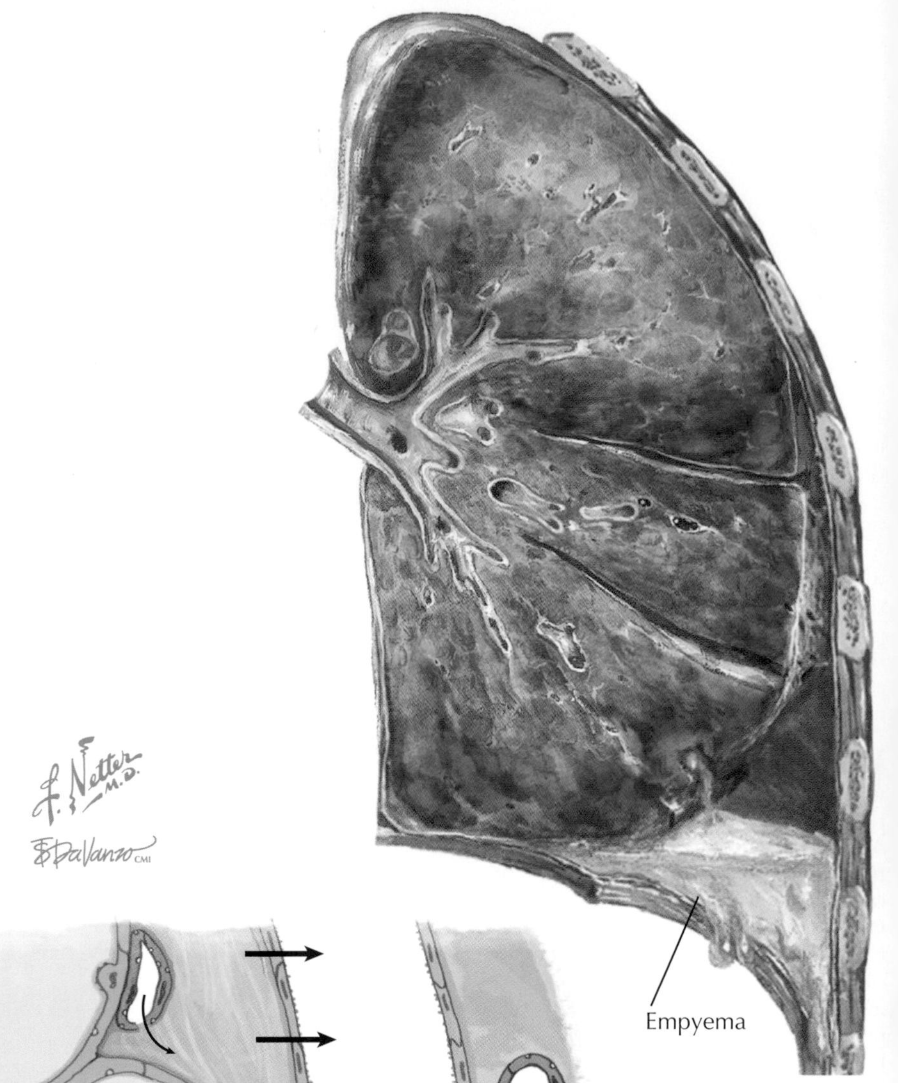

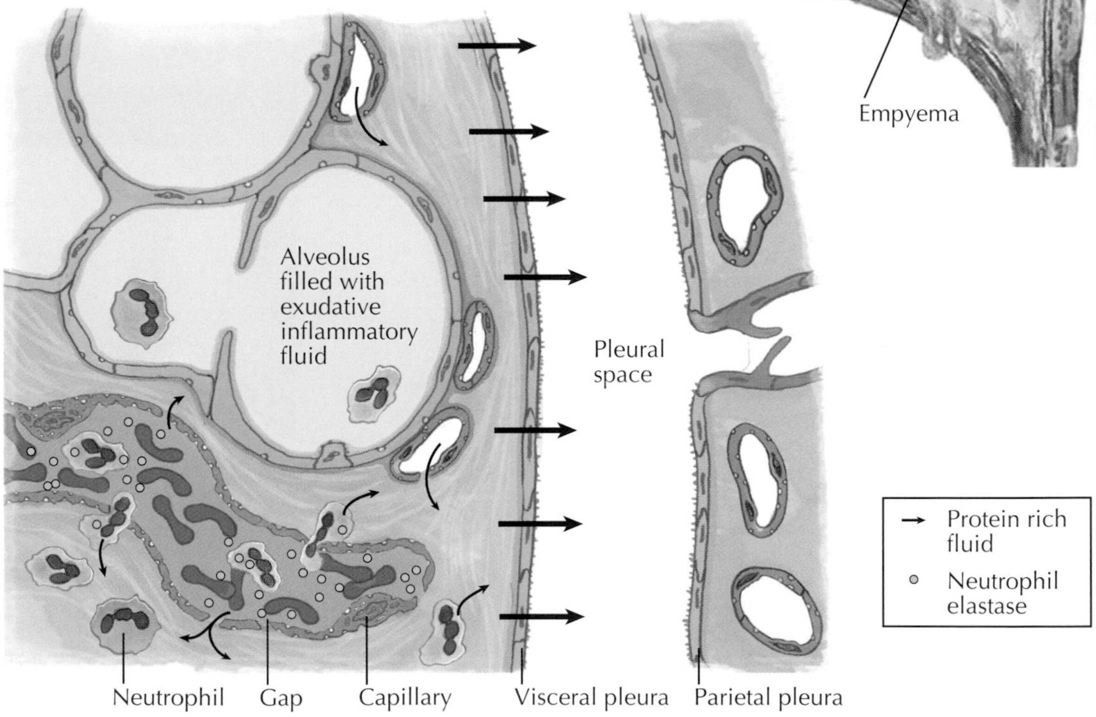

PLEURAL EFFUSION IN MALIGNANCY

The diagnosis of a malignant pleural effusion is established when malignant cells are identified in pleural fluid or in pleural tissue. However, in about 10% to 15% of patients with a known malignancy and a pleural effusion, malignant cells cannot be identified; these effusions are termed *paramalignant effusions*. Paramalignant effusions develop from local effects of the tumor (lymphatic obstruction), systemic effects of the tumor (pulmonary embolism), and complications of therapy (radiation pleuritis and effects of chemotherapy). Although carcinoma from any organ can metastasize to the pleura, lung cancer and breast carcinoma are responsible for approximately 60% of all malignant pleural effusions. Ovarian and gastric carcinoma are the third and fourth leading cancers to cause malignant effusions; lymphomas account for approximately 10% of all malignant pleural effusions.

Impaired lymphatic drainage, tumor-induced angiogenesis, and increased capillary permeability from vasoactive cytokines and chemokines contribute to the pathogenesis of the malignant effusion.

Patients with malignant pleural effusions most commonly present with dyspnea, with the degree dependent on the volume of pleural fluid and the underlying lung disease. A therapeutic thoracentesis provides temporary relief of dyspnea in most patients.

With lung cancer, the pleural effusion is typically ipsilateral to the primary lesion. With a non-lung primary lesion, there appears to be no ipsilateral predilection, and bilateral effusions are common. When a pleural effusion is massive, occupying the entire hemithorax, there is usually contralateral mediastinal shift, and malignancy is the cause in approximately 70% of patients. When there is complete opacification with absence of contralateral shift, the scenario suggests carcinoma of the ipsilateral mainstem bronchus (the density on chest radiographs represents complete lung collapse and a smaller pleural effusion); the initial diagnostic test should be bronchoscopy with biopsy of the endobronchial lesion.

A malignant effusion may appear serous, serosanguineous, or grossly bloody. The total nucleated cell count normally ranges from 1500 to 4000/μL and consists of lymphocytes, macrophages, and mesothelial cells. These effusions are predominantly lymphocytes (50%-75% of the nucleated cells) in about half of patients. Neutrophils tend to be less than 25% of the total nucleated cells. The prevalence of pleural fluid eosinophilia in malignant effusions ranges from 8% to 12%; therefore, finding pleural fluid eosinophilia (eosinophils >10% of the total nucleated cells) should not be considered a predictor of benign disease. The pleural fluid protein and lactate dehydrogenase levels are typically in the exudative range. The pleural fluid pH is less than 7.30, and the glucose is less than 60 mg/dL in approximately 30% of patients at presentation. A low pH and glucose level suggests significant involvement of the pleura. This inhibits glucose movement into the pleural space and efflux of the end products of glucose metabolism, CO_2 and lactic acid, resulting in pleural fluid acidosis. A low pH predicts decreased survival and a poorer response to pleurodesis.

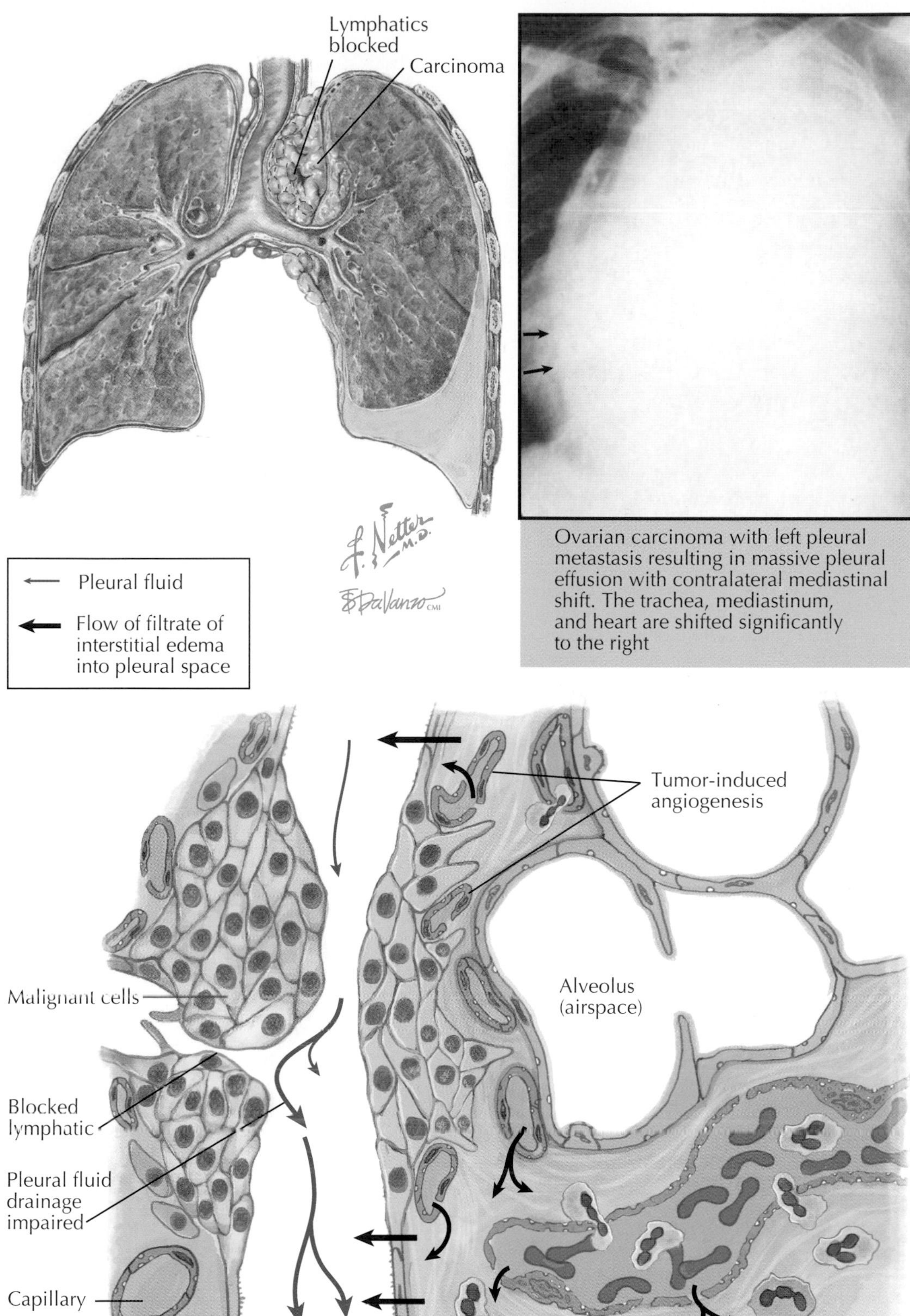

Ovarian carcinoma with left pleural metastasis resulting in massive pleural effusion with contralateral mediastinal shift. The trachea, mediastinum, and heart are shifted significantly to the right

The yield from diagnostic testing of a malignant pleural effusion correlates directly with the extent of disease. Pleural fluid cytology is more sensitive than percutaneous pleural biopsy because the latter is a blind sampling procedure. Thoracoscopy by an experienced operator will diagnose up to 95% of malignant pleural effusions. The diagnosis of a malignant pleural effusion signals a poor prognosis; therefore, with lung and gastric carcinoma, the survival is typically a few months. With breast cancer and lymphoma, a response to chemotherapy may result in a longer survival. In patients unresponsive to chemotherapy, relieving breathlessness by controlling the malignant pleural effusion substantially improves quality of life. If the lung is expandable, pleurodesis with talc is an option. With an unexpandable lung, placing an indwelling catheter as an outpatient with home drainage can manage the patient's breathlessness.

CHYLOTHORAX

A *chylothorax* is defined as the accumulation of chyle in the pleural space that results from disruption of the thoracic duct or one of its major tributaries. A total of 1500 to 2500 mL of chyle empties into the venous system daily from the thoracic duct, depending on the fat content of the diet. The formation of chylomicrons occurs from long-chain triglycerides in dietary fats that are transported to the cisterna chyli, which overlie the anterior surface of the second lumbar vertebrae to the right and posterior to the aorta. Although there are multiple variations in the course of the thoracic duct, the usual pathway is through the aortic hiatus of the diaphragm into the posterior mediastinum. The thoracic duct most commonly crosses from the right side of the vertebral column to the left between the 7th and 5th thoracic vertebrae as it ascends posterior to the aortic arch and empties into the junction of the jugular and subclavian veins.

There are multiple causes of chylothorax, with the most common being malignancy and surgical trauma. Surgical procedures that have been associated with chylothorax include esophageal resection, coronary bypass grafting, and radical neck dissection. Chylothorax has been associated with nonsurgical trauma, such as sudden hyperextension of the spine, seat belt injury, severe paroxysms of cough, and even stretching. Non-Hodgkin lymphoma is the most common malignancy associated with chylothorax. Other causes of chylothorax include lymphangioleiomyomatosis, tuberculosis, sarcoidosis, and tuberous sclerosis. Chylous ascites from abdominal malignancy, cirrhosis, or severe right-sided heart failure can result in chylothorax after movement of ascitic fluid transdiaphragmatically into the chest.

The symptoms associated with a chylothorax are related to the volume of pleural fluid and the status of the underlying lung. Therefore, the most common presenting symptom is dyspnea, which tends to be insidious in onset. On pleural fluid analysis in a nonfasting patient, the fluid will appear milky in character; the milky fluid may be serous if the patient has been fasting for at least 12 hours or bloody if trauma is involved. Chyle has a variable protein content, usually between 2.2 and 6 g/dL, and is lymphocyte predominant (usually >80% of the nucleated cells). A chylothorax is a protein discordant exudate with a lactate dehydrogenase level in the transudative range. A chylothorax has an elevated triglyceride concentration, typically greater than 110 mg/dL. If the level is less than 50 mg/dL in a patient who is not fasting, chylothorax can virtually be excluded. However, the definitive diagnostic test is the presence of chylomicrons.

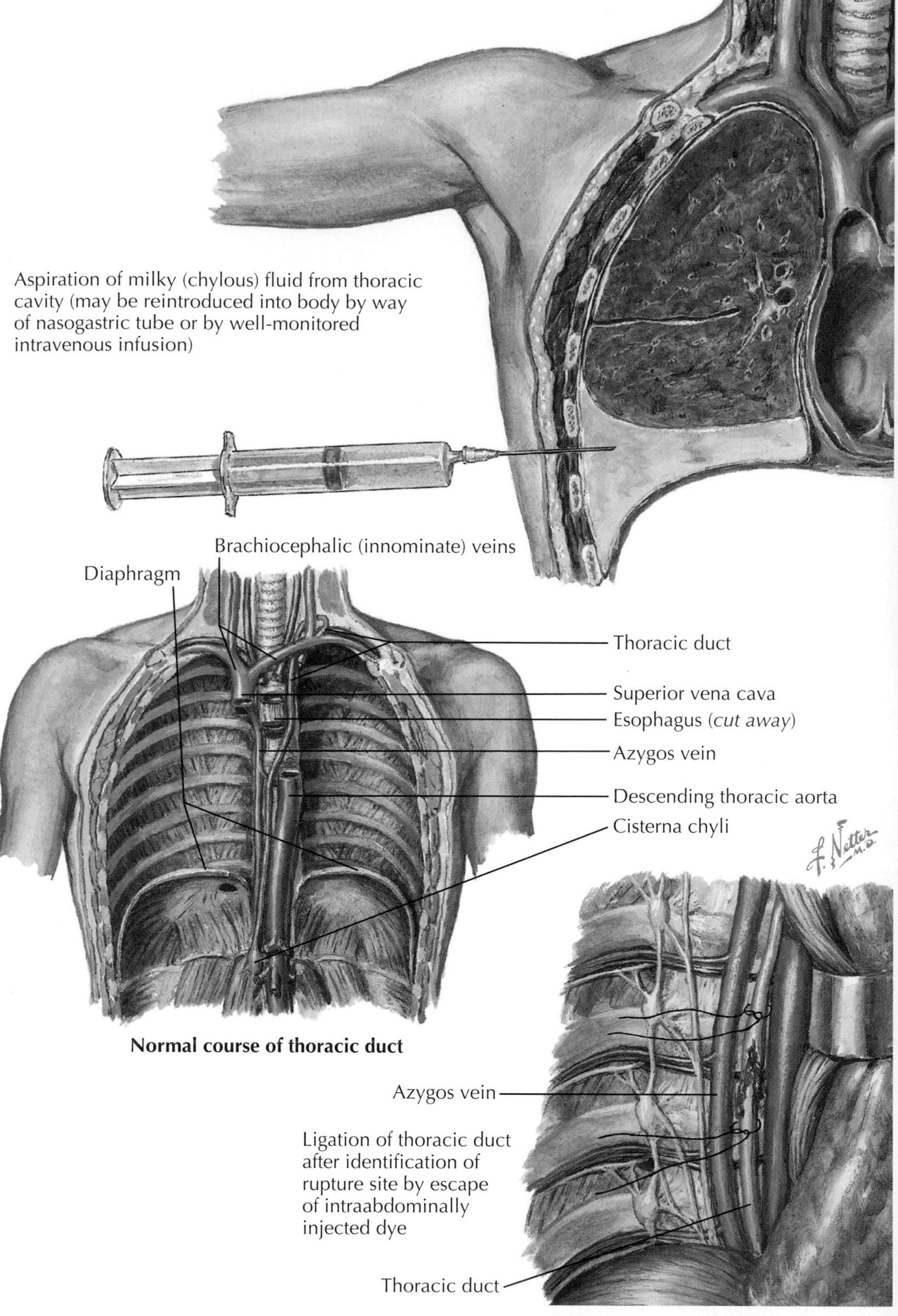

Normal course of thoracic duct

Management is focused on maintaining adequate nutrition and minimizing chyle production. Treatment of the underlying disease, such as lymphoma, should always be the initial treatment option. Repeat thoracenteses or chest tube drainage results in removal of large amounts of protein, fats, fat-soluble vitamins, electrolytes, and lymphocytes, promoting an impaired immune response and severe metabolic abnormalities. In traumatic chylothorax, the defect in the thoracic duct often closes spontaneously within 10 to 14 days, and conservative treatment is advocated. Chemical pleurodesis has been successful in patients who are not responsive to conservative therapy. Other measures that have been successful include thoracic duct embolization and administration of a somatostatin, such as octreotide. Thoracic duct ligation is considered to be the definitive treatment but is often technically problematic in some individuals.

RIB AND STERNAL FRACTURES

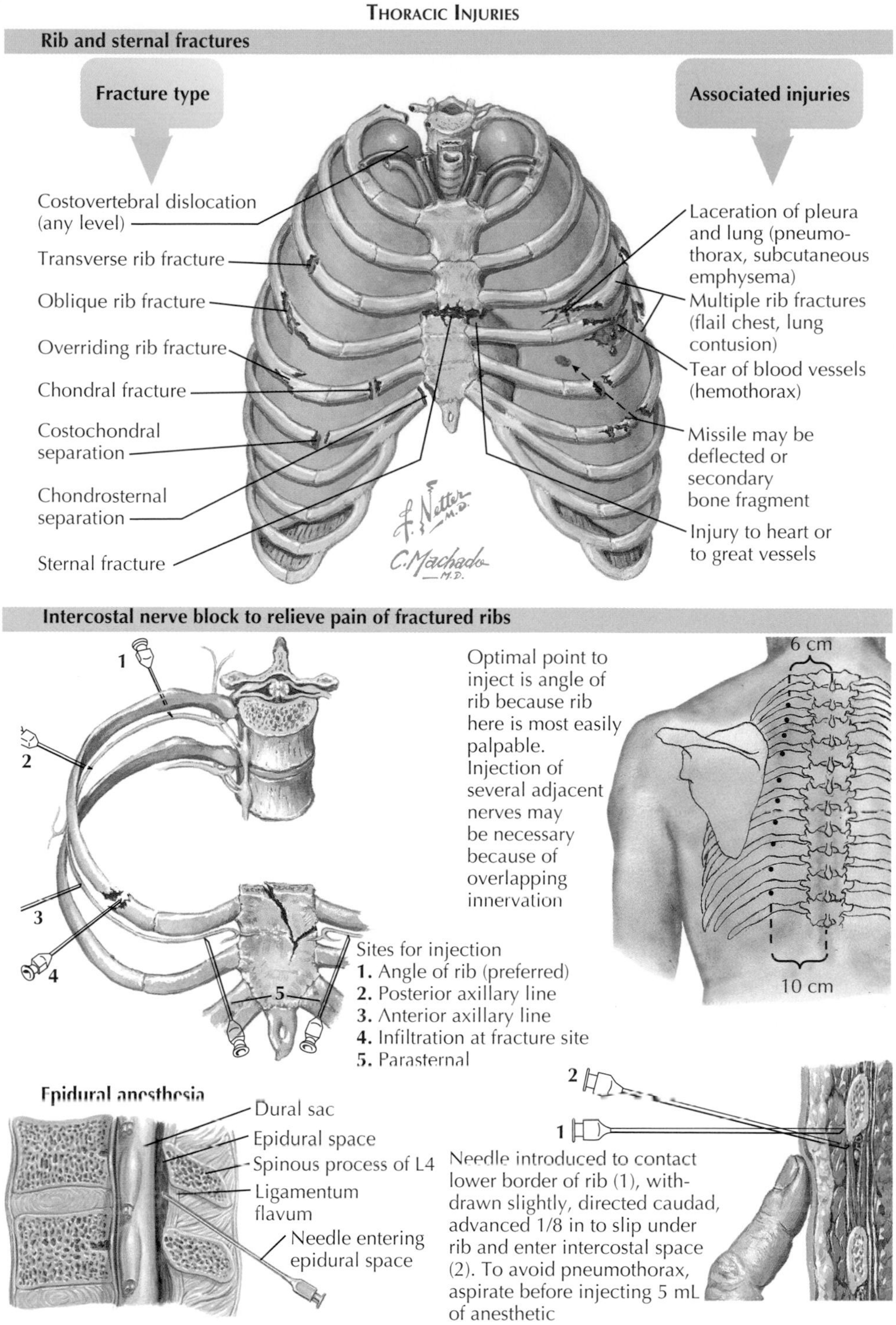

Thoracic injury is directly responsible for 25% of trauma deaths and contributes to the demise of another 25%. Most mortality directly attributable to chest trauma occurs in the prehospital setting, resulting from disruption of the great vessels, heart, or tracheobronchial tree. Of those who survive the initial insult, fewer than 15% sustain injury that necessitates operative intervention. Although tube thoracostomy is often the only procedure required initially for chest trauma, injuries to the thoracic cage and lung prolong hospitalization and may be the source of long-term morbidity and occasionally death.

A rib fracture is usually the result of a direct force applied to the chest wall. The pattern of rib fractures is primarily determined by the direction of the forces as well as vulnerability without protection of the shoulder girdle. Whereas frontal impact on the steering column from a motor vehicle crash usually produces upper anterior fractures that may have associated costochondral separations, a lateral impact results in middle and lower lateral rib fractures. Lateral and posterior fractures of the 8th, 9th, and 10th ribs are markers for concomitant intraperitoneal injury, notably the spleen on the left side and the liver on the right. Posterior 11th or 12th rib fractures may be associated with renal injury on the involved side.

Fracture configuration varies from single cortex involvement that may be difficult to identify radiographically to fragmented ribs that may penetrate adjacent intrathoracic structures. Fractures may be transverse or oblique, and the segments may override or be displaced inward, disrupting the adjacent intercostal artery or tearing the pleural and underlying lung.

Penetrating injuries, particularly gunshot wounds, may fragment the rib with a piece driven into the lung as a secondary missile. Ribs may also become disengaged from the sternum where they are attached by cartilaginous bridges or occasionally from the vertebral column from ruptured ligaments. Costochondral separation occurs at the rib-cartilage interface, and chondrosternal separation occurs at the cartilage-sternum juncture. The sternum may also become fractured at any point of contact along its course. Sternal fractures imply a major force to the anterior chest and thus should raise concern for underlying cardiac or great vessel injury.

Clinical suspicion of fractures of the ribs or sternum or cartilaginous separation is usually prompted by severe local tenderness or crepitus with respiration. Pain is more evident on inspiration, so patients tend to hypoventilate with significant rib fractures. An anteroposterior (AP) chest radiograph will usually confirm the diagnosis of rib fractures, but a lateral view is more sensitive for sternal fractures. Occasionally, oblique views of the ribs are necessary to identify isolated rib fractures. With multiple fractures, AP and lateral views of the chest are important to identify the location and extent of the fractures, as well as to exclude secondary pneumothorax or hemothorax or mediastinal hematoma caused by associated great vessel injury. A CT scan, usually obtained because of concern for major thoracic trauma, is much better at characterizing fractures and their associated complications.

The management of patients with rib and sternal fractures is fundamentally directed at pain control. The consequences of inadequate pain control are shallow breathing and poor coughing leading to atelectasis, retained secretions, and ultimately pneumonia. Elderly patients with multiple rib fractures are particularly at risk for this scenario, leading to pneumonia. Patients older than age 65 years with more than three rib fractures or any patient with more than five rib fractures should be hospitalized for pain management and pulmonary surveillance. In most trauma centers, epidural anesthesia is used preemptively in high-risk patients.

Intercostal nerve blocks, however, remain a valuable adjunct for treating patients with rib fracture pain. These nerve blocks should be used liberally in the emergency department for high-risk patients awaiting epidural placement and can be used to supplement intravenous opiates in hospitalized patients with multiple fractures. The technique consists of inserting a needle below the inferior border of the rib and injecting an anesthetic agent into the intercostal space containing the nerve. Typically, injections are required into one or two interspaces above and below the fractures to encompass overlapping innervation. Caution must be used in performing intercostal blocks because the underlying pleura can be violated, producing a pneumothorax and, rarely, an intercostal artery can be injured, producing a hemothorax. Additional benefit can be derived from direct injection into the fracture site. Patients must be encouraged to cough frequently and breathe deeply with an incentive spirometer (IS). An IS is also helpful to gauge patient compliance and optimize pain management.

Flail Chest and Pulmonary Contusion

Flail chest refers to instability of the chest wall caused by multiple segmented rib fractures or cartilage disruptions such that a portion of the bony chest wall loses its continuity from the remaining thoracic cage because of contiguous rib disruptions. A flail chest occurs in the setting of severe trauma, usually after a motor vehicle crash or fall from more than 20 feet. If the crushing blow is directly over the sternum, as with an impact by the steering column, the flail segment is produced by bilateral costochondral separations, and there may be an associated sternal fracture. Because of protective air bag systems in automobiles, however, lateral mid-chest flail segments are more common. In either location, it is evident on physical examination that the floating portion of the chest wall moves in and out with respiration in an opposite or paradoxical manner with respect to the remaining intact chest wall. This abnormality in ventilatory mechanics renders the respiratory effort inefficient and, when compounded by reduced tidal volume because of pain, may produce extensive lung collapse with hypoxia, hypercapnia, ineffective cough, and retention of secretions. Although the mechanical effects of a flail segment may appear impressive, the associated hypoxia is often exacerbated by underlying pulmonary contusion. Consequently, the management beyond pain control of flail chest is largely governed by the magnitude of concomitant pulmonary contusion. Although surgical stabilization of the chest wall for acute flail chest has been suggested in the past, randomized trials have not established an outcome benefit. Occasionally, a patient with persistent chest wall instability caused by nonunion will be a candidate for internal rib fixation with a plate. These patients include those with severe pain and respiratory compromise, typically caused by multiple, severely displaced rib fractures with overriding fragments.

The most common source of pulmonary dysfunction after chest trauma is direct injury to the lung (i.e., pulmonary contusion). Pulmonary contusions produce ventilation/perfusion (V/Q) mismatching, resulting in arterial hypoxemia. Because the force required to produce a lung contusion is severe, this lesion occurs predominantly from high-speed motor vehicle crashes, falls from great heights, or high-velocity missiles. The pathophysiology is complex, with the initial defect largely a reflection of direct mechanical disruption and alveolar collapse with hemorrhage. But a delayed component caused by the inflammatory response to injury is often more significant, with the secondary interstitial and interalveolar edema producing shunting and severe hypoxemia.

The multiphase pathophysiology of pulmonary contusion is mirrored in the clinical findings. Often the contusion is relatively subtle on the initial chest radiograph and the pulmonary symptoms are mild, but typically, the lesion extends and symptoms and signs progress over the ensuing 12 to 48 hours. Typical symptoms include dyspnea and chest pain, and common signs are tachypnea, tachycardia, pulmonary crackles, and variable signs of chest contusion or rib fracture. Hypoxemia, documented by arterial blood gas analysis, is often out of proportion to the extent of opacities on the chest radiographs. Consequently, prompt recognition of pulmonary contusion is critical to avoid sudden unexpected pulmonary failure. Serial physical examination, chest radiographs, and monitoring of oxygen saturation are important in high-risk patients, and endotracheal intubation should be considered early in patients manifesting progressive deterioration. The management of pulmonary contusion is largely supportive, using positive end-expiratory pressure to maintain oxygenation and avoiding excessive airway pressure with lower tidal volumes. Unless complicated by ventilator-associated pneumonia, the physiologic effects of pulmonary contusion usually resolve in 5 to 7 days. On the other hand, in multisystem-injured patients, pulmonary contusion is a risk factor for the development of adult respiratory deficiency syndrome.

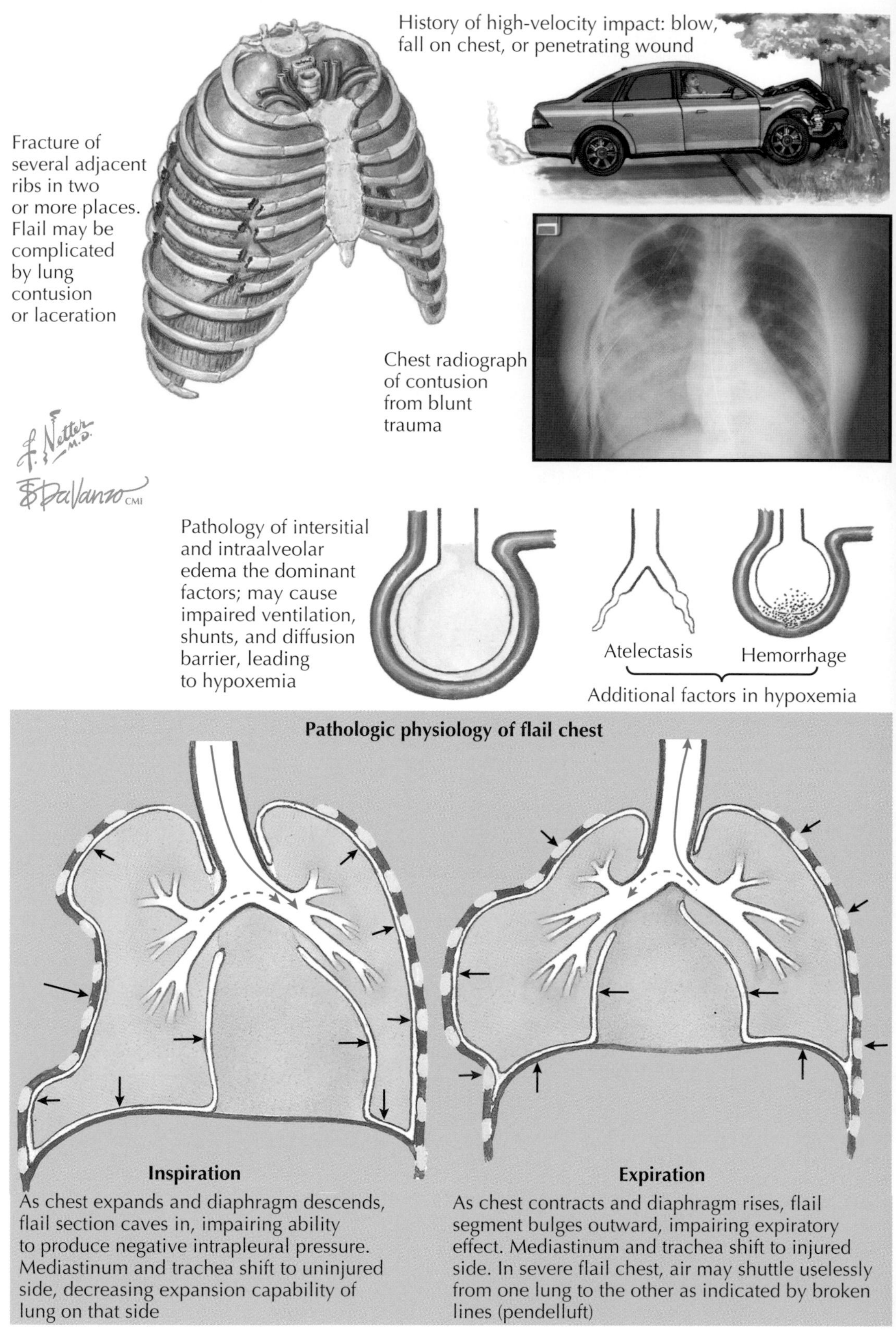

Fracture of several adjacent ribs in two or more places. Flail may be complicated by lung contusion or laceration

History of high-velocity impact: blow, fall on chest, or penetrating wound

Chest radiograph of contusion from blunt trauma

Pathology of intersitial and intraalveolar edema the dominant factors; may cause impaired ventilation, shunts, and diffusion barrier, leading to hypoxemia

Atelectasis Hemorrhage

Additional factors in hypoxemia

Pathologic physiology of flail chest

Inspiration

As chest expands and diaphragm descends, flail section caves in, impairing ability to produce negative intrapleural pressure. Mediastinum and trachea shift to uninjured side, decreasing expansion capability of lung on that side

Expiration

As chest contracts and diaphragm rises, flail segment bulges outward, impairing expiratory effect. Mediastinum and trachea shift to injured side. In severe flail chest, air may shuttle uselessly from one lung to the other as indicated by broken lines (pendelluft)

Tension Pneumothorax

Pathophysiology

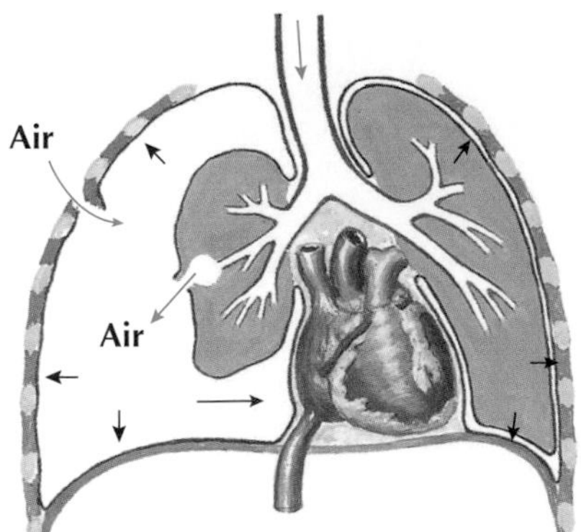

Inspiration

Air enters pleural cavity through lung wound or ruptured bleb (or occasionally via penetrating chest wound) with valvelike opening. Ipsilateral lung collapses, and mediastinum shifts to opposite side, compressing contralateral lung and impairing its ventilating capacity

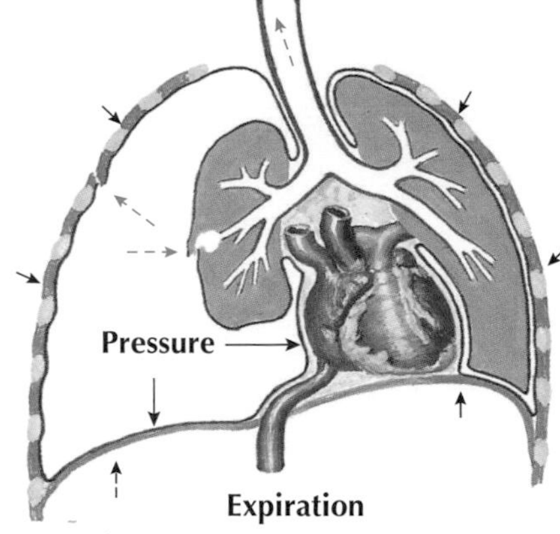

Expiration

Intrapleural pressure rises, closing valvelike opening, preventing escape of pleural air. Pressure is thus progressively increased with each breath. Mediastinal and tracheal shifts are augmented, diaphragm is depressed, and venous return is impaired by increased pressure and vena caval distortion

Clinical manifestations

Respiratory distress
Cyanosis
Tracheal deviation
Chest pain
Hyperresonance

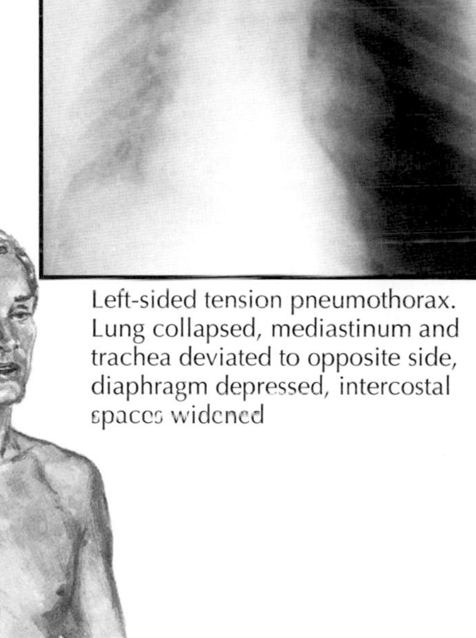

Left-sided tension pneumothorax. Lung collapsed, mediastinum and trachea deviated to opposite side, diaphragm depressed, intercostal spaces widened

Therapeutic maneuvers

Large-bore needle inserted for emergency relief of intrathoracic pressure. Finger cot flutter valve, Heimlich valve, or underwater seal should be attached

Incision in 5th interspace with introduction of thoracostomy tube attached to underwater-seal suction

To underwater seal

Pneumothorax

Pneumothorax is a collection of air within the pleural space; after trauma, pneumothorax is most commonly caused by a rib fracture tearing the visceral pleura of the lung, allowing air to escape during inspiration. Penetrating injuries (e.g., stab wounds, gunshot wounds) also frequently produce a pneumothorax via this mechanism. In these cases of penetrating trauma, 80% of patients will also have blood in the pleural space. Pneumothorax is usually identified on chest radiographs, although it may also be seen during chest or abdominal computed tomography scanning or during ultrasound examination of the abdomen after trauma (focal assessment with sonography for trauma [FAST] examination).

Other causes of traumatic pneumothorax include inadvertant puncture of the lung during central venous access or thoracentesis. The lung can also be ruptured by excessive positive airway pressure during mechanical ventilation, termed *barotrauma*. Spontaneous pneumothorax is usually caused by a ruptured bleb that is often precipitated by coughing. Irrespective of the cause, when the pleural pressure exceeds the normal subatmospheric pressure, the elastic recoil of the lung results in partial collapse. If air continues to flow into the pleural space, the lung collapses entirely and can no longer serve to exchange oxygen (O_2) and carbon dioxide (CO_2). A one-way valve typically occurs on the lung surface, and air is forced into the pleural space with each breath, which progressively increases the intrapleural pressure and may result in escape of air into the subcutaneous tissues, manifesting as diffuse upper torso swelling and palpable crepitus. Ultimately, if the intrapleural pressure continues to increase, a tension pneumothorax develops. This condition may occur rapidly when the patient is ventilated mechanically, increasing the airway pressure. Eventually, the pressure within the pleural cavity can shift the mediastinum and impede blood return to the right heart. Thus, clinical manifestations of tension pneumothorax reflect progressive impairment of pulmonary and myocardial function.

Patients with a tension pneumothorax become dyspneic or hypoxic if ventilated mechanically, with cyanosis and distended neck veins. Hyperresonance and lack of breath sounds on the involved side of the thorax cement the diagnosis without the need for radiographic confirmation. Electrocardiographic changes include (1) rightward shift in the QRS axis, (2) diminution in the QRS amplitude, and (3) inversion of precordial T waves. Tension pneumothorax is a life-threatening

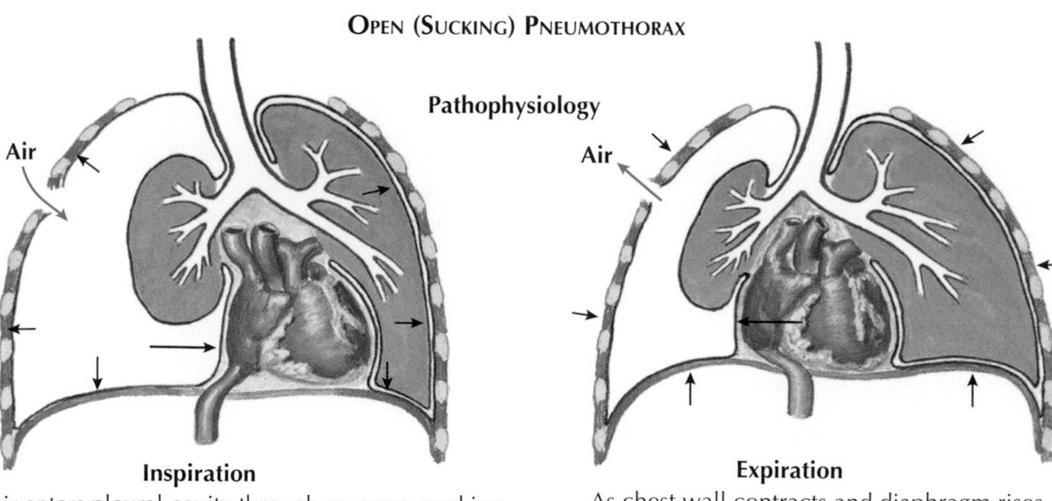

Inspiration
Air enters pleural cavity through an open, sucking chest wound. Negative pleural pressure is lost, permitting collapse of ipsilateral lung and reducing venous return to heart. Mediastinum shifts, compressing opposite lung

Expiration
As chest wall contracts and diaphragm rises, air is expelled from pleural cavity via wound. Mediastinum shifts to affected side, and mediastinal flutter further impairs venous return by distortion of venae cavae

Patient often cyanotic and in severe respiratory distress or in shock. Immediate closure of sucking wound imperative, preferably by petrolatum gauze pad, but if not available, by palm or anything at hand

Chest strapped over packing on top of petrolatum gauze. Thoracostomy tube attached to underwater-seal suction drainage indicated to promote reexpansion of lung

PNEUMOTHORAX *(Continued)*

emergency, and the air must be urgently released from the pleural cavity. If it is clinically suspected in a patient who is unstable, immediate treatment is indicated without any further diagnostic tests. In an intubated patient in the prehospital setting, air can be vented with a large-bore needle via the anterior second intercostal space in the midclavicular line. Subsequent definitive treatment with tube thoracostomy should follow. In the hospital, a tube thoracostomy is usually done via the fifth intercostal space at the anterior axillary line. Under these dire circumstances, the tube should be placed expeditiously using primarily a scalpel and scissors. After a limited chest wall preparation and local anesthesia, a 2-cm incision should be made into the intercostal space and the chest entered directly using heavy scissors. The tube should then be directed into the posterior sulcus to optimize subsequent drainage of blood or other pleural fluid.

Alternatively, air can accumulate within the pleural space because of an external wound that violates the parietal pleural, exposing it to the atmosphere. This form of pneumothorax is usually self-limited because the skin edges and adjacent chest wall soft tissue seal the opening. The notable exception is open chest wounds, in which the chest wall defect is sufficiently large to remain open, permitting air to move freely in both directions. Open pneumothoraces are usually caused by high-energy gunshot wounds (e.g., close-range shotgun wounds) or impalement during motor vehicle crashes. An open pneumothorax is often referred to as a *sucking chest wound* because of the sound made as a relatively large volume of air moves through the defect with respiratory effort. The lung on the involved side collapses upon exposure to atmospheric pressure, rendering it nonfunctional. Additionally, because air passes more easily into the chest on inspiration than it exits during expiration, an element of tension pneumothorax with mediastinal shift occurs. Ultimately, this impedes blood return to the heart, leading to clinical signs of cardiac as well as pulmonary dysfunction.

Prehospital management of an open pneumothorax is a partially occlusive dressing in which one corner of the bandage is free to permit escape of pleural air under pressure. In the hospital, treatment consists of applying a completely occlusive dressing, usually of petroleum gauze, followed by standard tube thoracostomy. Although a slash wound may occasionally be managed definitively in the emergency department, most patients with an open pneumothorax warrant prompt operative care for associated visceral injury as well as chest wall reconstruction. One approach to extension chest wall defects is cephalad transposition of the diaphragm.

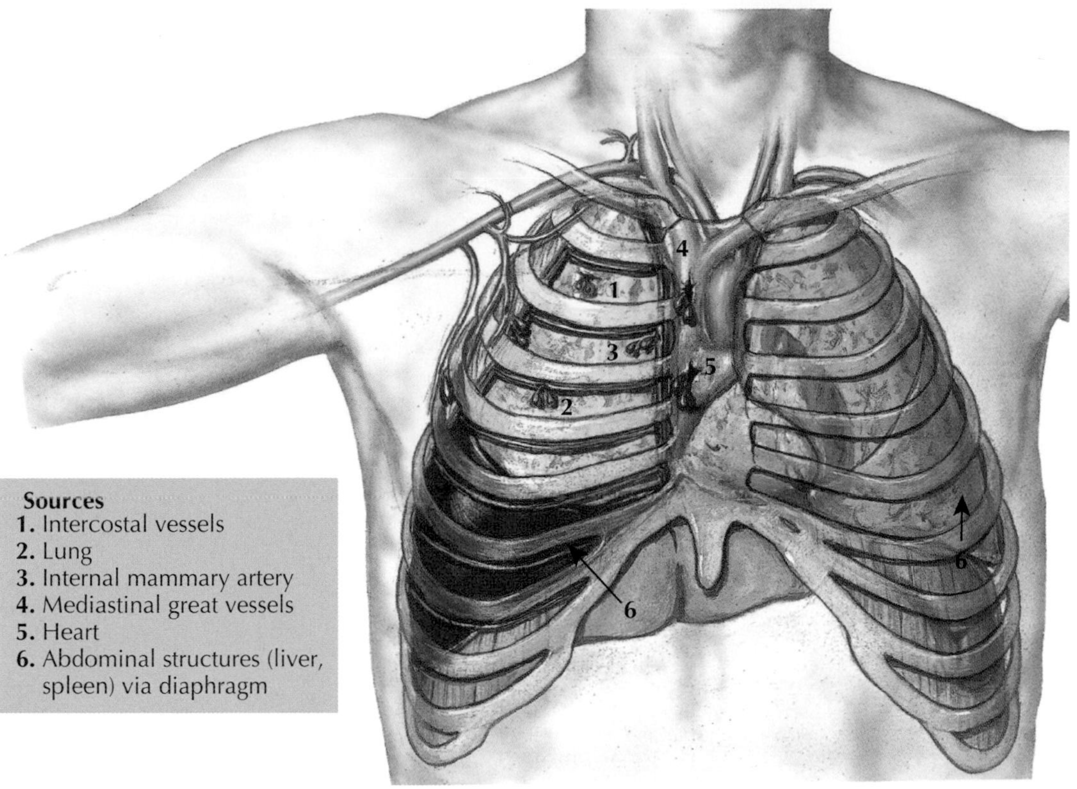

HEMOTHORAX

Hemothorax is bleeding into the pleural cavity; the source of bleeding can be from a variety of structures in the thorax or from the abdomen through a diaphragmatic injury. The most common cause of hemothorax after blunt trauma is the chest wall with disrupted parietal pleural allowing blood loss from torn intercostal vessels to enter the pleural cavity; after penetrating injuries, it is usually from the lung parenchyma. Persistent bleeding into the thorax suggests a systemic source, usually an intercostal or internal mammary artery, but occasionally a named thoracic vein (e.g., azygos, subclavian, or pulmonary) will produce ongoing blood loss. Typically, a hemothorax from a ruptured thoracic aorta, pulmonary artery, or heart is extensive at the time of emergency department arrival. Of note, occasionally, the source of major persistent bleeding in the thorax originates from the liver or spleen via an associated diaphragmatic injury.

The diagnosis of hemothorax is usually established by chest radiography or with the presumptive placement of a chest tube in a patient arriving in hemorrhagic shock. Hemothorax is recognized more frequently with computed tomography (CT) scanning because small collections are seen that are not apparent on chest radiography. Management is dictated by the size of the hemothorax and physiologic condition of the patient. In general, hemothoraxes can be considered minimal if they are smaller than 350 mL, moderate at 350 to 1500 mL, and massive above 1500 mL. Minimal hemothoraxes are usually first identified by CT scanning and can be treated expectantly. Moderate hemothoraxes warrant tube thoracostomy because this evacuates the blood completely; reexpands the lung, which tamponades chest wall bleeding; and permits monitoring of continued blood loss. A chest tube placed for moderate bleeding should be relatively large (e.g., 28 Fr in women and 32 Fr in men).

The tube should be placed after ample chest wall preparation and generous local anesthesia. An incision should be made in the midclavicular line at a relatively superior location on the chest wall (i.e., the fifth intercostal space) to avoid injury to the liver or spleen caused by a high-lying diaphragm. A gloved finger should be inserted into the pleural space to ensure proper positioning, and the tube should be directed into the lung apex with a blunt clamp. After it is in position, −20 cm H_2O is applied to the chest tube to evacuate the pleural cavity quickly. Finally, the tube should be sutured securely to the chest wall to avoid dislodgement during patient transport. Follow-up radiography is essential to ensure good tube placement and complete removal of the hemothorax. The initial management of a massive hemothorax is similar except that a large chest tube (i.e., 36 Fr) should be used. If the follow-up chest radiograph does not show complete blood evacuation, a second large-bore tube should be inserted.

Degrees and management

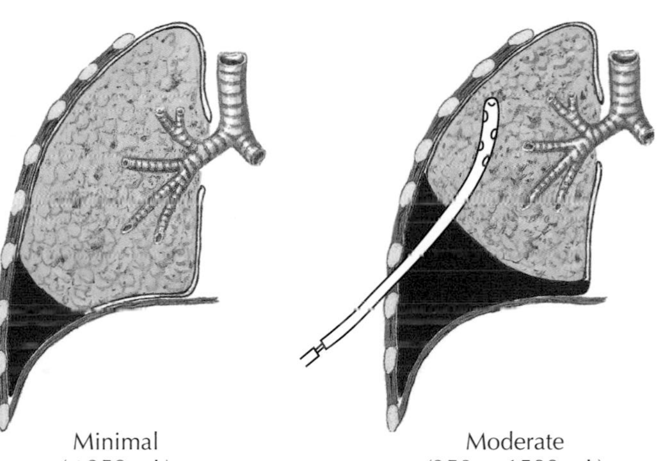

Minimal (≤ 350 mL)
Blood usually resorbs spontaneously with conservative management. Thoracentesis rarely necessary

Moderate (350 to 1500 mL)
Thoracentesis and tube drainage with underwater-seal drainage usually suffices

Massive (>1500 mL)
Two drainage tubes inserted because one may clog, but immediate or early thoracotomymay be necessary to arrest bleeding

The decision for emergent thoracotomy is largely determined by the patient's response to tube thoracostomy in conjunction with evidence of ongoing bleeding. In general, an initial return of more than 1500 mL or the failure to eliminate a hemothorax with two chest tubes, referred to as a *coked hemothorax*, warrants exigent thoracotomy. There is also general agreement that chest tube output greater than 250 mL/h for 3 successful hours requires thoracic exploration, although video-assisted thoracoscopy (VATS) may be reasonable in hemodynamically stable patients. Alternatively, angioembolization may be appropriate if the suspected source of persistent bleeding is an intercostal artery. If a patient fails to resorb a moderate hemothorax after 72 hours or if there is a delayed hemothorax refractory to tube thoracostomy, VATS is a very effective maneuver for definitive removal of the retained hemothorax.

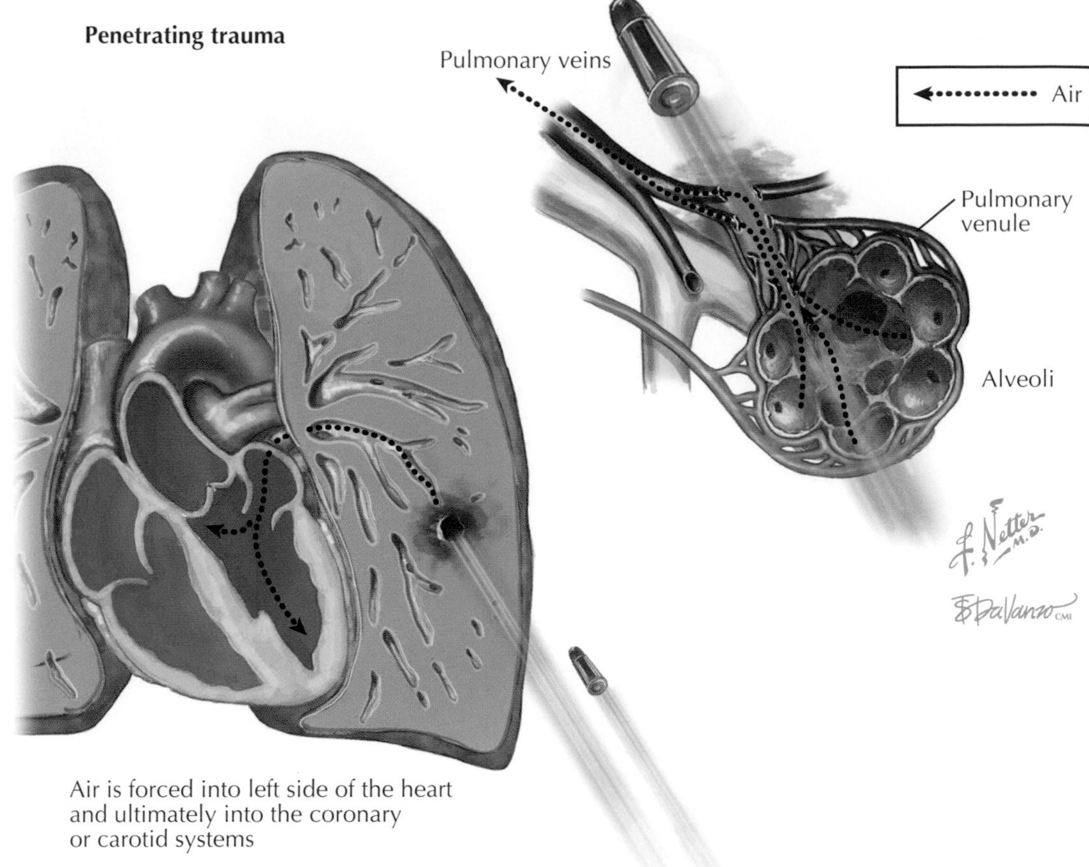

Air is forced into left side of the heart and ultimately into the coronary or carotid systems

Pulmonary Laceration

Rapid deceleration from blunt thoracic trauma may produce shearing forces that lacerate the lung. Other causes include missiles, knives, and fractured ribs that directly lacerate the lung and lung hyperinflation from such causes as blast injuries and diving accidents. Lung lacerations usually manifest as hemopneumothoraxes requiring early tube thoracostomy. A persistent air leak is common but typically seals as the lung becomes fully reexpanded. With more extensive injuries requiring endotracheal intubation and positive-pressure ventilation, however, there is a risk of life-threatening acute bronchovenous air embolism. The typical scenario is a patient who is hypovolemic and requires semi-urgent endotracheal intubation for moderate hypoxemia but develops acute cardiac deterioration. As pressure in the airway is increased, air is forced from disrupted terminal bronchi into an adjacent injured pulmonary vein, which conveys the air bubbles into the left side of the heart and ultimately into the coronary or carotid systems. The hypovolemic patient is more susceptible to air embolism because of decreased pulmonary venous pressure, thus increasing the gradient from the airway. Symptomatic coronary air embolus mandates resuscitative thoracotomy with pulmonary hilar cross-clamping and vigorous internal cardiac massage. Air should be vented from the left ventricle and ascending aorta. Ongoing air leak from the injured lung is usually managed with staple tractotomy (i.e., linear stapling is performed on both sides of the torn lung as an alternative to anatomic resection). Pulmonary tractotomy is particularly useful when required for persistent air leaks from multiple lobes caused by a gunshot wound, avoiding the necessity for emergent pneumonectomy, which is often poorly tolerated because of right ventricular failure.

Cavitation of the lung is a variant of pulmonary laceration that occurs after blunt trauma. The cavitation represents bursting of the lung parenchyma without disruption of the visceral pleural and is likely caused by a combination of increased airway pressure and a shearing stress, which exceed the elasticity of the lung. Bleeding into the lung occurs, causing a hematoma, which appears as a poorly defined density on chest radiography but becomes more defined within the next 2 weeks after injury. Cystic cavitation of the hematoma may then develop. Several terms have been used to describe this entity; perhaps the most widely recognized is *posttraumatic pneumatocele*. The initial chest radiograph typically shows a cavity with air or air and fluid with adjacent radiodensity caused by lung hemorrhage. The vast majority of pneumatoceles resolve uneventfully, but occasionally, a lung resection is required for secondary infection.

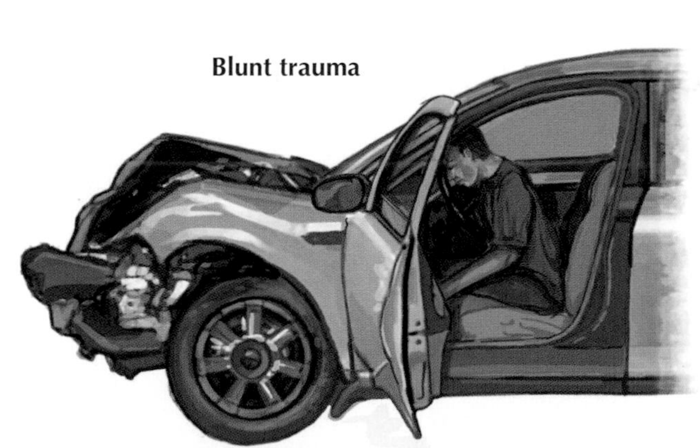

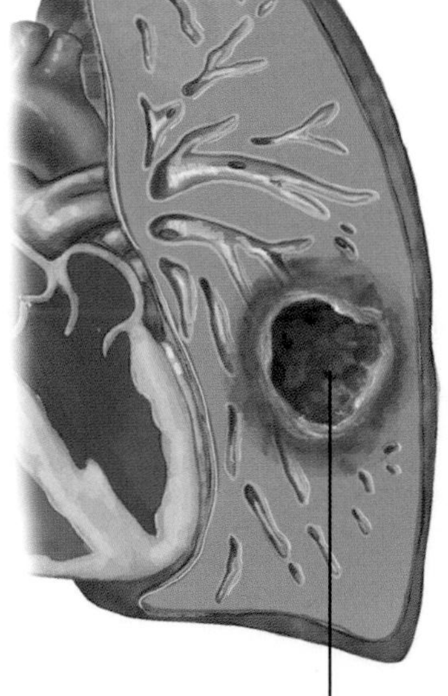

Blunt force trauma leading to pseudocyst formation and cavitation

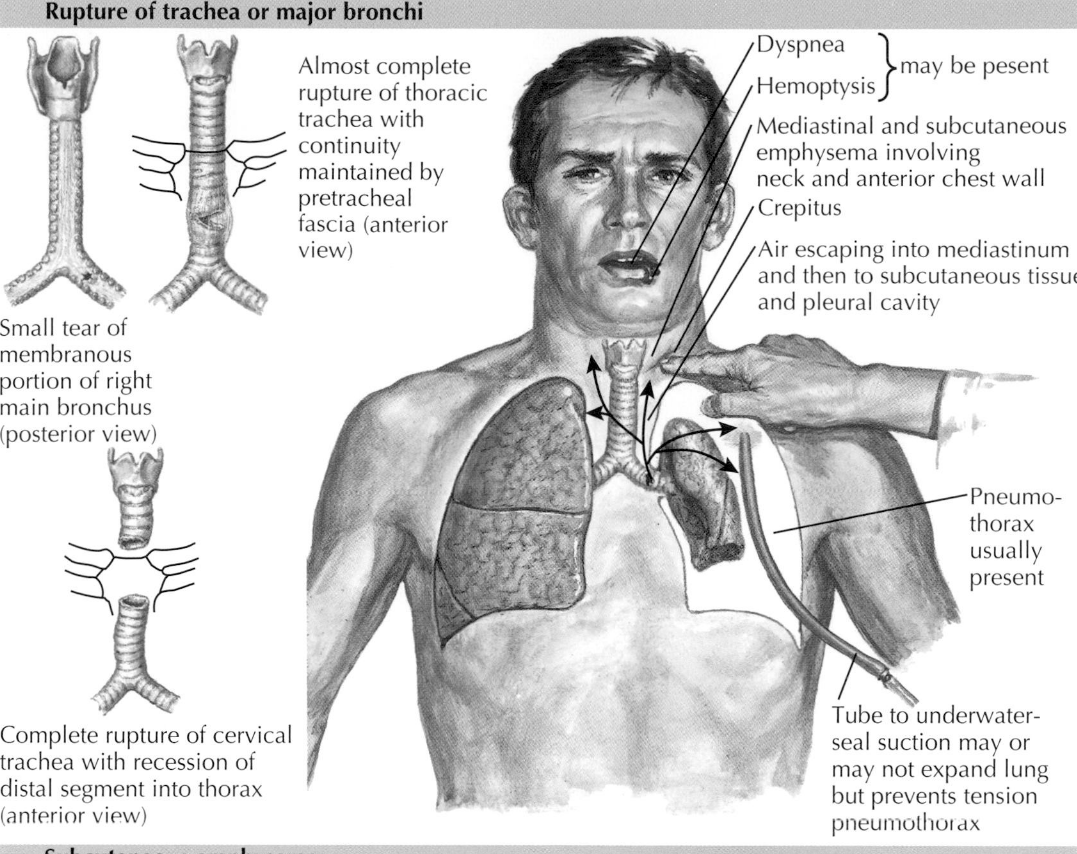
Rupture of trachea or major bronchi
Almost complete rupture of thoracic trachea with continuity maintained by pretracheal fascia (anterior view)
Small tear of membranous portion of right main bronchus (posterior view)
Complete rupture of cervical trachea with recession of distal segment into thorax (anterior view)
Dyspnea
Hemoptysis
may be pesent
Mediastinal and subcutaneous emphysema involving neck and anterior chest wall
Crepitus
Air escaping into mediastinum and then to subcutaneous tissue and pleural cavity
Pneumothorax usually present
Tube to underwater-seal suction may or may not expand lung but prevents tension pneumothorax

Tracheobronchial Rupture

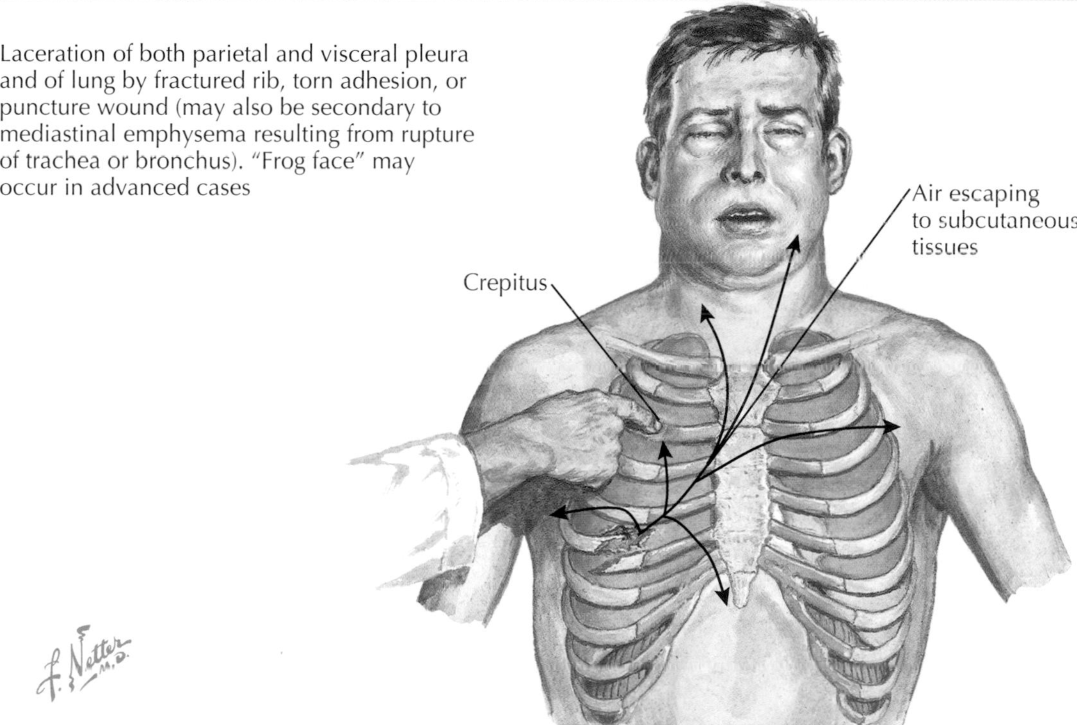
Subcutaneous emphysema
Laceration of both parietal and visceral pleura and of lung by fractured rib, torn adhesion, or puncture wound (may also be secondary to mediastinal emphysema resulting from rupture of trachea or bronchus). "Frog face" may occur in advanced cases
Air escaping to subcutaneous tissues
Crepitus

Rupture of the trachea or major bronchi is usually secondary to a nonpenetrating injury of the thorax resulting from a high-energy frontal impact motor vehicle crash. More than 80% of the ruptures are within 2.5 cm of the carina. The proposed mechanisms for this injury include (1) anteroposterior compression with subsequent widening of the transverse diameter that pulls the lungs apart, producing traction on the trachea at the carina; (2) compression of the trachea and major bronchi between the sternum and vertebral column in a patient with a closed glottis exceeds the elasticity of the membranous portion of the airway; and (3) rapid deceleration injury at a point of relative fixation of the carina produces shear forces. Tracheal lacerations usually occur at the junction of the membranous and cartilaginous trachea. Major bronchial rupture is typically unilateral and is more common on the right side. The severity of blunt trauma required for these tracheobronchial ruptures is usually associated with multisystem injuries of the head, abdomen, and extremities.

The clinical presentation appears in two distinct patterns, depending on whether there is free communication between the airway rupture and the pleural cavity. If there is free communication, a large pneumothorax is present, and despite tube thoracostomy, there is a persistent vigorous air leak and the lung cannot be reexpanded. Dyspnea is prominent because of the loss of functioning lung. If there is no communication with the pleural cavity, the air escaping via the tracheobronchial injuries forms impressive mediastinal and subcutaneous emphysema. On auscultation, Hamman sign may be evident (i.e., a crunching sound synchronized with the heart beat caused by mediastinal emphysema). In both cases, there may be significant hemoptysis as well. Air embolism is also a life-threatening consequence that must be promptly treated by emergency thoracotomy with cross-clamping of the pulmonary hilum on the affected side.

Prompt diagnosis of a tracheobronchial injury is critical, and bronchoscopy is the most accurate means of establishing the diagnosis and determining the need for urgent thoracotomy. If the tear is smaller than one-third the circumference, particularly when confined to the membranous portion, nonoperative management is appropriate if tube thoracostomy results in full expansion of the lung and there is no persistent air leak. Immediate repair of tracheobronchial injury is indicated. If more extensive injuries are not treated surgically, the bronchus heals by granulation, resulting in airway obstruction, atelectasis, and ultimately pulmonary infection. The details of thoracotomy and tracheobronchial repair are addressed elsewhere.

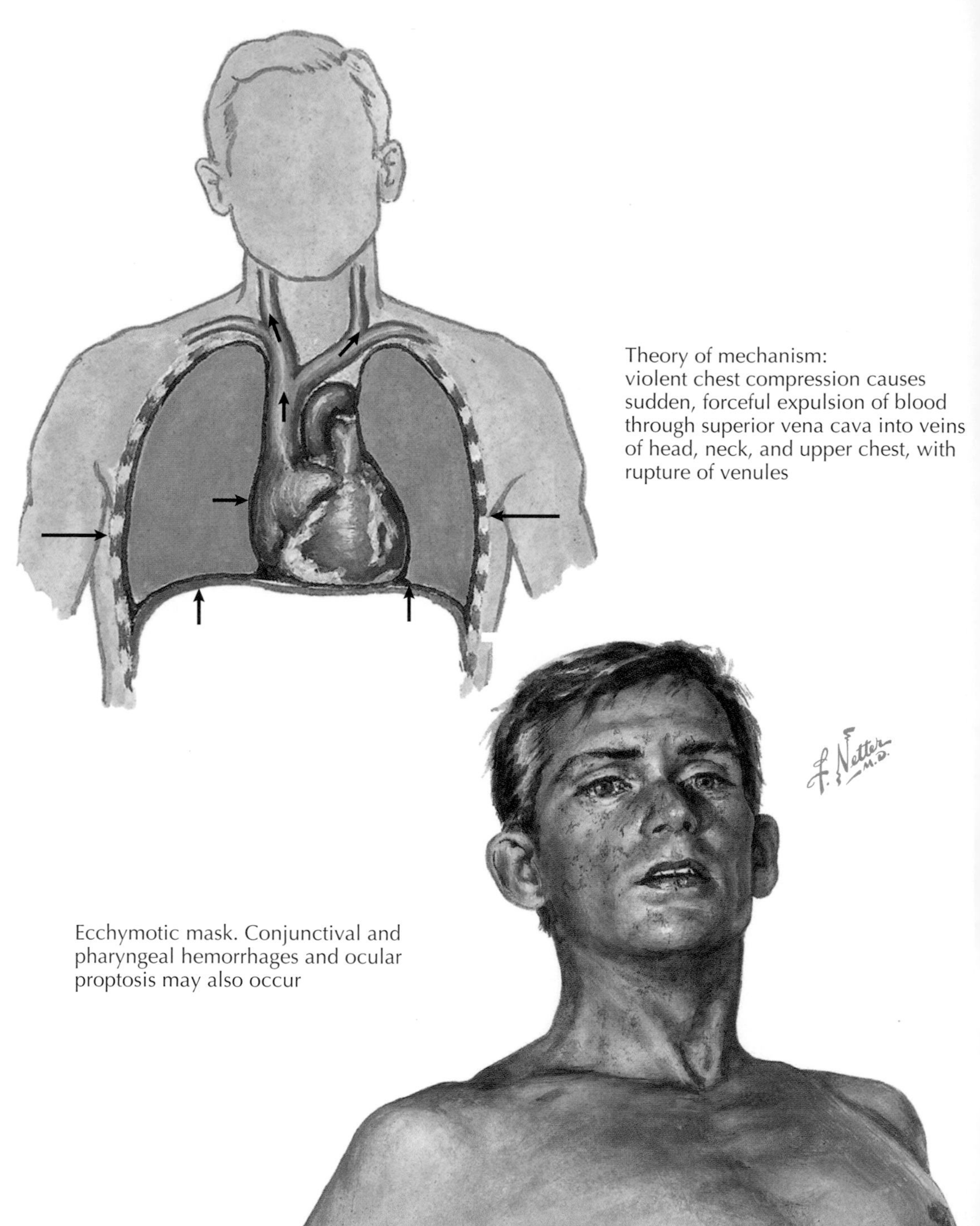

Theory of mechanism:
violent chest compression causes sudden, forceful expulsion of blood through superior vena cava into veins of head, neck, and upper chest, with rupture of venules
Ecchymotic mask. Conjunctival and pharyngeal hemorrhages and ocular proptosis may also occur

Traumatic Asphyxia

Traumatic asphyxia is a condition resulting from a severe sustained compressive force on the thorax. Ollivier is credited for the first autopsy description of a syndrome of cranial cyanosis, subconjunctival hemorrhage, and vascular engorgement of the head, which was observed in a person crushed to death by a panicked crowd in Paris. The syndrome was termed *masque ecchymotique*. This form of crush injury occurs in association with vehicle crashes, industrial accidents, uncontrolled crowd conditions and trampling, and any type of trauma characterized by a heavy object falling onto the chest, such as an individual working under a car that slips off the jack or a child pinned under a garage door. The syndrome is also seen with side wall collapse at an excavation site or may be seen with deep-sea divers from underwater explosions. The pathogenesis of traumatic asphyxia is attributed to a sudden compression of the heart between the anterior chest wall and vertebral column, generating a pressure surge in the right side of the heart that is decompressed by reverse blood flow into the superior vena cava and its major branches, which lack valves. The subsequent massive capillary engorgement and rupture throughout the head, neck, shoulders, and upper thorax results in stagnation of blood, which desaturates and results in the characteristic bluish discoloration of the skin. There may be intense swelling of the face and neck, as well as petechial hemorrhages of the skin of the face and conjunctiva. It is postulated that deep inspiration and transient airway obstruction exaggerate the superior vena cava hypertension. These events may occur as a reflex in the victim's anticipating the impact.

Traumatic asphyxia can be fatal, but the prognosis for those surviving to reach the hospital is good. It is critical to examine the patient for other potentially lethal associated injuries, such as pulmonary or cardiac contusion and injury to the spinal cord, brain, liver, or spleen. Rib fractures and visual changes are common. Approximately one-third of patients with traumatic asphyxia experience loss of consciousness or other neurologic findings. Interestingly, despite the alarming appearance, many patients have relatively few complaints. Occasionally, there is permanent loss of vision caused by retinal hemorrhage or transient vision changes from retinal edema. There is no specific treatment for traumatic asphyxia, but elevation of the head of the bed 30 degrees to minimize venous hypertension and supplemental oxygen to hasten absorption of air within the mediastinum are recommended. Ninety percent of patients who survive the first few hours after injury will recover, but survival rates vary depending on the prevalence and degree of associated injuries.

Diaphragmatic Injuries

The diaphragm is an arched muscle dividing the thorax and the abdomen and is interrupted by three major openings: the vena cava, esophagus, and aorta. The diaphragm is the main respiratory muscle, with inspiratory and expiratory functions. Diaphragmatic injuries may be caused by penetrating or blunt trauma; the mechanism influences the site and extent of injury. With gunshot wounds, the chances of right versus left side are roughly equal, and the wound from most handguns is small, usually smaller than 1 cm. In contrast, stab wounds involve the left side of the diaphragm more commonly because the right-handed assailant holds the weapon in the right hand and confronts the victim at close range. Knife wounds are also typically small, usually smaller than 2 cm. The left hemidiaphragm is injured two to three times more frequently than the right after blunt trauma. The difference is attributed to the protective effect of the liver that distributes a sudden increase in intraabdominal pressure more evenly across the right hemidiaphragm. Blunt diaphragm injuries are considerably larger than penetrating wounds and are usually larger than 5 cm in length and in many cases exceed 10 cm. During quiet respiration, the normal intraperitoneal pressures ranges from +2 to +10 cm H_2O, and the corresponding intrapleural pressure fluctuates from −5 to −10 cm; thus, a gradient exists varying from +7 to +20 cm H_2O. But with maximal inspiration, this gradient may exceed 100 cm H_2O. Consequently, there is high risk for abdominal viscera to herniate into the thorax. The risk is higher on the left side because the liver provides a barrier on the right, and herniation increases with the extent of the diaphragmatic defect. Ambroise Paré, in 1579, is credited with describing the first case of visceral herniation in a French artillery captain who sustained a gunshot wound to the left chest 8 months before a lethal colonic obstruction.

The diagnosis of diaphragmatic injury depends on the size of the diaphragm lesion. With larger defects, the presenting symptoms are usually pulmonary because of the volume of the pleural cavity occupied by the displaced intraabdominal viscera. On the other side, incarcerated stomach, colon, or small bowel may produce peritoneal signs. The most common finding on chest radiography is an apparent elevated hemidiaphragm and, when the left diaphragm is torn, a nasogastric tube is frequently seen in the thorax. Smaller defects produced by penetrating wounds, however, are frequently asymptomatic initially, and the chest radiographs are often normal. The most definitive diagnostic adjunct is laparoscopy or thoracoscopy, but multidetector computed tomography scanning and magnetic resonance imaging are becoming more accurate.

The operative management of patients with diaphragm injuries is largely dictated by the risk of associated abdominal injuries. In the acute phase, more than 50% of blunt trauma and more than 75% of penetrating trauma involve abdominal viscera. Thus, the operative approach is via the abdomen early after injury. In hemodynamically stable patients, laparoscopy may be used to evaluate the abdominal organs and, in the event of no hollow visceral injury, may suffice for definitive repair of the diaphragm. In the chronic phase with delayed visceral herniation, a thoracotomy is generally recommended to free the lung from adhesions and provide access to the diaphragm injury.

Diaphragmatic Injuries

Thoracoabdominal penetrating wounds

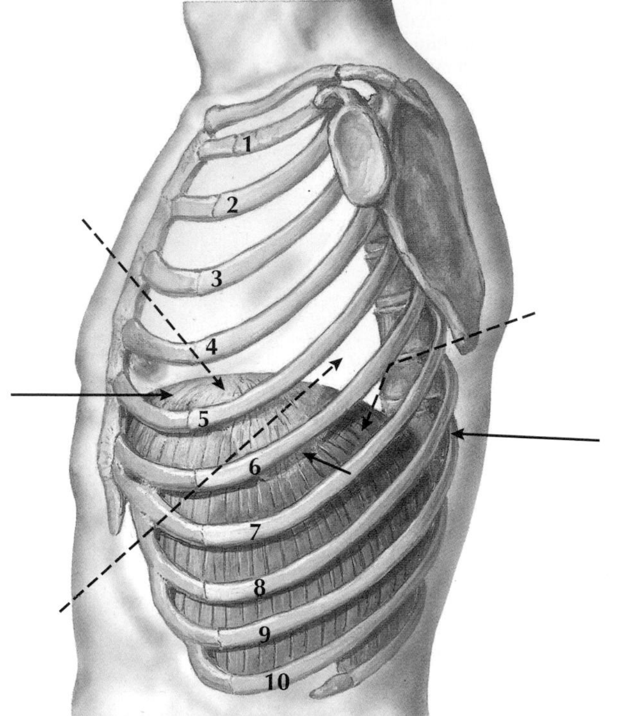

Diaphragmatic injury is suspected in any penetrating thoracic wound (gunshot, stab, or accidental perforation) at or below 4th intercostal space anteriorly, 6th interspace laterally, or 8th interspace posteriorly, although sharply oblique wounds or missiles deflected by ribs may also penetrate the diaphragm

Rupture of diaphragm

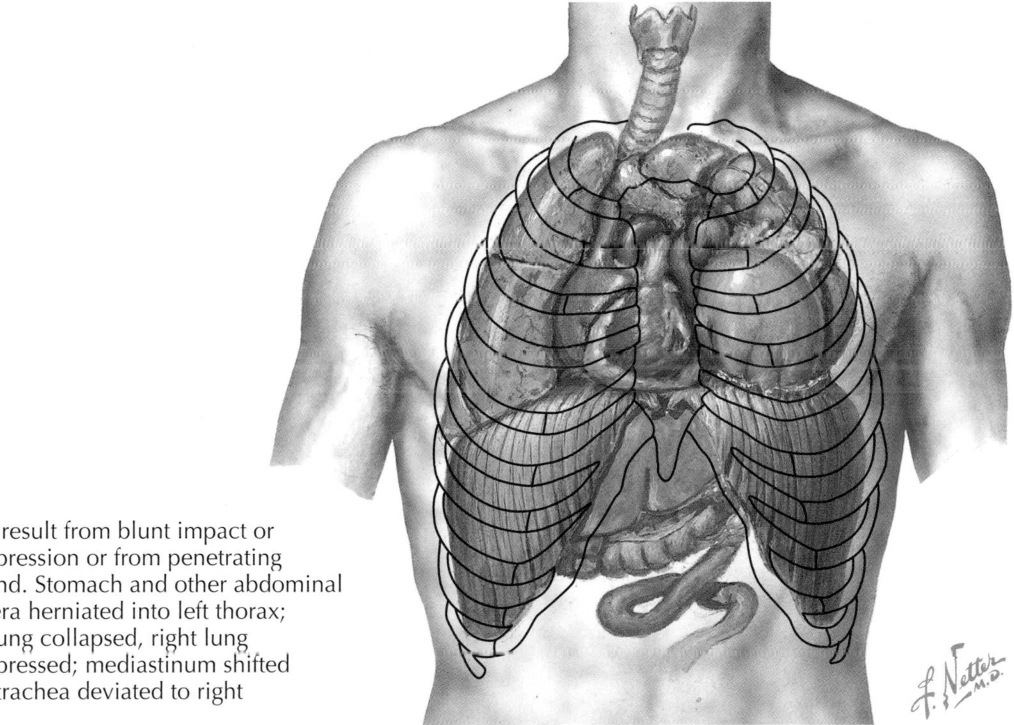

May result from blunt impact or compression or from penetrating wound. Stomach and other abdominal viscera herniated into left thorax; left lung collapsed, right lung compressed; mediastinum shifted and trachea deviated to right

RESPIRATORY DISTRESS SYNDROME

Respiratory distress syndrome (RDS) presents within 4 four hours of birth, usually in prematurely born infants. It used to be called *hyaline membrane disease* because hyaline membranes line the terminal airways of infants who are surfactant deficient. The hyaline membranes are formed by coagulation of plasma proteins that have leaked onto the lung surface through damaged capillaries and epithelial cells. The term *hyaline membrane disease* should only be used if there is histologic confirmation; therefore, the term *RDS* is now widely used.

EPIDEMIOLOGY

The risk of RDS is inversely proportional to the gestational age. It is more common in white than black infants and nearly twice as common in boys as girls. There is also the likelihood of familial recurrence in a subsequent prematurely born infant. Surfactant protein B deficiency results in lethal respiratory failure; it has an autosomal recessive inheritance. Delivery by cesarean section in the absence of previous labor also poses a risk, particularly if the birth occurs before 37 weeks of gestation. Precipitous delivery after maternal hemorrhage, asphyxia, or maternal diabetes is associated with a greater likelihood of RDS, and a second-born twin is at greater risk than the firstborn. Maternal conditions that are thought to have a sparing effect on the development of the disease are conditions associated with chronic intrauterine distress that lead to growth-retarded infants. There is no consensus on the impact of prolonged rupture of the membranes; an apparent sparing effect may be explained by greater use of antenatal corticosteroids. Antenatal administration of dexamethasone or betamethasone to women in preterm labor significantly reduces the risk of RDS and neonatal death.

PATHOLOGY

On gross examination, the lungs are found to be liver-like, and they generally sink in water or formalin. Under the microscope, much of the lung appears solid because of the tight apposition of most of the alveolar walls. Scattered throughout are dilated airspaces, respiratory bronchioles, alveolar ducts, and a few alveoli, some of whose walls are lined with pink-staining "hyaline" material containing fibrin and cellular debris. The capillaries are strikingly congested, and pulmonary edema and lymphatic distension may be present.

Epithelial necrosis in the terminal bronchioles at sites underlying the hyaline membranes suggests that a reaction to injury has taken place. Hypersecretion of tracheobronchial mucus is evident, and reparative proliferation of type II cells is seen in infants who die on the second or third day of life.

These changes are now rarely seen because prematurely born infants have usually received prophylactic surfactant (see below).

PATHOGENESIS

RDS is caused by immaturity of the lung with respect to surfactant synthesis or suppression of synthesis adequate to meet postnatal demands as, for example, by asphyxia. Surfactant deficiency results in failure of stabilization of small airways at end-expiration with consequent reduction of functional residual capacity. Each new inspiration requires the application of sufficient transpulmonary pressure to reinflate atelectatic airspaces. A high respiratory frequency and large applied pressures have to be used to maintain effective ventilation. Uneven distribution of inspired air and perfusion of nonventilated alveoli result in poor gas exchange characterized chiefly by hypoxemia. The infant grunts in an attempt to prolong end-inspiration, a pattern of breathing that can be shown experimentally to improve alveolar ventilation.

Pulmonary vascular resistance is increased by vasoconstriction caused by hypoxia, with a resulting increase in right-to-left shunts through the persistent fetal vascular pathways, ductus arteriosus, and foramen ovale. The hypoxemia is further aggravated because as much as 80% of the cardiac output may be shunted past airless lungs.

Wasted ventilation and ineffective perfusion initiate a train of events that accounts for most of the findings in RDS. Reduced oxygenation of the myocardium impairs cardiac output and perfusion of the kidneys, whose ability to maintain acid-base homeostasis is compromised. Poor perfusion of peripheral tissues contributes to lactic acidemia and a profound metabolic acidosis.

DIAGNOSIS

The onset of symptoms is within minutes of birth and always within hours of birth. Tachypnea, grunting, and

HYALINE MEMBRANE DISEASE

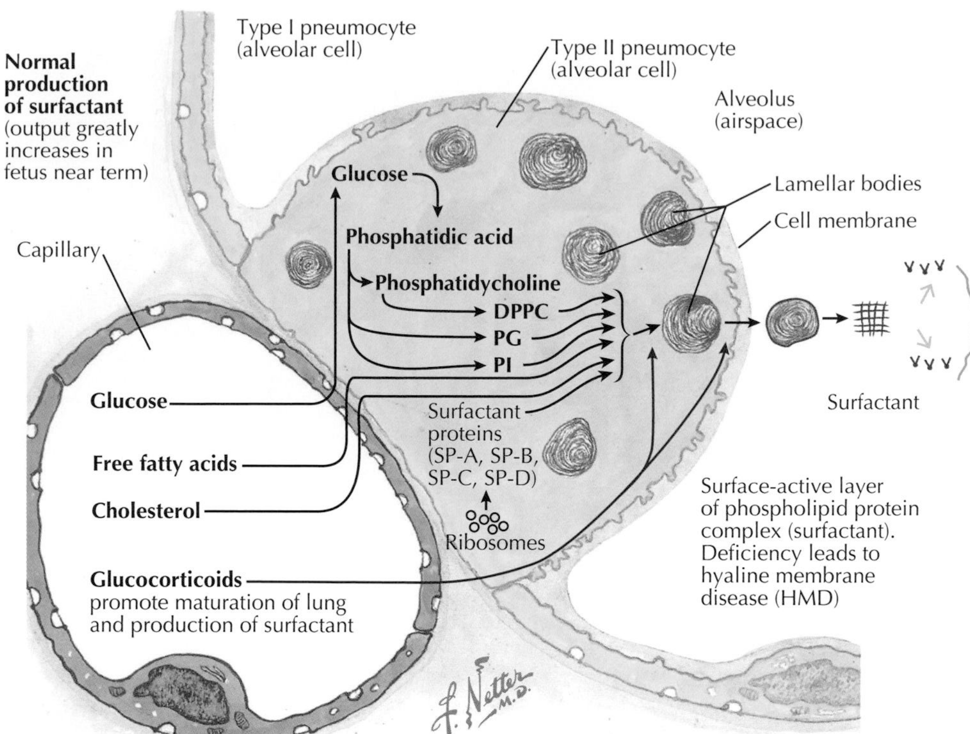

DPPC = dipalmitoylphosphatidylcholine; PG = phosphatidylglycerol; PI = phosphatidylinositol

Pathology of hyaline membrane disease

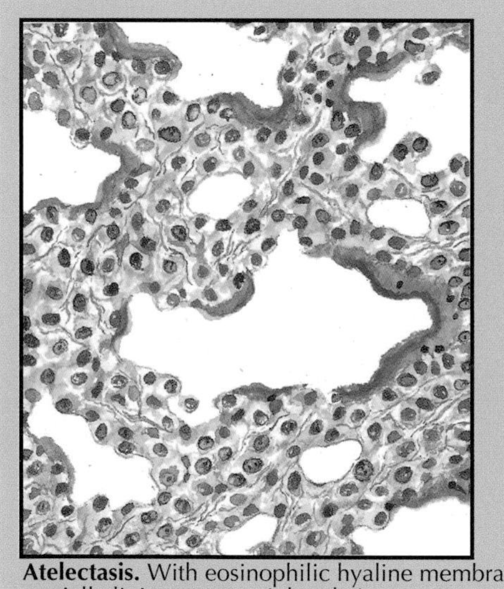

Atelectasis. With eosinophilic hyaline membrane partially lining most peripheral air space

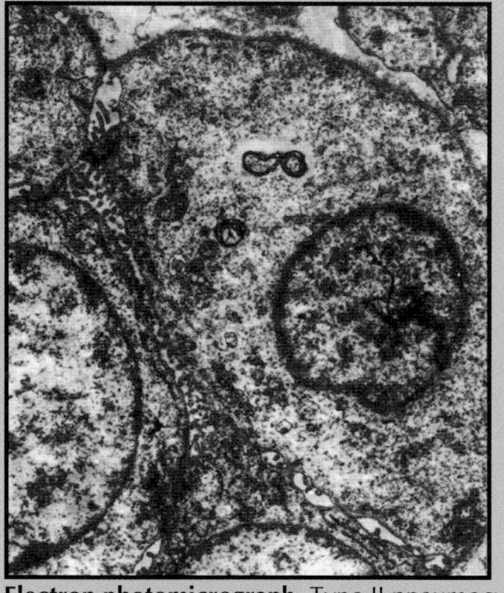

Electron photomicrograph. Type II pneumocyte practically devoid of lamellar bodies

Respiratory Distress Syndrome *(Continued)*

indrawing of the sternum, intercostal spaces, and lower ribs during inspiration are characteristic. Increasing cyanosis is a notable feature of the disease. In the absence of treatment with exogenous surfactant, the dyspnea worsens over the next 36 to 48 hours, and the infant becomes edematous. Surfactant synthesis then commences, and this is associated with spontaneous diuresis.

RADIOLOGIC FINDINGS

The earliest radiographic finding is a fine miliary mottling of the lungs. The air-filled tracheobronchial tree stands out in relief against the opacified lung roots, which often obscure the cardiothymic silhouette. The appearance may change depending on the lung volume at which the radiograph is taken. A good cry can aerate both lungs, and a deep inspiratory effort may produce a radiographic picture suggesting minimal disease. The miliary reticulogranularity of the lung parenchyma is usually present within minutes of birth.

During the course of the disease, chest radiographs may show a number of changes, including pulmonary interstitial emphysema, pneumomediastinum, and pneumothorax. In some infants, recovery is slow, with infants remaining ventilator and oxygen dependent for weeks and even months.

TREATMENT

Exogenous surfactant therapy is usually given. In many centers, this is administered within the first few minutes after birth (prophylactic surfactant). Both synthetic and natural surfactants have been used. Meta-analyses of the results of randomized trials have demonstrated that prophylactic surfactant reduces mortality and pneumothoraces. The results of other trials have demonstrated that it is better to give surfactant prophylactically rather than selectively (i.e., when RDS has developed) and early rather than late.

Of primary importance is the need to correct any blood gas abnormalities. Some babies may only require supplementary oxygen to keep arterial oxygen tensions at 50 to 70 mm Hg. Others, however, have an associated respiratory acidosis and need more respiratory support. Some centers prefer to use continuous positive airway pressure delivered by nasal cannulae, but others intubate and ventilate. Numerous forms of mechanical ventilation are available, including positive-pressure ventilation, patient-triggered ventilation, high-frequency jet ventilation, and high-frequency oscillation. Randomized trials have been undertaken, but to date, the form of respiratory support with the least chronic respiratory morbidity has not been identified.

COMPLICATIONS OF RESPIRATORY THERAPY

Infants may develop pulmonary interstitial emphysema and pneumothorax during the course of ventilatory therapy, although these complications are less common in infants who have received surfactant therapy. Infants who survive the first week or so of illness may become respirator and oxygen dependent. Typically, their lungs undergo a series of changes that are characterized by air trapping, atelectasis, fibrosis, cyst formation, and basilar emphysema. This condition was described by Northway and Rosan in 1967 and called *bronchopulmonary dysplasia* (BPD). Nowadays, infants who remain oxygen dependent for more than 28 days after birth are described as having BPD. The course is chronic, sometimes lasting months or years. Complete recovery is possible, but death from intercurrent illness is a continuing threat. At autopsy, the lungs are found to be heavy, hypercellular, and fibrotic, with squamous metaplasia of even the small airways. Because the cilia are gone, it is not surprising that secretions pool; either atelectasis or lobular emphysema is common. BPD has a multifactorial cause and may occur in very prematurely born infants exposed to high inspired oxygen concentrations and high airway pressures. Increasingly, however, it is now appreciated that BPD can occur in infants who initially had minimal or even no respiratory distress. Antenatal infection and inflammation contribute to the development of BPD, and there appears to be a genetic predisposition. Affected infants may experience chronic respiratory morbidity with lung function abnormalities and exercise intolerance even as adolescents.

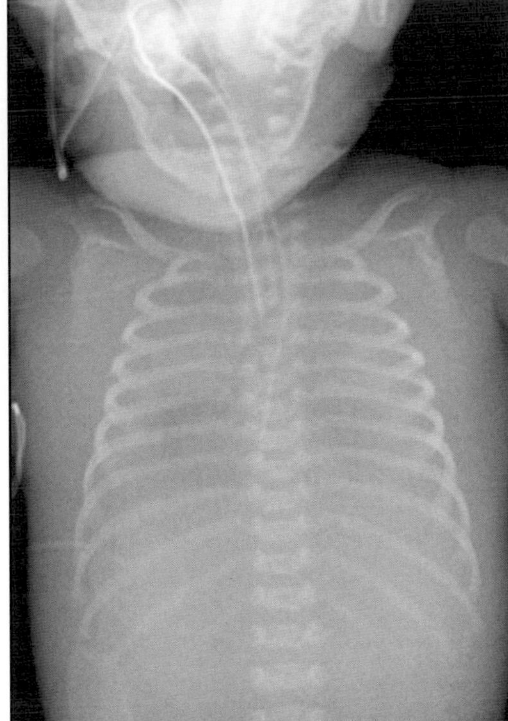

Respiratory distress syndrome. Radiographic findings include symmetric, reticulogranular changes throughout both lungs. The bronchial tree can often be visualized against the opacified lung

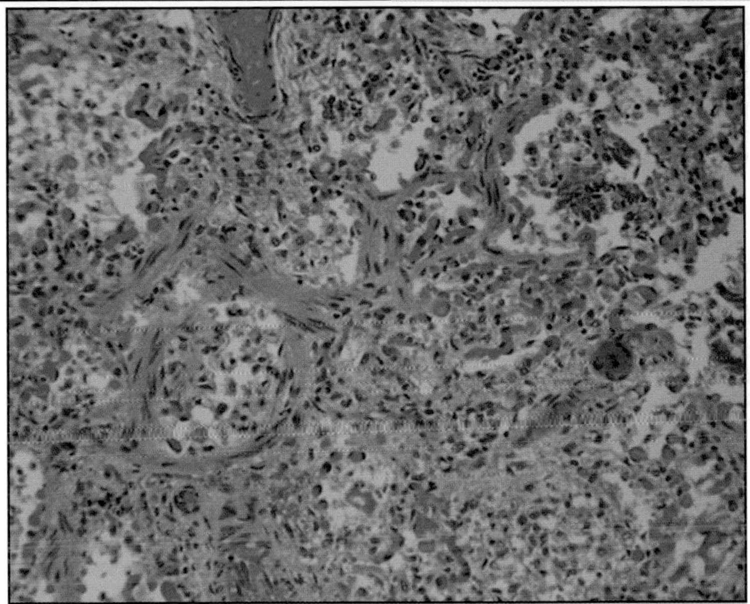

Bronchopulmonary dysplasia. The lung parenchyma shows markedly thickened alveolar septa with fibrosis and some muscle fibers. Hypertensive vascular disease and small patches of hyperinflated, emphysematous parenchyma trapped in between fibrotic areas also present in other sections

PROGNOSIS

When antenatal corticosteroids and prophylactic surfactant are used, the overall mortality rate from RDS has been reduced to between 5% and 10%.

ACUTE LUNG INJURY

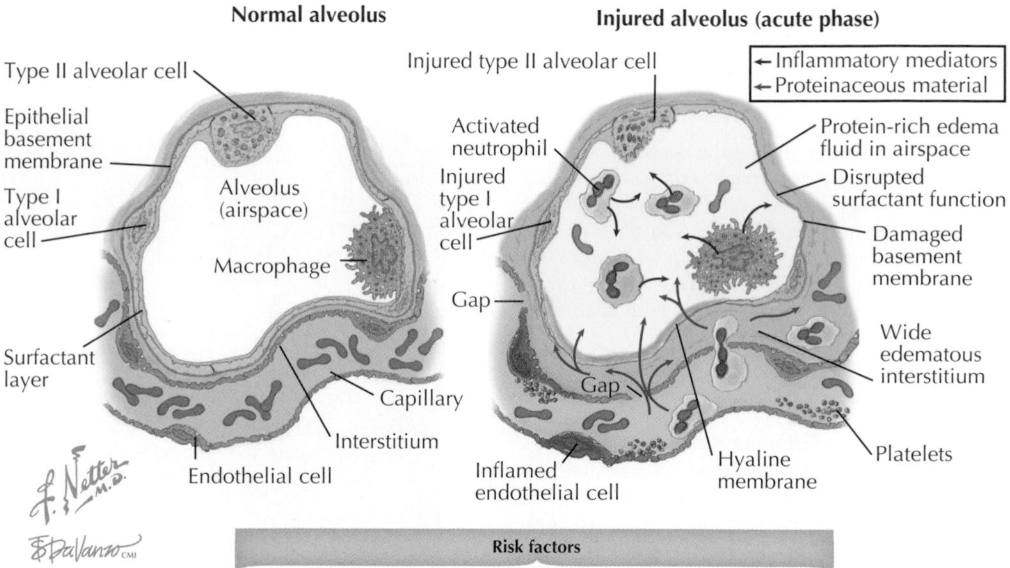

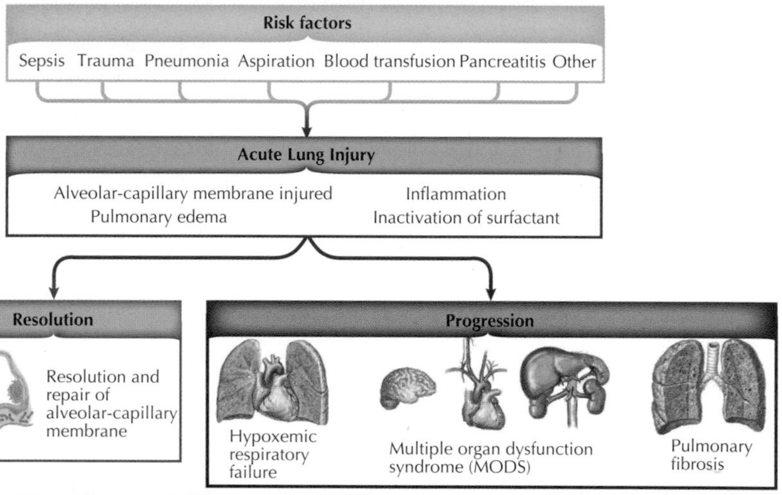

The syndrome now referred to as acute lung injury (ALI) is a condition defined by noncardiogenic pulmonary edema, originally described almost 50 years ago as Da Nang lung and subsequently as acute or adult respiratory distress syndrome (ARDS). The commonly used definition of ALI includes four elements: acute onset of symptoms, bilateral alveolar infiltrates on chest radiography, a PaO_2 (partial pressure of oxygen)/FIO_2 (fraction of inspired oxygen) ratio below 300 (<200 defines the more severe subset of the patients as ARDS), and no evidence of left atrial hypertension. Histologically, the syndrome is identified by the classic finding of diffuse alveolar damage, but few patients undergo lung biopsy during the course of their clinical illness.

EPIDEMIOLOGY

More than 200,000 patients are diagnosed with ALI each year in the United States alone. That number is projected to increase over time as the prevalence of risk factors that lead to ALI increases. The most common risk factors for the development of ALI are sepsis, trauma, pneumonia, aspiration of gastric contents, pancreatitis, and blood transfusion. The incidence of ALI or ARDS, the mortality rate, and the pathogenesis vary with the underlying risk factor. Other conditions that impact the incidence, pathogenesis, and mortality rate of ALI or ARDS include alcohol use, diabetes, acute kidney injury, obesity, age, gender, ethnicity, and genetics. Although the primary manifestation of ALI is hypoxemic respiratory failure, the syndrome is not necessarily limited to the lungs. Many patients develop multiple organ dysfunction syndrome, which further contributes to morbidity and mortality.

PATHOGENESIS

The hallmark of ALI is increased alveolar permeability caused by a failure of the alveolar-capillary membrane. The initial insult may be either direct (e.g., aspiration) or indirect (e.g., sepsis, nonpulmonary trauma), with the common end point being the initiation of an inflammatory cascade with the release of inflammatory mediators and activation of both the endothelium and circulating neutrophils. The subsequent damage to the alveolar-capillary membrane results in an influx of proteinaceous material into the alveolar space that impedes oxygen transport and decreases compliance. The ability of the injured alveolar epithelium to reabsorb alveolar fluid is rapidly overwhelmed, leading to further fluid accumulation. The influx of edema fluid and the injury to the alveolar epithelium (specifically type II cells) also impact surfactant function, which increases lung surface tension, allowing for further alveolar collapse and decreased lung compliance. In some patients, the inflammatory response is self-limited, and the alveolar-capillary membrane is able to be repaired. In other patients, the inflammation persists, and fibrotic lung injury ensues.

TREATMENT

Despite years of investigation, no pharmacologic intervention has improved the morbidity or mortality rate for patients with ALI. This is likely related to the heterogeneity of the patient population with the syndrome. Although no drugs impact mortality in patients with ALI, there have been significant advances in the management of these patients that have contributed to a decrease in mortality. The cornerstone of therapy for patients with ALI is low tidal volume ventilation with sufficient positive end-expiratory pressure (PEEP). A landmark trial published by the National Institutes of Health ARDS Clinical Trials Network showed that the mortality rate could be decreased from 40% to 31% using a tidal volume of 6 mL/kg predicted body weight and a plateau pressure limit of 30 cm H_2O. The mechanism responsible for this improvement is, at least in part, a modulation of the inflammatory cascade. Nosocomial infection is a significant cause of morbidity and mortality in patients with ALI, so attention to daily, routine care is critical to management. Elevation of the head of the bed to more than 40 degrees is associated with a decreased incidence of ventilator pneumonia, a common cause of death in patients with ALI.

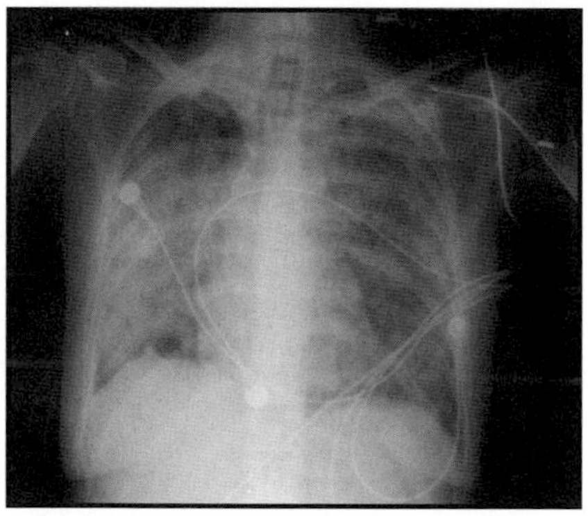

OUTCOMES

When the syndrome was originally described, the mortality rate was approximately 60%. More recently, the mortality rate is closer to 30% to 40%. With an apparent decrease in mortality, there has been a renewed focus on patients who survive ALI. The primary impairment of these patients was originally thought to be loss of pulmonary function, but it is now clear that neuromuscular and neuropsychiatric impairment are actually far greater issues.

AP portable chest radiograph of a patient with ARDS showing bilateral airspace disease

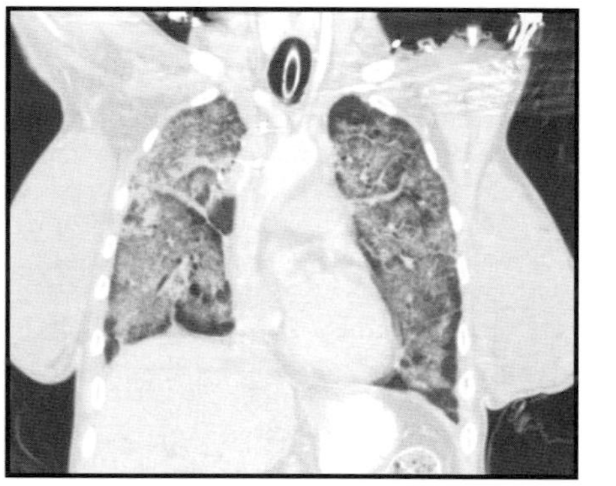

Coronal CT image of same patient illustrating bilateral, diffuse, heterogeneous alveolar filling

IDIOPATHIC INTERSTITIAL PNEUMONIAS

The idiopathic interstitial pneumonias (IIPs) are a subset of the acute and chronic lung disorders collectively referred to as interstitial lung diseases (ILDs) or diffuse parenchymal lung diseases. In 2002, the American Thoracic Society/European Respiratory Society consensus classification separated the IIPs into seven clinical-radiologic-pathologic entities: idiopathic pulmonary fibrosis (IPF), idiopathic nonspecific interstitial pneumonia (NSIP), respiratory bronchiolitis–associated ILD/desquamative interstitial pneumonia (RB-ILD/DIP), cryptogenic organizing pneumonia (COP), acute interstitial pneumonia (AIP), and lymphoid interstitial pneumonia (LIP). The various subgroups of the IIPs are often clinically indistinguishable (with the exception of COP and AIP).

IDIOPATHIC PULMONARY FIBROSIS

IPF is a specific form of chronic fibrosing interstitial pneumonia limited to the lung and associated with the histologic appearance of usual interstitial pneumonia (UIP) on surgical lung biopsy. IPF mainly affects people older than 50 years of age. The incidence of IPF is estimated at 6.8 cases per 100,000, and the prevalence is estimated to be 14.0 per 100,000. Cigarette smoking has been identified as a risk factor for developing IPF.

The clinical manifestations of IPF include dyspnea on exertion, nonproductive cough, and inspiratory crackles on physical examination. Digital clubbing and signs of cor pulmonale may be present in advanced disease.

The chest radiographs typically reveal diffuse bibasilar reticular opacities. However, the chest radiograph lacks diagnostic specificity. High-resolution computed tomography (HRCT) scanning is more sensitive and specific for the diagnosis of IPF. The characteristic HRCT features of IPF include patchy, predominantly basilar, subpleural reticular opacities; traction bronchiectasis and bronchiolectasis; and subpleural honeycombing. The presence of extensive ground-glass opacities, nodules, upper lobe or mid-zone predominance of findings, and significant hilar or mediastinal lymphadenopathy should question the radiographic diagnosis of IPF.

Pulmonary function tests often reveal restrictive impairment (decreased static lung volumes), reduced diffusing capacity for carbon monoxide (DL_{CO}), and arterial hypoxemia exaggerated or elicited by exercise.

The histologic appearance of the UIP pattern is essential to confirm this diagnosis. UIP is characterized by a heterogeneous, predominantly subpleural distribution of involvement (often distinguishable even on low-power magnification). There is temporal heterogeneity, with areas of end-stage fibrosis and "honeycombing" (thickened collagenous septa surrounding airspaces lined by bronchial epithelium) abutting areas of active proliferation of fibroblasts and myofibroblasts (termed *fibroblastic foci*). There is generally minimal interstitial inflammation, and if this is present in significant amounts, the histopathologic diagnosis should be reconsidered.

IPF patients have a distinctly poor prognosis with only a 20% to 30% survival at 5 years after the time of diagnosis. Acute deterioration in IPF—"acute exacerbations" with an abrupt and unexpected worsening of the underlying lung disease in the absence of any identifiable cause—may occur and portends a poor prognosis (mortality rate, 20%-86%). Lung transplantation is the only measure shown to prolong survival.

No specific drug treatment recommendations can be made. Treatment of patients with IPF with corticosteroids alone or with cytotoxic agents is of unproven benefit and causes substantial morbidity. *N*-acetylcysteine, pirfenidone, or bosentan show promise, but there is insufficient evidence to recommend their general use. Improved management of acute exacerbations may improve survival in patients with IPF. Pulmonary rehabilitation and oxygen therapy are useful adjuncts in treatment. In addition, where available, lung transplant should be recommended to qualified patients.

NONSPECIFIC INTERSTITIAL PNEUMONIA

NSIP is a histopathologic pattern commonly found in the context of another disorder, such as a connective tissue disease, chronic hypersensitivity pneumonitis, or drug-induced ILD. Idiopathic NSIP is a distinct clinical entity that occurs mostly in middle-aged women who have never smoked. It has been suggested that

Histologic and clinical classification of idiopathic interstitial pneumonias

Histologic patterns	Clinical-radiologic-pathologic diagnosis
Usual interstitial pneumonia	Idiopathic pulmonary fibrosis/crytogenic fibrosing alveolitis
Nonspecific interstitial pneumonia	Nonspecific interstitial pneumonia
Organizing pneumonia	Cryptogenic organizing pneumonia
Diffuse alveolar damage	Acute interstitial pneumonia
Respiratory bronchiolitis	Respiratory bronchiolitis interstitial lung disease
Desquamative interstitial pneumonia	Desquamative interstitial pneumonia
Lymphoid interstitial pneumonia	Lymphoid interstitial pneumonia

Idiopathic pulmonary fibrosis

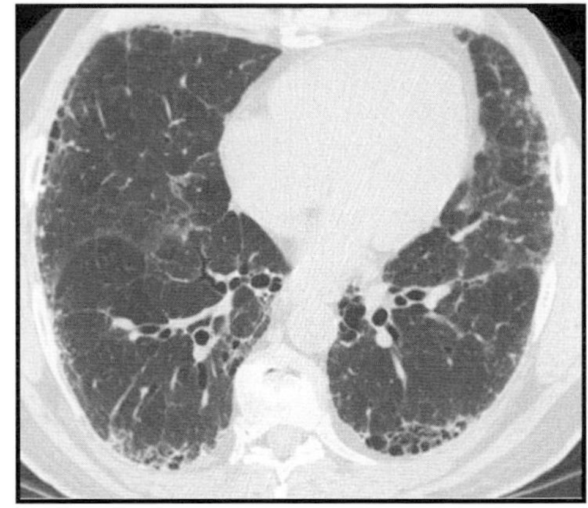

HRCT scan showing patchy, predominantly basilar, subpleural reticular opacities and subpleural honeycombing

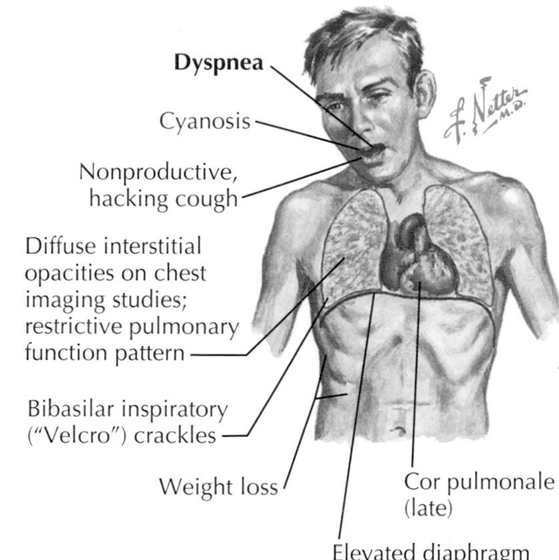

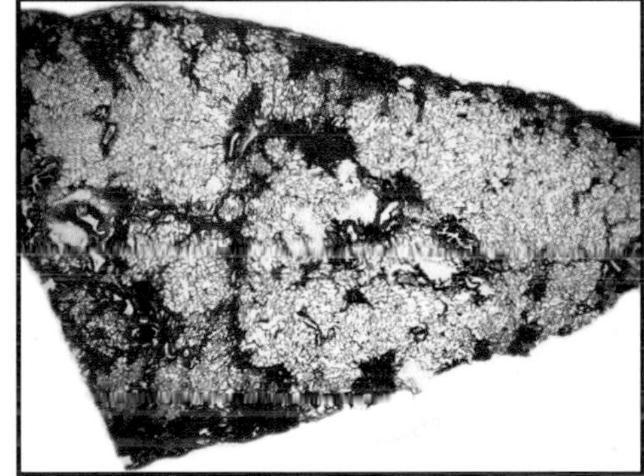

A low-power microscopic view that shows patchy fibrosis with remodeling of the lung architecture and a predominantly subpleural distribution

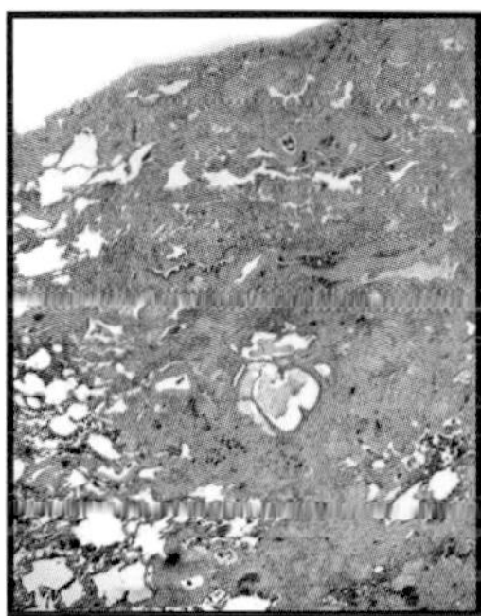

Patchy, subpleural fibrosis consists of dense collagenous scarring with remodeling of the lung architecture and small cystic changes

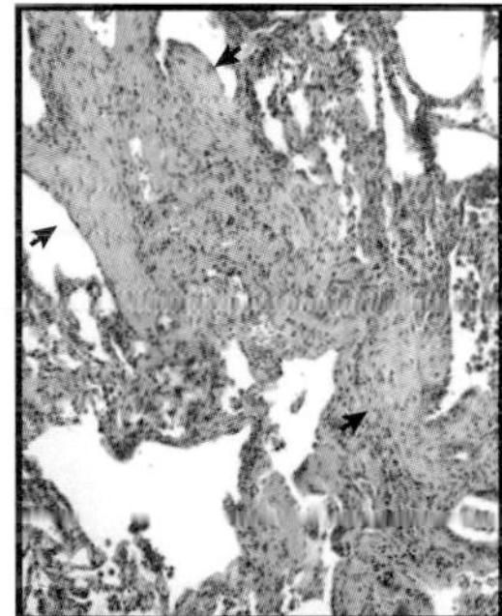

The dense collagenous fibrosis is juxtaposed with multiple fibroblastic foci (*arrows*) of loose organizing connective tissue

IDIOPATHIC INTERSTITIAL PNEUMONIAS *(Continued)*

idiopathic NSIP may be the lung manifestation of "undifferentiated connective tissue disease."

Dyspnea and cough are the most common symptoms. Serologic abnormalities (i.e., positive antinuclear antibodies or rheumatoid factor) are common. A restrictive pattern of pulmonary function abnormality is common.

Chest radiographic findings show primarily lower-zone reticular or hazy opacities. HRCT shows bilateral symmetric ground-glass opacities or bilateral airspace consolidation. A reticular pattern with traction bronchiectasis and volume loss is also common. Honeycombing is uncommon and when present should suggest another diagnosis.

Surgical lung biopsy is required to confirm the diagnosis of NSIP. The main histologic feature of NSIP is the homogeneous appearance of either inflammation or fibrosis. The lung injury pattern is characterized by varying degrees of inflammation and fibrosis ("fibrotic NSIP"). There is less temporal and spatial heterogeneity than in UIP and little honeycombing.

Patients with NSIP have a good prognosis, with most showing improvement after treatment with corticosteroids (often with a cytotoxic agent such as azathioprine). The 5-year mortality rate is estimated at 10% to 20%.

Nonspecific interstitial pneumonia

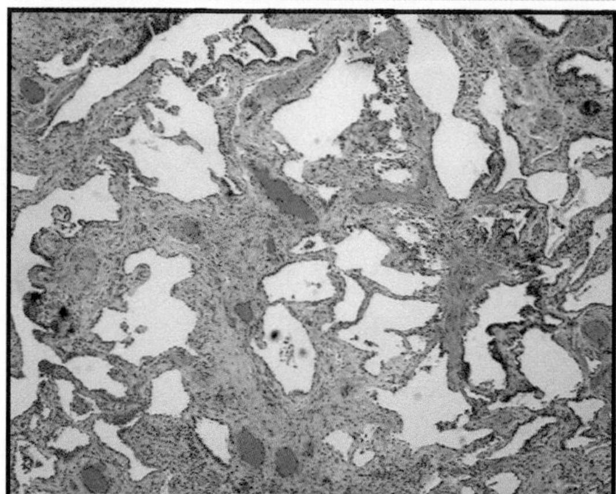

The fibrotic NSIP pattern is present showing the alveolar walls to be uniformly thickened by dense fibrosis. The architecture of the lung is relatively preserved, and the dense fibrosis is approximately of the same age. Fibroblastic foci are absent. Fibrotic NSIP can be difficult to reliably distinguish from UIP

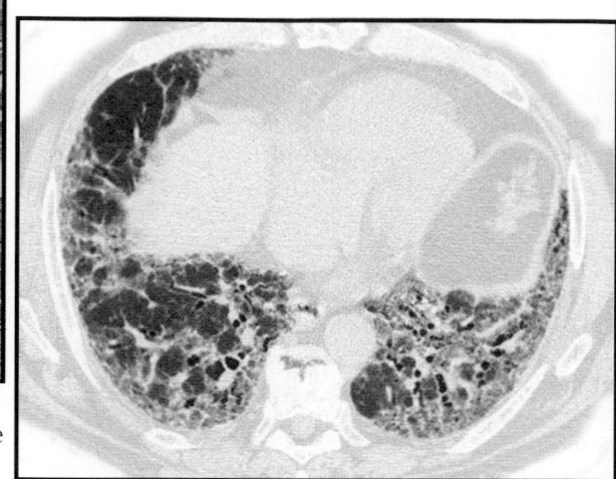

HRCT shows bilateral symmetric ground-glass opacities with traction bronchiectasis and volume loss. Honeycombing is absent

Respiratory bronchiolitis-associated ILD

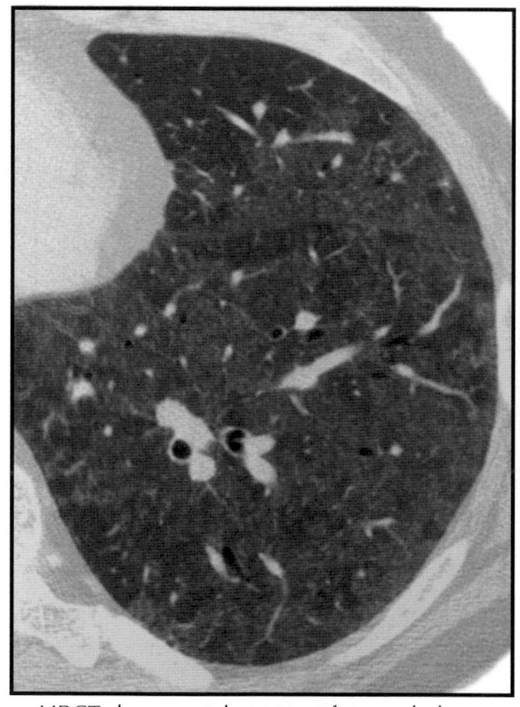

HRCT shows patchy areas of ground-glass opacities and a few poorly defined nodular opacities

Lymphoid interstitial pneumonitis

There is a diffuse lymphoid infiltrate with several reactive follicles that extend through the pulmonary interstitium. A mixture of lymphocytes and plasma cells is present in the interstitium

RESPIRATORY BRONCHIOLITIS–ASSOCIATED INTERSTITIAL LUNG DISEASES

RB-ILD is a clinical syndrome found in young adults (30-40 years old). Most are current or former cigarette smokers with a history of more than 30 pack-years of smoking. The clinical presentation is with cough and breathlessness on exertion, and crackles are found on chest examination.

Routine laboratory studies are not helpful. A mixed obstructive-restrictive pattern is found on lung function testing, and arterial hypoxemia is common.

The chest radiograph shows diffuse, fine reticular or nodular interstitial opacities, usually with normal-appearing lung volumes. HRCT scanning often reveals centrilobular nodules, ground-glass opacity, thickening of central and peripheral airways with associated centrilobular emphysema, and air trapping.

Pathologic criteria for the diagnosis of RB-ILD include the accumulation of pigmented alveolar macrophages within the lumina of respiratory bronchioles and alveolar ducts accompanied by chronic inflammation of the respiratory bronchiolar walls and both bronchiolar and peribronchiolar alveolar fibrosis causing architectural distortion. These features, at low magnification, are commonly patchy and confined to the peribronchiolar region.

Prolonged survival is common in patients with RB-ILD. However, symptomatic and physiologic improvement occurs in only a minority of patients (28% and 11% of cases, respectively). Neither smoking cessation nor immunosuppressive therapy is regularly associated with clinically significant benefit.

LYMPHOID INTERSTITIAL PNEUMONITIS

LIP is common in children but uncommon in adults. LIP is frequently associated with infection (HIV, Epstein-Barr virus, and human T-cell leukemia virus type 1), a serum protein abnormality (variable immunodeficiency and dysproteinemia), or autoimmune disorders (Sjögren syndrome, rheumatoid arthritis, systemic lupus erythematosus, polymyositis). LIP may occur before or after the diagnosis of the underlying process. LIP is part of a spectrum of pulmonary lymphoid proliferations that includes follicular bronchiolitis, nodular lymphoid hyperplasia, and low-grade malignant lymphoma. In fact, idiopathic LIP is rare, and many experts question if this entity should be a part of the IIPs.

The insidious onset of cough and dyspnea are the most common presenting symptoms of LIP. Weight loss, fevers, arthralgias, and pleuritic chest pain are other common findings. Physical examination may reveal crackles on chest examination.

Pulmonary function testing shows reduced lung volumes and diffusing capacity with preserved airflow. Marked hypoxemia may occur. Bronchoalveolar lavage may reveal increased numbers of lymphocytes.

IDIOPATHIC INTERSTITIAL PNEUMONIAS *(Continued)*

Desquamative interstitial pneumonia

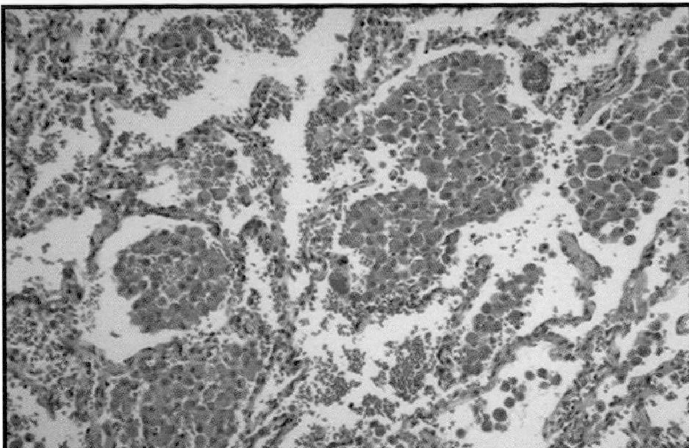

The lung is diffusely involved with prominent accumulation of alveolar macrophages. There is minimal fibrosis, and the lung architecture is well preserved. The alveolar macrophages contain finely granular brown pigment

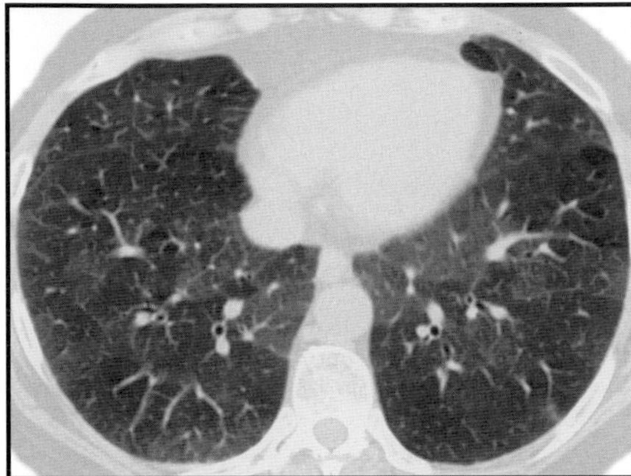

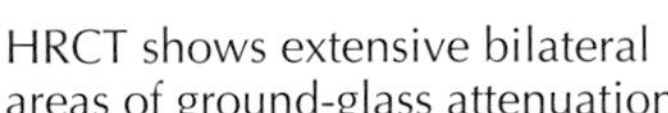

HRCT shows extensive bilateral areas of ground-glass attenuation

Acute interstitial pneumonia

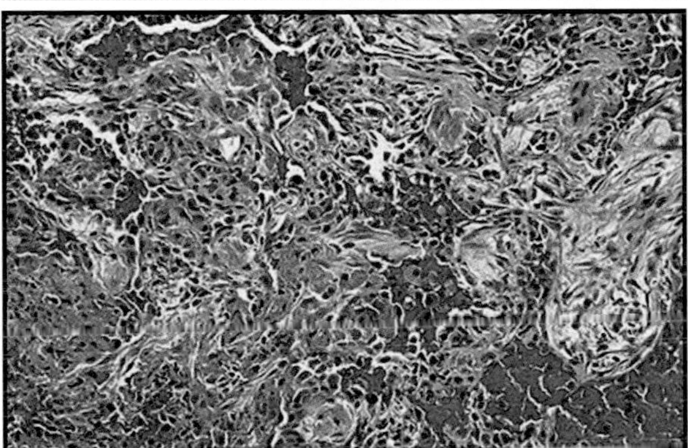

The interstitium is diffusely thickened by uniform, organizing fibrosis. The organizing fibrosis is located within the alveolar septal interstitium and within the airspace

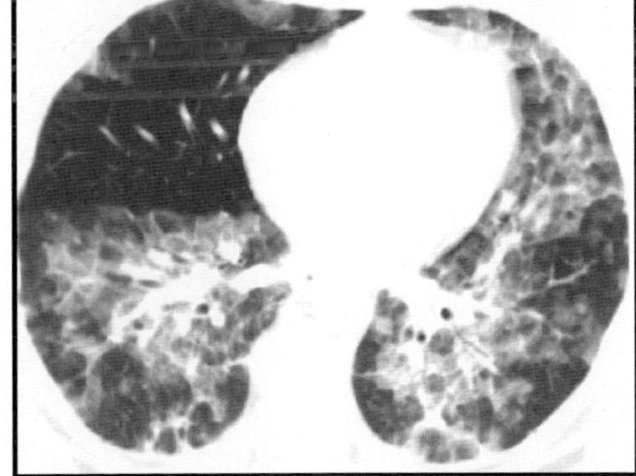

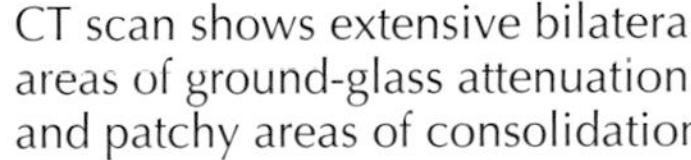

CT scan shows extensive bilateral areas of ground-glass attenuation and patchy areas of consolidation

LIP has a varied and nonspecific radiographic appearance. HRCT scanning is characterized by the presence of ground-glass attenuation, poorly defined centrilobular nodules, and thickening of the interstitium along the lymphatic vessels. Thin-walled cystic lesions have been described. Lymph node enlargement is more common.

The natural history and prognosis of LIP are poorly understood and highly variable. Corticosteroid therapy alone or in combination with other agents has been used to treat symptomatic patients with LIP, although its efficacy has not been established in a controlled trial.

ACUTE INTERSTITIAL PNEUMONIA

AIP is an uncommon fulminant form of lung injury that presents acutely (days to weeks from onset of symptoms). The clinicopathologic term is synonymous with the histopathologic pattern of idiopathic diffuse alveolar damage (DAD). Most patients have been previously healthy before the onset of the illness. There is no gender predilection.

A high index of suspicion is required to make this diagnosis. The onset is usually abrupt, although a prodromal illness lasting usually 7 to 14 days before presentation is common. Fever, cough, and shortness of breath are common clinical signs and symptoms. Tachypnea is present, and chest examination reveals crackles on auscultation. Routine laboratory studies are nonspecific and generally not helpful. Most patients have moderate to severe hypoxemia and develop respiratory failure.

The chest radiograph shows diffuse, bilateral, airspace opacities. CT scans show bilateral, patchy, symmetric areas of ground-glass opacities or occasionally airspace consolidation. A predominantly subpleural distribution may be seen.

Surgical lung biopsy is required to confirm the diagnosis, and the histologic presence of organizing DAD is usually present. The mortality rate is high, with the majority of patients dying within 6 months of presentation. If the patient recovers, substantial improvement in lung function and radiographic clearing may be seen. It is not clear whether corticosteroid therapy is effective in AIP. Mechanical ventilation is often required. The main treatment is supportive care.

DESQUAMATIVE INTERSTITIAL PNEUMONIA

DIP is a rare process that affects cigarette smokers in their fourth or fifth decades of life. Many cases previously called DIP are actually cases of RB-ILD. Clear evidence of cigarette smoke exposure is not always present in patients with DIP.

Most patients present with dyspnea. Lung function testing shows a restrictive pattern with reduced DL_{CO} and hypoxemia on arterial blood gas analysis.

The chest radiographs may be normal in up to 20% of cases. HRCT commonly shows bilateral symmetric areas of ground-glass opacification involving mainly the lower lung zones. Reticular opacities can be seen on CT in approximately 50% of patients.

The dominant histologic feature is intraalveolar macrophage accumulation. At low magnification, the process typically seems to affect the lung diffusely and appears uniform from field to field. There is often interstitial fibrosis present. Prussian blue staining for iron may reveal a finely granular hemosiderin pigment. Alveolar pneumocyte proliferation may be prominent along the thickened alveolar septa, but fibroblastic foci do not occur. Several histopathologic findings appear more often in patients with DIP compared with RB—extent of interstitial fibrosis, presence of lymphoid follicles, and eosinophilic infiltration.

Smoking cessation results in clinical improvement. The 5- and 10-year survival rates are 95% and 70%, respectively. Corticosteroid therapy appears to be associated with modest clinical benefit but usually not with resolution of disease. Progressive disease with eventual death may occur in subjects with DIP, especially with continued cigarette smoking.

Cryptogenic Organizing Pneumonia

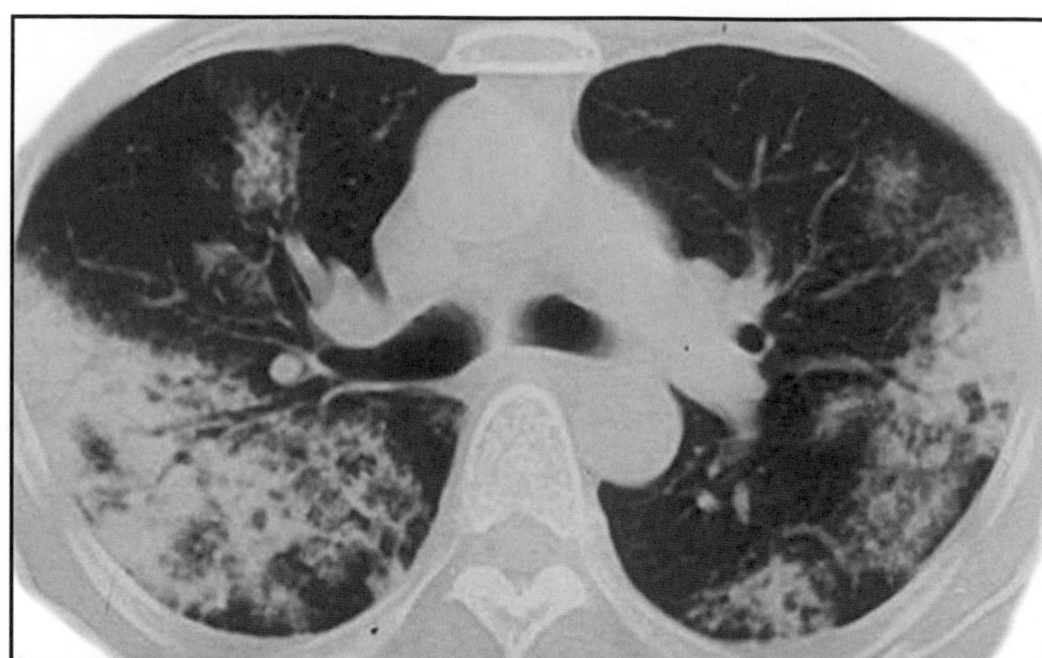
HRCT shows bilateral areas of consolidation. Although the consolidation has a patchy distribution, the lesions involve predominantly the subpleural and peribronchial regions. Areas of patchy ground-glass attenuation are present as well

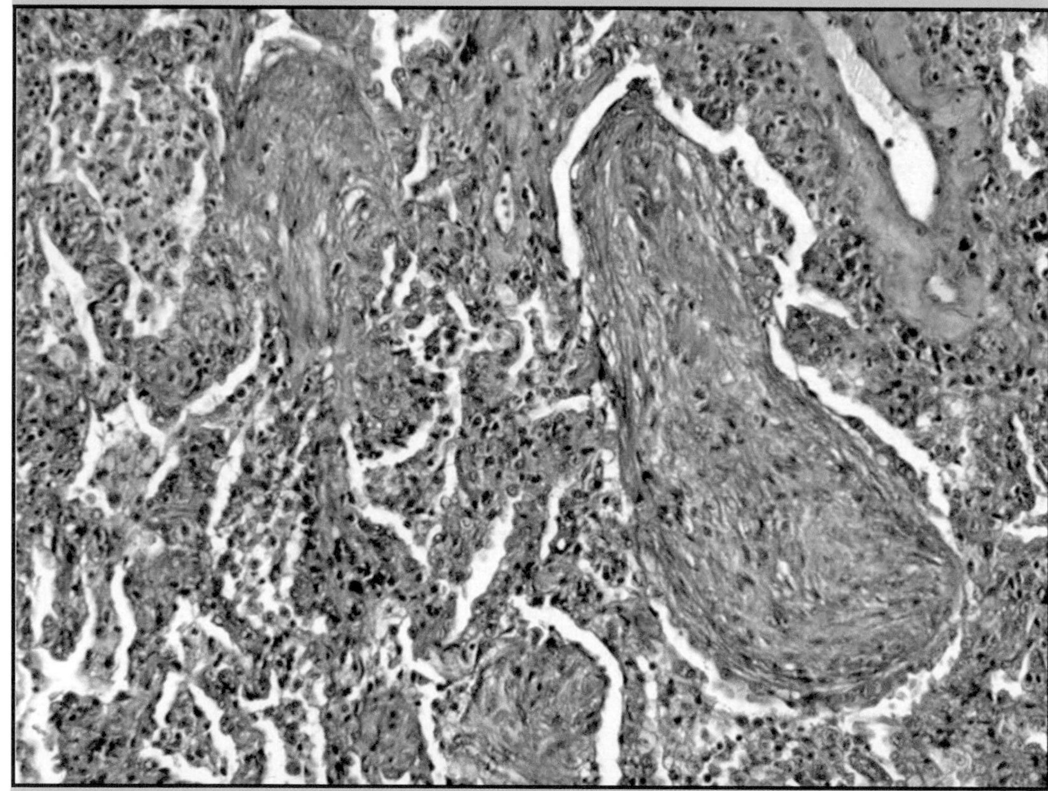
Intraluminal buds of granulation tissue consisting of loose collagen-embedded fibroblasts and myofibroblasts are present in the alveolar ducts and spaces

Cryptogenic organizing pneumonitis (COP) is a specific clinicopathologic syndrome of unknown cause. The incidence and prevalence of COP are unknown, but a cumulative incidence of six to seven per 100,000 hospital admissions was found at a major teaching hospital. The disease onset is typically in the fifth or sixth decades of life, with men and women being affected equally.

The clinical presentation of COP often mimics that of community-acquired pneumonia. In 50% of cases, the onset is heralded by a flulike respiratory illness that includes fever, malaise, fatigue, and cough. Almost three-fourths of patients have their symptoms for less than 2 months, and few have symptoms for more than 6 months before diagnosis. Weight loss of greater than 10 lb is seen in more than 50% of patients. Inspiratory crackles are frequently present on chest examination. A normal pulmonary examination is found in 25% of subjects.

Routine laboratory studies are nonspecific. A leukocytosis without increase in eosinophils is seen in approximately half of patients. The initial erythrocyte sedimentation rate is frequently elevated in patients with COP.

Pulmonary function is usually impaired with a restrictive defect being most common. Resting and exercise arterial hypoxemia is common.

The radiographic manifestations are quite distinctive. Bilateral, diffuse alveolar opacities in the presence of normal lung volume constitute the characteristic radiographic appearance in patients with COP. The alveolar opacities may rarely be unilateral. High-resolution computed tomography (HRCT) scans of the lung reveal patchy airspace consolidation, ground-glass opacities, small nodular opacities, and bronchial wall thickening and dilatation. These patchy opacities occur more frequently in the periphery of the lung and are often in the lower lung zone. The computed tomography (CT) scan may reveal much more extensive disease than is expected by review of the plain chest radiographs. Recurrent and migratory pulmonary opacities are common.

Histopathologic organizing pneumonia is a specific morphologic pattern of intraluminal fibrosis that is relatively nonspecific but may be characteristic of certain clinical syndromes. The lesion is characterized by excessive proliferation of granulation tissue within small airways (proliferative bronchiolitis) and alveolar ducts associated with chronic inflammation in the surrounding alveoli. Foamy macrophages are commonly seen in the alveolar spaces, presumably secondary to the bronchiolar occlusion. A uniform, temporally recent appearance to the changes without severe disruption of the lung architecture is a characteristic finding. The architecture of the lung is preserved, with no remodeling or honeycombing found.

Corticosteroid therapy is the most common treatment used in these patients. It results in clinical recovery in two-thirds of the patients. Early reduction in the dose or cessation of initial corticosteroid therapy may increase the risk of relapse.

Pulmonary Alveolar Proteinosis

Pulmonary alveolar proteinosis (PAP) is an uncommon disease characterized by filling of alveoli with a lipoproteinaceous material composed principally of the phospholipid surfactant and surfactant apoproteins. This amorphous material stains with periodic acid–Schiff (PAS) reagent. Impaired processing of surfactant by alveolar macrophages and diminished granulocyte macrophage-colony stimulating factor (GM-CSF) protein levels or function contributes to the pathogenesis of PAP. There is little inflammatory reaction in the surrounding lung, and the underlying lung architecture is preserved.

Three forms of PAP are recognized: acquired, congenital, and secondary. The vast majority of all cases of PAP (>90%) occur as a primary acquired disorder of unknown cause. The acquired form is seen in association with high-level dust exposures (e.g., silica, aluminum, or titanium), infection (e.g., *Nocardia*, *Pneumocystis jiroveci*, mycobacteria, and various endemic or opportunistic fungi), hematologic malignancies, and after allogeneic bone marrow transplantation for myeloid malignancies. The congenital form presents in the neonatal period and likely results from mutations in surfactant or the GM-CSF receptor gene. The secondary form develops in adulthood and is likely related to relative deficiency in GM-CSF and related macrophage dysfunction.

The typical age at presentation of an adult patient with PAP is 30 to 50 years, with a male predominance. Although some patients are asymptomatic, with only an abnormal chest radiograph at presentation, most patients have a cough (productive of mucoid or "chunky" gelatinous material) and dyspnea. In severely affected patients, constitutional symptoms of anorexia, weight loss, and fatigue appear. Physical examination may show tachypnea, cyanosis, crackles, tachycardia, and occasionally clubbing.

Laboratory abnormalities include polycythemia, hypergammaglobulinemia, and increased lactate dehydrogenase (LDH) levels. Elevated serum levels of lung surfactant proteins A and D (SP-A and SP-D) and several tumor markers (carcinoembryonic antigen [CEA], carbohydrate antigens sialyl Lewis-a [CA 19-9], and sialyl SSEA-1 [SLX]), have been found in bronchoalveolar lavage (BAL) and serum from some patients with PAP. Several serum biomarkers have been shown to correlate with disease severity, including LDH, SP-A, SP-D, Kerbs von Lungren 6 antigen (KL-6), and CEA.

A restrictive ventilatory defect is most common. Sometimes an isolated decrease in DL_{CO} (diffusing capacity for carbon monoxide), often out of proportion to the degree of reduced lung volume, may be found. The most marked abnormality is a reduced Pa_{O_2}, which may be profoundly lowered.

Chest radiographs show bilateral symmetric alveolar opacities located centrally in middle and lower lung zones, sometimes resulting in a "bat wing" distribution. Air bronchograms are rare. A thin lucent band may sharply outline the diaphragm and the heart consistent with sparing of the lung immediately adjacent to these structures. High-resolution computed tomography scanning (HRCT) reveals ground-glass opacification that typically spares the periphery. In addition, thickened intralobular structures and interlobular septa in typical polygonal shapes may give the "crazy paving" appearance. Crazy paving is not specific for PAP because it has been observed in patients with the acute respiratory distress syndrome, lipoid pneumonia, acute interstitial pneumonia, drug-related hypersensitivity reactions, and diffuse alveolar damage superimposed on usual interstitial pneumonitis.

When PAP is suspected, fiberoptic bronchoscopy to obtain BAL and, if possible, transbronchoscopic biopsy is the appropriate next step. Video-assisted transthoracic biopsy is required in the occasional patient with negative BAL and transbronchoscopic biopsy results. Characteristic BAL findings of PAP include opaque or milky appearance caused by abundant lipoproteinaceous material; cytologic examination of BAL reveals alveolar macrophages engorged with PAS-positive material. Transbronchial and open lung biopsies reveal filling of the terminal bronchioles and alveoli with flocculent and granular lipoproteinaceous material that stains pink with PAS stain.

The course of PAP is variable. The choice of treatment options for patients with PAP depends on the severity of symptoms and gas exchange abnormalities. For asymptomatic patients with little or no physiologic impairment (despite extensive radiographic abnormalities), a period of observation is recommended. For patients with severe dyspnea and hypoxemia, whole-lung lavage via a double-lumen endotracheal tube is recommended. The procedure should be done under general anesthesia. Only one lung is washed out at each session, and the contralateral lung receives oxygen as required. A few patients have improved after clearance of only one lung. Experimental therapy with GM-CSF has been used based on evidence that reduced GM-CSF effect contributes to PAP. Glucocorticoid therapy is not beneficial.

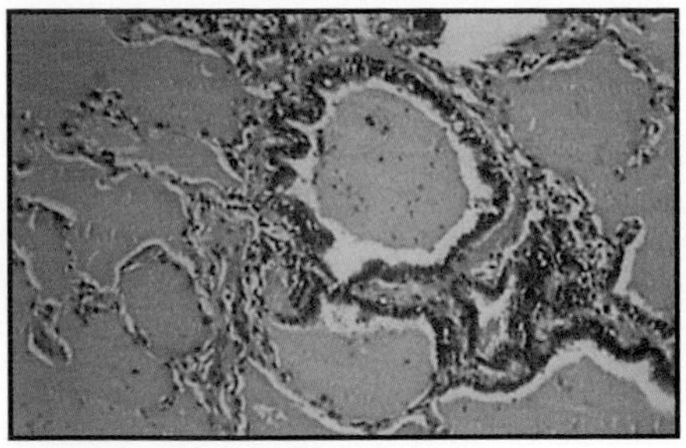

Alveoli and a small bronchus filled with eosinophilic fluid

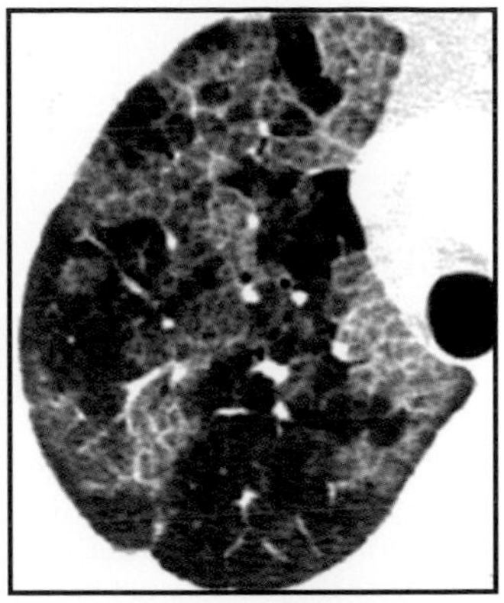

Widespread airspace disease in a geographic pattern. The "crazy paving pattern" (smooth interlobular opacities and ground-glass opacities) is visible

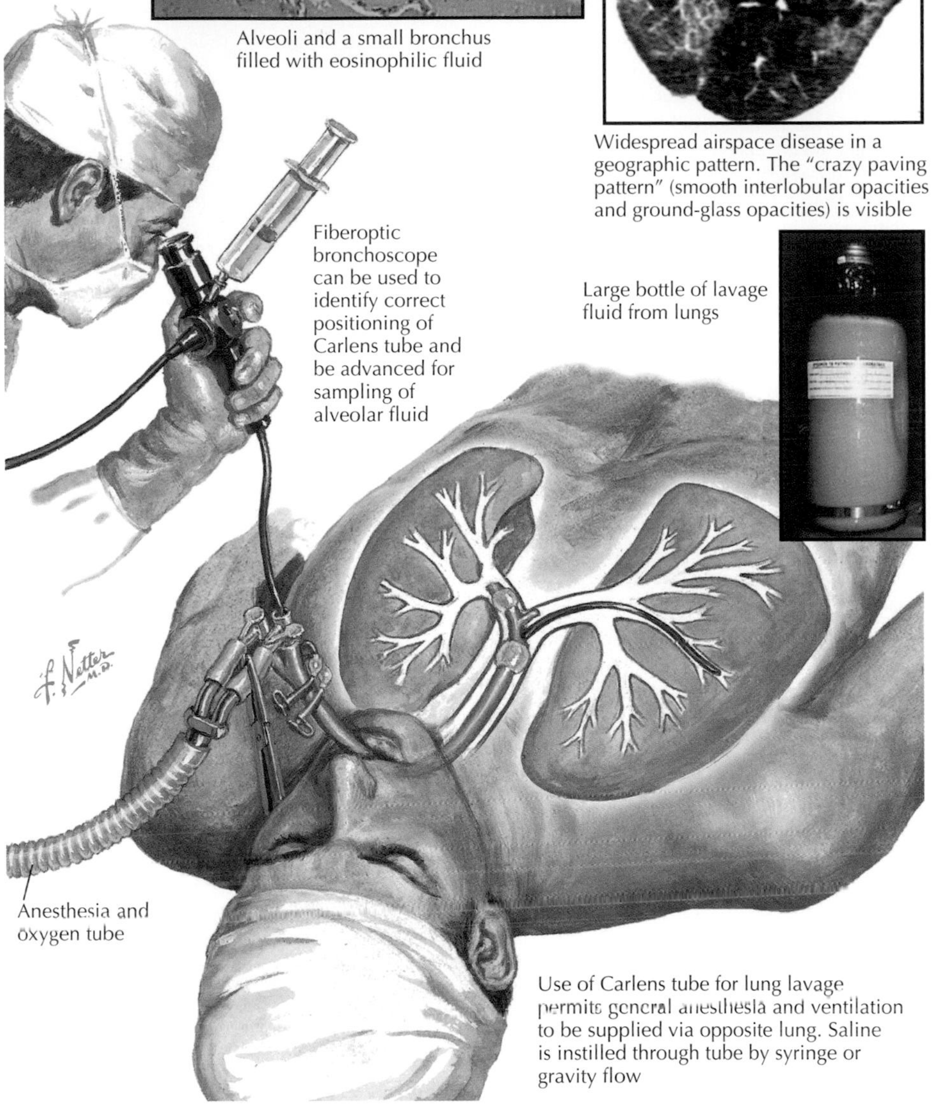

Fiberoptic bronchoscope can be used to identify correct positioning of Carlens tube and be advanced for sampling of alveolar fluid

Large bottle of lavage fluid from lungs

Anesthesia and oxygen tube

Use of Carlens tube for lung lavage permits general anesthesia and ventilation to be supplied via opposite lung. Saline is instilled through tube by syringe or gravity flow

Idiopathic Pulmonary Hemosiderosis

Idiopathic pulmonary hemosiderosis (IPH) is a disease of unknown origin, usually occurring in children, equally in both genders. Repeated episodes of pulmonary hemorrhage with resultant blood-loss anemia and eventual respiratory failure characterize the illness. In children, this disorder is associated with celiac disease and elevated IgA levels. Environmental exposure to molds, particularly *Stachybotrys chartarum*, has been suggested as a causative factor in infants with IPH, but the relationship remains unproven.

Bland pulmonary hemorrhages without immune complexes are typical histologic findings. A structural defect in the alveolar capillaries may predispose individuals to the condition. Neutrophilic infiltration (i.e., alveolar capillaritis or vasculitis) is not found. Repeated hemorrhages result in hemosiderin-laden alveolar macrophages and the deposition of free iron in pulmonary tissue; the latter may result in the development of lung fibrosis. Obliteration of alveolar capillaries may result in pulmonary hypertension. Hemosiderin-impregnated nodules are scattered in the parenchyma, along the lymphatics, and in the draining hilar lymph nodes. The role of immunologic injury in patients with IPH remains unclear.

The onset of IPH may be insidious or with an explosive episode of hemoptysis. In some patients, anemia, constitutional symptoms, cough, and radiographic changes precede frank hemoptysis. During acute bleeding episodes, crackles, wheezes, and rhonchi with dullness to percussion are noted over the involved lung areas. Later, dyspnea, tachypnea, hepatosplenomegaly, and clubbing of the fingers may be observed.

Routine laboratory data are remarkable only in the presence of marked iron deficiency. There is no evidence of coagulopathy, thrombocytopenia, hepatic dysfunction, or glomerulonephritis.

Physiologic abnormalities in IPH vary depending on the freshness of the hemorrhage, degree of fibrosis, and severity of vascular involvement. With acute hemorrhage, the vital capacity, flow rates, and arterial Po_2 may be diminished; however, the DL_{CO} (diffusing capacity for carbon monoxide) may be inappropriately high. As fibrosis ensues, a restrictive pattern with reduced DL_{CO} emerges. Irreversible pulmonary hypertension and right ventricular failure are hallmarks of the end stage of the disease.

During acute hemorrhagic episodes, the chest radiograph exhibits patchy or diffuse alveoli-filling shadows. These opacities may clear rapidly, only to appear in the same or other locations with subsequent bouts of hemorrhage. Air bronchograms are frequently obtained. High-resolution computed tomography (HRCT) scans show diffuse ground-glass or airspace-filling opacities most prominent in the middle and lower lung fields. With repeated episodes, a reticular interstitial pattern persists in the areas of prior hemorrhage. The hilar lymph nodes may become enlarged. In the later stages, right ventricular hypertrophy and enlarged pulmonary arteries are common. Perfusion lung scanning with technetium-99m (99mTc)–labeled albumin particles may show foci of high radioactivity in the lungs where radioactively tagged material has extravasated into the alveoli. In addition, active intrapulmonary bleeding can be visualized by pulmonary radioscintigraphy, in which autologous erythrocytes labeled with 51Cr or 99mTc are injected intravenously with subsequent recording of the radioactivity over the lungs.

IPH is a diagnosis of exclusion that is suggested by a history of recurrent episodes of hemoptysis, presence of an iron deficiency anemia, and typical radiographic abnormalities in a child with normal renal function. Sequential bronchoalveolar lavage (BAL) is useful because lavage aliquots are progressively more hemorrhagic. Hemosiderin-laden macrophages may be demonstrated by Prussian blue staining. BAL is most helpful in the diagnosis of diffuse pulmonary opacities without hemoptysis. In patients who do not experience the typical episodes of hemoptysis, lung biopsy is the only unequivocal means of establishing the diagnosis and may be accomplished by transbronchial or surgical lung biopsy techniques.

The prognosis in IPH is poor. Children and adolescents more frequently experience a rapid course and have a worse prognosis. In adults, the prognosis is more favorable. Corticosteroids and other immunosuppressive drugs may be effective during an acute episode. Chronic oral corticosteroids may decrease episodes of acute alveolar hemorrhage and delay progression to chronic fibrotic changes. In patients with severe respiratory failure, extracorporeal membrane oxygenation may prolong survival until immunosuppressive therapy becomes effective. In IPH patients with celiac disease, a gluten-free diet has been associated with remission of pulmonary symptoms.

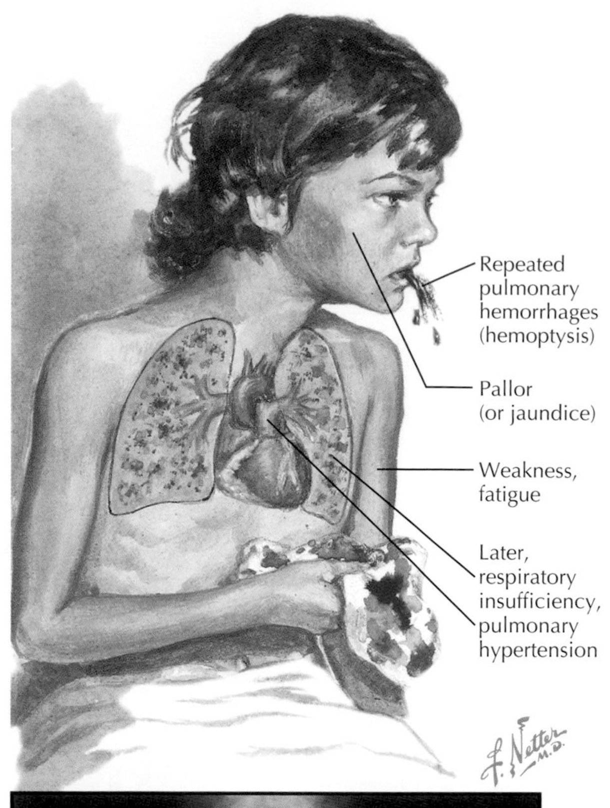

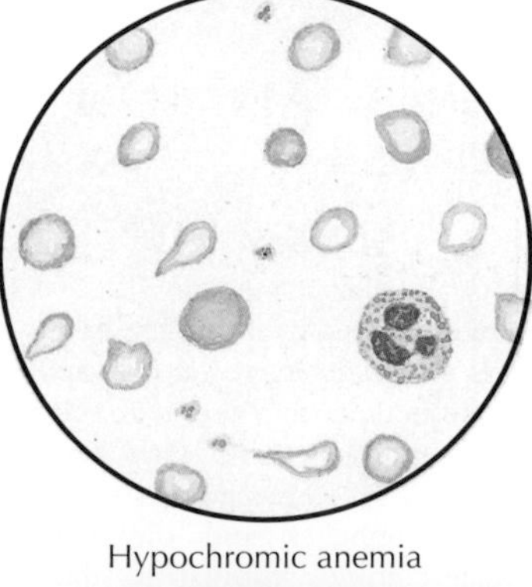
Hypochromic anemia

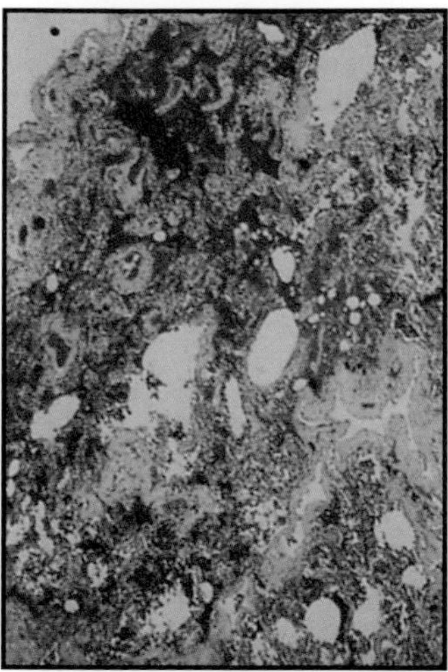
Fresh pulmonary hemorrhages

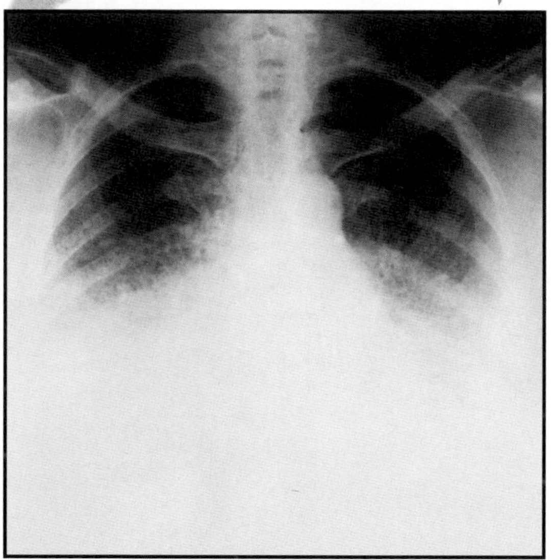
Fine reticular and mottled densities throughout both lungs. Diffuse fluffy shadows at both bases after acute hemorrhage

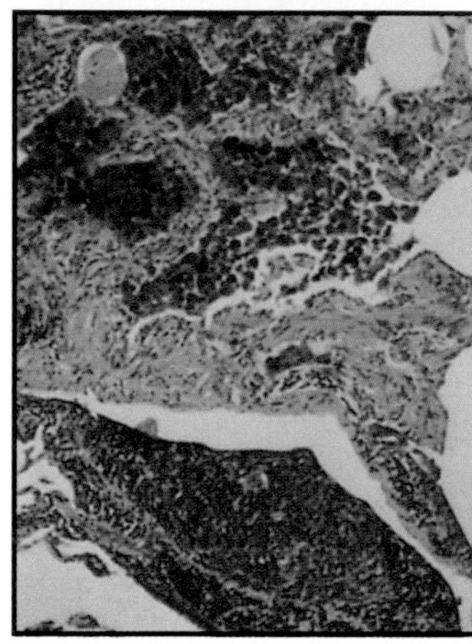
Intraalvolar macrophages full of hemosiderin plus septal fibrosis; lymphoid nodule at bottom

LYMPHANGIOLEIOMYOMATOSIS

Pulmonary lymphangioleiomyomatosis (LAM) is a diffuse, progressive lung disease that affects young women of childbearing age. It occurs as a sporadic disease (S-LAM) or with a tuberous sclerosis complex (TSC-LAM). The incidence and prevalence (two to five per million) of sporadic LAM are unknown. Whites are afflicted much more commonly than other racial groups.

Patients with S-LAM present with dyspnea or fatigue. Spontaneous pneumothorax occurs in almost two-thirds of cases. It is often recurrent, may be bilateral, and may necessitate pleurodesis for more definitive therapy. Hemoptysis occurs and may be life threatening. Chylothorax, caused by obstruction of the thoracic duct or rupture of the lymphatics in the pleura or mediastinum by proliferating smooth muscle cells, is characteristic of this disorder. Chyle is milky white in appearance, has a high triglyceride level (>110 mg/dL), and has chylomicrons. Chyloperitoneum (chylous ascites), chyluria, and chylopericardium have been reported. Renal angioleiomyomata, a characteristic pathologic finding in tuberous sclerosis, is also common in LAM (≤50% of subjects).

The physical examination can be unrevealing or may demonstrate end-expiratory crackles, hyperinflation, decreased or absent breath sounds, ascites, and intraabdominal or adnexal masses.

Pathologically, LAM is characterized by proliferation of atypical smooth muscle around the bronchovascular structures and within the pulmonary interstitium. The abnormal-appearing smooth muscle–like cells have loss of heterozygosity and inactivating mutations in the tuberous sclerosis complex-2 (16p13). In addition, there is diffuse, cystic dilatation of the terminal airspaces. Hemosiderosis is common and a consequence of low-volume hemorrhage caused by the rupture of dilated and tortuous venules.

Estrogen appears to play a central role in disease progression. The disease does not present before menarche and only rarely after menopause (usually in association with hormonal supplementation). The disease may accelerate during pregnancy and abate after oophorectomy.

LAM most commonly presents with obstructive physiology (reduced FEV_1 [forced expiratory volume in 1 second], reduced FEV_1/FVC [forced vital capacity] ratio) and gas trapping. Both a loss of elastic recoil and an increase in airflow resistance contribute to the observed airflow limitation. A markedly reduced DL_{CO} (diffusing capacity for carbon monoxide) is a characteristic feature. The alveolar-arterial oxygen difference is also increased. There is a diminished exercise performance with a reduced oxygen consumption and low anaerobic threshold in most patients.

The chest radiographic findings in patients with LAM are variable, ranging from normal early in the course of the disease to severely emphysematous-like changes in advanced disease. Pneumothorax may be an early feature, and chylous pleural effusion may develop at any time during the course. The thin-section high-resolution computed tomography (HRCT) scanning shows diffuse, homogeneous, small (<1 cm diameter), thin-walled cysts (100% of patients) and ground-glass opacities (59%) and can be pathognomonic in an appropriate clinical context. The most common abdominal findings include renal angiomyolipoma (54%), enlarged abdominal lymph nodes (39%), lymphangiomyoma (16%), ascites (10%), dilatation of the thoracic duct (9%), and hepatic involvement (4%).

In general, the diagnosis should be strongly suspected in any young woman who presents with emphysema, recurrent pneumothorax, or a chylous pleural effusion. LAM can be readily diagnosed by its characteristic histologic findings on surgical lung biopsy. Immunohistochemical stains specific for smooth muscle components actin or desmin and HMB-45 have been used to improve diagnostic sensitivity and specificity.

The most common reasons for hospitalization are for the management of spontaneous pneumothorax, chylothorax, or renal angiomyolipomas that are acutely bleeding or at risk for spontaneous hemorrhage. The prognosis is variable but generally poor, with about 22% to 62% of patients succumbing to progressive respiratory failure after 10 years from diagnosis. Long-term survival (>20 years after diagnosis) has been reported. Pregnancy and the use of supplemental estrogen are known to accelerate the disease process.

There is no proven role for corticosteroids, cytotoxic agents, oophorectomy, progesterone, tamoxifen, or luteinizing hormone–releasing hormone analogues in the treatment of patients with LAM. Lung transplantation should be considered for any failing patient. There have been reports of recurrent disease in transplanted lungs and the recurrent LAM cells within the donor lungs have been shown to be of recipient origin, suggesting metastatic spread.

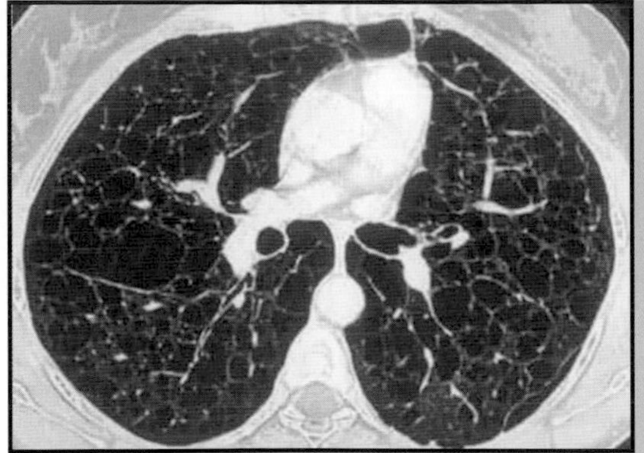

HRCT scan showing numerous thin-walled cysts bilaterally throughout the lung parenchyma.

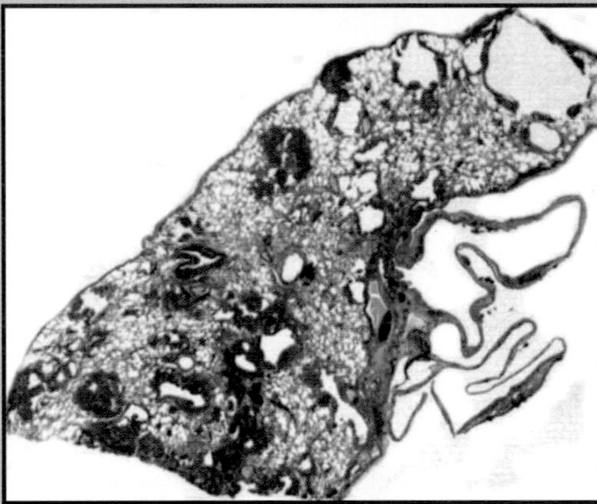

The lung shows cystic spaces with moderate amounts of LAM cells around the periphery of the spaces.

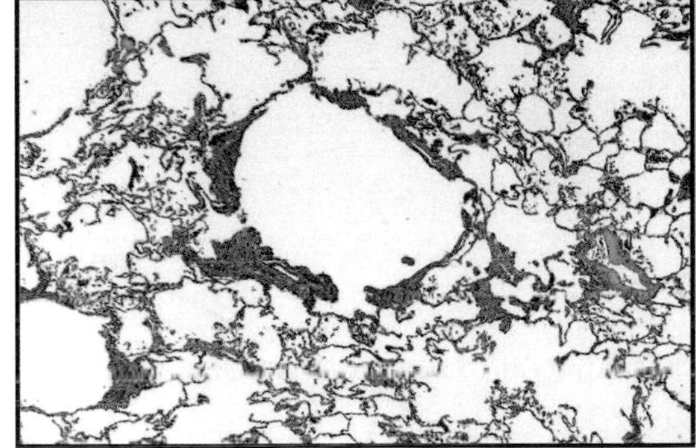

The lung shows cystic spaces with LAM cells around the periphery of the spaces. The cystic spaces contain no fluid or cellular content. The intervening lung parenchyma appears normal.

TUBEROUS SCLEROSIS

Tuberous sclerosis (TSC) is a rare autosomal dominant disorder. It affects men and women equally. Mental retardation, seizures, and facial angiofibroma (adenoma sebaceum) form the classic clinical triad. Up to 30% of female TSC patients have cystic lung changes consistent with LAM (TSC-LAM). In patients with TSC-LAM, peripheral blood DNA analysis reveals a single mutation in either *TSC1* or *TSC2*, and the LAM cells in the lung reveal a second hit (deletion) or loss of heterozygosity for the normal allele. Pulmonary involvement in TSC carries a poor prognosis.

Pulmonary Langerhans Cell Histiocytosis

Pulmonary Langerhans cell histiocytosis (PLCH) of the lung primarily affects young adults between the ages of 20 to 40 years. Whites are affected more commonly than individuals of African or Asian descent. The pathogenesis of PLCH is unknown. The near universal association of PLCH with cigarette smoking strongly implies a causative role.

The clinical presentation is variable, from an asymptomatic state (~16%) to a rapidly progressive condition. The duration of illness is usually less than 1 year before diagnosis. The most common clinical manifestations at presentation are cough (56%-70%), dyspnea (40%-87%), chest pain that is frequently pleuritic (10%-21%), fatigue (~30%), weight loss (20%-30%), and fever (15%). Pneumothorax occurs in about 25% of patients and is occasionally the first manifestation of the illness. Pulmonary hypertension is common. Hemoptysis occurs in approximately 13% of cases and should prompt consideration of superimposed infection or malignancy. In addition, diabetes insipidus, secondary to hypothalamic involvement, may be present in approximately 15% of patients and is believed to portend a worse prognosis. Cystic bone lesions are present in 4% to 20% of patients and may produce localized pain or a pathologic bone fracture. The physical examination findings are usually normal. Routine laboratory studies are nonspecific.

The radiographic features vary depending on the stage of the disease. The combination of ill-defined or stellate nodules (2-10 mm in size), reticular or nodular opacities, upper zone cysts or honeycombing, preservation of lung volume, and costophrenic angle sparing are highly specific for PLCH. High-resolution computed tomography (HRCT) lung scanning that reveals the combination of nodules and thin-walled cysts with a mid to upper zone predominance and interstitial thickening in a young smoker is so characteristic that it can be diagnostic of PLCH. Serial chest CT scanning suggests a sequence of progression from nodules to cavitating nodules to cystic lesions.

Physiologically, the most prominent and frequent pulmonary function abnormality is a markedly reduced DL_{CO} (diffusing capacity for carbon monoxide), but varying degrees of restrictive disease, airflow limitation, and diminished exercise capacity are described. Whereas predominantly nodular disease is usually associated with normal or restrictive pulmonary function tests, cystic disease is more likely to be associated with airflow limitation and hyperinflation. Limitations in activity and exercise intolerance out of proportion to pulmonary function abnormalities are commonly present. Gas exchange abnormalities, reflected by a worsening alveolar–arterial oxygen difference with increasing exercise, are seen in the majority of patients.

The finding of more than 5% Langerhans cells on bronchoalveolar lavage strongly suggests the diagnosis of PLCH. Transbronchial biopsy can be sufficient to make the diagnosis; however, a substantial number of false-negative or nondiagnostic biopsies may result from sampling error and insufficient tissue. Video thoracoscopic lung biopsy is generally definitive. Langerhans cells can be recognized by their characteristic staining for S-100 protein. Tissue immunostaining with the monoclonal antibody OKT-6 (CD1a) distinguishes Langerhans cells from other histiocytes and can be a useful adjunct in difficult cases. These cells also demonstrate staining with the monoclonal antibody MT-1.

Smoking cessation is the key treatment, resulting in clinical improvement in many subjects. Immunosuppressive therapies (i.e., glucocorticoids and cytotoxic agents) are of limited value. Lung transplantation should be considered in patients with advanced disease. Recurrence of the condition in the transplanted lung may occur. Estimated 5- and 10-year survival rates are 74% and 64%, respectively. Respiratory failure is the most common cause of death. The other major cause of death is malignancy, primarily of hematologic or epithelial origin.

Chest radiographic features

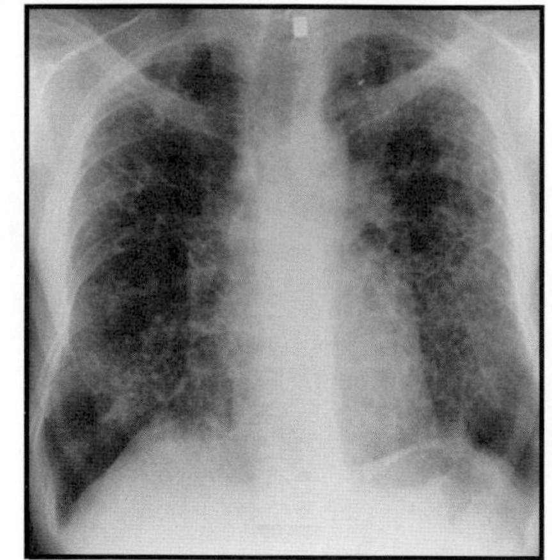

Reticular and nodular opacities are present in association with upper zone cysts, no volume loss, and sparing of the CPA

HRCT features

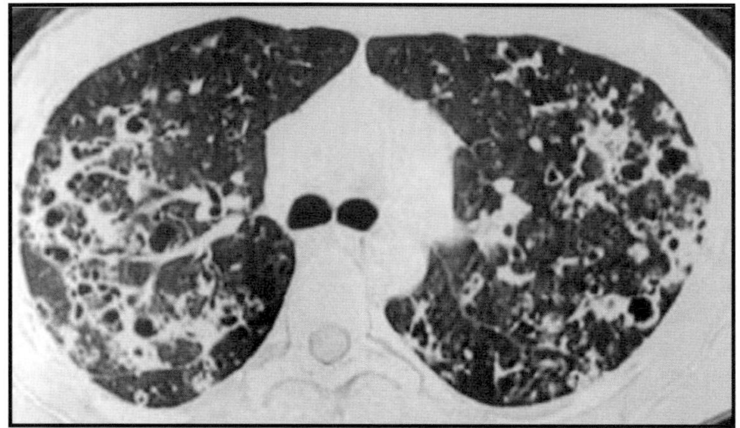

A combination of nodules and cysts (often bizarre-shaped), especially if present in a young smoker, is virtually diagnostic of PLCH. The lesions are usually equally distributed in the central and peripheral zones and follow a bronchovascular distribution

Histologic features

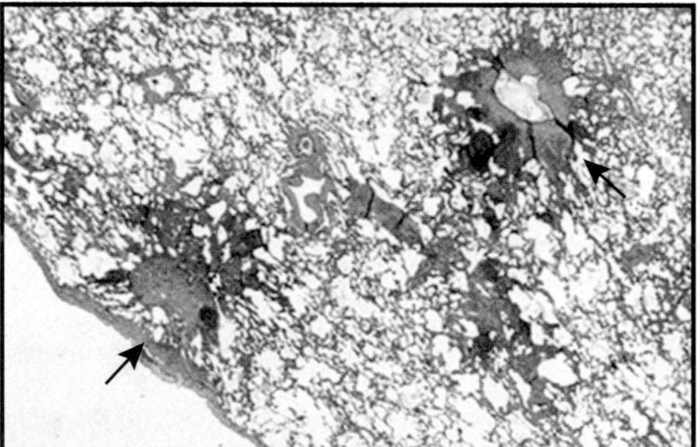

Low-power microscopy shows multiple stellate-shaped nodular infiltrates

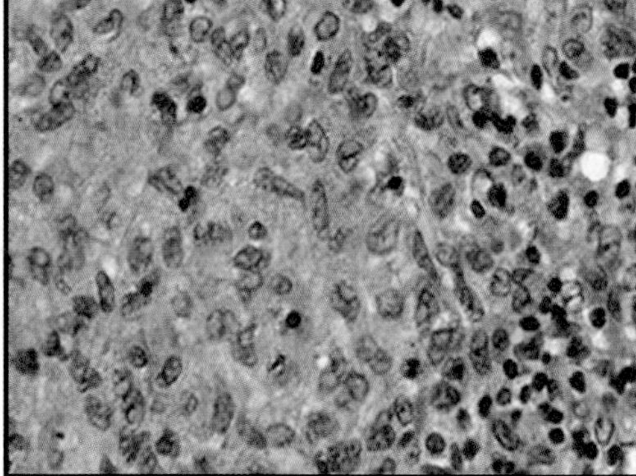

The cellular infiltrate consists of sheets of Langerhans cells, which have a uniform appearance consisting of moderate eosinophilic cytoplasm and prominent nuclear grooves. Scattered eosinophils are also present

SARCOIDOSIS

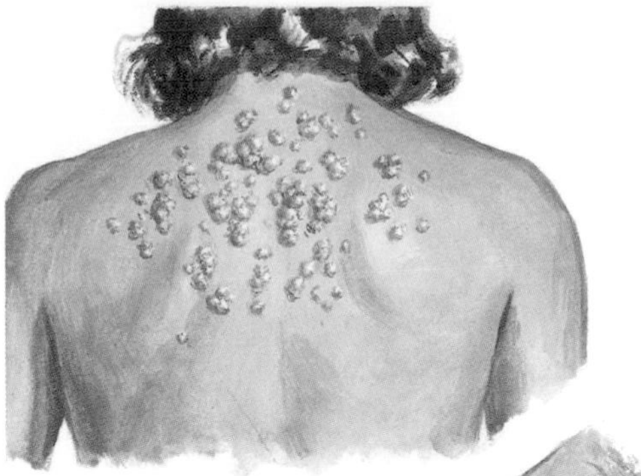

Sarcoidosis is a common disease of unknown origin characterized by the infiltration of many organs by noncaseating epithelioid granulomas. The lung is the most common organ affected by sarcoidosis. The skin, eye, and liver are also frequently involved. Sarcoidosis may affect many other organs, many of which are detailed in the next paragraph. Although in the United States sarcoidosis is most common in African Americans, the disease is also has a high prevalence in Northern Europeans and occurs worldwide. Women appear to contract the disease more often than men. The majority of patients are younger than 40 years of age at onset, although there is a second peak of increased incidence after age 50 years in women. There is a higher incidence of the disease in first-degree relatives (parents, siblings, and children) of sarcoidosis patients than the general population. This is in keeping with the belief that sarcoidosis represents an abnormal granulomatous response to an environmental exposure in genetically susceptible individuals. Sarcoidosis is rare in people younger than age 18 years. Sarcoidosis is often a benign condition that may run its entire course without detection. It is often discovered in asymptomatic patients on screening chest radiographs.

Sarcoidosis may present as a variety of clinical syndromes, which vary primarily depending on the distribution of granulomatous involvement of the affected organs (see Plate 4-155). These include (1) Löfgren syndrome (erythema nodosum with radiographic evidence of hilar lymph node enlargement, often with concomitant fever and joint [often ankle] arthritis); (2) cutaneous plaques and subcutaneous nodules; (3) Heerfordt syndrome (uveoparotid fever); (4) isolated uveitis; (5) salivary gland enlargement; (6) central nervous system (CNS) syndromes (usually seventh nerve palsy); (7) cardiomyopathy or cardiac arrhythmias; (8) hepatosplenomegaly (with or without hypersplenism); (9) upper airway involvement (sarcoidosis of the upper respiratory tract [SURT]); (10) hypercalcemia; (11) renal failure; (12) peripheral lymphadenopathy; and (13) various forms of pulmonary disease, including mediastinal adenopathy, interstitial lung disease, endobronchial involvement with airflow obstruction and wheezing, and pulmonary hypertension.

Pulmonary hypertension is a potentially life-threatening complication of sarcoidosis. Sarcoidosis associated pulmonary hypertension is classified in the miscellaneous category (class 5) according to the World Health Organization classification scheme. This is because there are multiple mechanisms that may cause pulmonary hypertension in sarcoidosis, including pulmonary venous hypertension from myocardial involvement, pulmonary fibrosis causing vascular distortion, hypoxemia from parenchymal sarcoidosis, compression of the vasculature from the thoracic lymphadenopathy of sarcoidosis, and direct granulomatous involvement of the pulmonary vasculature.

The radiographic presentations of sarcoidosis have been divided into five stages: (0) a normal chest radiograph, (I) bilateral hilar and right paratracheal lymph node enlargement, (II) persistence of lymph nodes with concomitant pulmonary infiltrations, (III) pulmonary infiltrations with no identifiable mediastinal adenopathy, and (IV) fibrocystic changes that are usually most prominent in the upper lobes. The fibrosis may be significant, with retraction of the hilar areas upward and unilateral deviation of the trachea. Occasionally, aspergillomas may develop in these fibrocystic spaces. Patients with radiographic stage I sarcoidosis are most often asymptomatic and usually have normal pulmonary function test results despite the universal presence of granulomas on lung biopsy specimens at this stage of the disease. With radiographically discernible pulmonary lesions, a restrictive pattern of dysfunction may emerge, with loss of lung volumes; decreased pulmonary compliance; hyperventilation; decreased diffusing capacity; and in the most severely afflicted patients, hypoxemia. In chronically scarred lungs, evidence of airway dysfunction usually appears, with decreased FEV_1 (forced expiratory volume in 1 second) and diminished flow rates at low lung volumes. Although dyspnea, pulmonary dysfunction, and prognosis are generally worse with higher radiographic stages, there is too much overlap for this to be useful to assess individual patients. It is clear that patients with stage IV radiographs include nearly all the patients with a very poor prognosis, although not all patients with stage IV radiographs will fare poorly.

Although chest computed tomography scanning is not required to assess the status of pulmonary sarcoidosis, it often clearly identifies mediastinal adenopathy. Furthermore, it may detect parenchymal disease that is not evident on chest radiographs. Parenchymal sarcoidosis is commonly located along the bronchovascular bundles and in subpleural locations.

Skin lesions

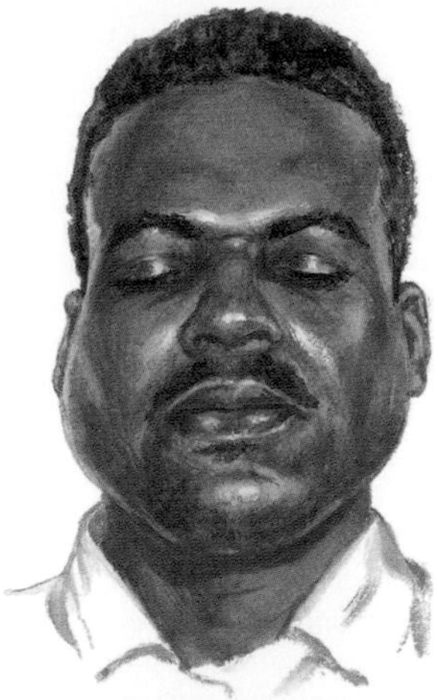

Bilateral parotid gland involvement

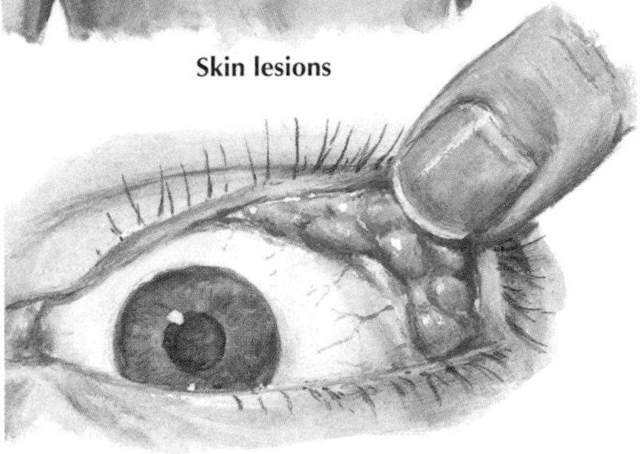

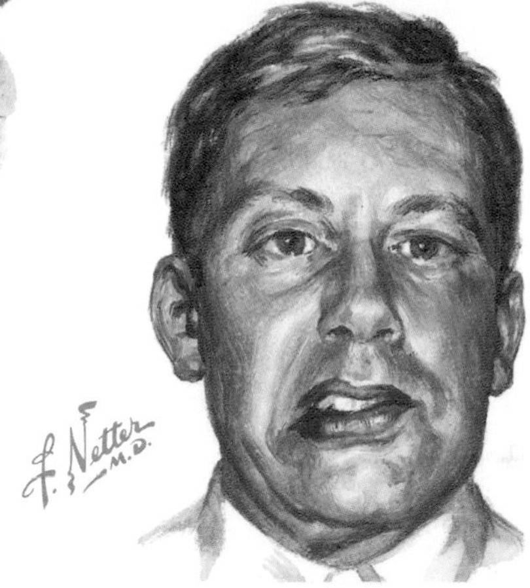

Lacrimal gland involvement

Paralysis caused by involvement of facial (VII) nerve

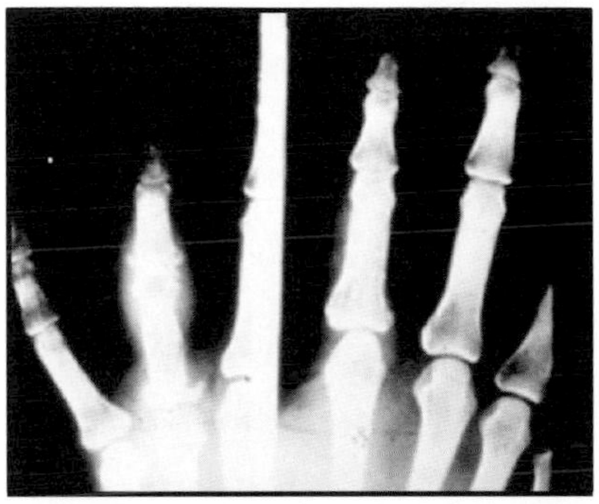

F. Netter M.D.

Bone destruction of terminal phalanges

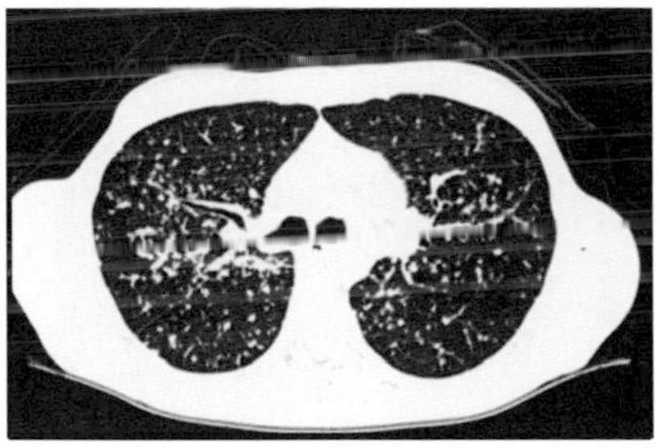

Chest computed tomography scan

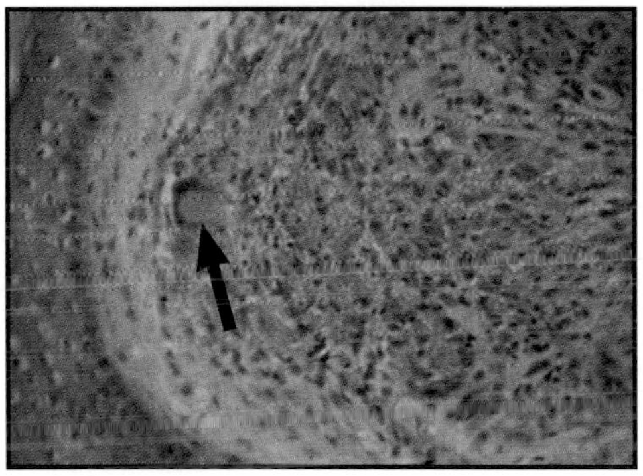

Biopsy of nodule. Reveals typical sarcoidal granuloma (dense infiltration with macrophages, epithelioid cells, and occasional multinucleated giant cells)

SARCOIDOSIS *(Continued)*

Noncaseating epithelioid granulomas, often accompanied by giant cells and rarely by small, calcified bodies (Schaumann bodies), are the fundamental pathologic lesions in sarcoidosis but are nonspecific (see Plate 4-156). However, these granulomas often cannot be differentiated from the granulomas of fungal infections, berylliosis, leprosy, brucellosis, hypersensitivity lung diseases, the occasional instances of tuberculosis when caseation and acid-fast bacilli are not apparent, and lymph nodes draining neoplastic tumors. Therefore, the diagnosis of sarcoidosis requires a compatible clinical picture and negative smears and cultures for organisms causing the diseases. Granulomas frequently develop in several organs, accounting for the multiple modes of clinical presentation when organ structure and function are impaired. In the majority of patients with disability, the organs primarily affected are the lungs, eyes, and myocardium.

The immunopathogenesis of sarcoidosis is not completely understood. The process probably begins with the interaction of unknown antigen(s) with antigen-presenting cells (APCs) such as dendritic cells and macrophages. It is postulated that these APCs process these antigens and present them via human leukocyte antigen class II molecules to T-cell receptors attached to T lymphocytes, usually of the CD4+ class. After these events occur, T cells are stimulated to proliferate, and cytokines including interleukin-2 and interferon-γ, are produced. These cytokines are thought to enhance production of macrophage-derived tumor necrosis factor-α (TNF-α). These cytokines and undoubtedly many others are responsible for granuloma formation.

Elevated levels of serum angiotensin-converting enzyme (ACE) have been observed in active sarcoidosis. However, the serum ACE level is thought not to be specific or sensitive enough for the diagnosis of sarcoidosis. The serum ACE level may be useful to measure disease activity in cases in which clinical methods of assessment are difficult or costly.

The diagnosis of sarcoidosis rests on the demonstration of noncaseating epithelioid granulomas in tissues subjected to biopsy (skin, lymph nodes, or lung) from a patient with a compatible clinical picture. As previously mentioned, the clinician must be vigilant that alternate potential causes of granulomatous inflammation have been reasonably excluded.

The majority of patients with sarcoidosis can expect a benign course with complete clearing or nondisabling persistence of radiographic and other clinical abnormalities. However, a small but significant number of patients will be disabled, and approximately 4% will die of their sarcoidosis, usually from respiratory failure. Less commonly, death occurs from sarcoid cardiomyopathy or CNS involvement. For unknown reasons, cardiac involvement is the major cause of death from sarcoidosis in Japanese individuals. Rarely, death may be the result of renal failure or from hemorrhage because of pulmonary aspergillomas that form in sarcoid bullae. African Americans tend to have more aggressive forms of sarcoidosis than whites.

Patients with active sarcoidosis usually respond well to corticosteroids. The usual course of therapy for acute pulmonary sarcoidosis is 20 to 40 mg/d prednisone equivalent for 6 to 12 months. Relapse is common after cessation of prednisone and may require reinstitution of treatment. Higher doses of corticosteroids are often required for cardiac involvement, disfiguring facial sarcoidosis (lupus pernio), and neurosarcoidosis. Prompt treatment with corticosteroids is indicated for patients with uveitis, CNS disease, hypercalcemia, cardiomyopathy, hypersplenism, and progressive pulmonary dysfunction, but only 10% of patients with sarcoidosis require mandatory treatment of this kind. Corticosteroids are not indicated in patients with asymptomatic hilar lymphadenopathy or minor radiographic pulmonary shadows or for asymptomatic elevations in serum liver function tests. The arthritis of Löfgren syndrome can usually be managed with nonsteroidal antiinflammatory agents.

Because prolonged corticosteroid therapy is hazardous, alternative medications to corticosteroids are often used for chronic sarcoidosis. In these instances, corticosteroids are often still required, but the addition of alternative medicines has a corticosteroid-sparing effect such that the maintenance corticosteroid dose can be reduced. Such medications include methotrexate, hydroxychloroquine, chloroquine, azathioprine, leflunomide, pentoxifylline, thalidomide, the tetracyclines, and infliximab.

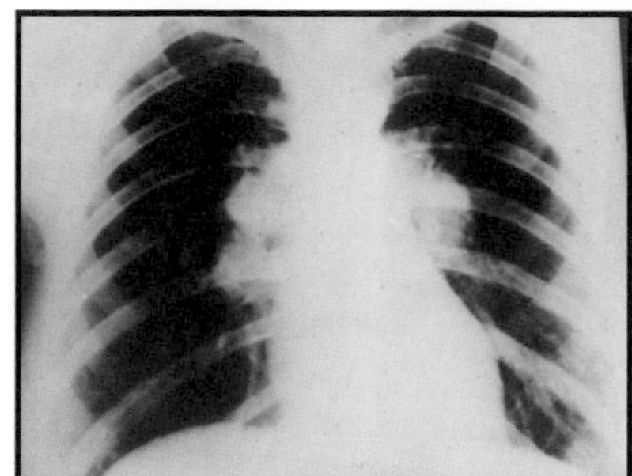

Radiologic stage I: Bilateral hilar lymph node enlargement

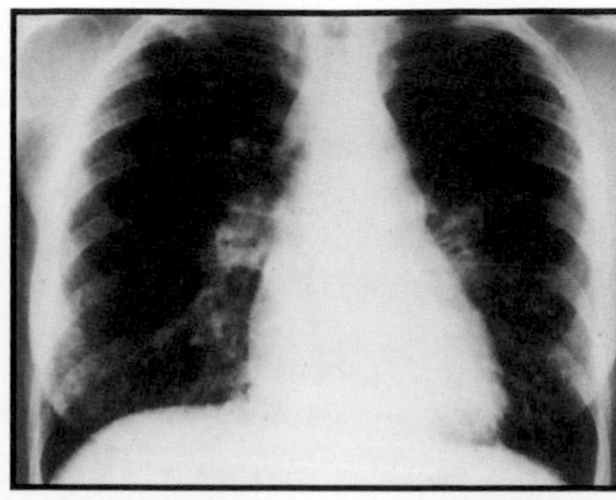

Stage II: Persistence of lymphadenopathy with reticular and nodular pulmonary infiltrations

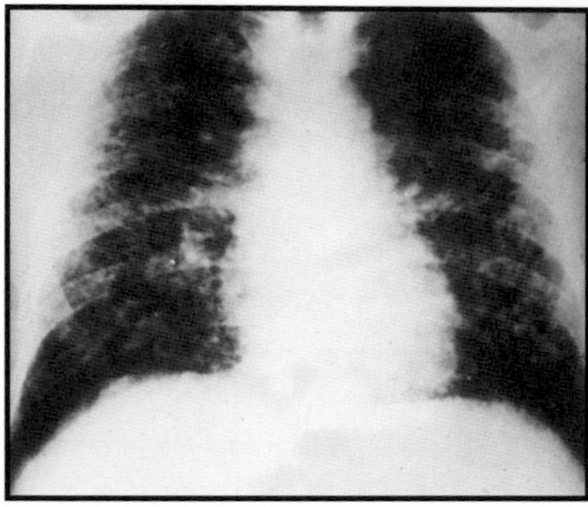

Stage III: Pulmonary infiltrations with no identifiable mediastinal lymphadenopathy

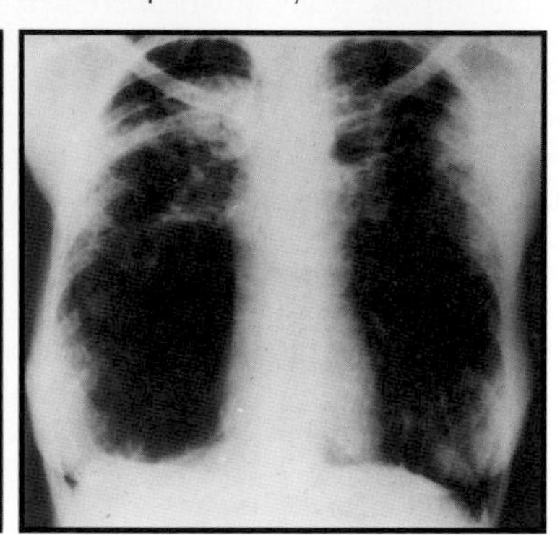

Stage IV: Fibrotic lungs with bullae

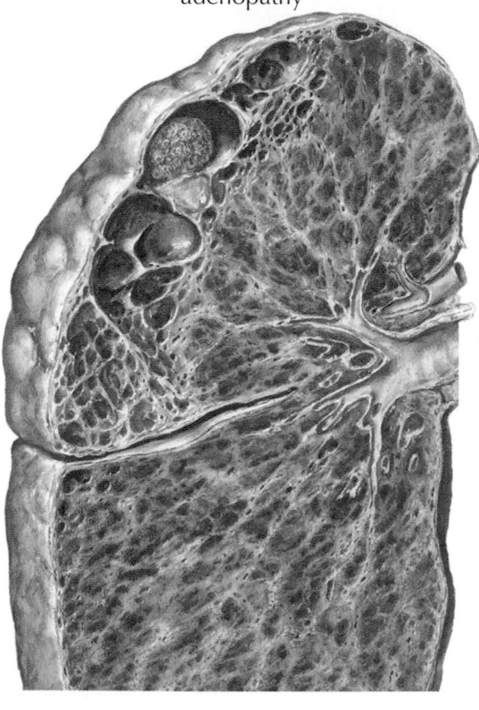

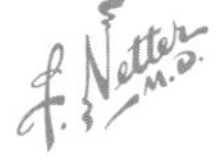

Sectioned lung in advanced sarcoidosis. Fibrosis in central zone with bullae near surface of upper lobe, one of which contains an aspergilloma

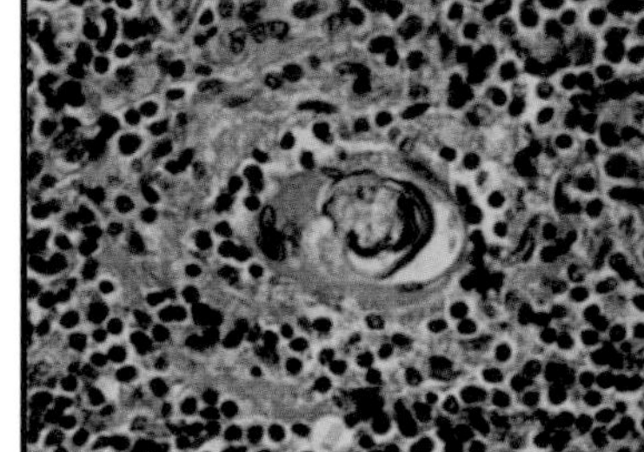

Schaumann's body (concentrically laminated, calcified body) in a mediastinal lymph node giant cell

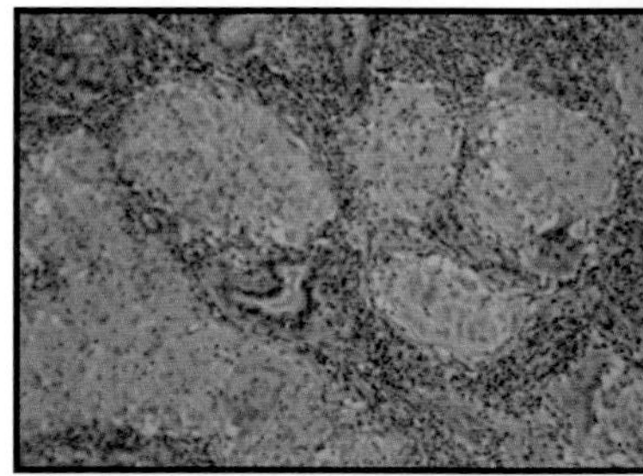

Typical epithelioid cell granulomas with occasional giant cells

Rheumatoid Arthritis

Rheumatoid arthritis (RA) is a systemic, autoinflammatory disorder defined by its characteristic attack on the diarthroidal joints. It affects approximately 1% of the adult U.S. population, with a two-to-one female predominance. When compared with the general population, overall mortality is increased, with the median survival decreased by 1 decade. A significant portion of the clinical impact of the disease is attributable to its extraarticular manifestations (ExRAs). ExRAs are common, the prevalence of clinically "severe" ExRA ranging up to 40%, and are dominated by cardiac, vascular, and pulmonary disorders.

Up to one-third of RA patients have respiratory symptoms, and up to two-thirds have chest imaging changes. Physiologic impairment occurs less frequently, but when present, it is a poor prognostic sign. Because the medications used to treat RA have been described to cause both direct pulmonary toxicity as well as increase the risk of infectious complications, both respiratory infection and drug-induced lung disease should always be considered in patients with new respiratory symptoms or signs. A large group of direct RA complications is also well recognized. These complications can be approached anatomically because they can affect all the compartments of the chest both in isolation or collectively.

RA can cause upper, lower, and distal airway disease. Arthritis of the cricoarytenoid joints, rheumatoid nodules of the upper airway, and vocal cord paresis all occur. Radiographic bronchiectasis has been described in up to one-third of patients, but clinically important disease appears much less frequently. Small airway disease with physiologic obstruction is common and presents with dyspnea, a nonproductive cough, or wheezing. Imaging with high-resolution computed tomography (HRCT) demonstrates centrilobular nodules, hyperinflation, and heterogeneous air trapping. Pathologically, both fibrosing (obliterative or constrictive bronchiolitis) and cellular (lymphocytic, follicular, and diffuse panbronchiolitis) types of small airways disease can be seen. Pleurisy, pleuritis, and effusions occur in approximately 5% of patients and may be the most common symptomatic intrathoracic manifestation of the disease. The effusions may precede, accompany, or follow the onset of joint involvement. Despite the preponderance of women with this disease, rheumatoid pleural effusions are more prevalent in men. They tend to be small and asymmetric and to wax and wane. Pleural fluid analysis generally reveals a low glucose level (<50 mg/dL), low pH (<7.30), high lactate dehydrogenase (LDH) level (>1000 IU/L), and high rheumatoid factor. When identified, effusions should not be assumed to be RA associated; empyema, sterile empyema, chylothorax, and congestive heart failure are all seen, but a fibrothorax with its physiologic restriction and trapped lung are rare. Isolated, pulmonary hypertension caused by a primary vasculopathy is exceedingly rare, but capillaritis or alveolar hemorrhage can occur. Rheumatoid (necrobiotic) nodules are found in up to 20% of patients, typically range from millimeters to centimeters in size, are usually asymptomatic, and can fluctuate in size over time. However, they can cavitate and be complicated by pneumothorax, hydropneumothorax, sterile empyema, and hemoptysis. Nodules identified on high-resolution computed tomography (HRCT) must be distinguished from malignant and infectious lesions. Caplan syndrome refers to conglomerations of nodules seen in patients with RA and pneumoconiosis.

Symptomatic interstitial lung disease (ILD) has been described in 10% of subjects, but prospective studies using HRCT have shown specific features of ILD in up to two-thirds. Similar to what is seen with pleural disease, ILD may precede, accompany, or follow the onset of joint involvement. Although all of the pathologic patterns described in the idiopathic interstitial pneumonias (usual interstitial pneumonia [UIP], nonspecific interstitial pneumonia [NSIP], organizing pneumonia, diffuse alveolar damage [DAD]) have been described in RA, unlike most other connective tissue diseases, on surgical lung biopsy a UIP pattern is more common than the NSIP pattern. The DAD pattern (i.e., Hamman-Rich syndrome), is quite uncommon but is impressive with its presentation as rapid and progressive respiratory failure that frequently results in death.

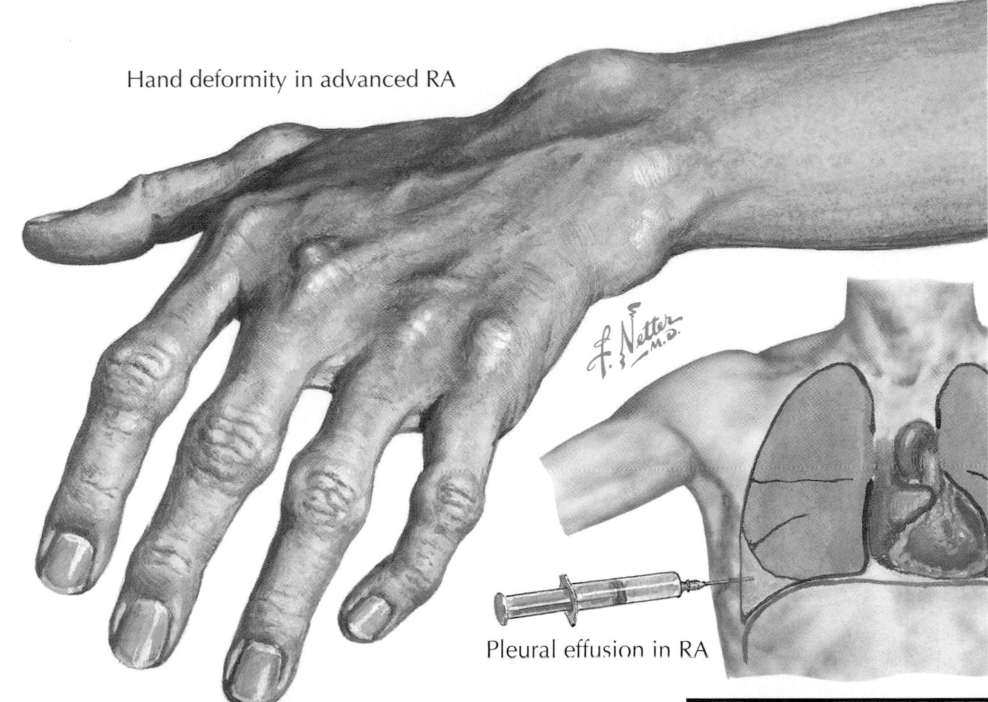

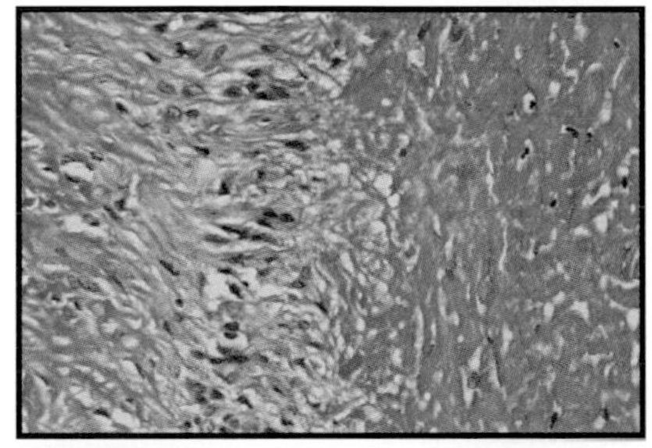

◀Portion of rheumatoid nodule. Fibrinoid necrosis on the right, palisading epithelial cells in the middle, dense collagen on the left

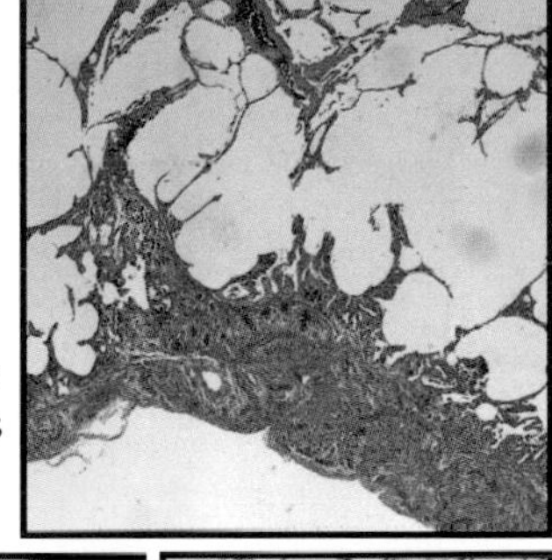

▶Histopathologic specimen showing chronic and fibrous pleural inflammation in rheumatoid arthritis

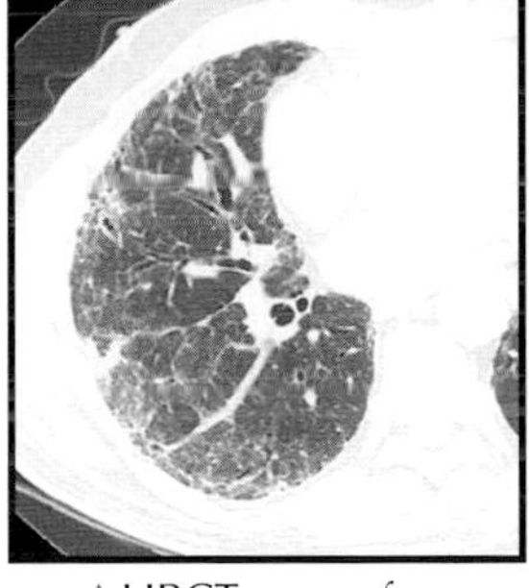

▲HRCT scan of radiographic UIP pattern fibrosis in RA

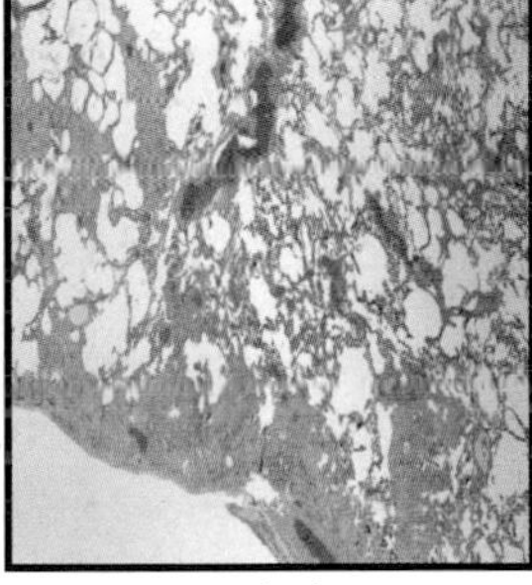

▲Histopathologic UIP pattern from a surgical lung biopsy in RA

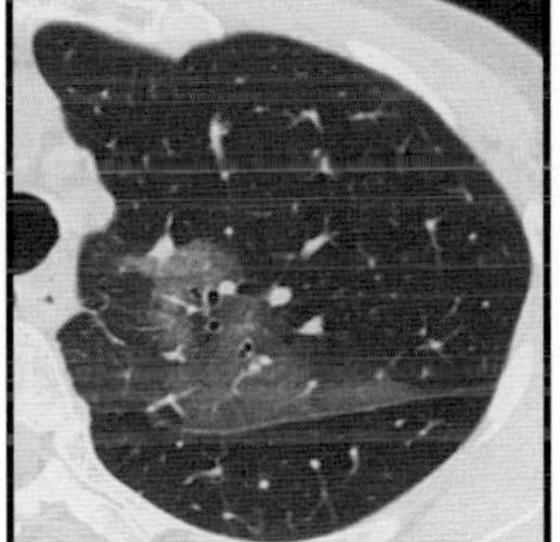

▲HRCT pattern of obliterative bronchiolitis with geographic air trapping

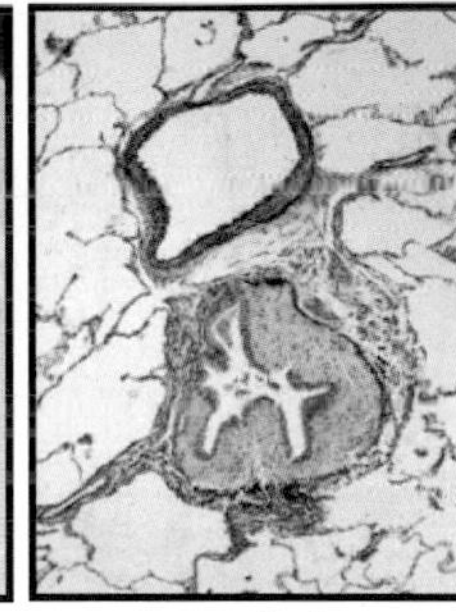

▲Histopathologic pattern of obliterative bronchiolitis. Bronchiole (*bottom*) shows considerable collagen accumulation surrounding and narrowing the lumen. The arteriole (*top*) is normal

SYSTEMIC SCLEROSIS (SCLERODERMA)

Systemic sclerosis (SSc) is a systemic autoimmune disorder that clinically involves the skin, gastrointestinal tract, musculoskeletal system, kidneys, heart, and lungs. Most patients are women in their fourth and fifth decades of life. Common presenting complaints include Raynaud phenomenon; tightening of the skin of the face, upper extremities, and thorax; dysphagia; cough; and dyspnea. A variety of clinical SSc subtypes exist; diffuse cutaneous, limited, and sine scleroderma are all defined by specific patterns of skin involvement. Some pulmonary abnormality can be identified in almost all patients, and certain phenotypes are more commonly associated with specific pulmonary complications than others. However, all known pulmonary manifestations have been described in each of the SSc subtypes, and one should not exclude a particular pulmonary disorder based solely on a clinical or serologic scleroderma phenotype.

A large number of pulmonary manifestations are recognized, with interstitial lung disease (ILD) and pulmonary hypertension being the most common as well as the leading causes of death. Chronic aspiration caused by esophageal dysmotility, airways disease, neuromuscular weakness, physiologic restriction secondary to a hide-bound chest, pleural effusions, pneumothorax, and lung cancer all cause clinically significant disease and occur commonly enough to be considered in SSc patients with respiratory symptoms. As in all connective tissue diseases (CTDs) the presence of infection or drug reaction should be an initial consideration in all patients with new or worsening respiratory signs or symptoms.

Pulmonary hypertension is the single leading cause of mortality. Although a pulmonary arteriopathy similar to that seen in idiopathic pulmonary arterial hypertension (IPAH) is the dominant mechanism, left ventricular diastolic dysfunction, chronic thromboembolic disease (generally associated with the presence of antiphospholipid antibodies), and loss of vascular bed as a consequence of ILD can all contribute. Dyspnea on exertion is the presenting symptom, and syncope is a poor prognostic sign. Chest imaging features on high-resolution computed tomography (HRCT) may give hints of pulmonary hypertension with the presence of pericardial disease, an enlarged main pulmonary artery, and mosaic attenuation. Given its ease of use, resting transthoracic echocardiography (TTE), with estimation of right ventricular systolic pressure (RVSP), is generally the first step in diagnosis; however, it regularly both overestimates and underestimates the presence or absence as well as the degree of pulmonary hypertension. When pulmonary hypertension is considered, right-sided heart catheterization remains the gold standard for diagnosis. With currently available treatments, survival rates at 1 year of 81% and at 2 years of 71% can be expected.

ILD is the most common pulmonary manifestation, with clinically significant disease observed in more than one-third of patients. Neither the extent nor severity of the skin disease correlates with the presence or severity of the pulmonary disease, and although it is seen more commonly in diffuse cutaneous disease (dcSSc), it also occurs in limited cutaneous disease (lcSSc) as well as in those without any skin involvement. Abnormalities on HRCT consistent with ILD are seen in a large majority of patients, and abnormal pulmonary physiology is reported in 45% to 100%, with a restrictive defect and a decreased diffusing capacity being the common findings. Because the most rapid decline in vital capacity occurs in the first 4 years of disease, those with a lower baseline forced vital capacity (FVC) are at higher risk of progressive lung disease. Although an isolated reduction in DL_{CO} (diffusing capacity for carbon monoxide) is an early and sensitive sign of SSc-ILD, this finding should also prompt evaluation for PH. Although bronchoalveolar lavage has been used to identify the presence of lung disease in SSc, HRCT has been found to be more sensitive. In contrast to RA and more in common with the other CTDs, nonspecific interstitial pneumonia (NSIP) is the most prevalent pathologic pattern seen on surgical lung biopsy. Treatment of patients with Ssc-ILD with cyclophosphamide has been shown to be associated with improvements in FVC, skin score, and quality of life.

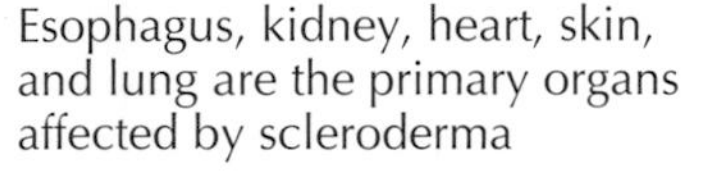
Esophagus, kidney, heart, skin, and lung are the primary organs affected by scleroderma

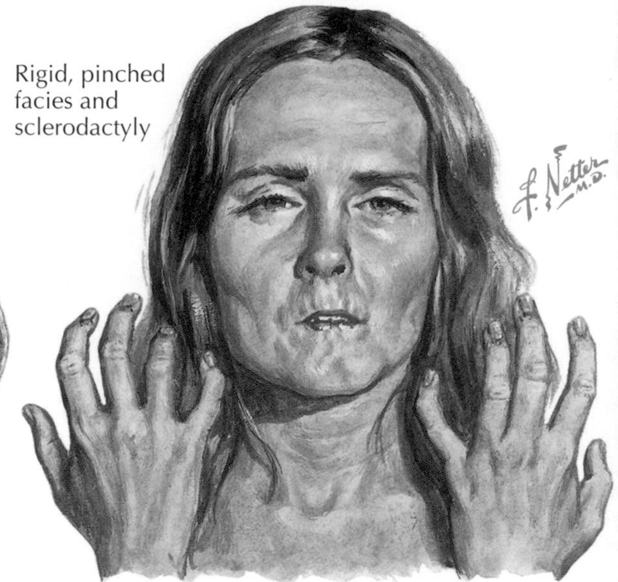

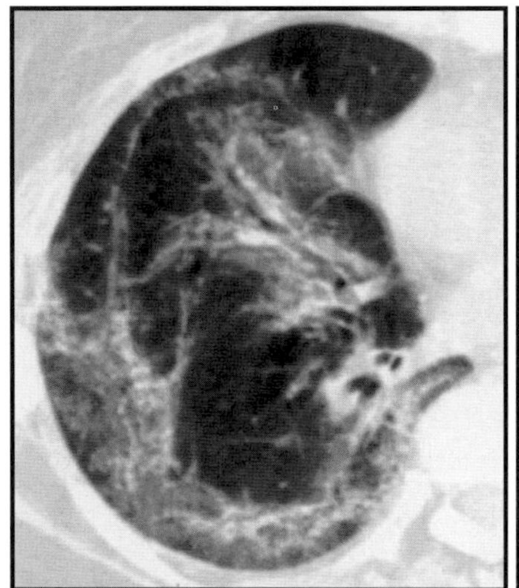
Transverse HRCT scan sections of the radiographic NSIP pattern in scleroderma

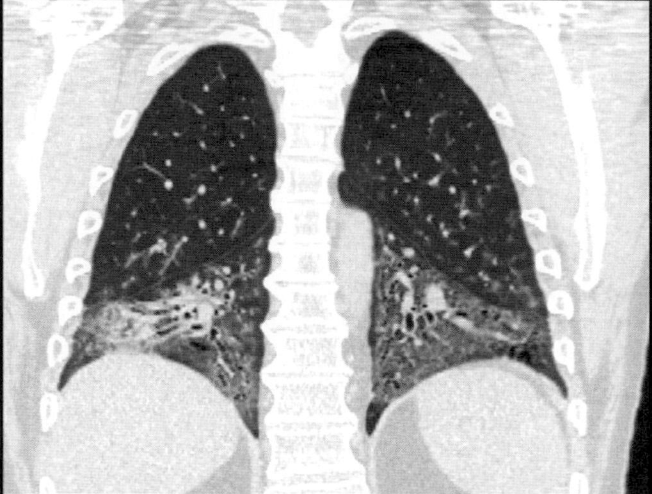
Coronal HRCT scan section of radiographic NSIP pattern highlighting the lower lobe predominance of the disease

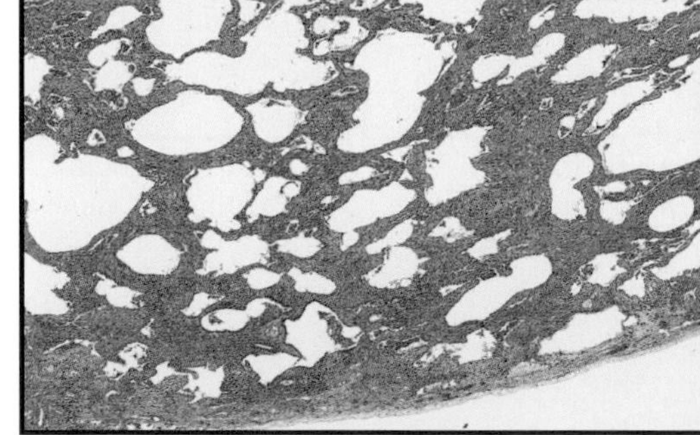
Histopathologic NSIP pattern from a surgical lung biopsy in scleroderma

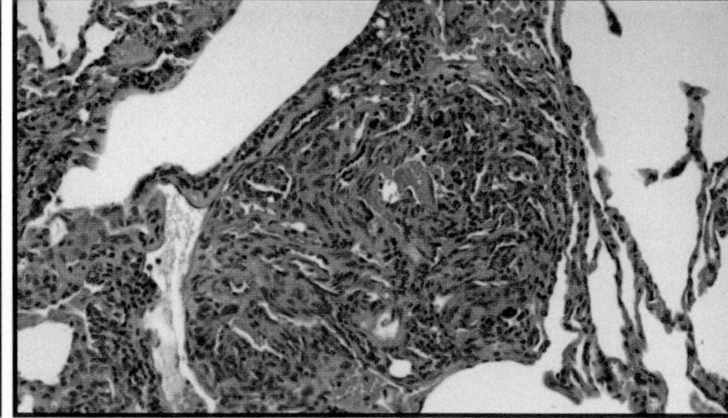
Plexiform lesion within a pulmonary artery in scleroderma-associated pulmonary hypertension

Systemic Lupus Erythematosus

Systemic lupus erythematosus (SLE) is a systemic autoinflammatory disorder that most commonly affects women of childbearing age. Hispanics and African Americans present earlier and with more active and aggressive disease than whites. When SLE is diagnosed after age 50 years, there is a lower female : male ratio; a higher incidence of neurologic, serosal, and pulmonary involvement; greater accumulated organ damage; and higher mortality.

The frequency and characteristics of pulmonary involvement depend on the clinical phenotype studied and the sensitivity of the investigative methods used. Infectious pneumonia remains the primary concern, particularly in those treated with corticosteroids or other immunomodulatory therapy, and infection should generally be the first consideration in patients presenting with new or worsening respiratory symptoms or abnormal chest imaging. Drug reactions are also important to consider because pulmonary toxicity has been noted with a number of medications commonly used to treat patients with SLE patients, including azathioprine, mycophenolate, cyclophosphamide, methotrexate, and nonsteroidal antiinflammatory drugs (NSAIDs).

Pulmonary physiologic abnormalities are common. A low diffusing capacity with or without a concomitant restrictive ventilatory defect is the most common finding. One-third or more will have isolated diffusion impairment. Airflow limitation, usually subclinical, is identified in the minority of patients. Chest imaging results are commonly abnormal. High-resolution computed tomography (HRCT) scan features of interstitial lung disease (ILD) are present in at least one-third of asymptomatic subjects with airway abnormalities seen in one-fifth. The most common abnormalities are a combination of ground-glass and reticular opacities in the middle and lower lung zones, with interlobular and intralobular lines, parenchymal bands, centrilobular nodularity, and focal consolidation less commonly observed. One-fifth of patients have otherwise unexplained mediastinal lymphadenopathy.

Pleural disease is believed to be the most common clinically relevant pulmonary manifestation. Up to one-third of patients present with pleuritis (symptoms of pleurisy with or without pleural effusion). The effusions are usually bilateral and small to moderate in size, although extremely large effusions may occur.

A variety of patterns of ILD have been described. The most common patterns observed include cellular, fibrotic, or mixed nonspecific interstitial pneumonia, although organizing pneumonia, and more rarely, diffuse amyloidosis, have been reported. Patterns of usual interstitial pneumonia and lymphoid interstitial pneumonia, particularly when secondary Sjögren syndrome is present, are also seen.

One of the more clinically severe pulmonary manifestations is diffuse alveolar hemorrhage (DAH). Respiratory failure may develop, and when it occurs, mechanical ventilation is frequently necessary. Rarely, DAH may be the presenting manifestation of SLE. Pathologic findings include intraalveolar hemorrhage and hemosiderin-laden alveolar macrophages with or without capillaritis (i.e., bland hemorrhage). A pathologic pattern of diffuse alveolar damage, with its hyaline membranes (and varying degrees of cellular interstitial infiltrates), is occasionally observed. The prognosis is variable; approximately half of patients die during their hospitalization. Survival depends on the degree of hypoxemia, the presence and severity of coincident extrapulmonary SLE manifestations, and the presence of infection. DAH can recur. Acute lupus pneumonitis is characterized by the abrupt onset of nonspecific symptoms, including dyspnea, cough, fever, pleuritic chest pain, and occasionally hemoptysis. Radiographic abnormalities are usually extensive and include diffuse ground-glass opacities and areas of consolidation. When surgical lung biopsy is performed, the histologic pattern has been described as DAD with or without alveolar hemorrhage and capillaritis.

The prevalence of pulmonary arterial hypertension in patients with SLE is unknown but is lower than that seen in scleroderma. In shrinking lung syndrome, patients present with dyspnea and elevated diaphragms on chest imaging. Measurement of transdiaphragmatic pressure suggests weakness as the cause. Progression is uncommon. With treatment, diaphragmatic motion may not normalize, and if it happens, it occurs only after several weeks of therapy.

Antiphospholipid antibodies (aPLs) are a family of acquired autoantibodies that bind serum proteins such as prothrombin, various protein-phospholipid complexes, and β-2 glycoprotein I. They can be found in up to two-thirds of SLE patients and are associated with vascular thrombosis; pregnancy morbidity; and several nonthrombotic intrathoracic complications, including PAH, DAH, adult respiratory distress syndrome, and cardiac valvular lesions. The two most well known and clinically important are the lupus anticoagulant (LA) and anticardiolipin antibodies (aCLs). Antiphospholipid syndrome (APS) refers to the combination of clinically important vascular events and the presence of the LA or aCL. Clinically significant small vessel occlusion in three or more organs may occur, a scenario referred to as *catastrophic APS* (CAPS). CAPS is often associated with physiologic stressors such as infection, neoplasm, and surgery. Respiratory failure is common, and mortality rates approach 50%. Lifelong anticoagulation is required, but recurrent thrombosis is common.

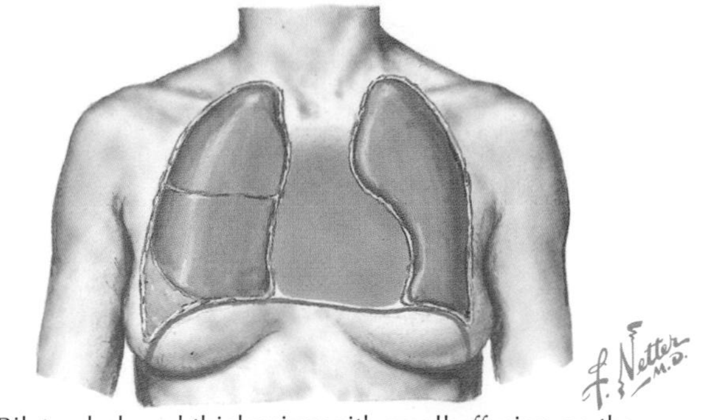

Bilateral pleural thickening with small effusion on the right. Globular cardiac silhouette suggests pericardial or cardiac involvement.

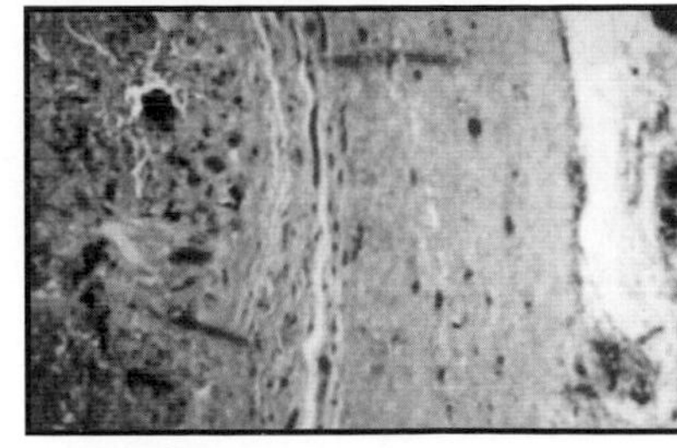
Marked pleural thickening with underlying pulmonary fibrosis.

Patogenesis of lupus (LE) cells and rosettes

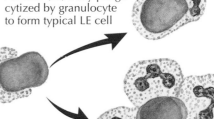

Polymorphonuclear leukocyte

Nucleus homogenized by LE factor (antinuclear antibody)

Homogenized nucleus extruded to form free nuclear (LE) body

Nuclear (LE) body phagocytized by granulocyte to form typical LE cell

Nuclear body encircled by granulocytes to form LE rosette

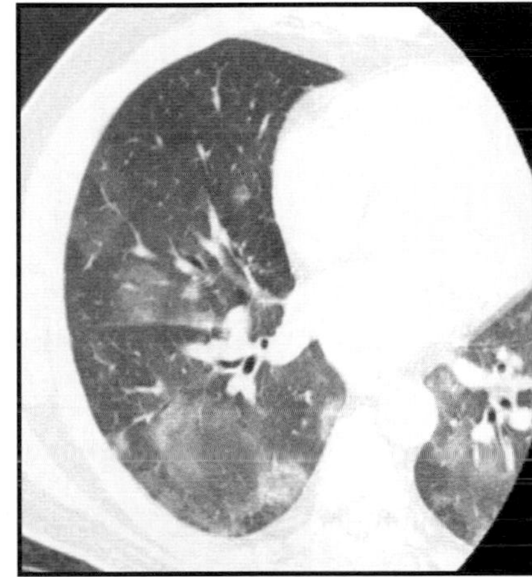
HRCT scan section of diffuse alveolar hemorrhage.

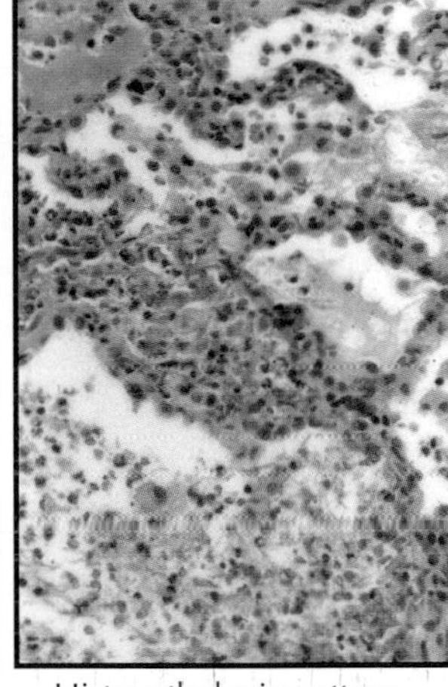
Histopathologic pattern of pulmonary capillaritis.

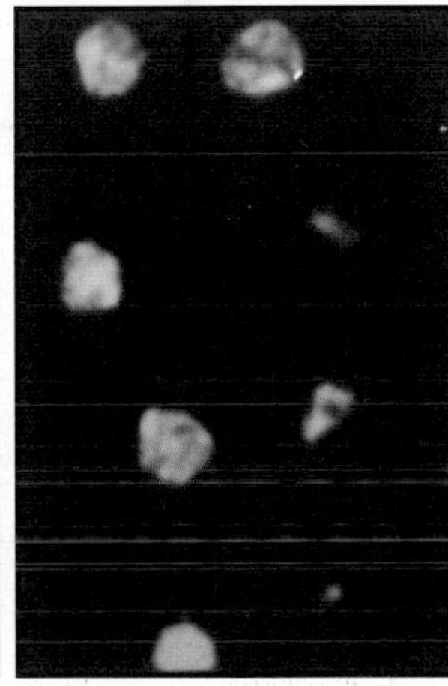
Antinuclear antibodies demonstrated by fluorescence.

Dermatomyositis and Polymyositis

Polymyositis and dermatomyositis are two of the idiopathic inflammatory myopathies, a group of rare systemic autoinflammatory disorders of unknown cause. They are characterized by proximal muscle weakness (most patients present with the subacute onset of weakness and myalgias), increased serum skeletal muscle enzymes, characteristic electromyography abnormalities, and the presence of inflammatory cell infiltrates in muscle tissue. Patients with dermatomyositis are defined by the additional presence of an exanthem, most commonly a purple discoloration of the eyelids (heliotrope rash) or a symmetric, palpable, erythematous rash over the extensor surfaces of the metacarpophalangeal and proximal interphalangeal joints of the fingers (Gottron papules). Extramuscular organ involvement is common, particularly the skin, joints, and lungs.

Pulmonary complications are a major cause of morbidity and mortality. These can be either primarily associated with the underlying autoinflammatory disorder or secondary to the muscle weakness. As with all autoimmune disorders, drug-induced disease and infection should always be an early consideration. Myositis specific findings include hypoventilation, aspiration pneumonia, and interstitial lung disease (ILD).

Hypoventilation and respiratory failure as a result of respiratory muscle weakness has been thought of as uncommon but has been reported in up to 20% of patients. There is often an associated reduction in the cough reflex with resulting basilar atelectasis and the inability to clear airway secretions. Both occur in patients with severe generalized weakness of the inspiratory and expiratory respiratory muscles. Chest imaging reveals small lung volumes, bibasilar infiltrates, and elevation of the diaphragm. Pulmonary physiology demonstrates reduced total lung capacity (TLC) with an increased residual volume, reduced forced vital capacity (FVC), and a preserved forced expiratory volume in 1 second (FEV_1) and FEV_1/FVC ratio. Maximal inspiratory and expiratory pressures are reduced. Aspiration pneumonia is also described in up to 20% of patients and is more common in patients with extensive muscle and skin disease. It is caused by pharyngeal and upper esophageal dysfunction of striated muscle with a loss of the normal swallowing mechanism and regurgitation. Not surprisingly, half of these patients have symptomatic dysphagia.

ILD has been reported in up to two-thirds of patients, depending on patient selection and the chosen diagnostic methods, and not all patients with identified abnormalities are symptomatic. Antisynthetase antibodies are found in most patients, and the presence of positive antiaminoacyl tRNA synthetase antibodies, of which the antihistidyl tRNA synthetase antibody (anti-Jo-1) is the most common, is frequently found. Similar to the other autoimmune disorders, the ILD may precede, appear simultaneously, or develop after the onset the muscle disease. Its presentation may be acute, chronic, and progressive or asymptomatic with only chest imaging abnormalities. Cough and dyspnea are the typical presenting symptoms. A restrictive ventilatory impairment with decreased TLC, functional residual capacity, residual volume, FEV_1, and FVC and reduced DL_{CO} (diffusing capacity for carbon monoxide) are generally seen. Chest imaging with high-resolution computed tomography (HRCT) is the most sensitive test for the detection of ILD and provides a description of the pattern and extent of the disease. The chest imaging patterns are identical to those found in idiopathic interstitial pneumonias with nonspecific interstitial pneumonia and organizing pneumonia patterns the most common. The natural history of ILD in myositis is not well understood but is considered to be a major risk factor for premature death. The pulmonary abnormalities associated with antisynthetase antibodies appear to show a clinically relevant response to immunosuppressive therapy.

Periorbital heliotrope discoloration and edema

Difficulty in swallowing caused by pharyngeal muscle weakness may lead to aspiration pneumonia

Weakness of diaphragm and intercostal muscle causes respiratory insufficiency or failure

Weakness of central muscle groups evidenced by difficulty in climbing stairs, rising from chairs, combing hair, and so on

Erythematous or violaceous scaly papules on dorsum of interphalangeal joints

F. Netter M.D.

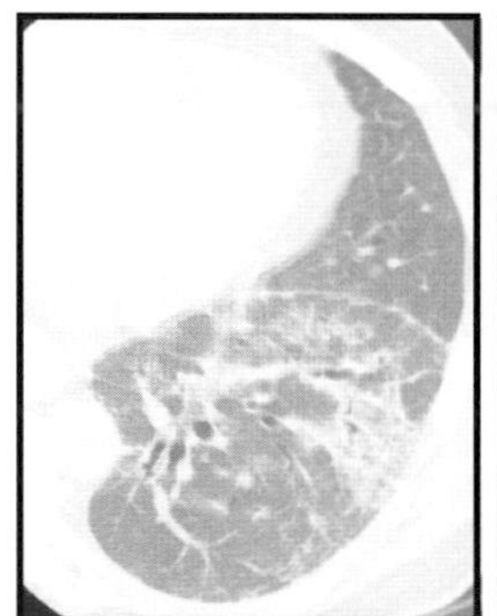
HRCT scan radiographic pattern of organizing pneumonia

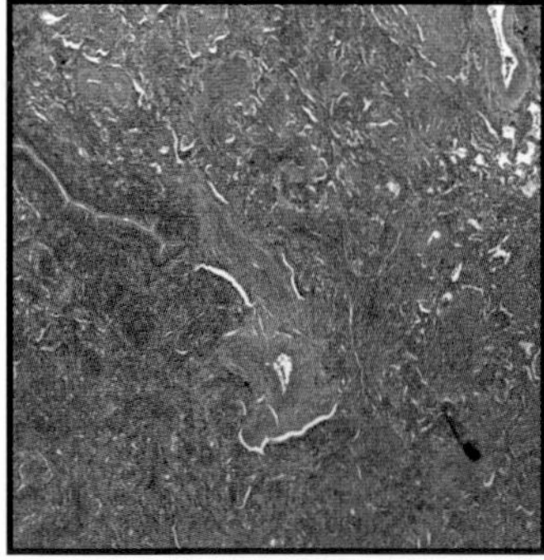
Histopathologic pattern of organizing pneumonia

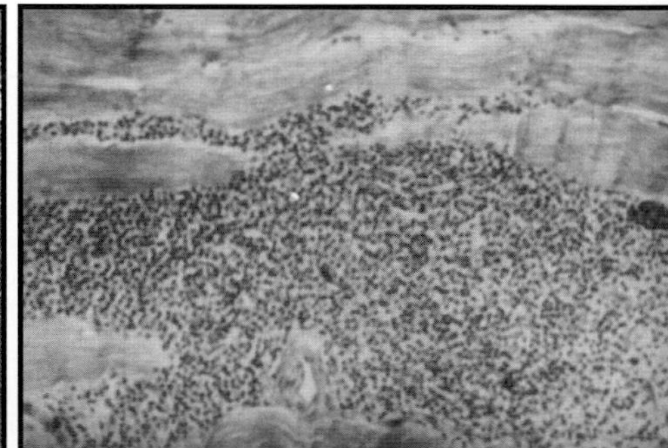
Longitudinal section of muscle showing intense inflammatory infiltration plus degeneration and disruption of muscle fibers

Pulmonary Vasculitis

The term *pulmonary vasculitis* describes a number of distinct disorders that are clinically and pathologically characterized by the destruction of blood vessels. Their diagnosis requires the identification of specific patterns of clinical, radiologic, laboratory, and pathologic abnormalities. Lung involvement is most commonly seen with the primary, idiopathic, small vessel, or antineutrophil cytoplasmic antibody (ANCA)–associated vasculitides: Wegener granulomatosis (WG), microscopic polyangiitis (MPA), and Churg-Strauss syndrome (CSS). However, primary, idiopathic medium and large vessel vasculitis, primary immune complex–mediated vasculitis, and secondary vasculitis may all present with lung involvement.

Vasculitis can be pathologically defined by the presence of cellular infiltration, vessel destruction, and associated tissue necrosis. The clinical features of each disease are determined by the site, size, and type of vessel involved and by the relative amounts of reversible cellular infiltration, vessel destruction, and tissue necrosis. The large vessels include the aorta and its largest branches (clinically affecting the extremities and head/neck). The medium-sized vessels refer to the main visceral arteries (e.g., renal, hepatic, coronary, mesenteric). The small vessels are the capillaries, venules, and arterioles.

Particular combinations of findings or clinical scenarios should suggest the possibility of vasculitis. These scenarios include diffuse alveolar hemorrhage (DAH), destructive upper airway lesions, cavitary or nodular disease on chest imaging, rapidly progressive glomerulonephritis (RPGN), palpable purpura on the skin, mononeuritis multiplex, pulmonary-renal syndromes, and other multisystem diseases. DAH occurs when the blood leaking from capillaries fills the alveolar space. Although hemoptysis, diffuse alveolar infiltrates, and a decrease in hematocrit are common, up to one-third of patients do not have hemoptysis, the alveolar infiltrates can be unilateral, and a decrease in hematocrit or hemoglobin can be difficult to document. DAH can be diagnosed with bronchoalveolar lavage as serially aspirated aliquots of fluid reveal a persistently bloody return. DAH is seen both with pathologic capillaritis (a cellular infiltrate of neutrophils in the capillaries and venules) and with normal vessels (bland hemorrhage). Destructive upper airway lesions include otherwise unexplained chronic refractory sinusitis, epistaxis, otitis, and significant ulcerative or destructive soft tissue or bony lesions. On chest imaging, a wide variety of nonspecific abnormalities may be seen. In particular, the presence of otherwise unexplained nodular or cavitary disease should raise one's suspicion. Nodular disease is found in 55% to 70% and cavitary disease in 35% to 50% of patients with WG. Clinically significant abnormalities in multiple organ systems either simultaneously or over time should raise suspicion. The most common example is the pulmonary-renal syndrome, which generally refers to patients with DAH and RPGN.

The ANCA-associated vasculitides, WG, CSS, and MPA, are grouped together because of common clinical features, pathologic involvement of the small vessels, similar responses to immunosuppressive interventions, and the common but not universal presence of ANCA positivity. Three indirect immunofluorescent staining patterns, cytoplasmic ANCA (C-ANCA), perinuclear ANCA (P-ANCA), and atypical ANCA, are described. Each pattern is associated with antibodies against intracellular antigen(s) found in neutrophils and monocytes.

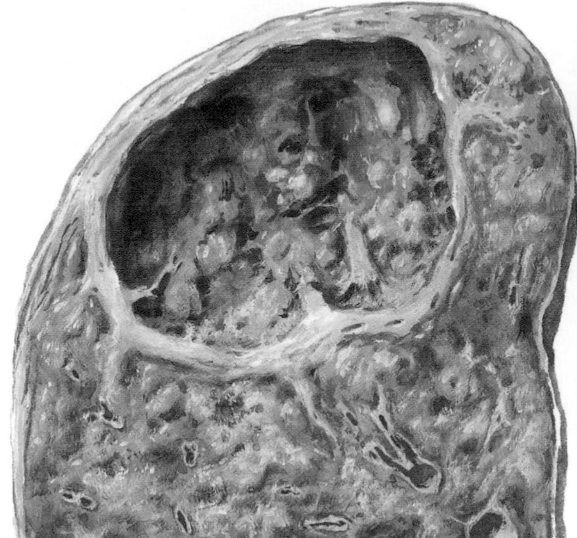

Wegener granulomatosis. Cavity in upper lobe of right lung lined with necrotic material

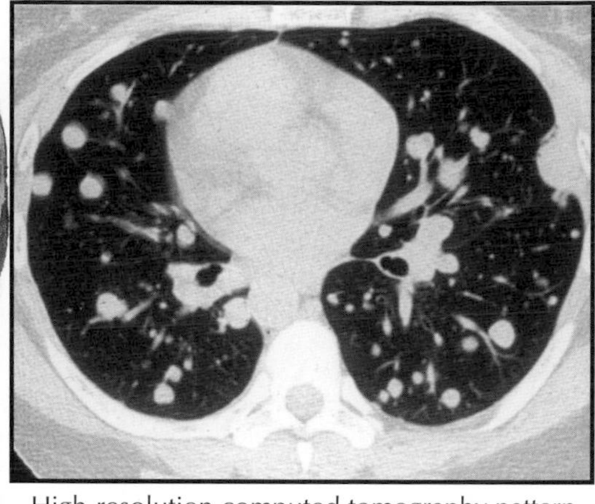

High-resolution computed tomography pattern of multiple, bilateral pulmonary nodules in Wegener granulomatosis.

Wegener granuloma. With giant cells (*arrow*)

Clinical manifestations of Wegener granulomatosis

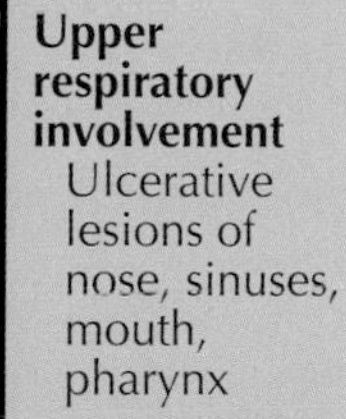

Upper respiratory involvement
Ulcerative lesions of nose, sinuses, mouth, pharynx

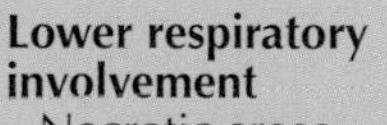

Lower respiratory involvement
Necrotic areas and cavitation in lungs; cough; dyspnea; hemoptysis; chest pain
F. Netter M.D.

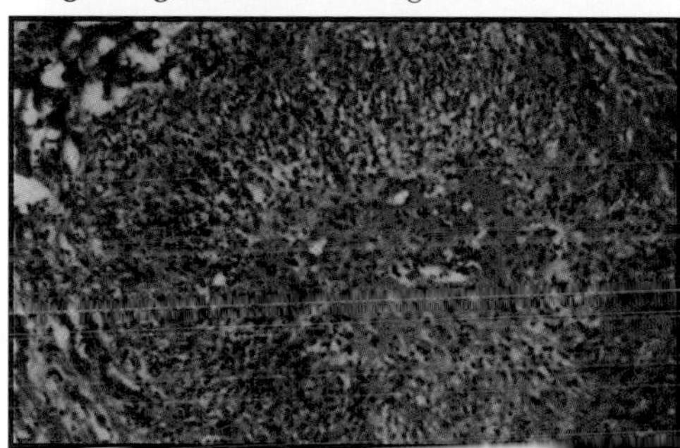

Severe arteritis. With destruction of vessel wall in Wegener granulomatosis

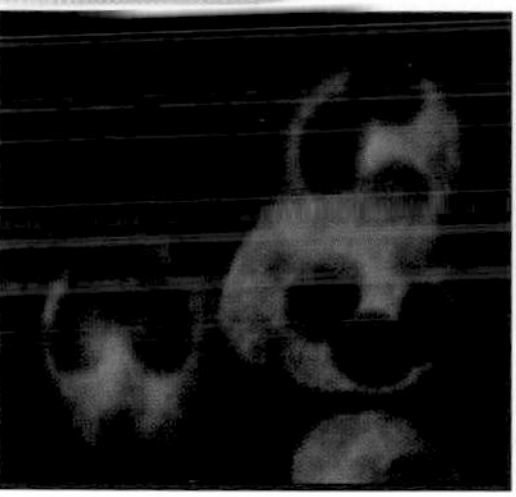

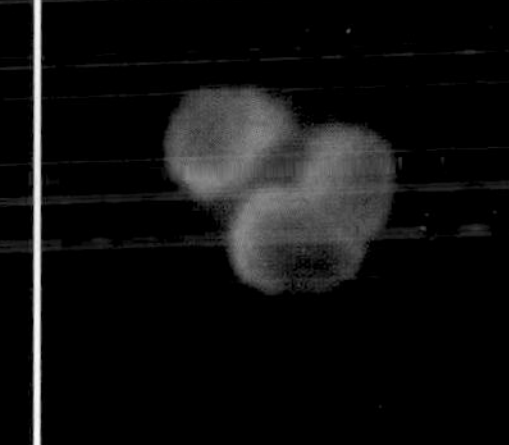

c-ANCA and p-ANCA staining pattern on left and right, respectively

With a number of caveats, C-ANCA is highly sensitive for active, systemic WG, with a specificity of approximately 90%. On the other hand, a positive P-ANCA lacks sensitivity and can be found in a wide variety of settings.

WG is the most common of the ANCA-associated vasculitides and is characterized by the triad of upper airway disease, lower respiratory tract disease, and glomerulonephritis. Pathologically, WG is characterized by a necrotizing vasculitis of the small and medium vessels, granulomatous inflammation, and geographic parenchymal necrosis. CSS is characterized by a triad of asthma, hypereosinophilia, and necrotizing vasculitis. There is also a three-phase presentation with an initial atopy, sinusitis, and asthma phase followed by an eosinophilic phase and then the vasculitic phase. ANCA positivity is less frequently seen than in WG. Pathologically, a necrotizing, small vessel vasculitis and an eosinophil-rich cellular infiltrate with necrotizing granulomas are seen. MPA is a clinicopathologic syndrome with essentially universal glomerulonephritis, although pulmonary involvement (DAH with pathologic capillaritis is the most common) is seen in up to 30% of patients. Pathologically, a focal, segmental necrotizing vasculitis and a mixed inflammatory infiltrate without granulomata are seen.

The goals of therapy in systemic vasculitis are focused on the early identification of disease or relapse, the prevention of disease-related mortality and morbidity, and the minimization of treatment-related complications. Before the institution of immunosuppressive therapy, the mortality rate of patients with systemic vasculitis was 75%, with a median survival of 5 months. The major breakthrough occurred when cyclophosphamide was added to corticosteroids, and this lowered the 5-year mortality to 12%.

Eosinophilic Pneumonia

Several pulmonary disorders are characterized by an abnormally elevated number of eosinophils in lung tissue, sputum, bronchoalveolar lavage (BAL) fluid, or peripheral blood. Because of overlapping clinical features, it can be difficult to distinguish among them. The first step in classification is to distinguish among primary pulmonary disorders and those in which the eosinophilia is secondary. For this, the importance of a detailed history cannot be overemphasized. In particular, the presence of pharmacologic, occupational, and environmental exposures, as well as details of family and travel history are crucial. Among the primary pulmonary eosinophilic disorders, acute and chronic eosinophilic pneumonia are the most common.

Acute eosinophilic pneumonia (AEP) is characterized by fevers, acute respiratory failure that often requires mechanical ventilation over days, diffuse pulmonary infiltrates, and pulmonary eosinophilia in a previously healthy individual. At presentation, it is often mistaken for overwhelming community-acquired pneumonia or acute lung injury without multisystem organ failure. Men between the ages of 20 and 40 years are most commonly affected. Although no clear cause has been identified, several reports have linked it to environmental exposures such as the initiation of tobacco smoking. The predominant chest symptoms are cough, dyspnea, and pleuritic chest pain. Constitutional symptoms of malaise, myalgias, and night sweats are common. Physical examination findings include fever and coarse crackles on chest auscultation. A key to establishing a diagnosis is the presence of more than 25% eosinophilia in BAL fluid. Lung biopsies show eosinophilic infiltration with acute and organizing diffuse alveolar damage. Oddly, peripheral blood eosinophilia is distinctly uncommon on presentation but often occurs 1 to 4 weeks after disease onset. Chest imaging is diffusely abnormal with high-resolution computed tomography (HRCT) showing bilateral random, patchy, ground-glass, or reticular opacities and small pleural effusions in up to two-thirds of patients. The effusions are also eosinophilic. If able to be performed, pulmonary physiology reveals a restrictive ventilatory defect with a reduced diffusion capacity. Most patients require admission to an intensive care unit with assisted ventilation. However, they are generally exquisitely responsive to corticosteroids within days of initiation of therapy and have an excellent prognosis with complete clinical recovery and without recurrence.

Chronic eosinophilic pneumonia (CEP) is characterized by both pulmonary and peripheral blood eosinophilia and is a much more indolent syndrome than AEP. The common patient is more often a woman in her mid-forties with asthma and atopy. Unlike AEP, acute respiratory failure is extremely rare, and patients present over weeks to months rather than days. Respiratory symptoms of cough, wheezing, and progressive dyspnea are the rule, and constitutional symptoms of low-grade fever, flulike symptoms, weight loss, and night sweats are common. Extrapulmonary diseases such as arthralgias, neuropathy, and skin disease are uncommon, and their presence suggests Churg-Strauss syndrome or hypereosinophilic syndrome (HES). Chest imaging is abnormal with bilateral, peripheral, often pleural-based opacities that are frequently migratory. This "photographic-negative pulmonary edema" imaging pattern on plain chest radiography and chest CT is considered diagnostic of CEP, but it is present in no more than 25% of patients. Peripheral blood and BAL eosinophilia are the rule. In more than 90% of patients, eosinophils account for about 30% of the total white blood cells in the peripheral blood and 60% of the cells in the BAL. IgE levels are almost always increased, as are the erythrocyte sedimentation rate and C-reactive protein. Lung pathology reveals an accumulation of eosinophils and histiocytes in the airspace and interstitium as well as focal areas of organizing pneumonia. Treatment is with corticosteroids, and the response is often prompt (within 48 hours) and dramatic with complete resolution of symptoms and laboratory and chest imaging abnormalities. However, unlike AEP, relapse is common with more than 50% of patients recurring with a reduction in the steroid dose. Many require therapy for 6 months or longer.

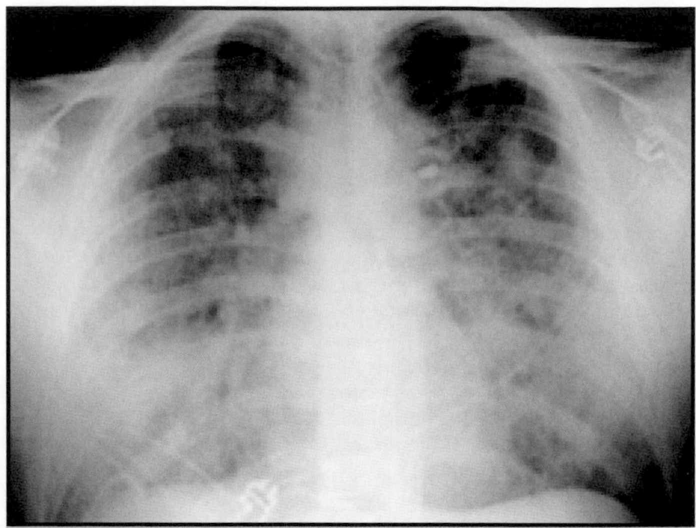
Plain chest radiograph of acute eosinophilic pneumonia

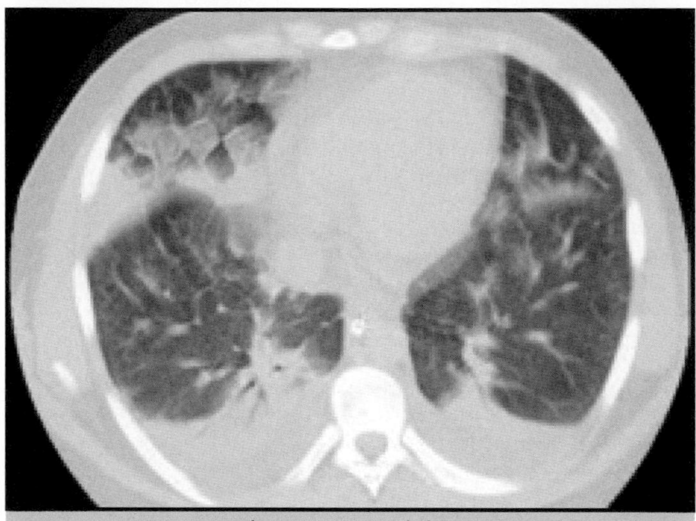
HRCT scan of acute eosinophilic pneumonia

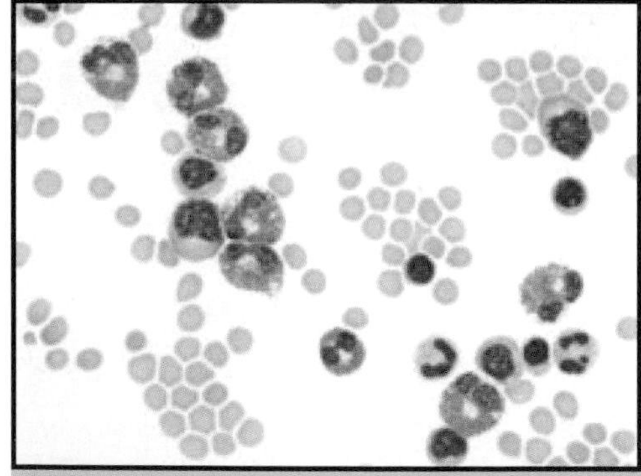
BAL cytology in with multiple eosinophils in eosinophilic pneumonia

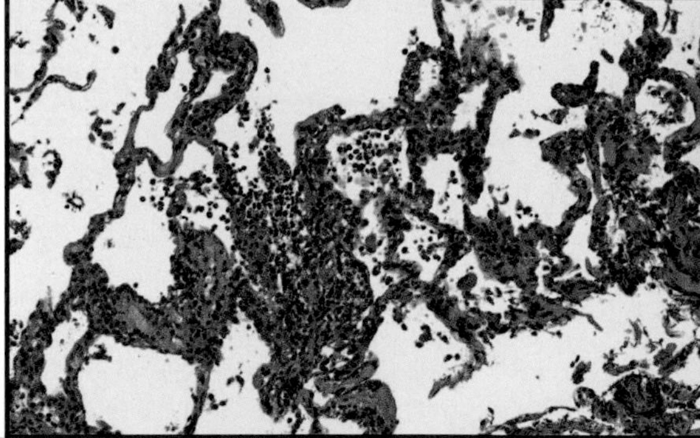
Histopathologic pattern in eosphilic pneumonia

Pulmonary Manifestations of Other Diseases

The lung is commonly affected by diseases of other organs and may be where the first manifestations of disease become apparent. The susceptibility of the lung in being affected by diseases of other organs is perhaps because of its capillary network that filters the blood, the intricate alveolar structure, and the lung's highly developed immunology.

Common examples of pulmonary disease caused by disease primarily of other organ systems are pleural effusion, pulmonary edema, lung restriction, and pulmonary vascular disease. Pleural effusions may be seen in heart failure, hypothyroidism, renal failure, and immunologic disease such as systemic lupus erythematosus. Acute respiratory distress syndrome may occur after sepsis and trauma or in association with pregnancy, such as with tocolytic therapy (treatment to inhibit premature labor) or with amniotic fluid embolism. Restrictive lung disease may be caused by extrapulmonary diseases such as muscular weakness; motor neuron disease and postpolio syndrome are examples. Restriction may also be caused by chest wall disease such as kyphoscoliosis. The pulmonary vasculature may be affected by emboli of tumor arising from malignancy, of fat after major trauma, and of amniotic fluid during parturition. The following discussion reviews in more detail lung manifestations of inflammatory bowel disease, hepatic disease, and pulmonary complications associated with hematopoietic stem cell transplantation (HSCT).

PULMONARY MANIFESTATIONS OF INFLAMMATORY BOWEL DISEASE

Lung disease associated with ulcerative colitis and Crohn disease has only recently been recognized. The manifestations are those of inflammation of the airways from the glottis to the terminal airways and disease of the lung parenchyma. The lung's embryologic origin from the foregut makes it attractive that there may be inflammatory linkages between the gut and the lung. The most common comorbid diseases reported in inflammatory bowel disease (IBD) are asthma or bronchitis and arthritis. Disease in airways may cause typical symptoms of airways disease, including cough; dyspnea or wheeze; and purulent sputum production, particularly if bronchiectasis is present. A very wide range of airways and parenchymal lung diseases has been reported to occur in association with IBD with a high prevalence of pulmonary function abnormalities being present in patients who have Crohn disease or ulcerative colitis. Up to two-thirds of patients with IBD have abnormal pulmonary function and one-quarter have a reduction in DLco.

Parenchymal inflammation may also be present in IBD patients and is manifest by lung infiltrates or opacities with varying patterns. More recently, high-resolution computed tomography (HRCT) findings have been described. These include evidence of small airways disease with expiratory CT images showing mosaic perfusion, and "tree-in-bud" opacities suggesting bronchiolitis or bronchiolectasis, bronchiectasis, and restrictive disease, with reticular infiltrates and appearances of fibrosis similar to idiopathic pulmonary fibrosis. The histologic abnormalities include organizing pneumonia and nonspecific interstitial pneumonia. Interstitial lung disease may also be seen in association with drug toxicity from medications used to treat IBD, such as sulfasalazine and mesalazine.

PULMONARY MANIFESTATIONS OF LIVER DISEASE: HEPATOPULMONARY SYNDROME

In the presence of severe liver disease, hepatopulmonary syndrome is present when there is clinical evidence of intrapulmonary shunt causing severe hypoxemia on exclusion of other causes of hypoxemia. Orthodeoxia and platypnea (i.e., worsening oxygen desaturation and breathlessness on assuming upright posture) are very common when hypoxia is severe.

In severe cases, a clinical picture of right-to-left shunt can be demonstrated by technetium-99m-labeled macroaggregated albumin scanning, in which radioactivity can be detected in the brain or liver after venous injection, reflecting the escape of the aggregates from the pulmonary vascular bed. Pulmonary and systemic vascular resistances are low with a hyperdynamic circulation present. The DLco is often reduced in the presence of normal lung volumes, and no airway obstruction is seen on pulmonary function testing.

Pulmonary vascular dilatations have been described in the vascular bed and on the pleural surface on histology and on pulmonary angiography, most of which occur near the gas-exchanging units, which causes hypoxemia. Interestingly, the presence of spider nevi appears to be associated with the syndrome. The capillaries themselves may have thickened walls, which further impair gas exchange. Anatomic arteriovenous malformations, however, are generally not found by either CT pulmonary angiography or formal right-sided heart catheterization pulmonary angiography.

The pathophysiology of the hepatopulmonary syndrome is that of vascular dilatation, presumably related to humoral abnormalities associated with severe liver disease. Nitric oxide–mediated mechanisms have been postulated to be the molecular basis of vascular dilatation and loss of hypoxic pulmonary

PULMONARY MANIFESTATIONS OF OTHER DISEASES *(Continued)*

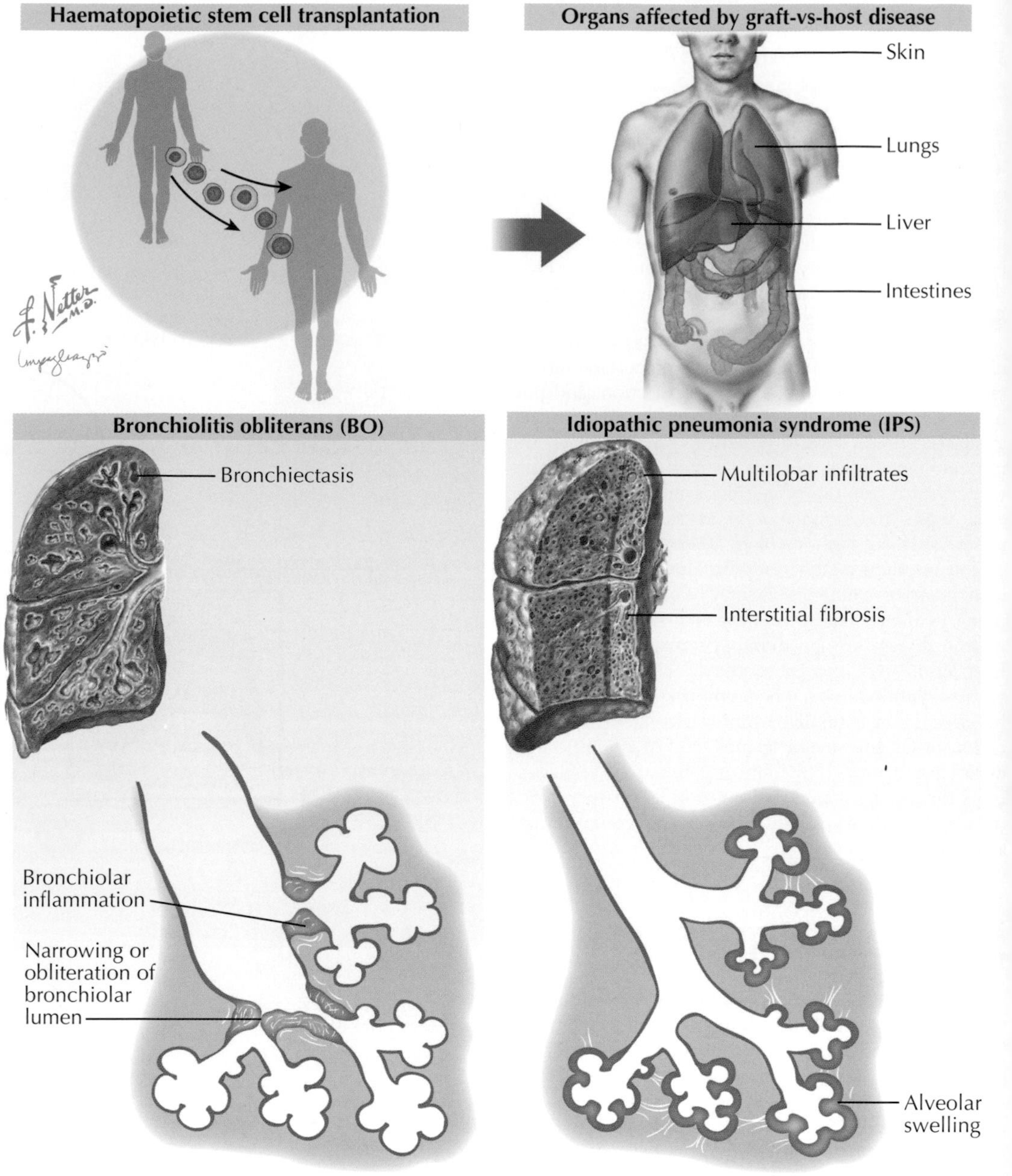

vasoconstriction. The mechanism of the hypoxia is multifactorial, but the dominant causes are ventilation/perfusion (V/Q) mismatch with an increase in low V/Q units, right-to-left shunting, and a "diffusion-perfusion" defect. The presence of dilated blood vessels at the precapillary and capillary levels along with an impaired hypoxic pulmonary vasoconstrictor response is the basis of the increase in low V/Q units and shunt. The combination of dilated vessels and increased cardiac output has been postulated to cause the "diffusion-perfusion" defect via an increased diffusion distance from the alveolus to the red blood cell with reduced transit time allowing insufficient time for equilibration.

Supportive treatment, particularly supplementary oxygen therapy, is the mainstay of management with no specific treatment aimed at altering the underlying hemodynamic abnormalities having been shown to be effective. The only effective treatment has been liver transplantation.

PULMONARY COMPLICATIONS AFTER HEMATOPOIETIC STEM CELL TRANSPLANTATION: BRONCHIOLITIS OBLITERANS AND IDIOPATHIC PNEUMONIA SYNDROME

HSCT is increasingly used to treat patients with a variety of hematologic and solid organ malignancies after high-dose radiation and chemotherapy, which has a side effect of ablating the bone marrow. It has also been used to treat nonmalignant hematologic disorders such as aplastic anemia and congenital immune deficiency syndromes. Subsequent to the initial few months after transplantation, when the pulmonary side effects are infection and drug toxicity, the most important long-term side effect of HSCT is graft-versus-host disease (GVHD).

The most common pulmonary manifestation of graft-versus-host disease is bronchiolitis obliterans, in which there is narrowing and obliteration of the bronchiolar lumen caused by peribronchiolar inflammation and fibrosis. Thus, rather than inflammatory infiltrate and fibrosis filling the lumen, airway narrowing and obstruction are caused by extrinsic constriction of the airway. This distinguishes bronchiolitis obliterans from cryptogenic organizing pneumonia, and it is therefore also known as *constricted bronchiolitis*. The severity and type of bronchiolar inflammation can be heterogeneous, ranging from acute to chronic inflammation but also eosinophilic inflammation being described. Fibrosis may be present in the subepithelial layer or the adventitial layer or may involve the entire thickness of the airway wall. Bronchiolitis obliterans is more commonly seen in allogeneic transplant recipients because GVHD is much more common in these patients compared with patients receiving autologous transplants. It can occur in up to 26% of patients with an incidence of approximately 10% per year.

Typical symptoms of bronchiolitis obliterans are dry cough, shortness of breath, and wheezing in conjunction with airway obstruction on spirometry. The diagnosis of bronchiolitis obliterans can be made clinically by the presence of typical symptoms and airway obstruction developing in a HSCT recipient, having excluded other causes of obstruction. Bronchoscopy with bronchoalveolar lavage is used to exclude infectious causes. Transbronchial biopsy has a low yield because of heterogeneous distribution of disease throughout the lung.

Treatment of patients with this disease remains a challenge. The presence of airflow obstruction is a significant risk factor for mortality in transplant recipients. The 10-year survival rate of patients with airflow obstruction is approximately 50% compared with at least 80% in those without obstruction. Currently, there is no convincing evidence that any treatment can alter the natural history of bronchiolitis obliterans complicating HSCT, although treatment with azithromycin may be promising. For any improvements to occur in the currently poor prognosis of patients with bronchiolitis obliterans, it is clear that early detection of small airways disease is required using sensitive, noninvasive tests. Spirometry is considered to be an insensitive indicator of small airways disease, and tests of ventilation distribution may prove to be sufficiently sensitive to detect early disease and allow earlier intervention.

Another pulmonary complication of HSCT is idiopathic pneumonia syndrome (IPS). IPS generally occurs days to weeks after HSCT but may occur many months afterward. IPS occurs in up to 15% of recipients. It has a high mortality rate with approximately 75% of patients dying from the disease.

The criteria for the diagnosis of the syndrome have been documented from a National Institutes of Health workshop. It is defined by evidence of widespread alveolar injury with (1) multilobar infiltrates on chest radiography or CT; (2) symptoms and signs of pneumonia; (3) evidence of abnormal physiology; and (4) absence of active lower respiratory tract infection from invasive sampling for bacteria, fungi, viruses (cytomegalovirus [CMV], respiratory syncytial virus, influenza virus, parainfluenza virus, and adenovirus), and *Pneumocystis jiroveci*.

A common histologic finding is that of interstitial pneumonitis or diffuse alveolar damage. The cause may be immunologic because it is strongly associated with acute GVHD; however, injury from radiation and drug-related conditioning and occult infection with CMV or metapneumovirus are also possible.

Sleep Medicine

Although we spend almost one-third of our lives asleep, very little time is spent in training health care workers about sleep. Primary disorders of sleep such as sleep apnea can significantly worsen quality of life and may increase mortality. Other medical disorders can worsen during sleep, such as chronic obstructive pulmonary disease, asthma, angina, or cardiac arrhythmias, leading to adverse consequences. Work and family demands often force individuals to sleep less or sleep at times of the day when their body wants to be awake.

There are 79 described primary sleep disorders. These include: (1) sleep-related breathing disorders (e.g., obstructive sleep apnea), (2) insomnia disorders, (3) parasomnias (e.g., somnambulism or REM [rapid eye movement] sleep behavior disorder), (4) circadian rhythm disorders (e.g., delayed sleep phase), (5) sleep-related movement disorders (e.g., restless legs syndrome or periodic limb movement disorder), and (6) hypersomnia disorders (e.g., narcolepsy). Some of these disorders can be diagnosed using a sleep-related history, including sleep logs or diaries and physical examination. However, many patients with sleep complaints often require formal sleep testing in the form of a polysomnogram (PSG) or sleep study.

PSG is the monitoring of physiologic signals from various organs and transduction of those signals to a recording device. PSGs can record 20 physiologic signals or more. Electroencephalographic leads are a necessary part of a PSG and are placed on the scalp based on the International 10/20 system. Electrooculographic (EOG) leads are placed slightly above and slightly below the outer canthus of each eye and referenced to an inert electrode placed behind the ear. Chin (genioglossus) electromyogram (EMG) leads are placed over the front of the chin, under the chin, or over the masseter muscle, and these are referenced to each other. Leg EMG leads are placed over the anterior tibialis muscles. A modified lead II of a standard electrocardiogram is used to monitor the heart signal.

For monitoring respiratory airflow, most sleep laboratories use either or both a nasal thermistor and a nasal cannula pressure transducer (NCPT). The thermistor works by sensing changes in temperature during ventilation. The NCPT measures the pressure change across the nasal inlet using a pressure-sensitive transducer and is more sensitive than temperature-based sensors. Currently, most sleep laboratories use both sensors.

Respiratory effort is usually measured with respiratory inductance plethysmography or impedance pneumography. Pulse oximetry is used to monitor oxygen saturation continuously throughout the night.

PSGs are usually conducted for one entire night. The studies are then "scored" using standardized criteria that define sleep stages (NREM [non–rapid eye movement] stage 1, NREM stage 2, NREM stage 3, and REM), respiratory events, limb movements, and cardiac events. From each PSG, one can determine sleep architecture, the presence of sleep-disordered breathing events, cardiac arrhythmias, and other sleep disruptions that may help explain the patient's sleep complaint.

Another common sleep test performed in a sleep center is a multiple sleep latency test (MSLT). An MSLT is usually performed the day after an overnight PSG and consists of a series of daytime naps, the first performed 2 hours after the completion of the PSG and subsequently every 2 hours thereafter. A total of four or five naps are performed, and they last for 20 to 35 minutes. The purpose of performing an MSLT is to determine objectively how sleepy someone is using the length of time it takes to fall asleep for the naps (mean sleep latency) and to assess whether the patient enters REM sleep during the naps. The presence of two or more naps with REM sleep is suggestive of narcolepsy in the appropriate clinic circumstance.

Electroculogram
Airflow sensor
Chin EMG
ECG
Effort belts
Pulse oximetry

Preparation of an awake patient for a PSG study to follow. EEG monitors have not yet been applied.

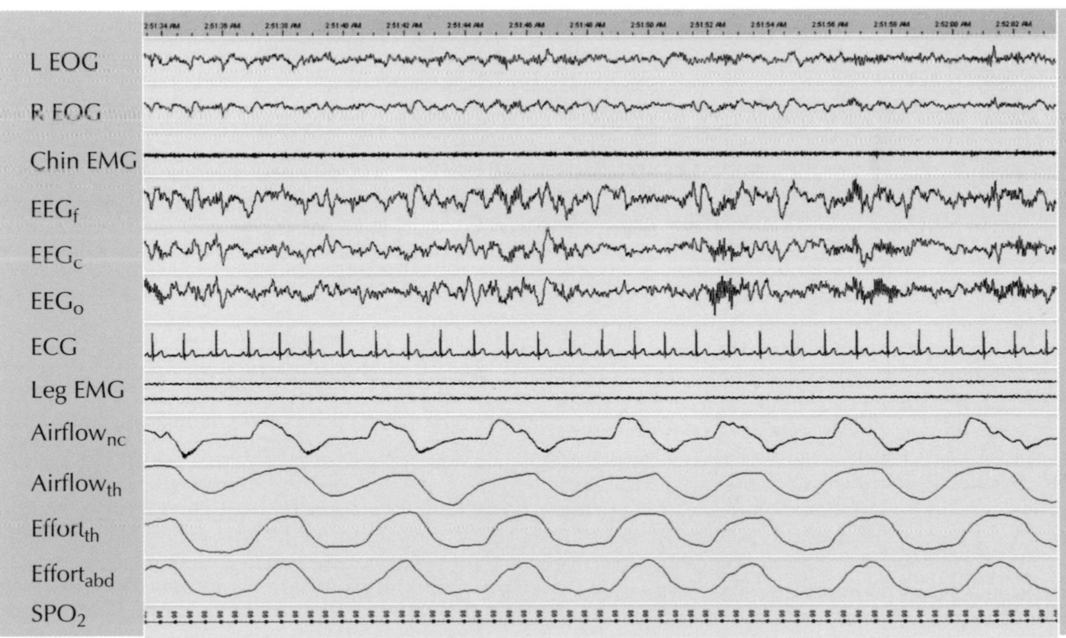

SLEEP-DISORDERED BREATHING

The most common sleep disorder screened for in sleep laboratories is obstructive sleep apnea (OSA). In OSA, the pharyngeal or hypopharyngeal airway collapses (apnea) or narrows to a degree to which ventilation is impeded (hypopnea), resulting in a decrease in oxygen levels or arousal from sleep. OSA is extremely common, affecting 1% to 2% of children and up to 10% of adults.

Risk factors for OSA in adults include male gender, obesity, small or narrow upper airway, and the post-menopausal state in women. In children, risk factors are obesity and enlarged tonsils or adenoids. Adult patients with OSA may complain of daytime sleepiness, nonrestorative sleep, chronic fatigue, insomnia, morning headaches, frequent nocturnal awakenings, and nocturia. Bed partners often bring the patient to medical attention because of loud, disruptive snoring and because they have witnessed apneas during sleep. Children with OSA may have similar complaints as adults or may have failure to thrive or attention deficit disorder.

A diagnosis of OSA is usually confirmed with a PSG, which will exhibit frequent apneas, hypopneas, or both during sleep. Patients with OSA can have hundreds of apneas, hypopneas, or respiratory effort–related arousals (RERAs) in one night. The severity of OSA is often determined by the apnea hypopnea index (AHI), which is the total number of apneas plus hypopneas divided by the total sleep time in hours. An AHI is considered normal if it is below 5 per hour and abnormal if it is above 10 per hour. A respiratory disturbance index (RDI) also includes RERAs in the numerator. The sleep-disordered breathing events can result in significant oxygen desaturation and dramatic changes in heart rate, blood pressure, cerebral artery pressure, and pulmonary artery pressures.

OSA is associated with a number of other medical disorders, including hypertension, pulmonary hypertension, stroke, gastroesophageal reflux, glucose intolerance, cardiac arrhythmias, and coronary disease. Treatment of OSA often improves the sequelae of some of these comorbid illnesses.

The options for treatment of OSA include surgery, weight loss, positive airway pressure devices, and dental appliances. For children, surgery is usually the treatment of choice, with tonsillectomy or adenotonsillectomy resulting in an 80% success rate. However, in adults, surgery is not as successful, so most adults with significant OSA are offered continuous positive airway pressure (CPAP), which is usually delivered via a nasal mask. Nasal CPAP works predominantly by acting as a pneumatic splint to maintain the patency of the airway throughout the respiratory cycle. The pressure is usually adjusted during a PSG to eliminate obstructive apneas, hypopneas, and snoring. CPAP is an extremely effective therapy and has been shown to reduce systemic blood pressure and pulmonary artery pressures, decrease subsequent hospitalizations, improve quality of life, and decrease sleepiness. Dental appliances for OSA have polymer inserts attaching to the upper and lower jaw and use the upper jaw as an anchor to protrude the lower jaw. These are not as effective as CPAP but are often preferred by patients and are a reasonable alternative for patients with milder degrees of OSA or those intolerant of CPAP.

Other forms of sleep-disordered breathing include central sleep apnea (including Cheyne-Stokes breathing), hypoventilation syndromes, and sleep-related hypoxemia. Central sleep apnea is defined by recurrent apneas during sleep associated with the lack of airflow and effort. This is usually seen in patients with central nervous system disorders, those with heart failure, or patients taking long-acting narcotic medications. Hypoventilation syndromes include congenital central alveolar hypoventilation syndrome, obesity hypoventilation syndrome, kyphoscoliosis, and neuromuscular disorders (e.g., muscular dystrophy). Many of these patients can be treated with noninvasive ventilation delivered via a nasal mask. Sleep-related hypoxemia may occur in a number of pulmonary disorders, including chronic obstructive pulmonary disease, cystic fibrosis, and idiopathic pulmonary fibrosis. Supplemental oxygen is typically prescribed after confirmation of low oxygen saturations made by nocturnal oximetry.

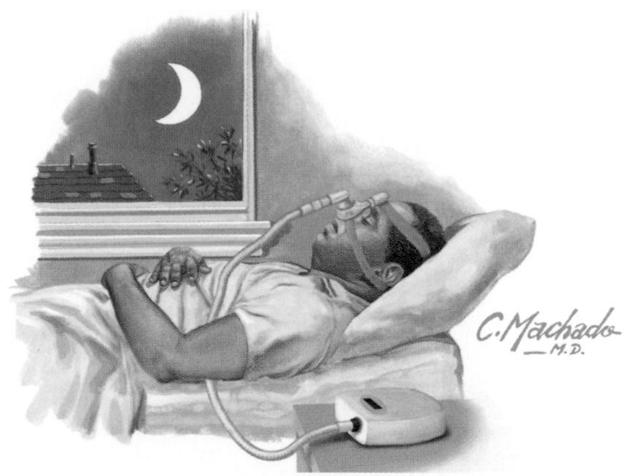

CONTINUOUS POSITIVE AIRWAY PRESSURE (CPAP)

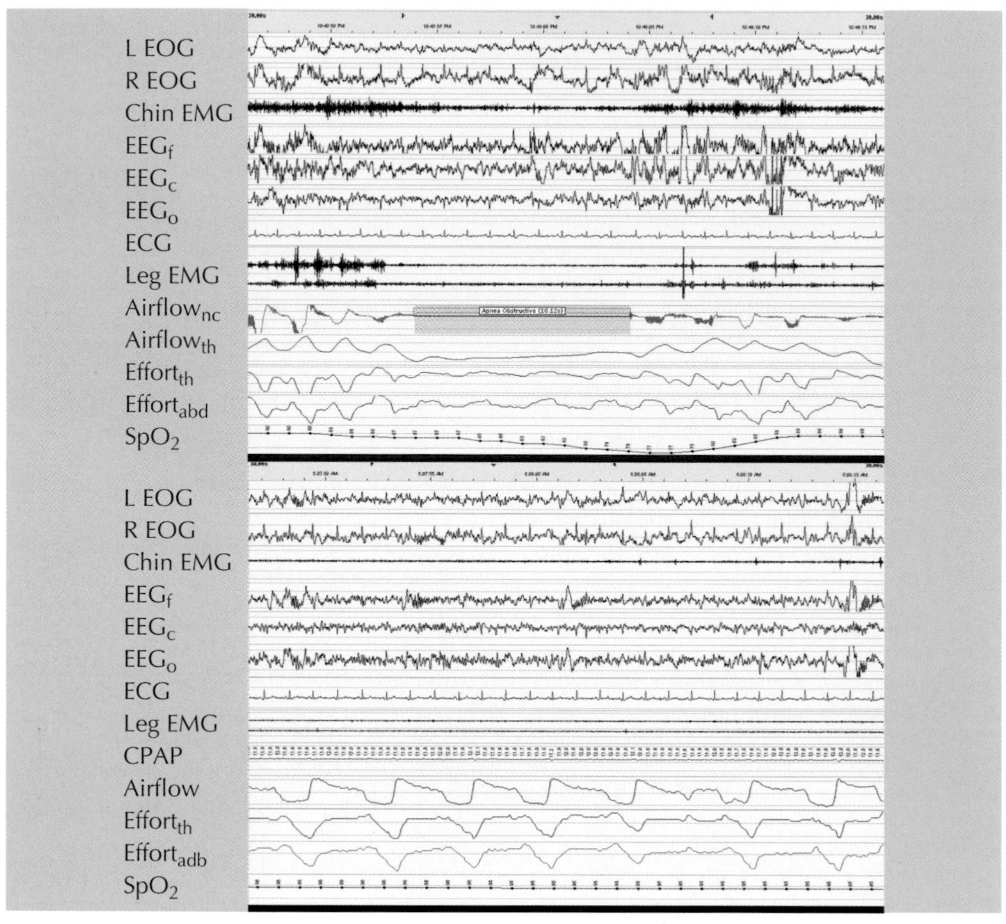

The upper half of this picture depicts an epoch out of a PSG showing an obstructive apnea (*pink highlight*); the lower half shows the same patient now asleep on CPAP with resolution of apneic events.

L EOG = left electrooculogram; R EOG = right eletrooculogram; Chin EMG = genioglossus electromyogram; EEG$_f$ = frontal electroencephalogram; EEG$_c$ = central electroencephalogram; EEG$_o$ = occipital electroencephalogram; EEG = lead 2 electrocardiogram; Leg EMG = anterior tibialis electromyograms, right and left legs; Airflow$_{th}$ = airflow as measured by a thermocouple; Airflow$_{nc}$ = airflow as measured by a nasal cannula; Effort$_{th}$ = thoracic effort belt; Effort$_{abd}$ = abdominal effort belt; SpO$_2$ = pulse oximetry

SECTION 5

THERAPIES AND THERAPEUTIC PROCEDURES

Pulmonary Pharmacology

Pulmonary pharmacology concerns the effects of drugs on the lungs and understanding how drugs used to treat patients with pulmonary diseases work. Much of this pharmacology concerns drugs used to treat obstructive airway diseases, such as asthma and chronic obstructive pulmonary disease (COPD).

Two types of drugs are used in the treatment of obstructive airway diseases:

- Relievers (bronchodilators) give immediate reversal of airway obstruction, largely by directly relaxing airway smooth muscle.
- Controllers (preventers) suppress the underlying disease process and provide long-term control of symptoms. These drugs include antiinflammatory treatments, such as corticosteroids.

Both asthma and COPD are characterized by airway narrowing secondary to a chronic inflammatory process. In asthma, eosinophilic (and sometimes neutrophilic) inflammation occurs throughout the respiratory tract, although the proximal airways are predominantly affected. In COPD, there is inflammation and narrowing of small airways (chronic obstructive bronchiolitis) and destruction of lung parenchyma (emphysema), resulting in loss of support for the airways, early closure on expiration, and air trapping.

Bronchodilators cause immediate reversal of airway obstruction as a result of a relaxing effect on airway smooth muscle. However, other pharmacologic effects of bronchodilator drugs on other airway cells (reduced microvascular leakage, reduced release of bronchoconstrictor mediators from inflammatory cells) may contribute to the reduction in airway narrowing. Three classes of bronchodilators are in current clinical use for the treatment of obstructive airway diseases: β_2-agonists, theophylline, and anticholinergics.

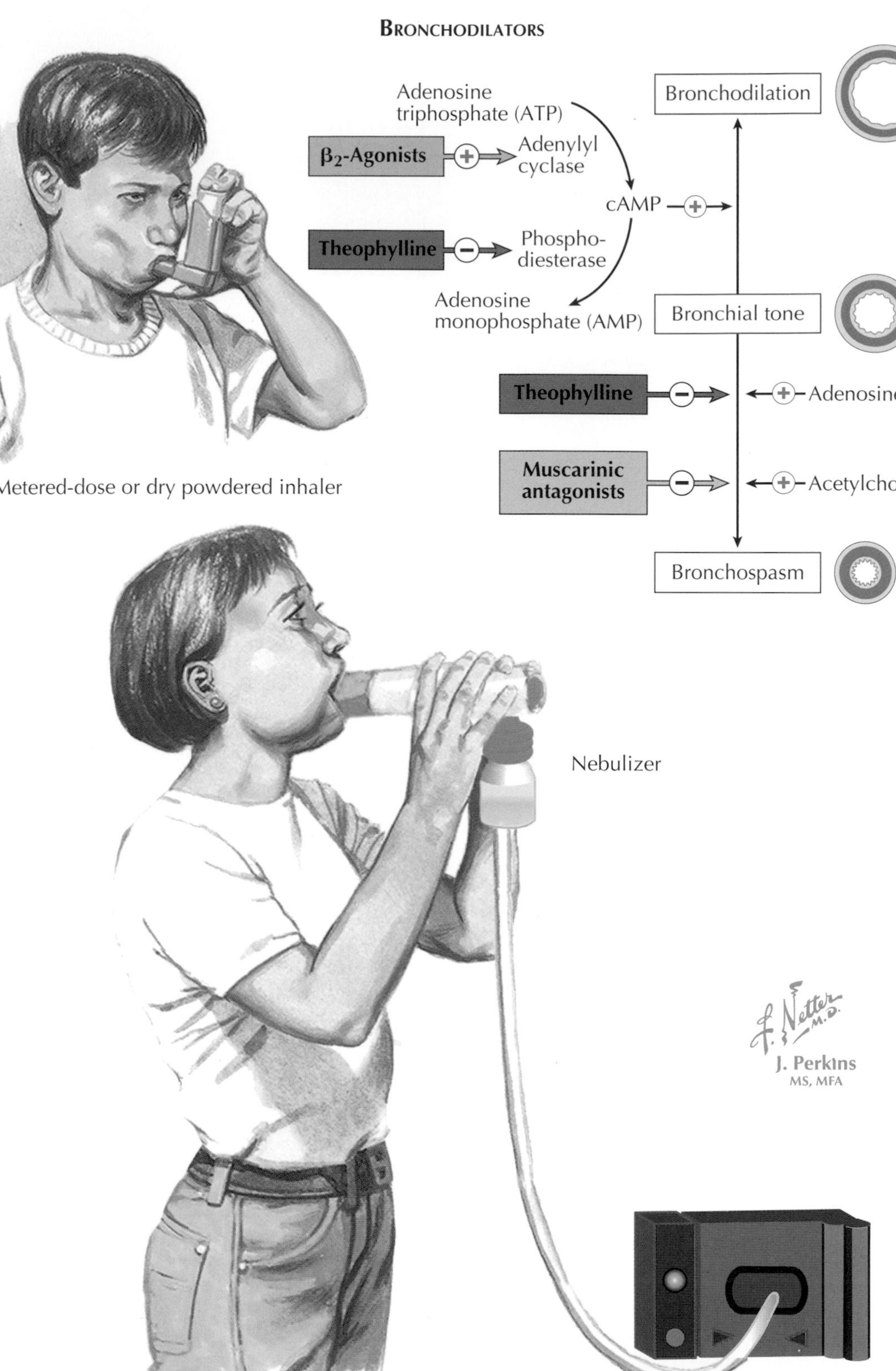

Metered-dose or dry powdered inhaler

β_2-Adrenergic Agonists

Inhaled β_2-agonists are the bronchodilator treatment of choice for patients with asthma because they are the most effective bronchodilators, reverse all known bronchoconstrictor mechanisms, and have minimal side effects when used correctly. Short-acting and nonselective β-agonists (e.g., isoproterenol) have no role.

Mode of Action

β_2-Agonists produce bronchodilatation by directly stimulating β_2-receptors on airway smooth muscle cells, which leads to relaxation of central and peripheral airways. β_2-agonists act as "functional antagonists" and reverse bronchoconstriction irrespective of the contractile agent; this is important in asthma because many bronchoconstrictor mechanisms (neural and mediators) are likely to constrict airways. In COPD, their major effect is reversal of cholinergic neural tone. Occupation of β_2-receptors by agonists results in the activation of adenylyl cyclase via the stimulatory G-protein (G_s), which increases intracellular cyclic AMP (cAMP), leading to relaxation through inhibition of the contractile machinery.

β_2-receptors are localized to several types of airway cells, and β_2-agonists may have additional effects. β_2-agonists may cause bronchodilatation, not only by a direct action on airway smooth muscle but also indirectly by inhibiting the release of bronchoconstrictor mediators from mast cells and of bronchoconstrictor neurotransmitters from airway nerves. β_2-agonists have an inhibitory effect on mast cell mediator release and microvascular leakage, suggesting they may inhibit acute inflammation. However, β_2-agonists do not have a significant inhibitory effect on the chronic inflammation of asthmatic airways and do not reduce airway hyperresponsiveness, which is a clinical manifestation of inflammation in asthma.

Pulmonary Pharmacology
(Continued)

Clinical Use

Short-acting inhaled β_2-agonists (e.g., albuterol, terbutaline) are the most widely used bronchodilators. Their duration of action is 3 to 4 hours (less in severe asthma). When inhaled from pressurized metered dose inhalers (pMDIs) in standard doses, they are convenient, easy to use, rapid in onset, and without significant side effects. They also protect against bronchoconstrictor stimuli such as exercise, cold air, and allergens. They are the bronchodilators of choice in acute severe asthma, in which the nebulized route of administration is as effective as intravenous use. The inhaled route of administration is preferable to the oral route because side effects are less common and because it may be more effective (better access to surface cells such as mast cells). Short-acting inhaled β_2-agonists should be used as required by symptoms and not on a regular basis; increased usage indicates a need for more antiinflammatory therapy.

Long-Acting Inhaled β_2-Agonists

The long-acting inhaled β_2-agonists (LABAs) salmeterol and formoterol are a significant advance in the treatment of patients with asthma and COPD. Both drugs have a bronchodilator action, protect against bronchoconstriction for more than 12 hours, and provide better symptom control (when given twice daily) than regular treatment with short-acting β_2-agonists (four times daily). Formoterol has a more rapid onset of action but is a fuller agonist than salmeterol, so tolerance is more likely. Inhaled long-acting β_2-agonists may be added to low or moderate doses of inhaled corticosteroids if asthma is not controlled, and this is more effective than increasing the dose of inhaled corticosteroids. Long-acting inhaled β_2-agonists should be used only in patients who are taking inhaled corticosteroids because these drugs do not have an antiinflammatory action and are potentially dangerous without corticosteroids. Combination inhalers with a long-acting β_2-agonist and corticosteroid (fluticasone/salmeterol, and budesonide/formoterol) are an effective and convenient way to control asthma and are useful in COPD.

Side Effects

Unwanted effects result from stimulation of extrapulmonary β-receptors and include tachycardia, tremors, and palpitations. Side effects are uncommon with inhaled therapy but more common with oral or intravenous administration.

Long-Term Safety

A large trial in the United States showed that salmeterol increased mortality in patients with asthma, but this was mainly in patients who were not using concomitant inhaled corticosteroids. This provides a strong argument for only prescribing long-acting β_2-agonists in a combination inhaler.

Tolerance

Continuous treatment with an agonist often leads to tolerance (desensitization), which may result from uncoupling or downregulation (or both) of the receptor. Tolerance of non-airway β-receptor responses (e.g., tremor, cardiovascular and metabolic responses) is readily observed. Loss of bronchodilator action is minimal, but there is some loss of bronchoprotective effect against, for example, exercise. This is incomplete and not progressive and does not appear to be a clinical problem.

THEOPHYLLINE (METHYLXANTHINES)

Worldwide, theophylline remains the most widely used antiasthma therapy because it is inexpensive, but the greater incidence of side effects with theophylline and

Methylxanthines

Theophylline also has antiinflammatory effects:
- Inhibits mast cell mediator release (by blocking adenosine A_2b receptors)
- Reduces eosinophils
- Reduces plasma exudation

Pulmonary Pharmacology
(Continued)

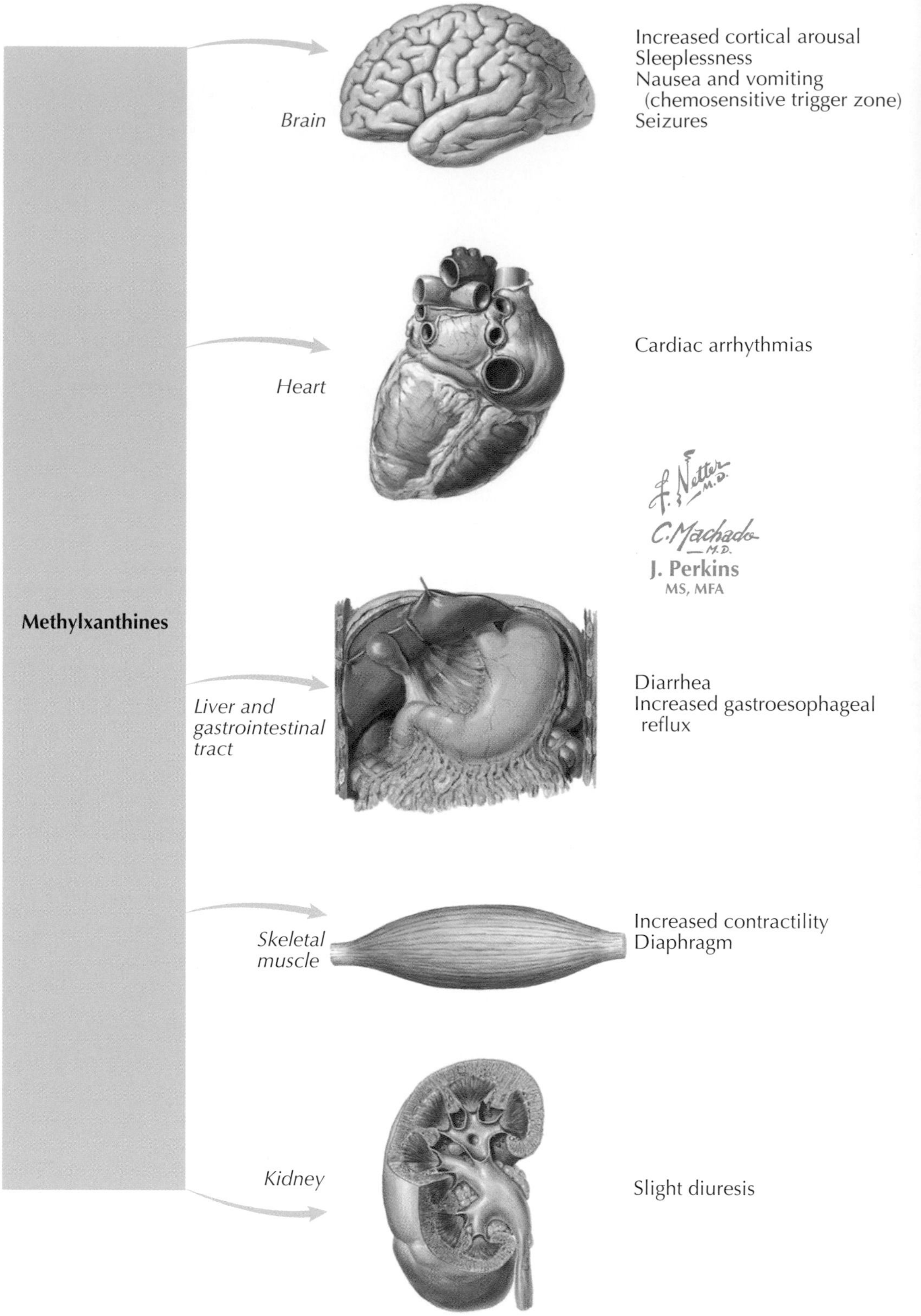

the greater efficacy of β_2-agonists and inhaled corticosteroids have reduced its use (see Plate 5-2). It still remains a useful drug in patients with severe asthma and COPD. There is increasing evidence that low-dose theophylline (plasma concentration, 5-10 mg/L) has an antiinflammatory or immunomodulatory effect and may be effective in combination with inhaled corticosteroids.

Mode of Action

Despite extensive study, it has been difficult to elucidate the molecular mechanisms of the antiasthma actions of theophylline. It is possible that any beneficial effect in asthma is related to its action on other cells (e.g., platelets, T lymphocytes, macrophages) or on airway microvascular leak and edema in addition to airway smooth muscle relaxation. Theophylline is a relatively ineffective bronchodilator, and high doses are needed for its bronchodilator action. Its antiasthma effect is more likely to be explained by other effects (e.g., immunomodulation). Several molecular modes of action have been proposed.

Inhibition of Phosphodiesterases

Phosphodiesterases (PDEs) break down cAMP in the cell; their inhibition leads to an increase in intracellular cAMP concentrations (see Plate 5-2). PDE inhibition is likely to account for the bronchodilator action of theophylline, but the degree of inhibition is relatively small at concentrations of theophylline within the therapeutic range. PDE inhibition also accounts for the side effects of nausea and headaches.

Adenosine Receptor Antagonism

Adenosine is a bronchoconstrictor in asthmatic patients via activation of mast cells (A_{2B} receptors). Adenosine antagonism may account for some side effects of theophylline (e.g., central nervous system [CNS] stimulation, cardiac arrhythmias, diuresis).

Histone Deacetylase Activation

Therapeutic concentrations of theophylline activate histone deacetylases in the nucleus, resulting in the switching off of inflammatory genes and enhancing the antiinflammatory action of corticosteroids, especially when there is corticosteroid resistance.

Clinical Use

In patients with acute asthma, intravenous aminophylline is less effective than nebulized β_2-agonists and should therefore be reserved for the few patients who fail to respond to β-agonists. (Aminophylline is a stable mixture or combination of theophylline and ethylenediamine, which confers greater solubility.) Theophylline is less effective as a bronchodilator than inhaled β_2-agonists and is more likely to have side effects. There is increasing evidence that low doses (giving plasma concentrations of 5-10 mg/L) may be useful when added to inhaled corticosteroids, particularly in more severe asthma. Theophylline is also useful as an additional bronchodilator in COPD, reducing hyperinflation and improving dyspnea.

Theophylline is readily and reliably absorbed from the gastrointestinal tract, but many factors affect plasma clearance, and thereby plasma concentration, that make the drug relatively difficult to use.

Methylxanthines: Adverse Effects

Side Effects

Adverse effects are usually related to plasma concentration and tend to occur when plasma levels exceed 20 mg/L, although some patients develop them at lower plasma concentrations. The severity of side effects may be reduced by gradually increasing the dose until therapeutic concentrations are achieved. The most common side effects are headache, nausea and vomiting, abdominal discomfort, and restlessness,

PULMONARY PHARMACOLOGY
(Continued)

which are likely caused by PDE inhibition and at higher concentrations cardiac arrhythmias and seizures caused by antagonists of adenosine A_1-receptors. Theophylline also has many interactions with other drugs because of alterations in liver enzyme metabolism.

ANTICHOLINERGICS

Atropine is a naturally occurring compound that was introduced for the treatment of asthma but because of side effects (particularly drying of secretions), less soluble quaternary compounds (e.g., ipratropium bromide) were developed.

Mode of Action

Anticholinergics are specific antagonists of muscarinic receptors and inhibit cholinergic nerve-induced bronchoconstriction. A small degree of resting bronchomotor tone is present because of tonic cholinergic nerve impulses, which release acetylcholine in the vicinity of airway smooth muscle, and cholinergic reflex bronchoconstriction may be initiated by irritants, cold air, and stress. Although anticholinergics protect against acute challenge by sulfur dioxide and emotional factors, they are less effective against antigen, exercise, and fog; they inhibit reflex cholinergic bronchoconstriction only and have no significant blocking effect on the direct effects of inflammatory mediators, such as histamine and leukotrienes. In COPD, cholinergic tone is the major reversible element of airway narrowing.

Clinical Use

Whereas ipratropium bromide and oxitropium bromide are administered three or four times daily via inhalation, tiotropium bromide is given once daily. In patients with asthma, anticholinergic drugs are less effective than β_2-agonists and offer less protection against various bronchial challenges. Nebulized anticholinergics are effective in acute severe asthma but less effective than β_2-agonists. Nevertheless, anticholinergic drugs may have an additive effect with β_2-agonists in acute and chronic treatment and should therefore be considered when control of asthma is inadequate, particularly when there are side effects with theophylline or inhaled β-agonists.

Anticholinergic drugs are the bronchodilators of choice in COPD, and once-daily tiotropium bromide is the most effective bronchodilator for COPD.

Side Effects

Inhaled anticholinergic drugs are well tolerated, and systemic side effects are uncommon because almost no systemic absorption occurs. Ipratropium bromide, even in high doses, has no detectable effect on airway secretions. Nebulized ipratropium bromide may precipitate glaucoma in elderly patients as a result of a direct effect of the nebulized drug on the eye; this is avoided by use of a mouthpiece rather than a face mask. Paradoxic bronchoconstriction with ipratropium bromide, particularly when given by nebulizer, was largely explained by the hypotonicity of an earlier nebulizer solution and by antibacterial additives such as benzalkonium chloride; this problem is avoided with current preparations. Dry mouth occurs in about 10% of patients taking tiotropium bromide but rarely requires discontinuation of treatment.

CORTICOSTEROIDS

Corticosteroids are the most effective therapy available for asthma (see Plates 5-5 and 5-6). Inhaled corticosteroids have revolutionized the management of patients

Pulmonary Pharmacology
(Continued)

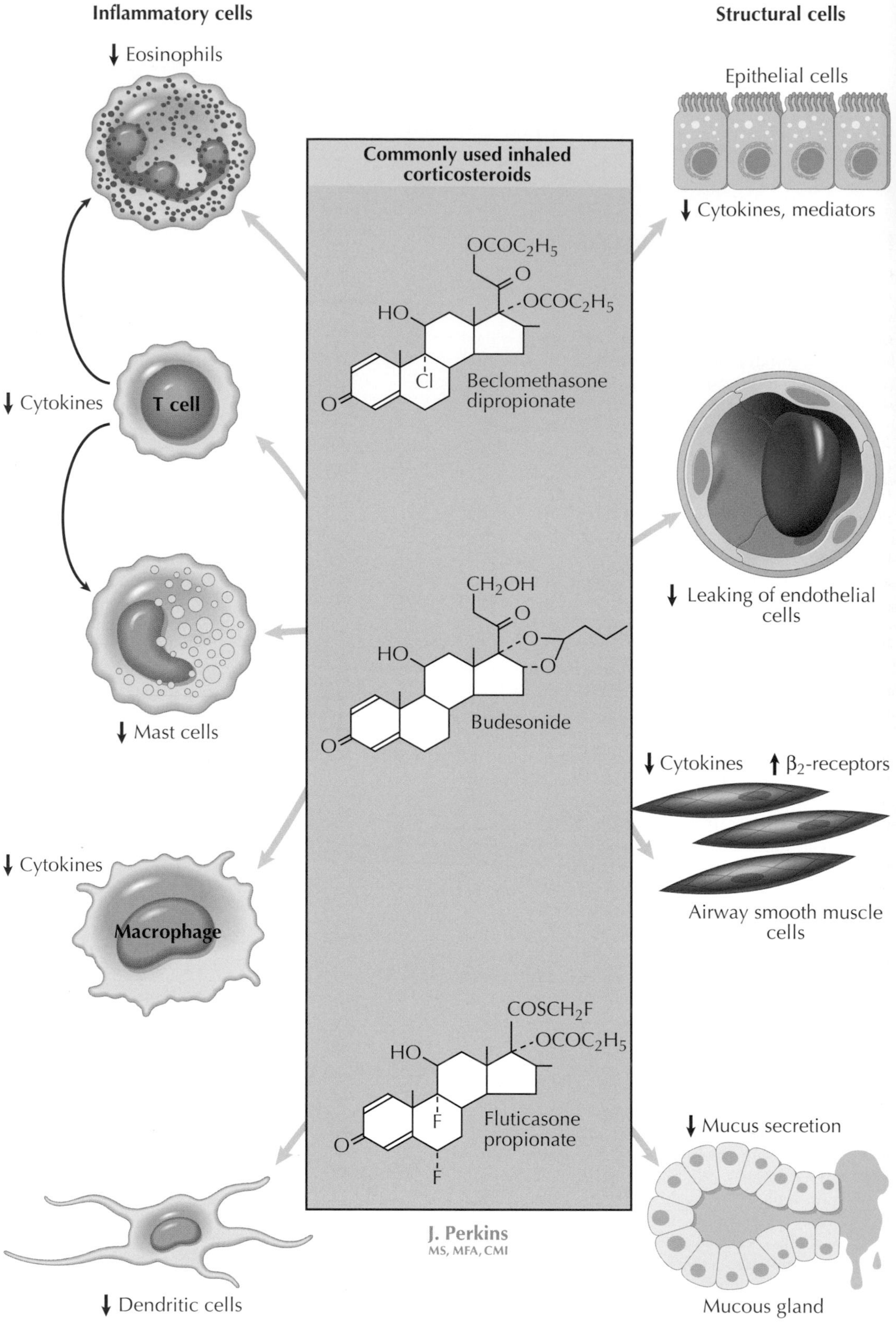

with chronic asthma and are now used as first-line therapy in all patients with persistent symptoms.

Mode of Action

Corticosteroids enter target cells and bind to glucocorticoid receptors in the cytoplasm. The corticosteroid-receptor complex is transported to the nucleus, where it binds to specific sequences on the upstream regulatory element of certain target genes, resulting in increased or decreased transcription of the gene and increased or decreased protein synthesis. Glucocorticoid receptors may also inhibit transcription factors, such as nuclear factor-κB and activator protein-1, which regulate inflammatory gene expression by a nongenomic mechanism. Corticosteroids inhibit acetylation of core histones and thereby inflammatory gene expression by recruiting histone deacetylase-2 to the activated transcriptional complex.

The mechanism of action of corticosteroids in asthma is most likely related to their antiinflammatory properties. Corticosteroids have widespread effects on gene transcription, increasing transcription of antiinflammatory genes and more importantly suppressing transcription of multiple inflammatory genes. At a cellular level, they have inhibitory effects on many inflammatory and structural cells that are activated in asthma. The inhibitory action of inhaled corticosteroids on airway epithelial cells may be particularly important; this results in a reduction in airway hyperresponsiveness, but in long-standing asthma, airway hyperresponsiveness may not return to normal because of irreversible structural changes in airways.

Clinical Use

Systemic corticosteroids are used in acute asthma and accelerate its resolution. There is no advantage with very high doses of intravenous corticosteroids (e.g., methylprednisolone, 1 g). Prednisolone or prednisone (40-60 mg orally) has an effect similar to intravenous hydrocortisone and is easier to administer.

Maintenance doses of oral corticosteroids are reserved for patients whose asthma cannot be controlled on other therapy; the dose is titrated to the lowest that provides acceptable symptom control. In any patient taking regular oral corticosteroids, objective evidence of corticosteroid responsiveness should be obtained before maintenance therapy is instituted. Short courses of oral corticosteroids (prednisolone, 30-40 mg/d for 1-2 weeks) are indicated for exacerbations of asthma; the dose may be tapered over 1 week after the exacerbation is resolved. (The tapering period is not strictly necessary, but patients find it reassuring.)

Inhaled corticosteroids are currently recommended as first-line therapy in all patients with persistent asthma. Inhaled corticosteroids, such as beclomethasone dipropionate, budesonide, fluticasone propionate, triamcinolone, mometasone furoate, and ciclesonide, act topically on the inflammation in the airways of asthmatic patients. They may be started in any patient who needs to use a β_2-agonist inhaler for symptom control more than twice a week. In most patients, inhaled corticosteroids are used twice daily; this improves compliance after control of asthma has been achieved. If a dose of more than 800 μg of budesonide or equivalent daily via MDI is administered, a spacer should be used to reduce the risk of oropharyngeal side effects and of absorption from the gastrointestinal tract. Inhaled corticosteroids at doses of 400 μg/d or less may be used safely in children.

Rarely, patients with severe asthma fail to respond to corticosteroids. Corticosteroid-resistant asthma is likely to be caused by several molecular mechanisms, including defective translocation of the glucocorticoid receptor as a result of activated kinases or reduced histone deacetylase-2 activity. COPD patients occasionally respond well to corticosteroids; these patients are likely to have undiagnosed asthma. Patients with COPD show a poor response to corticosteroids, and the inflammation is essentially steroid resistant. The steroid resistance in COPD appears to be caused by a marked

PULMONARY PHARMACOLOGY

(Continued)

reduction in histone deacetylase-2 in inflammatory cells, such as macrophages. Inhaled corticosteroids have no effect on the progression of COPD but reduce exacerbations in patients who have severe disease and frequent exacerbations. Inhaled corticosteroids do not reduce mortality in COPD, and recent evidence suggests that in high doses, they may increase the risk of developing pneumonia.

Side Effects *(see Plate 5-7)*

Corticosteroids inhibit cortisol secretion by a negative feedback effect on the pituitary gland. Hypothalamo–pituitary–adrenal axis suppression is dependent on dose and usually occurs when a dose of prednisone of more than 7.5-10 mg/d is used. Significant suppression after short courses of corticosteroid therapy is not usually a problem, but prolonged suppression may occur after several months or years; corticosteroid doses after prolonged oral therapy must therefore be reduced slowly. Symptoms of "corticosteroid withdrawal syndrome" include lassitude, musculoskeletal pains, and occasionally fever.

Side effects of long-term oral corticosteroid therapy include fluid retention, increased appetite, weight gain, osteoporosis, capillary fragility, hypertension, peptic ulceration, diabetes, cataracts, and psychosis. The incidence tends to increase with age.

Systemic side effects of inhaled corticosteroids have been investigated extensively. Effects such as cataract formation and osteoporosis are reported but often in patients who are also receiving oral corticosteroids. There has been particular concern about growth suppression in children using inhaled corticosteroids, but in most studies, doses of 400 μg or less have not been associated with impaired growth, and there may even be a growth spurt because asthma is better controlled.

The fraction of corticosteroid inhaled into the lungs acts locally on the airway mucosa and may be absorbed from the airway and alveolar surface, thereby reaching the systemic circulation. The fraction of inhaled corticosteroid deposited in the oropharynx is swallowed and absorbed from the gut. The absorbed fraction may be metabolized in the liver before it reaches the systemic circulation. Budesonide and fluticasone propionate have a greater first-pass metabolism than beclomethasone dipropionate and are therefore less likely to produce systemic effects at high inhaled doses. The use of a large volume spacer reduces oropharyngeal deposition, thereby reducing systemic absorption of corticosteroid.

- Initial studies suggested that adrenal suppression occurred only when inhaled doses of more than 1500 μg/d were used.
- More sensitive measurements of systemic effects include indices of bone metabolism (e.g., serum osteocalcin, urinary pyridinium cross-links), 24-hour plasma cortisol profiles and, in children, short-term growth of the lower leg, which may be affected by inhaled doses as low as 800 μg. The clinical relevance of these measurements is unclear. Nevertheless, it is important to reduce the risk of systemic effects by using the lowest dose of inhaled corticosteroid needed to control the asthma and by use of a large-volume spacer to reduce oropharyngeal deposition.

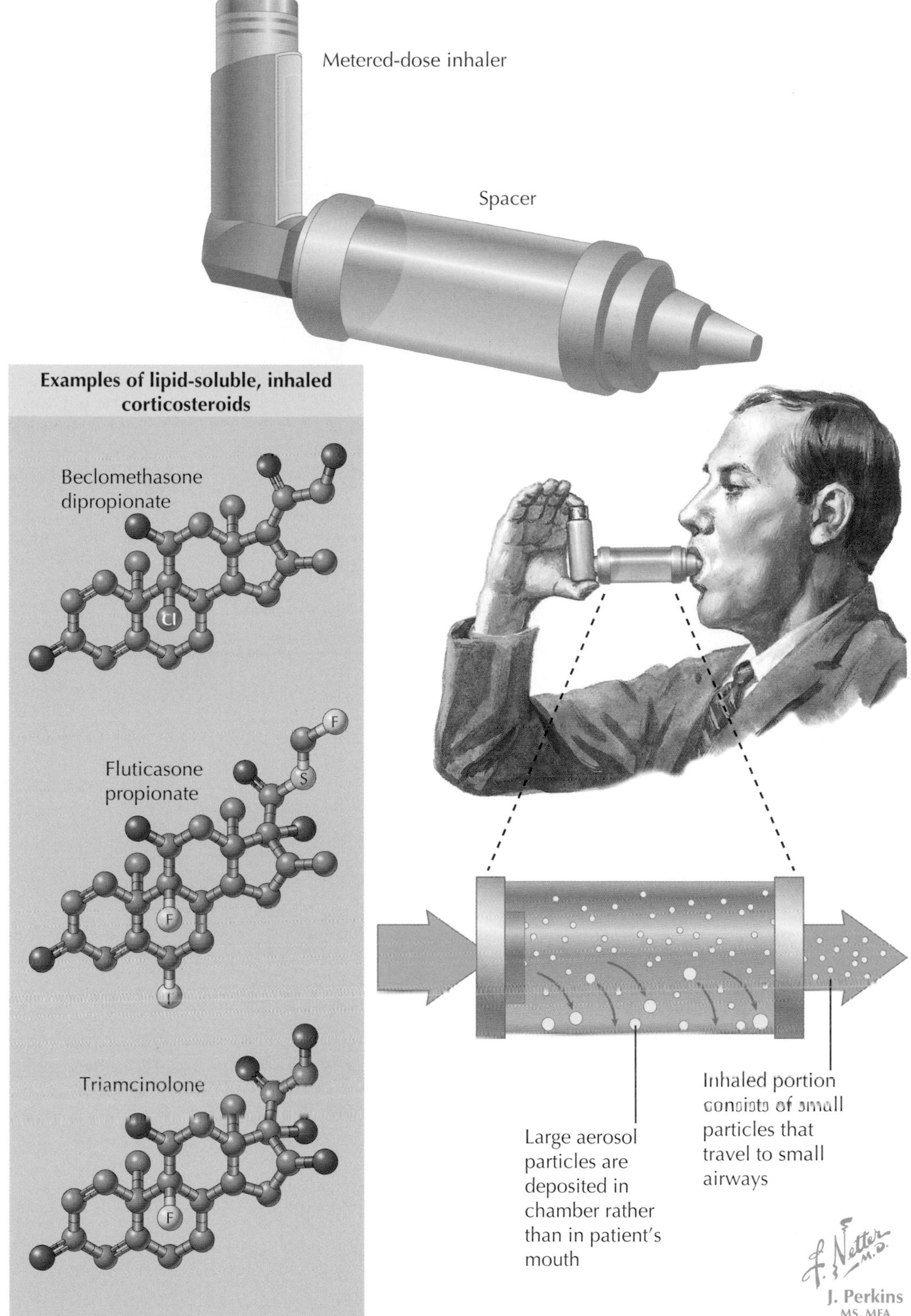

Inhaled corticosteroids may have local side effects caused by deposition of corticosteroid in the oropharynx. These side effects include oral thrush caused by overgrowth of *Candida* spp., throat irritation, and changes in voice caused by vocal cord irritation and weakness.

CROMONES

Cromones include cromolyn sodium and the structurally related nedocromil sodium.

Mode of Action

Initial investigations suggested that cromoglycate acts as a mast cell stabilizer, but this effect is weak in human mast cells. Cromones inhibit bronchoconstriction induced by sulfur dioxide, metabisulfite, and

PULMONARY PHARMACOLOGY
(Continued)

bradykinin, which are believed to act through activation of sensory nerves in the airways. Cromones have variable inhibitory actions on other inflammatory cells that may participate in allergic inflammation, including macrophages and eosinophils.

Cromoglycate blocks the early response to allergen (mediated by mast cells) and the late response and airway hyperresponsiveness, which are more likely to be mediated by macrophage and eosinophil interactions. The molecular mechanism of cromone action is not understood; evidence suggests they may block a type of chloride channel that may be expressed in sensory nerves, mast cells, and other inflammatory cells.

Clinical Use

Cromones are prophylactic treatments and must be given regularly. They protect against indirect bronchoconstrictor stimuli, such as exercise, allergens, and fog. Cromones are poorly effective compared with low doses of inhaled corticosteroids, and recent systematic reviews concluded that they provide little benefit in chronic asthma in children. Cromones are administered four times daily and may also be taken before exercise in children with exercise-induced asthma. There has been an increasing tendency to substitute low-dose inhaled corticosteroids for cromoglycate in adults and children, so they are now rarely used and are not recommended in most guidelines. There is no role for cromones in the management of patients with COPD.

Side Effects

Cromoglycate is one of the safest drugs available, and side effects are extremely rare. The dry-powder inhaler may cause throat irritation; coughing; and, occasionally, wheezing, but this is usually prevented by prior administration of a β-agonist inhaler. Very rarely, a transient rash and urticaria or pulmonary eosinophilia are seen; these result from hypersensitivity. Side effects are not usually a problem with nedocromil, although some patients have noticed a sensation of flushing after using the inhaler.

ANTILEUKOTRIENES

Antileukotrienes (leukotriene receptor antagonists) are less effective than inhaled corticosteroids in the control of asthma but have been widely used because they are effective by mouth and have few side effects (see Plates 5-8 and 5-9).

Mode of Action

Elevated levels of leukotrienes are detectable in bronchoalveolar lavage fluid, exhaled breath condensate, sputum, and urine of asthmatic patients. Cysteinyl-leukotrienes (cys-LTs) are generated from arachidonic acid by the rate-limiting enzyme 5-lipoxygenase. Cys-LTs are potent constrictors of human airways in vitro and in vivo, cause airway microvascular leakage in animals, and stimulate airway mucus secretion. These effects are all mediated in human airways via cys-LT_1 receptors. Montelukast and zafirlukast are potent cys-LT_1 receptor antagonists that markedly inhibit the bronchoconstrictor response to inhaled leukotrienes; reduce allergen-induced, exercise-induced, and cold air–induced asthma by about 50% to 70%; and inhibit aspirin-induced responses in aspirin-sensitive asthmatics almost completely. The only 5-lipoxygenase inhibitor clinically available is zileuton, the efficacy of which is similar to that of receptor antagonists. Antileukotrienes have also been shown to have weak antiinflammatory effects and reduce eosinophilic inflammation, which may be provoked by cys-LTs.

Clinical Use

Antileukotrienes may have a small and variable bronchodilator effect, indicating that leukotrienes may

ADVERSE EFFECTS OF CORTICOSTEROIDS

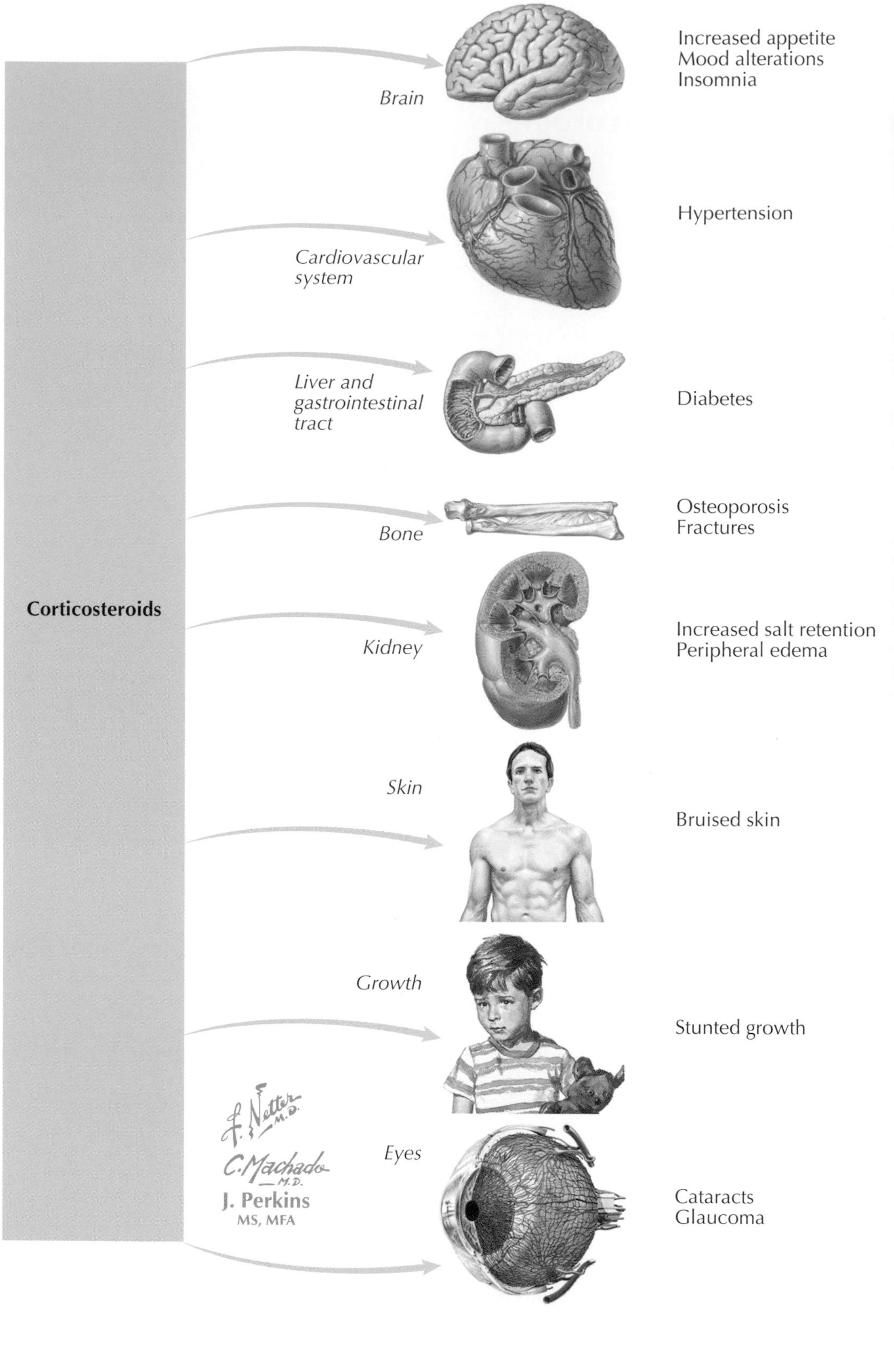

LEUKOTRIENES

PULMONARY PHARMACOLOGY

(Continued)

contribute to baseline bronchoconstriction in asthma. Long-term administration reduces asthma symptoms and the need for rescue β_2-agonists and improves lung function. However, their effects are significantly less than those with low-dose inhaled corticosteroids in terms of symptom control, improvement in lung function, and reduction in exacerbations. Antileukotrienes are not as effective as inhaled corticosteroids in the management of mild asthma and are not the preferred therapy. They may be useful in some patients whose asthma is not controlled on inhaled corticosteroids as an add-on therapy to inhaled corticosteroids but are less effective in this respect than a long-acting β_2-agonist or low-dose theophylline. They are effective in some but not all patients with aspirin-sensitive asthma. Patients appear to differ in their response to antileukotrienes, and it is impossible to predict which patients will respond best even when genetic polymorphisms of the leukotriene pathways are elucidated.

A major advantage of antileukotrienes is that they are orally active, and this is likely to improve compliance with long-term therapy. However, they are expensive, and a trial of therapy is indicated to determine which patients will benefit most.

Side Effects

Adverse effects are uncommon. Zafirlukast may produce mild hepatic dysfunction, so regular liver function tests are important. Several cases of Churg-Strauss syndrome (systemic vasculitis with eosinophilia and asthma) have been observed in patients taking antileukotrienes, but this is likely to be because a concomitant reduction in oral corticosteroids (made possible by the antileukotriene) allows the vasculitis to flare up.

ANTI-IgE THERAPY

Mode of Action

Omalizumab is a humanized recombinant monoclonal antibody that binds to circulating IgE and thus blocks it from activating high-affinity IgE receptors on mast cells and low-affinity IgE receptors on other inflammatory cells. This results in reduced responses to allergens. Over time, the blocking of IgE reduces its synthesis from B cells and results in a sustained reduction in IgE.

Clinical Use

Omalizumab reduces airway inflammation in patients with mild to moderate asthma and reduces the incidence of asthma exacerbations with improved control of asthma in patients maintained on reduced doses of inhaled corticosteroids. Omalizumab is most useful in patients with severe asthma who are not controlled with maximal doses of inhaled therapy because it reduces exacerbations and improves asthma control. Fewer than 30% of patients show a good response, and this is not predictable by any clinical features; therefore, a trial of therapy over 4 months is indicated. Omalizumab should be given only to patients with serum IgE levels of 20 to 700 IU/mL; above these levels, it is not possible to give enough antibody to neutralize IgE. The dose of omalizumab is determined by the serum IgE levels and is given either once or twice a month. Because of its high cost only patients at steps 4 (severe) and 5 (very severe) of the Global Initiative for Asthma (GINA) Guidelines who have frequent exacerbations are suitable for this therapy.

Side Effects

Omalizumab is well tolerated. Occasionally, local reactions occur at the injection sites, and very rarely, anaphylactic reactions have been seen.

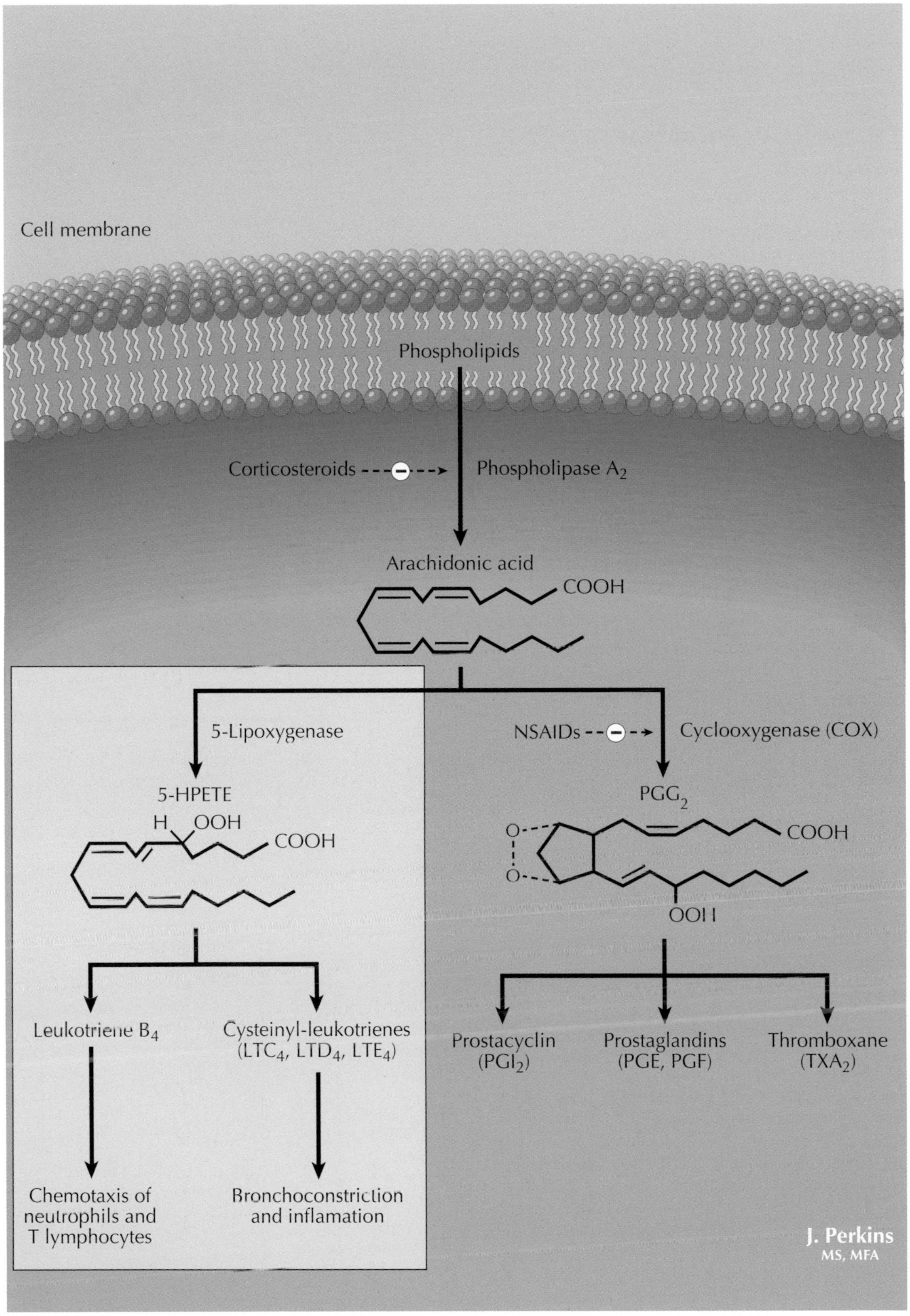

Pulmonary Pharmacology
(Continued)

IMMUNOSUPPRESSIVE AND CORTICOSTEROID-SPARING THERAPY

Immunosuppressive therapy has been considered in asthma when other treatments have been unsuccessful or when a reduction in the dosage of oral corticosteroids is required; it is therefore indicated in very few (<1%) asthmatic patients at present.

Methotrexate

Low-dose methotrexate, 15 mg weekly, has a corticosteroid-sparing effect in some patients with asthma, but side effects are relatively common and include nausea (reduced if methotrexate is given as a weekly injection), blood dyscrasia, hepatic damage, and pulmonary fibrosis. Careful monitoring (monthly blood counts and liver enzymes) is essential.

Gold

Gold has long been used in the treatment of patients with chronic arthritis. A controlled trial of an oral gold preparation (auranofin) demonstrated some corticosteroid-sparing effect in chronic asthmatic patients maintained on oral corticosteroids, but side effects (skin rashes and nephropathy) are a limiting factor.

Cyclosporine A

Low-dose oral cyclosporine A in patients with corticosteroid-dependent asthma is reported to improve control of symptoms, but in clinical practice, it is unimpressive, and its use is limited by severe side effects (nephrotoxicity, hypertension).

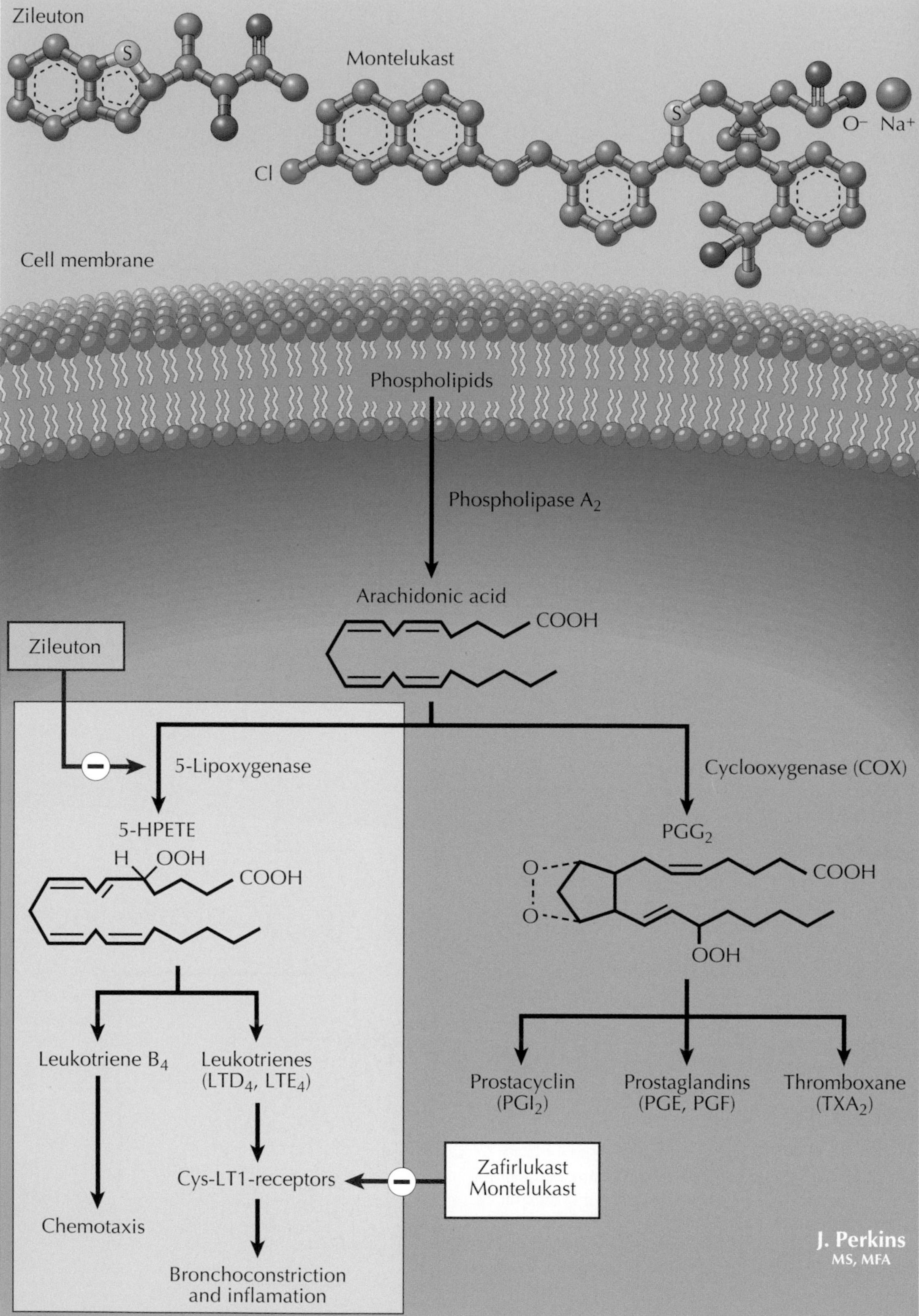

ANTITUSSIVES

Despite the fact that cough is a common symptom of airway disease, its mechanisms are poorly understood, and current treatment in unsatisfactory (see Plate 5-10). Because cough is a defensive reflex, its suppression may be inappropriate in those with bacterial lung infections. Before treatment with antitussives, it is important to identify underlying causal mechanisms that may require therapy. Treatments such as opioids may act centrally on the "cough center," but other treatments such as local anesthetics may act on airway sensory nerves.

Opiates have a central mechanism of action on the medullary cough center, but some evidence suggests that they may have additional peripheral action on cough receptors in the proximal airways. Codeine and dextromethorphan are commonly used, but there is little evidence that they are clinically effective. Morphine and methadone are effective but are only indicated in patients with intractable cough associated with bronchial carcinoma.

Asthma commonly presents as cough, and the cough usually responds to bronchodilators and inhaled corticosteroids. A syndrome characterized by cough in association with sputum eosinophilia but no airway hyperresponsiveness and termed *eosinophilic bronchitis* responds to inhaled corticosteroids and may be regarded as pre-asthma. Nonasthmatic cough does not respond to inhaled steroids but sometimes responds to cromones or anticholinergic therapy. The cough associated with postnasal drip of sinusitis responds to antibiotics, nasal decongestants, and intranasal steroids. The cough associated with angiotensin-converting enzyme inhibitors responds to withdrawal of the drug (or a switch to an angiotensin receptor antagonist) and to cromones. In some patients, there may be underlying gastroesophageal reflux, which leads to cough by a reflex mechanism and occasionally by acid aspiration. This cough responds to effective suppression of gastric acid with an H_2-receptor antagonist or more effectively to a proton pump inhibitor, such as omeprazole.

PULMONARY PHARMACOLOGY
(Continued)

Some patients have an intractable cough that often starts after a severe respiratory tract infection. When no other causes for this cough are found, it is termed idiopathic and may be caused by hyperesthesia of airway sensory nerves. This is supported by the fact that these patients have an increased responsiveness to tussive stimuli such as capsaicin. This form of cough is difficult to manage. It may respond to nebulized lidocaine, but this is not practical for long-term management, and novel therapies are needed.

There is a need to develop new, more effective therapies for cough, particularly drugs that act peripherally. There are close analogies between chronic cough and sensory hyperesthesia, so it is likely that new therapies are likely to arise from pain research.

DRUGS FOR DYSPNEA

Bronchodilators should reduce breathlessness, and chronic oxygen may have some effect, but in a few patients, breathlessness may be extreme. Drugs that have been shown to reduce breathlessness may also depress ventilation in parallel and may be dangerous in those with severe asthma and COPD. Some patients show a beneficial response to dihydrocodeine and diazepam, but these drugs must be used with caution. Slow-release morphine tablets may also be helpful in COPD patients with extreme dyspnea. Nebulized morphine may also reduce breathlessness in COPD and could act in part on opioid receptors in the lung.

VENTILATORY STIMULANTS

Several classes of drug stimulate ventilation and are indicated when ventilatory drive is inadequate rather than stimulating ventilation when the respiratory pump is failing. Nikethamide and ethamivan were originally introduced as respiratory stimulants, but doses stimulating ventilation are close to those causing convulsions, so their use has been abandoned. More selective respiratory stimulants have now been developed and are indicated if ventilation is impaired as a result of overdose with sedatives, postanesthetic respiratory depression, and in idiopathic hypoventilation. Respiratory stimulants are rarely indicated in patients with COPD because respiratory drive is already maximal, and further stimulation of ventilation may be counterproductive because of the increase in energy expenditure caused by the drugs.

Doxapram

At low doses (0.5 mg/kg intravenously), doxapram stimulates carotid chemoreceptors, but at higher doses, it stimulates medullary respiratory centers. Its effect is transient, and it must therefore be administered by intravenous infusion (0.3-3.0 mg/kg/min). The use of doxapram to treat ventilatory failure in patients with COPD has largely now been replaced by noninvasive ventilation. Unwanted effects include nausea, sweating, anxiety, and hallucinations. At higher doses, increased pulmonary and systemic pressures may occur.

COUGH SUPPRESSANTS (ANTITUSSIVE AGENTS)

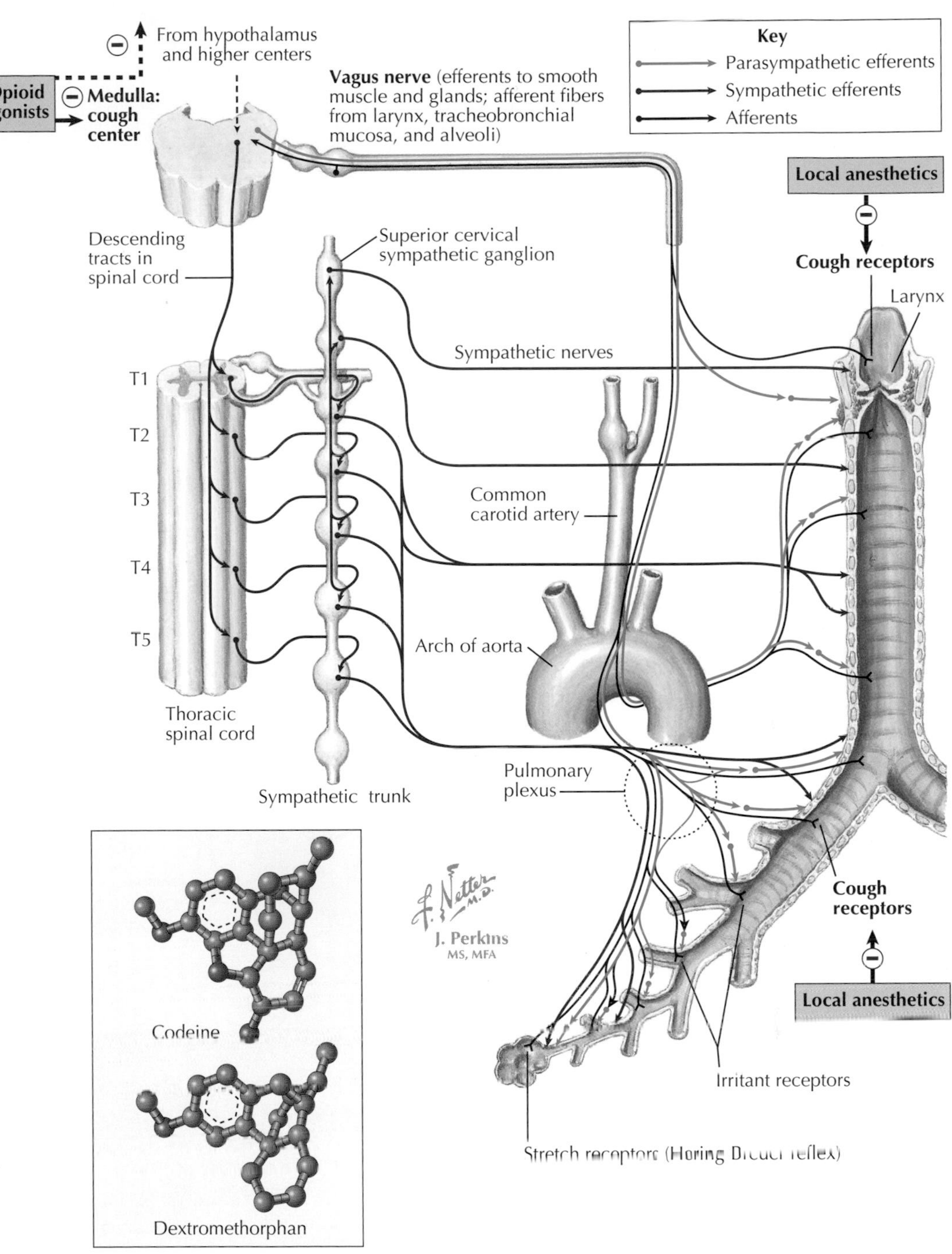

Doxapram is metabolized in the liver and should be used with caution if hepatic function is impaired.

Acetazolamide

The carbonic anhydrase inhibitor acetazolamide induces metabolic acidosis and thereby stimulates ventilation, but it is not widely used because the metabolic imbalance it produces may be detrimental in the face of respiratory acidosis. It has a very small beneficial effect in respiratory failure in COPD patients. The drug has proven useful in the prevention of high-altitude sickness.

Naloxone

Naloxone is a competitive opioid antagonist that is only indicated if ventilatory depression is caused by overdose of opioids.

Flumazenil

Flumazenil is a CNS benzodiazepine receptor antagonist and can reverse respiratory depression caused by overdose of benzodiazepines.

Protryptiline

Protryptiline has been used in the treatment of patients with sleep apnea syndromes, but its mode of action is unclear. It appears to stimulate activity of upper airway muscles via some central effect.

Modafinil

Modafinil is a nonamphetamine CNS stimulant occasionally used to treat drowsiness in patients with obstructive sleep apnea syndrome as an adjust to continuous positive airway pressure therapy. Side effects include insomnia, anxiety, and tachycardia.

Pulmonary Rehabilitation

Pulmonary rehabilitation is an evidence-based, multidisciplinary, and comprehensive intervention for patients with chronic respiratory diseases who are symptomatic and often have decreased daily life activities. Integrated into the individualized treatment of the patient, pulmonary rehabilitation is designed to reduce symptoms, optimize functional status, and reduce health care costs through stabilizing or reversing the manifestations of the disease.

Chronic obstructive pulmonary disease (COPD) is the fourth leading cause of death in the United States. In addition to impairing survival, COPD causes dyspnea that limits patients' daily function. Exercise intolerance is limited not only by lung function (including ventilatory and gas exchange abnormalities) but also by cardiac and skeletal muscle dysfunction. Exercise capacity, shortness of breath, and health status (disease-specific health-related quality of life) can be improved with pulmonary rehabilitation. The most important component of pulmonary rehabilitation is exercise training, including a lower extremity aerobic exercise program such as walking or stationary cycling. Strengthening and stretching programs are also incorporated. Supervised programs are usually 6 to 8 weeks in duration at least three times a week, but longer programs may be more effective. The goal is for the patient to continue exercising independently lifelong.

Other components of pulmonary rehabilitation include patient education, psychosocial counseling, and nutritional counseling. The goal of patient education is to assist the patient in incorporating health-enhancing behaviors such as adherence to prescribed medications and exercise. Use of inhaled medications is unique to patients with lung disease, and education should include teaching patients the skills of self-administration of such medications. Classes in anatomy and physiology of lung disease, respiratory medications, and oxygen therapy focus on improving patient understanding of their condition and its treatment. Other issues addressed include end-of-life considerations when appropriate and sexual counseling to assist patients in leading full lives.

Periods of increased respiratory symptoms (COPD exacerbations) are associated with impaired quality of life, worsening lung function, and urgent health care visits and hospitalizations. Education about COPD exacerbations incorporate timely recognition of changes in symptoms, how to contact health care professionals, and appropriate use of action plans for treatment. Collaborative self-management programs have been demonstrated to reduce hospitalizations.

Many patients with COPD demonstrate depressive symptoms, even if not clinical depression. Anxiety, partly related to the fear invoked by dyspnea, is also common. Psychosocial evaluation, including screening for depression and anxiety along with medications and counseling when appropriate, is incorporated in comprehensive pulmonary rehabilitation programs.

Weight loss can bee seen in patients with more severe COPD, and low body weight is a risk factor for mortality in COPD. In such patients, nutritional counseling, including intake of foods to maintain body weight and nutritional status, is of obvious importance. Patients with COPD may also present with weight gain caused by inactivity, and lowering body weight can improve exercise capacity.

Although most commonly applied to patients with COPD, patients with other respiratory disorders, including cystic fibrosis, asthma, bronchiectasis, and interstitial lung disease, may also be candidates for pulmonary rehabilitation.

C. Machado M.D.

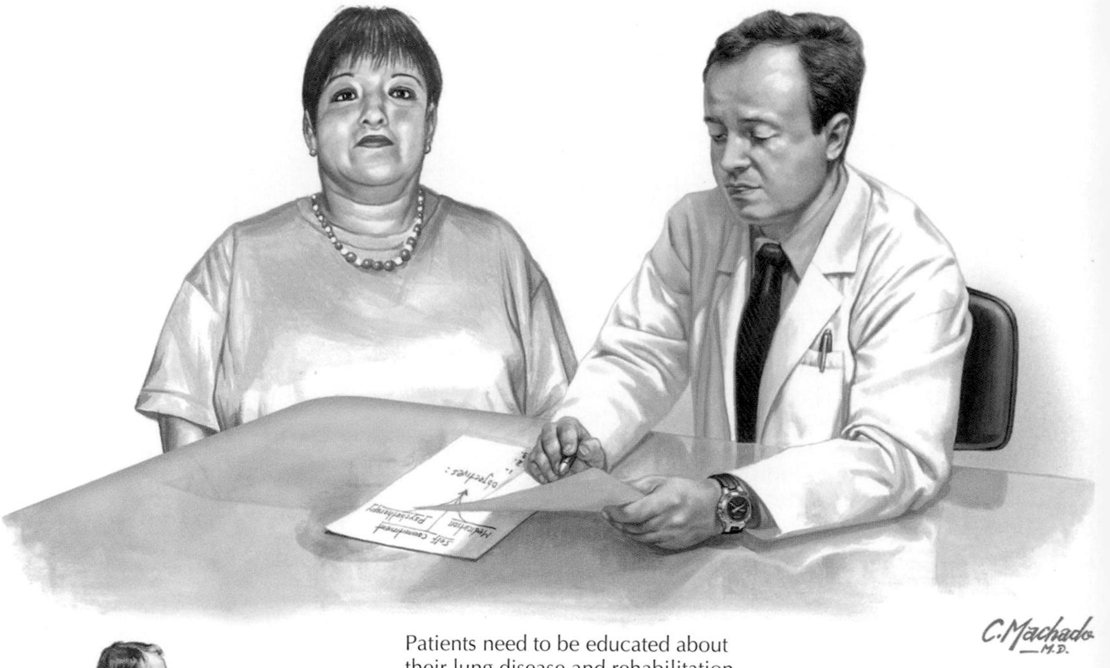

Patients need to be educated about their lung disease and rehabilitation

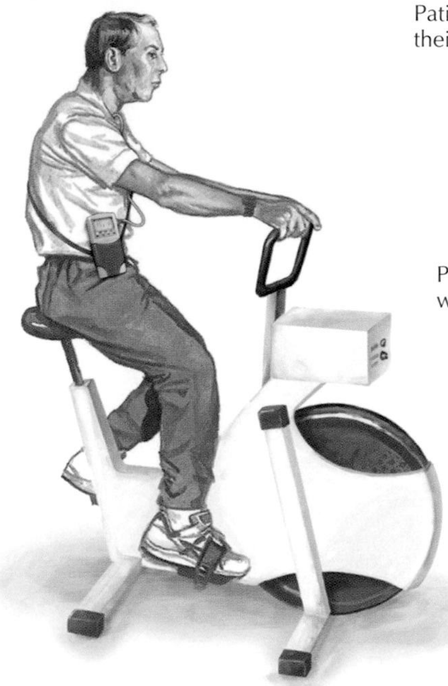

Patient rides exercise bike while wearing pulse oximeter

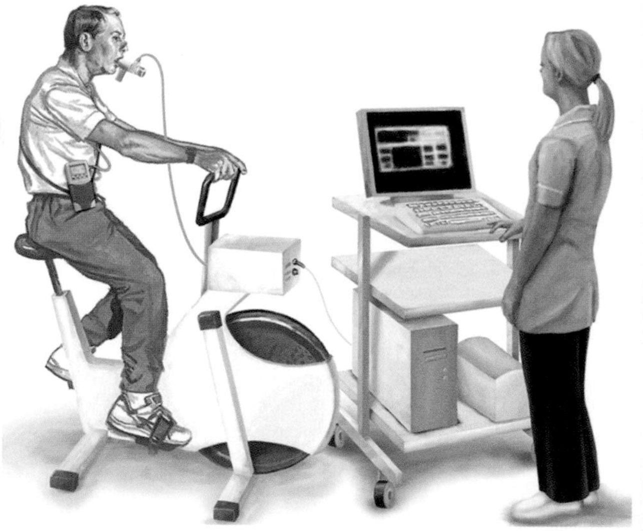

Patient exercises while wearing oxygen and being monitored by nurse or therapist

Oxygen Therapy in Acute Respiratory Failure

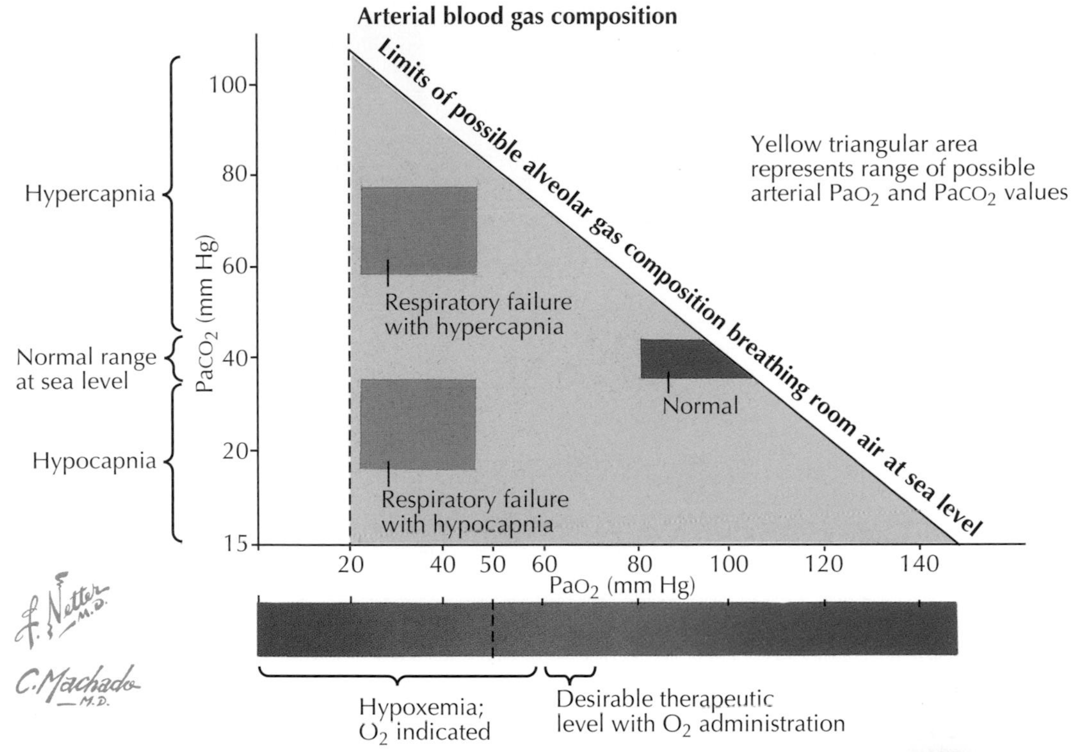

ARTERIAL BLOOD GAS COMPOSITION

Arterial blood gas (ABG) findings can be explained by the carbon dioxide: oxygen diagram shown at the top of the illustration. Because there is no uptake or excretion of nitrogen during respiration and the alveolar partial pressure of water vapor is a function of body temperature only, there is a reciprocal relationship between the alveolar P_{CO_2} and P_{O_2}, as indicated by the alveolar gas composition line. Because prolonged survival is not possible when the Pa_{O_2} is less than 20 mm Hg, the range of arterial gas tensions compatible with life is confined to the yellow triangle. Initial ABG values of air-breathing patients with decompensated chronic obstructive pulmonary disease (COPD) fall in the upper shaded blue area. With higher oxygen concentrations, the alveolar gas composition line is shifted to the right, and much higher Pa_{CO_2} values are possible.

Fortunately, because of the shape of the hemoglobin dissociation curve, only a small increase in oxygen tension is necessary to produce a marked increase in arterial oxygen content. In most patients, a 15-mm Hg increase in arterial oxygen tension can be produced by increasing the inspired oxygen fraction by only 4% to 7%. Administration of low oxygen concentrations (24%-35%) and low flows (1-3 L/min) can be achieved by use of a nasal cannula (see Plate 5-13). Care must be given to supplying enough oxygen to achieve adequate oxygenation (SaO_2 >90%) without causing too much CO_2 retention, which may occur during acute exacerbations in patients with severe COPD. Contrary to popular belief, CO_2 retention in COPD is caused by a worsening mismatch of ventilation and perfusion in the presence of excessive oxygen with a resulting increase in dead space ventilation, as well as an increased offloading of CO_2 by hemoglobin, rather than a reduced drive to breathe.

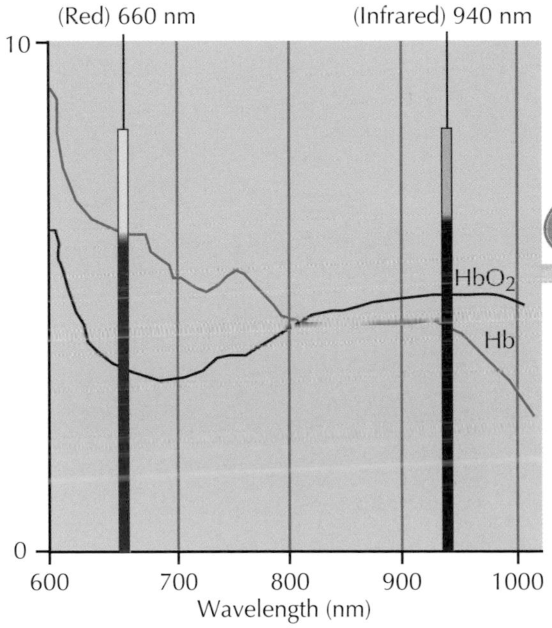

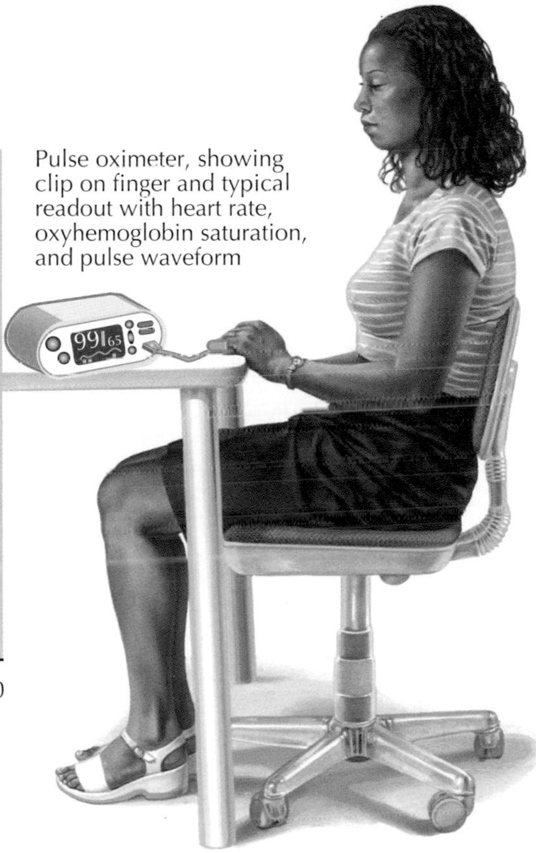

CARE AND MONITORING DURING OXYGEN THERAPY

Although measurement of AGBs is of prime importance in patients receiving oxygen for acute respiratory failure, a reduction in cardiac output, hemoglobin concentration, or local blood flow, a shift in position of the oxygen dissociation curve, or an increase in tissue requirements can result in inadequate oxygen delivery to the tissues even if the Pa_{O_2} is normal. Although there is no specific way to assess the level of tissue oxygenation, tissue hypoxia probably exists if the mixed venous P_{O_2} is less than 35 mm Hg. Monitoring and correcting abnormalities of cardiovascular function and hemoglobin concentration minimize tissue hypoxia.

Oxygen requirements may change during therapy, and a patient's respiratory, cardiovascular, and mental status should be evaluated often. Patients should be observed during sleep, when their breathing patterns may be different. Sedation should be avoided.

Pulse oximetry is a convenient and noninvasive method for monitoring oxyhemoglobin saturation; however, its limitations must be appreciated. The method does not allow direct measurement of P_{O_2}, P_{CO_2}, or pH, and accuracy may be affected by many factors, including skin pigmentation, adequate capillary blood flow, external light conditions, and alternative hemoglobin species such as carboxy- and methemoglobin. New pulse oximeters that use co-oximetry to determine the presence of these other hemoglobin species are being introduced into clinical practice.

Arterial blood gas composition

Yellow triangular area represents range of possible arterial PaO_2 and $PaCO_2$ values

Pulse oximeter, showing clip on finger and typical readout with heart rate, oxyhemoglobin saturation, and pulse waveform

The oximeter measures relative absorption of light at 660 nm and 940 nm to estimate the relative amount of saturated hemoglobin

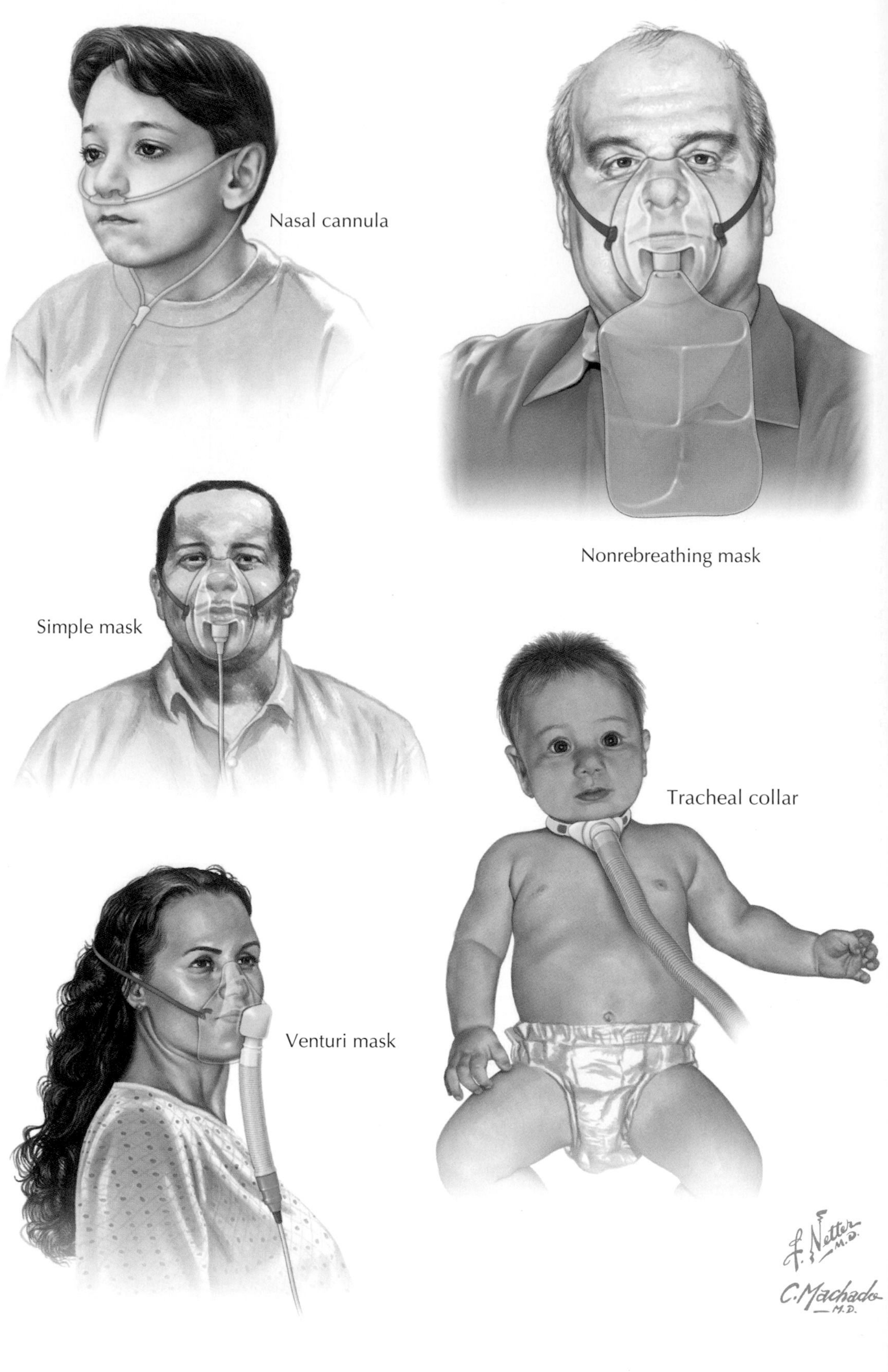

Nasal cannula

Nonrebreathing mask

Simple mask

Tracheal collar

Venturi mask

F. Netter M.D.

C. Machado M.D.

Methods of Oxygen Administration

Various types of oxygen delivery devices are available. With a flow rate of 6 to 10 L/min of 100% oxygen, it is possible to achieve inspired oxygen concentrations (FiO_2) of up to 95%. The actual FiO_2 depends on the system used and the oxygen flow rate relative to the patient's respiratory rate and tidal volume.

The *nasal cannula* (nasal prongs) is perhaps the most common mode of oxygen delivery and can provide 30% to 50% oxygen with flow rates of 6 to 8 L/min; higher flow rates may cause nasal irritation. The *simple mask* fits over the mouth and nose, and exhaled gas escapes via side ports. Carbon dioxide may accumulate if the oxygen flow rate is too low. Simple masks deliver an FiO_2 of 35% to 50% with a flow rate of 6 to 10 L/min.

The *partial rebreathing mask* is similar to the simple mask but has a reservoir bag. On inspiration, oxygen from the bag is mixed with air entering via the exhalation ports. The oxygen flow rate is adjusted so that the bag does not collapse with inspiration; most of the exhaled gas escapes via exhalation ports. Partial rebreathing masks deliver an FiO_2 of 50% to 70% with an oxygen flow rate of 6 to 10 L/min.

The *nonrebreathing mask* is a modification of the partial rebreathing mask and incorporates one-way valves between the mask and the reservoir bag and at the exhalation ports. Thus, oxygen is inspired only from the bag, and exhaled gas may escape via the ports. The oxygen flow rate is adjusted so that the bag does not collapse. The nonrebreathing mask can deliver an FiO_2 of up to 95%.

The *Venturi mask* is used to deliver a *fixed* low concentration (24%-40%) of oxygen. The *Venturi mask* works on the principle of air entrainment; 100% oxygen is directed through a tube in a center jet stream, which pulls in room air through side ports. The relative amounts of air and oxygen are determined by the size of the jet and side ports. Venturi masks deliver oxygen concentrations of 24%, 28%, 35%, or 40%. The amount of air entrained by the Venturi mask is high, and this flushes the environment around the patient's face—preventing rebreathing—and maintains a fixed oxygen concentration over a wide range of oxygen flow rates and independent of the patient's rate of ventilation, thus minimizing the danger of inadvertently supplying too much oxygen.

Disadvantages of the Venturi and other masks include difficulty with talking, eating, washing, expectoration, and administration of aerosol medications. The nasal cannula and Venturi mask are best suited for administering the low concentrations of oxygen necessary to minimize carbon dioxide retention in patients with chronic obstructive pulmonary disease. The nasal cannula is more comfortable and does not interfere with eating, washing, or expectorating. However, the actual FiO_2 depends on the amount of flow relative to the patient's demand and the amount of air taken in through the mouth or nose.

The *T tube* and *tracheostomy collar* (also available in a Venturi mode) are used to deliver supplementary oxygen to patients with tracheostomies (see Plate 5-21).

Oxygen Therapy in Chronic Respiratory Failure (Ambulatory and Home Use)

Supplemental oxygen was the first treatment shown to improve survival in patients with chronic obstructive pulmonary disease (COPD). A multicenter clinical trial published in 1980 demonstrated the benefit of oxygen used continuously compared with oxygen only administered nocturnally. The current recommendations for oxygen therapy in patients with COPD are (1) partial pressure of oxygen in arterial blood (Pao_2) of 55 mm Hg or below (or pulse oxygen saturation [Spo_2] ≤ 88%) or (2) Pao_2 of 56 to 60 mm Hg (Spo_2, 89%) with erythrocytosis (hematocrit >56 mL/dL) or cor pulmonale. Because of the benefits of oxygen, reimbursement is available from most medical insurance payers. The long-term benefit of oxygen in patients with less severe hypoxemia is unknown.

Three types of oxygen systems are available: (1) *gaseous* oxygen stored under high pressure in lighter weight aluminum or steel cylinders, (2) oxygen stored in *liquid* form, and (3) *concentrators* that are electrically powered and concentrate the oxygen in ambient air. To use oxygen 24 hours a day, patients need systems that will provide oxygen in the home and where they work during the day, at night, and during ambulation when out of the house during the day. Oxygen systems can reliably and conveniently provide oxygen in all of these circumstances. Smaller, lightweight oxygen systems are more appropriate for use during ambulation, and it has been recommended that systems designed for use during ambulation should weigh 5 lb or less. Each patient should be evaluated individually and provided with an oxygen system that best fills his or her needs. When prescribing oxygen, health care providers should order the flow rate of oxygen needed to ensure an Spo_2 of about 90%-92% at rest, during ambulation, and nocturnally. Home care oxygen suppliers, health care providers, and patients should carefully consider which oxygen system is best for each individual. The optimal oxygen system for each patient is the one that best fulfills that person's medical needs and allows him or her to pursue an independent and functional lifestyle with careful consideration of the oxygen flow rate and amount of time spent in various activities inside and outside the home.

Oxygen concentrators were originally designed for use in the home and are still widely used in that setting because of their reliability, durability, and low maintenance requirements. Newer units are smaller and quieter and can provide higher flow rates than previous models. Battery-powered concentrators can be used for mobility and are allowed for use on many commercial airliners.

Gaseous oxygen cylinders are available in a wide variety of sizes. Small cylinders are convenient and light enough for patients to carry over their shoulder. Larger cylinders contain more oxygen and provide a longer duration of use, but they are heavier and thus more difficult for patients to carry. Traditionally, gaseous cylinders had to be delivered to patients by a home care oxygen company. However, some oxygen systems now provide oxygen via concentrator while also filling a gaseous oxygen tank.

Liquid oxygen can be provided in a large tank for use during the day. Smaller liquid tanks weighing 5 lb or less can be filled by patients from the larger reservoir. One disadvantage of liquid oxygen is the need for delivery on a regular basis.

To reduce the amount of oxygen used by patients, oxygen conservers are commonly used in the home. These devices take advantage of the fact that oxygen is only needed during inspiration and is wasted during expiration. Moreover, only oxygen delivered during the early portion of inspiration reaches gas-exchanging alveoli.

Oxygen is most often delivered to the nares by an oxygen cannula. To be less obtrusive, the cannula can be embedded into eyeglass frames. Oxygen can also be delivered transtracheally (i.e., through a catheter placed through the neck into the trachea). Advantages of transtracheal oxygen include a reduction in the flow rates needed compared with a nasal cannula, elimination of nasal adverse effects, and the ability to conceal the catheter.

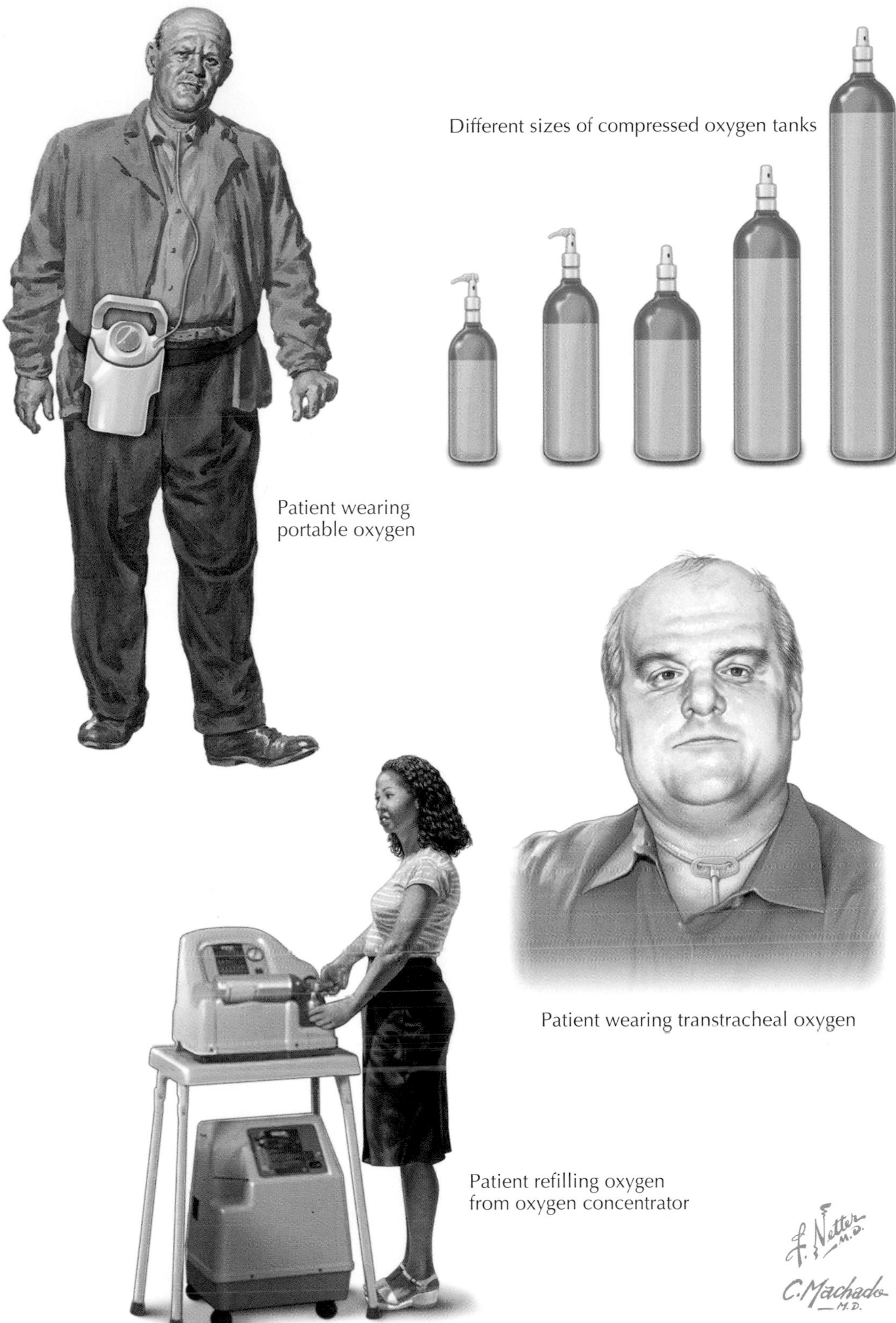

INTRODUCTION OF CHEST DRAINAGE TUBES

Pleural drainage tubes are inserted for evacuation of air or fluid from the pleural space in diseases such as pneumothorax, hemothorax, and empyema.

Placement of an intercostal tube or catheter for pneumothorax can be readily accomplished under local anesthesia, with or without an intercostal nerve block. Chest tube placement may be done at the bedside, but strict aseptic precautions should be observed. The second or third anterior intercostal space in the midclavicular line or the fourth or fifth intercostal space in the midaxillary line are the preferred sites for chest tube placement. To help select the optimal point of entry, chest radiographs should be reviewed unless the clinical situation is one of extreme urgency.

Anteriorly placed chest tubes in the second and third intercostal space must be placed at least two fingerbreadths lateral to the sternal border to avoid injury to the internal mammary vessels. Lateral tube placements must not be made too low in case there is penetration of the sloping diaphragmatic attachment where it joins the chest wall. The act of tube insertion *should not be forceful* but done with deliberate tactile control to avoid injuring the diaphragm or an enlarged heart if placed on the left side. Pleural access should always be on the superior surface of the rib to avoid the neurovascular bundle.

During the process of local anesthesia, needle aspiration and ready withdrawal of air or fluid should precede any tube insertion. Failure to find a free pleural space necessitates choosing another site for tube insertion. Because the parietal pleura can be quite sensitive, adequate local anesthesia is essential. The use of ultrasonography to select an appropriate insertion site has revolutionized pleural access. The site for tube insertion should be one that is away from adherent lung. Tubes placed to drain fluid should be directed posteriorly, but they should be directed anteriorly when placed to drain air.

Multifenestrated tubes should be checked carefully to be sure that all openings lie well within the pleural space. Thoracostomy tubes should be sutured to the skin, but such suture fixation cannot be depended on to hold the tube securely in place; for this purpose, careful binding with adhesive tape is required. All connections of the tube to the drainage system should be secured as well, and care should be taken to protect against traction and tube angulation.

Preferred sites
1. For pneumothorax (2nd or 3rd interspace at midclavicular line)
2. For hemothorax (5th interspace at midaxillary line)

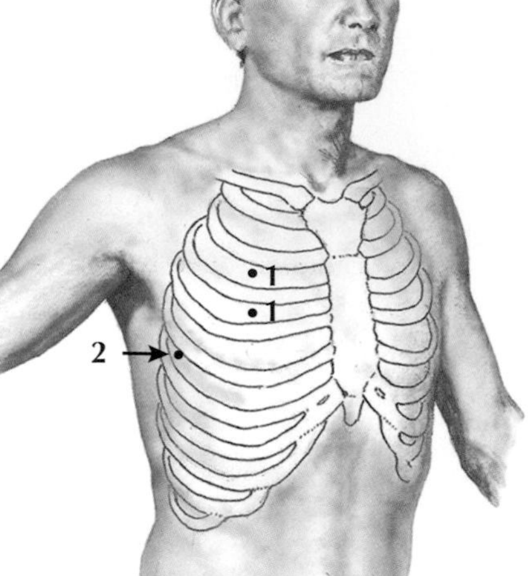

Hemostat technique

A. Skin incised and pleura entered by blunt dissection

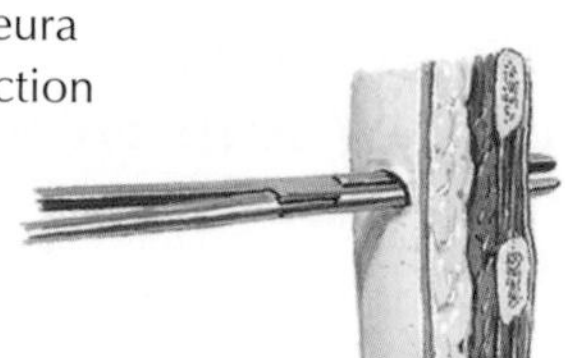

B. Tube inserted into pleural cavity

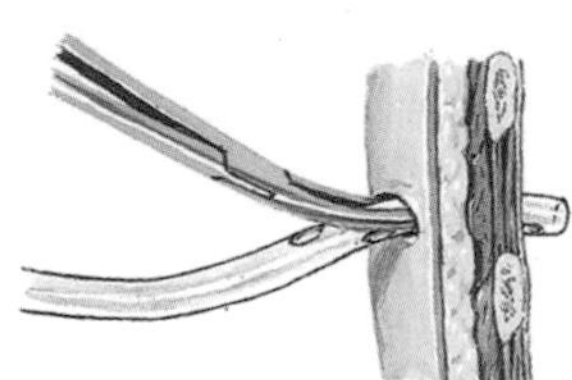

C. Tube attached to underwater seal (with suction if indicated)

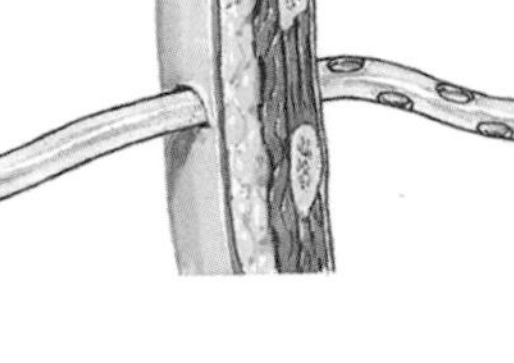

Note: For all techniques, local anesthesia is used; penetrate close to upper border of lower rib to avoid intercostal vessels. Aspirate first for free blood or free air (adherent lung)

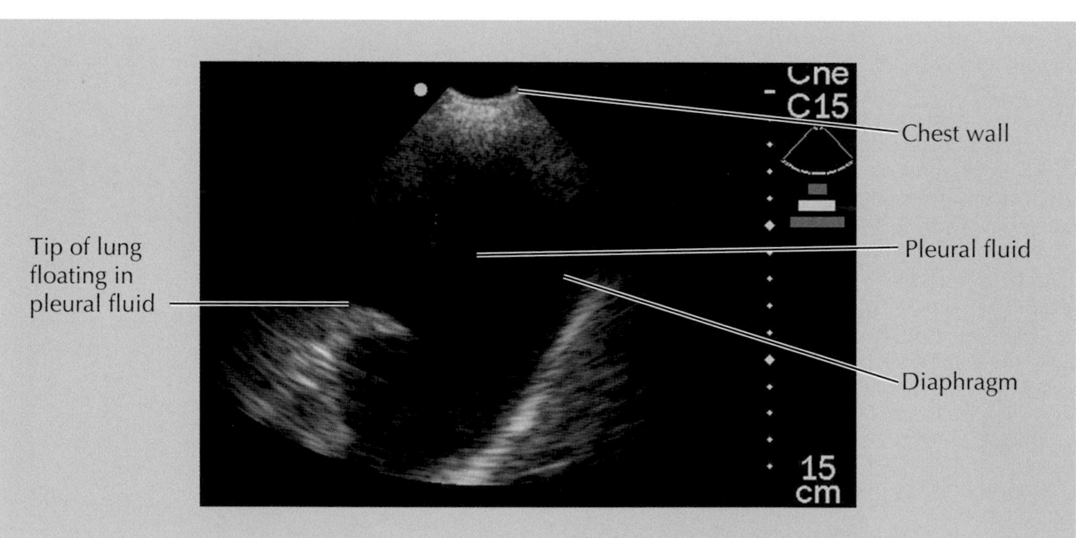

An underwater seal is attached to the tube and tube patency is present if an oscillating column within the tube is observed. Having the patient cough or sniff is the best way to demonstrate small oscillations of tube fluid; barely detectable tube fluid oscillation signifies either full lung expansion or tube blockage. Exacerbation of subcutaneous emphysema or an increasing pneumothorax with a tube in place usually signifies tube blockage or improper placement. Depending on the clinical situation, suction may also be applied to the tube.

After an intercostal tube has been inserted, its position and effectiveness must be checked by radiography as soon as possible.

Smaller tubes (8-14 Fr) can be used to drain pneumothoraces and simple pleural effusions. Larger tubes (>14 Fr) are typically required to drain empyema or hemothoraxes.

CHEST-DRAINING METHODS

Underwater-seal drainage of chest

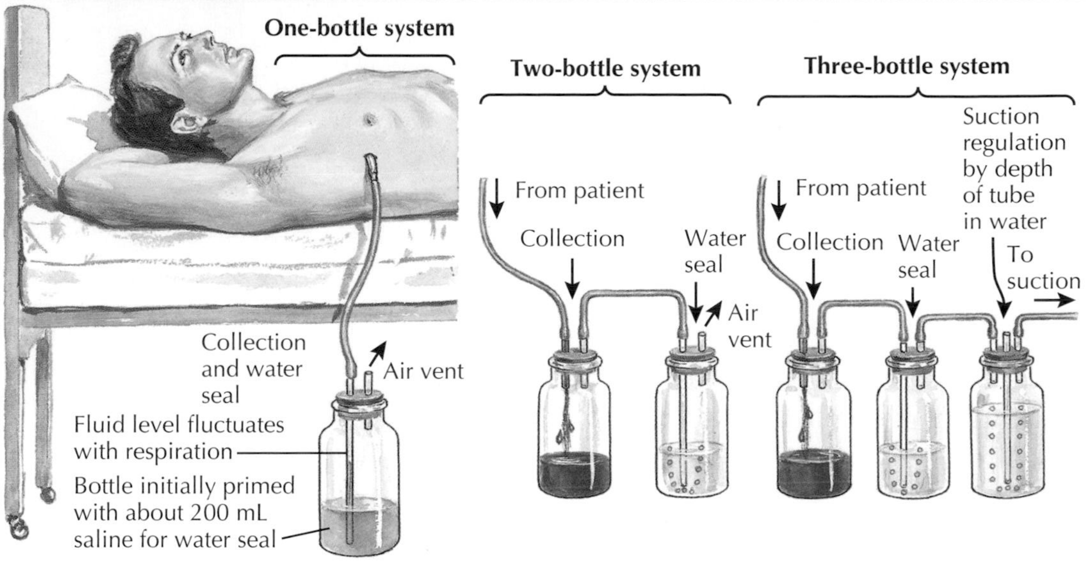

Heimlich valve

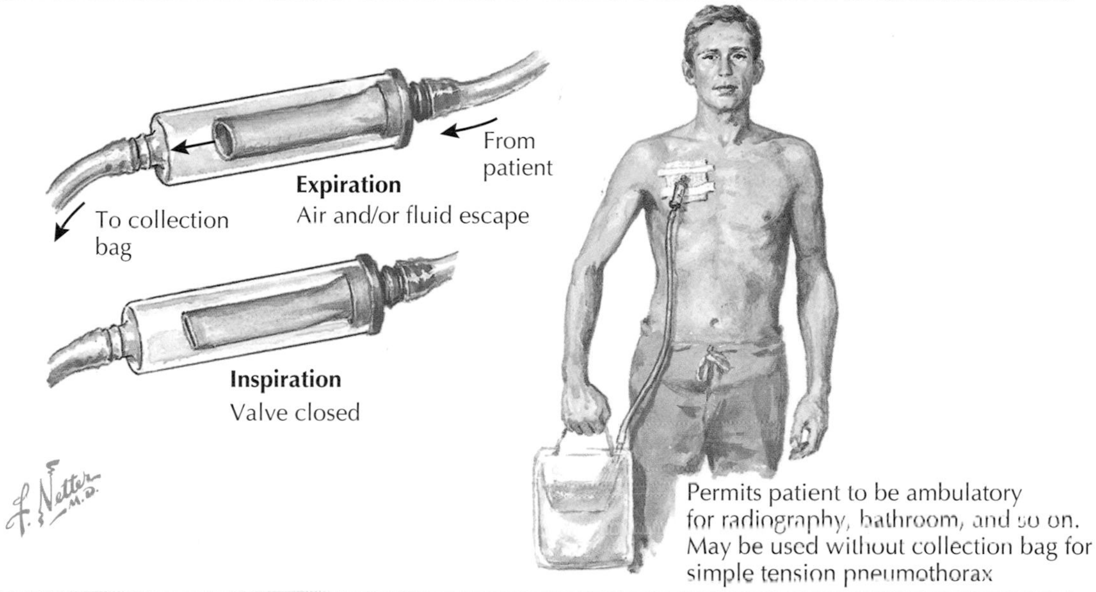

Subcutaneous chronic drainage catheter

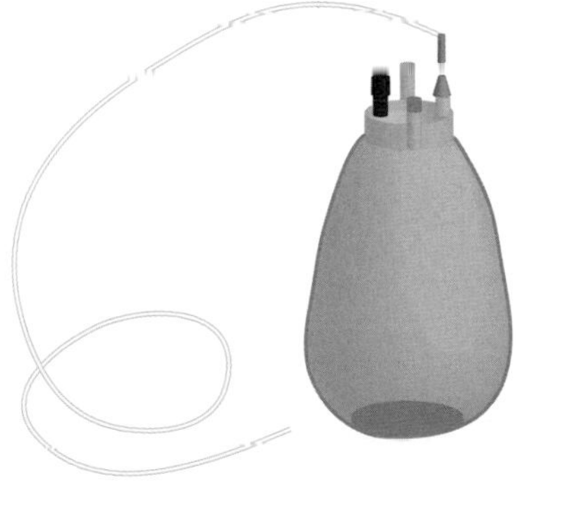

Disposable chest draining unit (three-bottle system)

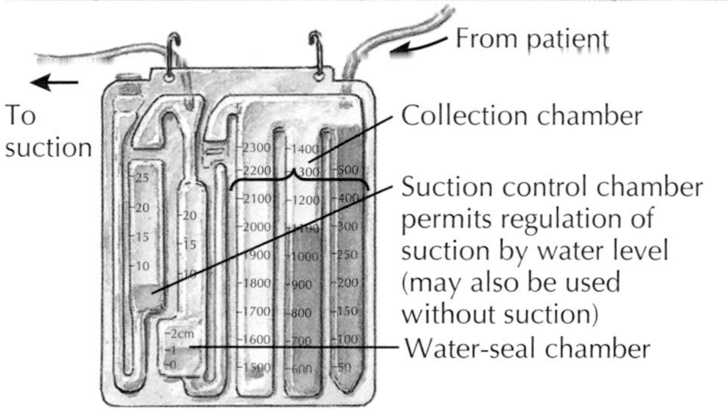

After an intercostal tube has been inserted, the pleural contents are evacuated into a chest drainage system. In the case of a pneumothorax, a one-way flutter valve (i.e., Heimlich valve) can also be used. The essential feature of the system is a means to permit escape of gas or fluid from the pleural space with no possibility of return using gravity or suction.

In recent years, disposable suction systems have become extremely popular, and some manufacturers have miniaturized these systems for true portability. It is important to understand the evolution of the now standard disposable suction systems. Initial drainage systems consisted of one bottle to drain fluid and act as a water-seal chamber. The water-seal chamber acts as a "pop-off" valve, preventing tension pneumothorax by allowing intrapleural air to leave the chest. When there is communication between airway opening (the mouth) and the pleural space, as in the case of a bronchopleural fistula, bubbles can be seen in the water-seal chamber of the chest tube. A drawback of the one-bottle system is that as drainage of fluid persisted, the increasing height of the fluid column increased the resistance for the evacuation of air. The two-bottle system separated the collection bottle from the water-seal bottle. By adding a third bottle, suction to the patient is regulated by the depth of the tube open to the atmosphere under water. As wall suction is increased, the meniscus drops until it reaches the bottom of the tube, and atmospheric air is then entrained. The disposable units incorporate these three bottles into one plastic container. When it is intended that the chest tube be connected to suction, one should always see bubbling in the suction chamber. Again, bubbling in the water-seal chamber indicates an air leak (communication between the airway opening and the pleural space) or a leak in the system. Some new disposable units are "dry," that is, suction is observed when a float is seen in the appropriate window.

If evacuation of fluid or air is impeded, there is a progressive increase in intrapleural pressure and further respiratory and circulatory compromise. This may occur in a number of ways. Soft chest drainage tubing may be occluded by kinking or outside pressure, or it may be of insufficient diameter to drain a large air leak. Dependent loops of tubing outside of the chest may contain fluid and result in significant back pressure and accumulation of intrapleural fluid or air. More than one drainage tube may be needed, especially in the case of larger air leaks.

In the case of pleural effusions, or in a patient who has had a recent pleurodesis, the chest tube can usually be removed when there is less than 100 to 200 mL of serous fluid draining in a 24-hour period. Occasionally, serosanguineous fluid may leak through the hole from which a tube has been removed, especially after coughing. This is not of concern because the leak almost always ceases spontaneously. If drainage occurs around a tube that is still in place, it suggests that the tip is no longer in communication with the intrapleural fluid, and needs to be stripped of fibrinous material, flushed with sterile saline, or removed. Infection caused by the presence of a drainage tube in the pleural space is unusual as long as sterile technique was used during insertion.

In certain situations, a tunneled, subcutaneous chest drain may be inserted to provide drainage of effusions for palliation. These devices allow patients to go home and can relieve symptoms of shortness of breath and chest pressure caused by chronic effusions.

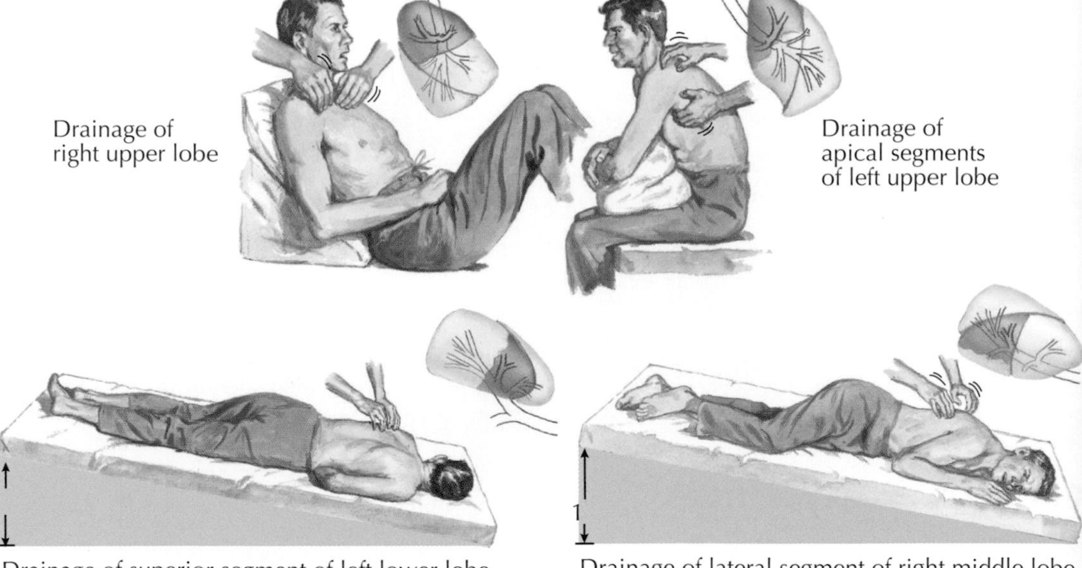

Drainage of right upper lobe

Drainage of apical segments of left upper lobe

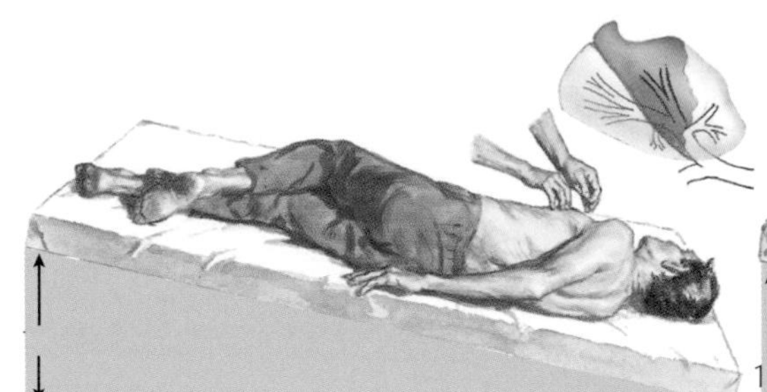

Drainage of superior segment of left lower lobe

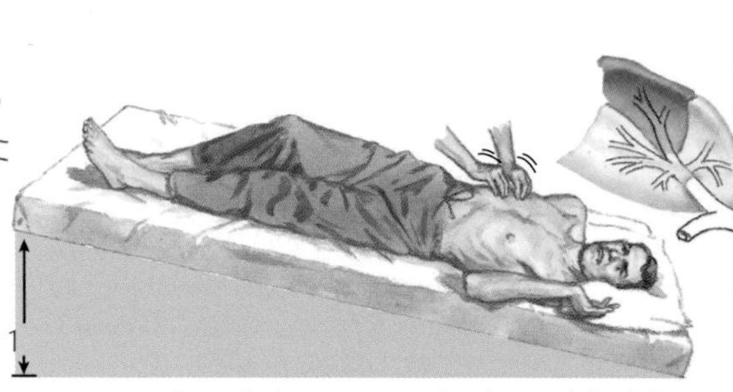

Drainage of lateral segment of right middle lobe

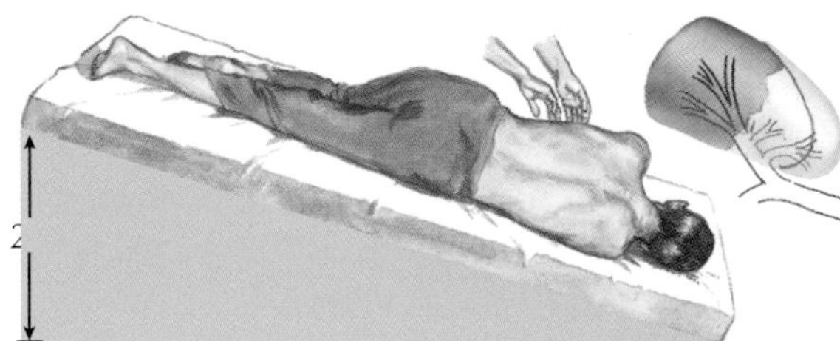

Drainage of inferior segment (lingula) of left upper lobe

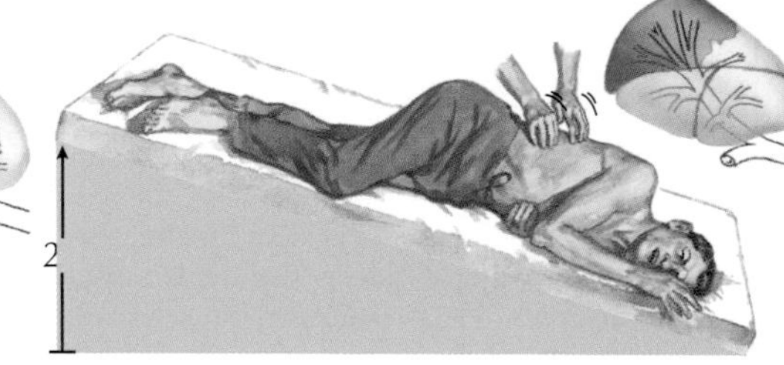

Drainage of medial segment of right middle lobe

Drainage of basal segments of left lower lobe

Drainage of basal segments of right lower lobe

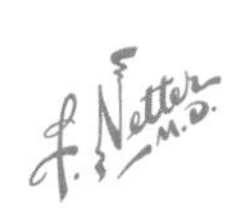

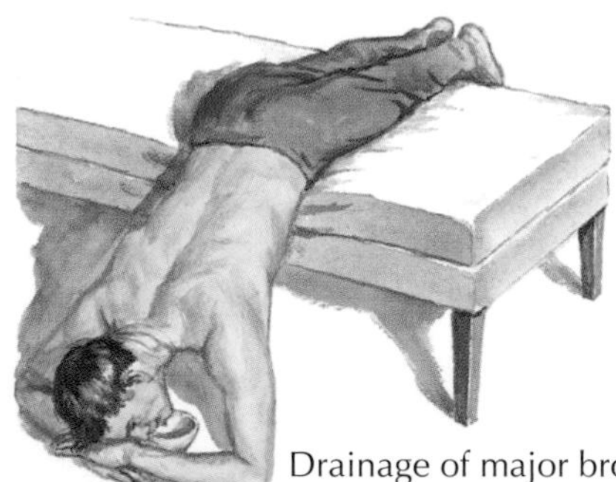

Drainage of major bronchi and trachea

Postural Drainage and Breathing Exercises

The accumulation of excess bronchial secretions is a major complicating factor in patients with chronic obstructive pulmonary disease, cystic fibrosis, or bronchiectasis and is particularly critical when the disease has advanced so far that both the cough mechanism and bronchociliary action are greatly impaired. The accumulated mucoid or mucopurulent secretions constitute a permanent source for the reactivation of bacterial infection. In addition, they can interrupt airflow and cause temporary or permanent airway obstruction.

Postural drainage, also called *gravitational drainage*, is the preferred and best-tolerated means for clearing the bronchial tree. Other techniques, such as suctioning or bronchial washing, cause considerable discomfort, often requiring local anesthetic and specialized paramedical personnel. Postural drainage can be practiced effectively in the patient's home with the assistance of a family member. Indeed, the fact that the patient is able to participate actively in his or her own therapy, rather than being merely a passive recipient, is also of value.

Adequate hydration is also important in facilitating drainage. Drainage is then accomplished by means of the following manual or electrically operated maneuvers to dislodge and help propel the trapped secretions toward the trachea: (1) percussion with rapid vibration tap, (2) tapping with cupped hands, and (3) high-frequency ultrasonography. These techniques are applied where drainage is most necessary, over either the anterior or the posterior chest wall, and are repeated during the time each position or posture is held by the patient.

Proper positioning of the patient, which is paramount, is done according to the distribution and configuration of the bronchopulmonary segments. To achieve maximal drainage of the apical segments of the upper lobe, for example, a slightly reclining upright position is the most effective. For drainage of the trachea and major bronchi, the right-angled head-down position should be assumed. The head-down (Trendelenburg) position should be used in draining the middle and lower pulmonary lobes.

Most patients tolerate these positions well, the exception being that the debilitated patient may initially experience difficulty in a achieving the right-angled head-down position. In such cases, this position should be attained very gradually and only to the degree of the individual's tolerance.

Postural drainage should be practiced at least twice a day. Each position should be held for 3 to 5 minutes. If at all possible, a family member should accompany the patient during the initial training for optimal preparation for assisting in home treatment.

The more recently developed high-frequency chest oscillation vest applies high-frequency vibrations throughout the chest wall. Patients typically wear the vest for 20 minutes twice a day. Vibrations can also be applied to the airways by breathing out through a small, handheld device that causes airway flutter. This may also facilitate removal of secretions. Autogenic drainage is another technique whereby patients breathe and "huff" cough at progressively larger lung volumes to facilitate movement of secretions from the smaller to the larger airways, where they can be more easily expectorated.

UPPER AIRWAY OBSTRUCTION AND THE HEIMLICH MANEUVER

"How many persons have perished, perhaps in an instant, and in the midst of a hearty laugh, the recital of an amusing anecdote, or the utterance of a funny joke, from the interception at the glottis of a piece of meat, a crumb of bread, a morsel of cheese, or a bit of potato, without suspicion on the part of those around of the real nature of the case!"

Although Gross wrote this comment in 1854, more than 100 years passed before Haugen, in 1963, used the term *café coronary* to describe sudden death—usually occurring in a restaurant—from food asphyxiation. Haugen and others advised that airway obstruction should immediately be suspected whenever an individual suddenly loses consciousness while dining and that, if death follows, one should question a diagnosis of "coronary" or "natural" causes.

In 1974, Heimlich first reported the results of animal studies on a new technique he proposed to relieve a completely obstructed airway. Over the next 2 years, Heimlich received reports of clinical experiences with the technique, documenting approximately 500 instances of successful resuscitative efforts, including 11 cases of self-resuscitation. His technique is now known as the Heimlich maneuver. Heimlich's work redirected attention to this important problem of food choking and foreign-body airway obstruction, including the need for immediate action.

The Heimlich maneuver is a technique whereby subdiaphragmatic compression creates an expulsive force from the lungs that is able to eject an obstructing object from the airway.

The anatomic basis for the Heimlich maneuver was established by observing that when a patient is in the lateral position during thoracotomy, pressure applied by the surgeon's fist upward into the abdomen below the rib cage causes the diaphragm to rise several inches into the pleural cavity. After studying airflow rates and pressures in conscious, healthy, adult volunteers, Heimlich concluded that the maneuver produced an average airflow of 205 L/min and pressure of 31 mm Hg, expelling an average of 945 mL of air in approximately 0.25 second. The projectile force thus generated propels nearly any obstruction from the airway.

Notably, chest thrusts and back slaps should not be used, as was once advocated. Chest thrusts produce less expelling force than the Heimlich maneuver, and back slaps may actually force an obstructing object deeper into the lungs.

To perform the Heimlich maneuver on an adult who is standing, the rescuer stands directly behind the victim.

1. The rescuer puts one arm around the victim's waist and makes a closed fist, positioning the thumb side of his or her fist just above the victim's navel and *well below the tip of the xiphoid process.*
2. The rescuer encircles the victim's waist with his or her free arm and clasps his or her closed fist.
3. The rescuer gives a single, sharp, quick inward and upward compression or "thrust." Sometimes a series of two or more thrusts may be necessary.

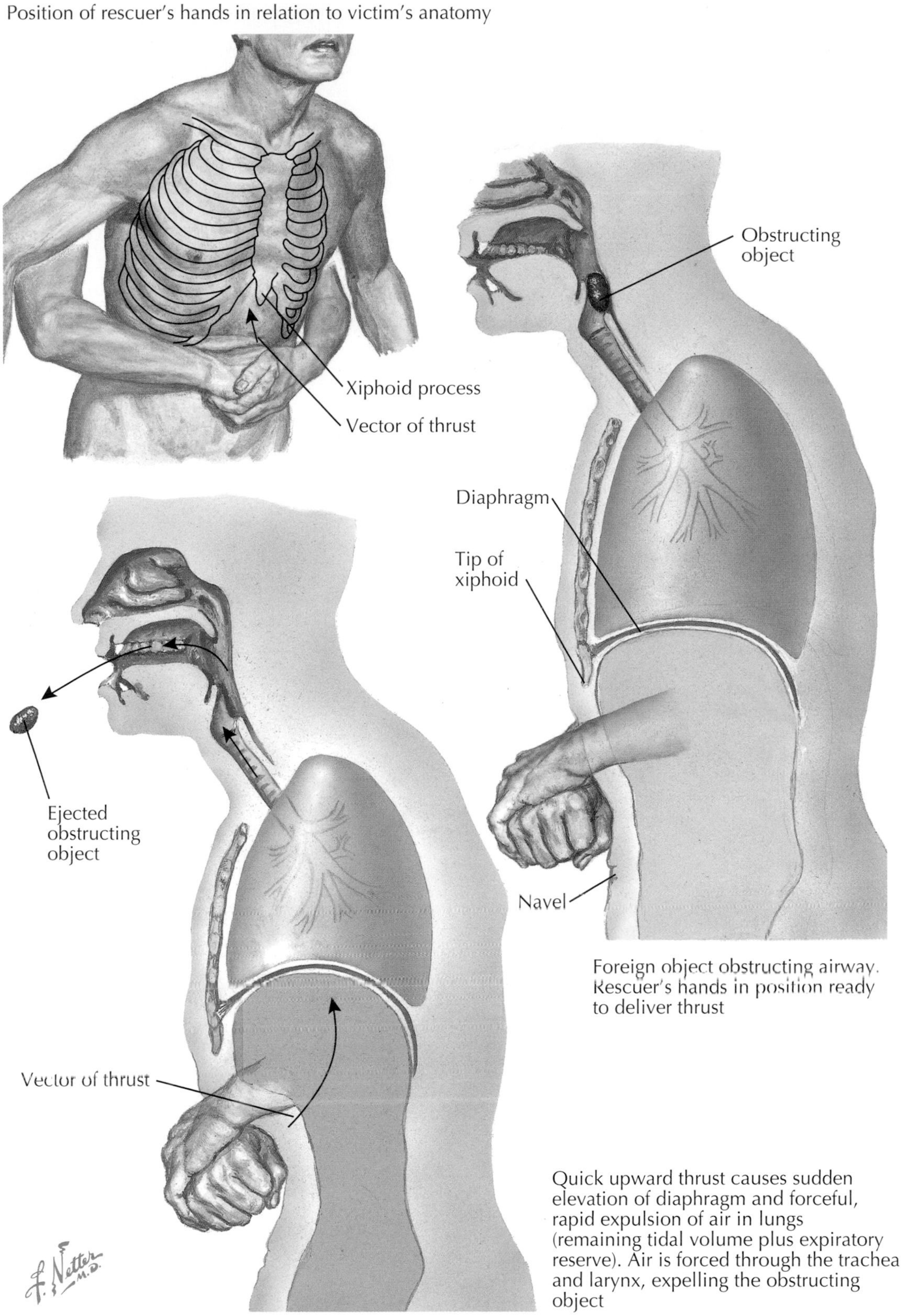

Position of rescuer's hands in relation to victim's anatomy

Foreign object obstructing airway. Rescuer's hands in position ready to deliver thrust

Quick upward thrust causes sudden elevation of diaphragm and forceful, rapid expulsion of air in lungs (remaining tidal volume plus expiratory reserve). Air is forced through the trachea and larynx, expelling the obstructing object

The compressions almost invariably cause the food bolus or foreign body to be ejected completely, or to "pop" out, or else propel the object into the mouth, where it is easily reached.

The Heimlich maneuver can also be performed in an adult victim who collapses to the floor supine. The rescuer simply kneels astride or straddles the victim and provides the maneuver via sharp inward and upward thrusts of the heel of the hand, maintaining a midline position. Adults may also apply the maneuver to themselves, either with their own fist, or by thrusting themselves over the edge of a chair, table, or other object to duplicate a rescuer's effort. In children, the rescuer applies the same technique using the index and middle fingers of one or both hands, depending on the child's size, either with the child supine, or held upright in the rescuer's lap. Infants should never be held upside down, and back blows should not be used.

Securing an Emergent Airway

Maintenance of a patent airway is a primary supportive and resuscitative maneuver, and every physician should be able to insert an oropharyngeal or nasopharyngeal airway, pass an endotracheal tube, and perform an emergency tracheotomy or cricothyrotomy. There are many causes of acute upper airway obstruction, including decreased pharyngeal muscle tone after loss of consciousness; acute inflammatory or infectious processes such as angioedema, epiglottitis, or Ludwig angina; and obstructing tumors or masses of the pharynx and larynx. Inhalation burns, laryngeal trauma, and foreign body aspiration can also lead to acute airway obstruction. Depending on the specific cause and severity of the airway compromise, different maneuvers and techniques may be implemented to secure an emergent airway.

Loss of consciousness is associated with relaxation of the pharyngeal musculature, causing the tongue to fall back and occlude the oropharynx. Simple repositioning with the neck extended and the mandible brought forward helps open the airway. If this fails, an oropharyngeal or nasopharyngeal airway can be used to reestablish the airway and allow for appropriate resuscitation measures to continue. For sustained ventilatory support, endotracheal intubation is required. The endotracheal tube may be introduced by the oropharyngeal or nasopharyngeal route. Oropharyngeal intubation is preferred, but nasopharyngeal intubation may be necessary in cases of posttraumatic cervical spine instability, impaired ability to open the mouth (trismus), or obstructing pathology affecting the tongue and floor of the mouth.

Whenever possible, endotracheal intubation is the procedure of choice for securing and maintaining a compromised airway. Unfortunately, this may not be feasible outside the hospital setting, and there will be times when endotracheal intubation fails despite multiple attempts in even the most experienced hands. In these situations, a surgical airway must be established, either by tracheotomy or cricothyrotomy. With the exception of young children and obese patients with poor anatomic landmarks, cricothyrotomy is preferred over tracheotomy in the emergent setting. Cricothyrotomy is performed by palpating the cricothyroid space in the midline of the neck and making a vertical incision through the overlying skin and soft tissue. A transverse stab incision is then made through the cricothyroid membrane with the point of the blade directed inferiorly to avoid laryngeal injury. A small endotracheal tube or any available tubular object is then inserted into the airway.

Cricothyrotomy carries the risk of permanent damage to the larynx and should be performed only in extreme emergencies when all other methods of providing an artificial airway have been exhausted. Serious bleeding may occur, and life-threatening subcutaneous emphysema has been reported. There is also the potential for adverse long-term sequelae, such as subglottic stenosis. For this reason, the cricothyrotomy should be converted to a formal tracheostomy by an experienced surgeon in the operating room after the patient has been stabilized. After the underlying condition or injury that caused the airway obstruction has been resolved and mechanical ventilation is no longer required, flexible fiberoptic laryngoscopy should be performed to assess the status of the upper airway before removing the tracheostomy tube.

Several temporizing measures have been described in an attempt to provide additional time to secure the airway without having to resort to emergent tracheotomy or cricothyrotomy. One example is "needle cricothyrotomy," in which a large-bore angiocatheter needle is used to cannulate the airway and deliver supplemental oxygen to the lungs. This technique carries the risk of inadvertently introducing air into the subcutaneous tissues of the neck, further complicating an already difficult situation. Ultimately, the potential morbidity and complications associated with emergent tracheotomy or cricothyrotomy are preferable to the anoxic brain injury or death that will occur if the airway is not secured.

Oropharyngeal airway

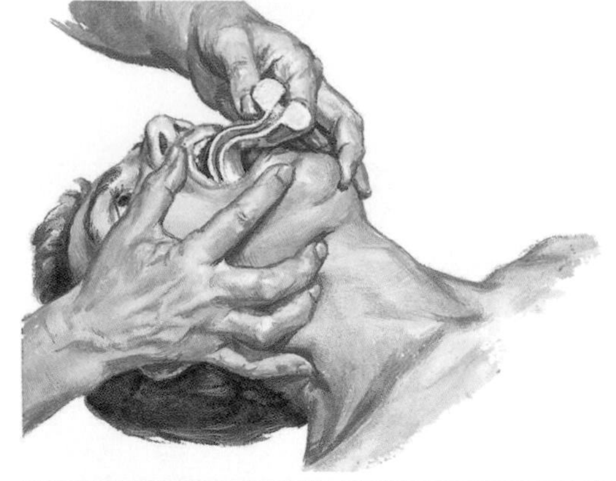

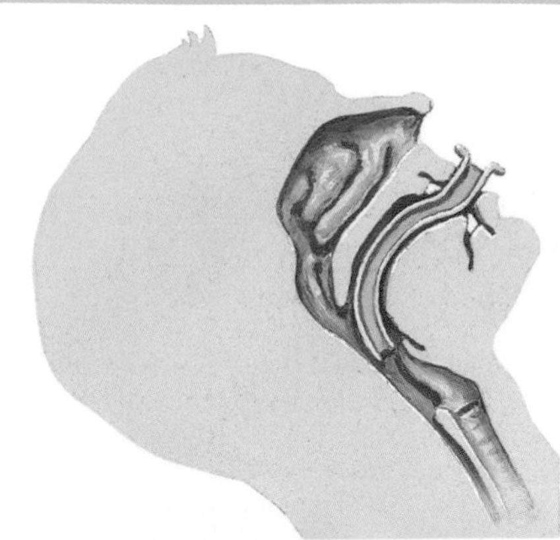

Nasopharyngeal airway

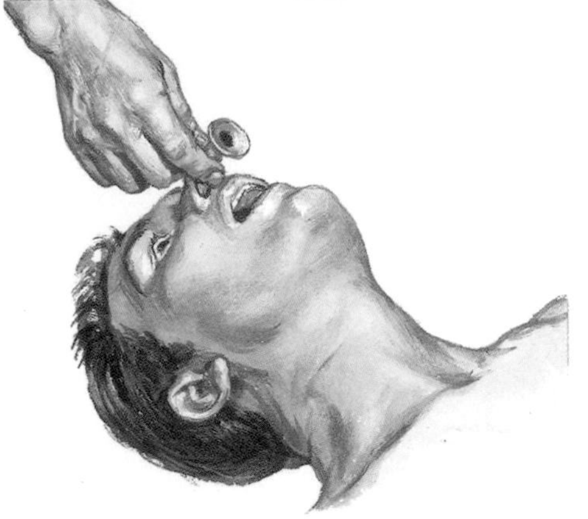

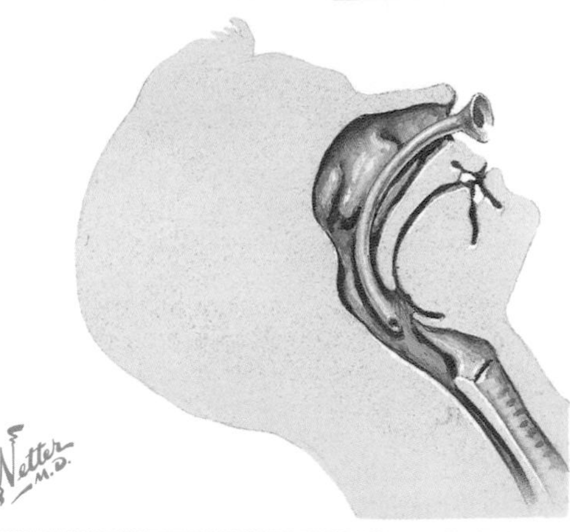

Cricothyrotomy

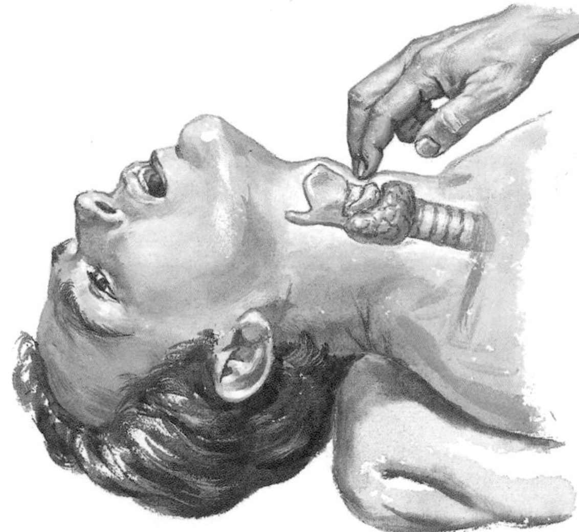

Cricothyroid membrane identified by palpating the transverse indentation between thyroid and cricoid cartilages

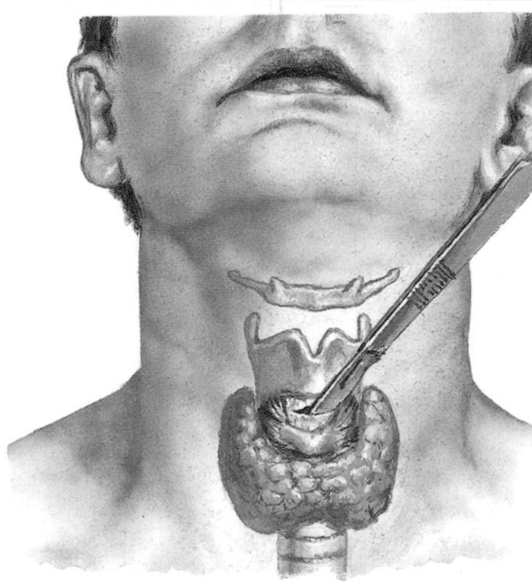

Skin and criocothyroid membrane incised with care not to injure the larynx or perforate the esophagus. Patency is then maintained by inserting the tube or, if not available, a distending object

A. Endotracheal tube introduced into larynx under direct vision with laryngoscope to avoid false passage into esophagus

B. Oral view

Endotracheal Intubation

Endotracheal intubation is a lifesaving procedure that requires familiarity with anatomy, physiology, pharmacology, and the necessary equipment required to perform the procedure.

Choice of the correct size of endotracheal tube is fundamental. The average man will accept a cuffed tube with an inner diameter of 8.0 or 8.5 mm. For women, the tube diameter is 0.5 to 1.0 mm smaller. Smaller tubes have more resistance to airflow and may not allow passage of a bronchoscope, but larger tubes may increase injury to the glottis and lower airway.

It is always best to be fully prepared with the necessary personnel and equipment before attempting endotracheal intubation. If a patient can be adequately oxygenated and ventilated with a bag-valve-mask, emergent intubation is not required. Necessary equipment includes an oxygen source and bag-valve-mask, suction, several sizes of endotracheal tubes and laryngoscopes, and any necessary medications. The light on the laryngoscope and the cuff of the endotracheal tube should always be tested before use.

Familiarity with various laryngoscopes is required. Whereas the curved McIntosh blade is positioned in the vallecula, the space between the base of the tongue and the epiglottis, laryngoscopes with straight blades (Miller) are designed to be placed posterior to the epiglottis. Proper positioning with the patient's neck flexed and head tilted slightly backward (the "sniffing position") is essential to provide a straight line from the oral cavity into the trachea.

To expose the larynx, the laryngoscope is held with the left hand, and the blade is first placed in the right side and then moved to the middle of the mouth, sweeping the tongue to the left. A straight blade is advanced along the posterior wall of the pharynx, distal to the epiglottis, and then gently lifted and withdrawn against the anterior wall, elevating the epiglottis until the larynx is clearly seen. A curved blade is moved along the base of the tongue until the tip is in the vallecula, and the tongue and epiglottis are lifted forward until the cords are in view. The laryngoscope should not be used to flex or extend the head by wrist movement because this may result in injury to the teeth. Introduction of an endotracheal tube should not be attempted unless the larynx is adequately exposed. A soft-metal stylet may facilitate intubation but should be removed after the tube passes the glottis so as not to injure the trachea.

Nasotracheal intubation is performed in a similar fashion except that the tube is inserted through the larger nostril, and a stylet cannot be used. When the tube reaches the pharynx, it may be grasped with a pair of curved forceps (Magill), with the balloon cuff being carefully avoided, and guided into the larynx and trachea.

After the tube has passed the vocal cords, it is advanced to a point approximately 2 to 3 cm proximal to the main carina. The low-pressure cuff is inflated with sufficient air to overcome any leak during forced ventilation. It should be tested intermittently with a gauge to ensure that the cuff pressure does not exceed 20 mm Hg. Adequate placement should be confirmed by auscultation of the lungs and epigastrium, visualization of chest rise, and the use of an end-tidal CO_2 detector. After the tube is correctly positioned, it should be adequately secured. It is sound practice to follow intubation with chest radiography to determine the tube's position.

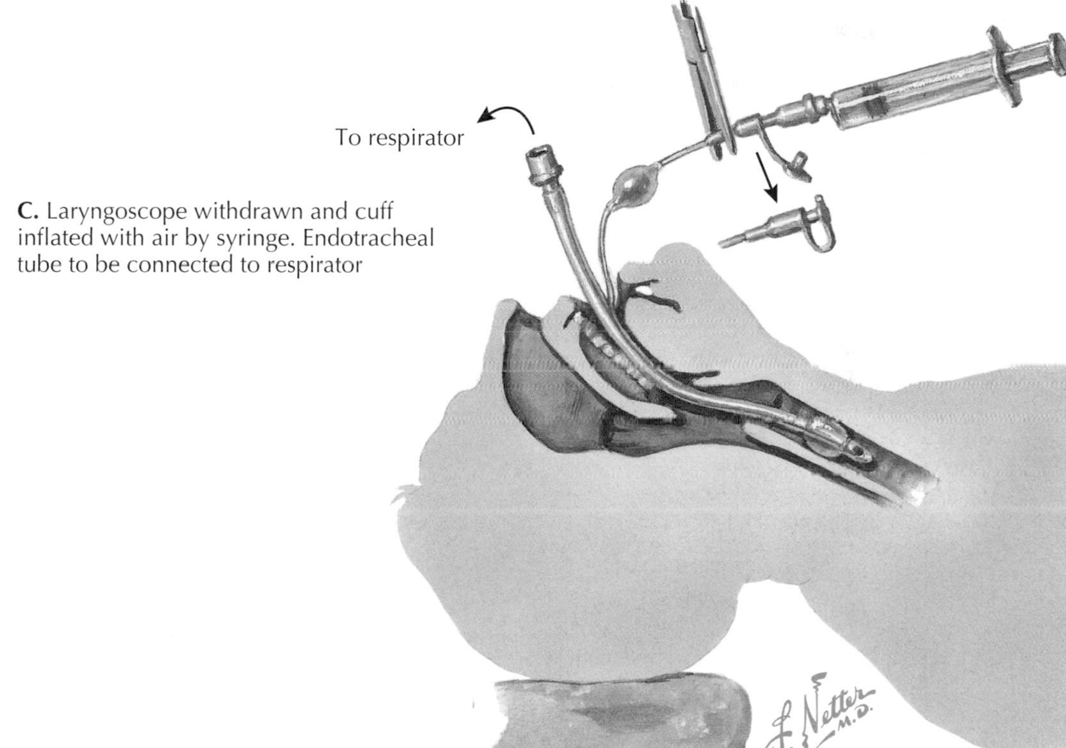

C. Laryngoscope withdrawn and cuff inflated with air by syringe. Endotracheal tube to be connected to respirator

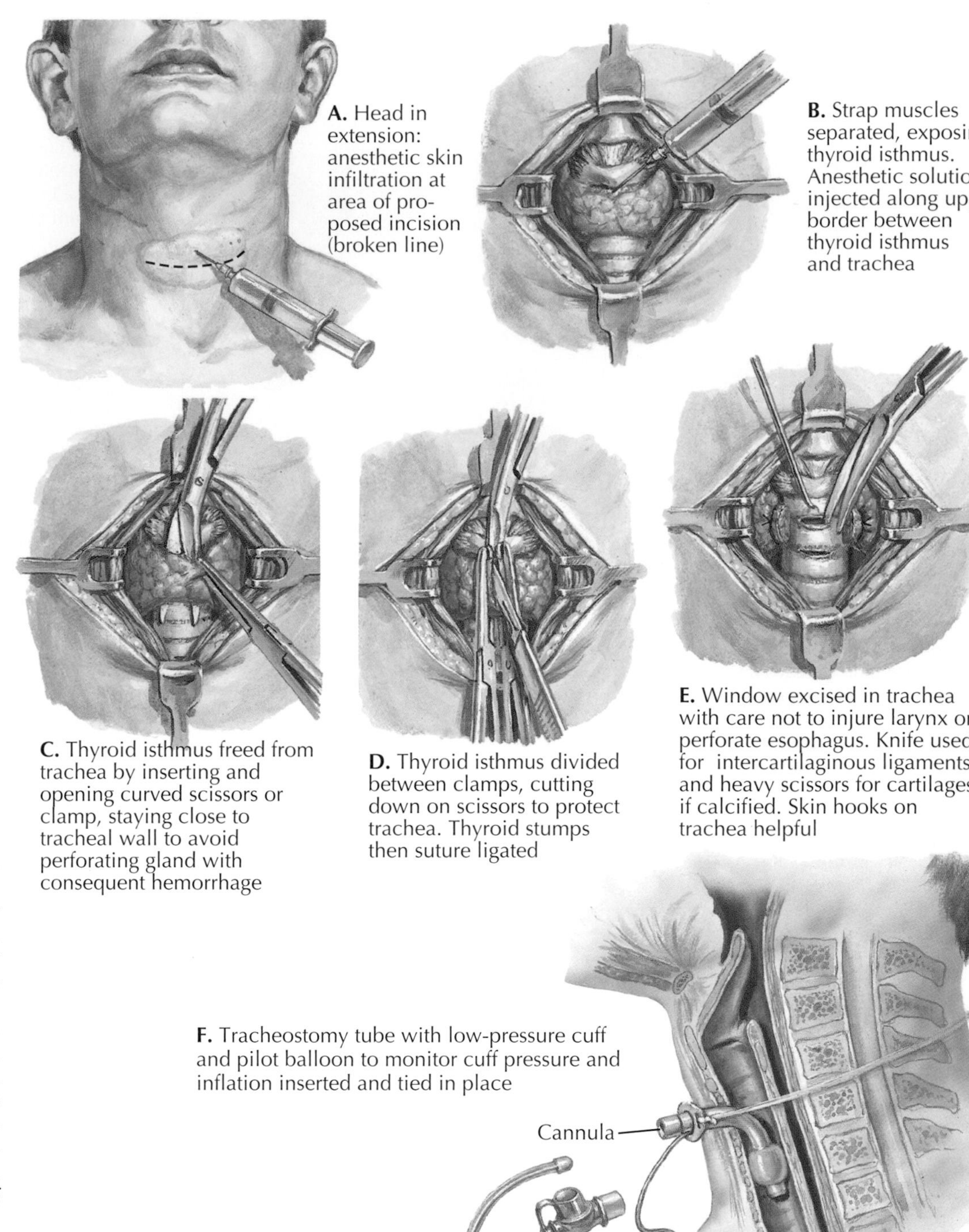

A. Head in extension: anesthetic skin infiltration at area of proposed incision (broken line)
B. Strap muscles separated, exposing thyroid isthmus. Anesthetic solution injected along upper border between thyroid isthmus and trachea
C. Thyroid isthmus freed from trachea by inserting and opening curved scissors or clamp, staying close to tracheal wall to avoid perforating gland with consequent hemorrhage
D. Thyroid isthmus divided between clamps, cutting down on scissors to protect trachea. Thyroid stumps then suture ligated
E. Window excised in trachea with care not to injure larynx or perforate esophagus. Knife used for intercartilaginous ligaments and heavy scissors for cartilages, if calcified. Skin hooks on trachea helpful
F. Tracheostomy tube with low-pressure cuff and pilot balloon to monitor cuff pressure and inflation inserted and tied in place
Cannula
Swivel connector
Obturator
G. Obturator removed and inner cannula inserted. Cuff inflated with care not to overinflate (some balloons automatically limit pressure). Mechanical ventilator may be connected if indicated, preferably via swivel connector to prevent undue rotation of tracheostomy tube as patient moves
Pilot balloon
F. Netter M.D.

Tracheostomy

Tracheostomy can be performed via an open surgical technique or via a percutaneous dilational technique. Percutaneous tracheostomy is becoming more popular because it is at least as safe as the surgical approach and is likely associated with fewer complications, primarily bleeding and infection. The choice between the two techniques typically depends on operator preference.

Key anatomic landmarks include the thyroid cartilage, cricoid cartilage, cricothyroid membrane, first and second tracheal rings, and sternal notch. The ideal insertion site for either technique is inferior to the first or second tracheal ring. Tracheostomies placed in the cricothyroid membrane have a higher incidence of tracheal stenosis, and those placed more inferiorly than the third or fourth ring may have a higher incidence of tracheoinnominate fistula formation.

With a surgical tracheostomy, the strap muscles are separated in the midline, exposing the isthmus of the thyroid gland. This usually overlies the second and third tracheal cartilaginous rings. If not retractable, the isthmus should be freed, divided, and ligated as illustrated. A Björk flap, an inferiorly based inverted U-shaped flap, is then created and sewn to the skin. A properly sized tracheostomy tube is then inserted and securely fixed.

Percutaneous dilational tracheostomy uses the same anatomic landmarks. After a small skin incision is made, blunt dissection is performed to the level of the trachea. A guidewire is placed via the modified Seldinger technique under bronchoscopic visualization, and the tract is dilated, most commonly with a initial punch dilator and then a single tapered dilator. The tracheostomy tube is then inserted and secured.

The classic silver-plated Jackson tracheostomy tubes have been replaced over the past decade by a variety of nonirritating plastic tubes. These have large-volume, low-pressure cuffs similar to endotracheal tubes, allowing for mechanical ventilation with minimal injury to the tracheal mucosa. Nonetheless, as with endotracheal tubes, cuff pressures should be followed, and kept below 20 mm Hg.

Tracheostomy has several benefits over translaryngeal intubation, including a requirement for less sedation, the ability to mobilize patients without fear of losing an airway, and perhaps more rapid weaning from mechanical ventilation and lower mortality rates. One-way valves (Passy-Muir) offer the ability to speak to some patients and can be of great psychological comfort to patients and their families.

Damage to the trachea from tracheostomy tubes can occur at the top of the tube, at the stoma, or at the level of the inflatable cuff. Erosion may occur into the esophagus, particularly if prolonged use of a nasogastric tube is also necessary, or into a major vessel with usually fatal results.

Morbidity of Endotracheal Intubation and Tracheostomy

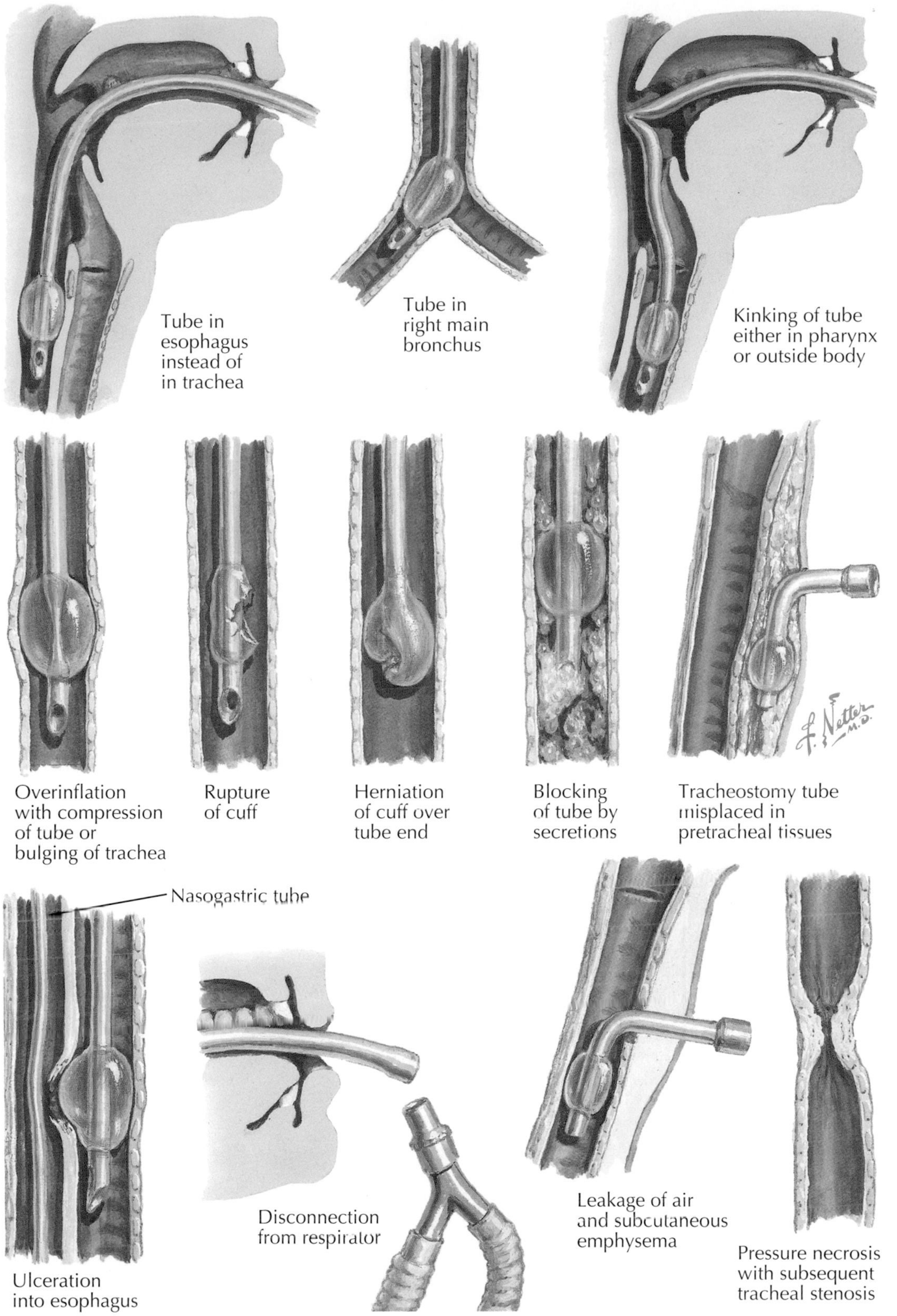

Nasotracheal tubes may be more easily inserted, less easily dislodged, and sometimes better tolerated than orotracheal tubes. However, they can cause nasal necrosis and maxillary sinusitis. "Blind insertion" may result in vocal cord trauma, which can be minimized by visualization, as with oral intubation. *Nasotracheal* tubes have small lumina, making suctioning and weaning from mechanical ventilation difficult. *Orotracheal tubes* are larger and more readily permit suctioning or bronchoscopy than nasotracheal tubes. However, they are less comfortable, more easily dislodged, and can be kinked or damaged by the patient's teeth.

Complications of intubation are caused by the pharmacologic and physiologic effects of medications and manipulation of the upper airway as well as mechanical injury from the laryngoscope, endotracheal tube, or stylet. Mechanical complications may include nasal, dental, or oropharyngeal trauma. Laryngospasm, laryngeal edema, aspiration of gastric contents, and intubation of the esophagus or right main bronchus may also occur. Additionally, tracheal injury, including rupture from the stylet may also be seen and is typically found at the junction of the posterior membrane with the cartilaginous trachea.

During mechanical ventilation, several problems may occur. *Obstruction* of the tube can be secondary to kinking, mucus plugging, blood clots, or slippage or overinflation of the cuff over the end of the tube. *Cuff leaks* caused by rupture may also occur, resulting in decreased minute ventilation and aspiration of secretions.

A serious complication of both tracheostomy and endotracheal intubation is the development of a *tracheoesophageal fistula*. A fistula should be suspected when air leaks, aspiration of saliva or secretions, or any signs of respiratory distress are noted. The diagnosis may be confirmed by bronchoscopy. The presence of a nasogastric tube may predispose to fistula formation caused by pressure necrosis between the trachea and esophagus.

Although occurring in fewer than 1% of patients with tracheostomy tubes, tracheoinnominate fistula may also occur; when untreated, it is associated with a mortality of 100%. The innominate artery typically traverses the trachea at the level of the ninth tracheal ring, although it may also do so between the sixth and thirteenth rings. Patients often present with peristomal bleeding or hemoptysis, which can be mild, moderate, or severe. If suspected, an emergent surgical consultation is required.

Acute and chronic problems may occur after *extubation*. An immediate complication is laryngospasm, which may require reintubation or tracheostomy. Minor problems such as sore throat and temporary hoarseness are frequent. Chronic problems include vocal cord incompetence, polyps, or ulcerations and development of a subglottic or tracheal stenosis or tracheomalacia. These can be diagnosed by indirect laryngoscopy or bronchoscopy. Common sites for stenosis and malacia include the area occupied by the cuff or tip of the endotracheal or tracheostomy tube as well as the superior tracheostomy stoma.

Bleeding and *subcutaneous emphysema* are more or less unique to tracheostomy. Bleeding at the incision site may be obvious or may occur internally with aspiration of blood. If the tracheostomy tube becomes dislodged, reinsertion is sometimes difficult, especially with a fresh tracheostomy. If a dislodged tracheostomy tube cannot be quickly and easily reinserted, endotracheal intubation or ventilation by mask may be required until an experienced surgeon is available. If a tracheostomy tube is inadvertently removed before the formation of a stoma (7-10 days after placement), replacement should *not* be attempted unless the airway is secured initially with an endotracheal tube.

Tube in esophagus instead of in trachea

Tube in right main bronchus

Kinking of tube either in pharynx or outside body

Overinflation with compression of tube or bulging of trachea

Rupture of cuff

Herniation of cuff over tube end

Blocking of tube by secretions

Tracheostomy tube misplaced in pretracheal tissues

Nasogastric tube

Ulceration into esophagus

Disconnection from respirator

Leakage of air and subcutaneous emphysema

Pressure necrosis with subsequent tracheal stenosis

F. Netter M.D.

ENDOTRACHEAL SUCTION

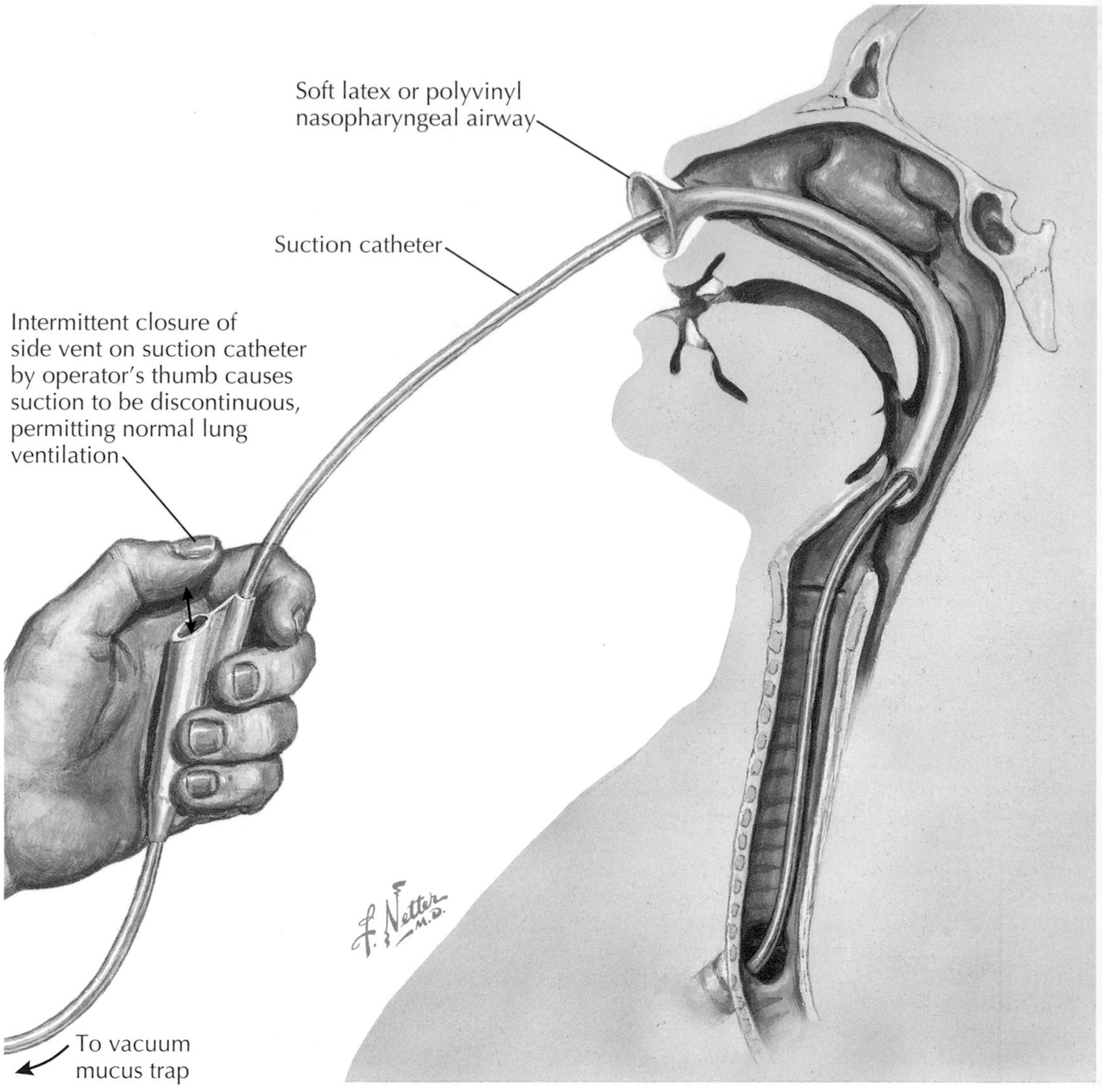

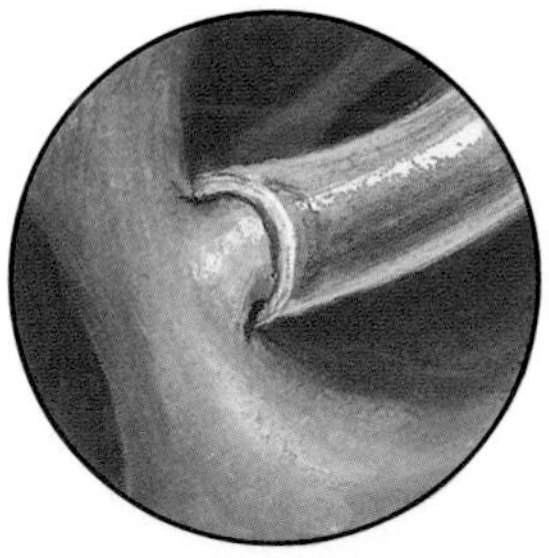

Nasotracheal suction aids in the removal of retained bronchopulmonary secretions in patients who are unable to expectorate sputum voluntarily. However, chest physiotherapy, including postural drainage, percussion, aided coughing, and vibratory positive expiratory pressure devices, can be quite effective and are more acceptable to alert and oriented patients. The major indication for nasotracheal suction is the semicooperative or obtunded patient who requires tracheobronchial toilet.

For nasotracheal suction, a soft latex or polyvinyl 32- or 34-Fr nasopharyngeal airway, lubricated with lidocaine jelly, is inserted into the nose and advanced so that its distal tip lies above the vocal cords. A 14-Fr suction catheter, held with a sterile-gloved hand, is then passed through the nasopharyngeal airway and advanced with each inspiratory phase of respiration. With passage through the vocal cords, the patient usually coughs. Introduction of the suction catheter in this way prevents trauma to the nasal mucosa and larynx and minimizes the deposition of upper airway secretions into the lung. Whereas approximately 90% of attempts to reach the tracheobronchial tree by this method are successful, the success rate for blind nasal passage ranges from 10% to 70% depending on the operator.

After passing the vocal cords, the catheter is advanced until it reaches the main bronchi. Because the right mainstem bronchus has a more vertical orientation than the left mainstem bronchus, the catheter more frequently enters the right-sided airways. The catheter is then withdrawn while the operator intermittently makes and breaks suction (set between 100 and 160 mm Hg) over a period of 15 to 25 seconds. The catheter is then removed and discarded after a single pass. Nasotracheal suctioning is generally effective in removing tracheal secretions. It also stimulates coughing, which facilitates clearance of secretions from the major bronchi. Nasotracheal suction of left-sided secretions usually is often ineffective, and bronchoscopic removal must be used.

Patients requiring mechanical ventilation often require "inline" suctioning because the presence of the endotracheal tube keeps the glottis patent, limiting the generation of sufficient intrathoracic pressure to adequately clear secretions. By minimizing disconnections from the ventilator, inline suctioning avoids derecruitment and reduces the risk of nosocomial infection. Hypoxemia may be minimized by limiting the duration of suctioning to 3 to 5 seconds and administering 100% oxygen for about 1 minute before the procedure.

Suctioning through a tracheostomy tube is performed in a similar fashion, using the inline method if the patient requires mechanical ventilation and the "sterile" technique if the patient is receiving supplemental oxygen via a humidified "trach collar." Clearly, because the airway is not a sterile environment, the procedure is not truly sterile; however, the operator should always try to minimize nosocomial infection by wearing sterile gloves and disposing of the suction tubing after each suctioning period.

It should be understood that all suction catheters traumatize the tracheobronchial mucosa in two ways: (1) by causing invagination of the mucosa into the end or side holes with consequent immediate ischemic necrosis of the area and (2) by direct physical contact, which results in delayed sloughing of ciliated epithelium many hours later. Erosions caused by suctioning permit colonization and penetration of the mucosa by pathogens as well as cessation of the host mechanism of mucociliary transport. Avoiding continuous suctioning and the use of a weaker vacuum tend to minimize the damage, but unfortunately, efficiency of secretion aspiration is also diminished.

Bronchoscopic view showing how mucosa may invaginate into side or end hole of ordinary suction catheter

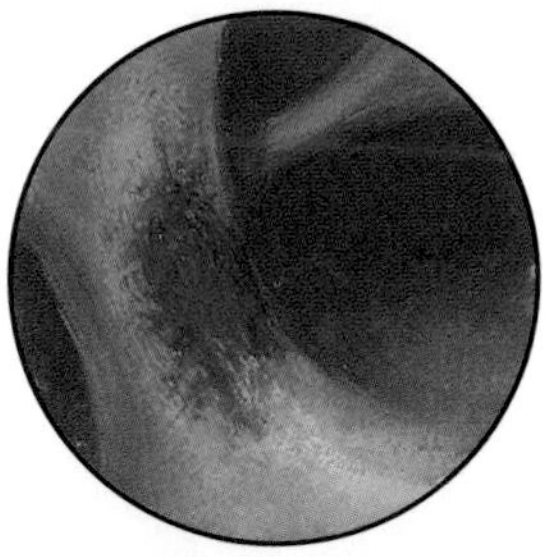

Hemorrhagic area at site of invagination after cessation of suction

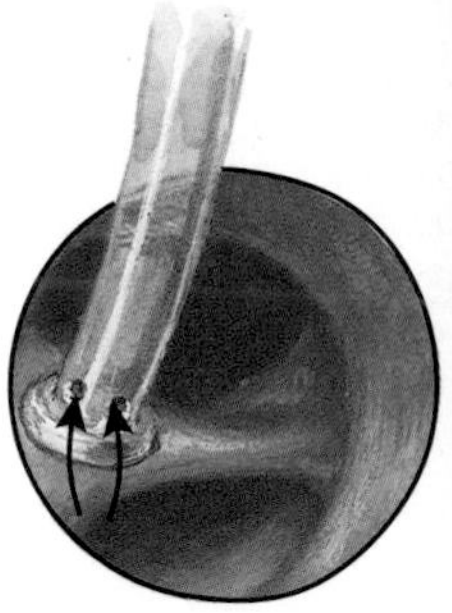

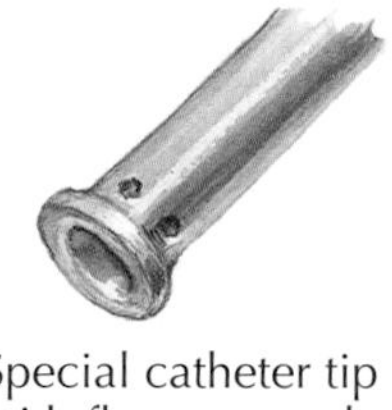

Flange prevents occlusion of small holes that serve as vents, and no invagination occurs even if end hole directly abuts wall (at bifurcation). Air cushion on way to small holes enhances protection

MECHANICAL VENTILATION

INDICATIONS AND GOALS OF THERAPY

Mechanical ventilation is used when patients cannot maintain adequate gas exchange because of neuromuscular impairment, cardiovascular failure, diffuse lung disease, or disordered respiratory drive. The goals of mechanical ventilation are to improve arterial oxygenation, decrease energy consumption, and facilitate carbon dioxide (CO_2) elimination so as to preserve adequate acid-base balance. Mechanical ventilation is continued until the condition responsible for respiratory failure improves and the patient can successfully resume adequate spontaneous respiration.

PRINCIPLES OF POSITIVE-PRESSURE MECHANICAL VENTILATION

To deliver a volume of gas into the lungs, a pressure difference (P_{tot}) must be applied across the respiratory system to overcome both the elastic recoil of the lung and chest wall (P_{el}) and the resistance of the anatomic and artificial (i.e., ventilator tubing, endotracheal tube) airways (P_{res}). This relationship can be approximated by the *equation of motion* for the respiratory system:

Eq 1 $$P_{tot} = P_{el} + P_{res}$$

or

Eq 2 $$Pressure = \frac{Volume}{Compliance} \times Flow \times Resistance$$

A ventilator can be set to control the flow applied and volume delivered during inspiration (right side of Eq 2), and the pressure applied by the ventilator is determined by the elastic recoil and resistance properties of the respiratory system. Because flow and volume are so closely related, this is conventionally called *volume-control ventilation*, even though most ventilators actually regulate flow. Alternatively, the ventilator can be set to apply a clinician-set airway pressure for a set time interval (left side of Eq 2). Flow and volume are then the dependent variables determined by respiratory system compliance and resistance, and this mode of ventilation is called *pressure-control ventilation*. Continuous positive end-expiratory pressure (PEEP) at 5 cm H_2O is routinely used to minimize atelectasis, but higher pressures are used to recruit collapsed alveoli in patients with acute respiratory distress syndrome (ARDS).

Modes of Ventilation

Mechanical ventilators must sense the patient's respiratory efforts and then interact with these efforts with a response selected by the clinician. Modes of ventilation refer to these different patterns of clinician-set responses to the patient's efforts. In full ventilatory support modes (*assist/control ventilation*), a full ventilator breath is delivered either at a set time after the last breath or in response to the patient's respiratory efforts as detected by changes in airway pressure or flow.

Alternatively, the clinician can set a minimum (backup) number of machine breaths triggered by the ventilator or the patient and allow the patient to have additional unsupported breaths above this backup rate without or with minimal machine support, a mode called *synchronized intermittent mandatory ventilation* (SIMV). Yet another option is *pressure support ventilation* (PSV), during which the patient triggers each breath but the ventilator provides only enough additional flow to maintain a clinician-set positive airway pressure. Both SIMV and PSV can be used to gradually reduce ventilatory support. PSV is often used during trials of spontaneous breathing to assess if mechanical ventilation can be discontinued.

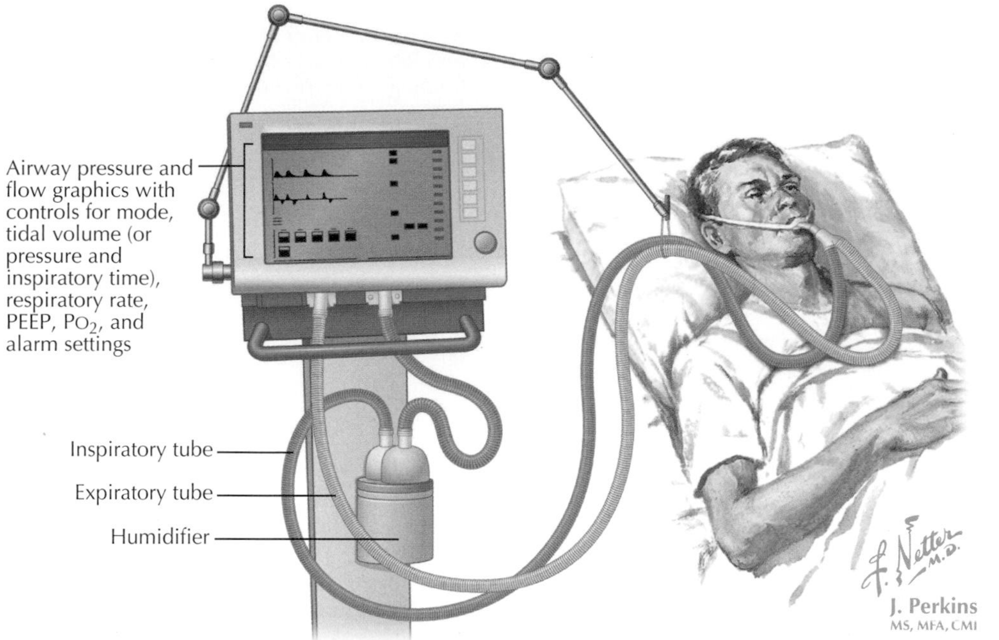

Airway pressure and flow graphics with controls for mode, tidal volume (or pressure and inspiratory time), respiratory rate, PEEP, PO_2, and alarm settings

Inspiratory tube

Expiratory tube

Humidifier

F. Netter M.D.

J. Perkins MS, MFA, CMI

Pressure and flow waveforms for volume-cycled ventilation

Peak P_{aw} | Peak P_A | Pressure | 0 | Inspiratory pause | Flow | 0 | P_{aw} | P_A

Schematic of pressure and flow during volume-cycled ventilation. The volume delivered is set by the operator; the resulting pressure is the dependent variable. The blue line shows ramped airway pressure (P_{aw}) applied during inspiration in response to a square-wave flow pattern shown in purple. The green line shows the change in alveolar pressure (P_A) with increasing lung volume. Application of a brief pause in flow at the end of inspiration allows demonstration of the plateau in P_{aw} and P_A.

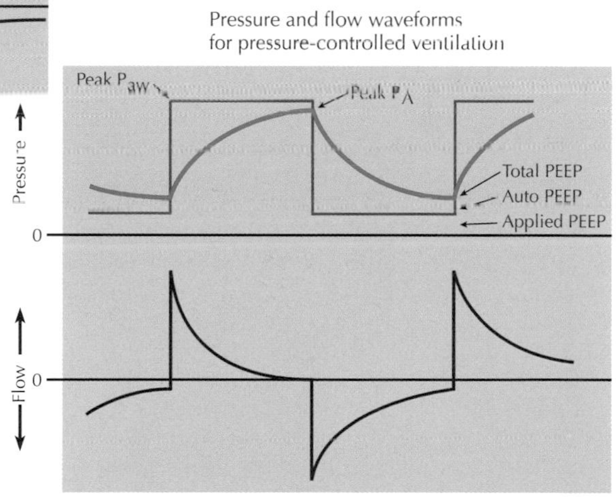

Pressure and flow waveforms for pressure-controlled ventilation

Peak P_{aw} | Peak P_A | Pressure | Total PEEP | Auto PEEP | Applied PEEP | 0 | Flow | 0

Schematic of pressure and flow during pressure-controlled ventilation. The inflation pressure is set by the operator, the resulting volume delivered is the dependent variable. The blue line shows the square wave of airway pressure (P_{aw}) applied during inspiration, generated by the decelerating flow pattern shown in purple. The green line shows the change in alveolar pressure (P_A). At the end of the expiratory phase, the total positive end-expiratory pressure (PEEP) remaining in the alveoli is equal to the applied PEEP plus any residual pressure (auto PEEP) that results from incomplete emptying of the lung.

Complications

After a patient has been placed on mechanical ventilation, the clinician must try to minimize the associated complications. Endotracheal and tracheotomy tubes bypass the anatomic barriers of the lung, putting patients at risk for ventilator-associated pneumonia (VAP), a serious and often fatal complication. Elevating the head of the bed 30 to 45 degrees appears to reduce aspiration and VAP incidence. Noninvasive ventilation using a tight-fitting nasal or full face mask may allow patients with chronic obstructive pulmonary disease exacerbations to avoid intubation and decrease the incidence of VAP. For patients with ARDS, use of low inspired lung volumes (6 mL/kg ideal body weight) improves outcomes by reducing additional lung injury, pneumothoraces, and hemodynamic compromise from excessive airway pressures. Because the rate of complications from mechanical ventilation increase with time, it is important to evaluate patients for liberation from mechanical ventilation on a daily basis.

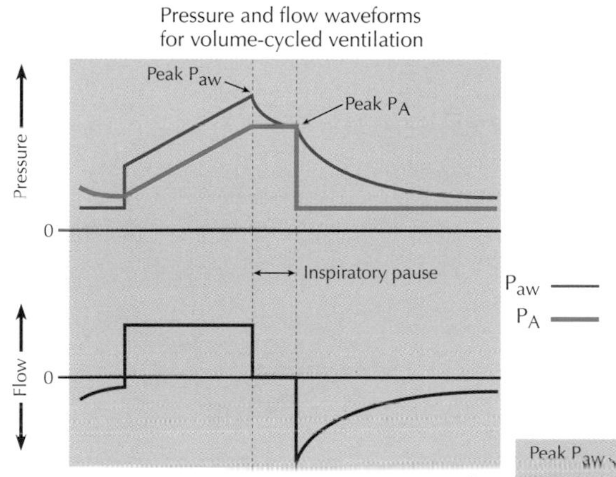

TRACHEAL RESECTION AND ANASTOMOSIS

Tracheal stenosis can be idiopathic but is most commonly the result of prior intubation or tracheostomy. Common areas of stenosis were previously located in the mid-trachea related to high-pressure, low-volume endotracheal tube cuffs; however, contemporary endotracheal appliances have low-pressure cuffs. Today stenotic lesions are typically found in the proximal or subglottic trachea at the site of a prior stoma. Mid- to distal tracheal resections are more likely performed as therapy for benign or malignant airway tumors. In most cases of symptom-producing stenosis of the trachea, conservative therapy, consisting of repeated dilatations, is either contraindicated or has proven to be ineffective. Consequently, surgical correction is necessary. The procedure of choice is resection of the stenotic tracheal segment with primary reconstruction via an end-to-end anastomosis (see illustration).

Resection and primary reconstruction are more easily accomplished if the lesion is in the cervical portion of the trachea than if it is within the mediastinum. In the former instance, the approach is via a transverse cervical incision; in the latter case, a full or partial (upper) median sternotomy or a fourth intercostal space right posterolateral thoracotomy may be required. Low intrathoracic tracheal lesions are more easily approached through a posterolateral thoracotomy, although some surgeons prefer a transpericardial approach accessing the trachea and main carina between the ascending aorta and superior vena cava through a sternotomy. Preoperative study of the location and extent of the lesion using both fiberoptic bronchoscopy and computed tomography is essential; the situation must be further evaluated at the time of surgery. Usually, the stenotic segment may be identified by the "hourglass" constriction of the outer tracheal wall. Nevertheless, the lumen must be examined via a transverse incision at the lower end of the constriction to determine whether the stenosis is circumferential or confined to the anterior and lateral cartilaginous walls of the trachea. Only the diseased region of the trachea should be dissected circumferentially to preserve the segmental blood supply of the remaining airway. For benign diseases, dissection should be directly on the airway cartilage to prevent injury to the recurrent laryngeal nerves that pass nearby in the tracheoesophageal groove. As the anastomosis is being completed, the surgeon assesses the reconstruction for tension. The patient's intraoperative position is adjusted by the anesthetist from full extension to partial neck flexion with pillows and blanket rolls to support the head. Additional length can be gained via release maneuvers. For extensive proximal tracheal resections, a suprahyoid or infrahyoid release may facilitate approximation of the divided tracheal ends. To relieve tension on an intrathoracic reconstruction, these cervical maneuvers provide minimal additional length. Releasing one or both inferior pulmonary ligaments as well as incision of the right-sided pericardial attachments to the atrium and inferior pulmonary vein is more efficacious.

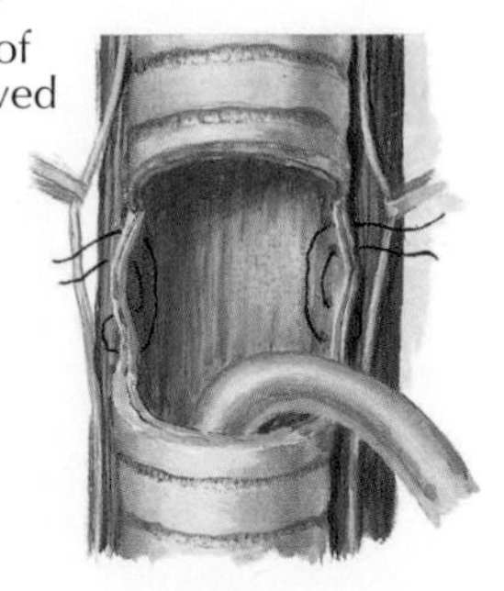

A. If only anterior and lateral walls of trachea are involved in stenosis, those portions are excised. A Stewart or Connell stitch is taken in each margin of intact posterior wall with care not to injure recurent laryngeal nerves

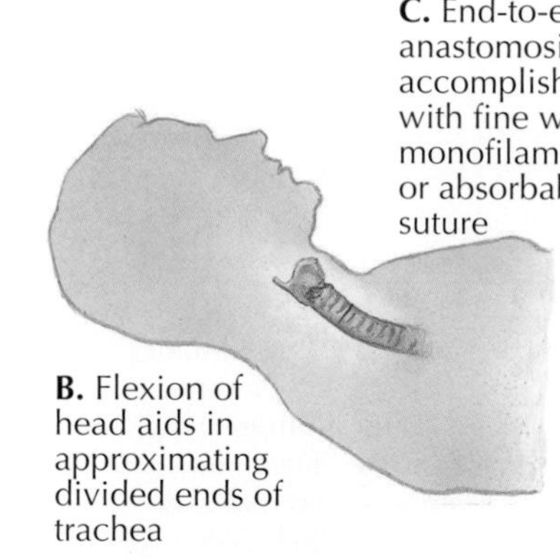

B. Flexion of head aids in approximating divided ends of trachea

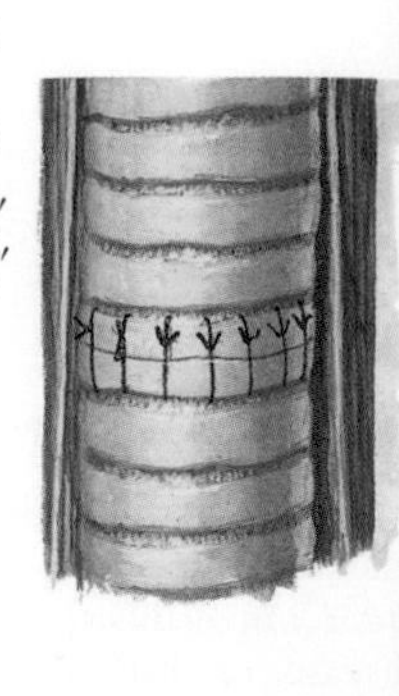

C. End-to-end anastomosis accomplished with fine wire, monofilament, or absorbable suture

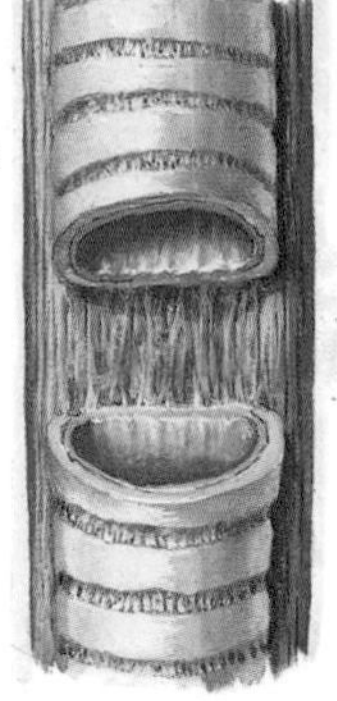

D. If entire circumference of trachea is involved, complete transection with excision of stenosed segment is necessary

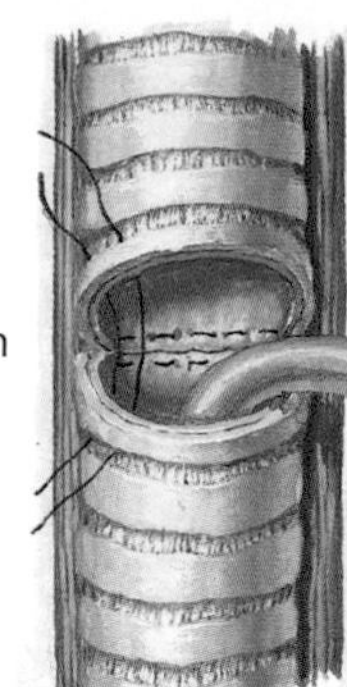

E. If only two or three rings require excision, approximation and suture may be accomplished with aid of head flexion

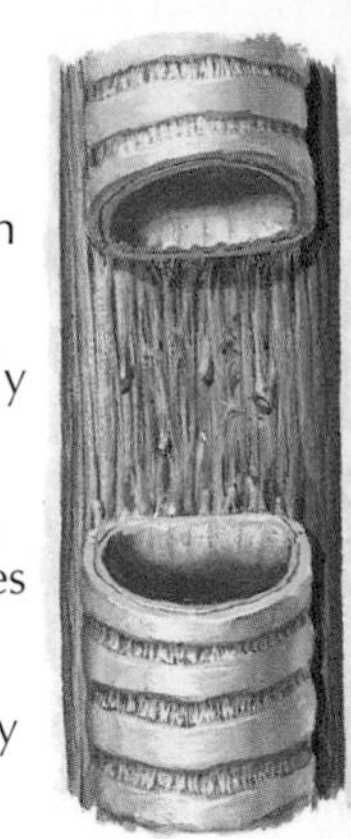

F. If more extensive excision is required, approximation may not be readily accomplished without undue tension on suture line, and measures to bring ends of trachea together become necessary

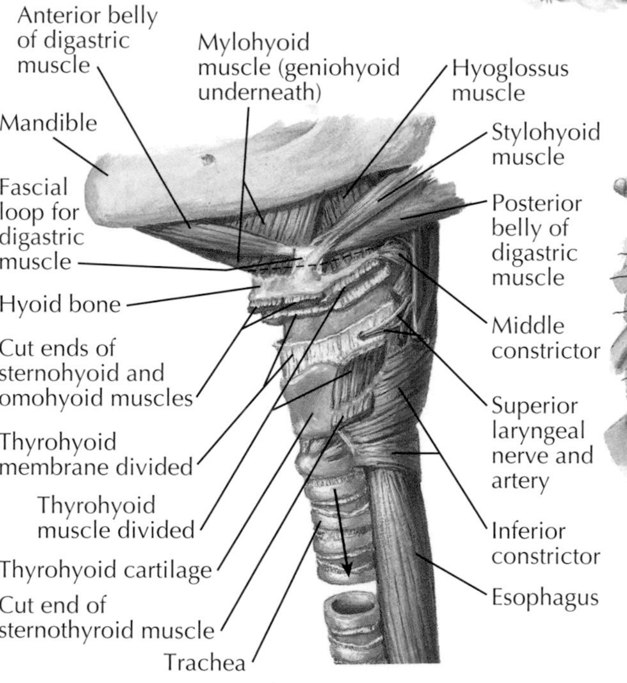

G. If upper tracheal relaxation is necessary, the larynx can be "dropped" by a suprahyoid release (dotted line), which involves cutting the muscles above the hyoid bone or an inferior hyoid release achieved by cutting the thyrohyoid muscle, thyrohyoid membrane, and upper fibers of the inferior constrictor, with care taken to avoid injury to the superior laryngeal artery and nerve

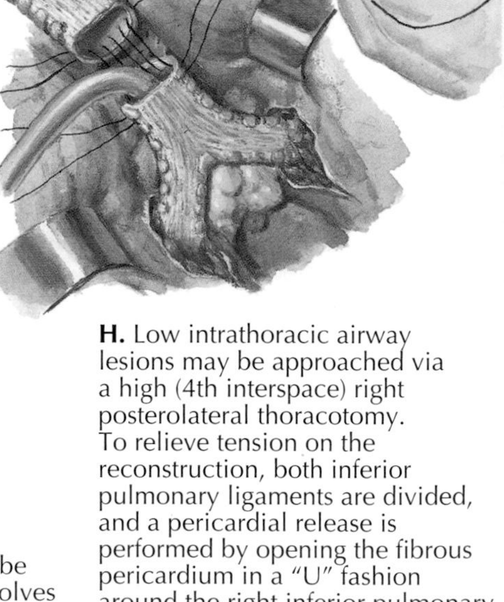

H. Low intrathoracic airway lesions may be approached via a high (4th interspace) right posterolateral thoracotomy. To relieve tension on the reconstruction, both inferior pulmonary ligaments are divided, and a pericardial release is performed by opening the fibrous pericardium in a "U" fashion around the right inferior pulmonary vein and dividing the frenulum of soft tissue attachments of the pericardium to the atrium

Removal of Mediastinal Tumors

Tumors of the mediastinum are a challenging group both diagnostically and in terms of treatment. A host of pathologic entities is involved, and for many of these, surgical excision is the treatment of choice. Recognition and identification of mediastinal abnormalities are almost always based on chest radiographs. Although the radiologic appearance is sometimes characteristic or (rarely) pathognomonic, most often it is the location within the mediastinum that is most influential in correct diagnostic interpretation.

Radiologic evaluation of the mediastinum depends on computed tomography (CT) imaging of the chest. If the chest, on lateral view, is divided into three roughly equal compartments in an anteroposterior plane, the most common tumors are as follows: (1) anterior/superior mediastinum—thymoma, germ cell tumors (mature teratoma, teratocarcinoma, yolk sac tumor), lymphoma, and intrathoracic thyroid extension (including substernal thyroid); (2) middle/visceral mediastinum—congenital bronchopulmonary foregut cysts and tumors of lymphoid involvement (Hodgkin and non-Hodgkin lymphomas and metastatic cancer); and (3) posterior mediastinum—tumors of neurogenic origin (neurofibroma) and esophageal lesions. Vascular tumors (aneurysms, anomalies, angiomas) may occur anywhere in the mediastinum.

The likelihood of malignancy is based on the location, the age of the patient, and the presence of symptoms. Two-thirds of mediastinal tumors are benign, but those in the anterior compartment are more likely to be malignant. The peak incidence of primary malignancy located in the mediastinum is between the second and fourth decades of life. Patients presenting with symptoms (localized or generalized) have a malignant process 85% of the time.

Most middle visceral and posterior compartment mediastinal tumors can be approached surgically by the standard posterolateral incision with the hemithorax entered at an appropriate level on the side of maximal projection of the lesion.

The illustration shows removal of a neurofibroma, the most common mediastinal tumor, which, characteristically, hugs the posterior costovertebral angle. Most such tumors are readily shelled out, and their blood supply is easily identified. The presence of an intraspinal component ("dumbbell" tumor) should be ruled out preoperatively by means of magnetic resonance imaging of the spine showing the intervertebral foramina. If present, a collaborative procedure with a neurosurgeon is necessary to control the intraspinal component, first avoiding potential cord compression or injury.

Although an anterior mediastinal lesion can be handled by the lateral approach, most surgeons prefer a median sternotomy, as shown. This is the preferred incision for thymic tumors, particularly in the presence of myasthenia gravis in which complete extirpation of all components of thymic origin is desired. When the tumor is large or densely adherent, this approach may present difficulties because the tumor lies between the operator and the vital structures from which it must be freed. A partial sternal splitting incision extended into an anterior thoracotomy (hemi-clamshell) or bilateral transverse sternothoracotomy (full clamshell) incision, on the other hand, is now quite commonly used (for bilateral lung transplantation), is reasonably rapid, and affords access to both pleural cavities.

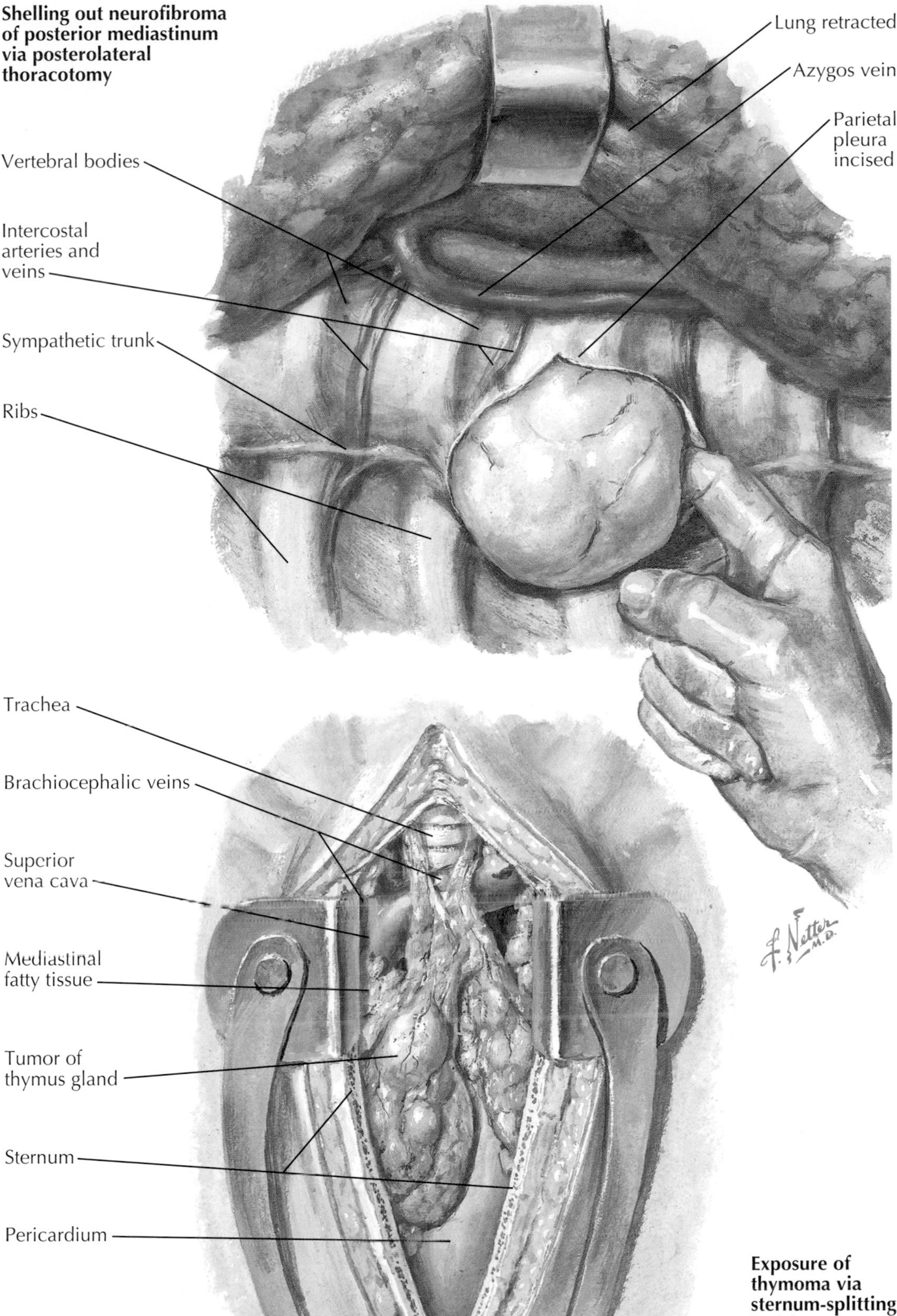

Sublobar Resection and Surgical Lung Biopsy

SEGMENTAL RESECTION

Resection of lung tissue anatomically less than a lobe is carried out for localized lesions such as benign tumors, granulomas, tuberculous foci, bronchiectasis, metastatic cancers, and others and to obtain tissue specimens required for the diagnosis of diffuse pulmonary disease processes. Recent evidence suggests anatomic segmentectomy may provide survival equivalent to lobectomy for small (≤2 cm) primary lung cancers in the absence of regional node involvement.

Segmentectomy requires a detailed anatomic knowledge of secondary and tertiary hilar structures. Intersegmental cleavage planes are best defined at operation when, by selective bronchial occlusion, adjacent portions of lung tissue are maintained, one inflated and the other atelectatic. Resection of only one or more segments has the advantage of removing only diseased structures and leaving healthy, functioning lung tissue that ordinarily would be removed if the excision involved the whole lobe. When the resection is for cancer, the oncologic principle of inclusion of regional draining lymphatics and nodes is preserved.

Segmental resection is commonly performed through the standard posterolateral thoracotomy incision, although video-assisted thoracoscopic surgery (VATS) segmentectomies are now acceptable. Depending on individual circumstances, the segmental bronchus is identified and approached first by palpation or the segmental artery first by dissection. Whenever feasible, it is preferable to locate and divide the arterial supply to the segment first because this minimizes chances of major bleeding during the procedure. The main pulmonary artery, or the continuing pulmonary artery, is identified in its proper anatomic location, and the perivascular sheath is entered. The segmental artery or arteries are located, carefully dissected free, and divided after appropriate proximal and distal ligation.

The segmental bronchus is closely adjacent and then may be palpated and dissected free. To ensure correct identification of the proper bronchus after it is dissected free, one carries out temporary atraumatic occlusion of this structure while the remainder of the lobe is being inflated by the anesthesiologist. After division and closure by stapling or by suture, a clamp is left on the distal portion of the severed bronchus, subsequently to be used for traction. If the draining vein or veins are seen, these are divided between ligatures. However, the veins are frequently identified only as branches in the intersegmental plane.

Separation of the intersegmental plane is performed either with a stapling device, which simultaneously controls the veins and parenchyma, or by blunt dissection with the fingers, working toward the pleural surface while exercising traction on the clamp attached to the distal divided bronchus. Venous branches on the segmental surface are grasped by small hemostats before cutting and subsequently ligated with fine suture material. These veins can serve as a helpful guide to the intersegmental plane as dissection proceeds.

Segmental resection

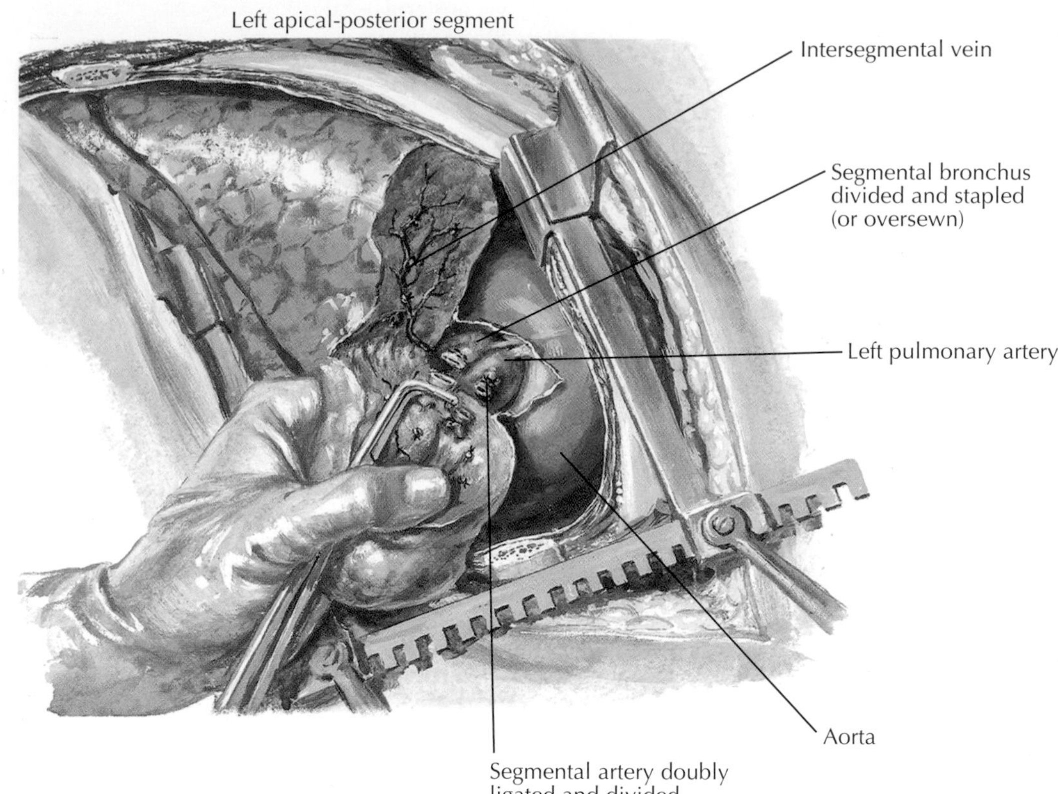

Wedge resection or open lung biopsy

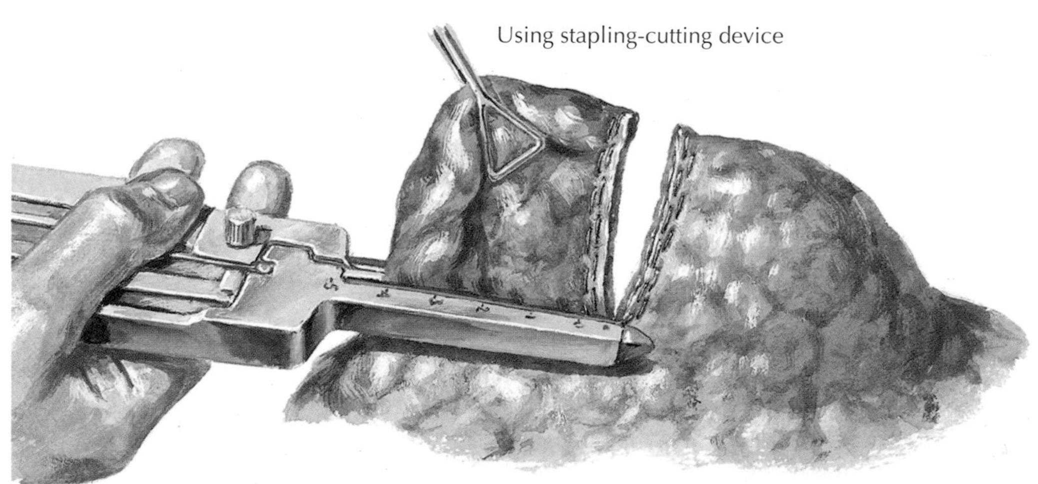

WEDGE RESECTION

Wedge resections are useful when one is dealing with small peripheral lesions or for diagnosis of a diffuse disease process. Less lung tissue is removed, as a rule, than with segmental resection, and the procedure is simpler, safer, and quicker.

Wedge resection has been made easier by the availability of stapling-cutting instruments that lay down two or three rows of staples on either side and divide lung tissue in between these rows. Bleeding is rarely a problem—requiring only one or two suture ligatures if it is present—and air leaks are negligible. These mechanical staplers have been modified for minimally invasive procedures so that most wedge resections can be performed by VATS, eliminating the morbidity of thoracotomy.

LOBECTOMY

Lobectomy is a more difficult procedure to perform than pneumonectomy, particularly in the presence of chronic inflammatory changes or where tumor (or involved lymph nodes) involves the lobar hilum. Not only must the critical lobar structures be individually identified and controlled by the surgeon, but the remaining structures must be painstakingly protected and preserved. Incomplete fissures may add to the problem, and the surgeon must possess a precise knowledge of hilar anatomy and common anomalies.

The standard approach is a posterolateral muscle-sparing thoracotomy. Video-assisted lobectomy is gaining popularity and is now routine in many centers. The key steps to performing a lobectomy involve mobilization of the lobe, dissection of the fissure, and vessel and bronchus division.

Dissection of the lobe can be complicated by an incomplete fissure. Pulmonary vein branches pass between bronchopulmonary segments and lobes, but pulmonary arterial branches generally follow the bronchial tree. An incomplete fissure may be congenital or the result of inflammation or a pathologic process extending across the fissure. Separating the lobes often requires sharp and blunt dissection and may require the use of a mechanical stapling device. Interlobar venous branches should be isolated and divided when encountered.

The key to anatomic pulmonary surgery is a detailed understanding of bronchopulmonary anatomy with careful dissection directly on the branch pulmonary arteries. Next, the perivascular sheath surrounding the pulmonary artery is entered and, with the lobe drawn downward and backward, each arterial branch is dissected free with a right-angle clamp as it is encountered. The segmental artery is then ligated close to its point of origin. After proximal ligation has been accomplished, it is usually possible to dissect distally along the branch so that placement of the distal tie will permit leaving a long proximal stump when the branch artery is divided. The first branch found is usually the apical posterior artery. Often segmental branch arteries have a common trunk, which can be ligated proximally while distal control is obtained of each segmental vessel.

The main artery is followed down the oblique fissure, exposing its anterior and posterior aspects. The lowermost branches to the upper lobe supply the lingula and come off anteriorly. Directly opposite, on the posterior aspect of the continuing left main pulmonary artery, the artery to the superior segment of the lower lobe takes origin, and this should be carefully preserved.

The lung is then retracted posteriorly for dissection of the superior pulmonary vein, which drains the upper lobe, including the lingula on the left side. This vein is proximally and distally ligated and divided. Alternatively, a vascular stapler may be used given sufficient length of the dissected vein.

After dissection of the fissures and vessels has been completed, the lung is left attached only by the bronchus, which is cleared by sweeping lymph nodes and connective tissue distally toward the specimen. An atraumatic bronchial clamp or noncutting stapler is then placed across the bronchus, and the anesthesiologist is asked to inflate the lung. Correct identification of the bronchus clamped is ensured when the lower lobe inflates and the upper remains collapsed. Despite the confidence of the surgeon in his or her dissection and perception of the anatomy, this simple maneuver, requiring only a few moments, may avoid considerable trouble later on. The stapling device is then fired across the bronchus close to its origin and the bronchus is amputated on the distal aspect of the anvil after stapling. The stump is then tested for an air leak.

Resection of the left upper lobe can be more difficult than a similar procedure on the right side. The main pulmonary artery is exposed as it emerges from beneath the arch of the aorta, and care is exercised to avoid the left recurrent nerve as it passes beneath the aortic arch. In contrast to the right side, the artery passes behind the bronchus. The arterial branches of the left main pulmonary artery may number five or more, and there are considerable variations in their location. If a problem situation is anticipated (e.g., bulky hilar lesion), the left main pulmonary artery should be freed up and an umbilical tape passed around it. Thus, if an arterial tear or hemorrhage occurs later on, it becomes a simple matter to place a vascular clamp or tourniquet across the vessel and gain control.

When an upper lobe lobectomy is performed for cancer, the mediastinum should be opened and all lymph nodes cleared to the carina (or beyond) if suspicion of lymphatic metastasis exists.

LOBECTOMY: LEFT UPPER LOBE

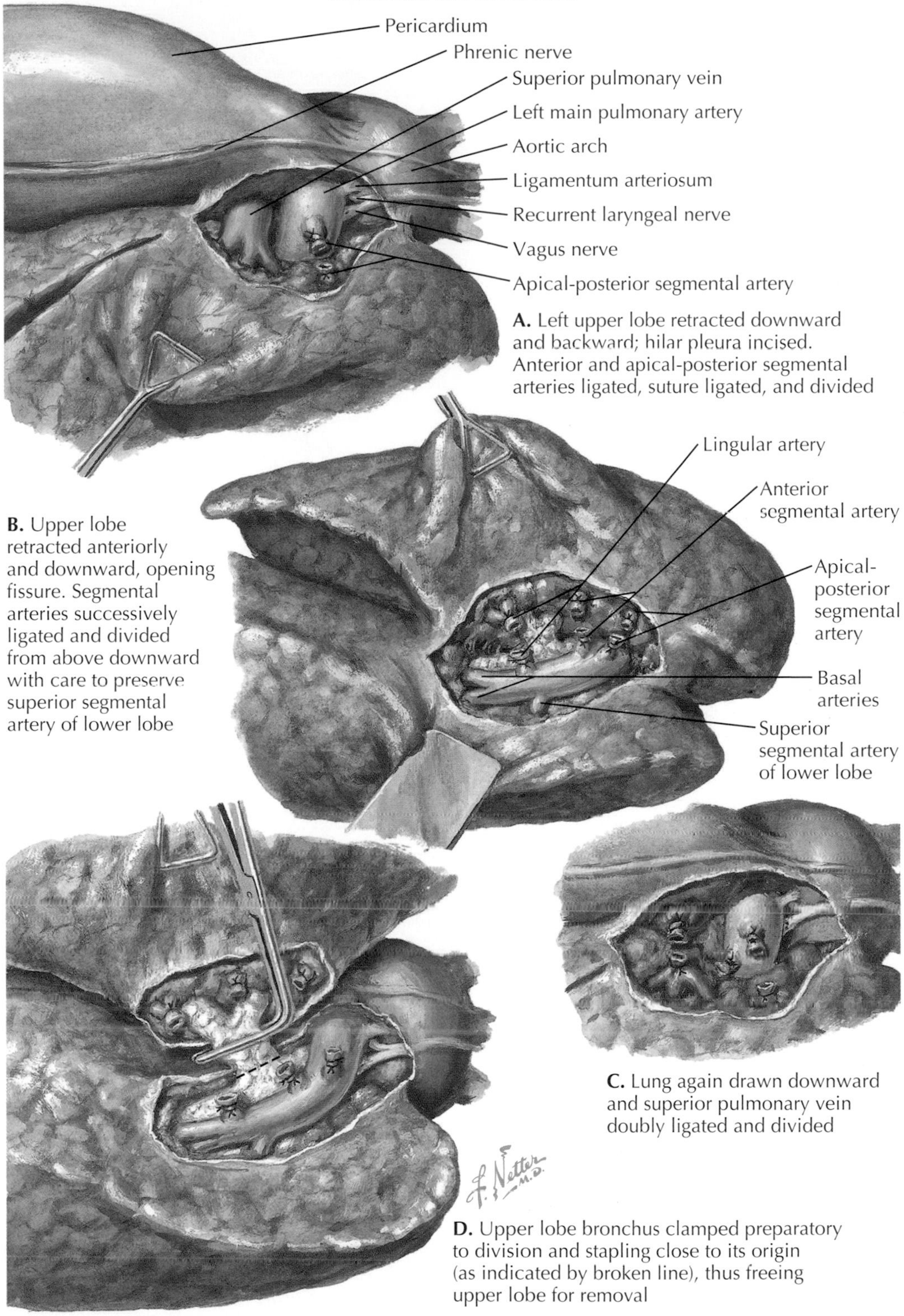

Pericardium
Phrenic nerve
Superior pulmonary vein
Left main pulmonary artery
Aortic arch
Ligamentum arteriosum
Recurrent laryngeal nerve
Vagus nerve
Apical-posterior segmental artery

A. Left upper lobe retracted downward and backward; hilar pleura incised. Anterior and apical-posterior segmental arteries ligated, suture ligated, and divided

Lingular artery
Anterior segmental artery
Apical-posterior segmental artery
Basal arteries
Superior segmental artery of lower lobe

B. Upper lobe retracted anteriorly and downward, opening fissure. Segmental arteries successively ligated and divided from above downward with care to preserve superior segmental artery of lower lobe

C. Lung again drawn downward and superior pulmonary vein doubly ligated and divided

F. Netter M.D.

D. Upper lobe bronchus clamped preparatory to division and stapling close to its origin (as indicated by broken line), thus freeing upper lobe for removal

Pneumonectomy (right lung)

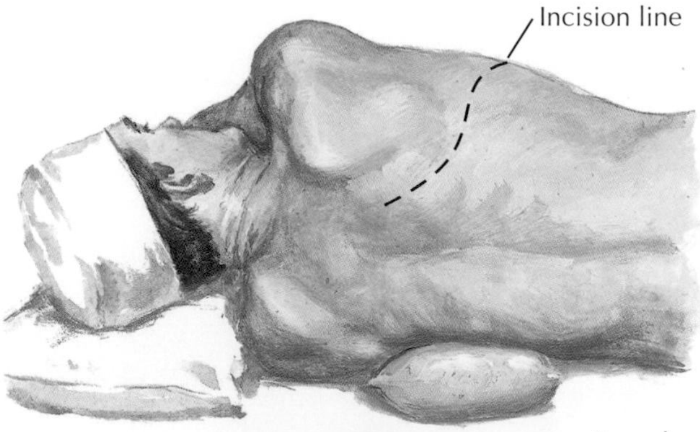

A. Patient in lateral recumbent position, inflatable bag or bolster under chest. Curved posterolateral ("hockey-stick") incision.

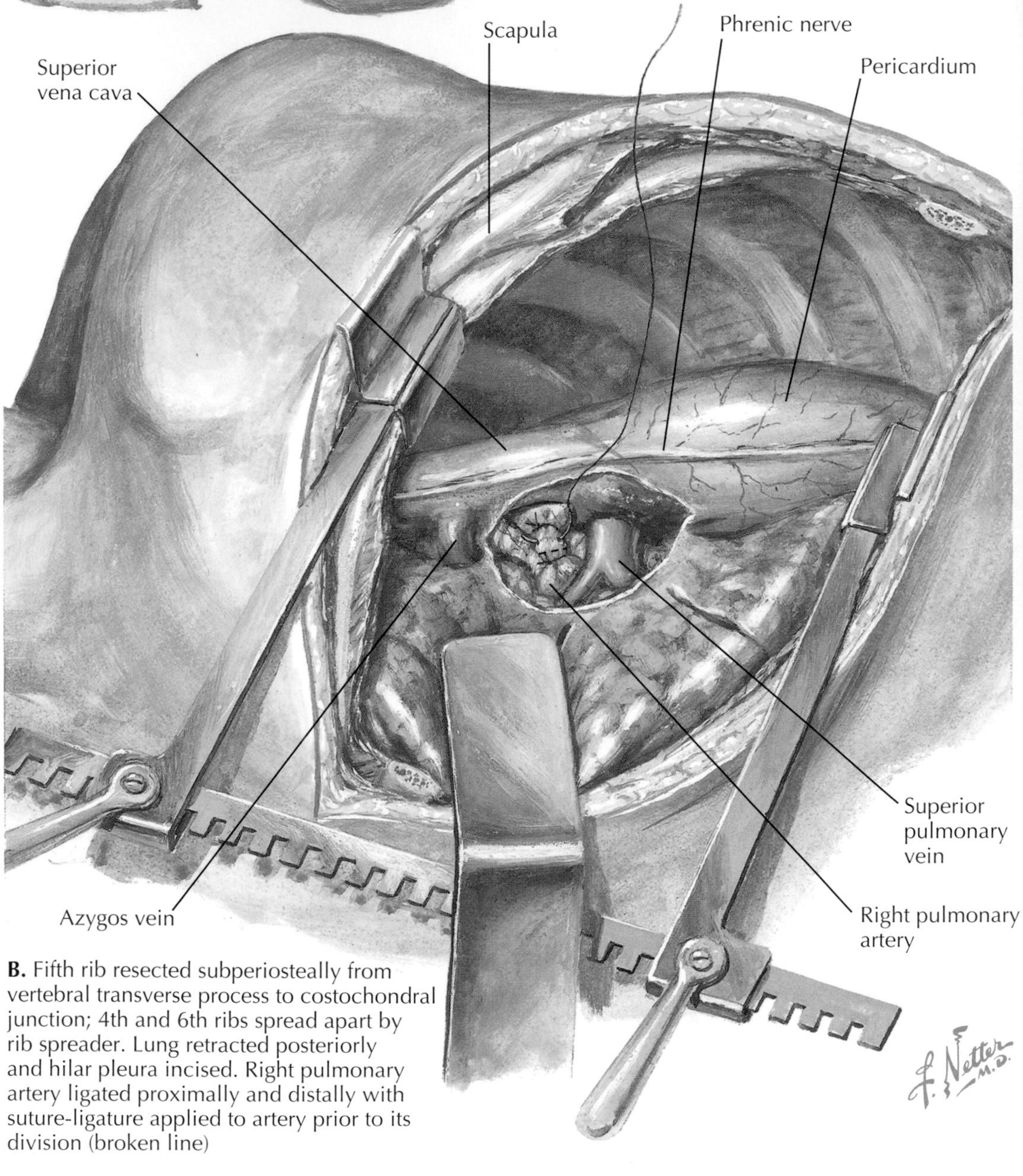

B. Fifth rib resected subperiosteally from vertebral transverse process to costochondral junction; 4th and 6th ribs spread apart by rib spreader. Lung retracted posteriorly and hilar pleura incised. Right pulmonary artery ligated proximally and distally with suture-ligature applied to artery prior to its division (broken line)

PNEUMONECTOMY

Pneumonectomy was first successfully performed in 1933 by Evarts Graham. The procedure was carried out for bronchogenic carcinoma in a fellow physician, James Gilmore, who eventually outlived his surgeon. The event is a milestone in surgical history. The technique of pneumonectomy has been improved and standardized in the intervening years, and the results are quite gratifying when the operation is carefully performed in appropriately selected cases. Current indications are chiefly as an operation for cure for lung cancer (usually centrally located) or for a destroyed lung as a result of infection or trauma. Palliative pneumonectomy is generally not warranted unless it is directed at alleviation of sepsis or control of recurrent hemorrhage. Before embarking upon resection of an entire lung, the surgeon must have a histologic diagnosis and a full assessment of the patient's cardiopulmonary reserve; little is gained if the pneumonectomized patient survives but has severe respiratory disability.

Pneumonectomy, as now practiced, is routinely performed via a standard posterolateral thoracotomy incision. The anterior approach has long been abandoned because of inadequate access to critical hilar structures; the posterior approach, with the patient in a face-down or prone position (once favored because it afforded better control of secretions from the operative side) is no longer required as a result of improvements in selective lung ventilation.

Posterolateral thoracotomy is performed with the patient securely fixed in a lateral recumbent position. An inflatable bag or bolster under the chest greatly improves access and exposure and is removed before closure of the incision. A curved incision is made, starting midway between the vertebral border of the scapula and the spine, clearing the angle of the scapula by one to two fingerbreadths and continuing forward in a transverse direction following the angle of the ribs to a submammary position. The standard incision involves division of the entire latissimus dorsi muscle, but the serratus anterior muscle can often be separated from its posterior border and detached from anterior rib insertions, preserving its function. If greater exposure is needed, especially cephalad, the skin incision is carried superiorly, and the lower fibers of the trapezius and rhomboid muscles are divided. With exposure of the subscapular space, the ribs are counted from the first rib downward. Entry through the fifth intercostal space along the superior border of the sixth rib is the standard approach to both pneumonectomy and any lobectomy. It affords good access for proximal control of any hilar vessel. Concern for optimal suprahilar exposure may necessitate a fourth interspace incision; an infrahilar lesion can be approached through the sixth space, although access to the proximal pulmonary artery may be compromised. Resection of a segment of rib (shingling) or rarely an entire rib, customarily the fifth, provides favorable exposure in older patients (who have less elastic chest walls) and allows for an airtight closure of the chest wall. Insertion of a rib spreader

PNEUMONECTOMY: RIGHT LUNG

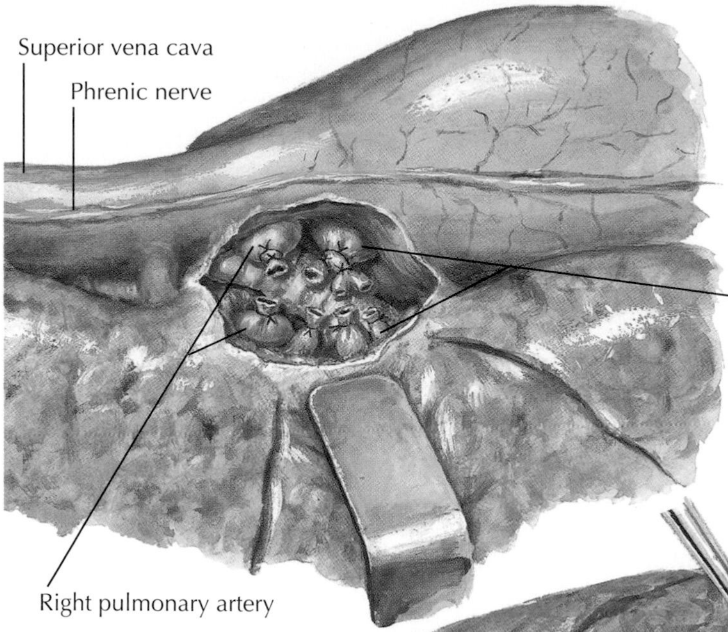

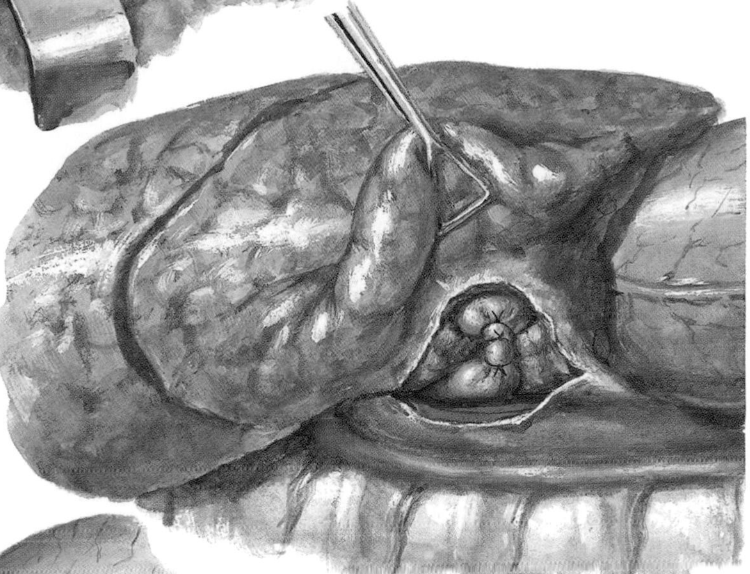

Lung retracted superiorly and inferior pulmonary ligament incised, exposing inferior pulmonary vein, which has been ligated and suture ligated (or secured with a vascular stapler) before division

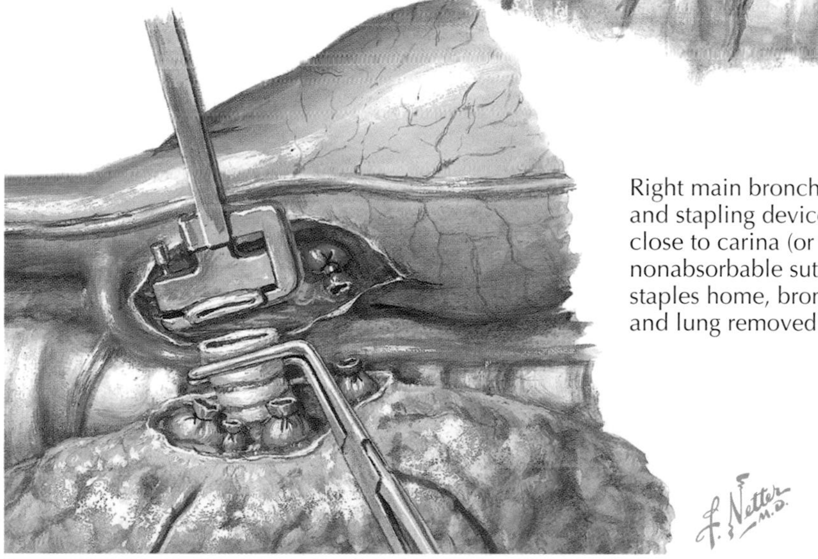

Right main bronchus clamped distally and stapling device placed across it close to carina (or closed by over-end, nonabsorbable sutures). After driving staples home, bronchus is divided and lung removed

PNEUMONECTOMY *(Continued)*

provides the exposure illustrated after any pleural adhesions present are divided.

The hilum is carefully studied by both visual examination and palpation for extension of tumor into the mediastinum—a sign of advanced disease that is not resectable. Infrequently, the pericardium must be opened to complete this assessment. The superior mediastinum is similarly explored via an incision through the parietal pleura dorsal to the superior vena cava. Suspicious lymph nodes may be removed and submitted for frozen section, and although nodes in this area may be removed with the lung, the presence of extensive mediastinal lymphatic spread predicts a poor prognosis and may influence the surgeon's decision whether to proceed with pneumonectomy.

After the lesion has been determined to be resectable for cure, hilar dissection is started. In general, the artery is divided first, followed by the vein, then the bronchus, although there are exceptions. First the lung is retracted posteriorly and inferiorly and the right main pulmonary artery exposed behind the lower superior vena cava. Division of the uppermost tributary of the right superior pulmonary vein may facilitate exposure. The perivascular sheath is entered, and the artery is freed up by sharp and blunt dissection using a right-angle or Semb clamp. The artery is then divided between ligatures or with a vascular stapler, leaving a long proximal stump.

The superior pulmonary vein is similarly freed up and divided, exposing the anterior aspect of the right main bronchus. Division of any or all critical hilar structures can be accomplished with suture or mechanical stapling devices.

The lung is then retracted superiorly and anteriorly to expose the inferior pulmonary vein along the superior margin of the inferior pulmonary ligament. This vessel also is exposed within its vascular sheath for a suitable extent and divided, leaving a long proximal stump, because slippage of the suture would cause catastrophic bleeding.

The right main bronchus is cleared and clamped after lymph nodes and areolar tissue have been swept distally onto the specimen. The bronchus is exposed to the level of the carina and a stapling device placed across it immediately below its origin. After the stapler has been fired, the bronchus is amputated distal to the line of staple closure and the lung removed from the chest. The bronchial stump is then tested under saline for air leakage by having the anesthesiologist apply positive airway pressure (20-25 cm H_2O) via the endotracheal tube. The stump should be buttressed with vascularized tissue such as pericardium, intercostal muscle, or parietal pleura. Postoperatively the hemithorax can be drained for a short period of time (often 24 hours) and then the space can be allowed to fill with fluid. Monitoring of the fluid level by chest radiographs is important if there is ever concern for a bronchopleural fistula because the level may decrease if a fistula has developed.

VIDEO-ASSISTED THORACOSCOPIC SURGERY

Video-assisted thoracoscopic surgery (VATS) has become a common tool for thoracic surgeons. It is useful in the evaluation and management of patients with pleural disease, benign and malignant pulmonary parenchymal neoplasms or diseases, mediastinal masses or adenopathy, and esophageal pathology and for resection of posterior mediastinal neurogenic tumors or conditions responsive to sympathectomy. A VATS operation is defined by use of two or more port incisions and video display of the involved hemithorax on operating room monitors, and it does not involve rib spreading. Most standard thoracic surgical instruments have been modified for thoracoscopic surgery.

Preparation for a thoracoscopic operation is similar to that for thoracotomy because the need for conversion to a conventional open surgical approach may arise. Reasons to convert include hemorrhage, extensive adhesions, inability to locate the lesion, a more extensive resection than planned, and the inability to proceed safely. Prophylaxis against deep venous thromboses with sequential compression devices and subcutaneous heparin is standard. The patient is placed in a maximally flexed lateral decubitus position. A double-lumen endotracheal tube or mainstem bronchial blocker is used to provide single-lung ventilation and allows the lung within the operative hemithorax to become fully atelectatic; insufflation is not commonly used.

Thoracic operating ports (Thoracoports) are shorter and blunter than laparoscopic ports and are not airtight. Use of a long-acting local anesthetic (e.g., bupivacaine) at the port sites results in decreased postoperative pain. A 30-degree, angled, rotating 5- or 10-mm videoscope is standard, with monitors placed on either side of the operating table at the level of the patient's head or pelvis depending on the location of the target lesion within the thorax. An angled videoscope allows superior visualization of the pleural space and central pulmonary vessels and bronchi without interfering with other endoscopic instrumentation. Flexible thoracoscopes allow even greater visualization and are becoming more common.

It is essential that the Thoracoports are triangulated relative to the operative lesion being addressed. The ports should face the lesion in an approximately 180-degree arc placed widely apart to prevent instrument crowding.

The thoracoscopic approach to resection of a pulmonary lobe is similar to the open approach. The hilar structures are individually dissected, and the vessels and bronchi are isolated and controlled. These structures can then be divided using endomechanical staplers of varying staple heights ranging from 2.0 to 4.5 mm, depending on the thickness of the tissue (e.g., pulmonary vessel, lung parenchyma, or bronchus).

Mechanical pleurodesis can be performed videoscopically to treat recurrent or persistent pneumothoraces by use of a rough object (e.g., Marlex mesh, coarse gauze sponge, electrocautery scratch pad). The rough material mounted on a ring forceps allows mechanical abrasion of the entire parietal pleural surface to create broad areas of pleural symphysis. Care should be taken at the apex because the subclavian vessels and stellate ganglion are superficially located. The pleura overlying the pericardium and diaphragm are commonly omitted from the process.

Locating a parenchymal lesion thoracoscopically can be more difficult than through an open incision. Methods to improve localization have been described. Subpleural lesions are often more visible in a fully atelectatic lung. A lung clamp or thoracoscopic ring forceps can be gently run across the lung to "palpate" the lesion. Preoperative computed tomography–guided needle localization can be used as well. The utility incision can also be enlarged and a lung clamp used to bring lung tissue to the incision for direct digital palpation. Anterior intercostal spaces are wider than posterior spaces, so palpation is often easier at an anterior incision.

At the completion of the operation, a standard chest tube or tubes are placed endoscopically, typically using the most inferior-anterior port site, and are positioned apically for air and posteriorly for dependent drainage. Smaller and softer closed-suction drains (e.g., Blake or Jackson-Pratt drains) may also be used. The lung can be reexpanded and checked for air leaks under thoracoscopic vision as well. If there is no evidence of air leak or excessive bleeding and the postoperative chest radiograph is within expectations, suction is discontinued, and the tubes are allowed to drain via gravity into the closed drainage unit with an underwater seal. If the course continues to be uneventful, the tubes are typically removed on the first postoperative day.

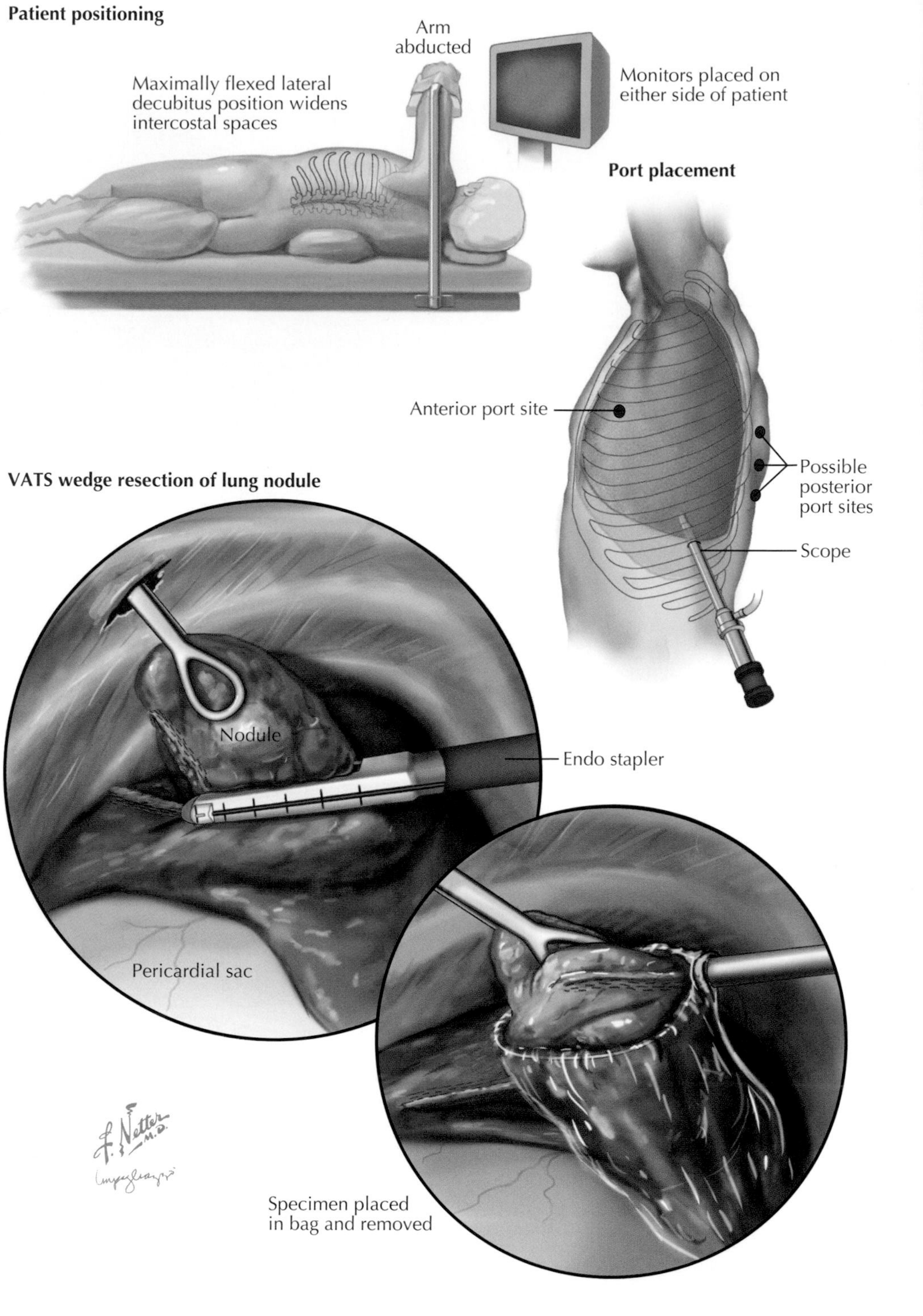

Patient positioning

Arm abducted

Maximally flexed lateral decubitus position widens intercostal spaces

Monitors placed on either side of patient

Port placement

Anterior port site

Possible posterior port sites

Scope

VATS wedge resection of lung nodule

Nodule

Endo stapler

Pericardial sac

Specimen placed in bag and removed

Lung Volume Reduction Surgery

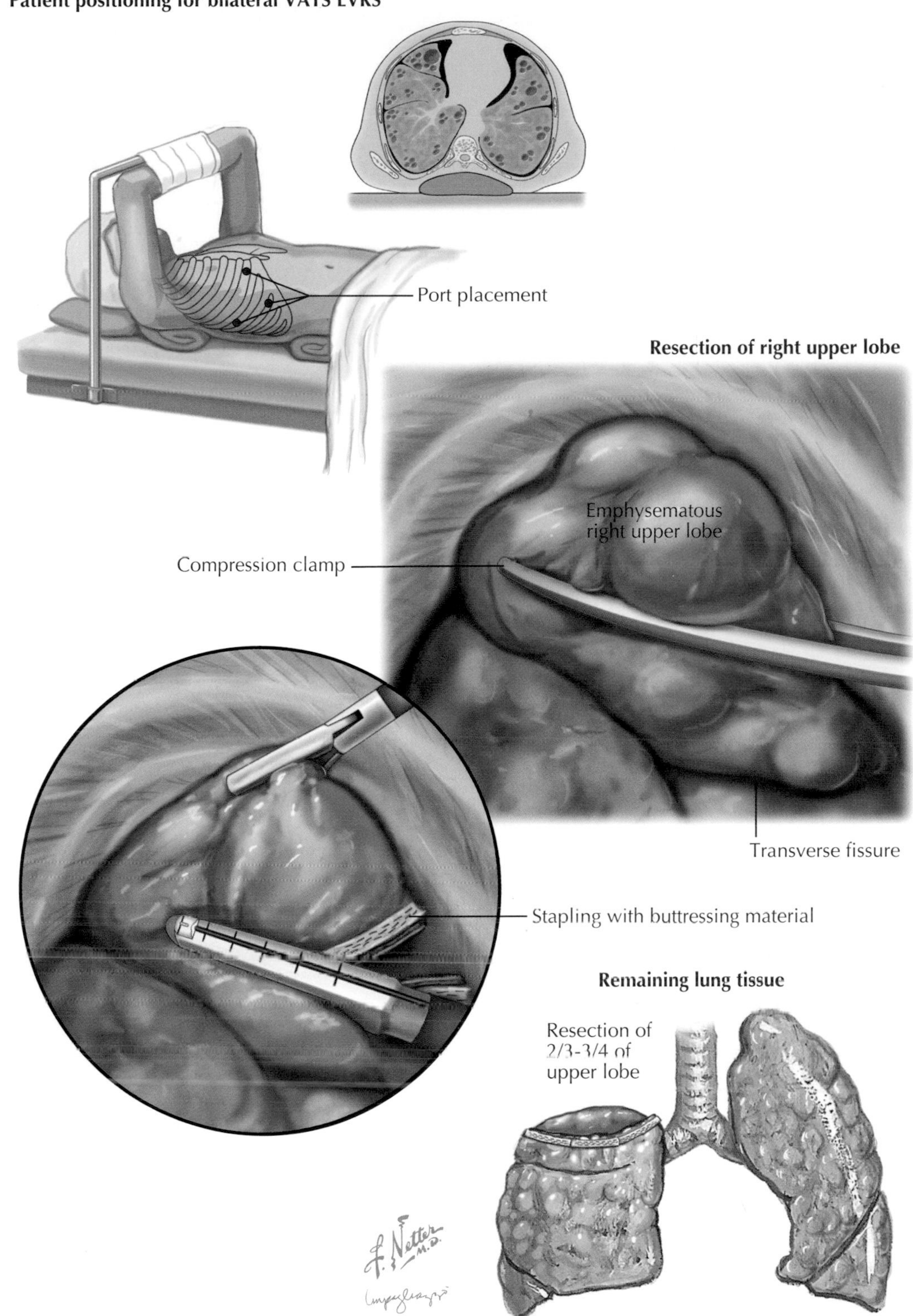

The goal of lung volume reduction surgery (LVRS) is to safely palliate dyspnea in patients with emphysema. Successful LVRS demands attention to the details of patient selection, preoperative preparation, intraoperative anesthetic and surgical technique, and multidisciplinary postoperative care. Expertise and effective communication among pulmonary medicine, thoracic surgery, thoracic anesthesia, pain management services, critical care medicine, respiratory therapy, and rehabilitation medicine departments are vital components to any LVRS program. In experienced centers, bilateral approaches yield nearly twice the physiologic benefit to unilateral LVRS without adversely affecting operative morbidity or mortality. Current practice favors stapled bilateral resection over plication or laser ablation to achieve lung volume reduction.

Bilateral LVRS is most commonly performed by median sternotomy or bilateral video-assisted thoracoscopic surgery (VATS). Via either approach, LVRS involves the resection of approximately two-thirds of the hyperinflated upper lobe using a series of intersecting staple lines. When performed through a sternotomy, the resection progresses from an anteromedial orientation and is completed posteriorly and laterally near the tip of the superior segment of the lower lobe. During VATS LVRS, the resection begins laterally and ends medially abutting the mediastinum. A buttressing material derived from either bovine pericardium or expanded polytetrafluoroethylene is commonly used to reinforce the staple lines and decrease the incidence of prolonged air leak after the procedure.

The National Emphysema Treatment Trial (NETT) was a multicenter, randomized, controlled trial that compared LVRS with maximal medical therapy in patients with severe emphysema. NETT enrolled patients with a variety of emphysema morphologies and has better defined who benefits and who does not benefit from LVRS. Patients with an extremely low forced expiratory volume in 1 second (FEV_1) with either a diffuse pattern of emphysema or a DL_{CO} (diffusing capacity for carbon monoxide) less than 20% predicted have excessive mortality after LVRS, as do patients with non–upper lobe emphysema and preserved exercise capacity. Conversely, patients not in these high-risk groups who undergo LVRS have a mortality risk not different from continued medical therapy but do have a greater chance for improvement in exercise capacity and in most cases a greater chance for sustained improvement in health-related quality of life. Moreover, those patients with upper lobe–predominant emphysema and low baseline exercise capacity enjoy a survival advantage after LVRS compared with patients who continue with only medical therapy. This is the only intervention for emphysema since the availability of portable supplemental oxygen to show a survival benefit.

Examination of NETT results with regards to approach to LVRS demonstrates an operative time for median sternotomy that was 20 minutes shorter then VATS but no difference in terms of air leak, days on the ventilator, or operative mortality. Patients undergoing bilateral VATS LVRS spent fewer days in the intensive care unit and on average 1 to 2 fewer days in the hospital. At 90 days after surgery, more VATS patients were at home and independent of additional nursing care. The functional outcomes of LVRS in terms of exercise capacity, FEV_1, 6-minute walk distance, and respiratory-specific quality of life were not different between the VATS and median sternotomy group. Total health care expenditure for both the hospitalization as well as 6 months of care after LVRS favored the VATS approach. On average, VATS patients expended $10,000 less than patients undergoing LVRS via a median sternotomy. Based on these experiences, it appears that LVRS is safe, reproducible, and effective by either median sternotomy or VATS. The complication rate is low and similar for both surgical approaches. Additionally, functional outcomes and durability between 3 and 5 years of follow-up are also similar between the two approaches. It does appear however, based on the only randomized data available, that VATS provides earlier recovery at a lower cost than median sternotomy for bilateral LVRS.

Lung Transplantation

Clinical lung transplantation was first attempted in the 1960s, but little success was achieved until the availability of more effective immunosuppressive drugs (cyclosporine) and improved surgical techniques in the early 1980s. The annual number of lung transplant procedures has increased steadily from fewer than 100 per year in the 1980s to more than 2700 transplants reported by 150 worldwide transplant centers in 2007. Lung transplantation is now an accepted therapy for all forms of advanced lung disease.

The most common indications for transplantation are diseases or conditions that produce extreme disability, are unresponsive to medical therapy, and are responsible for limited life expectancy. With the exception of a small number of cases of sarcoidosis and lymphangioleiomyomatosis, the original lung disease does not usually recur after lung transplantation. Emphysema accounts for half of all lung transplants performed each year, and pulmonary fibrosis and cystic fibrosis (CF) each account for 15% of cases annually. Candidate selection and listing are determined by distinct sets of disease-specific guidelines. Likewise, a number of standard donor criteria (e.g., age, size match, tobacco history) must be met in determining donor selection.

Currently, four types of lung transplantation procedures are performed. Single-lung transplantation is typically performed through a posterolateral thoracotomy incision and requires three anastomoses: the mainstem bronchus, pulmonary artery, and pulmonary veins or left atrium. The contralateral lung is not removed, so single-lung transplantation is not performed in patients with bilaterally infected lungs (e.g., patients with CF or bronchiectasis). Cardiopulmonary bypass is required if there is associated pulmonary hypertension. More than half of single-lung transplants are performed for emphysema, and an additional 30% are for fibrotic lung diseases, including sarcoidosis.

Bilateral lung transplantation was initially performed as an en bloc procedure with a distal tracheal anastomosis but is currently performed in a sequential fashion that is functionally equivalent to two single-lung transplantations completed during a single operation, most commonly through a transverse sternotomy ("clamshell") incision. It requires six anastomoses: both mainstem bronchi, both pulmonary arteries, and both sets of pulmonary veins. It is the procedure of choice for patients with bilaterally infected lungs (e.g., CF or bronchiectasis) and is also performed in certain patients with emphysema, primary pulmonary hypertension, and other diseases, especially if there is secondary pulmonary hypertension. Cardiopulmonary bypass is more likely to be needed in such cases. There has been a trend over the past decade in favor of bilateral transplants for nearly all indications. This has been driven by statistically superior late survival; 2007 data demonstrate the expected half-life of a single lung recipient as 4.6 years; a double lung recipient can expect a half-life of 6.6 years.

Heart-lung transplantation was initially the most common type of lung transplant procedure but is now performed infrequently (~75 cases in the United States in 2007). It is an en bloc procedure with right atrial, aortic, and distal tracheal anastomoses. It is performed in patients with advanced lung disease and coexistent irreparable cardiac disease usually associated with fixed pulmonary hypertension, such as those with Eisenmenger syndrome.

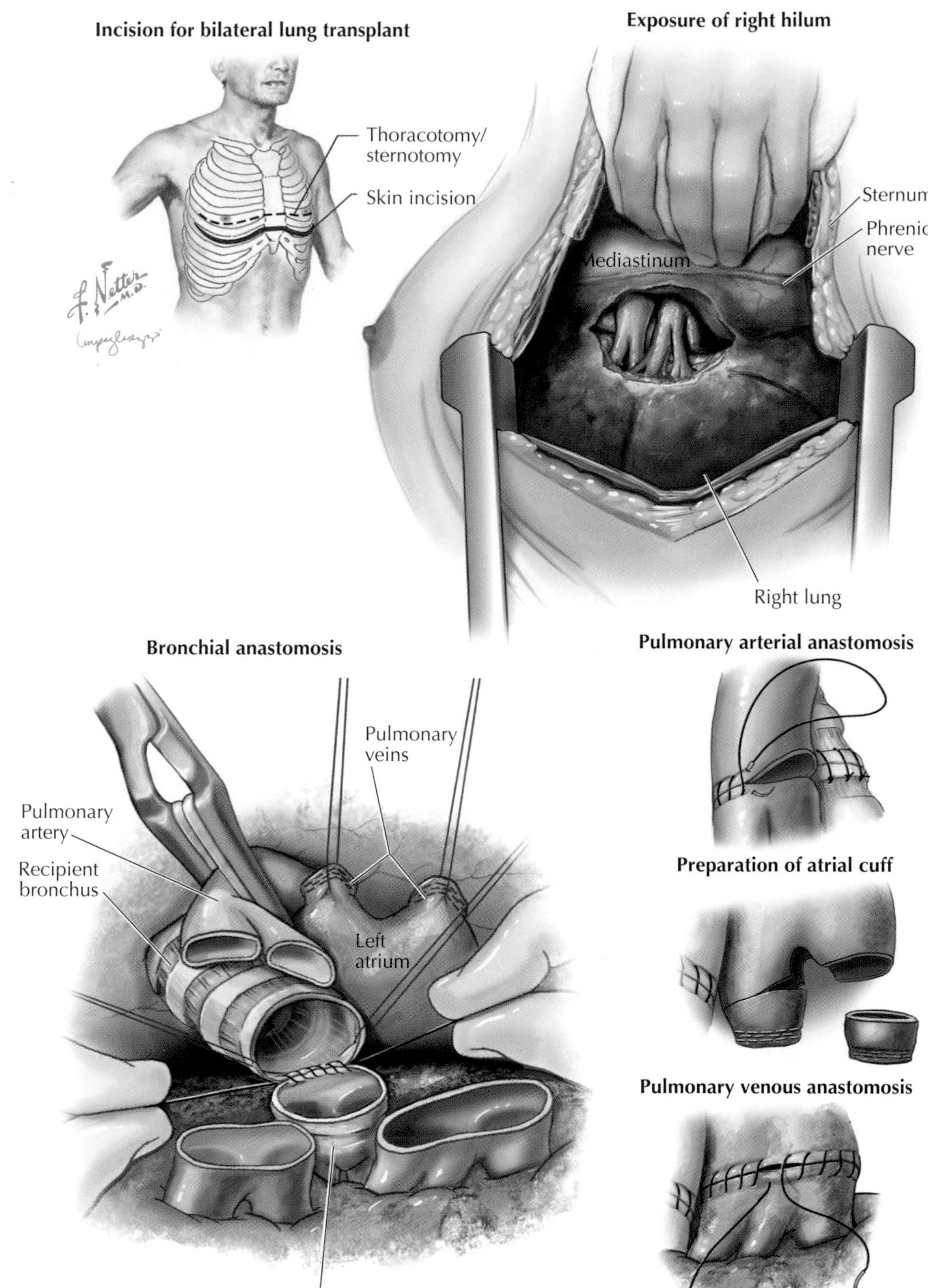

The most recently introduced lung transplant procedure is living donor lobar transplantation. This procedure involves the removal of a lower lobe from each of two living donors, with the implantation of one in each hemithorax of the recipient in a manner similar to bilateral sequential single lung transplantation.

Postoperative complications of lung transplant include airway ischemia, dehiscence, and stenosis. Three types of graft rejection may occur: primary graft dysfunction caused by acute lung injury from ischemia or reperfusion; acute cellular rejection, manifested by perivascular and interstitial lymphocytic infiltration; and chronic rejection, seen histologically as obliterative bronchiolitis. Infection is also a common complication and is caused not only by the immunosuppression required but also by the loss of the cough reflex as a result of denervation of the transplanted lungs. Bacterial, viral, and fungal pathogens are all seen, with cytomegalovirus (CMV), human herpesvirus, *Aspergillus* spp., and *Candida* spp. common. Prophylaxis against *Pneumocystis jiroveci*, CMV, and fungal organisms is used to reduce the incidence of infection.

Immunosuppression is the key to prolonged survival of transplanted patients but carries the risks of increased infection, especially with opportunistic organisms; increased malignancy; including posttransplant lymphoproliferative disorder; and drug toxicity, especially nephrotoxicity. Common induction regimens use OKT3 or antithymocyte globulin to acutely reduce circulating lymphocytes. Maintenance therapy usually involves an antiproliferative agent (calcineurin inhibitor), such as cyclosporine A or tacrolimus (FK506); an antimetabolite, such as mycophenolate mofetil or azathioprine; and a corticosteroid.

SELECTED REFERENCES

Section 1: Anatomy and Embryology

Abman SH: Recent advances in the pathobiology and treatment of persistent pulmonary hypertension of the newborn. Neonatology 91:283-290, 2007.

Adriaensen D, Brouns I, Pintelon I, et al: Evidence for a role of neuroepithelial bodies as complex airway sensors: comparison with smooth muscle-associated airway receptors. J Appl Physiol 101:960-970, 2006.

Adriaensen D, Scheuermann DW: Neuroendocrine cells and nerves of the lung. Anat Rec 236:70-85; discussion 85-76, 1993.

Akbari O, Stock P, Dekruyff RH, Umetsu DT: Mucosal tolerance and immunity: Regulating the development of allergic disease and asthma. Int Arch Allergy Immunol 130:108-118, 2003.

Andreeva AV, Kutuzov MA, Voyno-Yasenetskaya TA: Regulation of surfactant secretion in alveolar type II cells. Am J Physiol Lung Cell Mol Physiol 293:L259-L271, 2007.

Arey LB: *Developmental Anatomy*, 7th ed. Philadelphia, WB Saunders, 1965.

Avery ME, Fletcher BD: *The Lung and Its Disorders in the Newborn Infant*, 3rd ed. Philadelphia, WB Saunders, 1974.

Burri PH: Lung development and pulmonary angiogenesis. In Gaultier C, Bourbon J, Post M (eds): *Lung Disease*. New York, Oxford University Press, 1999, pp 122-151.

Cowan MJ, Gladwin MT, Shelhamer JH: Disorders of ciliary motility. Am J Med Sci 321:3-10, 2001.

Crelin ES: *Anatomy of the Newborn; An Atlas*. Philadelphia, Lea & Febiger, 1969.

Crelin ES: *Functional Anatomy of the Newborn*. New Haven, CT, Yale University Press, 1973.

Crystal RG, Randell SH, Engelhardt JF, et al: Airway epithelial cells: current concepts and challenges. Proc Am Thorac Soc 5:772-777, 2008.

Foot NJ, Orgeig S, Daniels CB: The evolution of a physiological system: The pulmonary surfactant system in diving mammals. Respir Physiol Neurobiol 154:118-138, 2006.

Godfrey S: Growth and development of the respiratory system. Functional development. In Davis A, Dobbing J (eds): *Scientific Foundations of Paediatrics*. Philadelphia, WB Saunders, 1974.

Guyton AC: *Textbook of Medical Physiology*, 4th ed. Philadelphia, WB Saunders, 1971.

Hamilton WJ, Boyd JD, Mossman HW: *Human Embryology*, 3rd ed. Baltimore, Williams & Wilkins, 1964.

Herzog EL, Brody AR, Colby TV, et al: Knowns and unknowns of the alveolus. Proc Am Thorac Soc 5:778-782, 2008.

Holt PG, Strickland DH, Wikstrom ME, Jahnsen FL: Regulation of immunological homeostasis in the respiratory tract. Nat Rev Immunol 8:142-152, 2008.

Hyman LH: *Comparative Vertebrate Anatomy*, 2nd ed. Chicago, University of Chicago Press, 1946.

Jeffery PK, Li D: Airway mucosa: Secretory cells, mucus and mucin genes. Eur Respir J 10:1655-1662, 1997.

Lambrecht BN, Hammad H: Biology of lung dendritic cells at the origin of asthma. Immunity 31:412-424, 2009.

Maeda Y, Cave V, Whitsett JA: Transcriptional control of lung morphogenesis. Physiol Rev 87:219-244, 2007.

Mountain CF, Dresler CM: Regional lymph node classification for lung cancer staging. Chest 111:1718-1723, 1997.

Patten BM: *Human Embryology*, 3rd ed. New York, McGraw-Hill, 1968.

Reid L, Meyrick B, Antony VB, et al: The mysterious pulmonary brush cell: A cell in search of a function. Am J Respir Crit Care Med 172:136-139, 2005.

Schnitzer JE: Caveolae: From basic trafficking mechanisms to targeting transcytosis for tissue-specific drug and gene delivery in vivo. Adv Drug Deliv Rev 49:265-280, 2001.

Stan RV: Structure of caveolae. Biochim Biophys Acta 1746:334-348, 2005.

Stenmark KR, Abman SH: Lung vascular development: Implications for the pathogenesis of bronchopulmonary dysplasia. Annu Rev Physiol 67:623-661, 2005.

Standring S (ed). *Gray's Anatomy*, 40th ed. Philadelphia, Elsevier, 2008.

Weinbaum S, Tarbell JM, Damiano ER: The structure and function of the endothelial glycocalyx layer. Annu Rev Biomed Engl 9:121-167, 2007.

Whitsett JA: Genetic disorders of surfactant homeostasis. Paediatr Respir Rev Suppl 1:S240-S242, 2007.

Section 2: Physiology

Barnes PJ: Histamine and serotonin. Pulm Pharmacol Ther 14: 329-339, 2001.

Black LF, Hyatt RE: Maximal respiratory pressures: Normal values and relationship to age and sex. Am Rev Respir Dis 99:696-702, 1969.

Bowler RP, Barnes PJ, Crapo JD: The role of oxidative stress in chronic obstructive pulmonary disease. J COPD 2:255-277, 2004.

Carey RM, Siragy HM: Newly recognized components of the renin-angiotensin system: Potential roles in cardiovascular and renal regulation. Endocr Rev 24:261-271, 2003.

Ciencewicki J, Trivedi S, Kleeberger SR: Oxidants and the pathogenesis of lung diseases. J Allergy Clin Immunol 122:456-468, 2008.

Cooper CB: The connection between chronic obstructive pulmonary disease symptoms and hyperinflation and its impact on exercise and function. Am J Med 119(suppl):S21-S31, 2006.

DuBois AB, Botelho SY, Bedell GN, et al: A rapid plethysmographic method for measuring thoracic gas volume: A comparison with nitrogen was about method for measuring functional residual capacity in normal subjects. J Clin Invest 35:322-326, 1956.

DuBois AB, Botelho SY, Comroe JH Jr: A new method for measuring airway resistance in man using a body plethysmograph: Values in normal subjects in patients with respiratory disease. J Clin Invest 35:327-355, 1956.

Filley GF, MacIntosh DJ, Wright GW: Carbon monoxide uptake and pulmonary diffusing capacity in normal subjects at rest and during exercise. J Clin Invest 33:530-539, 1954.

Finch CA, Lenfant C: Oxygen transport in man. N Engl J Med 286:407-415, 1972.

Fyhrquist F, Saijonmaa O: Renin-angiotensin system revisited. J Intern Med 264:224-236, 2008.

Gibson GJ, Pride NB: Lung distensibility. The static pressure-volume curve of the lungs and its use in clinical assessment. Br J Dis Chest 70:143-184, 1976.

Gillis CN, Pitt BR: The fate of circulating amines within the pulmonary circulation. Annu Rev Physiol 44:269-281, 1982.

Hyatt RE, Black LF: The flow-volume curve: A current perspective. Am Rev Respir Dis 107:191-199, 1973.

Hyatt RE, Flath RE: Relationship of airflow to pressure during maximal respiratory effort in man. J Appl Physiol 21:477-482, 1966.

Khoo MC: Determinants of ventilatory instability and variability. Respir Physiol 122(2-3):167-182, 2000.

Longobardo G, Evangelisti CJ, Cherniack NS: Effects of neural drives on breathing in the awake state in humans. Respir Physiol 129(3):317-333, 2002.

MacIntyre N, Crapo RO, Viegi G, et al: Standardisation of the single-breath determination of carbon monoxide uptake in the lung. Eur Respir J 26:720-735, 2005.

Macklem PT, Mead J: Resistance of central and peripheral airways measured by a retrograde catheter. J Appl Physiol 22:395-401, 1967.

Marshall RP: The pulmonary renin-angiotensin system. Curr Pharm Des 9:715-722, 2003.

Mead J, Turner JM, Macklem PT, et al: Significance of the relationship between lung recoil and maximum expiratory flow. J Appl Physiol 22:95-108, 1967.

Milic-Emili J, Henderson JA, Dolovich MB, et al: Regional distribution of inspired gas in the lung. J Appl Physiol 21:749-759, 1966.

Milic-Emili J, Mead J, Turner JM, et al: Improved technique for estimating pleural pressure from esophageal balloons. J Appl Physiol 19:207-211, 1964.

Miller MR, Hankinson J, Brusasco V, et al: Standardisation of spirometry. Eur Respir J26:319-338, 2005.

Nopmaneejumruslers C, Kaneko Y, Hajek V, et al: Cheyne-Stokes respiration in stroke: Relationship to hypocapnia and occult cardiac dysfunction. Am J Respir Crit Care Med 171(9):1048-1052, 2005.

Oglivie CM, Forster RE, Blakemore WS, et al: A standardized breath holding technique for the clinical measurement of the diffusing capacity of the lung for carbon monoxide. J Clin Invest 36:1-17, 1957.

Pride NB, Permutt S, Riley RL, et al: Determinants of maximum expiratory flow from the lungs. J Appl Physiol 23:646-662, 1967.

Pride NB: The assessment of airflow obstruction. Role of measurements of airways resistance and of tests of forced expiration. Br J Dis Chest 65:135-169, 1971.

Rahman I, Adcock IM: Oxidative stress and redox regulation of lung inflammation in COPD. Eur Respir J 28:219-242, 2006.

Rahn H, Fenn WO: Graphical analysis of the respiratory gas exchange: The O2-CO2 diagram. Am Physiol Soc 1955.

Riley RL, Cournand A: "Ideal" alveolar air and the analysis of ventilation-perfusion relationships in the lung. J Appl Physiol 1:825-847, 1949.

Rodman JR, Haverkamp HC, Gordon SM, Dempsey JA: Cardiovascular and respiratory system responses and limitations to exercise. In Weisman IM, Zeballos RG (eds): *Progress in Respiratory Research: Clinical Exercise Testing*. Basel, Karger, 2002, pp 1-17.

Roughton FJ, Forster RE: Relative importance of diffusion and chemical reaction rate in determining rate of exchange of gases in the human lung with special reference to true diffusing capacity of pulmonary membrane and volume of blood in the lung capillaries. J Appl Physiol 11:290-302, 1957.

Sippel RS, Chen H: Carcinoid tumors. Surg Oncol Clin North Am 15:463-478, 2006.

Smith TG, Robbins PA, Ratcliffe PJ: The human side of hypoxia-inducible factor. Br J Haematol 141:325-334, 2008.

Song G, Poon CS: Functional and structural models of pontine modulation of mechanoreceptor and chemoreceptor reflexes. Respir Physiol Neurobiol 143(2-3):281-292, 2004.

Stubbs SE, Hyatt RE: Effect of increased lung recoil pressure on maximal expiratory flow in normal subjects. J Appl Physiol 32:325-331, 1972.

Treppo S, Mijailovich SM, Venegas JG: Contributions of pulmonary perfusion and ventilation to heterogeneity in V(A)/Q measured by PET. J Appl Physiol 82:1163-1176, 1997.

Turner JM, Mead J, Wohl ME: Elasticity of human lungs in relation to age. J Appl Physiol 25:664-671, 1968.

Ward MP, Milledge JS, West JB: *High Altitude Medicine and Physiology*, 2nd ed. London, Chapman and Hall, 1995.

West JB, Dollery CT, Naimark A: Distribution of blood flow in isolated lung: relation to vascular and alveolar pressures. J Appl Physiol 19:713-724, 1964.

Woolcock AJ, Vincent NJ, Macklem PT: Frequency dependence of compliance as a test for obstruction in the small airways. J Clin Invest 48:1097-1106, 1969.

Section 3: Diagnostic Procedures

American Thoracic Society: Guidelines for methacholine and exercise challenge testing—1999. Am J Respir Crit Care Med 161:309-329, 2000.

American Thoracic Society/American College of Chest Physicians: ATS/ACCP Statement on cardiopulmonary exercise testing. Am J Respir Crit Care 167:211-277, 2003.

ATS/ERS Recommendations for Standardized Procedures for the Online and Offline Measurement of Exhaled Lower Respiratory Nitric Oxide and Nasal Nitric Oxide, 2005. Am J Respir Crit Care Med 171(8):912-930, 2005.

Bhalla M, McLoud TC: Pulmonary infections in the normal host. In *Thoracic Radiology: The Requisites*. St. Louis, Mosby, 1998, pp 122-130.

DeCamp MM Jr, Sodha NR: *Applied Anatomy of the Chest Wall and Mediastinum, Mastery of Surgery*, 5th ed. Philadelphia, Lippincott William & Wilkins, 2007, pp 556-570.

Dweik RA, Amann A: Exhaled breath analysis: The new frontier in medical testing. J Breath Res (3):300-301, 2008.

Eberhardt R, Anantham D, Ernst A, et al: Multimodality bronchoscopic diagnosis of peripheral lung lesions: a randomized controlled trial. Am J Respir Crit Care Med 176:36-41, 2007.

Fishman AP, Macklem PT, Mead J, Geiger SR (eds): The respiratory system. In *Handbook of Physiology*, vol III. Bethesda, MD, American Physiological Society, 1986.

Grob NM, Dweik RA: Exhaled nitric oxide in asthma. From diagnosis, to monitoring, to screening: Are we there yet? Chest 133(4):837-839, 2008.

Hammoud ZT, Anderson RC, Meyers BF, et al: The current role of mediastinoscopy in the evaluation of thoracic disease. J Thorac Cardiovasc Surg 118:894-899, 1999.

Hansell DM, Armstrong P, Lynch DA, McAdams HP (eds): Neoplasms of the lungs, airways, and pleura. In *Imaging of Diseases of the Chest*, 4th ed. Philadelphia, Elsevier Mosby, 2005, pp 864-872.

Horvath I, Hunt J, Barnes PJ, et al: Exhaled breath condensate: methodological recommendations and unresolved questions. Eur Respir J 26(3):523-548, 2005.

Kazerooni EA: High-resolution CT of the lungs. AJR Am J Roentgenol 177:501-519, 2001.

Kharitonov SA, Yates D, Robbins RA, et al: Increased nitric oxide in exhaled air of asthmatic patients. Lancet 343(8890):133-135, 1994.

Klein JS, Braff S: Imaging evaluation of the solitary pulmonary nodule. Clin Chest Med 29(1):15-38, 2008.

Lynch DA: Imaging of small airways disease and chronic obstructive pulmonary disease. Clin Chest Med 29(1):165-180, 2008.
MacIntyre N, Crapo RO, Viegi G, et al: Standardisation of the single-breath determination of carbon monoxide uptake in the lung. Eur Respir J 26:720-735, 2005.
Marom EM, Goodman PC, McAdams HP: Diffuse abnormalities of the trachea and main bronchi. AJR Am J Roentgenol 176:713-717, 2001.
Marom EM, Goodman PC, McAdams HP: Focal abnormalities of the trachea and main bronchi. AJR Am J Roentgenol 176:707-711, 2001.
Miller MR, Hankinson J, Brusasco V, et al: Standardisation of spirometry. Eur Respir J 26:319-338, 2005.
Muller NL: Imaging of the pleura. Radiology 186:297-309, 1993.
Pellegrino R, Viegi G, Brusasco V, et al: Interpretative strategies for lung function tests. Eur Respir J 26:948-968, 2005.
Pistolesi M, Miniati M, Milne ENC, et al: The chest roentgenogram in pulmonary edema. Clin Chest Med 6:315-344, 1985.
Proto AV, Speckman JM: The left lateral radiograph of the chest 1. Med Radiogr Photogr 55:30-74, 1979.
Proto AV, Speckman JM: The left lateral radiograph of the chest 2. Med Radiogr Photogr 56:38-64, 1980.
Ravin CE, Chotas HG: Chest radiography. Radiology 204:593-600, 1997.
Recommendations for standardized procedures for the on-line and off-line measurement of exhaled lower respiratory nitric oxide and nasal nitric oxide in adults and children—1999. This official statement of the American Thoracic Society was adopted by the ATS Board of Directors, July 1999. Am J Respir Crit Care Med 160(6):2104-2117, 1999.
Ruppel G: *Manual of Pulmonary Function Testing*, 9th ed. St. Louis, Mosby, 2009.
Schoepf UJ, Costello P: CT angiography for diagnosis of pulmonary embolism: State of the art. Radiology 230:329-337, 2004.
Siracuse JJ, DeCamp MM Jr: Surgical mediastinal lymph node sampling for staging of non-small cell lung cancer. Op Techniques in Thorac and Cardiovasc Surg 14(2):112-123, 2009.
Wanger J, Clausen JL, Coates A, et al: Standardisation of the measurement of lung volumes. Eur Respir J 26:511-522, 2005.
West JB: *Respiratory Physiology: The Essentials*, 8th ed. Baltimore, Williams and Wilkins, 2008.
Yasufuku K, Nakajima T, Chiyo M, et al: Endobronchial ultrasonography: Current status and future directions. J Thorac Oncol 2:970-979, 2007.

Section 4: Diseases and Pathology

Acevedo F, Baudrand R, Letelier LM, Gaete P: Actinomycosis: A great pretender. Case reports of unusual presentations and a review of the literature [review]. Int J Infect Dis 12(4):358-362, 2008.
Agarwal R: Allergic bronchopulmonary aspergillosis. Chest 135(3): 805-826, 2009.
Albert RK, Spiro SG, Jett JR (eds): *Clinical Respiratory Medicine*. Philadelphia, Mosby Elsevier, 2008.
Alberts WM: Diagnosis and management of lung Cancer: ACCP guidelines (2nd edition), Chest 132(suppl 3):1S-422S, 2007.
Allen GB, Parsons PE: Acute lung injury: Significance, treatment and outcomes. Curr Opin Anaesthesiol 18(2):209-215, 2005.
Allen GB, Parsons PE: Acute respiratory failure due to Acute respiratory distress syndrome and pulmonary edema. In Irwin RS, Rippe JM (eds). *Intensive Care Medicine*, 6th ed. Philadelphia, Lippincott Williams & Wilkins, 2008.
American Academy of Sleep Medicine: *International Classification of Sleep Disorders: Diagnostic and Coding Manual*, 2nd ed. Westchester, IL: American Academy of Sleep Medicine, 2005.
American Academy of Sleep Medicine: *The AASM Manual for the Scoring of Sleep and Associated Events*. Westchester, IL: American Academy of Sleep Medicine, 2007.
American Thoracic Society: An official ATS/IDSA statement: Diagnosis, treatment, and prevention of nontuberculous mycobacterial diseases. Am J Respir Crit Care Med 175:367-416, 2007.
American Thoracic Society: Diagnosis and initial management of nonmalignant diseases related to asbestos. Am J Respir Crit Care Med 170(6):691-715, 2004.
American Thoracic Society Guidelines: Targeted Tuberculin testing and treatment of latent tuberculosis infection. Am J Respir Crit Care Med 161:S221-5247, 2000.
American Thoracic Society, Centers for Disease Control and Prevention, and Infectious Diseases Society of America: Treatment of tuberculosis. Am J Respir Crit Care Med 167:603-662, 2003.
Antao VC, Pinheiro GA, Wassell JT: Asbestosis mortality in the USA: Facts and predictions. Occup Environ Med 66(5):335-338, 2009.
Anthonisen NR, Connett JE, Kiley JP, et al: Effects of smoking intervention and the use of an inhaled anticholinergic bronchodilator on the rate of decline of FEV 1: The Lung Health Study. JAMA 272:1497-1505, 1994.
Badesch DB, Abman SH, Simonneau G, et al: Medical therapy guidelines for pulmonary arterial hypertension. Updated ACCP evidence-based clinical practice guidelines. Chest 131:1917-1928, 2007.
Ballenger JJ, Snow JB (eds). Otorhinolaryngology: Head and Neck Surgery, 15th ed. Baltimore, Williams & Wilkins, 1996.
Banks DE, Shi R, McLarty J, et al: American College of Chest Physicians consensus statement on the respiratory health effects of asbestos. Results of a Delphi study. Chest 135(6):1619-1627, 2009.
Barnes PJ: Chronic obstructive lung disease. N Engl J Med 343(4):269-280, 2000.
Barnes PJ: The cytokine network in asthma and chronic obstructive pulmonary disease. J Clin Invest 118:3546-3556, 2008.
Barroso E, Hernandez L, Gil J, et al: Idiopathic organizing pneumonia: A relapsing disease. 19 years of experience in a hospital setting. Respiration 74:624-631, 2007.
Bartlett JG: Anaerobic bacterial infections of the lung and pleural space. Clin Infect Dis 16(suppl):S248, 1993.
Bateman ED, Hurd SS, Barnes PJ, et al: Global strategy for asthma management and prevention: GINA executive summary. Eur Respir J 31:143-178, 2008.
Baughman RP, Drent M: Sarcoidosis. Clin Chest Med 3:357-574, 2008.
Beccaria M, Luisetti M, Rodi G, et al: Long-term durable benefit after whole lung lavage in pulmonary alveolar proteinosis. Eur Respir J 23:526-531, 2004.
Beck JM, Rosen MJ, Peavy HH: Pulmonary complications of HIV infection. Report of the Fourth NHLBI Workshop. Am J Respir Crit Care Med 164:2120-2126, 2001.
Bernstein SM, Newell JD, Adamczyk D, et al: How common are renal angiomyolipomas in patients with pulmonary lymphangioleiomyomatosis? Am J Respir Crit Care Med 152:2138-2143, 1995.
Bjoraker JA, Ryu JH, Edwin MK, et al: Prognostic significance of histopathologic subsets in idiopathic pulmonary fibrosis. Am J Respir Crit Care Med 157:199-203, 1998.
Brown KK: Rheumatoid lung disease. Proc Am Thorac Soc 4(5):443-448, 2007.
Bulger EM, Edwards T, Klotz P, et al: Epidural analgesia improves outcome: After multiple rib fractures. Surgery 136:426-430, 2004.
Buller HR, Agnelli G, Hull RD, et al: Antithrombotic therapy for venous thromboembolic disease: The Seventh ACCP Conference on Antithrombotic and Thrombolytic Therapy. Chest 126(3 suppl)401S-428S, 2004.
Caminati A, Harari S: Smoking-related interstitial pneumonias and pulmonary Langerhans cell histiocytosis. Proc Am Thorac Soc 3:299-306, 2006.
Camus P, Colby T: The lung in inflammatory bowel disease. Eur Respir J 15(1):5-10, 2000.
Camus P, Piard F, Ashcroft T, et al: The lung in inflammatory bowel disease. Medicine (Baltimore) 72(3):151-183, 1993.
Canuet M, Kessler R, Jeung MY, et al: Correlation between high-resolution computed tomography findings and lung function in pulmonary Langerhans cell histiocytosis. Respiration 74:640-646, 2007.
Capron F, Ameille J, Leclerc P, et al: Pulmonary lymphangioleiomyomatosis and Bourneville's tuberous sclerosis with pulmonary involvement: The same disease? Cancer 52:851-855, 1983.
Carrington CB, Gaensler EA, Coutu RE, et al: Natural history and treated course of usual and desquamative interstitial pneumonia. N Engl J Med 298:801-809, 1978.
Castranova V, Vallyathan V: Silicosis and coal workers' pneumoconiosis. Environ Health Perspect 108(suppl 4):675-684, 2000.
Celli BR, MacNee W: ATS/ERS Task Force: Standards for the diagnosis and treatment of patients with COPD: a summary of the ATS/ERS position paper. Eur Respir J 23:932-946, 2004.
Cha SI, Fessler MB, Cool CD, et al: Lymphoid interstitial pneumonia: Clinical features, associations and prognosis. Eur Respir J 28:364-369, 2006.
Chakinala MM, Trulock EP: Pneumonia in the solid organ transplant patient. Clin Chest Med 26:113-121, 2005.
Chapman SW, Dismukes WE, Proia LA, et al: Infectious Diseases Society of America: Clinical practice guidelines for the management of blastomycosis: 2008 update by the Infectious Diseases Society of America. Clin Infect Dis 46(12):1801-1812, 2008.
Chastre J, Fagon JY: Ventilator-associated pneumonia. Am J Respir Crit Care Med 165:867-903, 2002.
Chien JW, Martin PJ, Gooley TA, et al: Airflow obstruction after myeloablative allogeneic hematopoietic stem cell transplantation. Am J Respir Crit Care Med 168(2):208-214, 2003.
Clark JG, Hansen JA, Hertz MI, et al: NHLBI workshop summary. Idiopathic pneumonia syndrome after bone marrow transplantation. Am Rev Respir Dis 147(6 Pt 1):1601-1606, 1993.
Cohen AJ, King TE Jr, Downey GP: Rapidly progressive bronchiolitis obliterans with organizing pneumonia. Am J Respir Crit Care Med 149:1670-1675, 1994.
Cohen AT, Tapson VF, Bergmann JF, et al: Venous thromboembolism risk and prophylaxis in the acute hospital care setting (ENDORSE study): a multinational cross-sectional study. Lancet 371:387-3894, 2008.
Cohen MM, Pollock-BarZiv S, Johnson SR: Emerging clinical picture of lymphangioleiomyomatosis. Thorax 60(10):875-879, 2005.
Collard HR, King TE Jr, Bartelson BB, et al: Changes in clinical and physiologic variables predict survival in idiopathic pulmonary fibrosis. Am J Respir Crit Care Med 168:538-542, 2003.
Cook DJ, Walter SD, Cook RJ, et al: Incidence of and risk factors for ventilator-associated pneumonia in critically ill patients: Results from a multicenter prospective study on 996 patients. Ann Intern Med 129:433-440, 1998.
Cordier JF: Cryptogenic organizing pneumonia. Clin Chest Med 25(4):727-738, vi-vii, 2004.
Craig PJ, Wells AU, Doffman S, et al: Desquamative interstitial pneumonia, respiratory bronchiolitis and their relationship to smoking. Histopathology 45:275-282, 2004.
Crausman RS, Jennings CA, Mortenson RL, et al: Lymphangioleiomyomatosis: The pathophysiology of diminished exercise capacity. Am J Respir Crit Care Med 153(4 Pt 1):1368-1376, 1996.
Crausman RS, Jennings CA, Tuder R, et al: Pulmonary histiocytosis X: Pulmonary function and exercise pathophysiology. Am J Respir Crit Care Med 153:426-435, 1996.
Crausman RS, King TE Jr: Primary pulmonary histiocytosis X. UpToDate 2009.
Crausman RS, Lynch DA, Mortenson RL, et al: Quantitative computed tomography (QCT) predicts the severity of physiological dysfunction in patients with lymphangioleiomyomatosis (LAM). Chest 109:131-137, 1996.
Daniil ZD, Gilchrist FC, Nicholson AG, et al: A histologic pattern of nonspecific interstitial pneumonia is associated with a better prognosis than usual interstitial pneumonia in patients with cryptogenic fibrosing alveolitis. Am J Respir Crit Care Med 160:899-905, 1999.
Daviskas E, Anderson SD, Ebert S, Young IH: Effect of increasing doses of mannitol on mucus clearance in patient with bronchiectasis. Eur Respir J 31:765-772, 2008.
De Roux A, Marcos MA, Garcia E, et al: Viral community-acquired pneumonia in nonimmunocompromised adults. Chest 125:1343-1351, 2004.
Donnell AE: Bronchiectasis. Chest 143:815-823, 2008.
Drumm ML, Konstan MW, Schluchter MD, et al: Gene Modifier Study Group. Genetic modifiers of lung disease in cystic fibrosis. N Engl J Med 353(14):1443-1453, 2005.
Eder W, Ege MJ, von Mutius E: The asthma epidemic. N Engl J Med 355:2226-2235, 2006.
Eliasson AH, Phillips YY, Tenholder MF: Treatment of lymphangioleiomyomatosis: A meta-analysis. Chest 196:1352-1355, 1989.
Expert Panel Report 3 (EPR-3): Guidelines for the Diagnosis and Management of Asthma-Summary Report 2007. J Allergy Clin Immunol 120(suppl):S94-S138, 2007.
Fagan KA, Badesch DB: Pulmonary hypertension associated with connective tissue disease. In Peacock AJ, Rubin LJ (eds): *Pulmonary Circulation*. London, Arnold Publishers, 2004, pp 181-190.
Fang W, Washington L, Kumar N: Imaging manifestations of blastomycosis: A pulmonary infection with potential dissemination [review]. Radiographics 27(3):641-655, 2007.
Farr BM, Kaiser DL, Harrison BW, Connolly CK: Prediction of microbial aetiology at admission to hospital for pneumonia from presenting clinical features. Thorax 44:1031-1035, 1989.
Farrell PM, Rosenstein BJ, White TB, et al: Cystic Fibrosis Foundation: Guidelines for diagnosis of cystic fibrosis in newborns through older adults: Cystic Fibrosis Foundation consensus report. J Pediatr 153(suppl 2):S4-S14, 2008.
Fathi M, Lundberg IE, Tornling G: Pulmonary complications of polymyositis and dermatomyositis. Semin Respir Crit Care Med 28(4):451-458, 2007.
Fedullo PF, Auger WR, Kerr KM, Rubin LJ: Chronic thromboembolic pulmonary hypertension. N Eng J Med 345:1465-1472, 2001.
Feikin DR, Schuchat A, Kolczak M, et al: Mortality from invasive pneumococcal pneumonia in the era of antibiotic resistance, 1995-1997. Am J Public Health 90:223-229, 2000.
Fishman AP, Elias JA, Fishman JA, et al (eds). *Fishman's Pulmonary Diseases and Disorders*, 4th ed. New York, McGraw-Hill, 2008.
Flagel BT, Luchette FA, Reed RL, et al: Half-a-dozen ribs: The breakpoint for mortality. Surgery 138:717-725, 2005.
Flaherty KR, Mumford JA, Murray A, et al: Prognostic implications of physiologic and radiographic changes in idiopathic interstitial pneumonia. Am J Respir Crit Care Med 168:543-548, 2003.
Fletcher C, Peto R: The natural history of chronic airflow obstruction. Br Med J 1(6077):1645-1648, 1977.
Flume PA, O'Sullivan BP, Robinson KA, et al: Cystic Fibrosis Foundation, Pulmonary Therapies Committee: Cystic fibrosis pulmonary guidelines: Chronic medications for maintenance of lung health. Am J Respir Crit Care Med 176(10):957-969, 2007.